Leukaemia

Leukaemia

and related disorders

Edited by J.A. Whittaker
MD, FRCP, FRCPath
Reader and Consultant Haematologist,
University of Wales College of Medicine,
Heath Park, Cardiff CF4 4XN

and J.A. Holmes
BSc, PhD, MRCP, MRCPath
Formerly Senior Lecturer and Consultant Haematologist,
Queen Elizabeth Medical Centre,
Birmingham B15 2TH

Third Edition

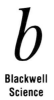

Blackwell Science

@ 1987, 1992, 1998 by
Blackwell Science Ltd
Editorial Offices:
Osney Mead, Oxford OX2 0EL
25 John Street, London WC1N 2BL
23 Ainslie Place, Edinburgh EH3 6AJ
350 Main Street, Malden
   MA 02148 5018, USA
54 University Street, Carlton
   Victoria 3053, Australia
10, rue Casimir Delavigne
   75006 Paris, France

Other Editorial Offices:
Blackwell Wissenschafts-Verlag GmbH
Kurfürstendamm 57
10707 Berlin, Germany

Blackwell Science KK
MG Kodenmacho Building
7–10 Kodenmacho Nihombashi
Chuo-ku, Tokyo 104, Japan

Set by Excel Typesetters Co., Hong Kong
Printed and bound in Great Britain
at the University Press, Cambridge

A catalogue record for this title
is available from the British Library

ISBN 0-86542-607-4

Library of Congress
Cataloging-in-publication Data

Leukaemia / edited by J.A. Whittaker and
J.A. Holmes. — 3rd ed.
         p.   cm.
      Includes bibliographical references
      and index.
      ISBN 0-86542-607-4
      1. Leukemia.   I. Whittaker, J.A.
      II. Holmes, J.A. (Jon A.)
      [DNLM: 1. Leukemia.
      WH 250 L6513 1998]
   RC643. L367   1998
   616.99′419—dc21
   DNLM/DLC
   for Library of Congress   97-31481
                                              CIP

First published 1987
Second edition 1992
Third edition 1998

The Blackwell Science logo is a
trade mark of Blackwell Science Ltd,
registered at the United Kingdom
Trade Marks Registry

DISTRIBUTORS

Marston Book Services Ltd
PO Box 269
Abingdon, Oxon OX14 4YN
(*Orders*:   Tel: 01235 465500
                 Fax: 01235 465555)

USA
Blackwell Science, Inc.
Commerce Place
350 Main Street
Malden, MA 02148 5018
(*Orders*:   Tel: 800 759 6102
                    781 388 8250
                 Fax: 781 388 8255)

Canada
Login Brothers Book Company
324 Saulteaux Crescent
Winnipeg, Manitoba R3J 3T2
(*Orders*:   Tel: 204 224-4068)

Australia
Blackwell Science Pty Ltd
54 University Street
Carlton, Victoria 3053
(*Orders*:   Tel: 3 9347 0300
                 Fax: 3 9347 5001)

For further information on
Blackwell Science, visit our website:
www.blackwell-science.com

Cover illustration based on a figure by
Barbara Bain in *Leukaemia Diagnosis*, 2nd
edition. With permission.

Contents

Colour plates appear between pp. 292 and 293

List of Contributors

C.C. Bailey MB, BSc, FRCP, FRCPCH, *Professor, Regional Director of Research and Development, Research School of Medicine, 24 Hyde Terrace, Leeds LS2 9LN, UK*

B.J. Bain MBBS, FRACP, FRCPath, *Senior Lecturer, Department of Haematology, Imperial College School of Medicine at St Mary's Hospital, London W2 1PG, UK*

F.G. Behm MD, *Department of Pathology and Laboratory Medicine, St Jude Children's Research Hospital, 332 North Lauderdale, Memphis, Tennessee 38105-2794, USA*

B. Bradley MB, ChB, PhD, MA, FRCPath, *Professor of Transplantation Sciences, University of Bristol Division of Transplantation Sciences, Southmead Health Services, Westbury-on-Trym, Bristol BS10 5NB, UK*

M.K. Brenner MB, PhD, FRCP, FRCPath, *Director, Division of Bone Marrow Transplantation and Cell and Gene Therapy Program, St Jude Children's Research Hospital, 332 North Lauderdale Street, Memphis, Tennessee 38105-2794, USA*

A.K. Burnett MD, FRCP (Glas), FRCP (Edin), FRCPath, *Professor of Haematology, University of Wales College of Medicine, Heath Park, Cardiff CF4 4XN, UK*

J. Burthem PhD, MRCP, *Clinical Lecturer, Department of Cell Science, John Radcliffe Hospital, Headington, Oxford OX3 9DU, UK*

D. Campana MD, PhD, *Department of Hematology–Oncology, St Jude Children's Research Hospital, 332 North Lauderdale, Memphis, Tennessee 38105-2794, USA*

R.A. Cartwright MA, MB, BChir, PhD, FFPHM, FFOM, *Director and Professor of Clinical Epidemiology, Leukaemia Research Fund Centre for Clinical Epidemiology, University of Leeds, Leeds LS2 9NG, UK*

D. Catovsky DSc (Med), FRCP, FRCPath, *Professor, Consultant Haematologist, Academic Department of Haematology and Cytogenetics, The Royal Marsden Hospital and Institute of Cancer Research, London SW3 6JJ, UK*

J.C. Cawley MD, PhD, FRCP, FRCPath, *Professor of Haematology, University Department of Haematology, Royal Liverpool Hospital, PO Box 147, Liverpool L69 3BX, UK*

J.A. Child MD, FRCP, FRCPath, *Consultant Haematologist, Department of Haematology, General Infirmary, Leeds LS1 3EX, UK*

H.S. Cuckle BA, MSc, DPhil, *Professor of Reproductive Epidemiology, Centre for Reproduction, Growth and Development, 26 Clarendon Road, Leeds LS2 9NZ, UK*

I.M. Franklin PhD, FRCP, FRCPath, *Professor of Transfusion Medicine, University of Glasgow,* and *Honorary Consultant, Bone Marrow Transplant Unit, Glasgow Royal Infirmary, Glasgow G4 0SF, UK*

C.G. Geary MA, MB, FRCP, FRCPath, *Consultant Haematologist, Department of Clinical Haematology, The Royal Infirmary, Manchester M13 9WL, UK*

J.M. Goldman DM, FRCP, FRCPath, *Professor of Leukaemia and Biology, Department of Haematology, Imperial College School of Medicine, Hammersmith Hospital, London W12 0NN, UK*

T.J. Hamblin DM, FRCP, FRCPath, *Professor of Immunohaematology, Southampton University,* and *Consultant Haematologist, Royal Bournemouth Hospital, Bournemouth BH7 7DW, UK*

J.A. Holmes BSc, PhD, MRCP, MRCPath, *Formerly Consultant Haematologist, Queen Elizabeth Medical Centre, Edgbaston, Birmingham B13 2TH, UK*

J. Hows MD, FRCP, FRCPath, *Professor of Clinical Haematology, University of Bristol Division of Transplantation Sciences, Southmead Health Services, Westbury-on-Trym, Bristol BS10 5NB, UK*

P. Johnson MA, MD, MRCP, *Senior Lecturer, ICRF Cancer Medicine Research Unit, St James' University Hospital, Leeds LS9 7TF, UK*

S.A.N. Johnson MB, BS, FRCPath, *Consultant Haematologist, Taunton and Somerset Hospital, Musgrove Park, Taunton TA1 5DA, UK*

S.E. Kinsey MD, MRCP, FRCPath, FRCPCH, *Consultant Paediatric Haematologist, Paediatric Haematology and Oncology, St James' University Hospital, Leeds LS9 7TS, UK*

J.S. Lilleyman DSc, FRCP, FRCPath, *Professor of Paediatric Oncology, St Bartholomew's and the Royal London School of Medicine and Dentistry, St Bartholomew's Hospital, London EC1A 7BE, UK*

D.C. Linch MB, BChir, FRCP, FRCPath, *Professor of Haematology, University College London Medical School, London WC1E 6HX, UK*

J.A. Liu Yin FRCP, FRCPath, *Consultant Haematologist and Director of Bone Marrow Transplant Programme, University Department of Haematology, Manchester Royal Infirmary, Manchester M13 9WL, UK*

C.A. Ludlam PhD, FRCP, FRCPath, *Consultant Haematologist, Department of Haematology, Edinburgh Royal Infirmary, Edinburgh EH3 9YW, UK*

A.T. Macheta BSc, FRCP, FRCPath, *Consultant Haematologist, Pathology Department, Furness General Hospital, Barrow-in-Furness LA14 4LF, UK*

K.A. MacLennan DM, FRCPath, *Reader in Tumour Pathology, Department of Histopathology, St James' University Hospital, Leeds LS9 7TF, UK*

E. Matutes MD, PhD, MRCPath, *Senior Lecturer and Consultant Haematologist, Academic Department of Haematology and Cytogenetics, The Royal Marsden Hospital and Institute of Cancer Research, London SW3 6JJ, UK*

J. Mehta MD, *Associate Professor of Medicine, Division of Hematology/Oncology, University of Arkansas for Medical Sciences, 4301 West Markham, Mail Slot 508, Little Rock, Arkansas 72205-9985, USA*

G.J. Morgan BSc, MB, BChir, PhD, MRCP, *Senior Lecturer and Honorary Consultant Haematologist, Department of Haematology, General Infirmary, Leeds LS1 3EX, UK*

J.A.F. Napier PhD, FRCPath, *Medical Director, Welsh Blood Service, Ely Valley Road, Talbot Green, Pontyclun CF72 9WB, UK*

A.J. Norton MB, BS, FRCPath, *Department of Histopathology, St Bartholomew's Hospital, London EC1A 7BE, UK*

D.G. Oscier MA, MB, BChir, FRCP, FRCPath, *Clinical Senior Lecturer in Haematology, Southampton University, and Consultant Haematologist, Royal Bournemouth Hospital, Bournemouth BH7 7DW, UK*

R.L. Powles BSc, MD, FRCP, FRCPath, *Professor of Haematologic Oncology and Head, Leukaemia and Myeloma Units, The Royal Marsden NHS Trust, Downs Road, Sutton SM2 5TT, UK*

S.J. Proctor FRCP, FRCPath, *Professor of Haematological Medicine, University of Newcastle upon Tyne, Department of Haematology, Royal Victoria Infirmary, Newcastle upon Tyne NE1 4LP, UK*

L.G. Robinson BSc, MRCP, Dip RCPath, *Lecturer in Haematology, University of Wales College of Medicine, Heath Park, Cardiff CF4 4XN, UK*

P.H. Roddie MRCP, MRCPath, *Senior Registrar in Haematology, Department of Haematology, Edinburgh Royal Infirmary, Edinburgh EH3 9YW, UK*

P. Selby MA, MD, FRCP, FRCR, *Professor of Cancer and Medicine, ICRF Cancer Medicine Research Unit, St James' University Hospital, Leeds LS9 7TF, UK*

P.R.A. Taylor MB, BS, *Associate Specialist, Department of Haematology, Royal Victoria Infirmary, Newcastle upon Tyne NE1 4LP, UK*

P.W. Thompson PhD, Dip RCPath, *Cytogeneticist, Medical Genetics Department, University of Wales College of Medicine, Heath Park, Cardiff CF4 4XN, UK*

J.A. Whittaker MD, FRCP, FRCPath, *Reader in Haematology, University of Wales College of Medicine, and Honorary Consultant, University Hospital of Wales, Heath Park, Cardiff CF4 4XN, UK*

D.A. Winfield FRCP, FRCPath, *Consultant Haematologist, Royal Hallamshire Hospital, Sheffield S10 2JF, UK*

Preface to the Third Edition

Since the second edition of this book was published in 1992, progress in our understanding of the leukaemias has continued at a rapid pace. These advances and the improvements in the clinical management of these disorders have necessitated a complete revision of the text. Significant contributions have been made by several new authors. While increasing the coverage of developments in the scientific knowledge of leukaemia, we have nevertheless determined that the book should be firstly a clinical text which we hope will continue to be of use to all those who care for patients, whether directly or indirectly. Once again, our intention has been to produce a broad view of the subject rather than a comprehensive reference text. However, because most physicians who manage patients with leukaemia also care for patients with related haematological malignancies, we have included several chapters covering myeloma and lymphoma.

Our thanks are due to the many people who have helped with the writing and production of this book and especially to Victoria Oddie and Jane Andrew at Blackwell Science who have so skilfully dealt with so many aspects of the book's publication.

J.A.W., J.A.H.
February 1998

Preface to the First Edition

Progress in both the scientific basis and clinical management of the spectrum of diseases which we call leukaemia has been rapid in recent years, so that we are now beginning to understand something of the events responsible for their initiation, while at the same time approaching treatment with increasing confidence of success. This book combines a review of the scientific developments with up-to-date descriptions of the diseases and their management and we hope it will be of use to all who have an interest in leukaemia and particularly to physicians responsible for patient management. While we have attempted to cover most topics, our intention has been to produce a broad view of the subject rather than a completely comprehensive reference text.

A carefully selected group of international authors, several from the USA, many from the UK and some from continental Europe, have provided manuscripts which we hope will speak for themselves. While we cannot claim that their contributions do not overlap, we have tried to avoid the repetition, or even conflict, which can bedevil multi-author texts. However, the decision to ask two authors to write on myelodysplasia, one concentrating on haemopoietic mechanisms and one on clinical aspects, was a conscious one and we have allowed these authors full latitude to interconnect.

Our thanks are due to our contributors, most of whom provided manuscripts promptly and in many cases willingly made alterations at what must have been irritatingly short notice; to Mr Peter Saugman and his staff at Blackwell Scientific Publications, without whom this book would not have been published; and in particular to our secretaries, Avril Porter and Margaret Power, who have cheerfully suffered the editorial process, answered hundreds of letters and retyped some sections of the text.

J.A.W., I.W.D.
December 1986

1 Epidemiology

R.A. Cartwright

Introduction

Leukaemia and its related conditions comprise a wide variety of malignancies; some, but not all, are clearly related in terms of their epidemiology. For the purposes of this review chapter, the major foci are the following conditions:

- acute myeloid leukaemia;
- myelodysplasia;
- chronic myeloid leukaemia;
- acute lymphoblastic leukaemia;
- chronic lymphoblastic leukaemia;
- non-Hodgkin's lymphoma;
- Hodgkin's disease;
- multiple myeloma.

This is a pragmatic choice, due partly to what is available in the world literature and partly to the relative frequency of these conditions. Many of these conditions are clearly composites of separate epidemiological subtypes—distinct in both their descriptive and aetiological epidemiology, but this aspect is rarely touched upon, and the few rare subtypes, such as hairy cell leukaemia, mycosis fungoides and acute T-cell leukaemia/lymphoma, are only mentioned briefly.

The epidemiology of these conditions presents particular difficulties, partly because of the diversity of the haematological malignancies encompassed and partly because of the temporal and geographical variation in criteria used both for diagnosing and recording these disorders.

Descriptive epidemiological investigations have often considered these diseases by using the criteria of the International Classification of Diseases (ICD) [1]. These classifications have changed with each edition of the manual for classification, and yet major conceptual advances, such as the link between the myeloid dysplastic group of conditions and the myeloid leukaemias, have not yet been adopted. Newer editions of the classification are slow to be adopted in many parts of the world.

The published national statistics for leukaemia and related conditions should be interpreted with particular caution. This is not only because of variation in diagnostic definitions, but also because the statistics may be influenced by problems of registration and by wide differences in the quality of case ascertainment. Such problems are particularly important when international comparisons are attempted. A good deal of epidemiological data are derived from cancer registries. However, the quality of such data varies considerably from registry to registry and from country to country. Cases ascertained from countries with population-based registries, centralized health services and complete lists of inhabitants must be assessed very differently from data from countries with few hospitals, numerous languages and no reliable schemes for recording births, deaths or the total population. Even in Britain where there is good cancer registration, the records for these conditions are deficient [2]. It is often left to the reader to assess the strength of routinely recorded registry information, because there is a lack of statistics or the statistics are incomplete.

Correlation or ecological analyses utilize descriptive data on leukaemias and make contrasts with the distribution of geographical or social features from routine data sources such as censuses. Because of the reservations expressed about data accuracy and completeness, these analyses should be viewed with caution, especially if they employ mortality rather than incidence data.

The two most commonly utilized analytical methods in epidemiology are the follow-up or cohort study and the case–control study. Cohort studies are more appropriate where the disease of interest has a relatively high incidence or where a particular exposure is being observed. The case–control study examines the frequency of exposure to a potential risk in patients with the disease and compares this with the same exposure in an appropriate comparison group. This method is better suited to the study of rarer diseases, such as the leukaemias and related diseases, where, in addition, pathways of pathogenesis may be both multiple with factors which may interact with each other, and have long latent intervals from exposure to diagnosis. Bias in such studies is a potential

1

limitation deriving from a number of sources, which include selection procedures of cases and controls and the exact nature of the exposure information [3].

Experimental work and clinical case reports have also made a significant contribution to the study of the epidemiology of these conditions. Today most new epidemiological approaches to aetiology rely heavily on an understanding of the relevant concepts that are currently accepted by the laboratory-based biologists working in this field. The term molecular epidemiology is used to refer to the study of the links between significant pathogenetic steps and the potential exposures causing these steps, which are investigated using basic epidemiological techniques.

Descriptive epidemiology

Descriptive statistics refer to recorded demographic variables including geographic distribution, age, sex, race or language type and social class, with respect to the disease group. Such statistics can also examine changes with time.

Incidence data are given here but, in fact, have only emerged recently and much accumulated knowledge has been derived from mortality statistics. Inferences about incidence based on mortality figures will be more accurate for the myeloid leukaemias, but overall are complicated by changes in survival; trends starting in the early 1970s.

Since 1966, incidence data from selected cancer registries worldwide have been summarized and published periodically [4]. This ongoing compilation records differences in the incidence of the haematological malignancies from those registries with reliable numerical estimates of the local population. Tables 1.1–1.5 give details of leukaemia distribution worldwide. No distinction is made between acute and chronic disease because the three-digit ICD classification is utilized [1]. Table 1.6 provides summary standardized rates by subtype and Table 1.7 gives data on the childhood leukaemias. These observed differences may be artificial, because of the constraints listed earlier, but other differences could be real; for example, they might be due to variations in genetic susceptibility, socioeconomic development and exposure to environmental carcinogens. Further examination of these differences can be pursued in other types of epidemiological studies. Unfortunately, reliable data specific to cell type are not available from many cancer registries.

A recent special investigation of these conditions from parts of England and Wales, which was started in 1984, has used

Country	Years	Sex	Age group (years)				
			0/1–4	20–24	40–44	60–64	70–74
Colombia (Cali)	1982–86	M	0.7	0.3	0.6	10.7	9.5
		F	0	0.9	1.2	5.2	5.1
Canada	1983–87	M	0.9	1.4	2.9	11.1	23.0
		F	0.7	1.1	2.6	7.2	13.7
USA: SEER (white population)	1983–87	M	0.9	0.9	2.6	10.7	22.9
		F	0.4	0.7	1.9	7.3	14.3
USA: SEER (black population)	1983–87	M	0.3	1.6	2.6	16.8	10.0
		F	0.3	0.7	2.8	5.7	13.7
China (Shanghai)	1983–87	M	0.7	0.9	2.2	4.2	5.1
		F	1.3	0.5	1.2	3.0	2.7
India (Bombay)	1983–87	M	0.6	0.9	1.4	5.9	9.6
		F	0.3	0.7	2.8	2.4	5.6
Israel (Jews)	1982–86	M	0.4	1.8	2.6	0	22.0
		F	0.9	0.4	3.4	0	18.4
Japan (Nagasaki)	1983–87	M	1.3	1.4	2.9	6.5	11.0
		F	0	0	2.6	3.2	8.1
Finland	1982–86	M	0.6	1.0	2.9	6.5	20.7
		F	1.3	0.7	1.8	6.1	12.2
Spain (Zaragoza)	1983–85	M	3.4	1.0	2.7	3.1	22.9
		F	0	1.1	2.7	2.7	1.9
UK (England and Wales)	1983–87	M	0.6	0.8	0.8	7.7	16.9
		F	0.6	0.7	2.1	5.7	9.7

Table 1.1 Incidence rates by sex and selected age group from certain indigenous populations (rate per 100 000 per year): myeloid leukaemia: acute myeloid leukaemia (AML) and chronic myeloid leukaemia (CML).

Table 1.2 Incidence rates by sex and selected age group from certain indigenous populations (rate per 100 000 per year): lymphatic leukaemia: acute lymphoblastic leukaemia (ALL) and chronic lymphoblastic leukaemia (CLL).

Country	Years	Sex	Age group (years)				
			0/1–4	20–24	40–44	60–64	70–74
Colombia (Cali)	1982–86	M	3.8	1.7	0	1.5	12.7
		F	5.0	0.7	1.2	3.0	5.1
Canada	1983–87	M	8.4	0.7	1.2	17.2	31.6
		F	6.8	0.4	1.2	7.2	15.8
USA: SEER (white population)	1983–87	M	5.5	0.9	1.3	13.7	28.9
		F	5.4	0.4	0.8	7.0	14.7
USA: SEER (black population)	1983–87	M	1.7	0.1	1.1	9.6	23.7
		F	2.5	0	0.8	4.9	9.1
China (Shanghai)	1983–87	M	2.8	0.4	0.1	2.2	3.9
		F	3.2	0.4	0.8	1.5	2.0
India (Bombay)	1983–87	M	2.3	0.7	0.5	2.0	6.4
		F	1.5	0.2	0.5	2.7	1.9
Israel (Jews)	1982–86	M	1.8	1.5	1.7	13.8	0
		F	2.9	0.8	0	4.5	9.2
Japan (Nagasaki)	1983–87	M	6.6	0	1.5	0	3.7
		F	4.3	0	1.3	4.8	2.7
Finland	1982–86	M	6.1	1.0	0.7	9.7	20.1
		F	6.5	0.3	0.8	3.5	9.8
Spain (Zaragoza)	1983–85	M	11.9	0	2.7	4.7	25.5
		F	9.0	0	0	6.9	11.2
UK (England and Wales)	1983–87	M	5.6	0.8	0.8	7.7	16.9
		F	4.8	0.4	0.5	3.4	7.9

Table 1.3 Incidence rates by sex and selected age group for certain indigenous populations (rate per 100 000 per year): non-Hodgkin's lymphoma (NHL).

Country	Years	Sex	Age group (years)				
			0/1–4	20–24	40–44	60–64	70–74
Colombia (Cali)	1982–86	M	1.0	0.6	2.6	13.8	19.0
		F	0.7	0.5	4.2	19.6	32.6
Canada	1983–87	M	1.3	2.3	11.5	41.7	67.3
		F	0.5	1.3	7.2	29.6	51.2
USA: SEER (white population)	1983–87	M	0.9	2.3	14.1	45.4	74.5
		F	0.5	1.4	7.8	31.7	56.2
USA: SEER (black population)	1983–87	M	0.3	1.6	7.1	26.4	39.2
		F	0.6	1.1	4.6	16.8	30.6
China (Shanghai)	1983–87	M	1.5	1.6	3.7	12.7	17.2
		F	1.1	0.7	1.4	7.2	7.6
India (Bombay)	1983–87	M	0.8	1.7	2.2	10.1	19.9
		F	0.3	0.8	1.2	6.7	15.5
Israel (Jews)	1982–86	M	1.7	1.3	13.1	36.9	33.0
		F	0.9	2.2	3.4	22.7	18.4
Japan (Nagasaki)	1983–87	M	1.3	1.4	10.3	15.1	29.4
		F	0	1.1	3.9	12.9	35.3
Finland	1982–86	M	1.3	1.9	5.7	28.8	48.5
		F	0.6	0.8	4.9	19.1	38.2
Spain (Zaragoza)	1983–85	M	0	3.1	4.1	18.6	35.7
		F	0	0	5.5	4.1	30.0
UK (England and Wales)	1983–87	M	0.9	1.6	7.5	23.7	39.6
		F	0.4	1.6	4.8	16.0	27.2

Country	Years	Sex	Age group (years)				
			0/1–4	20–24	40–44	60–64	70–74
Colombia (Cali)	1982–86	M	0.3	1.7	2.6	1.5	9.5
		F	0	0.5	1.8	2.6	2.5
Canada	1983–87	M	0.2	5.8	3.1	4.3	6.6
		F	0	4.1	2.1	2.8	3.7
USA: SEER (white population)	1983–87	M	0.1	5.7	3.9	4.1	4.8
		F	0	6.2	1.8	2.8	3.4
USA: SEER (black population)	1983–87	M	0	3.4	3.1	3.4	5.5
		F	0	1.5	1.0	2.5	1.3
China (Shanghai)	1983–87	M	0.3	0.4	0	1.0	0.8
		F	0.1	0.4	0.3	0.5	0.2
India (Bombay)	1983–87	M	0.3	0.5	0.9	3.2	3.9
		F	0.1	0.2	0.4	0.8	2.5
Israel (Jews)	1982–86	M	0.1	3.5	1.7	0	11.0
		F	0.1	3.5	2.6	0	9.2
Japan (Nagasaki)	1983–87	M	0	0	0	0	3.7
		F	0	0	0	0	0
Finland	1982–86	M	0	2.4	4.2	4.5	7.6
		F	0	2.8	0.8	2.5	3.6
Spain (Zaragoza)	1983–85	M	1.7	4.1	6.8	4.7	0
		F	0	4.3	0	4.1	1.9
UK (England and Wales)	1983–87	M	0.2	3.7	3.3	3.4	3.7
		F	0.1	3.3	1.6	2.2	2.5

Table 1.4 Incidence rates by sex and selected age group from certain indigenous populations (rate per 100 000 per year): Hodgkin's disease (HD).

Country	Years	Sex	Age group (years)				
			0/1–4	20–24	40–44	60–64	70–74
Colombia (Cali)	1982–86	M	0	0	0.6	7.7	15.9
		F	0	0	0	3.9	7.6
Canada	1983–87	M	0	0	1.1	14.6	33.9
		F	0	0	0.9	10.9	23.1
USA: SEER (white population)	1983–87	M	0	0	1.5	13.1	27.5
		F	0	0	0.8	10.0	18.2
USA: SEER (black population)	1983–87	M	0.3	1.6	3.4	27.4	54.7
		F	0	0.1	3.1	20.5	34.5
China (Shanghai)	1983–87	M	0	0	0	3.4	5.4
		F	0	0	0.7	3.0	2.7
India (Bombay)	1983–87	M	0	0	0.5	3.6	3.2
		F	0	0	0.4	3.5	4.3
Israel (Jews)	1982–86	M	0	0	3.5	18.5	33.0
		F	0	0	1.7	4.5	18.4
Japan (Nagasaki)	1983–87	M	0	0	0	6.5	14.7
		F	0	0	0	4.8	13.6
Finland	1982–86	M	0	0.2	1.5	15.6	21.0
		F	0	0	0.3	9.8	19.5
Spain (Zaragoza)	1983–85	M	0	0	0	7.8	10.2
		F	0	0	0	8.2	13.1
UK (England and Wales)	1983–87	M	0	0	0.9	11.4	25.2
		F	0	0	0.6	7.4	15.9

Table 1.5 Incidence rates by sex and selected age group from certain indigenous populations (rate per 100 000 per year): multiple myeloma (MM).

Table 1.6 Age-standardized world incidence rates for the leukaemias (rates per 100 000 per year).

Country	AML Male	AML Female	CML Male	CML Female	ALL Male	ALL Female	CLL Male	CLL Female
Brazil (San Paulo)	1.5	1.2	0.8	0.7	1.2	1.0	0.8	0.2
Columbia (Cali)	1.5	1.3	0.9	0.6	1.7	1.2	0.5	0.5
Canada (Alberta)	2.5	2.0	1.5	0.7	1.4	1.3	3.1	1.2
USA (San Francisco)								
White population	2.7	1.9	0.8	0.4	1.4	1.2	2.2	1.3
Black population	2.4	2.4	1.9	0.8	1.1	0.8	2.3	1.2
Japan (Hiroshima)	2.8	1.9	1.6	0.8	1.1	0.7	0.3	0.1
India (Bombay)	0.9	0.6	0.8	0.6	0.8	0.5	0.4	0.3
Israel (Jews)	1.9	1.5	0.9	0.5	1.3	1.1	2.3	1.5
Spain (Zaragoza)	1.1	1.0	0.3	0.1	0.7	0.8	0.7	0.3
UK (England and Wales)	1.7	1.3	0.8	0.4	1.4	1.1	1.6	0.7

Table 1.7 Age-standardized incidence rates of all types of childhood leukaemia (cases per 1 000 000 per year).

Country	Male	Female
Nigeria (Ibadan)	18.3	4.6
Brazil (San Paulo)	37.6	29.4
Columbia (Cali)	53.0	35.1
Costa Rica	62.6	56.0
Canada (Western Province)	47.9	39.6
USA (Los Angeles)		
Black population	31.6	23.9
White population	56.0	44.1
Hispanic population	52.7	43.6
Japan (Karagawa)	39.6	37.0
India (Bombay)	26.5	19.1
Israel (Jews)	37.6	27.5
Finland	48.0	36.4
Spain (Zaragoza)	49.1	43.8
UK (England and Wales)	41.8	32.9

Table 1.8 Age-specific incidence rates per 100 000 per year from a register of geographically based complete ascertainment estimates from parts of England and Wales based on 3310 cases, 1984–93: AML (M1–M7).

Age group (years)	Male rate	Female rate	Pooled rate
0–4	0.95	0.89	0.92
5–9	0.42	0.26	0.34
10–14	0.52	0.71	0.61
15–19	0.73	0.60	0.67
20–24	0.70	0.91	0.80
25–29	0.97	0.52	0.75
30–34	0.94	0.97	0.96
35–39	1.04	1.13	1.09
40–44	1.37	1.50	1.44
45–49	1.62	1.68	1.65
50–54	2.73	2.66	2.70
55–59	4.14	2.83	3.48
60–64	6.46	3.88	5.11
65–69	8.47	5.49	6.85
70–74	11.60	7.48	9.25
75–79	14.50	7.85	10.42
Uniform standardized rates	3.5	2.46	2.94

modern classifications and a mode of data collection independent of cancer registries [5]. Data on incidence from this source are given by age and sex in Tables 1.8–1.15. Some of these results vary somewhat from those published by the Office of Population Censuses and Surveys (OPCS) which are derived from cancer registries, as illustrated in Table 1.16. Further details of specific groups of interest are given in Tables 1.17 and 1.18. Table 1.19 provides estimated annual newly diagnosed case numbers for England and Wales based on recently collated data.

Age distribution in various populations

The specific types of conditions differ widely in their incidence by age.

Acute myeloid leukaemias and related acute leukaemias

Acute myeloid leukaemia (AML) represents the great majority of acute leukaemias in adults and there is an increasing incidence with increasing age, as shown in Tables 1.1 and 1.8. There, however, are some notable exceptions to this, for example in Ibadan, Nigeria, a childhood 'peak' of AML has been reported between the ages of 5 and 9 years, frequently occurring with chloroma and mainly affecting boys [6]. This pattern is seen elsewhere in developing countries in the tropics. However, it is conceivable that this excess of childhood

Table 1.9 Age-specific incidence rates per 100 000 per year from a register of geographically based complete ascertainment estimates from parts of England and Wales based on 3648 cases, 1984–93: MDS (all types).

Age group (years)	Male rate	Female rate	Pooled rate
0–4	0.06	0.04	0.05
5–9	0.04	0.02	0.03
10–14	0.06	0.02	0.04
15–19	0.05	0.12	0.08
20–24	0.08	0.14	0.11
25–29	0.09	0.19	0.14
30–34	0.14	0.25	0.19
35–39	0.20	0.33	0.26
40–44	0.39	0.59	0.49
45–49	0.62	0.93	0.77
50–54	1.12	1.07	1.10
55–59	3.12	1.94	2.52
60–64	6.60	3.86	5.17
65–69	11.48	6.67	8.88
70–74	21.41	9.63	14.68
75–79	35.07	18.92	25.17
Uniform standardized rates	5.03	2.80	3.73

Table 1.10 Age-specific incidence rates per 100 000 per year from a register of geographically based complete ascertainment estimates from parts of England and Wales based on 1114 cases, 1984–93: CML.

Age group (years)	Male rate	Female rate	Pooled rate
0–4	0.23	0.04	0.14
5–9	0.04	0.07	0.05
10–14	0.04	0.00	0.02
15–19	0.13	0.16	0.14
20–24	0.40	0.07	0.24
25–29	0.46	0.21	0.34
30–34	0.66	0.48	0.57
35–39	0.69	0.43	0.56
40–44	1.06	0.61	0.84
45–49	0.78	0.79	0.79
50–54	1.49	1.23	1.36
55–59	1.53	1.42	1.48
60–64	1.92	1.58	1.74
65–69	2.40	1.57	1.95
70–74	3.13	1.46	2.17
75–79	4.00	1.99	2.77
Uniform standardized rates	1.19	0.76	0.95

Table 1.11 Age-specific incidence rates per 100 000 per year from a register of geographically based complete ascertainment estimates from parts of England and Wales based on 1337 cases, 1984–93: ALL.

Age group (years)	Male rate	Female rate	Pooled rate
0–4	4.95	4.85	4.91
5–9	2.41	2.13	2.28
10–14	1.43	1.08	1.26
15–19	1.43	0.80	1.12
20–24	0.67	0.33	0.50
25–29	0.58	0.21	0.40
30–34	0.43	0.33	0.38
35–39	0.38	0.12	0.25
40–44	0.58	0.42	0.50
45–49	0.35	0.26	0.31
50–54	0.63	0.31	0.47
55–59	0.56	0.49	0.52
60–64	0.78	0.42	0.59
65–69	0.88	0.43	0.64
70–74	0.91	0.28	0.55
75–79	0.89	0.49	0.65
Uniform standardized rates	1.12	0.81	0.96

Table 1.12 Age-specific incidence rates per 100 000 from a register of geographically based complete ascertainment estimates from parts of England and Wales based on 3340, 1984–88*: CLL.

Age group (years)	Male rate	Female rate	Pooled rate
0–4	0.00	0.04	0.02
5–9	0.00	0.04	0.02
10–14	0.12	0.00	0.06
15–19	0.07	0.03	0.05
20–24	0.10	0.10	0.10
25–29	0.14	0.18	0.16
30–34	0.51	0.28	0.39
35–39	0.64	0.39	0.52
40–44	2.18	0.37	1.28
45–49	3.32	2.41	2.87
50–54	6.46	3.79	5.11
55–59	9.91	5.02	7.40
60–64	17.67	7.82	12.74
65–69	20.75	12.58	16.66
70–74	27.00	14.80	19.94
75–79	41.09	18.92	27.16
Uniform standardized rates	8.12	4.17	6.15

* Data not available after 1988.

myeloid leukaemia is only relative, due to the lack of common acute lymphoblastic leukaemia (ALL) in childhood.

AML rates also differ, being highest in certain Western countries and lowest in Asia (Table 1.6). The high rates seen in some populations of the Pacific rim, including Maori and related groups, are particularly interesting. The pattern in England and Wales is again heterogeneous, showing particularly high rates in parts of the east Midlands and southwest England [5].

Myelodysplastic syndrome

Information on the age-specific incidence of these conditions is strictly limited [7,8].

It appears that the age-specific incidence rates are greater in men and increase with age in a similar fashion to AML (Table 1.9).

Table 1.13 Age-specific incidence rates per 100 000 per year from a register of geographically based complete ascertainment estimates from parts of England and Wales based on 15 566 cases, 1984–93: NHL (all types and sites).

Age group (years)	Male rate	Female rate	Pooled rate
0–4	0.61	0.43	0.52
5–9	1.17	0.38	0.78
10–14	1.02	0.30	0.67
15–19	1.34	0.70	1.03
20–24	1.56	0.84	1.21
25–29	2.13	1.51	1.82
30–34	2.93	2.27	2.60
35–39	5.42	2.87	4.15
40–44	8.24	5.17	6.72
45–49	11.19	8.05	9.63
50–54	17.87	11.77	14.82
55–59	25.12	17.29	21.13
60–64	33.87	21.49	27.41
65–69	44.82	30.64	37.14
70–74	58.61	37.20	46.38
75–79	69.06	43.11	53.15
Uniform standardized rates	17.81	11.50	14.32

Table 1.14 Age-specific incidence rates per 100 000 per year from a register of geographically based complete ascertainment estimates from parts of England and Wales based on 3026 cases, 1984–1993: HD (all types).

Age group (years)	Male rate	Female rate	Pooled rate
0–4	0.21	0.02	0.12
5–9	0.60	0.16	0.39
10–14	1.15	0.48	0.82
15–19	2.67	2.87	2.77
20–24	3.87	3.91	3.89
25–29	3.86	2.84	3.36
30–34	3.38	2.38	2.89
35–39	3.23	2.04	2.64
40–44	3.02	1.60	2.32
45–49	2.62	1.18	1.90
50–54	2.99	1.41	2.20
55–59	2.88	1.50	2.18
60–64	2.48	1.70	2.08
65–69	3.35	1.41	2.30
70–74	3.09	2.40	2.70
75–79	2.74	1.66	2.08
Uniform standardized rates	2.63	1.72	2.16

Table 1.15 Age-specific incidence rates per 100 000 per year from a register of geographically based complete ascertainment estimates from parts of England and Wales based on 3323 cases, 1984–88*: MM.

Age group (years)	Male rate	Female rate	Pooled rate
0–4	0.00	0.00	0.00
5–9	0.00	0.00	0.00
10–14	0.00	0.00	0.00
15–19	0.03	0.00	0.02
20–24	0.03	0.00	0.02
25–29	0.00	0.04	0.02
30–34	0.27	0.16	0.22
35–39	0.39	0.36	0.37
40–44	1.25	0.94	1.10
45–49	2.95	1.86	2.40
50–54	4.97	3.08	4.03
55–59	8.87	5.57	7.18
60–64	14.67	9.16	11.91
65–69	19.19	13.31	16.25
70–74	28.03	17.19	21.76
75–79	34.90	22.04	28.47
Uniform standardized rates	7.22	4.61	5.92

* Data not available after 1988.

Chronic myeloid leukaemia

Chronic myeloid leukaemia (CML) tends to be a disease of middle life with a slowly increasing age trend within Western countries as shown in Table 1.10. Unfortunately much of the available tabulated information (Table 1.1) does not distinguish acute from chronic leukaemia.

Acute lymphoblastic leukaemia

Acute lymphoblastic leukaemia (ALL) occurs frequently in childhood and accounts for the sharp age peak for leukaemia in those under 5 years of age. This has been observed in white children for many years, but only since the early 1960s in non-white people in the USA and the Japanese [9,10]. Further data are given in Tables 1.6 and 1.7. The peak has been seen subsequently in Malaysian children [11], but in 1978 it was still absent in Papua New Guinea and parts of Central Africa [12]. Such a pattern must be due, in part, to environmental factors and changing socioeconomic conditions. It is now apparent that the childhood peak is due to an increase in the 'common' type of ALL. Recent data from parts of England and Wales indicates that the excess incidence, notably due to 'common' ALL, occurs at the ages of 2 and 3 (Table 1.17).

ALL varies worldwide, with the highest rates in childhood in Costa Rica (Table 1.7) and the lowest rates in Nigeria and Bombay. In England and Wales ALL also demonstrates county and administrative district heterogeneity [5]. Recent

Little is known of distributional data for the myelodysplastic syndrome (MDS). In the UK this data was complicated by diagnostic biases in the early 1980s [5]. Little data are available worldwide because cancer registries do not routinely collect this information, except for chronic myelomonocytic leukaemia (CMML).

Age group (years)	AML				ALL			
	OPCS: 1980–84		DCS: 1984–88		OPCS: 1980–84		DCS: 1984–88	
	Male	Female	Male	Female	Male	Female	Male	Female
0–4	0.30	0.47	1.18	0.94	4.39	4.04	5.10	5.54
15–24	0.64	0.43	0.82	0.83	1.10	0.51	1.25	0.57
35–44	1.06	1.04	1.25	1.39	0.25	0.21	0.36	0.21
55–64	3.83	3.23	5.77	3.65	0.66	0.65	0.75	0.48
65–74	8.02	6.78	10.82	7.16	0.89	1.20	0.91	0.43

Table 1.16 Comparison between a specialist leukaemia registry (Leukaemia Research Fund Data Collection Series (DCS)) and published (Office of Population Censuses and Surveys (OPCS)) incidence rates for selected leukaemias and selected age bands (rates per 100 000 per year).

Table 1.17 Age-specific incidence rates by age at diagnosis (0–14 years) for parts of England and Wales (rates per 100 000 per year) based on a total of 753 cases, 1984–93: ALL (all types).

Age (years)	Male rate	Female rate	Pooled rate
0	1.30	2.05	1.67
1	3.80	4.10	3.95
2	7.31	7.36	7.34
3	6.91	6.70	6.81
4	5.73	4.30	5.03
5	3.72	3.35	3.55
6	3.01	2.82	2.92
7	1.36	1.56	1.46
8	1.38	1.58	1.47
9	2.66	1.35	2.02
10	1.82	0.48	1.17
11	1.12	1.79	1.45
12	1.43	1.05	1.25
13	1.61	0.68	1.16
14	1.25	1.44	1.35

Table 1.19 Estimates of annual new case numbers in England and Wales based on data collected from 1984 to 1993: pooled ages 0–79 years.

Leukaemia/lymphoma	Male	Female	Total
AML	880	610	1 490
MDS	1 240	700	1 940
CML	290	190	480
ALL	280	200	480
CLL	4 060	2 000	6 060
NHL	4 380	2 850	7 230
HD	650	430	1 080
MM	3 900	1 900	5 800
Total	15 680	8 880	24 560

ecological analyses have linked this distribution with household radon gas levels [13] and quite markedly with the effects of rural isolation [14].

Chronic lymphocytic leukaemia

Chronic lymphocytic leukaemia (CLL) is rare before the age of 40, but increases steadily thereafter; this is shown in Table 1.12. Ninety per cent of patients with CLL are over 50 years of age and nearly two-thirds are over 60 years [15]. Table 1.2 indicates the rise of CLL in later life in all countries but the data are complicated by the inclusion of ALL.

CLL is the commonest type of leukaemia seen in Western countries, although its incidence is low in Far Eastern, African and South American populations (Table 1.2). This relative infrequency might be expected in developing countries with a low life expectancy when the disease is limited to middle and old age, but there are conspicuous anomalies which suggest that socioeconomic differences are only part of the explanation. In Japan, where the age distribution resembles that of Western populations, CLL is nearly absent, and among Japanese people living in Hawaii and the USA the incidence is much lower than in white people living in these same areas.

Among the black population, Africans have a very low inci-

Table 1.18 Age-specific incidence rates by age at diagnosis (15–29 years) for parts of England and Wales (rates per 100 000 per year) based on a total of 1067 cases, 1984–93: HD (all types).

Age (years)	Male rate	Female rate	Pooled rate
15	2.55	3.04	2.79
16	2.06	1.68	1.88
17	2.75	1.72	2.25
18	2.50	4.31	3.38
19	3.59	3.60	3.00
20	4.44	3.54	4.00
21	3.83	4.23	4.02
22	4.33	3.82	4.08
23	3.28	3.91	3.59
24	3.75	4.20	3.97
25	4.29	3.13	3.72
26	3.92	3.26	3.59
27	3.70	2.74	3.23
28	3.49	3.00	3.25
29	4.29	2.15	3.23

dence of CLL, although an exception may prove to be in younger multiparous black women but there are no competent epidemiological studies. Until recently, American black people have had a lower incidence than white Americans. However, this trend seems to be changing and in some parts of the USA, black people now have a higher incidence of CLL than white people, at least among males [10].

CLL in England and Wales has varied considerably in recorded incidence in recent years and displays true statistical heterogeneity by county [5]. However, the interpretation of this variation must rely heavily on nonbiological features, such as the rate at which the blood of older persons is routinely examined.

The high incidence of leukaemias and lymphomas among Jews has been frequently described. This is partly reflected in Table 1.4 for CLL. MacMahon & Koller [16] studied mortality data in Brooklyn, USA from 1943 to 1952, and were among the first to record a twofold excess for leukaemia in Jews compared with other ethnic groups. This relationship held for both men and women and at all ages. The tri-state leukaemia survey, 1959–62 [17], found a 2.4 relative risk associated with adult Jews compared with non-Jews. Russian Jews had a higher risk than other Russians or other Jews, and when compared to USA non-Jews their risk was fivefold. The prevalence of CLL was found by Bartal *et al.* [18] to vary with the country of origin of Jews in Israel, occurring more frequently among European-born Jews than in African and Asian Jews.

Non-Hodgkin's lymphoma

The worldwide distribution of non-Hodgkin's lymphoma (NHL) is shown in Table 1.3. This indicates the disease is particularly common in populations of Europe, America, Israel and Australasia and is rarer in South America, Africa, the Far East and rarer still in South Asia.

Recent UK rates given in Table 1.13 show the rarity in childhood, the male predominance at all ages and its increase with age.

Hodgkin's disease

Table 1.4 shows international variation in the rates of Hodgkin's disease (HD). Because of the unusual age-specific incidence rates showing the 'adolescent' peak at various ages between 15 and 29, these overall rate differences are difficult to interpret. Generally, Chinese and Japanese populations have some of the lowest rates while the rest of the world have very similar rates.

Recent UK data rates are similar to those in other parts of Europe. Table 1.14 shows the rarity of the condition both in childhood and in older people. Details of the recent adolescent peak are shown in Table 1.18, with the peak rates being in the early twenties.

Hodgkin's disease variation is complex, but rates in the Jewish population are high [4] and in the black populations lower than those in local white populations [19].

There is no obvious geographical variation within the UK at county or district levels [5].

Multiple myeloma

International data are sparse and given in Table 1.5. This shows the condition is usually absent in young persons. The exception is the US black population who have the highest rates. Asian populations have the lowest rates and most other populations have a similar and intermediate distribution. The UK rates are shown in Table 1.15.

One study on the subtypes of myeloma suggest that the IgA and IgG types are similar in incidence in terms of age and race [20].

Sex

There is a male predominance in most types of haematogenous malignancies which is generally observable throughout the world (Tables 1.1–1.7). The male:female ratio is highest in CLL (2:1) in the Western world. In ALL [5,21], interestingly, the childhood peak has a nearly equal distribution (Table 1.17) with only a slight male excess in teenagers before a small but consistent male excess occurs in older cases. The adolescent HD peak is also equally distributed between the sexes, with, if anything a slightly different and possibly excess pattern for females. Older HD has a marked excess of males, akin to NHL and multiple myeloma.

Detailed examination of the AML and myelodysplasia rates shows a roughly equal distribution between the sexes until the early fifties, when a male excess becomes marked. This is not seen in CML.

Secular trends

Acute myeloid leukaemia and related leukaemias

There was an increase in incidence and mortality of this form of leukaemia in England and Wales in the period 1961–78 but not in the period 1984–88.

Chronic myeloid leukaemia

Studies in Norway [22] show that age-specific rates for both acute and chronic leukaemias have been almost constant from 1957 to 1981, while in Denmark [23] the incidence of CLL and CML has remained unchanged from 1943 to 1977. However, in the same period there has been a steady increase in the incidence of acute leukaemia in patients over 50 years of age.

In the period 1984–88, CMML registrations have declined in parts of England and Wales [5]. This may be due to a diagnostic and classification change because CMML is now considered as, and grouped with, the myelodysplasias.

Myelodysplastic syndrome

There was a marked increase in the incidence of MDS from 1984 to 1988 [5], but this is very likely to be a result of the changes in diagnostic awareness and practice taking place during this period.

Acute lymphoblastic leukaemia

Stiller & Draper [24] observed an increase in Britain for leukaemia among children aged 0–4 years born after 1964. A statistically valid increase in childhood ALL in the Northwest of England has also been observed [25], with the rise beginning in about 1970 and being most marked in the 1–5-year age group.

Overall trends in registration for England and Wales show a steady increase in incidence of ALL for the age range 0–14 years in 1968–78 and a constant or declining mortality. No trends are deducible in the rare subgroup of adult ALL [26].

The changes in childhood ALL may be part of the continual shift in expression of the childhood peak, which was first noted in England in the late 1930s and in the USA shortly afterwards [27].

Chronic lymphocytic leukaemia

Incidence, as measured by registration rates, seems to be increasing, although there is no detectable trend in mortality. A recent review of CLL between 1984 and 1988 showed no secular trend [5].

Non-Hodgkin's lymphoma

There is an increasing awareness of the overall rise in incidence of NHL, which was first noted in the USA in the 1950s and has been detectable in the UK since the 1960s [28].

There is debate as to whether this might be an artefact due to the increasing awareness of the diagnosis, improvements in diagnosis and increased biopsy rates. However, estimates vary in the rate of increase, from 3 or 4% per annum to 10% [29]. Nevertheless, most authors agree that this rate is unlikely to be purely an artefact.

Hodgkin's disease

The changes in the rate of HD over the years have been complex. There may be a marked increase in childhood cases [25] and possibly fewer changes in the 15–29-year age group. However, there has been a marked decline in rates in the older cases [5]. This is possibly due to the rediagnosis and reclassification into NHL that has occurred over recent years.

This aspect of the epidemiology of HD, however, remains uncertain and further work is required to unravel any specific trends and changes.

Multiple myeloma

There may be an increase in incidence of multiple myeloma but this has been obscured by diagnostic variability.

Social class

Social class statistics in Britain are based on occupational data of the head of the household or, in the case of children, parental occupation, and so remain a crude social indicator. Since 1931 the standardized mortality ratio (SMR) has been consistently higher for leukaemias in social class I than social class V; data for women exhibit more fluctuations than those for men. Social class statistics based on male occupations are shown in Table 1.20. In 1971 four subcategories—lymphatic, myeloid, monocytic and other—were also analysed. For lymphatic and myeloid leukaemias, mortality was again generally positively correlated with social class, with higher SMRs found in higher social classes. For monocytic leukaemia there was no consistent gradient, while mortality for the remaining leukaemias showed a reverse gradient for men and single women which increased from social class I to V — mortality

Table 1.20 Standard mortality ratios by social class: males only.

Social class		Year			
		1931	1951	1961	1971
Leukaemia: all types					
I	(professional)	153	123	106	113
II	(management)	125	98	100	100
III	(skilled)	96	104	103	102
IV	(semiskilled)	94	93	97	104
V	(unskilled)	85	89	108	95
NHL: all types					
I	(professional)		138	110	147
II	(management)		104	96	101
III	(skilled)		103	101	96
IV	(semiskilled)		86	98	112
V	(unskilled)		91	114	106
HD: all types					
I	(professional)		142	101	113
II	(management)		110	107	103
III	(skilled)		100	107	104
IV	(semiskilled)		93	83	103
V	(unskilled)		87	109	91
MM: all types					
I	(professional)		188	143	122
II	(management)		101	101	105
III	(skilled)		104	104	107
IV	(semiskilled)		92	89	95
V	(unskilled)		76	110	108

being highest in social class V. This is difficult to interpret, as there could be a social class bias in diagnostic accuracy. Several studies in different parts of the world have suggested a higher incidence of childhood leukaemia among families of higher social class [30–32], which might reflect preferential treatment and diagnosis. The Manchester Children's Tumour Registry reported a similar distribution to the general population for socioeconomic status in ALL patients [33]. This has been weakly supported by a recent ecological study [14], in which the residents of areas of land defined by using data from the OPCS 1981 Census to house people of a 'higher' socioeconomic category, also contained more cases of certain leukaemias. In contrast, the distribution of cases of Hodgkin's disease is somewhat different [34]. Nothing is known of the social class distribution in MDS.

Clusters

Interest in the possibility that leukaemia and lymphoma might be the result of an infectious agent has been stimulated for many years by anecdotal descriptions of case aggregations in space and time, which have been variously described as 'clusters' or 'microepidemics'. Reports of leukaemia clusters go back to the last century, when the epidemiology of infectious diseases was an important focus of medical attention. However, scattered reports, for example a pair of cases in Kiev [35] in 1890 and a small cluster of leukaemia cases in young adults in Paris in 1923 [36], remained isolated in the literature until interest was again aroused in the 1950s, with the accumulating evidence suggesting a viral aetiology for leukaemia/lymphoma in many animal species.

It was not until 1964 that a method was suggested by Knox for a formal statistical approach for space–time clusters [37]. This method observes how frequently pairs of leukaemia cases occur together in time and space within a setting of defined critical limits. Observed pair frequencies are compared with what might be expected if case distribution was a random event following, say, a Poisson distribution. By applying this method to cases of childhood leukaemia diagnosed over a 10-year period in northeast England, Knox found a statistically significant excess in pairs of cases, with onset of disease within 2 months and resident at the time of diagnosis within 1 km [38]. Mantel further refined Knox's method, by applying a reciprocal transformation to separations which improved the statistical power [39]. Alternative statistical approaches have been devised by Pinkel & Nefzger [40] and David & Barton [41], and a number of workers were stimulated to look for clusters in defined populations using these methods.

Although occasional positive results have been reported, the level of statistical significance is generally unimpressive. Moreover, when such techniques have been applied to simulated data to study their sensitivity, they have proved to be generally inefficient, yielding inconclusive results [42]. A concept of brief latency is implicit in discrete space–time clusters and

techniques have largely developed extrapolating methods applicable to models of acute disease which may not be appropriate. Smith [43,44] devised a method which allowed for longer latent periods, but applied to data on all deaths from childhood leukaemia in Greater London from 1912 to 1965, no evidence of disease 'transmission' was found.

The inconsistencies of results are possibly attributable to the poor quality of data, problems of methodology and, particularly, to the inappropriateness of the space–time/infectious approach to disease transmission. More recently, Lewis re-evaluated some earlier studies for geographical space only using a 'nearest-neighbour' analysis. This technique does not require specified limits of time and space, and allows the data rather than the investigator to define the cluster, while the analysis evaluates the degree to which members of a population are clustered and is sensitive to departures from randomness in both directions [45]. This method produced significant clusters in Pinkel & Nefzger's data, suggesting a geographical relationship which did not also include a temporal one.

Recently considerable efforts have taken place to systematically rectify the deficiencies in previous methods. The methods have either been a non-boundary 'nearest-neighbour' technique, developed by Cuzick & Edwards [46] and Besag & Newell [47], or refinements on the use of Poisson distribution [48] or extension of a ward adjacency method used by Barnes *et al.* [49] by Alexander *et al.* [50].

When these methods are applied to the leukaemias to examine the generalized tendency for the diseases to cluster, CLL, for example, shows a tendency to cluster with each test [5]; this is possibly attributable to the heterogeneous local variations in recording for this condition. CML, however, shows no generalized tendency to cluster, neither does AML, while ALL shows some nearest-neighbour clustering but a substantial excess of neighbouring electoral wards have either high or low rates of the disease. This once more highlights the fact that local effects, but not necessarily local case contacts, are important for this condition.

Equally, with few exceptions [51], NHL and MM do not show much clustering, but Hodgkin's disease proves to be the exception. There is some data to suggest that not only does Hodgkin's disease vary in rate by areas of more or less isolation, but that its tendency to form clusters increases markedly in isolated rural areas [34], where possibly one in three cases occur as part of a cluster. Clustering has also been described in Hodgkin's disease in the USA [52].

The main alternative to detailed statistical analysis of leukaemia cases in defined populations has been the descriptive accounts of individual clusters. These are either *ad hoc* reports or attempts to use rates to comment on the disease. One of the first clusters to be studied in this way was the group of childhood leukaemia in Niles, Illinois, where eight cases of leukaemia were diagnosed in children under 15 years associated with a single school. This coincided with a 'rheumatic-like' illness among pupils in the same school, and it was suggested that the epidemiological features of this cluster indicated a relationship to infectious processes [53].

However, one of the most significant cluster reports originates from Albany, New York State, where an extensive network of cases and contacts between cases was investigated exhaustively [54]. Unfortunately, because little attention was given to constructing the total population at risk at the time, it is quite difficult to calculate or even infer the true and full significance of these striking observations. Many anecdotal reports of clusters have been published or (more often) recorded by health authorities since those times.

It is quite striking that most cluster reports, when they include a haematological malignancy, are dominated either by HD or childhood ALL.

Numerous investigations of individual case clusters of leukaemia and lymphoma in children and adults have been conducted since. More recently, close observation, using the methods of descriptive epidemiology, of sites of specific interest have highlighted some excesses over very long periods; an example is the area near the Sellafield nuclear reprocessing plant in Cumbria. This site has an excess of leukaemia/lymphoma in the age group 0–24 years from the 1950s until 1993 [55]. Closer examination of these sites indicates some local area excesses not confined to leukaemia which have no obvious explanation [56,57]. Recently, case–control methods have suggested that the parental occupations of residents in Cumbria might have some relevance to the cluster of cases near Sellafield [58]. However, this has been investigated thoroughly and it has been shown that this is unlikely to be the case [59].

The problem with the majority of close case association studies is the *post hoc* approach to the problem. Furthermore, many otherwise unbiased collections of data have been inadequate, in that they may have missed substantial numbers of cases.

It is therefore important to distinguish reports of cited or *post hoc* instances of clusters from those defined a priori by the newly assembled statistical techniques, which seek to uncover the natural tendency of the condition known as clustering.

The nearest-neighbour methods illustrate a point of major importance in the generalized clustering tests — that roughly 8% of all leukaemias cluster randomly. When 'true' case clusters occur among those random clusters, the same tests suggest that about 12% of cases cluster (i.e. 4% might be true clusters), then it is of great importance to distinguish one from another at this juncture. At present this is not possible.

An issue related to clustering is the possible seasonal excesses of these conditions by diagnostic date. The two haematological conditions which may well show some rare spatial clustering are the only two which also display possible diagnostic seasonality: ALL in children and HD. The best data are, however, with HD [34], although the full significance of this is not certain.

Aetiological factors

Ionizing radiation

The leukaemogenic effects of ionizing radiation have been thoroughly studied in atomic bomb survivors and those exposed diagnostically, therapeutically and occupationally. These studies show a relationship principally with the myeloid leukaemias in adults.

It should be recognized that those tissues which receive doses of irradiation are only one factor in assessing the probabilities of a leukaemogenic response. Generally, gamma rays have a leukaemogenic effect at high doses which is not so obvious at low doses, while X-rays appear to have effects at lower doses in certain circumstances. It is not known to what extent pure beta emitters have leukaemogenic effects in humans. However, most interest and current concern focuses on the effects of alpha emitters. Exposure to Thorotrast, the now redundant radioactive contrast medium, is a situation in which high-dose alpha exposures in lymph nodes and marrow occurs, and there is a suggestion that leukaemogenesis is a likely sequel [60]. What is not yet known is the effect of alpha sources in lower doses which might originate from medical procedures. There is some tenuous support for alpha exposures in the home causing leukaemia [61].

Atomic bomb survivors

Acute leukaemias were the first cancers reported in excess among atomic bomb survivors by the Atomic Bomb Casualty Commission at Hiroshima and Nagasaki [62]. However, chronic leukaemias show some differences, with CML being increased among Hiroshima survivors only and CLL being absent in both groups. The discrepancy in CML has been attributed to the physical differences in the radiation spectrum emitted by the two bombs; the Hiroshima bomb produced a mixture of gamma rays and neutrons and the Nagasaki bomb produced predominantly gamma rays. The dosimetry and the subsequent risk of leukaemia were reassessed in 1986 [63]. In addition, possible biological differences between the inhabitants of the two cities may be relevant. Experimental data have suggested that the age, genetic and physiological status of the host are important for the induction of radiation-related malignancies among survivors. A recent follow-up study showed that 83% of radiation-induced leukaemias occurred 5–21 years after exposure [64]; generally, the earlier the age of exposure, the shorter the latency. However, *in utero* exposure to high doses of radiation does not seem to have induced excess childhood cancers, including leukaemia [65]. Table 1.21 shows the incidence of leukaemia types in the life-span study cohort up to 1978 according to dose received. In all, 188 leukaemias occurred among the entire cohort of 110 000, representing a 20-fold excess over expected in some subgroups [66]. The incidence of different leukaemic types varied with

Table 1.21 Leukaemia incidence in life-span study cohort, 1950–78: Japanese atomic bomb survivors (110 000 residents).

Total air dose range (Gy)	Mean total marrow dose (Gy)	Incidence rate of leukaemia (100 000 per year)		
		Person-years	AML	CML
Unknown		56.73	7.0 (4)*	3.5 (2)*
4.00–6.00	2.77	20.97	85.8 (18)	14.3 (3)
2.00–3.99	1.47	49.83	34.1 (17)	20.1 (10)
1.00–1.99	0.76	76.29	19.7 (15)	3.9 (3)
0.5–0.99	0.38	102.50	5.9 (6)	4.9 (5)
0.01–0.49	0.06	921.42	3.3 (30)	2.3 (21)
<0.01	0	763.39	4.2 (32)	1.0 (8)
Not in city		626.20	2.1 (13)	0.2 (1)
Total		2617.35	5.2 (135)	2.0 (53)

* Number of cases are in parentheses.

Table 1.22 Annual incidence of various types of leukaemia by age in atomic bomb survivors who received 100+ rad (1+ Gy): Hiroshima and Nagasaki, 1950–78 (annual incidence rate (100 000 per year) for various ages at the time of the bomb).

Type of leukaemia	Age group (years)			
	<15	15–29	30–44	45+
Chronic granulocytic	14.5	7.3	15.5	15.5
Acute granulocytic	2.4	12.8	27.9	36.8
Acute lymphocytic	12.1	9.2	6.2	5.3

their age at exposure: CML with little age effect but ALL more frequently in younger persons and AML in older people—this is shown in Table 1.22.

Myelodysplastic states have also been found in survivors, while no excesses of Hodgkin's disease or NHL were found. Myeloma rates have been increased, however, in those heavily exposed [64,67].

Other groups exposed to nuclear fall-out

A total of 3072 (95.5%) participants from the armed forces in the American nuclear test 'Smoky', detonated in 1957, have now been followed up until 1979 and have shown a statistically significant increase in leukaemia incidence, (ten cases), and mortality, with a mean age at diagnosis of 41.8 years and a mean latency period of 14.2 years [68]. Controversy exists over whether children resident in the southern counties of Utah during the test period were at increased risk of developing cancers. An association between fall-out and childhood leukaemia mortality was suggested by Lyon *et al.* [69], but this claim has been refuted [70]. An excess of leukaemia incidence was noted among Utah Mormons living down-wind from the Nevada test site when compared with all other Mormons. The fivefold increase found in 1958–66 persisted to a lesser, although still significant, degree until 1980 [71]. A recent study has confirmed a dose-related excess particularly in those aged under 20 years and who died before 1964 [72].

Fall-out effects measured by the use of the strontium-90 levels which were distributed on the general population have been correlated by Archer [73], who took AML/ALL mortality from 1960 to 1969 by states in the USA. However, in a detailed study in Europe, no correlation was found for childhood leukaemia incidence and fall-out exposure [74]. Leukaemia was statistically increased in British forces participating in the atmospheric nuclear testing programme in the Pacific [75].

However, the results are difficult to interpret as there was no detectable 'dose response' and, furthermore, the leukaemia 'excess' is dependent on a particularly low leukaemia rate in the comparison group of other military personnel and disappears when a comparison is made with the population of England and Wales.

Little is known about whether the lymphomas and myelomas are in excess in such circumstances.

General population—irradiation exposure from natural sources

Regions with higher natural background levels in Europe and the USA have been weakly correlated with elevated leukaemia rates among local residents [76–78], while other studies have found no such excess in parts of the USA [79], Japan [80] and China [81]. Recently it has been shown that people living on thorium sands had greater numbers of cytogenetic abnormalities than a control group [82]. The situation regarding the possible hazards of inhaled radon gas is unclear, although there is some support for this as a potential hazard based on correlation studies and radiobiological theory [13,61]. Some elevation of leukaemia rates in Florida has been linked to higher levels of radium in drinking water, although the exposure data here are tenuous [83]. In general investigations correlating incidence with gamma ray exposures prove weakly negative [13,84], quite unlike those for radon gas.

General population—irradiation exposure from artificial sources

Much attention has been devoted to the proximity of childhood leukaemia to nuclear installations and several reports emanating from British governmental committees have resulted in the description of apparent childhood case excesses around three such installations in the UK [56,57,85,86]. This has resulted in considerable interest and further work in all areas, especially around Sellafield in Cumbria. The risk in that area appears to be limited to those children born and residing in the locality aged less than 25 [87] and not those attending school there [88]. In addition, it has been suggested that an association exists between certain parental occupations (including working at the nuclear reprocessing plant) and leukaemia risk in their children [58]. These results are based on small case numbers and have not been confirmed, as far as sources of irradiation are concerned, by similar studies elsewhere or by studies of associated populations [59,89].

Geographical studies in the USA and France have shown no association [90,91]. Further work on the geography of leukaemia mortality in Britain showed weak, inconsistent and unclear associations with sites of any nuclear installation [92], but similar weak links are recorded at sites where nuclear installations were either planned or were going to be built, but prior to their construction [93]. These observations are probably linked to the heterogeneous leukaemia distribution noted earlier [14] and could relate to various 'infectious agent' allergenic stimulation theories that are currently popular (see section on infections, p. 21). Recent reviews of the situation near to the reprocessing plant of Sellafield show that the excess of NHL and lymphoblastic leukaemia in those aged 0–24 is continuing [55]. The reasons still remain obscure.

Therapeutic and diagnostic radiation exposure

Apart from natural background sources of ionizing radiation, for which there is as yet little major evidence of a leukaemogenic effect, the other main sources of variable exposure to radiation are through therapeutic or diagnostic medical procedures. Several authors have attempted to relate the changing pattern of leukaemia mortality to the effects of ionizing radiation. Changing medical practices have played an important part in this assessment and patients receiving radiotherapy for such benign conditions as ankylosing spondylitis, thymic enlargement, ringworm, menorrhagia and tonsillitis, as well as for certain malignant conditions, have been studied. The Court Brown and Doll cohort of ankylosing spondylitis

sufferers [94] have received the most extensive follow-up [95]. Leukaemia and myeloma incidences are raised in this study with the exception of CLL, and a dose–response pattern has been demonstrated for leukaemia (Table 1.22).

The increased leukaemia rate achieves a maximum by about 10 years after irradiation and thereafter declines: very like the sequelae of the atomic explosion.

The causal link between marrow gamma irradiation in excess of 75 rad (0.75 Gy) received dose and subsequent adult leukaemias is well established. Table 1.23 gives details of other cohorts studied for their late consequences of irradiation [95–98]. The study of women treated by irradiation for metropathia showed a slight case excess of leukaemia and myeloma but the small study on fluoroscoped women showed no statistical excess having a mean marrow dose of 13 rad (0.13 Gy). A very large collaborative study on the late effects of irradiation for cervical carcinoma [98–100] showed a clear dose response linked to carcinoma of organs receiving well over 5 Gy, such as bladder or rectum. The marrow doses were widely variable (being largely in the pelvis), and although the overall estimated pelvic doses are moderate (1–3 Gy) the risk of leukaemia is low overall (observed/expected = 1.2) and does not exist for myeloma. However, careful examination of the data shows a high leukaemia rate in those with marrow exposure in the 2.5–5.0 Gy band but with less in higher exposure probably due to cell killing effects.

Generally, although the links with adult leukaemia (except CLL) are well established, there is less evidence relating to other haematogenic malignancies. No good data exist independently for MDS, although some of the original 'leukaemia' cases in the Japanese cohorts were MDS in transformation to AML. It might be inferred that MDS has a similar link with ionizing irradiation to the acute leukaemias of adult life.

	Observed	Expected	Observed/expected
1 Patients treated for ankylosing spondylitis (14 111 patients): mean marrow dose 320 rad (3.2 Gy)			
All causes	1795	1061.61	1.66
Leukaemia	31	6.47	4.79
2 Women treated for metropathia haemorrhagica (2067 patients): mean marrow dose 140 rad (1.4 Gy)			
Leukaemia	7	2.7	2.59
3 Women receiving fluoroscopic examinations of chest (1047 patients): mean marrow dose 13 rad (0.13 Gy)			
Leukaemia	2	1.2	1.67
4 Women treated for cervical cancer by irradiation (82 616 patients): pelvic marrow dose 100–300 rad (1–3 Gy)			
Leukaemia	77	65.83	1.2

Table 1.23 Studies of leukaemia incidence and mortality in populations exposed to low-level radiation: observed and expected deaths.

Consistent evidence throughout the published data has failed to link CLL or HD to ionizing irradiation exposure. Surprisingly, despite the relative commonness of NHL (at least at all sites and all histological types), the same attention has not been devoted to these conditions. There have been some weak and inconsistent associations reported between NHL and low linear energy transfer (LET) ionizing irradiation sources, but the consensus is that, at this group diagnostic level, a causal link is unlikely to exist [101]. An exception to this may be with high LET exposure as exemplified by Thorotrast exposure. Two of the cohorts of survivors reported an excess of B-cell NHL (but not CLL) [102]. However, thorotrast exposures confer greatest risks for the leukaemias (except CLL) [103].

Some studies show AML in excess in women treated for breast cancer by surgery and radiotherapy [104]. Similarly, Hodgkin's disease treated by radiation has produced excesses of AML in survivors in certain studies [105] and not others [106].

A review of the effects of diagnostic radiation in adults by Stewart *et al.* [107], and recently reconfirmed [108], showed an excess of myeloid leukaemias. A rigorous study of adult diagnostic exposures [101] has shown a slight risk for leukaemia (excluding CLL) and myeloma. Prenatal radiography was also studied by Stewart and linked with an increased risk of acute leukaemia during early childhood [109], but this excess has been attributed to selection bias, identifying women who already have characteristics that predispose their offspring to malignancy [110]. However, Bithell & Stewart [111] were able to show an increased risk with increasing number of X-ray films, which strengthens the hypothesis that the observed association was causal, and other authors confirm this association [112,113]. Paternal preconception X-ray exposures have also been shown to be associated with ALL and AML in the offspring [114,115], but this is likely to be a result of biases in the way the data were obtained [116]. Evans *et al.* [117] have estimated 1% of all leukaemia cases may be attributed to diagnostic X-rays.

There is no consensus about the possible harmful effects of postnatal childhood diagnostic irradiation, and major studies are still underway.

Myeloma is also linked to Thorotrast exposure; however, remarkably, there have been some consistent associations with low LET radiation from the major irradiation cohorts, with the exception of the cervical follow-up studies [118].

A case–control study of lymphoid leukaemias and lymphomas within the Yorkshire Health Region found a significant risk for lymphoid malignancies [119] among patients treated with Grenz ray therapy for eczema or dermatitis. Grenz rays are low energy and have little penetration and this observation awaits confirmation.

Occupational exposure

Classically, radium dial painters and underground miners are two groups heavily exposed to specific types of ionizing irradiation. Although they have developed various malignancies, leukaemia has not yet been shown to be in excess.

Radiologists were the first group of workers who were shown to exhibit a risk of leukaemia associated with chronic radiation exposure, which diminished as protection guidelines were enforced [120,121]. However, Chinese X-ray workers still appear to have a risk of the leukaemias other than CLL [122].

Recent interest in workers in nuclear power stations and other facilities has engendered much debate. This is because of the low total whole body gamma exposures involved and the unknown risks which might be associated with radioactive particulates. One intensive study in the 1960s and 1970s could reach little agreement about whether a leukaemia excess resulted from such exposure [123], but another analysis of the experience of 1722 shipyard nuclear workers indicated higher death rates from leukaemia, other haematological cancers and all cancers when compared with workers employed in non-nuclear occupations. This study stimulated the commencement of a major study of nuclear naval installations in the USA [124]. Subsequently several studies in various situations have found small, but statistically nonsignificant, excesses of leukaemia in exposed workforces [125–128]. By contrast, other studies found no such links [129,130]. These weak leukaemia excesses cannot, at this stage, be causally linked to radioactive emissions, not least because of the apparently low doses involved. All this evidence necessitates further investigations of other possible aetiological factors operating in these situations. Any excess numbers reported to be occurring in occupational situations are trivial compared with the total number of cases of the disease and do not present a public health problem. The studies may also suggest that the postulated hazards are unique to the geographical locality. If so, this indicates that further investigations may not assist in acquiring a greater understanding of the causes of most leukaemias.

The combined analysis of all the UK nuclear workers' cohorts has recently been published [131]. Over 75 000 workers were incorporated into this study. Mortality from leukaemia (excluding CLL) was positively associated with the cumulative external radiation dose, based on 49 deaths. No risks were recorded for MM, lymphomas or CLL. This is contrary to findings from America and, because of the relatively small case numbers, should not be regarded as a definitive result.

A study of the national UK radiation workers film badge doses has also taken place [132]. This cohort of over 95 000 persons overlapped with the nuclear industry study. It found, not surprisingly, similar results for leukaemia (excluding CLL), but also an association with myeloma but not for other lymphomas. Overall the rates of leukaemia in the cohort are lower than in the general public and the association in both these studies is one of trend with increasing dose.

Nonionizing radiation

The evidence relating chronic disease to most sources of non-ionizing radiations is inconclusive, but ultrasound, ultraviolet radiations and extremely low frequency electromagnetic radiation from domestic sources have attracted particular attention.

The use of ultrasound in medical diagnosis has greatly increased over the last three decades, particularly in obstetrics. The vast majority of all infants in the USA and UK will now have been exposed to ultrasound *in utero*, yet such exposures have not yet been shown to be entirely free of hazard. A few reports exist which suggest it is a potentially hazardous procedure; these include one which demonstrated that sister chromatoid exchange was significantly increased in freshly growing lymphoblast lines by exposure to diagnostic levels of ultrasound for 30 minutes [133]. However, data from a case–control study of childhood cancer have not revealed any significantly raised risk of the leukaemias in the exposed fetus following ultrasound examination in pregnancy [134].

The carcinogenic action of ultraviolet (UV) light might be more complex than first thought [135]. Evidence suggests that the part of the emission spectrum most damaging to DNA in skin cell is UVB, with a wavelength spectrum between 290 and 320 nm. Chronic exposure has been linked with skin cancers. However, an effect of UV irradiation on the immune system has been postulated, stimulated by experimental studies on transplanted immunogenic UV-induced tumours in mice [136] and the observed activity of circulating T cells in solarium-treated subjects [137]. CLL and skin cancer have frequently been found in the same patient in sequence or concurrently [138] and UV light may be an important common aetiological factor. These ideas have been elaborated in more detail recently and there are some scraps of epidemiological evidence to support possible links with NHL as well as CLL [28,139].

The effect of extremely low frequency alternating magnetic fields on cultured human cells has been studied by Tsoneva *et al.* [140], who found that certain magnetic fields gave a significantly increased mutagenic effect on cultured human peripheral blood lymphocytes. Chromosomal aberrations most commonly found were chromatoid gaps and breaks. *In vitro* studies have looked at calcium ion efflux from chick and cat brains exposed to extremely low frequency fields [141,142]. However, these observations led to work [143] which suggests a link between childhood cancers including leukaemia and magnetic fields. Attempts to repeat this controversial work have failed in the USA [144] and Britain [145]. These, and more recent work by Savitz [146,147], suffer from problems of dose measurements which makes the interpretation of each study very difficult [148]. Weak excesses were found in certain subgroups, of which some were statistically significant, while other studies have shown very little evidence of excess [149,150].

Recent investigations have revealed that great difficulties exist in assessing low frequency magnetic field exposures in the common environment. Major issues addressing how to assess past exposures meaningfully vary somewhat from country to country. The 'wire-code' methods used in North America have received some validation but are not useful in parts of Europe including the UK. Here it has been shown that proximity to overhead powerlines is a poor substitute for ambient household levels, although this and spot measurements have been used in more recent Scandinavian studies [151]. These studies show confusing and mixed results: spot measurements are poorly correlated with risk, while some 'historically' created measurements of proximity were associated with ALL. Because of this, and the fact that such studies did not assess directly other possible risk factors, it is not easy to interpret these results. The next generation of studies measuring more prolonged exposures in houses and elsewhere, along with investigations of other possible risk factors, are awaited from North America and Europe. Work is now underway using personal dosimeters and it is unlikely that this issue will be resolved until studies which make use of direct dosimetry are published. Recent overviews of data relating to childhood leukaemia and lymphoma, which assess the imperfections of previous studies, now exist [152].

The most consistent associations to date lie with wire-code estimates of ambient field strengths in North America and childhood leukaemia risks. Doubt has been cast upon these studies recently by the observation that a major social class bias might exist here [153].

Occupational exposure to nonionizing radiation has received separate attention. Milham suggested that occupations requiring people to work in an environment high in 'electrical' or 'magnetic' fields carry a higher risk of leukaemia [154] and an increased risk of death from leukaemia was found in 10 out of 11 occupations thought to be associated with such exposure. This observation prompted further reports on leukaemia morbidity and mortality among other workers also thought to be associated with electromagnetic fields, which reinforced the preliminary findings [155–157]. In a study by McDowall [156] the risk was found to be highest for AML and was particularly associated with telecommunication engineers. In an overview of many of these studies, Coleman & Beral [158] showed a 46% excess of AML, although this observation has not been supported by a recent large mortality study for the USA [159]. Unfortunately in all these studies there is no systematic evidence that the workers are in fact subjected to excessive electrical or magnetic fields. One further common factor may be exposure to noxious substances such as fumes from soldering, jointing and welding and, additionally, to solvent exposures.

More recently a Scandinavian study has suggested CLL is related to occupational electromagnetic field exposure [160] and a joint French–Canadian study produced some evidence for an AML excess at one of its power generation sites [161].

Both studies made extensive efforts to compute possible past exposure but did not take into account a wide range of possible confounders.

Occupational and chemical exposures

Occupational correlation studies using the descriptive epidemiology of the leukaemias give results that are neither consistent nor readily interpretable. Attempts have been made, for example, to correlate geographical patterns of occurrences and mortality with some manufacturing industries and occupations. Many of these studies are retrospective and rely on death certificates, which have serious limitations of both reliability and of the assumptions made about individual experience according to area of residence. Historically the occupational exposure of shoe manufacturers in Istanbul to high benzene levels and their consequential high levels of leukaemia is a significant observation [162].

Benzene

An unsubstantiated suggestion that benzene may be a leukaemogen was proposed in the late nineteenth century. Its immunosuppressive effects on haemopoietic and reticuloendothelial tissues implies an aetiological relationship for a range of lymphoid and myeloid malignancies. Early case reports did not appear until the 1920s [163], but recent studies of workers occupationally exposed to benzene have shown a fivefold increase in mortality risk for all types of leukaemia and a tenfold increase for myeloid leukaemias [164]. Recent updates of these data have shown an even stronger link between leukaemia and benzene [165]. Shoe workers in Istanbul, chronically exposed to benzene, showed excesses of various types of acute myeloid leukaemias, myelodysplastic states and chronic myeloid leukaemia [166].

A variety of cohort studies have now been published on this important topic, all of which show some magnitude of association of benzene with adult leukaemias. The risks vary considerably in different occupational circumstances, from non-significant but excessive risks to statistically significant tenfold excesses [167–172].

Other solvents

Interest has extended to exposure to other solvents, stimulating studies among such groups as chemists [173,174], rubber workers [175–177] and oil refinery workers [178–180]. Dry cleaning has been linked (via perchloroethylene) to risks of lymphomas [181].

Other occupations

There are other, often isolated, reports of occupational links with leukaemia. A few may prove to have real excesses, possibly among those exposed to diesel exhaust emissions [182–184], pathologists [185], wood industry workers [184] and welders [186]. This latter observation may be related to the 'electrically related occupations' observations made earlier. Myeloma has been linked to painters [187] and woodworkers [188]. Nickel refinery workers have an excess of myeloma and lymphoma [189].

These studies have often been poor in that they show the necessity for detailed analysis of type, intensity and duration of exposure to disentangle the various effects of different chemicals sufficiently sensitively to demonstrate possible relationships. In a case-control study of workers in the rubber industry, direct exposure to all solvents, including benzene, was 4.5 times as frequent in ALL cases as in matched controls [190]. Further analysis revealed that patients spent a greater proportion of their work experience in jobs with potential exposure to coal-tar-based solvents, again including benzene as well as xylene [191]. A similar risk for petroleum-based solvents was not apparent. The strongest association was with carbon disulphide (risk = 8.7), drawing attention to the common epidemiological problem of the interpretation of data from multiple simultaneous exposures. Many of the so-called 'other solvent' exposures could be benzene mixed with other substances of unknown potential hazard, for example in pressmen [192] and painters [193].

Agriculture and related exposures

There has been considerable interest in the possibility that agrichemical exposures might be linked with the leukaemias in some way. Early studies were conflicting [194–197] and emanated, for example, in the USA from geographic observations that suggested rates for some leukaemias were greater in the mid-West and related to areas of intense agriculture.

Many later studies have achieved some consistency, with the majority being supportive of a link with agrichemicals; such studies report from various parts of the USA [198,199], as well as Canada [200], New Zealand [201] and England [202]. Although all leukaemia types have been implicated, the most substantial links are with the chronic lymphoid types, particularly in farmers under the age of 65. These observations link up with further observations associating agrichemical use with NHL and myeloma.

Many papers link agrichemical exposure to both NHL and CLL [202,203]. This has been further linked, for example, to the increase in NHL incidence [204–206].

It has been suggested that hairy cell leukaemia is common in farmers [207]. Multiple myeloma is also strongly associated with farming exposure [118,187,208–210] and HD has been linked to agriculture [211].

There is no consensus of opinion about which chemicals, if any, might be implicated, although the chlorophenols, the chlorphenoxy herbicides and the hexachlorocychlohexanes, have all been weakly implicated as leukaemogens [212].

However, a large international study has shown no lymphoma excess amongst manufacturers [213].

Butchers and related occupations

Butchers and slaughterhouse workers could be exposed to animal viruses, and one study [214] has shown excess mortality from tumours of the haemopoietic and lymphatic systems; of 223 deaths, three were leukaemias, twice that expected. An excess of unspecified types of leukaemia among veterinary practitioners has also been noted [215].

Styrene exposures

Several reports have suggested risks of leukaemia as a result of exposure to styrene monomers and butadienes [216–218]. These exposures have to be distinguished from risks due to benzene inhalation, and a large cohort study has not found any leukaemia risk [219]. This has been challenged by more recent work [220].

Ethylene oxide exposure

Studies in Sweden [221] and the USA [222] show an excess of leukaemia, while two other studies do not [223,224]. Animal and *in vitro* studies, however, suggest that this substance may be potentially carcinogenic [212].

Parentally transmitted risks

Transplacental chemical or viral carcinogenesis has not yet been positively associated with the aetiology of childhood leukaemia. The Oxford Survey of Childhood Cancer [225] found a positive association between sedatives taken during pregnancy and subsequent malignancy in the offspring but most studies on this topic have found very few consistent results.

Evidence for nonleukaemogenic materno-fetal infections in man and also the model of feline leukaemia, where the infective agent can be spread congenitally to the developing fetus across the placenta, provided the impetus for a search for a similar effect in childhood leukaemia. Knox *et al.* [226] examined congenital rubella infections where a fetal exposure depends on the mother having escaped infection during her childhood. No evidence for any similarity to the congenital rubella syndrome was found in this study. Data from the Oxford Survey suggested a positive association between influenza during pregnancy and subsequent childhood cancer, including leukaemia. Three cases of ALL but no controls recorded chickenpox during the mother's pregnancy. The proportion of cases that could be attributable to virus infection is believed to be small [227], if it exists at all.

Several studies have attempted to link parental occupation with childhood leukaemia but findings have been conflicting and inconclusive. A number of these reports have been reviewed [228]. Nine studies have investigated leukaemia patients who had fathers with motor-vehicle-related occupations compared with cancer controls. Two showed significant excess odds ratios. In addition, machinists and other factory workers have been studied (three significant excesses); hydrocarbon exposure (two significant excesses in five publications); paint and pigment exposure (two significant excesses in eight studies); solvents and other chemical exposure (two significant excesses in eight studies) and two studies on medically related occupations (one significant excess).

Also, two studies related to nuclear reprocessing plant workers have shown a statistical excess of case fathers in one study [58] and not clearly in another [229]. A further study indicates that exposures to ionizing irradiation generally might be important, and that this exposure is especially so around the time of the conception of the child [230]. X-ray exposure of case fathers was described as excessive by Graham *et al.* [114] and Shu *et al.* [115].

The study reported by McKinney *et al.* [230] suggests that wood dust exposure in a parent might be implicated in childhood lymphoma/leukaemia and also confirmed a significant excess of solvent exposure in case fathers. A study from Spain found that women working at home exposed to fabric dust had an excess of offspring with ALL [231].

The interpretation of all these data must be limited. There is conflict in the data, the real meaning of the reported parental exposures are, often, highly suspect and, importantly, no biological mechanisms are yet known which could suggest any credible pathways of leukaemogenesis.

Parental exposure to ionizing irradiation has been dealt with earlier.

Environmental chemicals

Chronic exposure to certain chemicals as a consequence of occupational activities or environmental exposure has been shown to lead to the development of leukaemia.

There is some slight evidence accumulating that the dioxin-exposed people living around the Seveso chemical plant [232] show an excess of leukaemia mortality in men. This is contrary to the studies on chlorophenol manufacturers, who show no substantial excess leukaemia risk. Recent reanalysis shows an excess of NHL in those most exposed [233,234].

One study has unconvincingly linked residential pesticide use with childhood leukaemia [235].

Veterans of Vietnam have an excess of lymphomas, usually ascribed to exposures to defoliants, although the major excess is in the ex-navy personnel [236].

Cigarette smoking

Austin & Cole [237] have suggested that earlier cohort studies showed a continuing link between cigarette smoking and adult leukaemias. This was demonstrated in a very large cohort of US veterans [238,239]. The leukaemia excess is mainly for AML, with a large estimated population risk suggesting one in four of all cases of AML are the result of cigarette smoking.

Case–control studies have shown a less clear relationship, although Severson [240] noted an attributable risk for AML of 31%. There are several known or potential leukaemogens in cigarette smoking, including benzene, polonium-210 and various polycyclic aromatic hydrocarbons. No excesses linked to cigarette smoke have emerged with any other haematological malignancies, except weakly with NHL [241,242].

Hair dyes

Studies have suggested a leukaemogenic risk for both hair dye users [243,244] and for hairdressers [245]. This has been challenged [246]. Other studies have linked this exposure with NHL and even MM and HD [247].

Alcohol consumption

Alcohol ingestion in pregnancy has been linked with the risk of childhood AML [248], although direct risk data on adult leukaemia and lymphoma suggest that it is not a risk factor [249].

Diet

Other aspects of diet as risk factors have been inconclusive. A study linking processed meats and childhood leukaemia is unconvincing [250].

Past medical events including therapy

Medical history

Skin cancer. Investigators have reported the frequent association of leukaemia with other types of cancer and a number of authors have stressed a particular association with CLL. There is a significantly higher incidence of skin cancer in CLL patients [138,251,252], occurring simultaneously or in sequence. The same is true of NHL [139].

Second diseases. A particular example of an association between leukaemia and other cancers is when leukaemia occurs as a second primary malignancy, associated with treatment. (This topic is dealt with more fully in Chapter 12). AML has increasingly been reported following chemotherapy and/or radiotherapy for various haematological malignancies, solid tumors and non-malignant conditions. Until recently, the quantification of increased risk associated with each mode of treatment has been difficult, because epidemiological studies are often limited by small numbers of cases, lack of completeness of treatment data, use of poorly selected populations and/or an inadequate comparison group. An increased risk of leukaemia has been reported for irradiation alone, as discussed earlier, but it would appear that alkylating agents used in chemotherapy exert a dominant influence on the risks, while the combination of radiotherapy and chemotherapy may be synergistic [253]. The epipodophyllotoxins have been identified as particularly being linked to secondary AML [254].

An assessment of the available studies shows risks for leukaemia following chemotherapy in excess of tenfold and in some cases up to 100-fold. The studies have followed groups of cases, for example, of HD [105,255–257] and other haematological conditions such as CLL [258,259], as well as ovarian cancer [260], breast cancer [261] and certain nonmalignant conditions.

Generally, chemotherapy is the overwhelming source of risk. Leukaemia has a higher risk in those treated with multiple drugs and in the last 20 years.

Most of the leukaemias are AML with, rarely, ALL or biphenotypic leukaemias occurring [262].

Cases of rheumatoid arthritis and musculoskeletal diseases have been associated with the increased occurrence of acute myeloblastic leukaemia, lymphoma and myeloma, but these patients also receive immunosuppressants and azathioprine [263–265] and so the causal relationship is not clear from these studies. More recent studies, however, indicate a statistically valid three- to fourfold excess with myeloma and lymphoma [266,267].

Drugs

There is a clear link between chloramphenicol use and childhood leukaemia [268]. The suspicion that phenylbutazone might cause leukaemia in some patients has also been discussed since the first case reports were published in the late 1950s. Although there is little epidemiologically based evidence, the ability of phenylbutazone to suppress bone marrow function and possibly damage chromosomes has provided a biological basis for concern. In one case–control study [269] no association was found with prior phenylbutazone use — the small association observed was accounted for largely by an association with the prior disease rather than treatment. In another study a link was found with CLL [270].

Growth hormone therapy may be linked with childhood leukaemia [271]. One study appears unconvincingly to link marijuana use in pregnancy with subsequent childhood AML [272].

Transplants

Organ transplant recipients have been extensively followed by Penn in the Cincinnati (formerly Denver) Transplant Tumor Registry [273] and by Kinlen *et al.* in a collaborative UK–Australian study of renal transplant recipients [274]. Apart from skin malignancies, tumours of the reticuloendothelial system are the most commonly reported, with a 60-fold lymphoma excess, particularly large cell lymphomas, but leukaemias also occur, on average about 5 years after transplantation [275].

About 5% of all bone marrow transplant relapses had AML or ALL arising in the donated cells themselves [276]. Disturbances of immunity may either precede or be acquired after transplantation. Furthermore, occult viruses and/or drugs may lead to *de novo* leukaemia. Lymphoproliferative disease has also been reported following paediatric liver transplantation [277].

Finally a small study of blood recipients has also shown an excess of lymphomas [278].

Other medical conditions

An association between states of hypersensitivity and cancer has been shown, including an excess of allergies in childhood leukaemia [279]. Subsequent studies have usually reported no relationship or, in the case of adult leukaemias, a negative association between allergy and cancer [270,280,281]. Similarly cases of pernicious anaemia have a higher rate of AML [282], possibly in part due to a diagnostic bias as a result of difficulties in identifying some refractory anaemic states.

The tri-state leukaemia survey [283] searched for diseases occurring at least 1 year before diagnosis in 605 adult males with leukaemia and 668 controls. Out of 30 diseases studied, seven showed an excess among patients with leukaemia: infectious hepatitis, eczema, psoriasis, diabetes, arthritis and rheumatism, heart disease and ankylosing spondylitis. CLL in particular had a more frequent history of herpes zoster (relative risk (RR) = 1.95), while urticaria was positively associated with AML (RR = 2.93) and CML (RR = 2.95). A study of lymphoid cancer in Yorkshire, UK recorded a relative risk of 3.78 for eczema/dermatitis and lymphatic leukaemias and also a significantly increased risk associated with various allergies [119].

Excesses of CLL and AML have been demonstrated in rheumatoid arthritic cases [284] , possibly partly due to drug therapy.

BCG vaccination

BCG vaccination as part of the prevention programme for TB has been investigated following the suggestion that it may also afford 'protection' against leukaemia, although possibly enhancing the risk of developing a lymphoma. Hoover critically reviewed these studies in 1978 and concluded that there was little evidence that such vaccinations were 'effective' against leukaemia or other tumours. The Medical Research Council's clinical trial of the effects of BCG and vole bacillus vaccine began in 1950 and the trial population was followed through to the end of 1979 in respect of deaths from leukaemia [285]. Overall neither protection nor enhancement was apparent. A trivial early beneficial effect, followed by a later deleterious effect, was also discernible in a Puerto Rican trial [286]. Recent studies, however, have reopened this issue and suggested there are protective effects once more [287,288].

Chronic immune stimulation

There are a mixed variety of observations which suggest that myeloma, the lymphomas and CLL, in particular, might in some way be a consequence of chronic stimulation of the immune system.

This has been particularly investigated with myeloma where one study found less past chronic infection [289]. Another study found the opposite [290], whilst a more recent study showed very little indeed [291,292].

Early studies found an association between HD and tonsillectomy [293]. However, more recent work failed to support this conclusion [294,295].

A variety of weak relationships have been reported for CLL, NHL, HD and the leukaemias [202]. More recently, chronic fatigue syndrome has been weakly linked to NHL [296].

More convincingly, it has been suggested that childbearing has a protective effect for HD [297], and there has been a possibly related observation that breastfeeding might also be protective [298].

Inherited disorders

Congenital syndromes

Down's syndrome cases have an increased incidence of acute leukaemia, which is lymphoid in type in 70% of cases. It has been suggested that the increased risk, especially in children, is specifically associated with the presence of the extra 21 chromosome [299]. Down's AML cases present earlier than usual, while the ALL cases have a similar spectrum of incidence by age to ALL in normal children [300]. A number of instances of leukaemia in carriers of other congenital abnormalities of both somatic and sex chromosomes have been reported, but the rarity of such events makes their significance difficult to assess. Three rare congenital syndromes — Fanconi's anaemia, Bloom's syndrome and ataxia telangiectasia — are among the most thoroughly studied and are associated with a greatly increased incidence of leukaemia. They are, like Down's syndrome, associated with nonrandom chromosomal abnormalities [300,301,302]. ALL of types other than C-ALL has been described with microcephaly and immunodeficiency [303]. Relatives of parents with cystic fibrosis may have an increased risk of leukaemia [304].

Immune deficiency diseases

Gatti & Good [305] estimated that the frequency of malignancy in patients with primary immunodeficiency is approximately 10000 times greater than the general age-matched population. Each type of immunodeficiency has a distinctive constellation of malignancies associated with it: for example, lymphatic leukaemia with infantile X-linked agammaglobulinaemia; ataxia telangiectasia with ALL; common variable immune deficiency with CLL. Inherited disorders of immune regulation predispose both to the development of autoimmune diseases and lymphoid malignancies. Evidence for a genetic predisposition to autoimmune disease exists and the link with lymphoid neoplasia is persuasive, but this requires further clarification of the exact nature of the relationship. An immunodeficiency cancer registry was established in the USA in 1971. By 1978 data from 267 individuals with both genetically determined immunodeficiency and malignancy had been recorded from the USA and elsewhere. Lymphoreticular tumours were the most common (59% of the total), but 32 (12%) leukaemias were reported [306] with excesses of lymphoid as well as myeloid leukaemia [274,306].

There are extensively reported links between certain immunodeficient syndromes, both acquired and inherited, and the haematological malignancies. These include excesses in ataxia telangiectasia (NHL, CLL), Bloom's syndrome (NHL, AML, ALL), X-linked lymphoproliferation (NHL), Wiskott–Aldrich syndrome (HD, NHL, AML), severe combined immunodeficiency (NHL), common variable immunodeficiency (NHL, CLL), hyper IgM immunodeficiency (NHL) and selection IgH immunodeficiency (NHL) [307].

Familial aggregation

Leukaemias of childhood rarely occur in families except in identical twins who share a common placental circulation [308].

Many studies report familial excesses of adult leukaemias among blood relatives, in particular CLL and AML [309–311]. Also there may be a greater tendency for haematological or other malignancies to occur in the kindred of a case of leukaemia [202,312,313].

There is some weak evidence for an association with sharing of HLA haplotype [314] and also a link with specific alleles [315–318].

Infections and immune stimulation

There have been some recent epidemiological studies of viral involvement in leukaemogenesis of some note.

Human T-cell leukaemia virus I (HTLV-I) is clearly associated with an acute T-cell leukaemic syndrome [319] which is geographically circumscribed and well defined. Clustering of cases has been described [320]. Its epidemiology in the Caribbean is well documented [321].

HTLV-II was isolated from an intravenous drug abuser with a hairy cell leukaemia of a rare subtype. Little is known of its pathogenesis and epidemiology [322].

Human immunodeficiency virus (HIV) infection confirms a significant risk of subsequent lymphoma in roughly 3% of all reported AIDS cases [323] and in HIV-positive haemophiliacs [324].

Little else is known of any specific virus causally related to a leukaemia: Epstein–Barr virus (EBV) has never been directly linked with the leukaemic process, for example [325]. EBV is strongly related to paediatric HD [326] but less clearly with certain older cases [327]. Human herpesvirus (HHV-6) does not seem to be related to these malignancies [328] and the new Kaposi's agent is yet to be evaluated [329].

The search for human viruses akin to the bovine leukosis virus or feline leukaemia virus (FeLV) has failed and there are various lines of reasoning to suggest why a specific virus is unlikely [330].

However, there is an increasing volume of epidemiological evidence, with some biological and theoretical support that 'nonspecific' infections are implicated in childhood ALL. Such infections may be of two types: a nominal range of certain viruses, or any infection which might stimulate the immune system of the developing child at certain critical times.

The latter concept is part of the argument regarding the childhood peak of ALL formulated by Greaves [331]. He predicts that fewer allergenic stimuli in very early postnatal life, with later infection at a critical period, play a major role in precipitating the common ALL of the childhood peak. Limited support for this comes from a correlation study which shows for the first time that the childhood peak of ALL varies by the type of community: the peak is very pronounced in 'isolated' towns and villages and very much foreshortened in connurbations, which perhaps suggests a different spectrum of infections in different types of locality [14].

An alternative, and to some extent complementary, series of studies which originate from a report by Kinlen has raised the possibility that the migration of populations and population intermixing can, in certain circumstances, lead to an excess of leukaemias in young people [332].

Adolescent HD, like ALL, in some ways shows characteristics that might indicate that unidentified infectious agents are involved [333].

The other malignancies have not been associated with any viral agent.

Conclusion

Studies on the epidemiology of the haematological malignancies encompass diverse approaches and widely differing interpretations, yet the aetiology of these diseases still remains largely enigmatic. Other than cigarette smoking there are no obvious major occupational or environmental associations resulting in large numbers of cases. This suggests that host susceptibility and subtle changes in immune responses are important in these haematological neoplasms, and that such susceptibility and alterations in immune responses are confounding the relatively crude epidemiological observations which have in turn been made even more obscure in the past by poor case classifications and low case ascertainment. Several steps are certainly necessary in the pathogenesis of some malignancies and this has to be more clearly acknowledged. In addition, the latent intervals between exposures and onset need careful and further assessment. Important work on common infections and natural radiation exposures of many kinds has thrown open the debate, and it is possible that these agents will play major roles in the aetiology of the leukaemias and lymphomas; however, these speculations have yet to be confirmed by direct studies.

References

1 International Classification of Diseases (1978) *Manual of the International Statistical Classification of Diseases, Injuries and Causes of Death*. World Health Organization, Geneva.

2 Alexander F.E., Ricketts T.J., McKinney P.A. *et al.* (1989) Cancer registration of leukaemias and lymphomas: results of a comparison with a specialist registry. *Community Medicine*, **11**, 81–89.

3 Sackett D.L. (1979) Bias in analytic research. *Journal of Chronic Diseases*, **32**, 139–144.

4 International Agency for Research on Cancer (1987) *Cancer Incidence in Five Continents*, Vol. 5. IARC, Lyon, France.

5 Cartwright R.A., Alexander F.E., McKinney P.A. *et al.* (1990) *Leukaemia and Lymphoma. An atlas of distribution within areas of England and Wales 1984–1988*. Leukaemia Research Fund, London.

6 Oladipupo W.C.K. & Bamgboye E.A. (1983) Estimation of incidence of human leukaemia subtypes in an urban African population. *Oncology*, **40**, 381–386.

7 Cartwright R.A. (1992) Incidence and epidemiology of the myelodysplastic syndromes. In: *The Myelodysplastic Syndromes* (eds G.J. Mufti & D.A.G. Galton), pp. 23–53. Churchill Livingstone, Edinburgh.

8 Radlund A., Thiede T., Hansen S., Carlsson M. & Engquist L. (1995) Incidence of myelodysplastic syndromes in a Swedish population. *European Journal of Haematology*, **54**, 153–156.

9 Birch J.M., Marsden H.B. & Swindell R. (1980) Incidence of malignant disease in childhood: a 24-year review of the Manchester Children's Tumour Registry data. *British Journal of Cancer*, **42**, 215–223.

10 Editorial (1981) Leukaemia in black and white. *Lancet*, **ii**, 732–733.

11 Sinniah D. & Peng L.H. (1981) Malaysian childhood leukaemia, thirteen year review at the University Hospital, Kuala Lumpar. *Leukaemia Research*, **5**, 271–278.

12 Booth K. & Amato D. (1978) Leukaemia in Papua New Guinea. *Tropical and Geographical Medicine*, **30**, 343–349.

13 Alexander F.E., McKinney P.A. & Cartwright R.A. (1990) Radon and leukaemia. *Lancet*, **335**, 1336–1337.

14 Alexander F.E., Ricketts T.J., McKinney P.A. *et al.* (1990) Community lifestyle characteristics and risk of acute lymphoblastic leukaemia in children. *Lancet*, **336**, 1461–1465.

15 Gunz F.W. (1977) The epidemiology and genetics of the chronic leukaemias. *Clinics in Haematology*, **6**, 3–20.

16 MacMahon B. & Koller E.K. (1957) Ethnic differences in the incidence of leukaemia. *Blood*, **12**, 1–10.

17 Graham S. & Gibson R. (1970) Religion and ethnicity in leukaemia. *American Journal of Public Health*, **60**, 206–274.

18 Bartal A., Bentwich A., Manny N. & Izak G. (1978) Ethnical and clinical aspects of CLL in Israel. *Acta Haematologica*, **60**, 161–171.

19 Glaser S.L. (1991) Black white differences in Hodgkin's Disease incidence in the United States by age, sex, histology subtype and time. *International Journal of Epidemiology*, **20**, 68–75.

20 Herrington L.J., Demers P.A., Koepsell T.D. *et al.* (1992) Epidemiology of the M-component immunoglobulin types of multiple myeloma. *Cancer Causes and Control*, **4**, 83–92.

21 Adelstein A. & White G. (1976) Leukaemia 1911–1973: cohort analysis. *Population Trends*, **3**, 9–13.

22 Lund E. & Lie S.O. (1983) Incidence of acute leukaemia in Norway 1957–1981. *Scandinavian Journal of Haematology*, **31**, 488–494.

23 Hanson H.E., Karie H. & Jenson O.M. (1983) Trends in the incidence of leukaemia in Denmark 1943–1977. An epidemiologic study of 14 000 patients. *Journal of the National Cancer Institute*, **71**, 697–701.

24 Stiller C.A. & Draper G. (1981) Trends in childhood leukaemia in Britain. *British Journal of Cancer*, **45**, 543–554.

25 Blair V. & Birch J.M. (1994) Patterns and temporal trends in the incidence of malignant disease in children. Leukaemia and lymphoma. *European Journal of Cancer*, **30**, 140–149.

26 Toms J.R. (1982) *Trends in Cancer Survival in Great Britain 1960–1971*. Cancer Research Campaign, London.

27 Court Brown W.M. & Doll R. (1961) Leukaemia in childhood and young adult life. *British Medical Journal*, **1**, 981–988.

28 Cartwright R.A., McNally R. & Staines A. (1994) The increasing incidence of non-Hodgkin's Lymphoma (NHL): the possible role of sunlight. *Leukaemia and Lymphoma*, **14**, 387–394.

29 Devesa S. & Fears T. (1992) Non-Hodgkin's lymphoma time trends: United States and international data. *Cancer Research*, **52**(Suppl.), 5432–5440.

30 Browning P. & Gross S. (1968) Epidemiological studies of acute childhood leukaemia. *American Journal of Diseases of Children*, **116**, 576.

31 Saunders B.M., White G.S. & Draper G.J. (1981) Occupations of fathers of children dying from neoplasms. *Journal of Epidemiology and Community Health*, **35**, 245.

32 McWhirter W.R. (1982) The relationship of incidence of childhood lymphoblastic leukaemia to social class. *British Journal of Cancer*, **46**, 640–645.

33 Birch J.M. & Marsden H.B. (1981) Childhood leukaemia in north west England 1954–77. Epidemiology incidence and survival. *British Journal of Cancer*, **43**, 324–329.

34 Alexander F.E., Ricketts T.J., McKinney P.A. & Cartwright R.A. (1991) Community lifestyle characteristics and incidence of Hodgkin's disease in young people. *International Journal of Cancer*, **48**, 10–14.

35 Obrastzow H. (1890) Zwei falle von actuer leukamie. *Deutsche Medicinische Wochenschrift*, **16**, 1150–1153.

36 Aubertin C. & Grellety-Bosveil P. (1923) Contribution a l'etude de la leukemie aigue. *Archives Maladie de Coeur*, **16**, 693.

37 Knox E.G. (1964) Epidemiology of childhood leukaemia in Northumberland and Durham. *British Journal of Preventive Social Medicine*, **18**, 17–24.

38 Knox E.G. (1964) The detection of space–time interactions. *Applied Statistics*, **13**, 25–30.

39 Mantel N. (1967) The detection of disease clustering and a generalised regression approach. *Cancer Research*, **27**, 209–220.

40 Pinkel D. & Nefzger D. (1969) Some epidemiological features of childhood leukaemia in the Buffalo N.Y. area. *Cancer*, **12**, 351–358.

41 David F.N. & Barton D.E. (1966) Two space–time tests for epidemicity. *British Journal of Social and Preventive Medicine*, **20**, 44–48.

42 Chen R. & Mantel N. (1984) A study of 3 techniques for time–space clustering in Hodgkin's Disease. *Statistics in Medicine*, **3**, 173–184.

43 Smith P.G. (1978) Current assessment of case clustering of lymphomas and leukaemias. *Cancer*, **42**, 1026–1034.

44 Smith P.G. & Pike M.C. (1976) Epidemiology of childhood leukaemia in greater London: a search for evidence of transmission assuring a long latent period. *British Journal of Cancer*, **33**, 1–8.

45 Lewis M.S. (1980) Spatial clustering in childhood leukaemia. *Journal of Chronic Diseases*, **33**, 703–712.

46 Cuzick J. & Edwards R. (1990) Tests for spatial clustering in heterogeneous populations. *Journal of the Royal Statistical Society Series B*, **52**, 73–104.

47 Besag J. & Newell J. (1991) The detection of clusters in rare diseases. *Journal of the Royal Statistical Society Series A*, **152**, 367–368.

48 Potthoff R.F. & Wittinghill M. (1966) Testing for homogeneity: II. The Poisson distribution. *Biometrika*, **53**, 183–190.

49 Barnes N., Cartwright R.A. & O'Brien C. (1987) Spatial pattern in electoral wards with high lymphoma incidence in YRHA. *British Journal of Cancer*, **56**, 169–172.

50 Alexander F.E., Cartwright R.A. & McKinney P.A. (1990) Investigation of spatial clustering of rare diseases: childhood malignancies in North Humberside. *Journal Epidemiology and Community Health*, **44**, 39–46.

51 Kyle R.A., Herber L., Evatt B.L. & Clark W.H. (1970) Multiple myeloma: a community cluster. *Journal of the American Medical Association*, **213**, 1339–1341.

52 Glaser S.L. (1990) Spatial clustering of Hodgkin's disease in the San Francisco Bay area. *American Journal of Epidemiology*, **132**, 167–176.

53 Heath C.W. & Hatalik R.J. (1963) Leukaemia among children in a suburban community. *American Journal of Medicine*, **34**, 796–812.

54 Vianna N.J., Greenwald P., Brady J., Polar M.A. & Dwork A. (1972) Hodgkin's Disease: cases with features of a community outbreak. *American International Medicine*, **77**, 169–180.

55 Draper G.J., Stiller C.A., Cartwright R.A., Craft A.W. & Vincent T.J. (1993) Cancer in Cumbria and in the vicinity of the Sellafield nuclear installation 1963–90. *British Medical Journal*, **306**, 89–94, 761.

56 Black D. (1984) *Investigation of the Possible Increased Incidence of Cancer in West Cumbria*. HMSO, London.

57 Committee on Medical Aspects of Radiation in the Environment (COMARE) (1986) *First Report: the implications of the new data on the releases from Sellafield in the 1950s for the conclusions of the Report on the Investigation of the possible increased incidence of cancer in West Cumbria*. HMSO, London.

58 Gardner M.J., Snee M.P., Hall H.A. *et al.* (1990) Results of case-control study of leukaemia and lymphoma among young people near Sellafield nuclear plant in West Cumbria. *British Medical Journal*, **300**, 423–434.

59 Doll R., Evans J. & Darby S.C. (1994) Parental exposure not to blame. *Nature*, **367**, 678–680.

60 Strover B.J. (1983) Effects of Thorotrast in humans. *Health Physics*, **44**, 253–257.

61 Henshaw D.L., Eatough J.P. & Richardson R.B. (1990) Radon: a causative factor in the induction of myeloid leukaemia and other cancers in adults and children. *Lancet*, **335**, 1008–1012.

62 Beebe G.W. (1981) Atomic bomb survivors and problems of low dose radiation effects. Reviews and commentaries. *American Journal of Epidemiology*, **114**, 761–783.

63 Schull W.J., Shimizu Y. & Kato H. (1990) Hiroshima and Nagasaki: new doses, risks, and their implications. *Health Physics*, **59**, 69–75.

64 Kato H. & Schull W.J. (1982) Studies of the mortality of A bomb survivors. Mortality 1950–1978, part I: cancer mortality. *Radiation Research*, **90**, 395–432.

65 Yoshimoto Y., Neel J.V., Schull W.J. *et al.* (1990) *Frequency of Malignant Tumours During the First Two Decades of Life in the Offspring (F1) of Atomic Bomb Survivors*. Radiation Effects Research Foundation, Hiroshima, Japan.

66 Ichimaru M., Ishimaru T., Mikami M., Yamoda Y. & Ohkita T. (1981) *Incidence of Leukaemia in a Fixed Cohort of Atomic Bomb Survivors and Controls. Hiroshima and Nagasaki, October 1950–December 1978*. RERF Technical Report, pp. 13–81. Radiation Effects Reseach Foundation, Hiroshima, Japan.

67 Ichimaru M., Toranosuke I., Mikami M. & Matsunaga M. (1982) Multiple myeloma among atomic bomb survivors in Hiroshima and Nagasaki, 1950–76: relationship to radiation dose absorbed by marrow. *Journal of the National Cancer Institute*, **69**, 323–329.

68 Caldwell G.G., Kelley D., Zack M., Falk H. & Heath C.W. (1983) Mortality and cancer frequency among military nuclear test (Smoky) participants 1957 through 1979. *Journal of the American Medical Association*, **250**, 620–624.

69 Lyon J.L., Klauber M.R., Gardner J. & Udall K.S. (1979) Childhood leukaemias associated with fallout from nuclear testing. *New England Journal of Medicine*, **300**, 397–402.

70 Land C.E. & McKay F.W. (1984) Childhood leukaemia and fallout from the Nevada nuclear tests. *Science*, **223**, 139–144.

71 Johnson C.J. (1984) Cancer incidence in an area of radioactive fallout downwind from the Nevada test site. *Journal of the American Medical Association*, **251**, 230–236.

72 Stevens W., Thomas D.C., Lyon J. *et al.* (1990) Leukaemia in Utah and radioactive fallout from the Nevada test site. *Journal of the American Medical Association*, **264**, 585–591.

73 Archer V.E. (1987) Association of nuclear fallout with leukaemia in the US. *Archives of Environmental Health*, **42**, 263–271.

74 Darby S.C. & Doll R. (1987) Fallout radiation doses near Dounreay and childhood leukaemia. *British Medical Journal*, **294**, 603–607.

75 Darby S.C., Kendal G.M., Fell T.P. *et al.* (1988) A summary of mortality and incidence of cancer in men from the UK who participate in the UK's atmospheric test programming. *British Medical Journal*, **296**, 332–338.

76 Court Brown W.M., Spiers F.W., Doll R. *et al.* (1960) Geographical variation in leukaemia mortality in relation to background radiation and other factors. *British Medical Journal*, **1**, 1753–1759.

77 Flodin U., Fredrikson M., Axelson O. *et al.* (1986) Background radiation, electrical work and some other exposures associated with acute myeloid leukaemia in a case-referent study. *Archives of Environmental Health*, **41**, 77–84.

78 Fuortes L., McNutt L.A. & Lynch C. (1990) Leukaemia incidence and radioactivity in drinking water in 59 Iowa towns. *American Journal of Public Health*, **80**, 1261–1262.

79 Walter S.D., Meigs J.W. & Heston J.F. (1986) The relationship of cancer incidence to terrestrial radiation and population density in

Connecticut, 1935–1974. *American Journal of Epidemiology*, **123**, 1–14.

80 Sakka M. (1979) Background radiation and childhood cancer mortality. *Nippon Igaku Hoshasen Gakkai Zasshi*, **39**, 536–539.

81 Lu-xin W. & Jian-zhi W. (1994) Estimate of cancer risk for a large population continuously exposed to higher background radiation in Yangjiang, China. *Chinese Medical Journal*, **107**, 541–544.

82 Blot W.J., Xu Z-Y., Boice J.D. *et al.* (1990) Indoor radon and lung cancer in China. *Journal of the National Cancer Institute*, **82**, 1025–1030.

83 Lyman G.H., Lyman C.G. & Johnson W. (1985) Association of leukaemia with radium groundwater contamination. *Journal of the American Medicine Association*, **254**, 621–626.

84 Nambi K.S.V. & Soman S.D. (1990) Further observations on environmental radiation and cancer in India. *Health Physics*, **59**, 339–344.

85 Committee on Medical Aspects of Radiation in the Environment (COMARE) (1988) *Second Report: investigation of the possible increased incidence of leukaemia in young people near the Dounreay Nuclear Establishment, Caithness, Scotland*. HMSO, London.

86 Committee on Medical Aspects of Radiation in the Environment (COMARE) (1989) *Third Report: report on the incidence of childhood cancer in the West Berkshire and North Hampshire area, in which are situated the Atomic Weapons Research Establishment*. HMSO, London.

87 Gardner M.J., Hall A.J., Downes S. *et al.* (1987) Follow-up study of children born elsewhere but attending schools in Seascale, West Cumbria (schools cohort). *British Medical Journal*, **295**, 819–822.

88 Gardner M.J., Hall A.J., Downes S. *et al.* (1987) Follow-up study of children born to mothers resident in Seascale, West Cumbria (Birth cohort). *British Medical Journal*, **295**, 822–827.

89 McLaughlin J.R., King W.D., Anderson T.W., Clarke E.A. & Ashmore J.P. (1993) Paternal radiation exposure and leukaemia in offspring: the Ontario case-control study. *British Medical Journal*, **397**, 959–966.

90 Crump K.S., Ng T.H. & Cuddihy R.G. (1987) Cancer incidence patterns in the Denver metropolitan area in relation to the Rocky Flats plant. *American Journal of Epidemiology*, **126**, 127–135.

91 Hill C. & Laplandre A. (1990) Overall mortality and cancer mortality around French nuclear sites. *Nature*, **347**, 755–757.

92 Cook-Mozaffari P.J., Ashwood F.L., Vincent T. *et al.* (1987) *Cancer Incidence and Mortality in the Vicinity of Nuclear Installations, England and Wales 1959–1980*. Studies on Medical and Population Subjects, No. 51. HMSO, London.

93 Cook-Mozaffari P., Darby S. & Doll R. (1989) Cancer near potential sites of nuclear installations. *Lancet*, **ii**, 1145–1147.

94 Court Brown W.M. & Doll R. (1965) Mortality from cancer and other causes after radiotherapy for ankylosing spondylitis. *British Medical Journal*, **2**, 1327–1332.

95 Darby S.C., Doll R., Gill S.K. *et al.* (1987) Long term mortality after a single treatment course with X-rays in patients treated for ankylosing spondylitis. *British Journal of Cancer*, **55**, 179–190.

96 Smith P.G. & Doll R. (1976) Late effects of X-irradiation in patients treated for metropathia haemorrhagica. *British Journal of Radiology*, **49**, 224–232.

97 Boice J.D. & Manson R.R. (1981) Cancer mortality in women after repeated fluoroscopic examinations of the chest. *Journal of the National Cancer Institute*, **66**, 863–867.

98 Day N.C., & Boice J.D. (1983) *Second Cancer in Relation to Radiation Treatment for Cervical Cancer*. International Radiation Study Group on Cervical Cancer, IARC Scientific Publications, No. 52. WHO, Lyon.

99 Boice J.D. Jr, Blettner M., Kleinerman R.A. *et al.* (1987) Radiation dose and leukaemia risk in patients treated for cancer of the cervix. *Journal of the National Cancer Institute*, **79**, 1295–1311.

100 Boice J.D. Jr, Engholm G., Kleinerman R.A., *et al.* (1988) Radiation dose and second cancer risk in patients treated for cancer of the cervix. *Radiation Research*, **116**, 3–55.

101 Boice J.D., Michele M., Morin M.S. *et al.* (1991) Diagnostic X-ray procedures and risk of leukaemia, lymphoma and multiple myeloma. *Journal of the American Medical Association*, **265**, 1290–1294.

102 Visfeldt J. & Andersson M. (1995) Pathoanatomical aspects of malignant haematological disorders among Danish patients exposed to thorium dioxide. *APMIS*, **103**, 29–36.

103 Andersson M., Carstensen B. & Storm H.H. (1995) Mortality and cancer incidence after cerebral arteriography with or without Thorotrast. *Radiation Research*, **142**, 305–320.

104 Boiven J.F., Hutchinson G.B., Evans F.B. *et al.* (1986) Leukaemia after radiotherapy for first primary cancers of various anatomic sites. *American Journal of Epidemiology*, **123**, 993–1003.

105 Kaldor J.M., Day N.E., Clarke E.A. *et al.* (1990) Leukaemia following Hodgkin's disease. *New England Journal Medicine*, **13**, 322–327.

106 Pedersen-Bjergaard J., Specht L., Larsen S.O. *et al.* (1987) Risk of therapy-related leukaemia and preleukaemia after Hodgkin's disease. *Lancet*, **ii**, 83–88.

107 Stewart A., Pennyback W. & Barker R. (1962) Adult leukaemia and diagnostic X-rays. *British Medical Journal*, **5309**, 882–890.

108 Preston-Martin S., Thomas D.C., Yu M.C. *et al.* (1989) Diagnostic radiography as a risk factor for chronic myeloid and monocytic leukaemia. *British Journal of Cancer*, **59**, 639–644.

109 Stewart A. (1973) The carcinogenic effects of low level radiation. A reappraisal of epidemiologists' methods and observations. *Health Physics*, **24**, 223–240.

110 Miller R.W. (1972) Radiation induced cancer. *Journal of the National Cancer Institute*, **49**, 1221–1227.

111 Bithell J.F. & Stewart A.M. (1975) Pre-natal irradiation and childhood malignancy: a review of British data from the Oxford survey. *British Journal of Cancer*, **31**, 271–287.

112 Diamond E.L., Schmerler H. & Lilienfeld A.M. (1973) The relationship of intra-uterine radiation to subsequent mortality and development of leukaemia in children. *American Journal of Epidemiology*, **97**, 283–313.

113 Harvey E.B., Boice J.D., Haregman M. *et al.* (1985) Prenatal X-ray exposure and childhood cancer in twins. *New England Journal of Medicine*, **312**, 541–545.

114 Graham S., Levin M., Lilienfeld A. *et al.* (1966) Pre-conception intrauterine and postnatal irradiation as related to leukaemias. *National Cancer Institute Monograph*, **19**, 347–371.

115 Shu X-O., Gao Y-T., Brinton L.A. *et al.* (1988) A population-based case-control study of childhood leukaemia in Shanghai. *Cancer*, **62**, 635–644.

116 Shu X.O., Reaman G., Lampkin B. *et al.* (1994) Association of parental diagnostic X-ray exposure with risk of infant leukaemia. *Cancer Epidemiology, Biomarkers and Prevention*, **3**, 645–653.

117 Evans J.S., Wennberg J.E. & McNeil B.J. (1986) The influence of diagnostic radiography on the incidence of breast cancer and leukaemia. *New England Journal of Medicine*, **315**, 800–815.

118 Cuzick J. & De Stavola B. (1988) Multiple myeloma — a case-control study. *British Journal of Cancer*, **57**, 516–520.

119 Bernard S.M., Cartwright R.A. *et al.* (1984) Aetiologic factors in

lymphoid malignancies: a case-control epidemiological study. *Leukaemia Research*, **8**, 681–689.

120 March H.C. (1984) Leukaemia in radiologists. *Radiology*, **43**, 275–278.

121 Logue J.N., Barrick M.K. & Jessup G.L. (1986) Mortality of radiologists and pathologists in the radiation registry of physicians. *Journal of Occupational Medicine*, **28**, 91–99.

122 Wang J.-X., Inskip P.D., Boice J.D. Jr *et al.* (1990) Cancer incidence among medical diagnostic X-ray workers in China, 1950 to 1985. *International Journal of Cancer*, **45**, 889–895.

123 Yalow R.S. (1983) Reappraisal of potential risks associated with low-level radiation. *Annals of the New York Academy of Sciences*, **403**, 37–60.

124 Mauss E.A. (1983) Health effects of ionising radiation in the low dose range. *Annals of the New York Academy of Sciences*, **403**, 27–35.

125 Smith P.G. & Douglas A.J. (1986) Mortality of workers at the Sellafield plant of British Nuclear Fuels. *British Medical Journal*, **293**, 845–854.

126 Beral V., Fraser P., Carpenter L. *et al.* (1988) Mortality of employees of the Atomic Weapons Establishment 1951–1982. *British Medical Journal*, **297**, 757–770.

127 Checkoway H., Matthew R.M., Shy C.M. *et al.* (1985) Radiation, work experience, and cause specific mortality among workers at an energy research laboratory. *British Journal of Industrial Medicine*, **42**, 525–533.

128 Cragle D.L., McLain R.W. & Qualters J.R. (1988) Mortality among workers at nuclear fuels production facility. *American Journal of Industrial Medicine*, **14**, 379–401.

129 Gilbert E.S. & Marks S. (1979) An analysis of the mortality of workers in a nuclear facility. *Radiation Research*, **79**, 122–148.

130 Wilkinson G.S., Teitjen G.L. & Wiggs L.D. (1987) Mortality among plutonium and other radiation workers at a plutonium weapon facility. *American Journal of Epidemiology*, **125**, 231–250.

131 Carpenter L., Higgins C., Douglas A., Fraser P., Beral V. & Smith P. (1994) Combined analysis of mortality in three United Kingdom nuclear industry workforces, 1946–1988. *Radiation Research*, **138**, 224–238.

132 Kendall G.M., Muirhead C.R., MacGibbon B.H. *et al.* (1992) Mortality and occupational exposure to radiation: first analysis of the National Registry for Radiation Workers. *British Medical Journal*, **304**, 220–225.

133 Liebeskind D. (1979) Sister chromatid exchange in human lymphocytes after exposure to diagnostic ultrasound. *Science*, **25**, 1273–1275.

134 Cartwright R.A. & McKinney P.A. (1984) Ultra-sound examinations in pregnancy and childhood cancer: preliminary results from the inter-regional epidemiological study of childhood cancer. *Lancet*, **ii**, 999–1000.

135 Editorial (1982) Ultraviolet radiation, T lymphocyte and skin cancer. *Lancet*, **ii**, 530.

136 Fisher M.S. & Kripke M.L. (1982) Suppresser T lymphocytes control the development of primary skin cancers in ultra violet irradiated mice. *Science*, **216**, 1133–1134.

137 Hersey P. & Bradley M. (1983) Immunological effects of solarium exposure in human subjects. *Lancet*, **i**, 45–48.

138 Karchmer R.K. & Mellman J.A. (1974) Previous and simultaneous cancers in patients with leukaemia. *Journal of Chronic Diseases*, **27**, 5–13.

139 Adami J., Frisch M., Yven J. *et al.* (1995) Evidence of an association between non-Hodgkin's lymphoma and skin cancer. *British Medical Journal*, **310**, 1491–1495.

140 Tsoneva M.T. & Porcher P.R. (1975) Effect of magnetic fields on the chromosome set and cell division. VI. Lenin Higher Mechanical-electrotechnical Institute. Sofia Medical Faculty, Medical Academy, Sofia. *Genetika*, **ii**, 153–157.

141 Blackman C.F. & Shawnee G. (1982) Effects of ELF fields on calcium ion efflux from brain tissue *in vitro*. *Radiation Research*, **92**, 510–520.

142 Adey W.R. & Bawin S.M. (1982) Effects of weak amplitude modulated microwave fields on calcium efflux from awake cat cerebral cortex. *Bioelectromagnetics*, **3**, 297–307.

143 Wertheimer N. & Leeper E. (1979) Electrical wiring configurations and childhood cancer. *American Journal of Epidemiology*, **109**, 273–284.

144 Fulton J.F. & Cobb S. (1980) Electrical wiring configurations and childhood leukaemia in Rhode Island. *American Journal of Epidemiology*, **111**, 292–296.

145 Myers A., Clayden D., Cartwright S.C. & Cartwright R.A. (1990) Childhood cancer and overhead powerlines. *British Journal of Cancer*, **62**, 1008.

146 Savitz D.A., Wachtel H. & Barnes F.A. (1988) Case-control study of childhood cancer and exposure to 60-Hz magnetic fields. *American Journal of Epidemiology*, **128**, 21–38.

147 Savitz D.A., John E.M. & Kleckner R.C. (1990) Magnetic field exposure from electric appliances and childhood cancer. *American Journal of Epidemiology*, **131**, 763–773.

148 Cartwright R.A. (1989) Low frequency alternating electromagnetic fields and leukaemia: the saga so far. *British Journal of Cancer*, **60**, 649–651.

149 Severson R.K., Stevens R.G., Kaune W.T. *et al.* (1988) Acute non-lymphocytic leukaemia and residential exposure to power frequency magnetic fields. *American Journal of Epidemiology*, **128**, 10–20.

150 Coleman M.P., Bell C.M.J., Taylor H-L. *et al.* (1989) Leukaemia and residence near electricity transmission equipment: a case-control study. *British Journal of Cancer*, **60**, 793–798.

151 Feychting M. & Ahlbom A. (1993) Magnetic fields and cancer in children residing near Swedish high-voltage power lines. *American Journal of Epidemiology*, **138**, 467–481.

152 Washburn E.P., Orza M.J., Berlin J.A. *et al.* (1994) Critique of studies of EMF exposure. *Cancer Causes and Control*, **5**, 299–309.

153 Jones T.L., Shih C.H., Thurston D.H., Ware B.J. & Cole P. (1993) Selection bias from differential residential mobility as an explanation for associations of wire codes with childhood cancer. *Journal of Clinical Epidemiology*, **46**, 545–548.

154 Milham S. (1982) Mortality from leukaemia in workers exposed to electrical and magnetic fields. *New England Journal of Medicine*, **307**, 209.

155 Wright W.E. & Peters J.M. (1982) Leukaemia in workers exposed to electrical and magnetic fields. *Lancet*, **ii**, 1160–1161.

156 McDowall M.E. (1983) Leukaemia mortality in electrical workers in England and Wales. *Lancet*, **i**, 246.

157 Coleman M.C. & Bell J. (1983) Leukaemia incidence in electrical workers in England and Wales. *Lancet*, **i**, 246.

158 Coleman M. & Beral V. (1988) A review of epidemiological studies of the health effects of living near or working with electricity generation and transmission equipment. *International Journal of Epidemiology*, **17**, 1–13.

159 Loomis D.P. & Savitz D.A. (1990) Mortality from brain cancer and leukaemia among electrical workers. *British Journal of Industrial Medicine*, **47**, 633–638.

160 Floderus B., Persson T., Stenlund C., Wennberg A., Ost A. &

Knave B. (1993) Occupational exposure to electromagnetic fields in relation to leukaemia and brain tumours: a case-control study in Sweden. *Cancer Causes and Control*, **4**, 465–476.

161 Theriault G., Goldberg M., Miller A.B. *et al.* (1994) Cancer risk associated with occupational exposure to magnetic fields among electric utility workers in Ontario and Quebec, Canada and France 1970–1989. *American Journal of Epidemiology*, **139**, 550–572.

162 Aksoy M., Dincol K., Akgun T., Erdem S. & Dincol G. (1971) Haematological effects of chronic benzene poisoning in 217 workers. *British Journal of Industrial Medicine*, **28**, 296–302.

163 Delore P. & Borgomano C. (1928) Leukaemia aigue un cour de l'intoxication benzenique, sur l'origine toxique de certains leukemies aigues et leurs relations avec les anemies graves. *Journal Medicine Lyon*, **9**, 227–233.

164 International Agency for Research on Cancer ad-hoc Working Group on the Evaluation of Carcinogenic Risks to Humans (1987) *IARC Monographs on the Evaluation of Carcinogenic Risks to Humans: overall evaluations of carcinogenicity: an updating.* IARC, Lyon.

165 Rinsky R.A. & Young R.J. (1981) Leukaemia in benzene workers. *American Journal of Industrial Medicine*, **2**, 217–245.

166 Aksoy M. & Erdem S. (1975) On the problem of chemical leukaemogenesis. Extract. In: *International Symposium of Epidemiology. Milan, 4 September 1975.* 25th Congress of the Italian Haematological Society.

167 Wong O. (1987) An industry wide mortality study of chemical workers occupationally exposed to benzene. II. Dose response analyses. *British Journal of Industrial Medicine*, **44**, 382–395.

168 Olsen J.G., Hearn S., Cook R.R. *et al.* (1989) Mortality experience of a cohort of Louisianna chemical workers. *Journal of Occupational Medicine*, **31**, 32–34.

169 Yin S-N., Li G-L., Tain F-D. *et al.* (1987) Leukaemia in benzene workers: a retrospective cohort study. *British Journal of Industrial Medicine*, **44**, 124–128.

170 McCraw D.S., Joyner R.E., Cole P. *et al.* (1985) Excess leukaemia in a refinery population. *Journal of Occupational Medicine*, **27**, 220–222.

171 Bond G.G., McLaren E.A., Baldwin C.L. *et al.* (1986) An update of mortality among chemical workers exposed to benzene. *British Journal of Industrial Medicine*, **43**, 685–691.

172 Rinsky R.A., Smith A.B., Hornung R. *et al.* (1987) Benzene and leukaemia. An epidemiologic risk assessment. *New England Journal of Medicine*, **316**, 1044–1050.

173 Li F.P. & Fraumeni J.F. (1969) Cancer mortality among chemists. *Journal of the National Cancer Institute*, **43**, 1159–1164.

174 Olin R. (1978) The hazards of a chemical laboratory environment —a study of the mortality in 2 cohorts of Swedish chemists. *American Industrial Hygiene Association Journal*, **39**, 557–562.

175 Delzell E. & Monson R.R. (1981) Mortality among rubber workers. III. Cause specific mortality 1940–1978. *Journal of Occupational Medicine*, **23**, 677–684.

176 Delzell E. & Monson R.R. (1982) Mortality patterns among rubber workers. V. Processing workers. *Journal of Occupational Medicine*, **24**, 539–545.

177 McMichael A.J. & Andjelkovic D.A. (1975) Solvent exposure among rubber workers. *Journal of Occupational Medicine*, **17**, 234–240.

178 Rushton L. & Alderson M.R. (1981) Case-control study to investigate the association between exposure to benzene and deaths from leukaemia in oil refinery workers. *British Journal of Cancer*, **43**, 77–84.

179 Thomas T.L. & Waxweiler R.J. (1982) Mortality patterns among workers in three Texas oil refineries. *Journal of Occupational Medicine*, **24**, 135–141.

180 Conley C.L. & Misiti J. (1982) Mortality patterns among workers in three Texas oil refineries. *Journal of Occupational Medicine*, **24**, 135–141.

181 Blair A., Stewart P.A., Tolbert P.E. *et al.* (1990) Cancer and other causes of death among a cohort of dry cleaners. *British Journal of Industrial Medicine*, **47**, 162–168.

182 Rushton L., Alderson M.R. & Nagarajah C.R. (1983) Epidemiological survey of maintenance workers in London transport bus garages and Chiswick works. *British Journal of Industrial Medicine*, **40**, 340–345.

183 Schenker M.B., Smith T., Munoz A. *et al.* (1984) Diesel exposure and mortality among railway workers: results of a pilot study. *British Journal of Industrial Medicine*, **41**, 320–327.

184 Flodin U., Fredrikson M., Persson B. *et al.* (1988) Chronic lymphocytic leukaemia and engine exhausts, fresh wood, and DDT: a case-referent study. *British Journal of Industrial Medicine*, **45**, 33–38.

185 Harrington J.M. & Oakes D. (1984) Mortality study of British pathologists 1974–1980. *British Journal of Industrial Medicine*, **41**, 188–191.

186 Stern R.M. (1987) Cancer incidence among welders: possible effects of exposure to extremely low frequency electromagnetic radiation (ELF) and to welding fumes. *Environmental Health Perspectives*, **76**, 221–229.

187 Demers P.A., Vaughan T.L., Koepsell T.D. *et al.* (1993) A case-control study of multiple myeloma and occupation. *American Journal of Industrial Medicine*, **23**, 629–639.

188 Persson B., Dahlander A-M., Fredriksson M., Brage H.N., Ohlson C-G. & Axelson O. (1989) Malignant lymphomas and occupational exposures. *British Journal of Industrial Medicine*, **46**, 516–520.

189 Egedahl R.D., Carpenter M. & Homik R. (1993) An update of an epidemiology study at a hydrometallurgical nickel refinery in Fort Saskatchewan, Alberta. *Statistics Canada*, **5**, 291–302.

190 Arp E.W., Wolf P.H. & Checkoway H. (1983) Lymphocytic leukaemia and exposure to benzene and other solvents in the rubber industry. *Journal of Occupational Medicine*, **25**, 598–602.

191 Checkoway H. (1984) An evaluation of the association of leukaemia and rubber industry exposure. *American Journal of Industrial Medicine*, **5**, 239–249.

192 Paganini-Hill A., Glazer E., Henderson B.E. *et al.* (1980) Cause-specific mortality among newspaper web pressmen. *Journal of Occupational Medicine*, **22**, 542–544.

193 Wallace L.A. (1989) Major sources of benzene exposure. *Environmental Health Perspectives*, **82**, 165–169.

194 Milham S. Jr (1976) *Occupational Mortality in Washington State, 1950–1971*, Vols 1–3. Department of Health Education Washington, Public Health Service, US Government Printing Office, Washington DC.

195 Linos A., Kyle R.A., O'Fallon W.M. *et al.* (1980) A case-control study of occupational exposures and leukaemia. *International Journal of Epidemiology*, **9**, 131–135.

196 Donham K.J., Berg J.W. & Sawin R.S. (1980) Epidemiologic relationships of the bovine population and human leukaemia in Iowa. *American Journal of Epidemiology*, **112**, 80–92.

197 Donham K.J., Burmeister L.F., Van Lier S.F. *et al.* (1987) Relationships of bovine leukaemia virus prevalence in dairy herds and density of dairy cattle to human lymphocytic leukaemia. *Journal of Veterinary Research*, **48**, 235–238.

198 Burmeister L.F., Van Lier S.F. & Isacson P. (1982) Leukaemia and farm practices in Iowa. *American Journal of Epidemiology*, **115**, 720–728.

199 Blair A. & White D. (1985) Leukaemia cell types and agricultural practices in Nebraska. *Archives of Environmental Health*, **40**, 211–214.

200 Gallagher R.P., Thelfall W.J., Jeffries E. *et al.* (1984) Cancer and aplastic anaemia in British Columbia farmers. *Journal of the National Cancer Institute*, **72**, 1311–1315.

201 Pearce N.E., Sheppard R.A., Howard J.K. *et al.* (1986) Leukaemia among New Zealand agricultural workers. A cancer registry-based study. *American Journal of Epidemiology*, **124**, 402–409.

202 McKinney P.A., Alexander F.E., Roberts B.E. *et al.* (1990) Yorkshire case-control study of leukaemias and lymphomas: parallel multivariate analysis of seven disease categories. *Leukemia and Lymphoma*, **2**, 67–80.

203 Morrison H.I., Wilkins K., Semenciw R., Mao Y. & Wigle D. (1992) Herbicides and cancer. *Journal of the National Cancer Institute*, **84**, 1866–1874.

204 Pearce N. & Bethwaite P. (1992) Increasing incidence of non-Hodgkin's lymphoma: occupational and environmental factors. *Cancer Research*, **52**(Suppl.), 5496–5500.

205 Zahm S.H. & Blair A. (1992) Pesticides and non-Hodgkin's lymphoma. *Cancer Research*, **52**(Suppl.), 5485–5488.

206 Scherr P.A., Hutchison G.B. & Neiman R.S. (1992) Non-Hodgkin's lymphoma and occupational exposure. *Cancer Research*, **52**(Suppl.), 5503–5509.

207 Rask-Andersen A., Hagberg H., Hardell L. & Nordstrom M. (1995) Is hairy cell leukaemia more common among farmers? — A pilot study. *Oncology Reports*, **2**, 447–450.

208 Pearce N.E., Smith A.H., Howard J.K., Sheppard R.A., Giles H.J. & Teague C.A. (1986) Case-control study of multiple myeloma and farming. *British Journal of Cancer*, **54**, 493–500.

209 Brown L.M., Burmeister L.F., Everett G.D. & Blair A. (1992) Pesticide exposures and multiple myeloma in Iowa men. *Cancer Causes and Control*, **4**, 153–156.

210 Nandakumar A., Armstrong B.K. & De Klerk N.H. (1986) Multiple myeloma in Western Australia: a case-control study in relation to occupation, father's occupation, socioeconomic status and country of birth. *International Journal of Cancer*, **37**, 223–226.

211 Frenceschi S., Serraino D., Vecchia C.L., Bidoli E. & Tirelli U. (1991) Occupation and risk of Hodgkin's Disease in North-East Italy. *International Journal of Cancer*, **48**, 831–835.

212 International Agency for Research on Cancer and International Association of Cancer Registries (1987) *Cancer Incidence in Five Continents*. IARC Scientific Publication No.88. Lyon, France.

213 Saracci R., Kogevinas M., Bertazzi P-A. *et al.* (1991) Cancer mortality in workers exposed to chlorophenoxy herbicides and chlorophenols. *Lancet*, **338**, 1027–1032.

214 Johnson E.S. & Fischman H.K. (1982) Cancer mortality among butchers and slaughterhouse workers. *Lancet*, **i**, 913–914.

215 Blair A. & Hayes H.M. (1982) Mortality patterns among United States veterinarians 1947–1977: an expanded study. *International Journal of Epidemiology*, **11**, 391–397.

216 Monson R.R. & Fine L.J. (1978) Cancer mortality and morbidity among rubber workers. *Journal of the National Cancer Institute*, **61**, 1047–1053.

217 Downs T.D., Crane M.M. & Kim K.W. (1987) Mortality among workers at a butadiene facility. *American Journal of Industrial Medicine*, **12**, 311–329.

218 Ott M.G., Kolesar R.C., Scharnweber H.C. *et al.* (1980) A mortality survey of employees engaged in the development of manufacture of styrene-based products. *Journal of Occupational Medicine*, **22**, 445–460.

219 Wong O. (1990) A cohort mortality study and a case-control study of workers potentially exposed to styrene in the reinforced plastics and composites industry. *British Journal of Industrial Medicine*, **47**, 753–762.

220 Kolstad H.A., Lynge E., Olsen J. & Breum N. (1994) *Scandinavian Journal of Work, Environment and Health*, **20**, 272–278.

221 Hogstedt C., Aringer L. & Gustavsson A. (1986) Epidemiologic support for ethylene oxide as a cancer-causing agent. *Journal of the American Medicine Association*, **255**, 1575–1578.

222 Greenberg H.L., Ott M.G. & Shore R.E. (1990) Men assigned to ethylene oxide or other ethylene oxide related chemical manufacturing: a mortality study. *British Journal Industrial Medicine*, **47**, 221–230.

223 Gardner M.J., Coggon D., Pannett B. *et al.* (1989) Workers exposed to ethylene oxide: a follow-up study. *British Journal of Industrial Medicine*, **46**, 860–865.

224 Theiss A.M., Frentzel-Beyme R., Link R. *et al.* (1981) Mortality study on employees exposed to alkylene oxides (ethylene oxide/propylene oxide) and their derivatives. In: *Prevention of Occupational Cancer — International Symposium*. Occupational and Health Series No. 46, pp. 249–259. ILO, Geneva.

225 Kinnear-Wilson L.A. & Kneale G.W. (1981) Childhood cancer and pregnancy drugs. *Lancet*, **ii**, 314–315.

226 Knox E.G. & Stewart A.M. (1983) Foetal infection, childhood leukaemia and cancer. *British Journal of Cancer*, **48**, 849–852.

227 Bithell J.F. & Draper G.J. (1973) Association between malignant disease in children and maternal virus infections. *British Medical Journal*, **1**, 706–708.

228 Savitz D.A. & Chen J. (1990) Parental occupation and childhood cancer: review of epidemiologic studies. *Environmental Health Perspectives*, **88**, 325–337.

229 Urquart J.D., Black R.J., Muirhead M.J. *et al.* (1991) Results of a case control study of leukaemia and non-Hodgkin's lymphoma in children in Caithness near the Dounreay nuclear installation. *British Medical Journal*, **302**, 687–692.

230 McKinney P.A., Alexander F.E., Cartwright R.A. *et al.* (1991) The parental occupation of children with leukaemia in West Cumbria, North Humberside and Gateshead. *British Medical Journal*, **302**, 681–687.

231 Infante-Rivard C., Mur P., Armstrong B. *et al.* (1991) Acute lymphoblastic leukaemia among Spanish children and mothers' occupation: a case control study. *Journal of Epidemiology and Community Health*, **45**, 11–15.

232 Bertazzi P.A., Zocchetti C., Pesatori A.C. *et al.* (1989) Ten-year mortality study of the population involved in the Seveso incident in 1976. *American Journal of Epidemiology*, **129**, 1187–1200.

233 Bertazzi P.A., Pesatori A.C., Consonni D., Tironi A., Landi M.T. & Zocchetti C. (1993) Cancer incidence in a population accidentally exposed to 2,37,8-tetrachlorodibenzo-para-dioxin. *Epidemiology*, **4**, 398–406.

234 Bertazzi P.A., Zocchetti C., Pesatori A.C. *et al.* (1992) Mortality of a young population after accidental exposure to 2,3,7,8-tetrachlorodibenzodioxin. *International Journal of Epidemiology*, **21**, 118–123.

235 Lowengart R.A., Peters J.M., Ciccioni C. *et al.* (1987) Childhood leukaemia and parents' occupational and home exposures. *Journal of the National Cancer Institute*, **79**, 39–46.

236 Anonymous (1994) *Cancer. Health effects of herbicides used in Vietnam*, pp. 433–590. National Academy Press, New York.

237 Austin H. & Cole P. (1986) Cigarette smoking and leukaemia. *Journal of Chronic Diseases*, **39**, 417–421.

238 Kinlen L.J. & Roget E. (1988) Leukaemia and smoking habits among United States veterans. *British Medical Journal*, **287**, 657–659.

239 McLaughlin J.K., Hrubec Z., Linet M.S. *et al.* (1989) Cigarette smoking and leukaemia. *Journal of the National Cancer Institute*, **81**, 1262–1263.

240 Severson R.K. (1987) Cigarette smoking and leukaemia. *Cancer*, **60**, 141–144.

241 Linet M.S., McLaughlin J.K., Hsing A.W. *et al.* (1992) Is cigarette smoking a risk factor for non-Hodgkin's lymphoma or multiple myeloma? Results from the Lutheran Brotherhood cohort study. *Leukemia Research*, **16**, 621–624.

242 Brown L.M., Everett G.D., Gibson R., Burmeister L.F., Schuman L.M. & Blair A. (1992) Smoking and risk of non-Hodgkin's lymphoma and multiple myeloma. *Cancer Causes and Control*, **3**, 49–55.

243 Cantor K.P., Blair A., Everett G. *et al.* (1988) Hair dye use and risk of leukaemia and lymphoma. *American Journal of Public Health*, **78**, 570–571.

244 Markowitz J.A., Szklo M., Sensenbrenner I.L. *et al.* (1985) Hair dyes and acute non-lymphocytic leukaemia (ANLL). *American Journal of Epidemiology*, **122**, 523.

245 Spinelli J.J., Gallagher R.P., Band P.R. *et al.* (1984) Multiple myeloma, leukaemia and cancer of the ovary in cosmetologists and hairdressers. *American Journal of Industrial Medicine*, **6**, 97–102.

246 Grodstein F., Hennekens C.H., Colditz G.A., Hunter D.J. & Stampfer M.J. (1994) A prospective study of permanent hair dye use and hematopoietic cancer. *Journal of the National Cancer Institute*, **86**, 1466–1470.

247 Zahm S.H., Weisenburger D.D., Babbitt P.A., Saal R.C., Vaught J.B. & Blair A. (1992) Use of hair coloring products and the risk of lymphoma, multiple myeloma and chronic lymphocytic leukemia. *American Journal of Public Health*, **82**, 990–997.

248 van Duijn C.M., van Steensel-Moll H.A., Coebergh J-W.W. & van Zanen G.E. (1994) Risk factors for childhood acute non-lymphocytic leukemia: an association with maternal alcohol consumption during pregnancy. *Cancer Epidemiology, Biomarkers and Prevention*, **3**, 457–460.

249 Brown L.M., Gibson R., Burmeister L.F., Schuman L.M., Everett G.D. & Blair A. (1992) Alcohol consumption and risk of leukaemia, non-Hodgkin's lymphoma and multiple myeloma. *Leukemia Research*, **16**, 979–984.

250 Peters J.M., Preson-Martin S., London S.J., Bowman J.D., Buckley J.D. & Thomas D.C. (1994) Processed meats and risk of childhood leukemia (California, USA). *Cancer Causes and Control*, **5**, 195–202.

251 Gunz F.W. & Angus H.B. (1965) Leukaemia and cancer in the same patient. *Cancer*, **18**, 145–152.

252 Linos A. (1981) Leukaemia and prior malignant and hematologic diseases: a case-control study. *American Journal of Epidemiology*, **113**, 285–289.

253 Brenner B. & Carter A. (1984) Acute leukaemia following chemotherapy and radiation therapy — a report of 15 cases. *Oncology*, **41**, 83–87.

254 Whitlock J.A., Greer J.P. & Lukens J.N. (1991) Epipodophyllotoxin-related leukemia. *Cancer*, **68**, 600–604.

255 Curtis R.E. & Hankey B.F. (1984) Risk of leukaemia associated with first course of cancer treatment: an analysis of the surveillance epidemiology and end results program experience. *Journal of the National Cancer Institute*, **72**, 531–544.

256 Bovin J.A. & Hutchinson G.B. (1984) Second primary cancers following treatment of Hodgkin's disease. *Journal of the National Cancer Institute*, **72**, 233–241.

257 Cimino G., Papa G., Tura S. *et al.* (1991) *American Society of Clinical Oncology*, **9**, 432–437.

258 Teichmann J.V., Sieber S., Ludwig W.D. *et al.* (1986) Chronic myelocytic leukaemia as a second neoplasm in the course of chronic lymphocytic leukaemia. *Leukaemia Research*, **10**, 361–368.

259 Travis L.B., Curtis R.E., Hankey B.F. & Fraumeni J.F. (1992) Second cancers in patients with chronic lymphocytic leukaemia. *Journal of the National Cancer Institute*, **84**, 1422–1427.

260 Kaldor J.M., Day N.E., Petterson F. *et al.* (1990) Leukaemia following chemotherapy for ovarian cancer. *New England Journal of Medicine*, **322**, 1–6.

261 Haas J.F., Kittlemann B., Mehnert W.H. *et al.* (1987) Risk of leukaemia in ovarian tumour and breast cancer patients following treatment by cyclophosphamine. *British Journal of Cancer*, **55**, 213–218.

262 Chen S-J., Chen Z., Dene J. *et al.* (1989) Are most secondary acute lymphoblastic leukaemias mixed acute leukaemias? *Nouvelle Revue Française Hematologie*, **31**, 17–22.

263 Hazelman B.L. (1982) Comparative incidence of malignant disease in rheumatoid arthritis exposed to different treatment regimes. *Annals of the Rheumatic Diseases*, **41**(Suppl.), 12–17.

264 Eriksson M. (1993) Rheumatoid arthritis as a risk factor for multiple myeloma: a case-control study. *European Journal of Cancer*, **29**, 259–263.

265 Isomaki H.A., Haulinen T. & Joutsenlahti U. (1978) Excess risk of lymphomas, leukaemia and myeloma in patients with rheumatoid arthritis. *Journal of Chronic Diseases*, **31**, 691–696.

266 Tennis P., Andrews E., Bombardier C. *et al.* (1993) Record linkage to conduct an epidemiologic study on the association of rheumatoid arthritis and lymphoma in the province of Saskatchewan, Canada. *Journal of Clinical Epidemiology*, **46**, 685–695.

267 Gridley G., McLaughlin J.K., Ekbom A. *et al.* (1993) Incidence of cancer among patients with rheumatoid arthritis. *Journal of the National Cancer Institute*, **85**, 307–311.

268 Shu X-O., Gao Y-T., Linet M.S. *et al.* (1987) Chloramphenicol use and childhood leukaemia in Shanghai. *Lancet*, **ii**, 934–937.

269 Friedman G.B. (1982) Phenylbutazone, musculoskeletal disease and leukaemia. *Journal of Chronic Diseases*, **34**, 233–243.

270 Cartwright R.A., Bernard S.M., Bird C.C. *et al.* (1987) Chronic lymphocytic leukaemia: a case-control epidemiological study in Yorkshire. *British Journal of Cancer*, **56**, 79–82.

271 Stahnke N. & Zisel H.J. (1989) Growth hormone therapy and leukaemia. *European Journal of Pediatrics*, **148**, 591–596.

272 Robison L.L., Buckley J.D., Daigle A. *et al.* (1989) Maternal drug use and risk of childhood nonlymphoblastic leukaemia among offspring. *Cancer*, **63**, 1904–1911.

273 Penn I. (1984) Cancer in immunosuppressed patients. *Transplantation Proceedings*, **16**, 492–494.

274 Kinlen J.L. & Sheil A.G.R. (1979) Collaborative United Kingdom Australasian study of cancer in patients treated with immunosuppressive drugs. *British Medical Journal*, **2**, 1461–1466.

275 Kinlen L. (1992) Immunosuppressive therapy and acquired immunological disorders. *Cancer Research*, **52**(Suppl.), 5476–5478.

276 Boyd C.M., Ramberg R.C. & Thomas E.D. (1982) The incidence of

recurrence of leukaemia in donor cells after allogenic bone marrow transplantation. *Leukaemia Resarch*, **6**, 833–837.

277 Morgan G. & Superina R.A. (1994) Lymphoproliferative disease after pediatric liver transplantation. *Journal of Pediatric Surgery*, **29**, 1191–1196.

278 Blomberg J., Moller T., Olsson H., Anderson H. & Jonsson M. (1993) Cancer morbidity in blood recipients — results of a cohort study. *European Journal of Cancer*, **29A**, 2101–2105.

279 Manning M.D. & Carroll B.F. (1957) Some epidemiological aspects of leukaemia in children. *Journal of the National Cancer Institute*, **19**, 1087–1094.

280 Linet M.S., McCaffrey L.D., Hymphrey R.L. *et al.* (1986) Chronic lymphocytic leukaemia and acquired disorders affecting the immune system: a case-control study. *Journal of the National Cancer Institute*, **77**, 371–378.

281 McCormick D.P. & Anmann A.J. (1971) A study of allergy in patients with malignant lymphoma and chronic lymphocytic leukaemia. *Cancer*, **27**, 93–99.

282 Brinton L.A., Gridley G., Hrubec Z. *et al.* (1989) Cancer risk following pernicious anaemia. *British Journal of Cancer*, **59**, 810–813.

283 Gibson E. & Graham S. (1976) Epidemiology of diseases in adult males with leukaemia. *Journal of the National Cancer Institute*, **56**, 891–898.

284 Hakulinen T., Isomaki H. & Knekt P. (1985) Rheumatoid arthritis and cancer studies based on linking nationwide registries in Finland. *American Journal Medicine*, **78**(Suppl. 1A), 29–32.

285 Sutherland I. (1982) BCG and vole bacillus vaccination in adolescence and mortality from leukaemia. *Statistics in Medicine*, **1**, 329–335.

286 Snider O.E. & Constock G.W. (1978) Efficiency of BCG vaccination — prevention of cancer: an update brief communication. *Journal of the National Cancer Institute*, **60**, 785–788.

287 Haro A.S. (1986) The effect of BCG-vaccination and tuberculosis on the risk of leukaemia. *Developments in Biological Standardization*, **58**(Part A), 433–449.

288 Nishi M. & Niyake H. (1989) A case-control study of non-T cell acute lymphoblastic leukaemia of children in Hokkaido, Japan. *Journal of Epidemiology Community and Health*, **43**, 352–355.

289 Cohen H.J., Bernstein R.J. & Grufferman S. (1987) Role of immune stimulation in the etiology of multiple myeloma: a case-control study. *American Journal of Haematology*, **24**, 119–126.

290 Gramenzi A., Buttino I., D'Avanzo B. *et al.* (1991) Medical history and the risk of multiple myeloma. *British Journal of Cancer*, **63**, 769–772.

291 Doody M.M., Linet M.S., Glass A.G. *et al.* (1992) Leukemia, lymphoma and multiple myeloma following selected medical conditions. *Cancer Causes and Control*, **3**, 449–456.

292 Lewis D.R., Pottern L.M., Brown L.M. *et al.* (1994) Multiple myeloma among Blacks and Whites in the United States: the role of chronic antigenic stimulation. *Cancer Causes and Control*, **5**, 529–539.

293 Vianna N.J., Greenberg P. & Davies J.N.P. (1971) Tonsillectomy and Hodgkin's disease: the lymphoid tissue barrier. *Lancet*, **i**, 431.

294 Mueller N., Swanson M., Hsieh C-C. & Cole P. (1987) Tonsillectomy and Hodgkin's disease: results from companion population-based studies. *Journal of the National Cancer Institute*, **78**, 1–5.

295 Gledovic Z. & Radovanovic Z. (1991) History of tonsillectomy and appendectomy in Hodgkin's disease. *European Journal of Epidemiology*, **7**, 612–615.

296 Levine P.H., Peterson D., McNamee F.L. *et al.* (1992) Does chronic fatigue syndrome predispose to non-Hodgkin's lymphoma? *Cancer Research*, **52**(Suppl.), 5516–5518.

297 Kravdal O. & Hansen S. (1993) Hodgkin's disease: the protective effect of childbearing. *International Journal of Cancer*, **55**, 909–914.

298 Schu Z-O., Clemens J., Zheng W., Ying D.M., Ji B.T. & Jin F. (1995) Infant breastfeeding and the risks of childhood lymphoma and leukaemia. *International Journal of Epidemiology*, **24**, 27–32.

299 Rowley J.D. (1981) Downs syndrome and acute leukaemia: increased risk may be due to trisomy 21. *Lancet*, **i**, 1020–1022.

300 Robison L.L. & Neglia J.P. (1987) Epidemiology of Down syndrome and childhood acute leukaemia. In: *Oncology and Immunology of Down Syndrome* (eds E.E. McCoy & C.J. Epstein), pp. 19–32. Alan Liss, New York.

301 Miller R.W. (1967) Persons of exceptionally high risk of leukaemia. *Cancer Research*, **27**, 2420–2423.

302 Spector B.D., Filipovich A.H., Perry G.S. III *et al.* (1982) Epidemiology of cancer in ataxia-telangiectasia. In: *Ataxia-Telangiectasia: a cellular and molecular link between cancer, neuropathology, and immune deficiency* (eds B.A. Bridges & D.C. Harnden), pp. 121–129. Wiley, New York.

303 Seemanova E., Passarge E., Beneskova D. *et al.* (1985) Familial microcephaly with normal intelligence, immunodeficiency and risk for lymphoreticular malignancies: a new autosomal recessive disorder. *American Journal of Human Genetics*, **20**, 639–648.

304 Al-Jader L.N., West R.R., Goodchild M.C. *et al.* (1989) Mortality from leukaemia among relatives of patients with cystic fibrosis. *British Medical Journal*, **298**, 164.

305 Gatti R.A. & Good R.A. (1971) Occurrence of malignancy on immunodeficiency diseases. A literature review. *Cancer*, **28**, 89–98.

306 Spector B.D., Perry G.S. III, Kersey J. *et al.* (1978) Genetically determined immunodeficiency diseases (GDID) and malignancy; report from the Immunodeficiency Cancer Registry. *Clinical Immunology Immunopathology*, **11**, 12–29.

307 Strigini P., Carobbi S., Sansone R., Limbardo C. & Santi L. (1991) Molecular epidemiology of cancer in immune deficiency. *Cancer Detection and Prevention*, **15**, 115–126.

308 Hartley S.E. & Sainsbury C. (1981) Acute leukaemia and the same chromosome abnormality in monozygotic twins. *Human Genetics*, **58**, 408–410.

309 Cartwright R.A., Darwin C., McKinney P.A. *et al.* (1988) Acute myeloid leukaemia in adults: a case-control study in Yorkshire. *Leukaemia*, **2**, 687–690.

310 Linet M.S., Van Natta M.L., Brookmeyer R. *et al.* (1989) Familial cancer history and chronic lymphocytic leukaemia. A case-control study. *American Journal of Epidemiology*, **130**, 655–664.

311 Radovanovic Z., Markovic-Denic L.J. & Jankovic S. (1994) Cancer mortality of family members of patients with chronic lymphocytic leukemia. *European Journal of Epidemiology*, **10**, 211–213.

312 Gerncik A., Buser M., Temminck B. *et al.* (1987) High incidence of stomach cancer in relatives of patients with malignant lymphoproliferative disorders. *Cancer Detection and Prevention*, **1**(Suppl.), 121–129.

313 Linet M.S. & Blattner W.A. (1988) The epidemiology of chronic lymphocytic leukaemia. In: *Chronic Lymphocytic Leukemia* (eds A. Polliack & D. Catovsky), pp. 11–32. Harwood Academic Press, Chur, Switzerland.

314 Kato S., Tsuji K., Tsunematsu Y. *et al.* (1983) Familial leukaemia HLA system and leukaemia predisposition in a family. *American Journal of Diseases in Children*, **137**, 641–644.

315 D'Amaro H., Back F., van Rood J.J. *et al.* (1984) HLA-C associations with acute leukaemia. *Lancet*, **ii**, 1176–1178.

316 Taylor G.M., Robinson M.D., Binchy A. *et al.* (1995) Preliminary evidence of an association between HLA-DPBI*0201 and childhood common acute lymphoblastic leukaemia supports an infectious aetiology. *Leukemia*, **9**, 440–443.

317 Ludwig H. & Mayr W. (1982) Genetic aspects of susceptibility to multiple myeloma. *Blood*, **59**, 1286–1291.

318 Bodmer J.G., Oza A.M.M., Lister T.A. & Bodmer W.F. (1989) HLA-DP based resistance to Hodgkin's disease. *Lancet*, 1455–1456.

319 Blattner W.A. (1989) Retroviruses. In: *Viral Infections in Humans* (ed. A.S. Evans), 2nd edn, pp. 545–592. Plenum Medical Book Co., New York.

320 Gerard Y., Lepere J-F., Pradinaud R. *et al.* (1995) Clustering and clinical diversity of adult T-cell leukaemia/lymphoma associated with THLV-1 in a remote black population of French Guiana. *International Journal of Cancer*, **60**, 773–776.

321 Manns A., Cleghorn F.R., Falk R.T. & Hanchard B. (1993) Role of HTLV-1 in development of non-Hodgkin's lymphoma in Jamaica and Trinidad and Tobago. *Lancet*, **342**, 1447–1450.

322 Wiktor S.Z. & Blattner W.A. (1991) Epidemiology of HTLV-I. In: *The Human Retrovirus* (eds R.C. Gallo & G. Jay), pp. 121–129. Academic Press, Orlando.

323 Beral V., Peterman T., Berkelman R. & Jaffe H. (1991) AIDS-associated non-Hodgkin's lymphoma. *Lancet*, **337**, 805–809.

324 Ragni M.V., Belle S.H., Jaffe R.A. *et al.* (1993) Acquired immuno-deficiency syndrome-associated non-Hodgkin's lymphomas and other malignancies in patients with hemophilia. *Blood*, **81**, 1889–1897.

325 Finlay J., Luft B., Yousem S. *et al.* (1986) Chronic infectious mononucleosis syndrome, pancytopenia, and polyclonal B-lymphoproliferation terminating in acute lymphoblastic leukaemia. *American Journal of Pediatric Hematology/Oncology*, **8**, 18–27.

326 Armstrong A.A., Alexander F.E., Paes R.P. *et al.* (1993) Association of Epstein–Barr virus with pediatric Hodgkin's Disease. *American Journal of Pathology*, **142**, 1683–1688.

327 Jarrett R.F., Gallagher A., Jones D.B. *et al.* (1991) Detection of Epstein–Barr virus genomes in Hodgkin's disease: relation to age. *Journal of Clinical Pathology*, **44**, 844–848.

328 Clarke D.A., Alexander F.E., McKinney P.A. *et al.* (1990) The seroepidemiology of human herpesvirus-6 (HHV-6) from a case-control study of leukaemia and lymphoma. *International Journal of Cancer*, **45**, 829–833.

329 Moore P.S. & Chang Y. (1995) Detection of herpesvirus-like DNA sequences in Kaposi's sarcoma in patients with and those without HIV infection. *New England Journal of Medicine*, **332**, 1181–1191.

330 Editorial (1990) Childhood leukaemia: an infectious disease? *Lancet*, **ii**, 1477–1479.

331 Greaves M.F. (1989) Etiology of childhood acute lymphoblastic leukaemia: a soluble problem? In: *Acute Lymphoblastic Leukaemia. UCLA Symposium on Molecular and Cellular Biology* (eds R.P. Gale & D. Hoelzer), New Series Vol. 108, pp. 91–97. Academic Press, New York.

332 Kinlen J.L. (1988) Evidence for an infective cause of childhood leukaemia: comparison of a Scottish New Town with nuclear reprocessing sites in Britain. *Lancet*, **ii**, 1323–1326.

333 Alexander F.E., Ricketts T.J., McKinney P.A. & Cartwright R.A. (1991) Community lifestyle characteristics and lymphoid malignancies in young people in the UK. *European Journal of Cancer*, **27**, 1486–1490.

2 Morphology and Classification of Leukaemias

B.J. Bain

Introduction

The purpose of classification of leukaemias and other haematological neoplasms is to organize knowledge into a manageable form so that biologically meaningful entities can be recognized. This is fundamental in making further scientific advances. It also gives vital information about disease characteristics, including prognosis and likely responsiveness to treatment. Correct classification permits optimal patient management. Leukaemias are usually divided into myeloid and lymphoid, acute and chronic. This simple classification, based on lineage and on rate of disease progression when untreated, has some inherent problems. Biphenotypic leukaemias are now recognized and this necessitates a further category. Furthermore, the categories of chronic myeloid and chronic lymphoid leukaemias include a considerable number of very different diseases, some of which have quite a poor prognosis. Classifications of myeloid neoplasms also need to include the myelodysplastic syndromes, the myeloproliferative disorders and macrophage neoplasms. Classifications of chronic lymphoid leukaemias need to be related to classifications of lymphomas, because the same disease entity, for example adult T-cell leukaemia/lymphoma, may present as either a leukaemia or a lymphoma and furthermore, node-based lymphomas may have an 'overspill' of malignant cells into the peripheral blood. Therefore a somewhat expanded classification will be used here, as shown in Table 2.1.

Myeloid leukaemias and macrophage neoplasms

Acute and chronic myeloid leukaemias are diseases resulting from proliferation of a clone of neoplastic myeloid cells derived from a mutant stem cell which may be a pluripotent lymphoid-myeloid stem cell, a multipotent myeloid stem cell or a committed precursor cell. Although differentiation is essentially myeloid, in some types of myeloid leukaemia, for example chronic granulocytic leukaemia, at least some cells of the leukaemic clone preserve the potential for lymphoid differentiation. Acute leukaemias are characterized by a failure of maturation so that immature cells accumulate. This is also true, although to a lesser extent, in the myelodysplastic syndromes. In the myeloproliferative disorders, including the chronic myeloid leukaemias, there is an expanded population of haemopoietic cells with preservation of the capacity to differentiate and mature.

Neoplasms of the monocyte/macrophage lineage include not only acute and chronic leukaemias but also neoplastic proliferations in tissues. These may be localized or disseminated and acute or chronic in their clinical behaviour.

Acute myeloid leukaemia

Definitions and classification. Acute myeloid leukaemia (AML) is a disease resulting from the proliferation of a neoplastic clone of cells derived from a myeloid stem cell or committed progenitor cell. It is characterized by a marked imbalance of proliferation and maturation leading to an accumulation of blast cells and inadequate production of mature cells. The term 'acute non-lymphoblastic leukaemia' (ANLL), sometimes preferred in North America, is synonymous. AMLs are usually classified morphologically. The most widely used classification is that proposed by the French–American–British (FAB) cooperative group (Table 2.2) [2,3], which is based on the dominant cell type and the degree of maturation. The FAB classification also incorporates immunophenotyping, in order to identify acute megakaryoblastic leukaemia (M7 AML) and to differentiate AML with minimal evidence of myeloid differentiation (M0 AML) from acute lymphoblastic leukaemia (ALL). A more detailed classification which builds on the FAB morphological classification is the MIC (Morphologic–Immunologic–Cytogenetic) Classification which incorporates the results of cytogenetic analysis [4]. This is an open-ended classification which allows new categories to be added as they are recognized. Some established categories are shown in Table 2.3 [4,5]. The MIC classification leaves a proportion of

Table 2.1 Classification of haematological neoplasms.

Myeloid leukaemias and related disorders
Acute myeloid leukaemia
Myelodysplastic syndromes
Myeloproliferative disorders including chronic myeloid leukaemias
Histiocyte/macrophage neoplasms

Lymphoid leukaemias and lymphomas
Acute lymphoblastic leukaemia and lymphoblastic lymphoma
    B-lineage
    T-lineage
    NK-lineage
Other lymphoid leukaemias and lymphomas
    B-lineage
    T-lineage
    NK-lineage
Plasma cell dyscrasias

Biphenotypic leukaemias
Biphenotypic acute leukaemia
Other biphenotypic leukaemia

Table 2.2 The French–American–British (FAB) classification of AML. The criteria given apply to the bone marrow unless stated otherwise. (From Bain, 1995 [1].)

M1 (AML without maturation)
Blasts ≥90% of NEC; ≥3% of blasts positive for peroxidase or SBB; monocytic component ≤10% of NEC; granulocytic component ≤10% of NEC

M2 (AML with granulocytic maturation)
Blasts 30–89% of NEC; granulocytic component >10% of NEC; monocytic component <20% of NEC

M3 and M3 variant
Characteristic morphology

M4 (Acute myelomonocytic leukaemia)
Blasts ≥30% of NEC; granulocytic component (including myeloblasts) ≥20% of NEC

AND

EITHER	OR
BM monocytic component ≥20% of NEC and PB monocyte count ≥5 × 10⁹/l	BM resembling M2 but PB monocyte count ≥5 × 10⁹/l and lysozyme elevated
OR BM monocytic component ≥20% of NEC and lysozyme elevated*	*OR* BM resembling M2 but PB monocyte count ≥5 × 10⁹/l and cytochemical demonstration of monocytic component in BM
OR BM monocytic component ≥20% of NEC and cytochemical confirmation of monocyte component in BM†	

M5 (acute monocytic/monoblastic leukaemia)

    M5a (without maturation or acute monoblastic leukaemia)
    Monocytic component ≥80% of NEC; monoblasts ≥80% monocytic component

    M5b (with maturation or acute monocytic leukaemia)
    Monocytic component ≥80% of NEC; monoblasts <80% of monocyte component

M6 (erythroleukaemia)
Erythroblasts ≥50% blasts ≥30% of NEC

M7 (megakaryoblastic leukaemia)
Blasts demonstrated to be megakaryoblasts, for example by ultrastructural cytochemistry showing the presence of platelet peroxidase or by immunological cell marker studies showing the presence of platelet antigens

M0 (AML with minimal evidence of myeloid differentiation)
Peroxidase and SBB positive in <3% of blasts but blasts demonstrated to be myeloid by immunophenotyping

BM, bone marrow, NEC, non-erythroid cells; PB, peripheral blood.
* Lysozyme in serum or urine elevated threefold compared with normal.
† Positive for NASA esterase activity, with activity being inhibited by fluoride.

cases unclassified, because not all cases of AML have successful cytogenetic analyses. Since this classification was first proposed, there have been major advances in molecular genetics and there might now be the need for a MIC-M (Morphologic–Immunologic–Cytogenetic–Molecular Genetic) Classification. This would permit cases with a normal karyotype or failed cytogenetic analysis to be categorized with equivalent cases. For example, Ph-negative cases with a *BCR-ABL* rearrangement would be classified with Ph-positive cases, and cases lacking t(15;17)(q22;q11) but nevertheless with a *PML-RARα* rearrangement would be classified with other cases of M3 or M3v AML.

It could be possible to classify AML by immunophenotype alone but this approach has not been widely used. However, certain immunophenotypic profiles have been found to be typical of specific MIC subtypes of AML, for example M2/t(8;21) is usually CD34 positive and shows expression of HLA-DR and the pan-B marker CD19, in addition to myeloid markers such as CD13, CD33 and CD68 [7]. M3/t(15;17), in addition to myeloid markers including CD68 is CD9 positive, but usually HLA-DR and CD34 negative [8].

It would seem logical to attempt to classify AML according to whether the mutations which gave rise to the leukaemic clone arose in a pluripotent, multipotent or committed cell. Probably such a classification would identify categories of leukaemia with different biological properties and different responsiveness to treatment. However, in the majority of cases there are practical difficulties in identifying the nature of the clonogenic cell. Trilineage myelodysplasia indicates that the clonogenic cell is either a pluripotent or multipotent stem cell but morphology is unlikely to identify all such cases. A classification based on the presence or absence of evident multilineage involvement has been proposed [9], although it has not won

Table 2.3 The morphologic–immunologic–cytogenetic (MIC) classification of acute myeloid leukaemia [4,5].

Morphology	Cytogenetics	Comment
M2	t(8;21)(q22;q22)	Occasionally M1 or M4
M3 or M3v	t(15;17)(q22;q11)*	
M3	t(11;17)(q23;q21)	May be morphologically slightly atypical [6]
M4Eo	inv(16)(p13q22) or t(16;16)(p13;q22) or del(16)(q22)	Occasionally M2Eo or M4
M1	t(9;22)(q34;q11)	May also be M0, M2 or M4
M5	del(11)(q23) or t(11;V)(q23;V) (e.g. t(9;11)(p21;q23))	Usually M5a AML, sometimes M5b or M4, occasionally M1 or M2
M4	Trisomy 4	May also be M1 or M2
M2Baso or M4Baso	t(6;9)(p23;q34)†	Not all cases have basophilia; sometimes M1
M7	inv(3)(q21q26)†‡ or t(3;3)(q21;q26)†‡	May also be M0, M1, M2, M4, M5 or M6
M5	t(8;16)(p11;p13)*	Usually M5a, sometimes M5b or M4
M2Baso	del(12)(p11p13)	May also be M0 or M4Baso
M1	del(9)(q13q22)	
M7	t(1;22)(p13;q13)‖	
various	t(3;21)(q26;q22)†	
M1 or M4	t(1;3)(p36;q21)	
AML or malignant histiocytosis	i(12p)	Associated with and probably derived from mediastinal germ cell tumour

* Associated coagulation abnormality.
† Often secondary.
‡ Usually trilineage myelodysplasia.
‖ Occurs in infants.

general acceptance. An alternative approach is to categorize by the FAB or MIC classification but to also note the presence of trilineage myelodysplasia because, in most series of cases, this has been of prognostic importance.

It is also important to categorize AML according to whether it is primary or secondary and also whether there has been a preceding haematological abnormality, because such factors may alter the prognosis and influence therapy. The presence of relevant associated diseases (e.g. Down's syndrome, Li–Fraumeni syndrome or type 1 neurofibromatosis) should also be noted. Relevant associated and antecedent haematological diseases are those which predispose to leukaemia and which may also influence management. For example, Down's syndrome is associated with an increased incidence of AML which, in comparison with other cases of AML, has a different age distribution and a much higher incidence of the M7 subtype. The prognosis is better than is usual in AML and this should be considered in choice of treatment. Similarly, Fanconi's anaemia is associated with an increased incidence of AML and, because of the susceptibility to radiation-induced tissue damage, the diagnosis is relevant to choice of treatment. A suggested classification is shown in Table 2.4. It will be noted that there is some overlap between categories, for example between secondary AML and AML following myelodysplastic syndromes (MDS).

Acute myelofibrosis is a morphological variant of AML, often M7 AML. There are also some rare types of AML which are not included in the FAB and MIC classifications, for example acute leukaemia of Langerhans' cells [10] or dendritic cells [11] and acute mast cell leukaemia. In addition,

Table 2.4 Classification of AML according to antecedent history.

De novo AML

Secondary or therapy-related AML
  following exposure to alkylating agent and related drugs
  following exposure to topoisomerase II interactive drugs

AML with antecedent haematological disorder
  following myelodysplastic syndromes
  following aplastic anaemia (including Fanconi's anaemia)
  following paroxysmal nocturnal haemoglobinuria
  following myeloproliferative disorders
    following chronic granulocytic leukaemia (blast transformation)
    following polycythaemia rubra vera
    following idiopathic myelofibrosis
    following essential thrombocythaemia
  other antecedent haematological disorder (e.g. Shwachman–Diamond syndrome, Kostmann's syndrome)

AML with relevant associated disease or inherited predisposition to leukaemia
  Down's syndrome
  type 1 neurofibromatosis
  Li–Fraumeni syndrome

it should be noted that AML may present as a tumour of soft tissues, as either granulocytic or monocytic sarcoma. The bone marrow may be normal, but nevertheless such cases should be regarded as a variant of AML. Transient abnormal myelopoiesis which occurs in neonates with Down's syndrome is likely to represent transient acute leukaemia and may be regarded as a variant of AML [12].

Morphology and cytochemistry. The classification of AML requires the examination and differential counting of May–Grünwald–Giemsa (MGG) stained peripheral blood and bone marrow films, and the application of selected cytochemical reactions. Typical cytological and cytochemical features of the different subtypes of AML are shown in Plates 2.1–2.20 (between pp. 292 and 293).

The blood film usually shows normocytic normochromic anaemia, neutropenia and thrombocytopenia. Blast cells are present in the majority of cases and there may be occasional nucleated red cells. It is necessary to recognize myeloblasts, normal and abnormal promyelocytes and monoblasts in order to assess blood and bone marrow films. Myeloblasts (see Plate 2.2) are usually moderately large cells with a high nucleocytoplasmic ratio, a diffuse chromatin pattern and a variable number of nucleoli which vary in their size and prominence. The cytoplasm is usually weakly to moderately basophilic and may contain azurophilic crystalline inclusions known as Auer rods (see Plate 2.2). Myeloblasts, as defined by the FAB group [3], may have a small number of azurophilic granules but they lack the eccentric nucleus, chromatin condensation and Golgi zone which characterize the promyelocyte. Since leukaemic cells may have defective granule formation, cells which lack granules but which otherwise have the characteristics of promyelocytes should be classified as promyelocytes rather than as myeloblasts. Monoblasts (see Plates 2.9 & 2.12) are larger than myeloblasts with abundant cytoplasm which may be vacuolated, but they have few if any granules. The nucleus may be round or lobulated. There are often one or two prominent nucleoli. In hypergranular promyelocytic leukaemia (see Plate 2.7) the promyelocytes are much more heavily granulated than either normal promyelocytes or the promyelocytes of other types of AML. The granules are large, stain a bright purplish red and pack the cytoplasm, obscuring the nucleus. There may be giant granules or stacks of Auer rods. In the variant form of promyelocytic leukaemia (see Plate 2.8) the nucleus is bilobed with the two lobes being joined by a broad isthmus. Most variant promyelocytes in the peripheral blood have no granules visible by light microscopy, but in a minority of cells there are very fine granules or Auer rods or the cytoplasm has a pink blush. Some more typical hypergranular promyelocytes can usually be found in the bone marrow. The blood and bone marrow films of cases of AML should be examined for dysplastic features, all lineages being specifically evaluated.

The minimal panel of cytochemical reactions required for the diagnosis of acute leukaemia is: (i) either a myeloperoxidase or Sudan black B stain, and (ii) either a nonspecific esterase reaction, such as alpha naphthyl acetate esterase, or a combined esterase reaction, such as chloroacetate esterase plus alpha naphthyl acetate esterase [13,14]. When resources permit, the use of all four cytochemical stains is recommended. Alpha naphthyl butyrate esterase is an alternative to alpha naphthyl acetate esterase but although the former is more specific for the monocyte lineage the latter is preferred on technical grounds [13]. The usual pattern of cytochemical reactivity of leukaemic cells is summarized in Table 2.5 and illustrated in Plates 2.4, 2.6, 2.10 & 2.17.

It is important for the haematologist to recognize the typical cytological features of monoblasts, because some cases of AML show such limited cytoplasmic maturation that the usual cytochemical reactions are negative. The diagnosis then rests on the cytology together with the immunophenotype. Blasts in M7 AML sometimes show features suggestive of the megakaryocyte lineage (see Plate 2.18), such as cytoplasmic blebs, cytoplasmic staining characteristics resembling those of mature platelets or the presence of hyperchromatic nuclei with scanty cytoplasm ('bare' megakaryocyte nuclei). However in some cases there are no distinguishing characteristics (see Plate 2.20), the blasts resembling either myeloblasts or lymphoblasts. The diagnosis of M7 AML therefore requires the routine application of immunophenotyping. Immunophenotyping is also required to recognize M0 AML and to confirm the nature of rare leukaemias in which the blast cells are primitive erythroblasts.

The great majority of cases of AML can be diagnosed by

Table 2.5 Pattern of reaction with various cytochemical stains.

Myeloperoxidase and Sudan black B	Positive in primary granules of the neutrophil and eosinophil lineages from the promyelocyte to the mature granulocyte; positive in basophil precursors from the promyelocyte to the metamyelocyte; positive (in granules, Auer rods or both) in most leukaemic myeloblasts but usually negative in blasts of basophil lineage; Sudan black B may be positive in mast cells but myeloperoxidase is negative
Chloroacetate esterase	Positive in cells of neutrophil lineage from promyelocytes to mature neutrophils; positive in mast cells; positive (in granules, Auer rods or both) in most leukaemic myeloblasts; negative in normal eosinophils but may show aberrant activity in the eosinophils in M4Eo AML associated with inv(16)
Alpha naphthyl acetate esterase	Strongly positive in promonocytes and monocytes; positive in promonocytes and monocytes in acute and chronic leukaemias and positive in most leukaemic monoblasts; positive in platelets; strongly positive in some megakaryoblasts; weakly positive in myeloblasts
Alpha naphthyl butyrate esterase	As for alpha naphthyl acetate esterase except that platelets and megakaryoblasts show only a weak reaction

examination of the peripheral blood and bone marrow aspirate. However occasionally a trephine biopsy is needed for diagnosis. This is necessary if there is bone marrow fibrosis which prevents an adequate aspirate being obtained. This is particularly common in acute megakaryoblastic leukaemia (M7 AML) and in secondary leukaemia. A trephine biopsy is also necessary for the diagnosis of hypocellular AML, when a dilute nondiagnostic aspirate is often obtained. The trephine biopsy shows that although the marrow is hypocellular, a high proportion of the cells present are blast cells.

Summary and conclusions. It is recommended that all cases of AML:

1 should be categorized morphologically, according to the FAB classification;
2 should be studied cytogenetically and classified according to the MIC classification;
3 should have molecular genetic analysis carried out when cytogenetic analysis fails and when the presence of a specific cytogenetic abnormality would influence management;
4 should have the presence or absence of trilineage myelodysplasia noted;
5 should be categorized according to the presence or absence of antecedent haematological disease, relevant associated disease or exposure to known leukaemogens.

This categorization necessitates the use of:

1 cytochemistry to facilitate FAB classification;
2 immunophenotyping, at least in all cases which are not obviously myeloid from cytological and cytochemical features;
3 cytogenetic analysis in all cases;
4 molecular genetic analysis when specifically indicated.

The myelodysplastic syndromes

Definitions and classification. The myelodysplastic syndromes (MDS) are diseases resulting from partial or complete replacement of normal haemopoietic cells by a clone of neoplastic cells derived from a mutant multipotent or pluripotent haemopoietic stem cell. The neoplastic clone shows an imbalance between maturation (which is defective) and proliferation (which is usually preserved). Consequently, despite a bone marrow which is usually hypercellular or normocellular, there is cytopenia, for example anaemia, neutropenia or thrombocytopenia. A minority of cases have a hypocellular bone marrow. Haemopoiesis is morphologically dysplastic. In some cases the defect in maturation is severe and blast cells are increased. Although MDS is characterized by ineffective haemopoiesis and cytopenia, there may be effective production of cells of one or more lineage. Some cases have monocytosis, neutrophilia or thrombocytosis.

MDS has been classified by the FAB group [3,15] into five categories (Table 2.6). The two categories of refractory anaemia (RA) and refractory anaemia with ring sideroblasts (RARS) have a much better prognosis than the categories of refractory anaemia with excess of blasts (RAEB) and refractory anaemia with excess of blasts in transformation (RAEB-t). The prognosis of chronic myelomonocytic leukaemia (CMML) has been very variable between different series of patients. This is probably a result of inconsistent application of criteria for classification and exclusion of a varying proportion of cases with more pronounced myeloproliferative features (see below). Typical cytological findings of MDS are illustrated in Plates 2.21–2.31 (between pp. 292 and 293).

Although the FAB classification of MDS has aroused more

Table 2.6 The FAB Classification of the myelodysplastic syndromes [3,15].

Category	Peripheral blood			Bone marrow
Refractory anaemia (RA) or refractory cytopenia*	Anaemia*, blasts ≤1%, monocytes ≤1 × 10⁹/l		*and*	Blasts <5%, ring sideroblasts ≤15% of erythroblasts
Refractory anaemia with ring sideroblasts (RARS)	Anaemia, blasts ≤1%, monocytes ≤1 × 10⁹/l		*and*	Blasts <5%, ring sideroblasts >15% of erythroblasts
Refractory anaemia with excess of blasts (RAEB)	Anaemia, blasts >1%, monocytes ≤1 × 10⁹/l		*or*	Blasts ≥5%
			but	
	Blasts <5%		*and*	Blasts ≤20%
Chronic myelomonocytic leukaemia (CMML)	Monocytes >1 × 10⁹/l, granulocytes often increased, blasts <5%			Blasts up to 20%
Refractory anaemia with excess of blasts in transformation (RAEB-t)	Blasts ≥5%	*or*	Auer rods in blasts in blood or marrow *or*	Blasts >20% *but* <30%

* Or in the case of refractory cytopenia either neutropenia or thrombocytopenia.

controversy than the FAB classification of AML, it has nevertheless been quite widely accepted. The main problems with its application relate to overlap with the myeloproliferative disorders (MPD), particularly to difficulties in categorizing a case as CMML or as atypical chronic myeloid leukaemia (aCML). Both may have neutrophilia, monocytosis, anaemia, thrombocytopenia and dysplastic haemopoiesis. However eosinophilia and basophilia, which may occur in aCML, are quite uncommon in MDS, whereas a significant increase in immature granulocytes is uncommon in CMML. The sum of promyelocytes, myelocytes and metamyelocytes is usually less than 5% in CMML, whereas in aCML it is usually greater than 5% and quite often greater than 15% [16,17]. It should also be recognized that there are cases which do not fit neatly into definitions of MDS or MPD. For example, a case may have sideroblastic anaemia with marked thrombocytosis or there may be markedly dysplastic haemopoiesis with bone marrow fibrosis. Such cases may be designated 'overlap syndrome' or 'unclassified myelodysplastic/myeloproliferative disorder'. Childhood myelodysplastic/myeloproliferative disorders do not fit well into the FAB classification and will be considered separately (see below).

In addition to the FAB morphological classification, it is useful to consider cytogenetic abnormalities when assessing cases of MDS. Although few categories are well defined, there are some cytogenetic abnormalities which are particularly associated with one or two FAB categories of MDS and there are many which give prognostic information. The best defined morphological/cytogenetic category is the 5q– syndrome in which MDS, usually refractory anaemia, is associated with an interstitial deletion of the long arm of chromosome 5. The 5q– syndrome has a relatively good prognosis, whereas certain other cytogenetic abnormalities, such as complex karyotypes, inv(3)(q21q26) and t(6;9)(p23;q34), are associated with a poor prognosis. In characterizing the disease in an individual patient it is useful to think of both the karyotype and the FAB morphological category, because they have independent prognostic significance. Cases might be categorized, for example, as: RA/normal karyotype; RA/5q–; CMML/12p–; RAEB/–5, –7, 7q–.

In addition to a morphological/cytogenetic classification, it is important to classify MDS as primary or secondary. Those cases which are secondary to cytotoxic drugs have a much worse prognosis than *de novo* cases, even when they fall into the RA or RARS categories. When myelodysplastic features develop in patients with an antecedent haematological disorder (e.g. aplastic anaemia, paroxysmal nocturnal haemoglobinuria or chronic granulocytic leukaemia), the condition is often not classified as MDS. Nevertheless the significance is similar. The dysplastic features are a result of either the appearance or the evolution of a clonal disorder and indicate a worse prognosis and the likelihood of evolution to AML.

Immunophenotype is of little value in the classification of MDS, although it can be used to determine the lineage of any blast cells present.

When the FAB classification of MDS was first described, one of its aims was to define a group of patients with a disease which was less aggressive than AML and which did not warrant intensive therapy. However, it should be recognized that in the intervening years there have been marked improvements in the therapeutic results in intensively treated AML. It has also been found that the outcome in some cases of RAEB and RAEB-t, particularly in relatively young patients and in those with Auer rods, can be improved with similar treatment. The FAB classification should therefore now be regarded as a morphological categorization which gives prognostic information but which does not necessarily indicate the appropriateness of different forms of therapy. Decisions on therapy should be made using all available information, to determine the likely outcome with and without a specific form of therapy.

Morphology and cytochemistry. There are certain dysplastic features which are relatively specific for MDS and which are therefore of considerable value in diagnosis. These are hypogranular neutrophils (see Plates 2.21 & 2.23 between pp. 292 and 293), the acquired Pelger–Hüet anomaly (see Plates 2.21 & 2.22) in the peripheral blood and micromegakaryocytes (see Plate 2.30) in the bone marrow. Micromegakaryocytes, which are about the size of myeloblasts or even smaller, should be distinguished from large nonlobulated megakaryocytes (see Plate 2.27) which are characteristic of the 5q– syndrome but are less specific for MDS since they are seen, albeit in smaller numbers, in some normal bone marrows. Dyserythropoiesis, including the presence of ring sideroblasts (see Plates 2.28 & 2.29), is common in MDS but is less specific. The presence of increased blood or bone marrow blast cells and of Auer rods in blast cells is important in the diagnosis of MDS. A great variety of other dysplastic features can also occur and may be useful in diagnosis [18].

The cytochemical stains which are indicated in suspected MDS are: (i) a Perls' stain for iron which will demonstrate any ring sideroblasts, and (ii) either a myeloperoxidase or Sudan black B stain to identify any Auer rods. Auer rods are sometimes detected on an MGG stain, but cytochemical stains are more sensitive. It is important that Auer rods are detected whenever they are present, because their presence is one of the features considered in making decisions about treatment.

MDS can usually be diagnosed on the basis of peripheral blood and bone marrow aspirate features. Sometimes a trephine biopsy is useful. It may demonstrate abnormal topography such as: (i) ALIP or 'abnormal localization of immature precursors' (see Plate 2.31) when blasts and promyelocytes occur in clusters in an intertrabecular position; (ii) large poorly organized erythroid islands which may be in an abnormal position, adjacent to a trabeculum; (iii) megakaryocytes which are clustered or adjacent to a trabeculum. A trephine biopsy is useful in detecting megakaryocyte dysplasia but is less useful than blood and bone marrow films in detecting granulocyte dysplasia. Occasionally the diagnosis of MDS cannot be established despite assessment of a peripheral blood film, a bone marrow aspirate and a trephine biopsy. Supplementary techniques which can be useful include demonstration of clonality through investigation of X-linked polymorphisms (applicable to females) and cytogenetic analysis. In some cases of refractory anaemia with few dysplastic features, a diagnosis cannot be established with certainty but follow-up reveals the true nature of the condition.

Summary and conclusions. It is recommended that cases of MDS:
1 should be categorized morphologically according to the FAB classification;
2 should be studied and classified cytogenetically;
3 should be categorized as *de novo* or secondary.

This necessitates the application of cytochemical stains and cytogenetic analysis in all cases. The presence of antecedent haematological disease or relevant associated disease should also be noted. Decisions on the choice of therapy should be based on all relevant information, not simply on the morphological classification.

Chronic myeloid leukaemias

Definitions and classification. The chronic myeloid leukaemias (CML) are a heterogeneous group of diseases resulting from proliferation of a neoplastic clone of cells derived from a multipotent haemopoietic stem cell. The leukaemic clone preserves the capacity to differentiate and mature. Differentiation is predominantly to granulocytes, monocytes or both. The majority of cases of CML have distinctive haematological features and cytogenetic analysis demonstrates the presence of a Philadelphia (Ph) chromosome, an abbreviated chromosome 22 resulting from a translocation, t(9;22)(q34;q11); molecular genetic analysis demonstrates a characteristic *BCR-ABL* rearrangement. A minority of cases are Ph negative (Ph-) but have the same haematological features as the Ph-positive (Ph+) cases and demonstrate *BCR-ABL* rearrangement. A proposed classification of the CMLs and other myeloproliferative disorders is given in Table 2.7. It is suggested that 'chronic myeloid leukaemia' is used as a generic term and that cases with typical haematological features, which are demonstrated to have either Ph positivity or *BCR-ABL* rearrangement, are designated chronic granulocytic leukaemia (CGL). CGL can be further classified according to whether it is in chronic phase, accelerated phase or blast transformation. The morphological features of the CMLs and of systemic mastocytosis are illustrated in Plates 2.32–2.40 (between pp. 292 and 293).

Table 2.7 Classification of the chronic myeloid leukaemias and other myeloproliferative disorders.

Polycythaemia rubra vera (primary proliferative polycythaemia)
Essential thrombocythaemia
Primary or idiopathic myelofibrosis (myelofibrosis with myeloid metaplasia)
Systemic mastocytosis
Chronic myeloid leukaemias
    Chronic granulocytic leukaemia
        Ph positive
        Ph negative
    Atypical chronic myeloid leukaemia
    Chronic myelomonocytic leukaemia
    Chronic neutrophilic leukaemia
    Chronic eosinophilic leukaemia
    Chronic basophilic leukaemia
    Juvenile chronic myeloid leukaemia and other myelodysplastic/myeloproliferative disorders of childhood
    Chronic myeloid leukaemia following other myeloproliferative disorder (e.g. polycythaemia rubra vera or idiopathic myelofibrosis)
Unclassifiable myeloproliferative disorders

Morphology and cytochemistry. Diagnosis and classification of the CMLs requires careful peripheral blood differential white cell counts supplemented by examination of bone marrow aspirates and by cytogenetic and sometimes molecular genetic analysis.

Cytochemistry (the neutrophil alkaline phosphatase reaction) is of declining importance and immunophenotyping of no importance during the chronic phase of these diseases.

Chronic granulocytic leukaemia

Chronic granulocytic leukaemia (CGL) is characterized by an increased white cell count (usually more than 50×10^9/l), with a prominent increase in mature neutrophils and myelocytes (see Plate 2.32). Blasts and promyelocytes are increased but not out of proportion to more mature cells. The absolute basophil count is increased in almost all cases and the absolute eosinophil count in about 80% of cases. Monocytes are increased but proportionately less than neutrophils. The platelet count is usually normal or elevated. The bone marrow aspirate shows a very high myeloid:erythroid ratio (usually about 25:1). The average size and nuclear lobulation of megakaryocytes is reduced. The trephine biopsy shows a very marked increase of cellularity attributable to granulocytic or to granulocytic and megakaryocytic hyperplasia. During the chronic phase of the disease dysplastic features, other than in megakaryocytes and platelets, are absent. The neutrophil alkaline phosphatase (NAP) is reduced in about 95% of cases.

Atypical chronic myeloid leukaemia

Atypical chronic myeloid leukaemia (aCML), which is Ph- and *BCR-ABL* negative, has haematological features which differ somewhat from those of CGL. The white cell count at presentation tends to be lower. Basophilia and eosinophilia are less consistent findings and in most cases there is prominent monocytosis (see Plate 2.33). Dysplastic features may be present. Thrombocytopenia is more frequent and anaemia tends to be more severe. The bone marrow myeloid : erythroid ratio is increased but is usually less than 10 : 1. Mononuclear or binuclear micromegakaryocytes and other dysplastic features are present in some cases (see Plate 2.34).

Chronic myelomonocytic leukaemia

Chronic myelomonocytic leukaemia (CMML) (see Plates 2.35 & 2.36), which is also classified as one of the myelodysplastic syndromes, differs from atypical CML in that basophilia and eosinophilia are rare and peripheral blood granulocyte precursors are less prominent. The white cell count tends to be lower. CMML, as defined by the FAB group, has an absolute monocytosis and this is usually also true of atypical CML. Both conditions may also show dysplastic features in one or more lineages, so that distinguishing between them is done largely on the basis of the differential count.

Whether aCML and CMML represent distinct entities or merely two ends of a spectrum remains to be established. It should be noted that not only do transitions occur between CMML and the other MDS, but that aCML may also be part of the evolution of MDS, for example refractory anaemia [19]. Assessment of the clinical, haematological, cytogenetic and molecular genetic characteristics of a larger number of cases classified by agreed criteria will be necessary to clarify whether these are really two diseases. What is already clear is that both differ from *BCR-ABL*-positive CGL.

Chronic neutrophilic leukaemia

Neutrophilic leukaemia is a rare Ph- condition in which there is a prominent increase in neutrophils without any significant increase in peripheral blood granulocyte precursors. Granulocytes are sometimes but not always dysplastic. There may be heavy neutrophil granulation.

Chronic eosinophilic leukaemia

Chronic eosinophilic leukaemia is a rare Ph- condition characterized by an increase of eosinophils and their precursors in the blood and bone marrow but with blast cells being less than 30% of bone marrow cells. The eosinophils often show abnormalities such as vacuolation, degranulation, smaller granules than normal, hypolobulation and hyperlobulation. These cytological abnormalities are not specific for eosinophilic

leukaemia, and they have also been seen in some cases of reactive eosinophilia and in the idiopathic hypereosinophilic syndrome (a condition of unknown cause which, at least in some cases, probably represents a myeloproliferative disorder). If the percentage of blast cells is not increased it can be difficult to distinguish eosinophilic leukaemia from reactive eosinophilia. Cytogenetic analysis is indicated in such cases, because the demonstration of a clonal karyotypic abnormality confirms the diagnosis of leukaemia. In women it may also be possible to demonstrate clonality by molecular genetic analysis. In some cases only a period of follow-up permits the diagnosis of eosinophilic leukaemia to be made.

Chronic basophilic leukaemia

Basophilic leukaemia is usually found to be Ph+ and should therefore be regarded as a variant of CGL. Ph- cases should be categorized separately.

Juvenile chronic myeloid leukaemia

Juvenile chronic myeloid leukaemia is confined to children and will be discussed below.

Summary and conclusions (chronic myeloid leukaemias)

Diagnosis and classification of the chronic myeloid leukaemias requires:
1 a white cell differential count and assessment of cytological features of peripheral blood cells;
2 bone marrow aspiration for cytogenetic analysis, to assess megakaryocyte morphology and to exclude a disproportionate increase of blast cells.

Cases which are Ph- may require, in addition, molecular genetic analysis (e.g. reverse transcriptase-polymerase chain reaction (RT-PCR)) to determine whether or not the *BCR-ABL* rearrangement is present and to confirm a diagnosis of Ph- CGL. Assessment of the neutrophil alkaline phosphatase activity is unnecessary if the more specific cytogenetic and molecular genetic analyses are available.

Myelodysplastic/myeloproliferative disorders of childhood

Definitions and classification. The myelodysplastic/myeloproliferative syndromes of childhood differ from those of adults, in that chronic granulocytic leukaemia (Ph+ or Ph-) is rare. However a condition not seen in adults, designated juvenile chronic myeloid leukaemia (see Plates 2.37 & 2.38 between pp. 292 and 293), occurs in children. The distribution of the myelodysplastic syndromes differs from that in adults in that RARS is quite uncommon while CMML and RAEB-t are proportionately more common than in adults [20]. Myeloproliferative features, such as hepatomegaly, splenomegaly, leucocytosis, neutrophilia and monocytosis, are much more common in childhood MDS than in adult MDS and the use of the umbrella term 'myelodysplastic/myeloproliferative disorders of childhood' is therefore suggested.

The application of the FAB classification is less useful than in adults because there is less correlation with prognosis. In one series of patients an aggressive course was seen even in those with RA, an apparently favourable subtype [21]; others have observed a somewhat better prognosis in RA, although the survival is still inferior to that of adults with RA [20]. A high proportion of childhood cases fall into the CMML category but within this broad group there appear to be conditions with very variable clinical and haematological features, natural history and prognosis. Most distinct among these is juvenile CML. It has been suggested [22] that the FAB classification of MDS, when applied to children, should be modified as shown in Table 2.8, juvenile chronic myeloid leukaemia being defined as MDS, usually of CMML category, with a haemoglobin F percentage above 10%. The infant monosomy 7 syndrome is defined by Passmore *et al.* [22] as MDS with monosomy 7 and with onset under the age of 4 years. They categorized cases with an elevated haemoglobin F percentage and monosomy 7 as infantile monosomy 7 syndrome. However, because children with juvenile CML who are initially cytogenetically normal may subsequently develop monosomy 7 this categorization could be debated, and others have not taken this view [23]. The choice of 4 years of age as a diagnostic cut-off point is also arbitrary because, although most cases occur in young children, 10% of reported cases have occurred in children over the age of 5 years [23].

Juvenile chronic myeloid leukaemia

If juvenile myeloid leukaemia is defined as childhood MDS with an elevated haemoglobin F percentage, it is found to be a recognizable syndrome [22]. Clinically it is common for there to be hepatomegaly, splenomegaly, lymphadenopathy and a rash. Immunoglobulin concentration is often increased. Patients are predominantly male with a median age of onset of 3–4 years. Haematologically, most cases fall into the FAB category of CMML. The Ph chromosome is not present. Many cases are cytogenetically normal at presentation but some show trisomy 8 or other clonal abnormality. If cases with

monosomy 7 are not arbitrarily excluded, then about a quarter of cases may show this abnormality [23].

Cytogenetically abnormal cases are sometimes excluded from the juvenile CML category, but there is no obvious justification for this. In juvenile CML not only is haemoglobin F elevated but there are also other features suggesting a reversion to haemopoiesis with fetal characteristics. Haemoglobin A_2 and carbonic anhydrase are reduced, as is the ratio of I:i antigen. Juvenile CML does not have a propensity to transform to AML but nevertheless the prognosis is poor with the median survival being less than a year. Onset in the first 6 months of life is associated with a better prognosis [23].

Infantile monosomy 7 syndrome

As for juvenile CML, infants with MDS and monosomy 7 are predominantly male but the median age of onset is less than 1 year. Hepatosplenomegaly is common and about half of affected infants have lymphadenopathy. The majority fall into the FAB category of CMML and a minority into the RAEB category. There is a propensity to transform to AML, but nevertheless the prognosis is better than that of juvenile CML and some cases respond to intensive chemotherapy. In the series reported by Passmore *et al.* [22], the median survival was about 3 years, intermediate between the survival of RAEB/RAEB-t and other cases of CMML. The justification for regarding the infant monosomy 7 syndrome as a distinct entity is less convincing than the justification for isolating juvenile CML. Monosomy 7 is a common secondary event in many different types of childhood MDS [23] and in some series of cases there has been no clear difference between those with and without monosomy 7 syndrome [21,24]. Nevertheless, until further series of fully characterized patients have been studied, it seems reasonable, at least provisionally, to adopt the classification proposed by Passmore *et al.* [22]. It might be useful, in further series of patients, if cases with the features of juvenile CML who also had monosomy 7 were analysed separately, so that disease characteristics in this group could be defined more clearly.

Other recommendations with regard to classification

The childhood myelodysplastic/myeloproliferative syndromes should also be classified as primary or secondary (to

---

Table 2.8 Modified FAB Classification for myelodysplastic/myeloproliferative syndromes of childhood [22].

Juvenile chronic myeloid leukaemia	MDS with haemoglobin F > 10% but without monosomy 7
Infant monosomy 7 syndrome	MDS with monosomy 7 syndrome and onset before 4 years of age
Refractory anaemia	
Refractory anaemia with ring sideroblasts	Defined as for adults but excluding any cases meeting the
Refractory anaemia with excess of blasts	definition of juvenile CML or infant monosomy 7 syndrome
Refractory anaemia with excess of blasts in transformation	

Table 2.9 Supplementary classification of childhood myelodysplastic/myeloproliferative syndromes.

De novo myelodysplastic/myeloproliferative disorder

Secondary myelodysplastic/myeloproliferative disorder

Myelodysplastic/myeloproliferative disorder associated with congenital (inherited or genetic) condition predisposing to leukaemia
  Down's syndrome
  Fanconi's anaemia
  Dyskeratosis congenita
  Shwachman's syndrome
  Kostmann's syndrome
  Neurofibromatosis type 1
  Familial predisposition to AML and MDS (sometimes associated with cerebellar ataxia)
  Familial platelet storage pool disorder
  Other

Myelodysplastic/myeloproliferative disorder associated with antecedent acquired haematological disorder
  Acquired aplastic anaemia
  Cyclical or idiopathic neutropenia

---

chemotherapy). The presence of any relevant congenital or inherited abnormality or antecedent haematological disease should be noted, as shown in Table 2.9. In addition, it has been recommended that a prognostic score is assigned [22]. This is of some importance in view of the imperfect correlation of the FAB classification with prognosis.

Morphology and cytochemistry. Differential counts and assessment of peripheral blood and bone marrow morphological features are required. Neutrophilia, marked monocytosis and trilineage myelodysplasia are common in all the childhood myelodysplastic/myeloproliferative syndromes. Some cases have eosinophilia and basophilia, and myeloblasts are usually present in the peripheral blood in small numbers. Circulating nucleated red blood cells are often much more numerous than in MDS in adults and the bone marrow may show erythroid hyperplasia. Auer rods and ring sideroblasts are not common. Isolated thrombocytopenia and megakaryocyte and platelet dysplasia are often particularly prominent in MDS associated with Down's syndrome. With the exception of the iron stain, cytochemistry (including the neutrophil alkaline phosphatase score) is not useful in the diagnosis or classification.

Summary and conclusions. The childhood myelodysplastic/myeloproliferative disorders:
1 should have cytogenetic analysis and determination of haemoglobin F percentage performed in all cases;
2 should be classified by a modified FAB classification;
3 should be classified as primary or secondary;
4 should have relevant antecedent or associated diseases noted;
5 should have a prognostic score assigned.

Table 2.10 Neoplasms of monocyte or macrophage/histiocyte lineage.

Acute monocytic/monoblastic leukaemia (M5 AML)
Malignant histiocytosis
True histiocytic lymphoma
Langerhans' cell leukaemia
Langerhans' cell histiocytosis ('histiocytosis X')
  Eosinophilic granuloma
  Letterer–Siwe disease
  Hand–Schüller–Christian disease
Dendritic cell leukaemia
Interdigitating cell sarcoma

Monocyte/macrophage neoplasms

Definitions and classification. Neoplasms known to be of monocyte or macrophage/histiocyte lineage are summarized in Table 2.10. It can be seen that there is some overlap with the classification of AML. Diagnosis of some of these disorders can be difficult. In the past it has often been difficult to determine lineage and to separate neoplastic and reactive macrophage proliferation. For example, the many cases once diagnosed as 'reticulum cell sarcoma' or 'histiocytic lymphoma' are now known to be mainly lymphoid, usually of B-lineage. However there remain a small group of cases when a neoplasm of monocyte/macrophage origin has a 'lymphomatous' presentation; such cases are usually classified as 'true histiocytic lymphoma'. In the past some reactive conditions have been misclassified as neoplastic, while the neoplastic nature of other disorders has only recently been recognized. Many cases previously diagnosed as malignant histiocytosis or as histiocytic medullary reticulosis are now known to have been reactive macrophage proliferations, often as a consequence of viral infection. However there does remain a small number of cases in which there is a neoplastic proliferation of cells of monocyte/macrophage lineage, the cells being somewhat more mature than those of M5 AML. The designation malignant histiocytosis is appropriate for such cases. Some have been associated with t(8;16)(p11;p13) and others with mediastinal germ cell tumour and an isochromosome of 12p. The converse problem is seen with histiocytosis X, more recently designated Langerhans' cell histiocytosis. For many years the nature of this condition was uncertain, but the recent demonstration that the histiocytes are clonal [25] indicates a neoplastic disorder.

It will be seen that in order to make a diagnosis of a neoplasm of monocyte/macrophage lineage, it is necessary to be sure: (i) that the condition is neoplastic and not reactive and (ii) that the neoplastic cells belong to the mononuclear phagocyte lineage.

Some monocyte/macrophage neoplasms are disseminated, have an acute clinical course and are usually classified as acute leukaemia. This is so in the FAB M5 category of AML and in the rare and recently recognized Langerhans' cell leukaemia

[10]. Malignant histiocytosis is also disseminated and has an acute clinical course. It differs from M5 AML in that some macrophage differentiation is apparent and the marrow may not be heavily infiltrated at presentation. Other monocyte/macrophage neoplasms may be localized at presentation but have an aggressive clinical course. This is the situation in soft tissue tumours which are likely to be classified as monocytic sarcoma if diagnosed by a haematologist or as true histiocytic lymphoma if they present with lymph node enlargement and are diagnosed by a histopathologist.

Langerhans' cell histiocytosis shows a spectrum of malignancy with eosinophilic granuloma being localized and low grade, whereas Letterer–Siwe disease is generalized and aggressive. These may be regarded as benign and malignant neoplasms respectively.

Morphology, cytochemistry and immunophenotyping. The cytological and cytochemical features of monocytes and monoblasts have been dealt with above. Macrophages have more voluminous cytoplasm than monocytes and may show some phagocytic activity. However marked phagocytosis suggests a reactive rather than a neoplastic proliferation of macrophages. Langerhans' cells show some similarities to monocytes. They may be very large cells with lobulated nuclei and voluminous cytoplasm.

In cytological preparations macrophages are positive for nonspecific esterase and acid phosphatase and are often positive with myeloid monoclonal antibodies such as CD13 and CD33 and with more selective monoclonal antibodies such as CD4, CD14, CD11c and CD68. In tissue sections immunophenotyping is useful in macrophage identification. Positive reactions may be obtained for lysozyme, alpha 1 antitrypsin, S100, peanut agglutinin, vimentin and with CD68 and MAC-387 monoclonal antibodies. Langerhans' cells in cytological preparations may be positive for CD4, CD11c and CD14; they differ from other histiocytes in being positive for CD1. In paraffin-embedded tissues positive reactions may be obtained for S100, and with peanut agglutinin and CD68 monoclonal antibodies. The interdigitating reticulum cell is also S100, CD1 and CD4 positive.

Langerhans' cells can be specifically identified by the demonstration of Birbeck granules on ultrastructural examination.

Summary and conclusions. The diagnosis of neoplasms of monocyte/macrophage lineage is complex and, depending on the clinical and pathological features in an individual patient, may require:
1 cytology;
2 cytochemistry;
3 histology;
4 immunocytochemistry;
5 immunohistochemistry;
6 cytogenetic analysis;
7 electron microscopy;
8 exclusion of other diseases.

Lymphoid leukaemias and lymphomas

The lymphoid leukaemias and lymphomas may be assigned to B-cell, T-cell or NK-cell lineages. They may be immunophenotypically immature or mature. Those with an immature phenotype comprise the acute lymphoblastic leukaemias and the lymphoblastic lymphomas. Those with a mature phenotype comprise the chronic lymphoid leukaemias and the non-Hodgkin's lymphomas. Diseases characterized by phenotypically immature cells generally have an acute clinical course. Those characterized by phenotypically mature cells usually have a chronic course. High-grade lymphomas, for example Burkitt's lymphoma or centroblastic lymphoma, have immunophenotypically mature cells (i.e. expressing surface membrane immunoglobulin) but run an acute course.

It is recommended that the lymphoid leukaemias are classified as advised by the FAB and MIC groups [3,26,27] and lymphomas either as advised by the Kiel group [28] or by the REAL (Revised European–American Lymphoma) Classification [29], which may be seen in some ways as a simplification of the Kiel Classification and in other ways as an expansion.

Acute lymphoblastic leukaemia and lymphoblastic lymphoma

Definition and classification. Acute lymphoblastic leukaemia (ALL) and lymphoblastic lymphoma have cells which are phenotypically very similar, but the diseases differ in the pattern of tissue infiltration. The clinical, haematological and pathological features therefore differ. Both may be of either B-lineage or T-lineage, but ALL is more often of B-lineage and lymphoblastic lymphoma is more often of T-lineage. In ALL the bone marrow is heavily infiltrated and there are commonly also neoplastic cells in the peripheral blood. In lymphoblastic lymphoma the disease initially presents in the thymus, lymph nodes, soft tissue or other organs. The bone marrow may subsequently be infiltrated. Because ALL may also involve lymph nodes and, in the case of T-lineage ALL, the thymus there is some overlap between these two categories of disease. Cases are arbitrarily classified as ALL if the bone marrow blast cell percentage is greater than 25–30% and as lymphoblastic lymphoma if blast cells are absent or less than 25–30%. It should be noted that ALL with an L3 morphology (see below), because of its mature B-cell immunophenotype, might be more appropriately regarded as the leukaemic phase of a high-grade lymphoma. However it is conventionally classified with ALL.

Most cases of ALL are of either B-lineage or T-lineage, but cases with a NK phenotype have also been recognized [30].

Classification of ALL may be based on morphology,

immunophenotype or karyotype, or the three modalities may be combined as in the MIC Classification [27]. The FAB Classification [3] is a purely morphological classification which does not distinguish between B- and T-lineage ALL. When ALL or lymphoblastic lymphoma is diagnosed histologically, use of either the Kiel [28] or the REAL [29] Classification is appropriate; both distinguish between B- and T-lineage cases.

Morphology and cytochemistry. The blasts of ALL are usually small to medium in size. The larger blasts have a diffuse chromatin pattern while smaller blasts may show some chromatin condensation. The cytoplasm may contain vacuoles or, occasionally, a few azurophilic granules. Cytoplasmic vacuoles are indicative of a better prognosis [31]. The most generally accepted morphological classification of ALL is that of the FAB group [3]. Cases are classified as L1, L2 and L3 (see Plates 2.41–2.44 between pp. 292 and 293). The blasts of L1 ALL are mainly round, small to medium in size with a high nucleocytoplasmic ratio. Their cytological features are fairly uniform. The blasts of L2 ALL are generally larger, more pleomorphic, with a more variable but lower nucleocytoplasmic ratio and sometimes prominent nucleoli. In L3 ALL the blasts are of medium size with strongly basophilic cytoplasm and heavy cytoplasmic vacuolation. The recognition of L3 ALL is important since there is a strong correlation of these cytological features with a mature B-cell phenotype and with Burkitt's lymphoma-associated chromosomal translocations. L1 and L2 ALL do have some biological differences but these are not of any major importance. Immunophenotype and, to an even greater extent, karyotype are more relevant to the biology of ALL than morphological features.

The bone marrow aspirate shows cells of similar morphology to those in the peripheral blood, generally constituting the majority of bone marrow cells. Classification as L1, L2 or L3 ALL should be based on the bone marrow morphology, not that of the peripheral blood. The trephine biopsy shows a diffuse infiltrate with a 'packed marrow pattern' of infiltration. The mitotic rate is high.

With the advent of immunophenotyping, the role of cytochemistry in the diagnosis of ALL has declined. Sudan black B and myeloperoxidase reactions are useful in excluding AML, particularly in cases with the cytological features of L2 ALL. (Although Sudan black B positivity has been reported in ALL, it is likely that such cases are actually biphenotypic and Sudan black B positivity can be regarded as strong evidence of myeloid differentiation.) Block positivity with a periodic acid-Schiff (PAS) reaction (see Plate 2.44) is characteristic of ALL, particularly B-lineage ALL, but is not pathognomonic. It indicates a better prognosis [32]. Focal positivity with acid phosphatase is typical of T-lineage ALL but is likewise not pathognomonic.

A presumptive diagnosis of ALL, based on morphology and cytochemistry, should be confirmed by immunophenotyping. Neither the PAS nor acid phosphatase reactions are necessary when immunophenotyping is available.

Summary and conclusions. It is recommended that all cases with a provisional diagnosis of ALL should be assessed:
1 cytologically;
2 immunophenotypically;
3 cytogenetically;
and should be classified by the FAB and MIC classifications. Molecular genetic analysis may be applied selectively or, depending on the speed with which results of cytogenetic analysis can be provided, may be carried out in all cases in order to identify poor prognosis cytogenetic abnormalities.

Other lymphoid leukaemias and lymphomas

It is recommended that the chronic lymphoid leukaemias are classified as recommended by the FAB Group and that the lymphomas should be classified by either the Kiel [28] or the REAL Classification [29]. Both of these lymphoma classifications recognize the importance of immunophenotype in addition to cytology and histology. They are both compatible with the FAB Classification of lymphoid leukaemias [26], although there are some distinct entities recognized by the FAB Group (e.g. chronic lymphocytic leukaemia and prolymphocytic leukaemia) which are not distinguished from each other in the Kiel and REAL Classifications.

Non-Hodgkin's lymphoma will be discussed in Chapters 17–19 and the morphology and classification of chronic lymphoid leukaemias in this chapter. However it should be noted that immunophenotype is crucial in the classification of chronic lymphoid leukaemias [33]. A morphological classification should therefore be regarded as provisional until it has been confirmed by immunophenotype, supplemented when necessary by cytochemistry, histology and cytogenetic and molecular genetic analysis. Even quite experienced haematologists are sometimes wrong in a diagnosis based solely on morphology.

B-lineage chronic lymphoid leukaemias

Chronic lymphocytic leukaemia

Definition and classification. Chronic lymphocytic leukaemia (CLL) is much commoner than any other B-lineage or T-lineage lymphoproliferative disorder. It may be defined as a disease caused by a monoclonal proliferation of B-lymphocytes with specific cytological and immunophenotypic features [26,34]. An association with trisomy 12 and with chromosomal rearrangements with a 13q14 breakpoint is recognized. In the REAL and Kiel Classifications, CLL is grouped with B-prolymphocytic leukaemia and small lymphocytic lymphoma into a single category.

Morphology and cytochemistry. The lymphocytes of CLL are more uniform in size and cytological features than normal lymphocytes (see Plate 2.45 between pp. 292 and 293). The nucleocytoplasmic ratio is high. Chromatin is usually coarsely clumped but sometimes it is more uniformly condensed. Nucleoli are either inapparent or small and inconspicuous. The cytoplasm is scanty and weakly to moderately basophilic. Sometimes there are cytoplasmic crystals or globular inclusions, both representing immunoglobulin secretion. Some cases show a minimal degree of plasmacytoid differentiation, cells having basophilic cytoplasm and a poorly developed Golgi zone. The presence of up to 10% prolymphocytes (larger cells with a prominent nucleolus) is compatible with a diagnosis of CLL. Cells are mechanically fragile and therefore 'smear cells' or 'smudge cells' are often present. Although smear cells may also be seen in other lymphoproliferative diseases and in reactive lymphocytosis, they are most characteristic of CLL and often give a clue to this diagnosis before the lymphocyte count is greatly elevated.

A condition designated by the FAB group CLL, mixed cell type [26], has either an admixture of prolymphocytes (between 10 and 55%) or has a greater degree of pleomorphism than is usual in CLL (see Plate 2.46 between pp. 292 and 293).

In CLL the bone marrow aspirate does not usually give any more information than can be gained from examination of the peripheral blood. Trephine biopsy, however, is diagnostically useful since the pattern of infiltration differs from that in the commoner lymphomas. Infiltration is interstitial, nodular or diffuse (the term 'diffuse' in this context indicating a 'packed marrow' pattern).

Cytochemistry is not useful in the diagnosis of CLL.

Prolymphocytic leukaemia

Definition and classification. Prolymphocytic leukaemia (PLL) is a rare condition. It may be defined as a disease caused by a monoclonal proliferation of B-lymphocytes with specific cytological features and with an immunophenotype similar to that of non-Hodgkin's lymphoma (NHL) [26]. In the REAL and Kiel Classifications it is grouped with CLL and small lymphocytic lymphoma as a single category.

Cytology and cytochemistry. The cells of PLL are larger than those of CLL and usually show more variation in size and cytological features. The typical prolymphocyte has moderately plentiful cytoplasm and a large nucleus with a prominent vesicular nucleolus (see Plate 2.47 between pp. 292 and 293). Occasional cases have cytoplasmic crystals or azurophilic granules. Cases may have predominantly typical prolymphocytes or there may be a range of cell size, with the smaller cells having a smaller and less prominent nucleolus. There is generally no difficulty in distinguishing PLL from CLL or mixed cell type, but if necessary the percentage of prolymphocytes can be counted; cases with more than 55% prolymphocytes are classified as PLL [35].

The bone marrow aspirate shows cells similar to those in the peripheral blood. The trephine biopsy shows infiltration which may be interstitial, interstitial-nodular, interstitial-diffuse or diffuse. In good quality sections it is apparent that the cells are larger than those of CLL and have identifiable nucleoli.

Cytochemistry is not useful in the diagnosis of PLL.

Hairy cell leukaemia

Definition and classification. Hairy cell leukaemia (HCL) is a rare condition. It may be defined as a disease caused by the monoclonal proliferation of a late B cell with specific cytological and immunophenotypic features [26,36]. In the Kiel Classification it is grouped with CLL and PLL in a single category, but in the REAL Classification it is recognized as an entity.

Morphology and cytochemistry. Hairy cells may be absent or infrequent in the peripheral blood. In such cases the bone marrow aspirate (and trephine biopsy) are very important in the diagnosis. Hairy cells are larger than the cells of CLL with voluminous weakly basophilic cytoplasm which has an irregular or 'hairy' margin (see Plate 2.48 between pp. 292 and 293). In occasional cases moderately basophilic paired linear structures are apparent in the cytoplasm; these represent the ribosomal lamellar complex which is a feature, although not pathognomonic, of hairy cell leukaemia. The nucleus may vary in shape from round to oval, dumbbell or peanut shaped or lobed. Nuclear chromatin is more delicate than in CLL. There may be a small, inconspicuous nucleolus. Sometimes the characteristic 'hairs' are more apparent in the thicker part of the film.

The characteristic pancytopenia and, in particular, the severe monocytopenia, are useful morphological clues to a diagnosis of hairy cell leukaemia.

A bone marrow aspirate is usually hypocellular but contains at least a few hairy cells, even in cases in which none have been detected in the peripheral blood. The trephine biopsy is much more useful in diagnosis. It shows an infiltrate which is focal or diffuse but usually extensive. Neoplastic cells are characteristically spaced apart and, particularly in paraffin-embedded specimens, the cytoplasm is shrunken so that the cell appears to be surrounded by a space. Reticulin is characteristicaly increased.

Cytochemistry is useful in the diagnosis of HCL. Hairy cells almost always show tartrate-resistant acid phosphatase activity, which is much less common in other lymphoproliferative disorders. The wider application of immunophenotyping and trephine biopsy has rendered cytochemistry of less importance in the diagnosis of hairy cell leukaemia. Nevertheless, the demonstration of tartrate-resistant acid phosphatase activity is still diagnostically useful, because many laboratories which see only small numbers of patients with HCL do not have the necessary panel of antibodies [36] to make a specific immunophenotypic diagnosis.

Hairy cell leukaemia variant

Definition and classification. The variant form of HCL [37] is even less common than the classical form. It may be defined as a disease caused by monoclonal proliferation of a late B cell with specific cytological features and with an immunophenotype which shows some similarities, but is not identical, to that of HCL [36]. Recognition of the inferior response to new therapeutic modalities makes it important to distinguish the variant form of HCL from classical HCL.

Morphology and cytochemistry. In comparison with HCL, the white cell count is usually higher, severe monocytopenia is lacking and circulating neoplastic cells are much more numerous. Cells have abundant, weakly basophilic, 'hairy' cytoplasm which resembles that of the classical hairy cell (see Plate 2.49 between pp. 292 and 293). The nucleus is round and has a large prominent nucleolus resembling that of a prolymphocyte.

The bone marrow is often more easily aspirated than in hairy cell leukaemia and more numerous neoplastic cells are present in the aspirate. The trephine biopsy shows an interstitial infiltration but does not usually show the 'spaced' pattern which is characteristic of hairy cell leukaemia.

Tartrate-resistant acid phosphatase activity is usually not detected. Immunophenotyping is useful in distinguishing between HCL and the variant form, but if the specific panel of antibodies is not available then cytochemistry is helpful in making the distinction.

Splenic lymphoma with villous lymphocytes

Definition and classification. Splenic lymphoma with villous lymphocytes (SLVL) may be defined as a disease caused by proliferation of a monoclonal B cell with specific cytological features and with an immunophenotype similar to that of NHL [26,38]. An association with t(11;14)(q13;q32) is recognized but this translocation is much less common in SLVL than in mantle cell lymphoma. SLVL is considerably less common than CLL, with which it was commonly confused in the past. It is not specifically identified in the Kiel Classification but is recognized in the REAL Classification, being assigned to the provisional category of splenic marginal zone lymphoma, with or without villous lymphocytes.

Morphology and cytochemistry. The cells of SLVL are small mature lymphocytes (see Plate 2.50 between pp. 292 and 293). They are somewhat more pleomorphic than the cells of CLL, tend to be larger and show more cytoplasmic basophilia. Nuclei are round or oval, chromatin is clumped and some cases have visible nucleoli. Some cells have hairy or 'villous' cytoplasmic projections, sometimes but not always at one pole of the cell. A minority of cells show plasmacytoid differentiation. Smear cells are not a feature. There may be some increase in rouleaux formation and in background staining as a consequence of secretion of a paraprotein. SLVL is most likely to be confused with CLL or, in the cases with nucleoli, with the variant form of hairy cell leukaemia.

The bone marrow aspirate may show similar cells to those in the peripheral blood but is sometimes normal. The trephine biopsy is more often abnormal, the infiltrate being nodular or diffuse.

Cytochemistry is not useful in the diagnosis of SLVL. The tartrate-resistant acid phosphatase reaction is usually negative.

Follicular lymphoma

Definition and classification. Centroblastic/centrocytic (follicular) lymphoma is defined histologically [28,29], but a characteristic cytology and immunophenotype [26] is also recognized. There is a strong association with t(14;18)(q32;q21). Circulating neoplastic cells are not infrequently present, either at diagnosis or during the course of the disease. The leukaemic phase of follicular lymphoma is less common than CLL but it is not a rare condition. Follicular lymphoma is a specific category in the Kiel and REAL Classifications, being designated respectively centroblastic/centrocytic lymphoma and follicular centre lymphoma, follicular.

Morphology and cytochemistry. Follicular lymphoma cells are small lymphocytes with condensed chromatin and scanty cytoplasm (see Plate 2.51 between pp. 292 and 293). Often they are smaller than the cells of CLL and have even less cytoplasm. They may be slightly angular and some nuclei are cleft or lobulated. The chromatin shows a more even condensation than is seen in CLL. Sometimes a small nucleolus is apparent. Although most cases can be distinguished cytologically from CLL cells, the differences can be very subtle and immunophenotyping is then necessary to make the distinction.

In patients with circulating lymphoma cells the bone marrow aspirate shows similar cells but does not give any further diagnostically useful information. The bone marrow trephine biopsy is more useful and infiltration may be detected even in cases in which no abnormal cells have been detected in the peripheral blood or the bone marrow aspirate. The characteristic pattern of infiltration is paratrabecular. A follicular infiltrate is quite uncommon. The cells in the bone marrow, like those in the peripheral blood, are usually centrocytes alone even though lymph node biopsy shows both centrocytes and centroblasts.

Cytochemistry is not useful in the diagnosis of follicular lymphoma.

Lymphoplasmacytoid lymphoma

Definition and classification. Lymphoplasmacytoid lymphoma may be defined as a disease caused by a monoclonal proliferation of a late B cell with cytological features intermediate between those of a lymphocyte and a plasma cell. In many cases a monoclonal paraprotein is secreted. It is recommended that the REAL Classification should be followed in classifying lymphomas with plasmaytoid differentiation, rather than the Kiel Classification. Cases which resemble CLL but which show a trivial degree of plasmacytoid differentiation should therefore be classified as CLL and only cases with marked plasmacytoid differentiation should be classified as lymphoplasmacytoid lymphoma.

Morphology and cytochemistry. There is usually a range of cells from lymphocytes to mature plasma cells (see Plate 2.52 between pp. 292 and 293). However often the majority of cells are plasmacytoid lymphocytes—cells with a somewhat eccentric nucleus, with cytoplasmic basophilia but without the cytological features of mature plasma cells. Cells sometimes contain globular inclusions or crystals.

The blood film may also have features indicative of the presence of a paraprotein such as increased rouleaux formation, increased background staining and sometimes red cell agglutination or cryoglobulin precipitation.

The bone marrow aspirate contains similar cells. The trephine biopsy shows interstitial, focal of diffuse infiltration. Cells show plasmacytoid features and Dutcher bodies and Russell bodies are sometimes apparent.

Cytochemistry is not useful in the diagnosis of lymphoplasmacytoid lymphoma.

Mantle cell lymphoma

Definition and classification. Mantle cell lymphoma (previously also designated lymphoma of intermediate differentiation or diffuse centrocytic lymphoma) is defined histologically [29,39], but a characteristic immunophenotype and a strong association with t(11;14)(q13;q32) is recognized. The bone marrow is often infiltrated and neoplastic cells are present in the peripheral blood in a significant minority of cases. This lymphoma is recognized in the FAB Classification ('intermediate lymphoma'), the Kiel Classification ('diffuse centrocytic lymphoma') and the REAL Classification ('mantle cell lymphoma').

Morphology and cytochemistry. The cells of mantle cell lymphoma are usually larger and more pleomorphic than those of CLL (see Plate 2.53 between pp. 292 and 293). They vary in their size, nucleocytoplasmic ratio and nuclear characteristics. Nuclear shape and the degree of chromatin condensation vary from cell to cell. There are usually some cells with irregular, cleft or lobulated nuclei and some with visible nucleoli. The cytoplasm is weakly or moderately basophilic. The differential diagnosis is with CLL, mixed cell type, and with follicular lymphoma. It can also sometimes be difficult to distinguish cases with marked pleomorphism and moderate cytoplasmic basophilia from reactive lymphocytosis, for example that associated with a viral infection.

The bone marrow aspirate shows similar cells to those in the peripheral blood. Trephine biopsy shows infiltration in the majority of cases. The pattern of infiltration differs from that in follicular lymphoma, because paratrabecular infiltration is not usually seen [40]. Infiltration is generally focal or diffuse.

Cytochemistry is not useful in the diagnosis of mantle cell lymphoma.

Summary and conclusions

It is recommended that all cases with a provisional diagnosis of CLL or other B-lineage chronic lymphoid leukaemia should:
1 be assessed cytologically;
2 be immunophenotyped;
3 be categorized according to the FAB Classification.

Bone marrow aspiration and trephine biopsy histology is usually also indicated. Lymph-node histology, cytochemistry, cytogenetic analysis and molecular genetic analysis should be applied selectively.

T-lineage chronic lymphoid leukaemias

The chronic lymphoid leukaemias of T-lineage are all rare conditions.

T-lineage prolymphocytic leukaemia

Definition and classification. T-lineage prolymphocytic leukaemia (T-PLL) is even less common than B-lineage PLL (B-PLL). It is defined on the basis of morphological and immunophenotypic features [26]. An association with inversion (14)(q11q32) and trisomy 8q is recognized. In many cases the diagnosis can be made on morphological grounds, but some cases cannot be distinguished morphologically from B-PLL and immunophenotyping is always essential for confirmation of the diagnosis. The small cell morphological variant of T-PLL is sometimes referred to as T-CLL. However this is not recommended, because all cases of T-PLL, as defined by the FAB group, share the same immunophenotypic, cytogenetic and clinical features and, furthermore, the term 'T-CLL' has been used to refer to a variety of conditions including large granular lymphocyte leukaemia.

T-PLL is a specific entity in the REAL Classification but not the Kiel Classification.

Morphology and cytochemistry. Some cases are morphologically very similar to B-PLL. In other cases the cells are more pleomorphic, they are irregular in shape and have some irregular or hyperchromatic nuclei (see Plate 2.54 between pp. 292 and 293). Cytoplasmic basophilia is often greater than in B-PLL. A small cell variant is recognized in which cells are not only smaller but have less cytoplasm and a much less prominent nucleolus. Sometimes the small cell variant shows cytoplasmic 'blebs'.

The small cell variant does not differ in clinical, haematological or cytogenetic features from other cases of T-PLL, so it should be regarded as part of the morphological spectrum of this condition rather than as a distinct disease.

The bone marrow is infiltrated by similar cells to those seen in the peripheral blood. Patterns of infiltration on trephine biopsy are similar to those seen in B-PLL.

Strong focal acid phosphatase and nonspecific esterase activity is common, but immunophenotyping is diagnostically more useful than cytochemistry.

Sézary's syndrome

Definition and classification. Sézary's syndrome and mycosis fungoides are part of the spectrum of cutaneous T-cell lymphomas. They are defined on the basis of clinical, histological, cytological and immunophenotypic features [26]. Pautrier's microabscesses (neoplastic lymphocytes within the epidermis), which are usually regarded as essential for the diagnosis, are not confined to this group of disorders and they are seen, for example, in some cases of adult T-cell leukaemia/ lymphoma. Nevertheless they are useful in making this diagnosis. Circulating neoplastic cells are present, by definition, in Sézary's syndrome. They are sometimes also present in mycosis fungoides; the likelihood of their presence increases with the stage of the disease.

Cutaneous T-cell lymphomas are a specific category in both the Kiel and the REAL Classifications where they are designated, respectively, small cell, cerebriform and mycosis fungoides/Sézary's syndrome.

Morphology and cytochemistry. Sézary's cells vary in cytological features between cases and even in a single case. Some patients have predominantly small cells, some have predominantly large cells and some have a mixture. Small Sézary cells (see Plate 2.55 between pp. 292 and 293) can be difficult to recognize on light microscopy. They are similar in size to normal lymphocytes with scanty cytoplasm and a high nucleocytoplasmic ratio. The nuclear outline is irregular and the nuclear surface appears grooved; these features are indicative of the convoluted or cerebriform nucleus which is more easily recognized on ultrastructural examination. Some nuclei are hyperchromatic. Some of the larger cells show a row or ring of cytoplasmic vacuoles.

On light microscopy large Sézary cells (see Plate 2.56) are more strikingly abnormal than small Sézary cells. They are two to three times the size of a normal lymphocyte with a hyperchromatic, lobulated and infolded nucleus. Cytoplasm is more abundant than in the small Sézary cell.

Bone marrow infiltration is present in only a minority of cases and may be absent even in some cases with circulating lymphoma cells. Patterns of infiltration seen on trephine biopsy are focal or diffuse.

A PAS stain may show PAS-positive cytoplasmic inclusions which account for the presence of cytoplasmic vacuoles. However cytochemistry is not important in the diagnosis.

Adult T-cell leukaemia/lymphoma

Definition and classification. Adult T-cell leukaemia/lymphoma (ATLL), although mainly a disease of Japan and the West Indies, is being increasingly recognized in diverse parts of the world (from Australian aboriginals to Brazil, Chile and the Aleutian population of Canada). It is therefore important to be alert for this rare disease in almost any ethnic group. The disease may be defined as developing as a consequence of proliferation of a clone of neoplastic T cells with specific cytological and immunophenotypic features [26], occurring in HTLV-I positive subjects and showing clonal integration of HTLV-I in the neoplastic cells. About 90% of cases have circulating neoplastic cells, the remaining 10% having a lymphomatous presentation. ATLL is a specific category in the REAL Classification, but in the Kiel Classification cases are not specifically identified and fall into three or more histological categories.

Because of the therapeutic implications it is important to distinguish the acute form of ATLL from smouldering and chronic forms. All cases show clonal integration of HTLV-I in a clone of morphologically atypical T cells. The Lymphoma Study Group, Japan [41], has suggested the classification summarized in Table 2.11. Others have suggested slightly different criteria for separating 'pre-ATLL' from chronic ATLL [42].

Morphology and cytochemistry. The neoplastic cells of the acute form of ATLL are highly pleomorphic (see Plate 2.57 between pp. 292 and 293). They vary in size, shape, nucleocytoplasmic ratio and degree of chromatin condensation and cytoplasmic basophilia. The most typical cells are moderately large with hyperchromatic, polylobulated nuclei. Nucleoli are often prominent. Some of the nuclei have a 'flower' shape. Occasional cells have less cytoplasm and a more compact infolded nucleus and thus resemble Sézary cells. Some cells may have features of blast cells. Marked pleomorphism with at least some cells having polylobulated nuclei is the most useful feature in diagnosis. In the chronic and smouldering forms of ATLL the majority of cells are small mature lymphocytes with incised or lobulated nuclei, but there are occasional typical ATLL cells such as 'flower cells'. Neutrophilia is common in acute ATLL.

The bone marrow aspirate and trephine biopsy show infiltration which is usually interstitial and may be quite subtle. It is usually much harder to make a specific diagnosis from examination of the bone marrow than from the peripheral blood.

Cytochemistry is not useful in the diagnosis of ATLL.

Large granular lymphocyte leukaemia

Large granular lymphocyte leukaemia is a disease that results from proliferation of a clone of lymphocytes with morphological and/or immunophenotypic features identifying a relationship to normal large granular lymphocytes. The term 'large granular lymphocyte leukaemia', which is recommended by the MIC Group and by the REAL Group, is preferred to the FAB Group's term 'T-CLL' and the Kiel designation 'T lineage,

Table 2.11 Subclassification of ATLL.

Category	Peripheral blood lymphocytes	Tissue infiltration	Biochemistry
Smouldering ATLL	Lymphocyte count < $4 \times 10^9/1$ and either ≥5% abnormal lymphocytes or histological proof of lung or skin infiltration	Lung or skin may be infiltrated but no infiltration of lymph nodes, liver, spleen, gastrointestinal tract or central nervous system and no ascites or pleural effusion	LDH up to 1.5 the upper limit of normal; no hypercalcaemia
Chronic ATLL	Lymphocyte count > $4 \times 10^9/l$ and T-lymphocytes > $3.5 \times 10^9/l$ with morphologically abnormal cells and occasional frank ATLL cells (such as flower cells); (in most cases there are ≥5% abnormal lymphocytes)	Lung, skin, lymph nodes, liver and spleen may be infiltrated but no infiltration of gastrointestinal tract or central nervous system and no ascites or pleural effusion	LDH up to twice the upper limit of normal, no hypercalcaemia
Lymphoma-type ATLL	Lymphocyte count < $4 \times 10^9/l$ and ≤1% abnormal lymphoid cells	Histologically demonstrated lymphoma	May have elevated LDH or hypercalcaemia
Acute ATLL		All other cases	

low grade, lymphocytic lymphoma', since the latter terms are ambiguous.

Large granular lymphocyte leukaemia may be of either T-lineage or NK-cell lineage [26,28,43]. In the T-lineage cases the cells are CD3+ and show rearrangement of T-cell receptor genes, neither of which are seen in the NK group. Clonality of the T-lineage cases can be demonstrated by molecular genetic analysis of T-cell receptor genes, but clonality of the NK cases cannot be demonstrated unless there is a clonal cytogenetic abnormality or, in females, an X-linked polymorphism detectable by molecular genetic analysis. This can cause some diagnostic problems if the disease is not obviously 'malignant'. There are clinical and haematological differences between T-lineage and NK cases, but the morphology does not differ. If clonality has not been demonstrated and it is not clear whether the disorder is neoplastic or reactive, the term 'lymphoproliferative disorder of large granular lymphocytes' can be used.

Morphology and cytochemistry. The neoplastic cells usually closely resemble normal large granular lymphocytes (see Plate 2.58 between pp. 292 and 293). They are large lymphocytes with prominent azurophilic granules. Occasional cases have smaller cells, cells with scanty granules or atypical cells which are larger with less chromatin condensation or more cytoplasmic basophilia.

Some T-lineage cases are markedly neutropenic and others are severely anaemic, sometimes with macrocytosis, or have thrombocytopenia. Anaemia, thrombocytopenia and mild neutropenia are common in NK cases and some cases have severe neutropenia [43].

The bone marrow aspirate shows cells of similar morphology to those in the peripheral blood. Trephine biopsy shows sparse focal or interstitial infiltration. Because the granules are not apparent, it is much more difficult to make a specific diagnosis from the trephine biopsy than from the peripheral blood.

The differential diagnosis of large granular lymphocyte leukaemia is with a reactive increase in large granular lymphocytes, for example caused by chronic viral infection or following splenectomy. Morphology is usually not of any use in making the distinction, so studies of clonality and cytogenetic analysis are indicated if the diagnosis is in doubt.

Cytochemistry is not useful in the diagnosis of large granular lymphocyte leukaemia.

Summary and conclusions

It is recommended that all cases with a provisional diagnosis of T-lineage chronic lymphoid leukaemia should:

1 be assessed cytologically;
2 be immunophenotyped;
3 be categorized according to the FAB and MIC Classifications.

Bone marrow aspiration and trephine biopsy usually contribute less diagnostic and prognostic information than in B-lineage chronic lymphoid leukaemias. Histological examination (of lymph node, skin or other tissue) and cytogenetic and molecular genetic analysis should be applied selectively. In addition, cases of ATLL require measurement of serum lactate dehydrogenase (LDH) and calcium concentrations.

Plasma cell dyscrasias

The term plasma cell dyscrasia includes multiple myeloma, plasma cell leukaemia, monoclonal gammopathy of undeter-

Table 2.12 Plasma cell dyscrasias.

Malignant
Multiple myeloma
Solitary plasmacytoma
    Solitary plasmacytoma of bone
    Extramedullary plasmacytoma
Plasma cell leukaemia
Lymphoplasmacytoid lymphoma (including Waldenström's
    macroglobulinaemia)
Heavy-chain diseases

'Benign'
Asymptomatic
Monoclonal gammopathy of undetermined significance (MGUS)—also
    known as benign monoclonal gammopathy (BMG)

Causing disease
Cold haemagglutinin disease
Primary amyloidosis
Light-chain deposition disease
Heavy-chain deposition disease
Type I and II cryoglobulinaemia
POEMS syndrome (*polyneuropathy, organomegaly, endocrinopathy,*
    m-protein, *skin changes syndrome*)
Some cases of acquired angio-oedema

---

mined significance and a variety of less common conditions which are listed in Table 2.12 [44]. Lymphoplasmacytoid lymphoma is also often included under the heading of plasma cell dyscrasia. The plasma cell dyscrasias, although all neoplastic, may be clinically either malignant or benign. The group classified as 'benign' may be completely asymptomatic or may produce disease as a consequence of production of a monoclonal immunoglobulin known as a paraprotein. This may be either a complete immunoglobulin, a light chain (kappa or lambda) or a heavy chain (gamma, alpha or mu) or both an immunoglobulin and either a heavy chain or a light chain.

Multiple myeloma

Definition and classification. Multiple myeloma (MM) may be defined as a disease caused by the proliferation, at multiple sites in the bone marrow and sometimes elsewhere, of a clone of neoplastic cells showing plasma cell differentiation. In the great majority of cases there is secretion of a monoclonal immunoglobulin or a free light chain. The disease can be further classified, according to the paraprotein secreted, as IgG, IgA, IgD, IgE, Bence Jones (only light chain secreted) or non-secretory MM.

Morphology and cytochemistry. The peripheral blood usually shows a normocytic normochromic anaemia, increased rouleaux formation and increased background staining. Sometimes there are circulating plasma cells or plasmacytoid lymphocytes, usually in small numbers.

Since there are usually only small numbers of circulating myeloma cells, diagnosis usually requires bone marrow aspiration. Because myeloma cells are not necessarily either very numerous in a bone marrow aspirate or morphologically very abnormal, diagnosis also requires consideration of clinical and haematological features and detection and quantification of any paraprotein present in serum or urine. The bone marrow shows a very variable degree of plasma cell infiltration, ranging from 5 to 10% to almost complete marrow effacement. Myeloma cells may be cytologically very similar to normal plasma cells or may show a variable degree of dysplasia (see Plate 2.59–2.61 between pp. 292 and 293). Abnormal features may include multinuclearity, asynchrony between nuclear and cytoplasmic maturation and gigantism. Myeloma cells may contain secretory globules or, less often, crystals. The cytoplasm is usually strongly basophilic with a paranuclear paler area but is sometimes pink or 'flaming'. Plasmablasts with a primitive chromatin structure and a prominent nucleolus may be present and sometimes comprise the majority of cells.

The trephine biopsy shows infiltration which may be interstitial, focal or diffuse. Abnormal cytological features, including the presence of Russell bodies or Dutcher bodies, may be apparent. Because of the patchy nature of the bone marrow involvement in MM, the trephine biopsy sometimes permits a diagnosis when the aspirate is nondiagnostic and, less often, the reverse may also be true. Sometimes it is necessary to repeat the aspiration and trephine biopsy at another site or to biopsy a radiologically abnormal site in order to confirm the diagnosis.

Cytochemistry is not useful in the diagnosis of multiple myeloma.

Summary and conclusions. It is recommended that all cases of suspected MM should have:
1 bone marrow aspiration and trephine biopsy;
2 serum protein electrophoresis for detection and quantification of any serum paraprotein;
3 estimation of concentrations of normal serum immunoglobulins;
4 examination of urine by a sensitive technique for detection of Bence Jones protein and quantification of any paraprotein detected;
5 skeletal survey;
6 blood count and biochemical screening including estimation of serum calcium and creatinine concentration.

Immunophenotyping can be applied selectively, with demonstration of light-chain restriction being mainly of use when the percentage of plasma cells in the bone marrow is low. Cytogenetic analysis and molecular genetic analysis is not necessary in routine practice.

Plasma cell leukaemia

Definition and classification. Plasma cell leukaemia is a disease caused by the proliferation in the bone marrow and appearance in the circulating blood of a clone of neoplastic cells showing plasma cell differentiation. Conventions differ as to whether the term is applied only to *de novo* cases [26] or whether cases of MM terminating in plasma cell leukaemia [45] are also included. The latter seems preferable, but *de novo* cases should then be specifically identified.

Morphology and cytochemistry. The cytological features of circulating neoplastic cells are very variable, ranging from plasmacytoid lymphocytes, through recognizable but dysplastic plasma cells, to plasmablasts (see Plate 2.62 between pp. 292 and 293). Sometimes plasmablasts are very primitive cells which are barely recognizable as belonging to the plasma cell lineage. In these cases morphology must be supplemented by immunophenotyping to make the diagnosis. Plasmablasts may be indistinguishable cytologically from immunoblasts but the immunophenotype differs.

Monoclonal gammopathy of undetermined significance

Definition and classification. Monoclonal gammopathy of undetermined significance (MGUS) is an asymptomatic condition in which there is proliferation of a clone of cells showing plasma cell differentiation with secretion of a paraprotein, usually an immunoglobulin but sometimes a Bence Jones protein. MGUS is distinguished from multiple myeloma on the basis of the lack of any evidence of disease (e.g. anaemia, lytic lesions or pathological fractures), the number of plasma cells in the bone marrow and the amount of paraprotein secreted [44]. The designation MGUS is preferred to 'benign monoclonal gammopathy', because the behaviour of the clone of cells does not necessarily remain 'benign'. A significant proportion of patients subsequently develop overt multiple myeloma, other lymphoproliferative disorder, light-chain-associated amyloidosis or other serious tissue damage as a consequence of the paraprotein secreted.

Morphology and cytochemistry. There are no circulating plasma cells. The bone marrow shows an increase of plasma cells but these are less than 10%, most often less than 5%. There may be a minor degree of cytological atypia. The trephine biopsy shows a slight interstitial increase of plasma cells but no large focal lesions.

Summary and conclusions. Distinguishing between MGUS and multiple myeloma sometimes requires the full range of investigations listed under multiple myeloma. However it should be noted that MGUS is very common in elderly people who should not be subjected to unnecessary investigations because of the incidental detection of a serum paraprotein. These investigations should therefore be applied selectively, depending on the clinical features of individual cases.

Biphenotypic leukaemias

Definition and classification. Biphenotypic leukaemias are those showing both myeloid and lymphoid differentiation or differentiation to both T- and B-lineages. Since neoplastic cells often express inappropriate antigens, it is important to have a fairly rigorous definition of biphenotypic leukaemia. This is likely to lead to the recognition of a relatively small number of patients with a disease which is biologically different from AML or ALL. Regarding a case as biphenotypic because of the expression of only one inappropriate antigen, or because of expression of a marker which is lineage related rather than lineage specific, leads to large numbers of patients with AML or ALL being misclassified and blurs the whole distinction between these two diseases. Such cases are best regarded as lymphoid antigen-positive AML or myeloid antigen-positive ALL.

The application of a scoring system which gives greatest weight to the cell markers which are most strongly linked to specific lineages is recommended. One such scoring system, applicable to biphenotypic acute leukaemia, is shown in Table 2.13 [46]. Differentiation to different lineages may be synchronous or asynchronous. Both forms should be regarded as biphenotypic as long as there is evidence that they have the same clonal origin. For example, children with t(4;11)(q21;q23) may present with ALL and relapse as M5 AML. The recognition of biphenotypic leukaemia is important because of the common association with adverse cytogenetic abnormalities and the likelihood of a poor prognosis.

Biphenotypic leukaemias so far recognized are mainly acute leukaemia but chronic granulocytic leukaemia undergoing a lymphoblastic transformation could be regarded as biphenotypic. Other biphenotypic leukaemias are occasionally recognized [48]. It is important to differentiate asynchronous

Table 2.13 A scoring system for the diagnosis of biphenotypic acute leukaemia [46].

Points scored	B-lymphoid	T-lymphoid	Myeloid
2	CD79a* CD22 CyIg‡	CD3	MPO†
1	CD19 CD10	CD2 CD5	CD13 CD33
0.5	TdT‖	TdT‖ CD7	CD14, CD15, CD11b, CD11c

Biphenotypic acute leukaemia is recognized when the score for more than one lineage is more than 2.
* CD79a (mb-1) [47] was not included in original publication but its inclusion is now recommended (E. Matutes, personal communication).
† Demonstrated cytochemically or immunologically.
‡ Cytoplasmic immunoglobulin.
‖ Terminal nucleotidyl transferase.

biphenotypic acute leukaemia from secondary therapy-induced leukaemia and to differentiate biphenotypic leukaemia from the stimulation of proliferation of another lineage (e.g. eosinophils) by cytokines secreted by cells of the leukaemic clone.

Morphology and cytochemistry. Cytological features may be those of AML (mainly M1, M2, M4, or M5) or ALL (mainly L2 but sometimes L1). Sometimes there is a mixture of large and small blast cells with somewhat different cytological features.

Cytochemistry can be important in identifying biphenotypic acute leukaemia, because peroxidase activity provides strong evidence of myeloid differentiation. However immunophenotyping is essential for the diagnosis. Cytochemical reactions which are not truly lineage specific, such as PAS-block positivity or focal acid phosphatase activity, are not helpful.

Summary and conclusions. Cases of suspected biphenotypic acute leukaemia should be assessed:
1 cytologically;
2 cytochemically;
3 immunophenotypically;
4 cytogenetically.

There is no general agreement about whether all cases of acute leukaemia should be investigated by a standard panel of monoclonal antibodies to exclude biphenotypic leukaemia. If an association with unfavourable cytogenetic features and a suspected poor prognosis is confirmed for larger numbers of well-characterized cases, such investigation may become standard.

References

1 Bain B.J. (1995) *Blood Cells: A Practical Guide*, 2nd edn. Blackwell Science, Oxford.
2 Bennett J.M., Catovsky D., Daniel M.T. *et al.* (1976) Proposals for the classification of the acute leukaemias (FAB cooperative group). *British Journal of Haematology*, **33**, 451–458.
3 Bennett J.M., Catovsky D., Daniel M.T. *et al.* (1985) Proposed revised criteria for the classification of acute myeloid leukemia. *Annals of Internal Medicine*, **103**, 626–629.
4 Second MIC Cooperative Study Group (1988) Morphologic, immunologic and cytogenetic (MIT) working classification of the acute myeloid leukaemias. *British Journal of Haematology*, **68**, 487–494.
5 Mittleman F. & Heim S. (1992) Quantitative acute leukaemia cytogenetics. *Genes, Chromosomes and Cancer*, **5**, 57–66.
6 Licht J.D., Chomienne C., Goy A. *et al.* (1995) Clinical and molecular characterization of a rare syndrome of acute promyelocytic leukemia associated with translocation 11;17. *Blood*, **85**, 1083–1094.
7 Kita K., Shirakawa S., Kamada N. & the Japanese Cooperative Group of Leukemia/Lymphoma (1994) Cellular characteristics of acute myeloblastic leukemia associated with t(8;21)(q22;q22). *Leukemia and Lymphoma*, **13**, 229–234.
8 Erber W.N., Asbahr H., Rule S.A. & Scott C.S. (1994) Unique

immunophenotype of acute promyelocytic leukaemia as defined by CD9 and CD68 antibodies. *British Journal of Haematology*, **88**, 101–104.
9 Hayhoe F.G.J. (1988) Classification of acute leukaemias. *Blood Reviews*, **2**, 186–193.
10 Srivastava B.I.S., Srivastava A. & Srivastava M.D. (1994) Phenotype, genotype and cytokine production in acute leukemia involving progenitors of dendritic Langerhans' cells. *Leukemia Research*, **18**, 499–512.
11 Santiago-Schwarz F., Coppock D.L., Hindenberg A.A. & Kern J. (1994) Identification of malignant counterpart of the monocyte-dendritic cell progenitor in acute myeloid leukemia. *Blood*, **84**, 2054–3062.
12 Bain B.J. (1994) Transient leukaemia in newborn infants with Down's syndrome. *Leukemia Research*, **18**, 723–724.
13 International Council for Standardization in Haematology (1993) Recommended procedures for the classification of acute leukaemias. *Leukemia and Lymphoma*, **11**, 37–49.
14 Bain B.J. (1995) Routine and specialized techniques in the diagnosis of haematological neoplasms. *Journal of Clinical Pathology*, **48**, 501–508.
15 Bennett J.M., Catovsky D., Daniel M.T. *et al.* (1982) Proposals for the classification of the myelodysplastic syndromes. *British Journal of Haematology*, **51**, 189–199.
16 Shepherd P.C.A., Ganesan T.S. & Galton D.A.G. (1987) Haematological classification of the chronic myeloid leukaemias. *Baillière's Clinical Haematology*, **1**, 887–906.
17 Galton D.A.G. (1992) Haematological differences between chronic granulocytic leukaemia, atypical chronic myeloid leukaemia, and chronic myelomonocytic leukaemia. *Leukemia and Lymphoma*, **7**, 343–350.
18 Bain B.J. (1990) *Leukaemia Diagnosis: a guide to the FAB classification*, pp. 44–47. Gower Medical Publications, London.
19 Oscier D.G. (1994) Atypical chronic myeloid leukaemia. Is it a separate entity? *Leukemia Research*, **18**(Suppl.), 37.
20 Hasle H. (1994) Myelodysplastic syndromes in childhood — classification, epidemiology, and treatment. *Leukemia and Lymphoma*, **13**, 11–26.
21 Tuncer M.A., Pagliuca A., Hicsonmez F.G., Yetgin S., Ozsoylu S. & Mufti G.J. (1992) Primary myelodysplastic syndrome in children: the clinical experience in 33 cases. *British Journal of Haematology*, **82**, 347–353.
22 Passmore S.J., Hann I.M., Stiller C.A. *et al.* (1994) Pediatric myelodysplasia: a study of 68 children with a new prognostic scoring syndrome. *Blood*, **85**, 1742–1750.
23 Luna-Fineman S., Shannon K.M. & Lange B.J. (1995) Childhood monosomy 7: epidemiology, biology, and mechanistic implications. *Blood*, **85**, 1985–1995.
24 Miyauchi J., Asada M., Sasaki M. *et al.* (1994) Mutations of the N-*ras* gene in juvenile chronic myelogenous leukemia. *Blood*, **83**, 2248–2254.
25 Willman C.L., Busque L., Griffith B.B. *et al.* (1994) Langerhan-cell histiocytosis (histiocytosis X) — a clonal proliferative disease. *New England Journal of Medicine*, **331**, 154–160.
26 Bennett J.M., Catovsky D., Daniel M-T. *et al.* (1989) Proposals for the classification of chronic (mature) B and T lymphoid leukaemias. *Journal of Clinical Pathology*, **42**, 567–584.
27 First MIC Cooperative Study Group (1986) Morphologic, immunologic, and cytogenetic (MIC) working classification of acute lymphoblastic leukaemias. *Cancer Genetics and Cytogenetics*, **23**, 189–197.

28 Stansfeld A., Diebold J., Kapanci Y. *et al.* (1988) Updated Kiel classifiction for lymphomas. *Lancet*, **i**, 292–293, 373.

29 Harris N.L., Jaffe E.S., Stein H. *et al.* (1994) A Revised European–American classification of lymphoid neoplasms: a proposal from the International Lymphoma Study Group. *Blood*, **84**, 1361–1392.

30 Ichikawa M., Kawai H., Komiyama A. *et al.* (1991) Functional p75 interleukin-2 receptor expression on fresh blast cells in childhood acute lymphoblastic leukemia with natural killer properties. *American Journal of Hematology*, **36**, 259–264.

31 Lilleyman J.S., Hann I.M., Stevens R.F., Richards S.M., Eden O.B., Chessels J.M., Bailey C.C., on behalf of the United Kingdom Medical Research Council Working Party on Childhood Leukaemia (1992) Cytomorphology of childhood lymphoblastic leukaemia: a prospective study of 2000 patients. *British Journal of Haematology*, **81**, 52–57.

32 Lilleyman J.S., Britton J.A., Andersen L.M., Richards S.M., Bailey C.C., Chessels J.M on behalf of the Medical Research Council Working Party on Childhood Leukaemia (1994) Periodic acid Schiff reaction in childhood lymphoblastic leukaemia. *Journal of Clinical Pathology*, **47**, 689–692.

33 The General Haematology Task Force of BCSH (1994) Immunophenotyping in the diagnosis of chronic lymphoproliferative disorders. *Journal of Clinical Pathology*, **47**, 871–875.

34 Matutes E., Owusu-Ankomah K., Morilla R. *et al.* (1994) The immunological profile of B-cell disorders and proposal of a scoring system for the diagnosis of CLL. *Leukemia*, **8**, 1640–1645.

35 Melo J.V., Catovsky D. & Galton D.A.G. (1986) The relationship between chronic lymphocytic leukaemia and prolymphocytic leukaemia. I. Clinical and laboratory features of 300 patients and characterisation of an intermediate group. *British Journal of Haematology*, **63**, 377–387.

36 Matutes E., Morilla R., Owusu-Ankomah K., Houlihan A., Meeus P. & Catovsky D. (1994) The immunophenotype of hairy cell leukemia (HCL). Proposal for a scoring system to distinguish HCL from B-cell disorders with hairy or villous lymphocytes. *Leukemia and Lymphoma*, **14**(Suppl. 1), 57–62.

37 Cawley J.C., Burns G.F. & Hayhoe F.G.H. (1980) A chronic lymphoproliferative disorder with distinctive features: a distinct variant of hairy cell leukaemia. *Leukemia Research*, **4**, 547–559.

38 Matutes E., Morilla R., Owusu-Ankomah K., Houlihan A. & Catovsky D. (1994) The immunophenotype of splenic lymphoma with villous lymphocytes and its relevance to the differential diagnosis with other B-cell disorders. *Blood*, **83**, 1558–1562.

39 Raffeld M. & Jaffe E. (1991) bcl-1, t(11;14), and mantle-cell derived lymphomas. *Blood*, **78**, 259–263.

40 Obeso G., Sanz E.R., Rivas C. *et al.* (1994) B-cell follicular lymphomas: clinical and biological characteristics. *Leukemia and Lymphoma*, **16**, 105–111.

41 Shimoya M. & members of the Lymphoma Study Group (1984–87) (1991) Diagnostic criteria and classification of adult T-cell leukaemia-lymphoma: a report from the Lymphoma Study Group (1984–87) *British Journal of Haematology*, **79**, 428–437.

42 Ikeda S., Momita S., Kinoshita K-I. *et al.* (1993) Clinical course of human T-lymphotropic virus type I carriers with molecularly detectable monoclonal proliferation of T lymphocytes defining a low- and high-risk population. *Blood*, **82**, 2017–2024.

43 Loughran J.P. (1993) Clonal diseases of large granular lymphocytes. *Blood*, **82**, 1–14.

44 Bain B.J., Clark D.M. & Lampert I. (1993) *Bone Marrow Pathology*, pp. 189–203. Blackwell Scientific Publications, Oxford.

45 Kyle R.A., Maldonado J.E. & Bayrd E.D. (1974) Plasma cell leukemia; report on 17 cases. *Archives of Internal Medicine*, **133**, 813–818.

46 Buccheri V., Matutes E., Dyer M.J.S. & Catovsky D. (1993) Lineage committment in biphenotypic acute leukaemia. *Leukemia*, **7**, 919–927.

47 Buccheri V., Mihaljevic B., Matutes E., Dyer M.J.S., Mason D.Y. & Catovsky D. (1993) mb-1: a new marker for B-lineage lymphoblastic leukemia. *Blood*, **82**, 853–857.

48 Inhorn R.C., Aster J.C., Roach S.A. *et al.* (1995) A syndrome of lymphoblastic lymphoma, eosinophilia, and myeloid malignancy associated with t(8;13)(p11;q11): description of a distinctive clinicopathologic entity. *Blood*, **85**, 1881–1887.

3 Cytogenetics

P.W. Thompson

Introduction

The first evidence that cytogenetic changes in human cancer were nonrandom events came in 1960 when Nowell & Hungerford reported a small marker chromosome, termed the Philadelphia chromosome (Ph), in the peripheral blood of patients with chronic myeloid leukaemia (CML) [1]. Despite the importance of this discovery, the limitations of the cytogenetic techniques available at the time prevented any further progress in determining the role of karyotypic change in tumour pathogenesis, and it was not until the introduction of chromosome banding in the early 1970s that the situation changed [2]. Whereas previously chromosomes could only be classified in groups according to their size and shape, with banding techniques it became possible to identify accurately individual chromosomes and their structural abnormalities. This led to an increased interest in cancer cytogenetics and many different types of malignancies were examined for chromosomal aberrations. From these studies it soon became clear that consistent and often disease-specific abnormalities were a characteristic feature, and nonrandom chromosomal changes have since been found in all cancers examined in sufficient detail [3].

Clonal chromosomal abnormalities are seen in most patients with leukaemia and lymphoma, and a large number of consistent changes have been reported [4,5]. In the 1970s the more common changes, particularly the myeloid ones, were discovered, and the first concerted effort to evaluate the role of these abnormalities was made in 1977 at the First International Workshop on Chromosomes in Leukaemia [6]. Five subsequent workshops have since been held [7–9]. In the 1980s further improvements in culturing techniques, and the use of synchronization of cells to produce high resolution banding, resulted in many other consistent abnormalities being found. Efforts were also made to determine a 'working classification' based on cytomorphology, immunology and cytogenetics (MIC) [10–12].

It is now well established that many of the cytogenetic changes show such a close association with a particular subtype of leukaemia or lymphoma that they are clearly of both diagnostic and prognostic significance, and can be used in determining treatment protocols. For this reason it is important that there is good communication between the cytogenetics laboratory and the referring clinicians, and that results are reported as quickly as possible.

In addition to their value at diagnosis, cytogenetic studies can also be used to monitor residual disease. The finding of new abnormalities is usually an unfavourable sign associated with clinical progression.

A recent exciting development for cytogenetic studies is the transition of *in situ* hybridization from a research method into a powerful diagnostic technique. This potentially allows the rapid screening of both interphase and metaphase cells [13,14].

As well as helping in patient management decisions, it should not be forgotten that the chromosomal changes found by cytogeneticists have been used to target regions of interest for the molecular biologists. This work started with the t(9;22)(q34;q11) in CML and the t(8;14)(q24;q32) in Burkitt's lymphoma, and has now reached the stage where the breakpoints of the majority of the consistent rearrangements have been characterized. As a result, a number of genes potentially involved in the malignant process have been identified, and molecular diagnostic tests for the more common changes have been developed.

A great deal of published information now exists on cytogenetic abnormalities in haematology. In addition to the workshops mentioned above, there have been several recent disease-specific reviews [15–19], and a more comprehensive overview is given in three excellent books [4,5,20].

Cytogenetic techniques

There are a wide variety of culturing, harvesting, slide-making and banding protocols available to the cytogeneticist for the study of haematological malignancies, and only a brief summary is given below. A more extensive description of the principles and practices involved can be found in a number of manuals and publications [5,20,21].

Bone marrow aspirate is the preferred tissue for the study of most haematological disorders. If bone marrow is not available, then peripheral blood can be used provided there are sufficient circulating blast cells. Two important exceptions are chronic lymphocytic leukaemia (CLL), where peripheral blood is required, and the lymphomas, where a sample from the lymph node is more informative.

The bone marrow sample should be placed into sterile, heparinized culture medium and sent to the laboratory as soon as possible. Excessive delay could lead to an overgrowth of normal nonmalignant cells. Most laboratories will establish a number of different cultures for each sample to ensure the cytogenetically abnormal clone can be detected. For a standard culture, bone marrow is added to basal medium contaning fetal calf serum, l-glutamine and the antibiotics penicillin and streptomycin. The final cell concentration should be approximately 10^6 cells/ml, as too high a concentration will lead to poor cell growth and too low may result in insufficient chromosome spreads for analysis. The sample is then incubated at 37°C for 24 hours. For the last hour of culture colcemid is added to arrest the cells at metaphase, the stage at which the chromosome structure is discernible by light microscopy. After centrifugation the cells are resuspended in a hypotonic solution (usually 0.075 M KCl) to swell the chromosomes, and are then treated with three changes of a fixative (3 parts methanol to 1 part glacial acetic acid) which removes the lipids from the cell membranes and most of the nonhistone proteins.

Chromosome preparations for cytogenetic analysis are made by allowing a drop of the fixed material to run down a microscope slide. As the slide dries, the remnants of the cell membranes rupture and the chromosomes spread out on the slide. The preparations are then treated to produce banding of the chromosomes. The most common technique is to partially digest the chromatin with the protease enzyme trypsin and then stain with Giemsa.

Important variations in culture technique include, the use of direct cultures where there is only a short incubation (1 hour), synchronization of cultures to give longer chromosomes, and an increased time of exposure to colcemid which increases the number of cells in metaphase. In practice the techniques employed will depend on the reason for referral, for example, a direct culture may be the best method for studying childhood acute lymphoblastic leukaemia (ALL) [22], but it is of no use in acute promyelocytic leukaemia where the t(15;17) can only be detected after an overnight incubation [23]. It is generally considered that a cytogenetic study should involve the full analysis of a minimum of 20 metaphases [24].

Cytogenetic terminology

Chromosome changes are designated by the International System for Human Cytogenetic Nomenclature (ISCN), and a supplement for use in cancer cytogenetics was published in 1991 [25]. The normal diploid human karyotype of 46 chromosomes consists of 22 autosomal pairs numbered 1–22 in decreasing order of size, and the sex chromosomes. The centromere is a primary constriction along the length of a chromosome which divides it into a long arm (q) and a short arm (p). A range of techniques can be used to achieve a unique pattern of alternating light and dark bands for each chromosome, so allowing individual identification. Each band is given a specific number.

The chromosome rearrangements most often seen in leukaemia are: translocations (designated by the letter t) where there is an exchange of material between two or more chromosomes; deletions (del) where a chromosomal segment is missing; and inversions (inv) which involve two breaks in the same chromosome with a 180 degree rotation of the interstitial segment. Numerical changes also occur, and the gain of a chromosome (or trisomy) is indicated by a plus sign in front of the extra chromosome, while the loss of a chromosome (or monosomy) is indicated by a minus sign before the missing chromosome.

For example, the karyotype of a Philadelphia (Ph)-chromosome-positive case is written 46,XY,t(9;22)(q34;q11), indicating the normal chromosome number (46) in a male (XY) who has a translocation between chromosomes 9 and 22 (t(9;22)) with the breakpoint on the long arm of chromosome 9 at band 34 and the long arm of the 22 at band 11 ((q34;q11)).

Chronic myeloid leukaemia

CML was the first malignant disorder in which a consistent chromosomal abnormality was defined when Nowell & Hungerford identified the Ph chromosome in 1960 [1]. The cytogenetic defect was subsequently shown to be a reciprocal translocation between chromosomes 9 and 22, t(9;22)(q34;q11) (Fig. 3.1a) [26]. Many detailed studies have since investigated the diagnostic and prognostic significance of this and other changes in CML [5,27–29]. The consistency of the Ph chromosome, and the extensive data gained on its role in CML, made it the ideal model for the early investigations on gene rearrangements in leukaemia, and its molecular mechanisms are now well understood.

Chronic phase

Approximately 90% of cases of CML are Philadelphia chromosome positive (Ph+), and in the majority of patients it results from the standard translocation between chromosomes 9 and 22. In roughly 5–10% of cases it results from a complex rearrangement involving at least three chromosomes including 9 and 22 (Fig. 3.1b) [5,27–29]. There is no difference in the clinical and haematological picture between cases with a standard or a complex translocation.

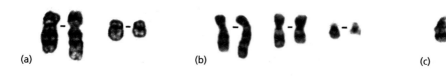

Fig. 3.1 Partial karyotypes showing: (a) the standard Ph chromosome translocation t(9;22)(q34;q11); (b) a complex Ph chromosome resulting from a three-way translocation t(9;11;22)(q34;q14;q11); (c) an isochromosome 17q. The abnormal chromosomes are on the right of each pair.

Table 3.1 Nonrandom chromosomal abnormalities in CML and other myeloproliferative disorders.

Disease	Abnormality	% of patients
CML chronic phase	t(9;22)(q34;q11)	90
CML blastic phase	t(9;22)(q34;q11) with +8, +Ph, i(17q), +19	75
Polycythaemia vera	del(20q), +8, +9, del(13q) abnormalities of 1q	40
Myelofibrosis	+8, +9, −7, del(13q), abnormalities of 1q, del(20q)	50

The Ph chromosome is usually present in all cells examined in the marrow, and remains throughout the course of the disease. There are a few reports of patients with Ph+ and chromosomally normal cells having a longer survival [30,31], but most large studies have failed to show any prognostic advantage of this type of clonality.

At diagnosis of Ph+ CML, between 10 and 20% of cases have additional cytogenetic abnormalities. The most frequent changes include an extra copy of the Ph chromosome (+Ph), loss of the Y chromosome and trisomy 8. These changes are generally thought to be of no clinical significance, and can be transitory in nature [29]. One report does suggest that these patients do have a poorer prognosis than those with the Ph chromosome alone, although the difference is not seen until 2 years postdiagnosis [32].

The finding of an additional abnormality during the course of the chronic phase is, on the other hand, an unfavourable sign usually indicative of impending blast crisis.

Intensive chemotherapy can produce a transient decrease in the Ph+ population, but fails to have any effect on survival [33]. Treatment with alpha interferon (IFNα) in chronic phase can lead to a complete haematological response and loss of the Ph chromosome in the marrow [34]. The exact relationship between these two events is not yet clear, but it does appear that there is an increased survival in patients who show a cytogenetic response [35]. Regular cytogenetic assessment thus forms an integral part of the studies evaluating the effects of IFNα.

Blastic phase

In over 75% of patients in accelerated and/or blastic phase, additional cytogenetic abnormalities are found (Table 3.1). These changes, which are presumably involved in disease progression, can precede other clinical signs of the blastic phase by 2–4 months. The most common changes found are trisomy 8, an extra Ph chromosome, an isochromosome for the long arm of chromosome 17 (i(17q)) (Fig. 3.1c) and trisomy 19. These can occur singly or in combination, giving a modal chromosome number of 47–50 [5,29,36]. The i(17q) in CML is exclusive to the blastic phase. The prognostic value of karyotypic

evolution in predicting the blast crisis of CML illustrates the importance of cytogenetic monitoring in this disorder.

A number of studies have tried to correlate chromosomal changes and phenotype in blast crisis, but the only clear association is the i(17q) with myeloid characteristics. Prognosis appears to be independent of the types of abnormalities found [5,37].

Philadelphia-chromosome-negative chronic myeloid leukaemia

About 10% of patients diagnosed as CML fail to show the Ph chromosome in their marrow (Ph−). Molecular investigations of these cases has shown that approximately 25–50% have a submicroscopic rearrangement involving chromosomes 9 and 22. These patients, termed Ph− BCR+, are clinically indistinguishable from Ph+ CML. The remaining patients present clinical problems. Although it is probable that some have been misdiagnosed, there does appear to be a group who morphologically have classical CML, despite having neither cytogenetic or molecular evidence of a rearrangement (Ph− BCR−) [38].

Myeloproliferative disorders

Consistent chromosomal abnormalities occur in a proportion of cases of myeloproliferative disorders (MPD), but due to their lack of specificity within the subgroups, the role of cytogenetic studies at diagnosis cannot be definitive (Table 3.1). Prognostically, the chromosome changes seen are of little value, although a complex karyotype may be related to a poor outcome [39], and there is some evidence that clonal evolution during the course of MPD is also an unfavourable sign [40]. Many of the changes found are also common to the other myeloid disorders.

Polycythaemia vera

Chromosomal abnormalities in polycythaemia vera (PV) are seen in about 40% of cases during the course of the disease and in 15% of cases at diagnosis (Table 3.1). The most common abnormality is a deletion of the long arm of chromosome 20 (del(20)(q11)) found in 27% of patients. Other abnormalities include trisomy 8, trisomy 9, del(13q), and partial trisomy for the long arm of chromosome 1 [4,5]. One recent study has suggested that patients with a chromosomally abnormal clone at the time of diagnosis of PV had a poorer survival than did those with only normal metaphases [41].

Myelofibrosis

Abnormalities are seen in approximately 50% of patients with myelofibrosis. The changes are similar to those in PV, although del(20) is less frequent (10%), and monosomy 7 is also found [4,5].

Essential thrombocythaemia

A normal karyotype is seen in the vast majority of cases with essential thrombocythaemia, and no consistent changes have been reported [7].

Acute myeloid leukaemia

Cytogenetic studies are an essential part of the diagnosis of patients with acute myeloid leukaemia (AML). Chromosome abnormalities are seen in 60–80% of patients, and a number of them correlate with a particular FAB group. Most of the common changes have been well documented, however, rarer consistent changes (<1% of AML cases) that also have clinical implications are still being reported. The most frequent findings are shown in Table 3.2.

Structural abnormalities

t(8;21)(q22;q22)

A translocation between chromosomes 8 and 21 was the first cytogenetic abnormality found in AML (Fig. 3.2a) [42]. It is the most common structural abnormality in *de novo* AML, occurring in 10% of cases [43,44]. It is usually associated with the FAB group M2 where it is seen in 40% of karyotypically abnormal cases [43], but has also been reported in M4 and M1. Morphologically, the cells may show high numbers of Auer rods, and the blasts are strongly myeloperoxidase positive. [44]. The t(8;21) is particularly common in children (in one study occurring in 17% of cytogenetically abnormal cases), but is rarely found in elderly patients. It is occasionally found in therapy-related AML.

Variant translocations, although unusual, can occur in a

Table 3.2 Nonrandom chromosomal abnormalities in AML.

FAB group	Abnormality	% of patients
M2	t(8;21)(q22;q22)	40
M3	t(15;17)(q22;q21)	90+
M4Eo	inv(16)(p13q22)	?100
M5, M4	t/del(11q)	35
Various	+8	13
	−7	9
	−5 or del(5q)	6
	t(9;22)(q34;q11)	3
	t(3;3)(q21;q26) or inv(3)(q21q26)	2
	t(6;9)(p23;q34)	2
	+4, +11, +13, +21	<1
	i(17q), t(8;16)(p11;p13)	<1
	t(1;22)(p13;q13)	<1

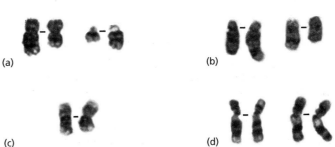

Fig. 3.2 Partial karyotypes showing the common cytogenetic rearrangements in AML. (a) t(8;21)(q22;q22) associated with M2. (b) t(15;17)(q22;q21) associated with M3. (c) inv(16)(p13q22) associated with M4Eo. (d) t(9;11)(p21;q23) associated with M5. The abnormal chromosomes are on the right of each pair.

similar manner to the Ph chromosome in CML [3]. Secondary chromosomal changes frequently accompany the t(8;21). Most cases show sex chromosome loss, with up to 85% of males losing the Y chromosome, and 73% of females the inactive X chromosome. An interstitial deletion of the long arm of chromosome 9 is another consistent finding. In adults, the t(8;21) has a favourable prognosis compared with AML as a whole [45,46]. However, it has recently been reported that in children, despite a high complete remission rate, survival was very poor [47]. The translocation results in the fusion of the two genes AML1 at 21q22 and ETO at 8q22 [48].

t(15;17)(q22;q21)

A clear correlation exists between a translocation of chromosomes 15 and 17 and acute promyelocytic leukaemia (APL) (Fig. 3.2b). First reported in 1977 [49], the translocation is exclusive to APL, and is found in nearly every case of both the hypergranular and microgranular forms [50]. Variant translocations have been reported, and trisomy 8 is a frequent secondary change [5]. The molecular mechanisms of the trans-location, which include a disruption of the retinoic acid receptor-alpha on chromosome 15, are well understood [51]. Patients with the t(15;17) have bleeding problems, in particular, disseminated intravascular coagulation. However, survival is generally good once remission is achieved, and recent treatment regimens with all *trans* retinoic acid have further improved prognosis [52].

inv(16)(p13q22)

An association between an abnormality of chromosome 16 and acute myelomonocytic leukaemia with eosinophilia was first reported in 1983 [53]. The rearrangement has subsequently been shown to be usually an inversion of chromosome 16 (Fig. 3.2c), with a translocation between the chromosome 16 homologues also being found, t(16;16)(p13;q22) [54]. Nearly all patients with AML M4Eo show an abnormality of chromosome 16, with associated atypical eosinophils, containing large irregular granules. Increased numbers of bone marrow eosinophils, although common, are not always present. The inv(16) is not exclusive to M4Eo, it has also been reported in other AML subtypes, myelodysplastic syndrome (MDS) and in blast crisis CML with bone marrow eosinophilia [55,56].

The inv(16) is a prognostically favourable finding in both adult and paediatric AML [45,54]. In one large study [54], 78% of patients achieved a complete remission, compared with 36% of other patients with acute myelomonocytic leukaemia. Median survival was also longer: 65 weeks compared with 29 weeks. A high risk of central nervous system involvement in patients with the inv(16) has been reported in some studies. The breakpoints and molecular pathology of the inversion have been determined [55].

Abnormalities of 11q

Another cytogenetic–morphological correlation exists between abnormalities of the long arm of chromosome 11 and acute monocytic leukaemia [57]. Both translocations and deletions can occur, and a number of different chromosomes have been involved in exchanges with 11q, particularly 6, 9, 17 and 19 [58]. Up to 35% of cases with M5 have been reported with 11q abnormalities [57], and at the Fourth International Workshop [8] two-thirds of cases with chromosome 11 rearrangements belonged to the M5 subgroup.

In some cases the breakpoint on chromosome 11 has been reported as q13–14, however, they are mostly at q23 and involve the MLL gene also implicated in ALL (see below). In general an abnormality of 11q is common in young patients, particularly in those under 1 year of age where it is accompanied by a high white blood cell count (WBC) and a poor outlook. In adults 11q23 abnormalities are associated with a poor prognosis [59]. The translocation t(9;11)(p21;q23) is the

most frequent rearrangement involving 11q23 (Fig. 3.2d) and is of particular interest as it is found in both *de novo* and secondary AML. In a recent paediatric study, in *de novo* AML the translocation t(9;11) conferred a favourable outlook, whereas prognosis was poor when it was present in secondary AML [60].

Other structural abnormalities

As well as the abnormalities outlined above, there are some less frequent structural cytogenetic changes worthy of comment. The Ph chromosome is present in 3% of AML patients, typically with an M1 and M2 phenotype. In contrast with CML, the Ph chromosome disappears during remission [5,61]. Normal or elevated platelet counts with abnormalities of megakaryocytopoiesis are associated with rearrangements of the long arm of chromosome 3, either an inversion, inv(3)(q21q26), or a translocation between both chromosomes 3, t(3;3)(q21;q26) [62,63]. There is a predominance of female patients, and the prognosis is extremely poor [63]. A translocation t(6;9)(p23;q34) is accompanied by raised levels of basophils in the marrow, and associated with a young age at presentation, FAB subtypes M1 and M4, and a poor response to therapy [64,65]. A translocation t(8;16)(p11;p13) is usually associated with erythrophagocytosis and a poor outcome [66]. The t(1;22)(p13;q13) is exclusive to childhood acute megakaryoblastic leukaemia. At presentation, patients are of a young age (median 6 months), have a low leucocyte count, organomegaly and bone marrow fibrosis. The prognosis is extremely poor [67].

Numerical abnormalities

Trisomy 8

Aneuploidy is another mechanism of chromosome imbalance in AML. The most common aneuploidy is trisomy for chromosome 8, which occurs in approximately 13% of cases. It has been reported in all subtypes of AML, and can be the sole change, or it can occur in combination with other abnormalities [68]. Trisomy 8 carries an intermediate prognosis.

Monosomy 7

Monosomy for chromosome 7 is seen in approximately 4% of cases of *de novo* AML [68]. It is most usually seen in M1, but it has been reported in all subtypes. Treatment is complicated by infections caused by a deficiency of chemotaxis in the granulocytes [69]. The prognosis for patients with monosomy 7 in AML, and any other myeloid disorder, is poor.

A distinct subset of paediatric patients who have lost a chromosome 7 have 'childhood monosomy 7 syndrome'. They present with either MDS which subsequently evolves to secondary AML, or with *de novo* AML. Anaemia is common and there is a marked excess of males [70,71]. There is some evidence for a familial element to the disorder [72]. Clinically, these children present a problem with their failure to respond to chemotherapy, and the lack of success of allogeneic bone marrow transplantation [73]. Distinguishing between childhood monosomy 7 syndrome and juvenile CML is difficult because of the similar clinical picture and poor prognosis, however, only about 25% of patients with juvenile CML have monosomy 7 [71].

Other aneuploidies

The other consistent, although rarer (<1%), trisomies seen in AML are 4, 11, 13 and 21. Trisomy 4 is a recent finding in AML [74], and it has been suggested that it may be caused by environmental factors. To date, despite a number of published reports, this cannot be substantiated. Trisomy 4 is usually seen in M2 and M4 and appears to have no independent prognostic significance [75]. Trisomy 11 is characterized by a stem/progenitor cell immunophenotype, previous MDS, an old age at presentation and an unfavourable prognosis [76]. Trisomy 13 usually occurs in elderly males and the leukaemia can be undifferentiated or biphenotypic, expressing both lymphoid and myeloid markers. Prognosis is poor with a low complete remission (CR) rate [77]. Trisomy 21 as the only abnormality in AML has no cytogenetic–clinicopathological associations [78].

Myelodysplastic syndrome

A number of reports on large patient cohorts have shown the value of cytogenetic analysis in primary MDS (for reviews see refs [12,16,79,80]). The published frequency of chromosomal abnormalities varies widely from 35 to 75%. These differences may be the result of a number of factors including: the standard of cytogenetic analysis, the diagnostic criteria of the referral centre and the inclusion of patients with secondary MDS. In a recent review of over 3000 reported cases, karyotypic abnormalities were seen in 48% of patients [79]. The most common chromosomal changes found are shown in Table 3.3.

The frequency of clonal abnormalities differs between the FAB subtypes. Noël *et al.* [16] quote a figure of 45% for refractory anaemia, 33% for refractory anaemia with ring sideroblasts, 61% for refractory anaemia with excess of blasts, 62% for refractory anaemia with excess of blasts in transformation and 33% for chronic myelomonocytic leukaemia. Diagnostically, there are no firm correlations between recurring cytogenetic changes and FAB subtypes. Many of the abnormalities also occur in other myeloid disorders.

The 5q– syndrome

In 1974 Van den Berghe *et al.* [81] first defined the '5q– syndrome'. It occurs in elderly women with macrocytic anaemia, normal or elevated platelets, hypolobulation of megakaryo-

Table 3.3 Nonrandom changes found in chromosomally abnormal MDS patients. (Adapted from Mufti, 1992 [79], with permission.)

Chromosomal abnormality	% of patients
Aneuploidy	
+8	19
–7	15
–5	5
Deletions	
5q–	27
11q–	7
12p–	5
20q–	5
7q–	4
13q–	2
Others	
i(17q)	5
t(1;7)(q10;p10)	2
t(3;3)(q21;q26)	2
or inv(3)(q21q26)	

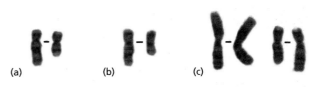

(a)   (b)   (c)

Fig. 3.3 Partial karyotypes showing: (a) an interstitial deletion of chromosome 5 del(5)(q13q33); (b) a deletion of the long arm of chromosome 7; (c) the t(1;7)(q10;p10). The abnormal chromosomes are on the right of each pair.

cytes, and a deletion of the long arm of chromosome 5. The prognosis is favourable and there is a low risk of leukaemic transformation. The breakpoints of the deletion can vary, although in more than 90% of cases they are interstitial, involving bands q12–q14 (proximal) and q31–q33 (distal) (Fig. 3.3a). The common deleted segment in over 98% of cases is 5q31 [82]. It should be noted that a 5q– chromosome in the karyotype does not necessarily mean that a patient has '5q– syndrome'. The above clinical criteria should also be fulfilled before such a classification is made.

Abnormalities of chromosome 7

Monosomy for all of chromosome 7 or part of the long arm is seen in 19% of karyotypically abnormal cases of primary MDS, and is normally associated with a rapidly fatal outcome (Fig. 3.3b) [12].

Trisomy 8

Trisomy 8 occurs in all MDS subtypes, either singly or with other abnormalities, and appears to carry a poor prognosis.

Table 3.4 Prognostic significance of cytogenetic studies in MDS.

Favourable prognosis	Unfavourable prognosis
Normal karyotype	Complex karyotype
	All abnormal metaphases
del(5q), del(20q)	−7/del(7q), +8, i(17q)
	Karyotypic evolution

Table 3.5 Nonrandom chromosomal abnormalities in childhood ALL.

Phenotype	Abnormality	% of total ALL
Pre-B	t(1;19)(q23;p13)	5–6
Early B precursor, common, pre-B	t(9;22)(q34;q11)	2–5
Early B precursor, mixed	t(4;11)(q21;q23)	2
B	t(8;14)(q24;q32)	3
T	t(11;14)(p13;q11)	1
Mostly common	del(6q)	4–13
Mostly common	t/del(9p)	7–12
Mostly common	t/del(12p)	10–12

Other abnormalities

A deletion of the long arm of chromosome 11 is often associated with refractory anaemia with ring sideroblasts, where it may be found in up to 20% of cases [83]. A deletion of 12p occurs in approximately 15% of cases of chronic myelomonocytic leukaemia [84].

The prognostic value of cytogenetic studies in MDS is well established, although there is still a need for more data on some of the specific chromosomal rearrangements (Table 3.4). In broad terms, patients who present with a normal karyotype have a longer survival than those with an abnormal one, particularly if it is complex [85], and patients with only normal metaphases do better than those with both normal and abnormal metaphases, who in turn do better than those with only abnormal metaphases [86]. Of the consistent changes, del(5q) and del(20q) have a favourable prognosis, and −7/del(7q), trisomy 8 and an isochromosome (17q) have a poor prognosis [87,88]. Karyotypic evolution, either the appearance of a chromosomally abnormal clone in a patient with a previously normal karytoype, or additional changes in an abnormal clone, occurs in 15–30% of primary MDS cases and is associated with a short survival and accelerated disease [89,90].

Secondary myelodysplastic syndrome/acute myeloid leukaemia

The frequency and types of karyotypic change in secondary MDS and secondary AML are very similar, and the two disorders can be considered together for the purpose of interpretation.

The abnormality rate in secondary MDS/AML is higher than in *de novo* MDS or AML, ranging from 66 to 97%, and although single changes are found, the karyotype is more often a complex hypodiploid one [12,91,92]. Furthermore, variability and instability, often to an extreme degree, can be encountered. Abnormalities of chromosomes 5 and/or 7 are by far the most common changes, occurring in up to 90% of cases [91]. Other changes include, +8, −17, −18, +21 and −21, and anomalies involving 3q, 6p, 11q, 12p, 17p, 17q and 21q. Ring and dicentric chromosomes are also occasionally observed. The specific structural changes of *de novo* AML are rarely seen in secondary AML [12,19].

The prognosis of secondary MDS/AML patients is invariably poor [12]. There has been a recent report that the small group of patients who have a karyotypic abnormality associated with primary AML also carry the concomitant prognosis [93].

Acute lymphoblastic leukaemia

Cytogenetic analysis in acute lymphoblastic leukaemia (ALL) is hindered by the morphology of the leukaemic metaphases, which consist of poorly spread chromosomes that fail to produce a clearly defined banding pattern. Extensive efforts have been made to overcome this problem, and although recent technical advances have led to some improvement, the banding resolution achieved still falls short of that possible in the other leukaemias [22]. The awareness of the clinical value of chromosomal studies in ALL has meant that despite the above difficulties, most laboratories are now capable of finding abnormalities in up to 80% of patients, with some reporting a figure of over 90% [94,95].

A number of ALL-specific chromosomal changes have been reported, some of which correlate with distinct morphological or immunological subtypes (Table 3.5) [18,96]. Cytogenetic studies in ALL can be of independent prognostic value, in particular, they can identify patients who have a poor response to treatment (Table 3.6). ALL is mainly a disease of the young, and consequently most published cytogenetic data is based on studies on children [18,96]. What little data there is available on adult ALL suggests that the karyotype–survival correlations in children also apply to older patients [97–100]. ALL can be categorized cytogenetically, by either chromosome number (ploidy) or by structural rearrangements.

Numerical abnormalities

Chromosome number was the original classification used to illustrate the importance of cytogenetic studies in ALL, and it is still a valid method today (for more comprehensive reviews see Pui *et al.* [96] and Raimondi [18]) (Table 3.6) (Fig. 3.4). Furthermore, patients originally categorized by this method have had a long-term follow-up, allowing assessment of factors such as late relapse [101,102].

Table 3.6 Event-free survival after intensified chemotherapy in different cytogenetic subgroups. (Adapted from Rivera *et al.*, 1991 [105], © 1991 *The Lancet* Ltd.)

Cytogenetic classification	4-year event-free survival (%)*
Ploidy	
Hyperdiploid >50	84 (6)
Hyperdiploid 47–50	77 (11)
Normal diploid	87 (10)
Pseudodiploid	63 (7)
Hypodiploid <45	46 (19)
Structural	
B-cell lineage	
t(1;19)(q23;p13)	79 (21)
t(9;22)(q34;q11)	36 (21)
t(9p;V)	47 (20)
t(11q23;V)	56 (21)
t(12p;V)	83 (12)
T-cell lineage	
t(7q35;V)	43 (23)
t(14q11;V)	50 (25)
Non-specific lineage	
del(6q)	74 (15)
del(9p)	49 (12)
del(12p)	95 (6)

* Figures in parentheses are standard error.

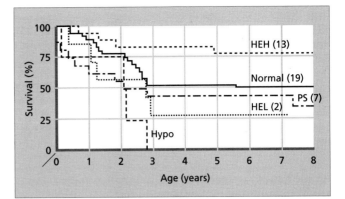

Fig. 3.4 Event-free survival by ploidy group in childhood ALL. HEH = high hyperdiploidy; HEL = low hyperdiploidy; Hypo = hypodiploidy; PS = pseudodiploids. Numbers in parentheses are equivalent to numbers of patients who are event free at 6 years. (From Secker-Walker *et al.*, 1989 [101], with permission.)

Hyperdiploidy >50 chromosomes

Hyperdiploidy with greater than 50 chromosomes accounts for approximately 25% of cases of ALL diagnosed in children. Clinically, this group is associated with favourable indicators, including a low WBC, expression of CD10, and an age range from 2 to 10 years. Both children and adults show an excellent response to treatment [97,101–105]. The most common gains are 4, 6, 10, 14, 17, 18, 20, 21 and X. Structural chromosome abnormalities are found in 62% of cases, and include ALL-specific translocations. Patients with numerical changes only, have a better prognosis than those with numerical and structural rearrangements [103].

Hyperdiploidy 47–50 chromosomes

This group constitutes 15% of cases in children and has been associated with an intermediate prognosis [104]. Extra copies of chromosomes 8, 10 and 21 are most frequently seen, and structural abnormalities are present in 76% of cases. Intensive treatment therapies can result in a favourable prognosis [105].

Pseudodiploidy 46 chromosomes

Pseudodiploidy, or 46 chromosomes with stuctural and/or numerical changes, is now the most common ploidy group in childhood ALL. Most patients have a structural abnormality, usually a translocation [106]. Numerical abnormalities are rarely seen. Pseudodiploidy was originally given an intermediate prognosis, but here again intensive therapy can improve outcome [105,107].

Hypodiploidy <46 chromosomes

Hypodiploidy with less than 46 chromosomes occurs in 6–7% of children with ALL. The chromosome number is usually 45, and chromosome 20 loss the most common finding [108,109]. Hypodiploid cases have a poor response to treatment. Within the hypodiploid category are a small number of patients (<1% of total ALL) with a near haploid karyotype [110]. These have a clone with one copy of each chromosome, usually a second sex chromosome and 21 chromosome, and can also have two copies of 10, 14 and 18. A hyperdiploid cell line is usually present which has a duplication of all of the chromosomes in the near haploid cell line. Patients with a near haploid karyotype have a poor prognosis.

Normal chromosomes

Patients with no detectable cytogenetic abnormality show an intermediate prognosis with conventional treatment and a good prognosis with intensive therapy [105,107]. When classifying cases into this group there is always the possibility that cytogenetic analysis has failed to detect the abnormal clone.

Structural abnormalities

The benefit of the improvement in chromosome resolution in ALL in the 1980s was reflected in the finding of many consistent structural abnormalities, and there are now well over 30 disease-specific changes [18,96]. The most common structural

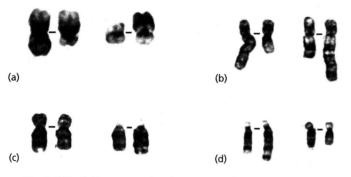

(a)

(b)

(c)

(d)

Fig. 3.5 Partial karyotypes showing common changes in lymphoid disorders: (a) t(1;19)(q23;p13) associated with pre-B ALL; (b) t(4;11)(q21;q23) associated with ALL; (c) t(8;14)(q24;q32) associated with B-ALL and Burkitt's lymphoma; (d) t(14;18)(q32;q21) associated with follicular lymphoma. The abnormal chromosomes are on the right of each pair.

rearrangements seen in ALL are translocations [107]. Both random and nonrandom clonal translocations are seen in roughly equal proportions. A number of the nonrandom translocations have both diagnostic and prognostic significance (Table 3.6).

t(1;19)(q23;p13)

The t(1;19)(q23;p13) is the most common translocation in paediatric ALL, occurring in 5–6% of cases [111,112]. It is closely linked to a pre-B immunophenotype, where it is seen in 25% of cases, but can also be found in other subtypes [112,113]. The rearrangement is seen in two forms, either as a balanced translocation between chromosomes 1 and 19, t(1;19)(q23;p13) (25%) (Fig. 3.5a), or in an unbalanced form with two normal chromosomes 1 and an abnormal 19 with extra chromosome 1 material on the short arm, der(19),t(1;19)(q23;p13) (75%). At the molecular level, the t(1;19) in both forms results in the fusion of the genes E2A on chromosome 19 and PBX1 on chromosome 1. The presence of the t(1;19) has been shown to be the causative factor for the poor response to treatment of patients with pre-B ALL [114], although there is now evidence that more intensive treatment protocols can improve prognosis [105,107,112]. A recent study group has shown that patients with the unbalanced form of the translocation have a significantly better outcome than those with the balanced form [115].

Philadelphia chromosome

A t(9;22) is found in 3–5% of children and 15–25% of adults with ALL. It is normally accompanied by a high WBC, B-lineage immunophenotype and, in children, an older age at presentation. An increased frequency of central nervous system (CNS) involvement has also been suggested. In both children and adults the t(9;22) is an independent prognostic

indicator, with patients responding poorly to conventional and intensive treatment [99,116]. In a study by Fletcher *et al.* [116], 4-year event-free and overall survivals were 81 and 88% respectively in children lacking the t(9;22), contrasting with figures of 0 and 20% respectively for children with the t(9;22). In adults, a report has shown that lineage commitment may have prognostic implications [99]. Patients whose lymphoid and myeloid cells were Ph+ had a longer event-free survival than those in whom only the lymphoid lineage was involved (a median survival of 35 months compared to less than 6 months).

The clinical problem of distinguishing between Ph+ ALL and lymphoid blast crisis of CML can usually be resolved cytogenetically. In contrast to CML where the Ph chromosome persists throughout the course of the disease, when a Ph+ ALL patient enters remission the Ph chromosome disappears. In addition, the chromosome changes characteristic of the blast crisis of CML are not seen in Ph+ ALL at diagnosis.

Molecular studies have shown two subtypes of Ph+ ALL. The BCR-ABL gene rearrangement can either produce the p210 protein seen in CML, or it can be in a different position and result in a novel p190 protein. In adults the two breakpoints are found in equal numbers, while in children the majority have the p190 fusion protein [116]. There is no difference in treatment outcome between the two types. Analysis with DNA probes for the t(9;22) indicate that it may be present in as many as 30% of cases of adult ALL [117].

Translocations involving 11q23

Rearrangements of 11q23 are another consistent finding in ALL. The most common of these is the t(4;11)(q21;q23) (Fig. 3.5b). This accounts for 2% of paediatric ALL, and is associated with female sex, a high WBC, CNS involvement, and is very common in children under the age of 1 year [118,119]. The translocation is unusual in that it is also associated with heterogeneity of cell lineage. The usual classification is B-precursor ALL (pre-B or early pre-B), but there are a number of reported cases with myelomonocytic or mixed lineage characteristics, indicating that the t(4;11) originates in a stem cell with the capacity to differentiate in both myeloid and lymphoid directions [120,121]. Prognosis is poor for infants and children aged 10 years or older regardless of the treatment regimen used [118]. In adults, where the abnormality is seen in 3–6% of cases, prognosis is also poor, with an event-free survival shorter than that of children [100].

A further 3% of childhood ALL cases have abnormalities of 11q23, including the t(1;11)(p32;q23), t(10;11)(p14–15;q23), and the t(9;11)(p21;q23) and t(11;19)(q23;p13) more usually found in AML. As a group they tend to show the same clinical characteristics, including poor prognosis, as the t(4;11) [122].

Visible cytogenetic abnormalities of 11q23 are seen in between 42 and 66% of cases of infant ALL [58]. The gene

MLL (ALL-1, HRX, HTRX) is altered in translocations of 11q23, and the use of DNA probes for this region has resulted in an increased detection rate of abnormalities at this locus in infant ALL to 70–80% [58,123]. In multivariate models of risk factors in infant ALL, the alteration of the MLL gene is the most important variable negatively affecting prognosis [119,123].

t(8;14)(q24;q32)

The t(8;14) (Fig. 3.5c) and its variants found in Burkitt's lymphoma are also seen in most cases of B-cell ALL with an L3 morphology. Extramedullary disease is frequent in this group [124]. Prognosis used to be considered very poor in ALL patients with this translocation, however new treatment regimens have improved the outcome [105,125].

Abnormalities at the T-cell receptor loci

Chromosomal changes at the T-cell receptor loci, 14q11, 7q34 and 7p15, are seen in approximately 50% of cases of T-cell ALL [18,126]. The most common consistent abnormalities of 14q11 are the translocations t(11;14)(p13;q11), t(10;14)(q24;q11), t(8;14)(q24;q11), t(1;14)(p32;q11), and a paracentric inversion of chromosome 14, inv(14)(q11q32). Rearrangements of the genes on chromosome 7 are less frequently seen, although specific changes have been reported. A report by Pui *et al.* [127] on paediatric patients with T-cell ALL found the presence of an abnormal karyotype (75% of cases) conferred an increased risk of treatment failure.

Other rearrangements

The other most frequent structural alterations in ALL involve the long arm of chromosome 6 and the short arm of chromosomes 9 and 12. These changes can occur singly or in conjunction with other abnormalities and are not restricted to any one lineage. A deletion involving bands q15 or q21 is the usual rearrangement of chromosome 6, and as a group these patients show no specific features and have a favourable prognosis [128]. The abnormalities of 12p are more varied [129], with quite a few consistent changes documented, for example dic(9;12)(p11;p12). This group also shows no specific characteristics and has a very good prognosis. A study on children who had abnormalities of 9p showed that, compared to patients without the rearrangement, they were older at presentation, had a higher WBC, a greater frequency of splenomegaly and an increased risk of extramedullary relapse [130]. There is conflicting data on the prognosis of children with this change from two studies using intensive treatment regimens. One showed an event-free survival no different from the cohort as a whole (*n* = 11) [107], whereas the larger study showed it to be worse (*n* = 38) [104].

Chronic lymphoproliferative disorders

The importance of chromosomal abnormalities in the chronic lymphoproliferative disorders (CLD) has yet to be determined. It has long been known that nonrandom changes do occur, and that they consistently involve the immunoglobulin heavy-chain locus at 14q32 in B-cell disorders, and the T-cell receptor alpha-chain locus at 14q11 in T-cell disorders [4,5]. Unfortunately, the problems caused by the low mitotic index of the malignant cells makes cytogenetic analysis very time consuming, and the lack of specificity of the changes seen makes interpretation difficult; not only can the same abnormalities be found in different CLDs, but they may also be seen in the lymphomas.

Chronic lymphocytic leukaemia

Despite constituting approximately 30% of all leukaemias, cytogenetic analysis is not yet considered to be an essential part in the diagnosis of chronic lymphocytic leukaemia (CLL). This is partly due to the problems mentioned above. However, the commercial availability of reliable B-cell mitogens in recent years has greatly helped in determining the role of chromosomal abnormalities in this disorder, and a number of large studies have been reported [131–133]. The majority of centres find an abnormality rate of 50% or greater. Originally, trisomy 12 was the most common change, being found in one-third of patients, with the other frequent changes being structural abnormalities of chromosome regions 13q14, 14q32 and 11q23. More recent papers report structural abnormalities of 13q14 to be more frequent[17,134]. The use of fluorescence *in situ* hybridization (FISH) techniques has resulted in the detection of chromosomal changes in a higher percentage of CLL cases (see below), and one report which used cytogentic, interphase FISH and comparative genome hybridization studies found an abnormality rate of 66% [135].

A number of significant clinical conclusions can be drawn from the cytogenetic data (Fig. 3.6).
1 Patients with a normal karyotype do better than those with an abnormal karyotype.
2 Patients with a single abnormality do better than those with a complex karyotype.
3 A high percentage of cytogenetically abnormal cells is associated with a poor survival.

Clonal karyotypic evolution is seen in approximately 15% of cases with CLL [136–138], and there are conflicting reports on its association with disease progression.

Multiple myeloma

Stimulation of cell division by the addition of cytokines to long-term cultures of bone marrow samples from myeloma patients has helped in detection of the malignant clone, and cytogenetic abnormality rates of over 50% have been achieved

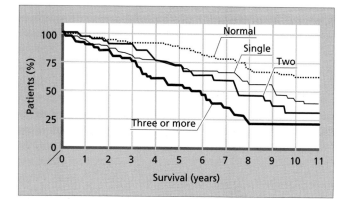

Fig. 3.6 Overall survival according to the number of chromosomal aberrations in CLL: none (normal karyotype; *n* = 173), single (*n* = 113), two (*n* = 52) or three or more (*n* = 53). Survival was measured from the time of diagnosis. (From Juliusson *et al.*, 1990 [131], by permission of *The New England Journal of Medicine*, © 1990 Massachusetts Medical Society.)

[139,140]. Structural rearrangements frequently involve chromosomes 1 (p and q arm), 14q32 and 19p13 [139,141]. A number of consistent translocations of 14q32 have been found, as has a translocation between chromosomes 1 and 16. The abnormality rate increases with stage [139,140], and in one large study patients with an abnormal karyotype had a 2.5-fold greater chance of death than those with a normal one [139].

Lymphoma

The short-term cytogenetic culture of lymph-node biopsy material is now a well-documented technique that allows reliable and accurate chromosome analysis in the lymphomas [142–144]. Yet despite its potential the method has not been widely incorporated by diagnostic cytogenetic laboratories. Clonal abnormalities are now found in over 90% of patients, and cytogenetic studies can provide useful clinical information [143,144]. In non-Hodgkin's lymphoma (NHL) many consistent primary and secondary rearrangements have been reported for both B- and T-cell lineages, and clear cytogenetic-clinical associations exist [9]. In Hodgkin's disease no specific changes have yet been noted.

The preferential involvement of selected chromosome regions in rearrangements seen in the CLD also occurs in lymphoma. Over 70% of B-cell lymphomas have translocations at the immunoglobulin heavy-chain receptor at 14q32, while in the T-cell subtypes the T-cell receptor gene at 14q11 is usually involved [9,145,146].

Both structural and numerical abnormalities have been found, and three translocations have been characterized in detail.

t(8;14)(q24;q32)

Abnormalities involving the chromosome region 8q24 are seen in nearly all cases of Burkitt's lymphoma [147]. In 75% of patients it is due to a translocation between chromosomes 8 and 14, t(8;14)(q24;q32) (Fig. 3.5c), and in the remaining patients it results from one of two variant translocations, involving either chromosome 2, t(2;8)(p12;q24), or chromosome 22, t(8;22)(q24;q11). These translocations have also been described in B-cell ALL, and occasionally in other high-grade lymphomas [9,147].

t(14;18)(q32;q21)

The t(14;18) (Fig. 3.5d) is seen in more than 75% of patients with follicular lymphoma [144,148], and is also found in 28% of cases of high-grade lymphoma, and in CLL.

t(11;14)(q13;q32)

This translocation is found in small cell lymphocytic lymphoma, CLL, multiple myeloma and mantle cell lymphoma [149].

Other abnormalities

Although cytogenetic changes are seen in most cases of lymphoma, only one recently reported abnormality appears to be exclusive to a histological subtype, the t(2;5)(p23;q35) found in anaplastic large cell lymphoma [145,150]. Other frequent changes that show little specificity include trisomy 3 and structural rearrangements of chromosomes 3 and 6p. A further group of abnormalities that are secondary in nature include structural abnormalities of 1p, 1q, 6q, 7p, 7q and 17p, and trisomies 7 and 18 [143,144].

There have been only a few detailed studies on the prognostic implications of chromosomal changes in lymphoma. A recent publication on follicular lymphoma found that they could give information on survival and risk of transformation [143]. A high percentage of abnormal metaphases (>90) and a complex karyotype was associated with a poor prognosis; abnormalities of 1p12–21, 6q23–26 and 17p conferred a significantly shorter survival, and patients with the latter two changes also had the greatest risk of transformation to diffuse large cell lymphoma. A study of 434 non-Hodgkin's (NHL) lymphoma patients [15] showed a complex karyotype and abnormalities of 1q21–23 shortened median survival, and breaks at 6q21–25 decreased the probability of achieving remission.

Bone marrow transplantation

Cytogenetic studies have been shown to be a valuable technique in monitoring patients who have undergone allogeneic bone marrow transplantation. Two methods are available. Firstly, if a clonal abnormality was present at diagnosis it can be used post-transplant as a marker for the return of the malignant cell population. Secondly, in patients who have a donor of a different sex, analysis of the sex chromosomes will show the origin of the cells examined [151–154].

Early cytogenetic studies helped to resolve some of the problems associated with monitoring bone marrow transplant (BMT) patients. Analysis in sex-mismatched BMT donors has demonstrated that mixed haematopoietic chimaerism is compatible with long-term disease-free survival [155], and chromosome analysis confirmed the rare, but well-documented, event of leukaemic relapse in donor cells [156,157].

The recent development of DNA-based tests for mixed chimaerism has diminished the role of cytogenetic studies in BMT [158], and there have been very few recent publications on their use. The new tests include restriction fragment length polymorphism (RFLP) and minisatellites which show a sensitivity of 5–10%, the polymerase chain reaction (PCR) using RFLPs or variable number tandem repeats (VNTRs) which has a sensitivity of 0.1–1%, and PCR amplification of microsatellites which has a sensitivity of 0.01–0.1%. These all compare favourably to karyotypic analysis which has a sensitivity of only 12–20% [158]. In addition, FISH studies with probes for the sex chromosomes or disease-specific rearrangements are also more sensitive [159].

The clear advantage of cytogenetic studies is that all of the chromosomes are analysed, not just a few markers. For example, the DNA-based techniques will show the presence of mixed chimaerism, whereas a chromosome analysis may also be able to reveal if the host cells are malignant or not.

Cytogenetics has provided the greatest benefit in patients who have been transplanted for CML, where the Ph chromosome can be used as a marker for monitoring engraftment and disease status. The recurrence of Ph+ host metaphases in the marrow is usually indicative of a future relapse and, importantly, the cytogenetic changes seen may precede other clinical symptoms by anything from a few months to several years. This phenomenon has been termed 'cytogenetic relapse' [160]. There is usually a gradual increase in Ph+ host cells, until the disease returns (usually when >50% of cells are Ph+). On rare occasions, a Ph+ clone, which disappears in subsequent analyses, can be detected [151,154]. These transient clones are only seen in the first year after BMT, and presumably arise from nonpluripotential cells. A low percentage of Ph+ cells are sometimes seen immediately after BMT, but these are usually lost from the marrow within a few months, and are thought to be damaged cells [151,154].

Serial cytogenetic studies can also be applied to patients who have had a BMT for acute leukaemia, where again the reappearance of the abnormal clone can precede other clinical signs of relapse, but only by a few weeks [152].

Two recent surveys have demonstrated that relapse rates were higher and leukaemia-free survival lower in patients with cytogenetic abnormalities traditionally associated with a poor prognosis [161,162].

Fluorescence *in situ* hybridization

In the past few years fluorescence *in situ* hybridization (FISH) has become a valuable diagnostic technique to help study cytogenetic changes in haematological disorders [13,14]. *In situ* hybridization describes the method whereby nucleic acid sequences and labelled probe DNA are denatured and then allowed to reanneal together to form hybrid molecules. It allows the identification of cytogenetic changes in both metaphase chromosomes and interphase nuclei. A brief outline of the technique will be given below, but for more information there are a number of publications which comprehensively cover the methodology [163–165].

The probe DNA is usually labelled by nick translation with digoxygenin- or biotin-incorporated nucleotides. The cells, which are fixed to a microscope slide, and the probe DNA are denatured, the probe is then added to the slide and hybridization occurs overnight in a humidified chamber at 37°C. There then follows a series of posthybridization washes in a formamide and/or salt solution (SSC) which remove unbound and nonspecifically bound probe. Fluorescence detection of the probe will depend on the hapten used: for digoxygenin it is via the use of antibodies conjugated with a fluorochrome, and for biotin, fluorochrome-conjugated avidin is used. A counterstain is added to allow the identification of the chromosomes or nuclei, and the slides are examined using an epifluorescence microscope.

Various types of probes are available for FISH studies. Locus-specific sequences such as the alphoid, or satellite, centromeric repeats are now available for all chromosomes. They produce strong site-specific signals, and are of particular use in determining the copy number of chromosomes [166,167] (see Plate 3.1a between pp. 292 and 293). Chromosome paints that hybridize along the whole length of a chromosome are also available, and are used to detect structural rearrangements in metaphase chromosomes (see Plate 3.1b) [168]. Any sequence of interest in the genome can be cloned into vectors and used for FISH studies, and probes can be obtained for the breakpoint regions of a number of consistent cytogenetic abnormalities, allowing their identification in metaphase and interphase cells [169–177]. Their use is based on two methods of analysis. Firstly, if a probe spans the breakpoint, cells with the rearrangement will show three signals instead of two [171]. Secondly, dual-colour FISH allows different colour probes to be used for the regions involved in a translocation, and in cells with the abnormality one of each pair of signals will colocalize [173].

A very recent advance in malignancy cytogenetics, which is

yet to be fully developed, is the technique of comparative genome hybridization (CGH) [178]. In CGH the complete genomic DNA of the malignant cells is used as a FISH probe, and is hybridized to normal metaphase spreads. This will result in a fluorescence signal on all of the chromosomes; however, regions that are overexpressed (e.g. trisomies) will give a stronger signal, and regions that are underexpressed (e.g. monosomies) will give a weaker one.

Fluorescence *in situ* hybridization has been shown to be a sensitive and reliable method for the detection of chromosome abnormalities. It has a number of potential advantages over standard cytogenetic studies:

1 it can be performed on interphase cells;
2 it is not dependent on metaphase quality for an accurate result;
3 a large number of cells can be quickly examined for a probe;
4 blood and bone marrow smears can be used, which removes the need for cell culture;
5 it can be combined with immunophenotyping and morphology to demonstrate which cell lineages are involved.

There are drawbacks with the technique. The most important being that at patient presentation a test with a specific probe will give information on that abnormality alone, whereas a cytogenetic study gives information on all of the chromosomes. Another problem arises when determining low-level clones of malignant cells, where false-positive results from nonmalignant cells may cause problems in interpretation.

Myeloid disorders

The most common aneuploidies associated with myeloid disorders are monosomy 7 and trisomy 8, and a number of interphase FISH studies have been carried out using centromeric probes to detect these [167,179–181]. One study on trisomy 8 [167] attempted to evaluate the technique in 203 cases with a myeloid disorder. They found a sensitivity of 90.2%, with 55/61 cytogenetically positive cases also identified by FISH, and a specificity of 98.6%, with 140/142 cytogenetically negative cases being negative with FISH. The technique also detected trisomy where a normal karyotype was seen by conventional analysis, and was of use in patients with an inconclusive cytogenetic result.

Unique sequence probes are available for the most frequent abnormalities found in AML, t(8;21) [169], t(15;17) [170], inv(16) [171] and t/del(11q23) [172].

The pioneering work on interphase FISH studies on structural abnormalities in malignancy was concentrated on detection of the Philadelphia chromosome, and a number of probe sets can now be obtained [173,182,183]. They are of particular use in identifing cases which are Ph⁻ but BCR-ABL⁺ [173,183], in cases where there is a variant translocation [183], and where the rapid monitoring of large numbers of cells is required after therapy.

Lymphoid disorders

Probes are also available for some of the chromosome regions consistently involved in ALL, t(9;22) [173,174], t(4;11) [172], abnormalities of 14q32 [176] and 8q24 [177]. The probes for the t(9;22) give unambiguous results in the analysis of BCR-ABL [174], and have also detected the rearrangement in a Ph⁻ case of *de novo* ALL [184]. In childhood ALL it is the total chromosome number that has prognostic implications, therefore studies with a single probe at diagnosis are of little relevance. However, such studies have been used to detect minimal residual disease by using a probe for a numerical change previously identified by G-banding [185–188].

The difficulty with cytogenetic studies in B-CLL has focused attention on the potential of interphase FISH in this disorder. A large number of published reports demonstrate that the use of a centromeric probe for chromosome 12 is an effective and reliable method on cultured cells and direct blood smears [162,189–191]. They also show that interphase FISH is a more sensitive technique for the detection of this abnormality than conventional cytogenetics. In one study [191], of 18 cases of trisomy 12 detected by FISH, only 12 were identified by metaphase chromosome analysis. Two studies have looked for deletions of the retinoblastoma gene (RB-1) region at 13q14 [175,192], and again FISH detected more positive cases for this deletion than conventional cytogenetic studies. When interphase studies are carried out with probes for the other commonly involved chromosomes regions in B-CLL, 11q23 and 14q32, the true frequency of chromosomal abnormalities in this disorder may become known.

Minimal residual disease

A potential use for FISH is in monitoring for minimal residual disease and response to treatment, where nuclei and metaphase cells can be rapidly scored for fluorescence signals. Some of the initial results suggest this may be a useful method, but as yet the limited data does not allow an accurate assessment [185–188,193]. The main problem in analysing results is in distinguishing between leukaemic cells with an abnormality and false-positive results from normal cells. Tests that are more sensitive than FISH for detecting minimal residual disease also exist, although unlike FISH these do not allow the size of the clone to be determined.

References

1 Nowel P.C. & Hungerford D.A. (1960) A minute chromosome in human granulocytic leukemia. *Science*, **132**, 1497.
2 Caspersson T., Zech L. & Johansson C. (1970) Differential binding of alkylating fluorochromes in human chromosomes. *Experimental Cell Research*, **60**, 315–319.
3 Mitelman F. (ed.) (1991) *Catolog of Chromosome Aberrations in Cancer*, 4th edn. Wiley-Liss, New York.

4 Heim S. & Mitelman F. (eds) (1995) *Cancer Cytogenetics*, 2nd edn. Wiley-Liss, New York.

5 Sandberg A.A. (ed.) (1990) *The Chromosomes in Human Cancer and Leukemia*, 2nd edn. Elsevier, New York.

6 First International Workshop on Chromosomes in Leukemia (1978) Chromosomes in acute nonlymphocytic leukemia. *British Journal of Haematology*, **39**, 311–316.

7 Third International Workshop on Chromosomes in Leukemia (1981) Report on essential thrombocythaemia. *Cancer Genetics and Cytogenetics*, **4**, 138–142.

8 Fourth International Workshop on Chromosomes in Leukemia (1984) A prospective study of acute nonlymphocytic leukemia. *Cancer Genetics and Cytogenetics*, **11**, 249–360.

9 Fifth International Workshop on Chromosomes in Leukemia-Lymphoma (1987) Correlation of chromosome abnormalities with histologic and immunologic characteristics in non-Hodgkin's lymphoma. *Blood*, **70**, 1554–1564.

10 First MIC Cooperative Study Group (1986) Morphologic, immunologic, and cytogenetic (MIC) working classification of acute lymphoblastic leukemias. *Cancer Genetics and Cytogenetics*, **23**, 189–197.

11 Second MIC Cooperative Study Group (1988) Morphologic, immunologic, and cytogenetic (MIC) working classification of the acute myeloid leukemias. *Cancer Genetics and Cytogenetics*, **30**, 1–15.

12 Third MIC Cooperative Study Group (1988) Recommendations for a morphologic, immunologic, and cytogenetic (MIC) working classification of the primary and therapy-related myelodysplastic disorders. *Cancer Genetics and Cytogenetics*, **32**, 1–10.

13 Le Beau M.M. (1993) Detecting genetic changes in human tumor cells: have scientists 'gone fishing?' *Blood*, **81**, 1979–1983.

14 Bentz M., Dohner H., Cabot C. & Lichter P. (1995) Fluorescence *in situ* hybridization in leukemias: 'The FISH are spawning!'. *Leukemia*, **8**, 1447–1452.

15 Offit K., Wong G., Filippa D.A., Tao Y. & Chaganti R.S.K. (1991) Cytogenetic analysis of 434 consecutively ascertained specimens of non-Hodgkin's lymphoma: clinical correlations. *Blood*, **77**, 1508–1515.

16 Noël P., Tefferi A., Pierre R.V., Jenkins R.B. & Dewald G.W. (1993) Karyotypic analysis in primary myelodysplastic syndromes. *Blood Reviews*, **7**, 10–18.

17 Oscier D.G. (1994) Cytogenetic and molecular abnormalities in chronic lymphocytic leukaemia. *Blood Reviews*, **8**, 88–97.

18 Raimondi S.C. (1993) Current status of cytogenetic research in childhood acute lymphoblastic leukemia. *Blood*, **81**, 2237–2251.

19 Walker H., Smith F.J. & Betts D.R. (1994) Cytogenetics in acute myeloid leukaemia. *Blood Reviews*, **8**, 30–36.

20 Rooney D.E., Czepulkowski B.H. (eds) (1992) *Human Cytogenetics. A practical approach. Vol II. Malignancy and acquired abnormalities*, 2nd edn. IRL Press, Oxford.

21 Gosden J.R. (ed.) (1994) *Chromosome Analysis Protocols*. Humana Press, Totowa, New Jersey.

22 Williams D.L., Harris A., Williams K.J., Brosius M.J. & Lemonds W. (1984) A direct bone marrow chromosome technique for acute lymphoblastic leukemia. *Cancer Genetics and Cytogenetics*, **13**, 239–257.

23 Berger R., Bernheim A., Daniel M.T., Valensi F. & Flandrin G. (1983) Cytological types of mitoses and chromosome abnormalities in acute leukemia. *Leukemia Research*, **7**, 221–236.

24 Knutsen T., Bixenman H.A., Lawce H. & Martin P.K. (1991) Chromosome analysis guidelines preliminary report. *Cancer Genetics and Cytogenetics*, **52**, 11–17.

25 Mitelman F. (ed.) (1991) *Guidelines for Cancer Cytogenetics. Supplement to an International System for Human Cytogenetic Nomenclature*. S. Karger, Basel.

26 Rowley J.D. (1973) A new consistent chromosomal abnormality in chronic myelogenous leukaemia identified by quinacrine fluorescence and Geimsa staining. *Nature*, **243**, 290–293.

27 Rowley J.D. (1986) The Philadelphia chromosome translocation. In: *Genetic Rearrangements in Leukaemia and Lymphoma* (eds J.M. Goldman & D.G. Harnden), pp. 82–99. Churchill Livingstone, London.

28 Sandberg A.A., Gemmill R.M., Hecht B.K. & Hecht F. (1986) The Philadelphia chromosome: a model of cancer and molecular cytogenetics. *Cancer Genetics and Cytogenetics*, **21**, 129–146.

29 Hagemeijer A. (1987) Clinical abnormalities in CML. *Baillière's Clinical Haematology*, **1**, 963–981.

30 Brandt L., Mitelman F., Panani A. & Lenner H.C. (1976) Extremely long duration of chronic myeloid leukaemia with Ph¹ negative and Ph¹ positive bone marrow cells. *Scandinavian Journal of Haematology*, **16**, 321–325.

31 Singer C.R.J., McDonald G.A. & Douglas A.S. (1984) Twenty-five year survival of chronic granulocytic leukaemia with spontaneous karyotype conversion. *British Journal of Haematology*, **57**, 309–313.

32 Sokal J.E., Gomez G.A., Baccarani M. *et al.* (1988) Prognostic significance of additional cytogenetic abnormalities at diagnosis of Philadelphia chromosome-positive chronic granulocytic leukemia. *Blood*, **72**, 294–298.

33 Sharp J.C., Joyner M.V., Wayne A.W. *et al.* (1979) Karyotypic conversion in Ph¹-positive chronic myeloid leukaemia with combination chemotherapy. *Lancet*, **i**, 1370–1372.

34 Talpaz M., Kantarjian H.M., McCredie K.B., Keating M.J., Trujillo J. & Gutterman J. (1987) Clinical investigation of human alpha interferon in chronic myelogenous leukemia. *Blood*, **69**, 1280–1288.

35 Kantarjian H.M., Deisseroth A., Kurzrock R., Estrov Z. & Talpaz M. (1993) Chronic myelogenous leukemia: a concise update. *Blood*, **82**, 691–703.

36 Heim S. & Mitelman F. (1987) Multistep cytogenetic scenario in chronic myeloid leukemia. In: *Advances in Viral Oncology* (ed. G. Klein), pp. 53–76. Raven Press, New York.

37 Anastasi J., Feng J., Le Beau M.M., Larson R.A., Rowley J.D. & Vardiman J.W. (1995) The relationship between secondary chromosomal abnormalities and blast transformation in chronic myelogenous leukemia. *Leukemia*, **9**, 628–633.

38 Costello R., Lafage M., Toiron Y. *et al.* (1995) Philadelphia chromosome-negative chronic myeloid leukaemia: a report of 14 new cases. *British Journal of Haematology*, **90**, 346–352.

39 Nowell P.C., Besa E.C., Stelmach T. & Finan J.B. (1986) Chromosome studies in preleukemic states. *Cancer*, **58**, 2571–2575.

40 Miller J.B., Testa J.R., Lindgren V. & Rowley J.D. (1985) The pattern and clinical significance of karyotypic abnormalities in patients with idiopathic and postpolycythaemic myelofibrosis. *Cancer*, **55**, 582–591.

41 Diez-Martin J.L., Graham D.L., Petitt R.M. & Dewald G.W. (1991) Chromosome studies in 104 patients with polycythemia vera. *Mayo Clinical Proceedings*, **66**, 287–299.

42 Rowley J.D. (1973) Identification of a translocation with quinacrine fluorescence in a patient with acute leukemia. *Annales Genetique (Paris)*, **16**, 109–112.

43 Rowley J.D. & Testa J.R. (1983) Chromosome abnormalities in malignant hematologic disorders. In: *Advances in Cancer Research*

(eds G. Klein & S. Weinhouse), pp. 103–148. Academic Press, New York.

44 Swirsky D.M., Li Y.S., Matthews J.G., Flemans R.J., Rees J.K.H. & Hayhoe F.G.J. (1984) 8;21 translocation in acute granulocytic leukaemia: cytological, cytochemical and clinical features. *British Journal of Haematology*, **56**, 199–213.

45 Bitter M.A., Le Beau M.M., Rowley J.D., Larson R.A., Golomb H.M. & Vardiman J.W. (1987) Association between morphology, karyotype, and clinical features in myeloid leukemias. *Human Pathology*, **18**, 211–225.

46 Swansbury J.G., Lawler S.D., Alimena G. *et al.* (1994) Long-term survival in acute myelogenous leukemia: a second follow-up of the Fourth International Workshop on Chromosomes in Leukemia. *Cancer Genetics and Cytogenetics*, **73**, 1–7.

47 Martinez-Climent J.A., Lane N.J., Rubin C.M. *et al.* (1995) Clinical and prognostic significance of chromosomal abnormalities in childhood acute myeloid leukemia de novo. *Leukemia*, **9**, 95–101.

48 Nucifora G. & Rowley J.D. (1995) AML1 and the 8;21 and 3;21 translocations in acute and chronic myeloid leukemia. *Blood*, **86**, 1–14.

49 Rowley J.D., Golomb H.M., Vardiman J., Fukuhara S., Dougherty C. & Potter P. (1977) Further evidence for a non-random chromosomal abnormality in acute promyelocytic leukemia. *International Journal of Cancer*, **20**, 869–872.

50 Larson R.A., Kondo K., Vardiman J., Butler A.E., Golomb H.M. & Rowley J.D. (1984) Evidence for a 15;17 translocation in every patient with acute promyelocytic leukemia. *American Journal of Medicine*, **76**, 827–841.

51 Lavau C. & Dejean A. (1994) The t(15;17) translocation in acute promyelocytic leukemia. *Leukemia*, **8**, 1615–1621.

52 Tallman M.S. & Rowe J.M. (1994) Acute promyelocytic leukemia: a paradigm for differentiation therapy with retinoic acid. *Haematological Oncology*, **8**, 70–78.

53 Arthur D.C. & Bloomfield C.D. (1983) Partial deletion of the long arm of chromosome 16 and bone marrow eosinophilia in acute nonlymphocytic leukemia: a new association. *Blood*, **61**, 994–998.

54 Larson R.A., Williams S.F., Le Beau M.M., Bitter M.A., Vardiman J.W. & Rowley J.D. (1986) Acute myelomonocytic leukemia with abnormal eosinophils and inv(16) or t(16;16) has a favourable prognosis. *Blood*, **68**, 1242–1249.

55 Liu P.P., Harja A., Wijmenga C. & Collins F.S. (1995) Molecular pathogenesis of the chromosome 16 inversion in the M4Eo subtype of acute myeloid leukemia. *Blood*, **85**, 2289–2302.

56 Mitelman F. & Heim S. (1992) Quantative acute leukemia cytogenetics. *Genes Chromosomes and Cancer*, **5**, 57–66.

57 Berger R., Bernheim A., Sigaux F., Daniel M.T., Valensi F. & Flandrin G. (1982) Acute monocytic leukemia chromosome studies. *Leukemia Research*, **6**, 17–26.

58 Pui C-H., Kane J.R. & Crist W.M. (1995) Biology and treatment of infant leukemias. *Leukemia*, **9**, 762–769.

59 Stasi R., Poeta G., Masi M. *et al.* (1993) Incidence of chromosome abnormalities and clinical significance of karyotype in *de novo* acute myeloid leukemia. *Cancer Genetics and Cytogenetics*, **67**, 28–34.

60 Sandoval C., Head D.R., Mirro J. Jr, Behm F.G., Ayers G.D. & Raimondi S.C. (1992) Translocation t(9;11)(p21;q23) in pediatric de novo and secondary acute myeloblastic leukemia. *Leukemia*, **6**, 513–519.

61 Raza A., Minowada J., Barcos M., Rakowski I. & Preisler H.D.

(1984) Ph¹-positive acute leukemia. *European Journal of Cancer and Clinical Oncology*, **20**, 1509–1516.

62 Bitter M.A., Neilly M.E., Le Beau M.M., Pearson M.G. & Rowley J.D. (1985) Rearrangements of chromosome 3 involving bands 3q21 and 3q26 are associated with normal or elevated platelet counts in acute nonlymphocytic leukemia. *Blood*, **66**, 1362–1370.

63 Fonatsch C., Gudat H., Lengfeldre E. *et al.* (1994) Correlation of cytogenetic findings with clinical features in 18 patients with inv(3)(q21q26) or t(3;3)(q21;q26). *Leukemia*, **8**, 1318–1326.

64 Pearson M.G., Vardiman J.W., Le Beau M.M. *et al.* (1985) Increased numbers of marrow basophils may be associated with a t(6;9) in ANLL. *American Journal of Haematology*, **18**, 393–403.

65 Lillington D.M., MacCullum P.H., Lister A.T. & Gibbons B. (1993) Translocation t(6;9)(p23;q34) in acute myeloid leukemia without myelodysplasia or basophilia: two cases and a review of the literature. *Leukemia*, **7**, 527–531.

66 Heim S., Avanzi G.C., Billstrom R. *et al.* (1987) A new specific chromosomal rearrangement, t(8;16)(p11;p13), in acute monocytic leukaemia. *British Journal of Haematology*, **66**, 323–326.

67 Carrol A., Civin C., Schneider N. *et al.* (1991) The t(1;22)(p13;q13) is nonrandom and restricted to infants with acute megakaryoblastic leukemia: a Paediatric Oncology Group study. *Blood*, **78**, 748–752.

68 Heim S. & Mitelman F. (1986) Numerical chromosome abberations in human neoplasia. *Cancer Genetics and Cytogenetics*, **22**, 99–108.

69 Ruutu P., Ruutu T., Vuopio P., Kosunen T.U. & de la Chapelle A. (1977) Defective chemotaxis in monosomy 7. *Nature*, **265**, 146–147.

70 Weiss K., Stass S., Williams D. *et al.* (1981) Childhood monosomy 7 syndrome: clinical and *in vitro* studies. *Leukemia*, **1**, 97–104.

71 Luna-Fineman S., Shannon K.M. & Lange B.J. (1995) Childhood monosomy 7: epidemiology, biology, and mechanistic implications. *Blood*, **85**, 1985–1999.

72 Carroll W.L., Morgan R. & Glader B.E. (1985) Childhood bone marrow monosomy 7 syndrome: a familial disorder? *Journal of Paediatrics*, **107**, 578–580.

73 Borgstrom G.H., Teerenhovi L., Voupio P. *et al.* (1980) Clinical implications of monosomy 7 in acute nonlymphocytic leukemia. *Cancer Genetics and Cytogenetics*, **2**, 115–126.

74 Sandberg A.A., Morgan R., Jani Sait S.N. *et al.* (1987) Trisomy 4: an entity within acute nonlymphocytic leukemia. *Cancer Genetics and Cytogenetics*, **26**, 117–125.

75 Thompson P.W., Thompson E.N. & Whittaker J.A. (1989) Four cases of acute leukemia with trisomy 4. *Cancer Genetics and Cytogenetics*, **43**, 211–217.

76 Slovak M.L., Traweek S.T., Willman C.L. *et al.* (1995) Trisomy 11: an association with stem/progenitor cell immunophenotype. *British Journal of Haematology*, **90**, 266–273.

77 Baer M.R. & Bloomfield C.D. (1992) Trisomy 13 in acute leukemia. *Leukemia and Lymphoma*, **7**, 1–6.

78 Cortes J.E., Kantarjian H., O'Brien S., Pierce S., Freireich E.J. & Estey E. (1995) Clinical and prognostic significance of trisomy 21 in adult patients with acute myelogenous leukemia and myelodysplastic syndrome. *Leukemia*, **9**, 115–117.

79 Mufti G.J. (1992) Chromosomal deletions in the myelodysplastic syndrome. *Leukemia Research*, **16**, 35–41.

80 Morel P., Hebbar M., Lai J-L. *et al.* (1993) Cytogenetic analysis has strong independent prognostic value in *de novo* myelodysplastic syndromes and can be incorporated in a new scoring system: a report on 408 cases. *Leukemia*, **7**, 1315–1323.

81 Van den Berghe H., Cassiman J-J., David G., Fryns J-P., Michaux J-L. & Sokal G. (1974) Distinct haematological disorder with deletion of long arm of No. 5 chromosome. *Nature*, **251**, 437–438.

82 Pedersen B. & Jensen I.M. (1991) Clinical and prognostic implications of chromosome 5q deletions: 96 high resolution studied patients. *Leukemia*, **5**, 566–573.

83 Mecucci C., Van Orshoven A., Vermaelen K. *et al.* (1987) 11q-chromosome is associated with abnormal iron stores in myelodysplastic syndromes. *Cancer Genetics and Cytogenetics*, **27**, 39–44.

84 Groupe Français de Cytogénétique Hématologique (1986) Cytogenetics of chronic myelomonocytic leukemia. *Cancer Genetics and Cytogenetics*, **21**, 11–30.

85 Pierre R.V., Catovsky D., Mufti G.J. *et al.* (1989) Clinical–cytogenetic correlations in myelodysplasia (preleukemia). *Cancer Genetics and Cytogenetics*, **40**, 149–161.

86 Larripa I., Labal de Vinuesa M., Bengiò R. & Slavutsky I. (1987) Chromosome studies in human hematologic diseases: II. Myelodysplastic syndromes. *Hematologica*, **72**, 399–403.

87 Jacobs R.H., Cornbleet M.A., Vardiman J.W., Larson R.A., Le Beau M.M. & Rowley J.D. (1986) Prognostic implications of morphology and karyotype in primary myelodysplastic syndromes. *Blood*, **67**, 1765–1772.

88 Yunis J.J., Lobell M., Arnesen M.A. *et al.* (1988) Refined chromosome study helps define prognostic subgroups in most patients with primary myelodysplastic syndrome and acute myelogenous leukaemia. *British Journal of Haematology*, **68**, 189–194.

89 Horiike S., Taniwaki M., Misawa S. & Abe T. (1988) Chromosome abnormalities and karyotypic evolution in 83 patients with myelodysplastic syndrome and predictive value for prognosis. *Cancer*, **62**, 1129–1138.

90 Geddes A.D., Bowen D.T. & Jacobs A. (1990) Clonal karyotype abnormalities and clinical progress in the myelodysplastic syndrome. *British Journal of Haematology*, **76**, 194–202.

91 Le Beau M.M., Albain K.S., Larson R.A. *et al.* (1986) Clinical and cytogenetic correlations in 63 patients with therapy related myelodysplastic syndromes and acute nonlymphocytic leukemias: further evidence for characteristic abnormalities of chromosome nos. 5 and 7. *Journal of Clinical Oncology*, **4**, 325–345.

92 Johansson B., Mertens F., Heim S., Kristoffersson V. & Mitelman F. (1991) Cytogenetics of secondary myelodysplasia (sMDS) and acute nonlymphocytic leukemia (sANLL). *European Journal of Haematology*, **47**, 17–27.

93 Fenaux P., Lai J.L., Quiquadon I. *et al.* (1991) Therapy related myelodysplastic syndrome with no 'unfavourable' cytogenetic findings have a good response to intensive chemotherapy: a report on 15 cases. *Leukemia and Lymphoma*, **5**, 117–125.

94 Stewart E.L. & Secker-Walker L.M. (1986) Detection of the chromosomally abnormal clone in acute lymphoblastic leukemia. *Cancer Genetics and Cytogenetics*, **23**, 25–35.

95 Williams D.L., Raimondi S., Rivera G., George S. & Berard C.W. (1985) Presence of clonal chromosomal abnormalities in virtually all cases of acute lymphoblastic leukemia. *New England Journal of Medicine*, **313**, 640–641.

96 Pui C.-H., Crist W.M. & Look A.T. (1990) Biology and clinical significance of cytogenetic abnormalities in childhood acute lymphoblastic leukemia. *Blood*, **76**, 1449–1463.

97 Bloomfield C.D., Secker-Walker L.M., Goldman A.I. *et al.* (1987) Six-year follow-up of the clinical significance of karyotype in acute lymphoblastic leukemia. *Cancer Genetics and Cytogenetics*, **40**, 171–185.

98 Secker-Walker L.M. (1990) Prognostic and biological importance of chromosome findings in acute lymphoblastic leukemia. *Cancer Genetics and Cytogenetics*, **49**, 1–13.

99 Secker-Walker L.M. & Craig J.M. (1993) Prognostic implications of breakpoint and lineage heterogeneity in Philadelphia-positive acute lymphoblastic leukemia: a review. *Leukemia*, **7**, 147–151.

100 Pui C.-H. (1992) Acute leukemia with the t(4;11)(q21;q23). *Leukemia and Lymphoma*, **7**, 173–179.

101 Secker-Walker L.M., Chessells J.M., Stewart E.L., Swansbury G.J., Richards S. & Lawler S.D. (1989) Chromosomes and other prognostic factors in acute lymphoblastic leukaemia: a long term follow-up. *British Journal of Haematology*, **72**, 336–342.

102 Dastugue N., Robert A., Payen C. *et al.* (1992) Prognostic significance of karyotype in a twelve-year follow-up in childhood acute lymphoblastic leukemia. *Cancer Genetics and Cytogenetics*, **64**, 49–55.

103 Pui C.-H., Raimondi S.C., Dodge R.K. *et al.* (1989) Prognostic importance of structural abnormalities in children with hyperdiploid (>50 chromosomes) acute lymphoblastic leukemia. *Blood*, **73**, 1963–1967.

104 Raimondi S.C., Roberson P.K., Pui C.-H., Behm F.G. & Rivera G.K. (1992) Hyperdiploid (47–50) acute lymphoblastic leukemia in children. *Blood*, **79**, 3245–3252.

105 Rivera G.K., Raimondi S.C., Hancock M.L. *et al.* (1991) Improved outcome in childhood acute lymphoblastic leukaemia with reinforced early treatment and rotational combinational chemotherapy. *Lancet*, **337**, 61–65.

106 Williams D.L., Harber J., Murphy S.B. *et al.* (1986) Chromosomal translocations play a unique role in influencing prognosis in childhood acute lymphoblastic leukaemia. *Blood*, **68**, 728–731.

107 Lampert F., Harbott J., Ritterbach J. *et al.* (1991) Karyotypes in acute childhood leukemias may lose prognostic significance with more intensive and specific chemotherapy. *Cancer Genetics and Cytogenetics*, **54**, 277–279.

108 Pui C.-H., Williams D.L., Raimondi S.C. *et al.* (1987) Hypodiploidy is associated with a poor prognosis in childhood acute lymphoblastic leukemia. *Blood*, **70**, 247–253.

109 Betts D.R., Kingston J.E., Dorey E.L. *et al.* (1990) Monosomy 20: a nonrandom finding in childhood acute lymphoblastic leukemia. *Genes Chromosomes and Cancer*, **2**, 182–185.

110 Gibbons B., MacCallum P., Watts E. *et al.* (1991) Near haploid acute lymphoblastic leukemia: seven new cases and a review of the literature. *Leukemia*, **5**, 738–743.

111 Carroll A.J., Crist W.M., Parmley R.T., Roper M. & Finley W.H. (1984) Pre-B cell leukemia associated with chromosome translocation 1;19. *Blood*, **63**, 721–724.

112 Raimondi S.C., Behm F.G., Robertson P.K. *et al.* (1990) Cytogenetics of pre-B cell acute lymphoblastic leukemia with emphasis on prognostic implications of the t(1;19). *Journal of Clinical Oncology*, **8**, 1380–1388.

113 Troussard X., Rimokh R., Valensi F. *et al.* (1995) Heterogeneity of t(1;19)(q23;p13) acute leukaemias. *British Journal of Haematology*, **89**, 516–526.

114 Crist W.M., Carroll A.J., Shuster J.J. *et al.* (1990) Poor prognosis of children with pre-B acute lymphoblastic leukemia is associated with the t(1;19)(q23;p13): a Pediatric Oncology Group study. *Blood*, **76**, 117–122.

115 Secker-Walker L.M., Berger R., Fenaux P. *et al.* (1992) Prognostic significance of the balanced t(1;19) and unbalanced der(19)t(1;19) translocations in acute lymphoblastic leukemia. *Leukemia*, **6**, 363–369.

116 Fletcher J.A., Lynch E.A., Kimball V.M., Donnelly M., Tantravahi R. & Sallan S.E. (1991) Translocation t(9;22) is associated with extremely poor prognosis in intensively treated children with acute lymphoblastic leukemia. *Blood*, **77**, 435–439.

117 Westbrook C.A., Hooberman A.L., Spino C. *et al.* (1992) Clinical significance of the BCR-ABL fusion gene in adult acute lymphoblastic leukemia: a cancer and leukemia group B study (8762). *Blood*, **80**, 2983–2990.

118 Pui C.-H., Frankel L.S., Carroll A.J. *et al.* (1991) Clinical characteristics and treatment outcome of childhood acute lymphoblastic leukemia with the t(4;11)(q21;q23): a collaborative study of 40 cases. *Blood*, **77**, 440–447.

119 Pui C.-H., Carroll A.J., Raimondi S.C., Shuster J.J., Crist W.M. & Pullen D.J. (1994) Childhood acute lymphoblastic leukemia with the t(4;11)(q21;q23): an update. *Blood*, **83**, 2384–2385.

120 Heim S., Bekassy A.N., Garwitz S. *et al.* (1987) New structural chromosomal rearrangements in congenital leukemia. *Leukemia*, **1**, 16–23.

121 Strong R.C., Korsmeyer S.J., Parkin J.L., Arthur D.C. & Kersey S.H. (1985) Human acute leukemia cell line with the t(4;11) chromosomal rearrangement exhibits B lineage and monocytic characteristics. *Blood*, **65**, 21–31.

122 Kaneko Y., Maseki N., Takasaki N. *et al.* (1986) Clinical characteristics in acute lymphoblastic leukemia with 11q23 translocations. *Blood*, **67**, 484–491.

123 Cimino G., Rapanotti M.C., Rivolta A. *et al.* (1995) Prognostic significance of ALL-1 gene rearrangements in infant acute leukemias. *Leukemia*, **9**, 391–395.

124 Berger R. & Bernheim A. (1985) Cytogenetics of Burkitt's lymphoma-leukaemia: a review. In: *Burkitt's Lymphoma: a human cancer model.* (eds G. Lenoir, G. O'Connor & C.L.M. Olweny), pp. 65–80. Scientific Publication, No. 60. IARC, Lyon.

125 Murphy S.B., Bowman W.P., Abromowitch M. *et al.* (1986) Results of treatment of advanced stage Burkitt's lymphoma and B-cell (sIg+) acute lymphoblastic leukemia with high-dose fractionated cyclophosphamide and coordinated high-dose methotrexate and cytarabine. *Journal of Clinical Oncology*, **4**, 1732–1739.

126 Raimondi S.C., Behm F.G., Roberson P.K. *et al.* (1988) Cytogenetics of childhood T-cell leukemia. *Blood*, **72**, 1560–1566.

127 Pui C.-H., Behm F.G., Singh B. *et al.* (1990) Heterogeneity of presenting features and their relation to treatment outcome in 120 children with T-cell acute lymphoblastic leukemia. *Blood*, **75**, 174–179.

128 Hayashi Y., Raimondi S.C., Look A.T. *et al.* (1990) Abnormalities of the long arm of chromosome 6 in childhood acute lymphoblastic leukemia. *Blood*, **76**, 1626–1630.

129 Raimondi S.C., Williams D.L., Callihan T., Peiper S., Rivera G.K. & Murphy S.B. (1986) Nonrandom involvement of the 12p12 breakpoint in chromosome abnormalities of childhood acute lymphoblastic leukemia. *Blood*, **68**, 69–75.

130 Murphy S.B., Raimondi S.C., Rivera G.K. *et al.* (1989) Nonrandom abnormalities of chromosome 9p in childhood acute lymphoblastic leukemia: association with high-risk clinical features. *Blood*, **74**, 409–415.

131 Juliusson G., Oscier D.G., Fitchett M. *et al.* (1990) Prognostic subgroups in B-cell chronic lymphocytic leukemia defined by specific chromosomal abnormalities. *New England Journal of Medicine*, **323**, 720–724.

132 Ross F.M. & Stockhill G. (1987) Clonal chromosome abnormalities in chronic lymphocytic leukemia patients revealed by TPA stimulation of whole blood cultures. *Cancer Genetics and Cytogenetics*, **25**, 109–121.

133 Castoldi G.L., Lanza F. & Cuneo A. (1987) Cytogenetic aspects of B-cell chronic lymphocytic leukemia: their correlation with clinical stage and different polyclonal mitogens. *Cancer Genetics and Cytogenetics*, **26**, 75–84.

134 Peterson L.C., Lindquist L., Church S. & Kay N.E. (1992) Frequent clonal abnormalities of chromosome 13q14 in B-cell chronic lymphocytic leukemia: multiple clones, subclones and nonclonal alterations in 82 midwestern patients. *Genes Chromosomes and Cancer*, **4**, 273–280.

135 Bentz M., Huck K., du Manoir S. *et al.* (1995) Comparative Genomic Hybridization in chronic B-cell leukemias shows a high incidence of chromosomal gains and losses. *Blood*, **85**, 3610–3618.

136 Nowell P.C., Moreau L., Growney P. & Besa E.C. (1988) Karyotypic stability in chronic B-cell leukemia. *Cancer Genetics and Cytogenetics*, **33**, 155–160.

137 Juliusson G., Friberg K. & Garhton G. (1988) Consistency of chromosome aberrations in chronic B-lymphocytic leukemia. *Cancer*, **62**, 500–506.

138 Oscier D., Fitchett M., Herbert T. *et al.* (1991) Karyotypic evolution in B-cell chronic lymphocytic leukaemia. *Genes Chromosomes and Cancer*, **3**, 16–20.

139 Lai J.L., Zandecki M., Mary J.Y. *et al.* (1995) Improved cytogenetics in multiple myeloma: a study of 151 patients including 117 patients at diagnosis. *Blood*, **85**, 2490–2497.

140 Smadja N.V., Louvet C., Isnard F. *et al.* (1995) Cytogenetic study in multiple myeloma at diagnosis: comparison of two techniques. *British Journal of Haematology*, **90**, 619–624.

141 Taniwaki M., Nishida K., Takashima T. *et al.* (1994) Nonrandom chromosomal rearrangements of 14q32.3 and 19p13.3 and preferential deletion of 1p in 21 patients with multiple myeloma and plasma cell leukemia. *Blood*, **84**, 2282–2290.

142 Yunis J.J., Oken M.M., Kaplan M.E., Ensurd B.S., Howe R.H. & Theologides A. (1982) Distinctive chromosomal abnormalities in histological subtypes of non-Hodgkin's lymphoma. *New England Journal of Medicine*, **307**, 1231–1236.

143 Tilley H., Rossi A., Stamatoullas A. *et al.* (1994) Prognostic value of chromosomal abnormalities in follicular lymphoma. *Blood*, **84**, 1043–1049.

144 Pirc-Danoewinata H., Chott A., Onderka E. *et al.* (1994) Karyotype and prognosis in non-Hodgkin's lymphoma. *Leukemia*, **8**, 1929–1939.

145 Trent J.M., Kaneko Y. & Mitelman F. (1989) Report of the committee on structural chromosome changes in neoplasia. Human Gene Mapping 10: Tenth International Workshop on Human Gene Mapping. *Cytogenetics and Cell Genetics*, **51**, 533–562.

146 Griesser H., Tkachuk D., Reis M.D. & Mak T.W. (1989) Gene rearrangements and translocations in lymphoproliferative diseases. *Blood*, **73**, 1402–1415.

147 Dalla-Favera R., Bregni M., Erickson J., Patterson D., Gallo R.C. & Croce C.M. (1982) Human c-*myc* oncogene is located on the region of chromosome 8 that is translocated in Burkitt's lymphoma cells. *Proceedings of the National Academy of Sciences, USA*, **79**, 7824–7827.

148 Weiss L.M., Warnke R.A., Sklar J. & Cleary M.L. (1987) Molecular analysis of the t(14;18) chromosomal translocation in malignant lymphomas. *New England Journal of Medicine*, **317**, 1185–1189.

149 Van den Berghe H., Parloir C., David G., Michauk J.L. & Sokal G.

(1979) A new characteristic karyotypic abnormality in lympho-proliferative disorders. *Cancer*, **44**, 188–195.

150 Schlegelberger B., Himmler A., Gödde E., Grote W., Feller A.C. & Lennert K. (1994) Cytogenetic findings in peripheral T-cell lymphomas as a basis for distinguishing low-grade and high-grade lymphomas. *Blood*, **83**, 505–511.

151 Zaccaria A., Rosti G., Testoni N. *et al.* (1987) Chromosome studies in patients with a Philadelphia chromosome-positive chronic myeloid leukemia submitted to bone marrow transplantation—results of a European cooperative study. *Cancer Genetics and Cytogenetics*, **26**, 5–13.

152 Zaccaria A., Rosti G., Testoni N. *et al.* (1987) Chromosome studies in patients with acute nonlymphocytic or acute lymphocytic leukemia submitted to bone marrow transplantation—results of a European cooperative study. *Cancer Genetics and Cytogenetics*, **26**, 51–58.

153 Lawler S.D., Baker M.C., Harris H. & Morgenstern G.R. (1984) Cytogenetic studies on recipients of allogeneic bone marrow using the sex chromosomes as markers of cellular origin. *British Journal of Haematology*, **56**, 431–443.

154 Walker H., Singer C.R.J., Patterson J., Goldstone A.H. & Prentice H.G. (1986) The significance of host haemopoietic cells detected by cytogenetic analysis of bone marrow transplants. *British Journal of Haematology*, **62**, 385–391.

155 Petz L.D., Yam P., Wallace B. *et al.* (1987) Mixed hematopoietic chimerism following bone marrow transplantation for haematological malignancies. *Blood*, **70**, 1331–1337.

156 Schmitz N., Johannson W., Schmidt G., von der Helm K. & Löffler H. (1987) Recurrence of acute lymphoblastic leukemia in donor cells after allogeneic transplantation associated with a deletion of the long arm of chromosome 6. *Blood*, **70**, 1099–1104.

157 Palka G., Calabrese G., Di Girolamo G. *et al.* (1991) Cytogenetic survey of 31 patients treated with bone marrow transplantation for acute nonlymphocytic and acute lymphoblastic leukemias. *Cancer Genetics and Cytogenetics*, **51**, 223–233.

158 McCann S.R. & Lawler M. (1993) Mixed chimaerism; detection and significance following BMT. *Bone Marrow Transplantation*, **11**, 91–94.

159 Kögler G., Wolf H.H., Heyll A., Arkesteijn G. & Wernet P. (1995) Detection of mixed chimerism and leukemic relapse after allogeneic bone marrow transplantation in subpopulations of leucocytes by fluorescent *in situ* hybridization in combination with the simultaneous immunophenotypic analysis of interphase cells. *Bone Marrow Transplantation*, **15**, 41–48.

160 Apperley J.F., Jones J., Hale G. *et al.* (1991) Bone marrow transplantation for patients with chronic myeloid leukaemia: T-cell depletion with Campath-1 reduces the incidence of graft-versus-host disease but may increase the risk of leukaemic relapse. *Bone Marrow Transplantation*, **1**, 53–66.

161 Ferrant A., Doyen C., Delannoy A. *et al.* (1995) Karyotype in acute myeloblastic leukemia: prognostic significance in a prospective study assessing bone marrow transplantation in first remission. *Bone Marrow Transplantation*, **15**, 685–690.

162 Gale R.P., Horowitz M.M., Weiner R.S. *et al.* (1995) Impact of cytogenetic abnormalities on outcome of bone marrow transplants in acute myelogenous leukemia in first remission. *Bone Marrow Transplantation*, **16**, 203–208.

163 Wilkinson D.G. (ed.) (1992) *In situ Hybridization: a practical approach*. Oxford University Press, New York.

164 Lichter P. & Cremer T. (1992) Chromosome analysis by non-isotopic *in situ* hybridization. In: *Human Cytogenetics: a practical approach*. Vol. I. (eds D.E. Rooney & B.H. Czepulkowski), pp. 157–192. Oxford University Press, New York.

165 Choo K.H.A. (ed.) (1994) *Methods in Molecular Biology 33. In situ hybridization protocols*. Humana Press, Totowa, New Jersey.

166 Perez Losoda A., Wessman M., Tianinen M. *et al.* (1991) Trisomy 12 in chronic lymphocytic leukemia: an interphase cytogenetic study. *Blood*, **78**, 775–779.

167 Jenkins R.B., Le Beau M.M., Kraker W.J. *et al.* (1992) Fluorescence *in situ* hybridization: a sensitive method for trisomy 8 detection in bone marrow specimens. *Blood*, **79**, 3307–3315.

168 Lichter P., Cremer T., Borden J., Manuelidis L. & Ward D.C. (1988) Delineation of individual human chromosomes in metaphase and interphase cells by *in situ* suppression hybridization using recombinant DNA libraries. *Human Genetics*, **80**, 224–234.

169 Goa J., Erickson P., Gardiner K. *et al.* (1991) Isolation of a yeast artificial chromosome spanning the 8;21 translocation breakpoint t(8;21)(q22;q22.3) in acute myelogenous leukemia. *Proceedings of the National Academy of Science, USA*, **88**, 4882–4886.

170 Warrell R.P., de The' H., Wang Z.Y. & Degos L. (1994) Acute promyelocytic leukemia. *New England Journal of Medicine*, **329**, 177–189.

171 Dauwerse J.G., Wessels J.W., Giles R.H. *et al.* (1993) Cloning the breakpoint cluster region of the inv(16) in acute nonlymphocytic leukemia M4Eo. *Human Molecular Genetics*, **2**, 1527–1534.

172 Kearney L., Bower M., Gibbons B. *et al.* (1992) Chromosome 11q23 translocations in both infant and adult acute leukemias are detected by *in situ* hybridization with a yeast artificial chromosome. *Blood*, **80**, 1659–1665.

173 Tkachuk D.C., Westbrook C.A., Andreef M. *et al.* (1990) Detection of the bcr-abl fusion in chronic myelogenous leukemia by *in situ* hybridization. *Science*, **250**, 559–562.

174 Bentz M., Cabot G., Moos M. *et al.* (1994) Detection of chimeric BCR-ABL genes on bone marrow samples and blood smears in chronic myeloid and acute lymphoblastic leukemia by *in situ* hybridization. *Blood*, **83**, 1922–1928.

175 Stilgenbauer S., Döhner H., Bulgay-Mörschel M., Weitz S., Bentz M. & Lichter P. (1993) Retinoblastoma gene deletion in chronic lymphocytic leukemias: a combined metaphase and interphase cytogenetic study. *Blood*, **81**, 2118–2124.

176 Taniwaki M., Matsuda F., Jauch A. *et al.* (1994) Detection of 14q32 translocations in B-cell malignancies by *in situ* hybridization with yeast artificial chromosome clones containing the human IgH gene locus. *Blood*, **83**, 2962–2969.

177 Veronese M.L., Ohta M., Finan J., Nowell P.C. & Croce C.M. (1995) Detection of myc translocations in lymphoma cells by fluorescence *in situ* hybridization with yeast artificial chromosomes. *Blood*, **85**, 2132–2138.

178 Kallioniemi A., Kallioniemi O-P., Sudar D. *et al.* (1992) Comparative genome hybridization for molecular cytogenetic analysis of solid tumours. *Science*, **258**, 818–821.

179 Bentz M., Schröder M., Herz M., Stilgenbaur S., Lichter P. & Döhner H. (1993) Detection of trisomy 8 on blood smears using fluorescence *in situ* hybridization. *Leukemia*, **7**, 752–757.

180 Baurmann H., Cherif D. & Berger R. (1993) Interphase cytogenetics by fluorescence *in situ* hybridization (FISH) for characterization of myeloid disorders. *Leukemia*, **7**, 384–391.

181 Kibbelar R.E., Mulder J.W.R., Dreef E.J. *et al.* (1993) Detection of monosomy 7 and trisomy 8 in myeloid neoplasia: a comparison of banding and fluorescence *in situ* hybridization. *Blood*, **82**, 904–913.

182 Anastasi J., Le Beau M.M., Vardimar J.W. & Westbrook C.A. (1990) Detection of bcr-abl fusion in chronic myelogenous leukemia by *in situ* hybridization. *Science*, **250**, 559–562.

183 Chen Z., Morgan R., Berger C.S., Pearce-Birge L., Stone J.F. & Sandberg A.A. (1993) Identification of masked and variant Ph (complex type) translocations in CML and classic Ph in AML and ALL by fluorescence *in situ* hybridization with the use of bcr/abl cosmid probes. *Cancer Genetics and Cytogenetics*, **70**, 103–107.

184 van Rhee F., Kasprzyk A., Jamil A. *et al.* (1995) Detection of the BCR-ABL gene by reverse transcription/polymerase chain reaction and fluorescence *in situ* hybridization in a patient with Philadelphia chromosome negative acute lymphoblastic leukaemia. *British Journal of Haematology*, **90**, 225–228.

185 Anastasi J., Thangavelu M., Vardiman J.W. *et al.* (1991) Interphase cytogenetic analysis detects minimal residual disease in a case of acute lymphoblastic leukemia and resolves the question of origin of relapse after bone marrow transplantation. *Blood*, **77**, 1087–1091.

186 Anastasi J., Vardiman J.W., Rudinsky R. *et al.* (1991) Direct correlation of cytogenetic findings with cell morphology using *in situ* hybridization: an analysis of suspicious cells in bone marrow specimens of two patients completing therapy for acute lymphoblastic leukemia. *Blood*, **77**, 2456–2462.

187 Heerma N.A., Argyropoulos G., Weetman R., Tricot G. & Secker-Walker L.M. (1993) Interphase *in situ* hybridization reveals minimal residual disease in early remission and return of the diagnostic clone in karyotypically normal relapse of acute lymphoblastic leukemia. *Leukemia*, **7**, 537–543.

188 Nylund S.J., Ruutu T., Saarinen U., Larramendy M.L. & Knuutila S. (1994) Detection of minimal residual disease using fluorescence *in situ* hybridization: a follow-up study in leukemia and lymphoma patients. *Leukemia*, **8**, 587–594.

189 Anastasi J., Le Beau M.M., Vardiman J.W., Fernald A.A., Larson R.A. & Rowley J.D. (1992) Detection of trisomy 12 in chronic lymphocytic leukemia by fluorescence *in situ* hybridization to interphase cells: a simple and sensitive method. *Blood*, **79**, 1796–1801.

190 Escudies S.M., Pereira-Leahy J.M., Drach J.W. *et al.* (1993) Fluorescence *in situ* hybridization and cytogenetic studies of trisomy 12 in chronic lymphocytic leukemia. *Blood*, **81**, 2702–2707.

191 Que T.H., Marco J.G., Ellis J. *et al.* (1993) Trisomy 12 in chronic lymphocytic leukemia detected by fluorescence *in situ* hybridization: analysis by stage, immunophenotype, and morphology. *Blood*, **82**, 571–575.

192 Döhner H., Piltz T., Fischer K. *et al.* (1994) Molecular cytogenetic analysis of RB-1 deletions in chronic B-cell leukemias. *Leukemia and Lymphoma*, **16**, 97–103.

193 Zhao L., Chang K-S., Estey E.H., Hayes K., Deisseroth A.B. & Liang J.C. (1995) Detection of residual leukemic cells in patients with acute promyelocytic leukemia by the fluorescence *in situ* hybridization method: potential for predicting relapse. *Blood*, **85**, 495–499.

4   Immunophenotyping

D. Campana and F.G. Behm

Introduction

Haematological malignancies were first characterized immunophenotypically after the development of heterologous antisera against human haemopoietic cells [1]. The first reagents to be used included antisera to T cells, immunoglobulin (Ig) heavy and light chains, common acute lymphoblastic leukaemia (ALL) antigen, major histocompatibility complex (MHC)-Class II molecules and terminal deoxynucleotidyl transferase (TdT). At the same time, the selective capacity of T-lineage cells to form 'rosettes' with sheep erythrocytes was exploited to identify T-ALL blasts, while B-cell chronic lymphocytic leukaemia (B-CLL) cells were found to form rosettes with mouse erythrocytes [1].

With the development of monoclonal antibody (MAb) technology, the increasing commercial availability of these reagents, and the refinement and simplification of immunophenotyping techniques, the immunological study of malignant cells has become a routinely used tool in the clinical management of leukaemia and lymphoma. The selection of clinically useful reagents has been facilitated through periodic International Workshops on Leucocyte Differentiation Antigens [2–7], in which newly developed MAbs have been extensively studied and related to clusters of differentiation (CD). The MAbs within each CD recognize the same antigen, as determined by immunoprecipitation and/or binding inhibition experiments. Thus they have a similar, although not always identical, reactivity with cells and tissues. One hundred and sixty-six CDs have been defined so far [2–7].

There has been remarkable progress not only in the number of reagents available but also in the sensitivity and accuracy of antibody binding detection. Double and triple marker staining techniques, which allow the precise investigation of the phenotype of cell subsets, have become common procedures [8–11]. Modern flow cytometers can precisely analyse not only fluorescence labelling but also cell size and granularity with a single laser system. Thus, sophisticated immunophenotypic studies can be carried out on morphologically defined cell subpopulations. Flow cytometry, because of its speed and informative power, has become the 'gold standard' among immunophenotyping techniques. Other staining methods, such as immunoperoxidase and immunoalkaline phosphatase [12,13], as well as immunogold [10,14], allow a visual correlation between antibody binding and the cellular morphology to which haematologists are more accustomed. However, these techniques are clearly less suitable for double and triple marker analysis, antigen quantitation and analysis of a large number of cells.

The clinically relevant objectives of leukaemia and lymphoma cell marker analysis are:

1 to establish the lineage affiliation of neoplastic cells;

2 to identify prognostic indicators which may aid in treatment decisions;

3 to define leukaemia-associated phenotypic features which may be used to detect minimal residual disease.

Thus, the information gained via appropriate immunophenotyping techniques may play a crucial role in selecting the optimal therapeutic strategy for individual patients.

Normal lymphohaemopoietic differentiation

Phenotypic development of lymphoid cells

If B- and T-cell progenitors are to differentiate and become mature lymphocytes, their Ig and T-cell receptor (TCR) genes must undergo productive rearrangement. The expression of molecules critical for these processes, TdT and the products of the recombinase genes RAG1 and RAG2, is highest at the earliest stages of lymphoid development [8,9,15–19]. If such gene rearrangements are successful, a variety of phenotypic and proliferative changes take place. These occur in the central lymphoid organs, which are the bone marrow for B cells and the thymus for T cells.

B-lineage

Immature B-lineage cells which lack surface immunoglobulins are CD22 [20], CD19 [20–22], CD79 [23] and CD10+ (Fig. 4.1) [8,20,22,24]. The most immature cells express CD34 and nuclear TdT, while the most mature subset is characterized by cytoplasmic expression of mu heavy chains (Fig. 4.1) [8,20,25]. Several other B-cell-associated antigens are expressed in these progenitor cells, as shown in Fig. 4.1. When normal B-cell differentiation is completed successfully, Ig light chains kappa or lambda are coupled to the mu heavy chains and monomeric Ig molecules are inserted into the cell membrane (Fig. 4.1). This stage is preceded by the surface expression of mu chains with pseudolight chains, λ5 and VpreB [26,27]. Subsequently, B cells migrate to the peripheral lymphoid organs, although B-lymphocyte traffic in the opposite direction has also been demonstrated [28]. Thus, surface IgM (sIgM)+ lymphocytes found in the bone marrow are a mixed population of early and mature B lymphocytes. TdT expression gradually diminishes during development and is absent in most cμ+ pre-B cells and virtually all sIg+ B cells [8,16].

Many early B-cell progenitors, including pre-B cells, have a high rate of proliferation, as indicated by their expression of Ki67 and incorporation of bromodeoxyuridine [29]. Prolifera-

tion ceases when sIg is expressed [25,29,30]. Most sIg+ lymphocytes in the bone marrow and peripheral blood are in G₀, but their cell division cycle may restart in the peripheral lymphoid organs.

T-lineage

T cells undergo stepwise phenotypic and proliferative changes that parallel the synthesis and expression of TCR proteins. TCR chains are assembled with the CD3 chains in the rough endoplasmic reticulum before membrane insertion of the full TCR/CD3 complex [31]. Thus, immature T cells may express individual TCR or CD3 chains exclusively in cytoplasm (Fig. 4.2), as demonstrated in suspensions of fetal and infant thymocytes labelled with CD3 MAbs. Such samples contain three distinct cell subpopulations: membrane CD3 (mCD3)–, mCD3+dim and mCD3+bright [32,33]. In the mCD3– cells, cytoplasmic CD3 (cCD3) and membrane CD7 are detectable in virtually all cells, while CD2, CD5, CD4 and CD8 are expressed heterogeneously [34–40] (Fig. 4.2). The expression of TCR proteins can also be used to identify intermediate stages of differentiation in such immature cells. The most undifferentiated cells lack TCR protein expression, while more differentiated cells express either TCRα or TCRβ chains (Fig. 4.2). In the mCD3+dim cell population, which represents most of the cortical thymocytes, most cells express CD7, CD2, CD5 and CD1a, as well as CD4 and CD8, simultaneously [34,35,40] (Fig. 4.2). The vast majority of these cells in fetal and postnatal thymus express TCRαβ proteins in association with CD3 molecules on the cell membrane [32,39,41] (Fig. 4.2). Finally, mature mCD3+bright thymic cells resemble peripheral blood T cells and express either CD4 or CD8 in addition to CD7, CD2 and CD5 [34,35,40] (Fig. 4.2). Spontaneous dividing activity in mCD3– and mCD3+dim thymocytes is high and intermediate, respectively [29,42]. Such activity is absent in the mCD3+bright cell population [29,42].

TCRγδ cells comprise a minor proportion of maturing thymocytes and T-lymphocytes in peripheral tissues [43,44]. Patients with complete DiGeorge syndrome, who lack a thymic gland and TCRαβ lymphocytes, have normal numbers

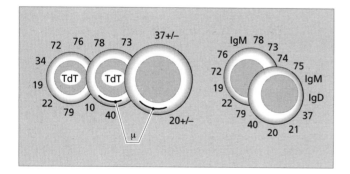

Fig. 4.1 Some of the phenotypic changes which occur during human B-cell development. The numbers shown correspond to different CDs. Immature B cells also express *RAG-1* and *RAG-2* genes.

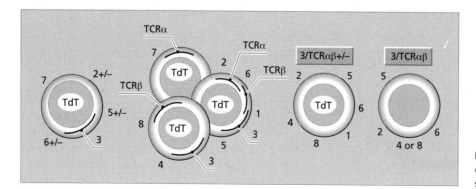

Fig. 4.2 TCR protein and cell marker differentiation in the thymus. The numbers shown correspond to different CDs.

Table 4.1 Immunophenotypic features of primitive haemopoietic progenitor cells.

Reference	CD34	HLA-DR	CD38	Thy1	Rho123	CD71
Huang & Terstappen [62]	+	+	–	+	NA	NA
Craig *et al.* [63]	+	NA	Dull	+	Dull	Dull
Verfaillie *et al.* [64]	+	–	NA	NA	NA	NA
Brand *et al.* [65]	+	–	NA	NA	NA	–
Baum *et al.* [66]	+	NA	NA	+	Dull	NA

NA = not assessed.

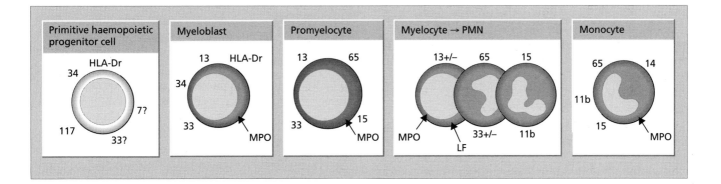

Fig. 4.3 Some of the phenotypic changes which occur during myeloid differentiation. The numbers shown correspond to different CDs. HLA = human leucocyte antigen; LF = lactoferrin; MPO = myeloperoxidase; PMN = polymorphonuclear neutrophils.

of TCRγδ cells, implying that the thymic microenvironment is not essential for their development [45].

Phenotypic development of nonlymphoid haemopoietic cells

The immunophenotypic development of myeloid cells is accompanied by morphological changes (Fig. 4.3). Myeloblasts strongly express myeloid associated markers such as CD13 and CD33 [46–48], as well as MHC-Class II [49] and CD34 [50,51]. Expression of the latter molecules decreases with cell differentiation and becomes undetectable in myelocytes and metamyelocytes. These changes are paralleled by an increase in CD15 and CD65. Monocytes strongly express CD14 [52] and CD11b [53] molecules. The detection of two intracellular molecules, myeloperoxidase and lactoferrin, may advance the immunological definition of myeloid cells. These molecules can now be detected by specific antibodies after cell permeabilization. Myeloblasts and promyelocytes are myeloperoxidase positive but lactoferrin negative [54]. A similar pattern of expression is found in monocytes [54].

Erythroid progenitor cells are distinguishable by the strong expression of glycophorin [55,56], whereas megakaryocytes and platelets exhibit CD41 (gpIIb/IIIa) [57,58], CD42a (gpIX) [57,58], CD42b (gpIb) [57–59] and CD61 (gpIIIa) [57,58,60,61].

Immunophenotypic features of primitive haemopoietic progenitor cells

The identification and characterization of haemopoietic stem cells is limited by a lack of well-defined and objective assays for self-renewal activity. Reported studies have usually relied on sorting specific subsets of bone marrow or cord blood cells and subsequently assessing their growth and differentiation *in vitro*. A general consensus is that primitive haematopoietic progenitor cells are CD34+ (Table 4.1). Huang & Terstappen have shown enrichment of cells with self-renewal capacity within the CD34+, HLA-Dr+, CD38– subset [62]. Lansdorp and collegues found similar growth abilities within the CD34+, Thy1+ cells that express CD38 and CD71 dimly [63]. Some investigators have used CD34 positivity and MHC-Class II negativity as important criteria [64,65], while others have considered CD34+ cells negative for CD19, CD13 and CD33 to be the most distinguished features [66].

Classification of acute leukaemia

Selection of reagents and methods

Among the many antibodies available, only a few appear to have a lineage-restricted reactivity in normal and leukaemic haemopoietic cells. These include CD79 for B cells, CD3 for T cells and antimyeloperoxidase for myeloid cells. These mole-

Table 4.2 Immunological classification of ALL.

Subtype	CD19	CD79	CD22*	cIgμ	sIgM	sIgκ or sIgλ	CD7	CD3*	Frequency (%)
Early Pre-B	+	+	+	–	–	–	–	–	60–65
Pre-B	+	+	+	+	–	–	–	–	20–25
Transitional Pre-B	+	+	+	+	+	–	–	–	1–2
B	+	+	+	+	+	+	–	–	2
T	–	–	–	–	–	–	+	+	15–18

* Cytoplasmic or surface expression.

cules appear to be strongly linked to the developmental programme of the individual lineages and are the most useful in leukaemia immunophenotyping. These reagents should allow successful lineage identification of blasts in nearly all cases of acute leukaemia and blast crisis of chronic granulocytic leukaemia. Other useful antibodies, albeit less specific, include CD19, CD22, CD5, CD7, CD13, CD33, glycophorin and CD61 (reviewed in ref. [67]).

Many important markers for leukaemia diagnosis are exclusively or predominantly intracellular and can be detected only via cell membrane permeabilization. Firstly, most CD79 antibodies recognize cytoplasmic domains of either the mb1 (CD79α) or the B29 (CD79β) components of the B-cell antigen receptor complex [23,68]. Secondly, some MAbs of the CD22 cluster react with epitopes which may also be undetectable in unpermeabilized cells [20,69–71]. The proportion of cases in which blast cell CD22 is detectable without membrane permeabilization is not clear, and disparate results have been reported [20,69–72]. These discrepancies may be due to the heterogeneous reactivity of individual MAbs within the CD22 cluster [73]. A third example is represented by the reactivity of CD3 MAbs. Due to their cytoplasmic location in immature T cells (see above), the molecules recognized by these reagents often are undetectable on the cell membrane of T-ALL blasts but are seen in blast cell cytoplasm in virtually all T-ALLs [37,38,74–76]. Myeloperoxidase and nuclear TdT can be detected only in permeabilized cells. Finally, intermediate stages of B- and T-cell differentiation, marked by the cytoplasmic expression of Ig and TCR chains, respectively, can be identified only by labelling with the corresponding antibodies after membrane permeabilization [77,78] (Figs 4.1 & 4.2).

In the past, intracellular antigens were optimally detected by staining cytospins or smears, because cell-permeabilization methods to stain cell suspensions for flow cytometric analysis were too harsh on cell morphology. More recently developed reagents, however, allow intracytoplasmic staining in suspension with optimal preservation of the cell morphology. These include Ortho Permeafix (Ortho, Raritan, NJ, USA) [79] and Fix & Perm (Am de Grube, Vienna, Austria; Caltag, San Francisco, CA, USA) [54].

B-lineage acute lymphoblastic leukaemia

Between 80 and 90% of newly diagnosed cases of ALL are B-lineage (Table 4.2). Typically, leukaemic cells are CD19+, CD22+ and CD79+ [21,23,71,80,81]. The B-lineage association of these leukaemias is not only demonstrated by the expression of B-cell markers but also by the rearrangement of IgH genes in virtually all cases [82]. The majority of cases have blasts that express CD10 (the common ALL antigen) and are termed 'common' ALL [83]. B-lineage ALL cases which lack CD10 expression are sometimes called 'null' ALL [84]. The cut-off point for distinguishing these two entities is arbitrarily established in individual laboratories, and is usually 10%. It is debatable whether null ALL represents a more immature stage of differentiation than 'common' ALL [85]. There is a strong association between the null phenotype and 11q23 abnormalities [86,87]. Another characteristic feature of the latter leukaemias is the high rate of expression of CD15 [87,88]. Common and null ALL are collectively termed 'early pre-B ALL'. Other molecules commonly expressed by these cells include CD24, CD72, HLA-Dr and nuclear TdT; about 80–85% of these cases are CD34+ [67]. Most cases are CD45+, although a subset express this molecule very weakly or not at all. The latter phenomenon is strongly associated with hyperdiploidy (>50 chromosomes) [89].

In 20–30% of B-lineage ALL there is further evidence of B-cell differentiation in the synthesis and accumulation of cytoplasmic mu heavy chains: such leukaemias are named 'pre-B-ALL' [77] (Table 4.2). The correct proportion of blasts with cytoplasmic mu chains necessary to diagnose pre-B ALL is also arbitrary, and the 10% cut-off value is commonly used. The majority of pre-B ALLs are CD10+. CD20 is expressed in approximately 40% of pre-B ALL cases, while CD34 is found in approximately 60% of these cases. Although rearrangement of light-chain genes can be demonstrated in many of these cases, kappa and lambda proteins are not detectable. About 25% of pre-B ALL have either the balanced form of t(1;19)(q23;p13) or its unbalanced form, der(19)t(1;19)(q23;p13) [90,91].

Leukaemic lymphoblasts that express cytoplasmic *and* surface mu heavy chains without kappa or lambda light chains have been called 'transitional pre-B ALL', implying an intermediate stage of differentiation between pre-B and mature B [92]. In these cases, the mu heavy chains are thought to be transported to the cell membrane by pseudolambda light chains. This ALL subtype is rare, comprising approximately 1% of childhood acute leukaemias. Unlike B-ALL (see below), transitional pre-B cases usually lack L3 morphology and translocations involving the chromosome 8q24. Indeed, no unique chromosomal abnormality is found in these cases. Most transitional pre-B ALL are CD10+, TdT+, and CD34+ [92].

The blasts in a few (<5%) B-lineage ALL cases express surface IgM and either kappa or lambda light chains; these cases are known as 'B-ALL' [93,94]. Occasionally, IgD or IgA are also expressed in addition to IgM. Childhood B-ALL consists of two distinct entities. The more common form is characterized by L3 morphology, extramedullary disease, chromosomal translocations t(8;14), t(8;22) or t(2;8), and blasts lacking PAS-reactive granules, TdT and CD34. These cases are usually the leukemic phase of Burkitt's lymphoma. A more uncommon type of B-ALL lacks extramedullary masses at presentation and translocations of the 8q24 chromosome, and displays FAB L1 or L2 morphology [95,96]. These blasts contain PAS-positive granules and may express TdT and CD34. Intensity of surface Ig expression is usually higher in the L3 type.

T-lineage acute lymphoblastic leukaemia

T-ALL blasts consistently express cytoplasmic or membrane CD3 molecules as well as membrane CD7 [36–38,74–76,81] (Table 4.2). CD2, CD5, CD6 and nuclear TdT are found in over 90% of cases, while CD1a, CD4, CD8, CD10 and CD21 are heterogeneously expressed, and HLA-Dr is uncommonly found [67]. CD45 is expressed in all cases, usually to a greater extent than in B-lineage ALL.

In the vast majority of T-ALL cases, TCRβ, TCRγ and TCRδ genes are rearranged or deleted [75,78,97–99]. The availability of MAbs to the individual chains of the TCR has allowed the investigation of the stages of TCR development in T-ALL at the protein level. In our study, leukaemic cells in 40 of 68 T-ALL cases lacked membrane CD3/TCR expression (mCD3−) [100]. In 20 of these mCD3− cases TCRαβ proteins were expressed in the cells' cytoplasm: in 17 samples, leukaemic blasts expressed TCRβ chains, in one case they expressed TCRα chains, and in two cases blasts expressed both TCRα and TCRβ chains. In the other 20 mCD3− T-ALLs blasts did not show membrane or cytoplasmic reactivity with anti-TCRα or TCRβ MAbs. In the remaining 28 T-ALLs studied (41%), blasts expressed membrane CD3/TCR chains: in 23 cases, CD3 molecules were associated with the αβ form of the TCR, while the remaining five cases expressed TCRγδ. In all 68 cases studied, leukaemic cells were generally strongly CD7+, with the exception of three mCD3+/TCRαβ+ cases in which blasts expressed CD7 weakly and heterogeneously. No clear correlation between stages of

TCR differentiation and expression of other surface markers could be found.

It has been suggested that mTCRγδ is more frequently seen than mTCRαβ in T-ALL, whereas TCRαβ would be more frequent in T-lymphoblastic lymphoma [101]. In our study, such TCRγδ predominance in mCD3+ T-ALL was not found [100]. From these data it appears that blasts expressing mTCRγδ can be found in approximately one-fifth of mCD3+ T-ALL cases. Considering that TCRγδ-bearing cells normally represent less than 1% of fetal and infant thymocytes, the relatively high proportion of TCRγδ T-ALLs may reflect a higher susceptibility to leukaemogenesis in the TCRγδ lineage.

In addition, the possibility of an exclusive cytoplasmic expression of TCRγδ chains in cases with no membrane TCRγδ expression has been tested. While no cytoplasmic TCRδ expression was observed among 40 mCD3− and 23 mCD3+ TCRαβ+ T-ALL cases studied, two of nine mCD3− and two of seven mCD3+TCRαβ+ cases expressed cytoplasmic TCRγ chains [100]. One of the mCD3−, TCRγ+ cases also expressed cytoplasmic TCRβ chains and one of the five mCD3+, TCRγδ+ cases expressed TCRβ chains. These observations revealed the promiscuous expression of TCR protein in T-ALL which is not seen during normal T-cell development.

Acute myeloid leukaemia

Malignant blast cells in virtually all acute myeloid leukaemia (AML) cases express myeloperoxidase, CD13 and/or CD33 [46,54,81,102–108] (Table 4.3). Attempts to correlate myeloid-associated antigen expression with FAB grouping have only partially succeeded. CD34 is more commonly expressed in cases with less differentiated morphology, while most FAB M3 and M5 cases are CD34− [50,51,102] (Table 4.3). MHC-Class II antigens are found in both CD34+ and CD34− groups of AML, including AMLs with M4 and M5 features, but are negative in the majority of M3 cases [102] (Table 4.3). The expression of CD13, CD15, CD65 and CD33 is not related to FAB subgroups [46,102–104]. CD117 (c-kit) is also expressed in many AML cases, with the exception of the M3 subtype [54,109].

Leukaemias whose blasts react with CD14 antibodies usually have monocytic morphology (FAB M4 or M5) [46,52,102–104]. Monocytic differentiation of AML is also suggested phenotypically by CD11c [53], and CD4 expression [106]. Virtually all these cases are CD34−, and most lack CD117 [54]. A few cases may contain blasts expressing CD34 and CD14, but double-marker studies have shown that these constitute two separate cell subpopulations [67]. Identical methods have also demonstrated that blasts expressing TdT or CD7 are generally CD14− [67]. An additional sign of monocytic differentiation is the high membrane expression of Fc receptors [107]. These receptors have a high affinity for mouse immunoglobulins, particularly of IgG2 isotype, and cause the high frequency of nonspecific labelling seen in these cases. Thus, nonspecific Fc binding must be rigorously excluded.

Table 4.3 Immunophenotype according to FAB classification in AML.*

FAB group	HLA-DR	CD33	CD13	CD15	CD11b	CD14
M1	70†	70	76	22	35	8
M2	91	71	85	55	62	12
M3	7	94	76	14	15	2
M4	95	85	71	70	81	63
M5	92	92	45	75	89	57

* Cases compiled from refs [103,104,158] and St Jude Children's
Research Hospital. Most cases of AML are MPO+ [58,108].
† Percentage of positive cases.

Often a subpopulation of leukaemic blasts appears positive with CD41a due to adherence of platelets or cell-surface absorption of glycoprotein IIb/IIIa.

Finally, cases of acute erythroid leukaemia can be identified with antibodies antiglycophorin A [55,56], while cases of acute megakaryocytic leukaemia react with CD41b, CD42a and CD61 [57,60,61]. These subtypes are rare among acute leukaemias: in a large series, blasts in only three out of 500 cases exhibited such markers (two cases were glycophorin A positive and one was CD61+) [81].

'Mixed' and 'hybrid' leukaemias

In a minority of acute leukaemia cases (<5%), blast cells have immunophenotypic features which may be difficult to interpret. Among these are those 'mixed' leukaemias in which two separate blast populations express lymphoid and myeloid markers. Such leukaemias are extremely rare (four of 500 cases in one report [81]) and should be documented with double marker analysis. The term 'mixed' or 'biphenotypic' leukaemia has also been applied to cases in which blasts simultaneously express 'myeloid' and 'lymphoid' associated markers. Some investigators have proposed a scoring system to help classify these cases [110], which, however, rarely represent a diagnostic problem.

A proportion of ALLs are consistently found to express CD13, CD33 and/or CD15 [111–119]. In most of these cases, the expression of a variety of lymphoid-associated antigens and the rearrangement of Ig or TCR genes strongly indicate a lymphoid origin. In a proportion of AML cases, blasts may express 'lymphoid-associated' markers [106]. These include TdT [13,120] and CD7 [121]; in most of these cases, the blast cells are morphologically immature and the majority are CD34+ [67,122]. TdT is expressed by >60% of blasts in 20–30% of cases [13,120], although Adriaansen *et al.* have recently reported that a larger percentage of cases contain a smaller subpopulation of TdT+, CD13+ and/or CD33+ leukaemic cells [123]. CD7 expression is seen in 5–10% of AMLs [105,121]. Two other markers inappropriately expressed in AML blasts are CD19 and CD56 [124–126], frequently found in cases with the t(8;21)(q22;q22) abnormality [127].

The existence of mixed lineage leukaemias has generated a great deal of debate and opened speculations about the fidelity of lineage commitment in progenitor cells. Some investigators have proposed that biphenotypic leukaemic lymphoblasts could be the result of a leukaemia-associated misprogramming of differentiation [128], while others have suggested that these cases manifest a phase of unrestricted gene expression that normally occurs during differentiation of haematopoietic progenitor cells [129]. To further elucidate this issue, CD13 expression was studied in two B-lineage ALL cell lines under different culture conditions [130]. These cells lacked CD13 expression when collected from patients at diagnosis, but acquired the antigen after *in vitro* culture. It was observed that CD13 expression in these leukaemias could be abrogated by culturing the cells on bone marrow-derived stromal layers. Stroma-mediated suppression of CD13 required direct contact with stromal elements, was due to inhibition of gene transcription, and was reversed by removing cells from stroma. These results suggest that CD13 expression is influenced by the cells' relation with the bone marrow microenvironment. Abnormal response to microenvironmental signals could explain the expression of CD13 seen in some cases of ALL.

Acute undifferentiated leukaemia

Several reports have described acute leukaemia cases as 'unclassifiable' or 'undifferentiated' because of the difficulty in interpreting the immunophenotype [131–133]. It has been proposed that the 'acute undifferentiated leukaemia' (AUL) classification should be reserved for cases that have received thorough phenotypic analysis and that express phenotypic 'immaturity' features and lack lineage-associated markers [107,134].

Nine cases of AUL have been encountered during the diagnostic investigation of 750 cases of acute leukaemias [134]. In seven of these cases the blasts were HLA-Dr+, CD34+ and TdT+; in one case they were HLA-Dr+, TdT+ and CD7+; in the remaining case, blasts were HLA-Dr+ only. The diagnosis of AUL was based on the expression of such immaturity features together with the absence of cytoplasmic and membrane CD22, CD3, CD13 and Ig as well as membrane CD19, CD10, CD37, CD2, CD33, CD14, glycophorin A and CD61. The TCR-β, –γ and –δ genes were in germline configuration in seven cases studied, while IgH genes were rearranged in two of seven cases. In four of seven cases, a minority of blasts showed peroxidase activity detectable by electron microscopy.

Relation of cell markers to treatment outcome

Acute lymphoblastic leukaemia

The first markers used to identify clinically significant groups of ALL were surface Ig expression and E-rosette formation. In early treatment protocols, patients with B-ALL and T-ALL, whose lymphoblasts had either of these markers, had a poorer clinical outcome than others [93,135,136]. More recent investigations have incorporated a vast array of monoclonal antibodies in a search for leukaemia immunophenotypes predictive of clinical behaviour. However, conclusions from these studies are largely dependent on the individual treatment regimen and are often influenced by the patient cohort. For example, patients with B-ALL and the t(8;14) translocation have a dismal prognosis with standard antimetabolite therapy but respond well to intensive short-term chemotherapy including high-dose cyclophosphamide, cytarabine and methotrexate, plus repeated intrathecal chemotherapy [137].

In some series, children with early pre-B ALL had significantly better disease-free survival rates than patients with pre-B ALL, B-ALL and T-ALL [138]. Children whose leukaemic blasts do not express CD10 generally fare worse than CD10+ cases [139,140], an observation that may be explained by the strong association between CD10 negativity, 11q23 abnormalities, and age less than 1 year, which are known to be unfavourable prognostic features [141]. CD34 expression [142] and lack of CD45 expression [89] have been correlated with favourable treatment outcome in childhood ALL.

Earlier studies found the pre-B immunophenotype to be a high-risk feature with independent prognostic significance [143,144]. However, it has become apparent that it is the higher incidence of chromosomal translocations, in particular the t(1;19) present in 25% of pre-B ALL, that confers the poorer prognosis [145,146]. Some investigators have also found that effective treatment can offset the negative impact of chromosomal rearrangements in this phenotypic variant of ALL [146,147]. By contrast, patients with transitional pre-B ALL have an excellent response to chemotherapy [92].

The rare cases of B-ALL in which blasts have FAB L1 or L2 cytology and lack the t(8;14) chromosomal translocations of Burkitt's lymphoma usually do not have the typical lymphomatous presentation, with abdominal, pelvic or Waldeyer's ring masses, observed in most patients with B-ALL [95,96]. These non-Burkitt types of B-ALL may follow the clinical course of the sIg-negative B-lineage ALLs.

T-lineage ALL comprises approximately 15–18% of cases of childhood ALL [138,147] (see Table 4.2). T-ALL is characterized by a high initial leucocyte count at diagnosis and mediastinal masses in one-half of the patients [138]. Children with T-ALL generally have a poorer prognosis than early pre-B and pre-B types of ALL [148,149]. However, in multivariate analysis, the effect of T-cell phenotype is lost when correction is made for age and leucocyte counts [147,150].

Attempts to identify subsets of T-ALL with prognostically relevant cell markers have yielded conflicting results. Subclassifications of T-ALL according to the level of thymic differentiation have been proposed [34,151]. However, studies which have used these classifications have failed to show rela-

tionships between age, sex, race, leucocyte counts, event-free survival and stage of thymocyte maturation [152–154]. In a study of 120 children with T-ALL, four presenting features were found to confer an increased risk of failure: age greater than 15 years, FAB L2 blast morphology, abnormal karyotype and surface membrane CD3 expression [153]. As in B-lineage ALL, the expression of CD10 in T-ALL has been associated with better clinical outcomes [147,155]. It has also been reported that T-ALLs in which blasts are CD2– and do not form rosettes with sheep erythrocytes have an unfavourable prognosis in adults [156,157].

In several investigations, myeloid antigen expression in ALL has been associated with a low rate of complete clinical remission or a shortened survival [113–116]. In two of these studies, many of the cases lacked lymphoid-associated antigens on the leukaemic blasts [113] or had blasts which reacted with antimyeloperoxidase antibodies [114]; these cases may more appropriately be classified as minimally differentiated myeloid leukaemias. Others have not found any adverse clinical outcomes in cases of ALL with myeloid marker expression [117–119,147].

Acute myeloid leukaemia

The expression of different myeloid-associated antigens in AML has not been found to correlate with age, sex, myeloperoxidase activity, platelet count or presence of infections [158]. A lower complete remission rate or shorter survival has been identified with leukaemic blast expression of CD9, CD11b, CD13, CD14, CD17 or CD34 [46,159–162]. Patients with AML whose blasts lack the CD15 antigen may have a lower complete remission rate [163]. Others have found a greater likelihood of complete remission when AML blasts lack CD34 [164]. Of note, a recent study of 267 children with AML failed to identify any prognostically independent immunophenotypic marker [165].

Blasts of AML may simultaneously express myeloid- and lymphoid-associated antigens (see above and refs [127,165–169]). Lymphoid antigens expressed in AML include CD2, CD5, CD7, CD10 and CD19 [121,122,124,127,128,169,170]. The expression of TdT in a high proportion of blasts was considered to be an adverse prognostic feature in earlier studies of AML [120,171,172], although its predictive value in modern chemotherapy regimens is controversial [159,173].

Phenotype of lymphoproliferative disorders

The neoplastic cell populations found in chronic lymphoproliferative disorders reflect the processes of lymphocyte activation and proliferation in the peripheral lymphoid organs, and the complex variety of accompanying phenotypic changes [174,175]. The aim of cell marker analysis of chronic lymphoid leukaemias and lymphomas is to complement the clinical,

Table 4.4 Predominant immunophenotypes of mature B-cell leukaemias.

Marker	CLL	PLL	HCL	SLVL
CD19	+	+	+	+
CD20	+	+	+	+
CD37	+	+	+	+
sIg	+/−	+	+	+
FMC7	−	+	+	+
CD5	+	−	−	−
CD11c	−	−	+	+/−
CD22	−	+	+*	+
CD23	+	−	−	−
CD25	−	−	+	−
B-ly-7	−	−	+	+/−

CLL = chronic lymphocytic leukaemia; HCL = hairy cell leukaemia; PLL = prolymphocytic leukaemia; SLVL = splenic lymphoma wth villous lymphocytes.
* Typically, high expression.

morphological and histological classification of the disease. This essentially consists of establishing the lineage association and the clonality of the neoplastic cells.

The immunophenotypic patterns of the most common B-lineage chronic lymphoproliferative disorders are summarized in Table 4.4. Cells typically express CD19, CD79, CD20 and CD37, whereas TdT is absent [174–178]. The level of expression of immunoglobulins on the cell membrane is heterogeneous and often weak. Therefore, the investigation of Ig expression after cell permeabilization is often more successful in proving the clonality of B-CLL cells. Similarly, CD22 is detectable in cytocentrifuge preparations in virtually all cases, but its membrane expression may be extremely weak or, in most B-CLL cases, undetectable.

Attempts to correlate phenotypic features with particular histological types or haematological classifications have only partially succeeded. Nevertheless, some subtypes have characteristic immunophenotypic features (Table 4.4). For example, B-ly-7, CD25, CD11c and HC-2 expression, together with high-level expression of CD22, are typical of hairy cell leukaemia [177], while CD23 and CD5 expression with extremely weak CD22 expression and surface Ig is characteristic of B-CLL [176].

Typically expressed markers in T-cell lymphoproliferative disorders are CD2, CD3 and TCR chains. CD3 and TCR molecules often accumulate in the cytoplasm and are weakly expressed on the cell membrane. In addition, natural killer (NK) associated markers such as CD16 and CD57 are usually found in T-chronic lymphocytic leukaemia (T-CLL) [179]. The majority of T-CLLs are CD8+, CD4− whereas the neoplastic cells in T-prolymphocytic leukaemia (T-PLL) and in adult T cell leukaemia/lymphoma (ATLL) are commonly CD4+, CD8−, although cases with different phenotypes have been described [179,180]. In T-CLL, CD7 is usually weakly expressed or nega-

tive and CD25 is absent. In contrast, in most T-PLL cases cells are strongly CD7+ and CD25−, while in ATLL cells are usually CD7+/− and CD25++ [179,180]. The phenotypic features of the neoplastic cells in T-cell non-Hodgkin's lymphoma (T-NHL) are heterogeneous and CD4+, CD8−, CD4−, CD8+ or CD4+, CD8+ cases have been reported [179].

In children, predominant lymphoproliferative disorders are non-Hodgkin's lymphomas, among which Burkitt's lymphoma, T-cell lymphoblastic lymphoma and diffuse large cell lymphoma predominate. In a recent report of 69 childhood cases of the latter disease, 25 were classified as B cell, 23 as T cell and 21 of indeterminate lineage [181]. Twenty-seven of the 69 cases were CD30 (Ki-1)-positive, and most of these showed histological features of anaplastic large-cell lymphoma. In this series, B-cell lineage was associated with a more favourable outcome.

Detection of minimal residual disease in acute leukaemia

The selection of therapeutic strategies in acute leukaemia depends on the patients' remission status. However, the current way of assessing such status, i.e. the morphological examination of peripheral blood and bone marrow smears, is limited in sensitivity. Experiments using artificial mixtures of leukaemic and normal cells have shown that a leukaemic cell component comprising less than 5% of cells is difficult to identify, even by experienced haematologists (reviewed in ref. [182]).

The sensitivity and precision of residual disease detection may be improved by several methods including enzymatic amplification using polymerase chain reaction (PCR) of molecular abnormalities, and of Ig and TCR genes (reviewed in ref. [182]). In addition, immunological methods offer a rapid and reliable option to investigate residual disease in a proportion of patients with acute leukaemia.

Leukaemia-associated phenotypes and methods

Single antibodies are not suitable for distinguishing neoplastic from normal lympho-haematopoietic cells, as the same antigens can be found on leukaemic cells and their normal counterparts [16,183]. Possible exceptions to this rule are the chimaeric proteins that result from gene fusions such as *BCR-ABL*, *E2A-PBX1*, *ALL1-AF4* and *TEL-AML1*. Specific antibodies against these tumour-associated antigens would, in principle, allow single-colour flow cytometric studies, but such reagents are not yet available in a form suitable for immunofluorescence staining of patients' samples with the exception of one monoclonal antibody recognizing the E2A-PBX1 nuclear protein [184]. Although CD10 and TdT have been used to identify ALL cells, the results have generally been disappointing [185–187] because these markers are also expressed by normal B-cell precursors found in marrow and, although

Table 4.5 Immunophenotypic combinations used to study MRD in patients with acute leukaemia.

Disease	Phenotype	Frequency (%)†	Frequency in normal marrow (% positive cells ± SD)‡
B-lineage ALL*	TdT-CD10 (or CD19–CD34)/CD13	7	0.02 ± 0.01
	TdT-CD10 (or CD19–CD34)/CD33	8	0.03 ± 0.02
	TdT-CD10 (or CD19–CD34)/CD65	7	0.02 ± 0.01
	TdT-CD10 (or CD19–CD34)/CD21	10	0.02 ± 0.01
	TdT-CD10 (or CD19–CD34)/CD56	9	<0.01
	TdT/cytoplasmic μ/CD34	14	0.03 ± 0.01
	KOR-SA3544/CD10	10	<0.01
	p53§	3	<0.01
T-lineage ALL	TdT/cytoplasmic CD3	90	<0.01
AML*	CD34/CD56	20	<0.01
	CDw65/CD34/TdT	15	<0.01
	p53§	10	<0.01

* Approximately 50–60% of cases have at least one leukemia-associated phenotype.

† Greater than 10% positive leukaemic lymphoblasts.

‡ Reduced level of expression of these phenotypes by normal cells makes it possible to distinguish one leukaemic cell among 10 000 normal marrow cells.

§ Cases with mutated p53 in which the p53 protein is highly expressed (E. Coustan-Smith & D. Campana, unpublished observations).

rarely, in peripheral blood. Thus, the current strategy of detecting residual disease by immunological methods relies on the expression of combinations of leucocyte markers which are found on malignant cells but not in normal peripheral blood and bone marrow cells [188–190].

Screening of multiple cytocentrifuge preparations by fluorescence microscopy affords a sensitivity of the order of one leukaemic cell among 10 000 normal haematopoietic cells [190,191]. Flow cytometry allows a maximum sensitivity of detection of one target cell in 10^6 after prolonged purging of the fluidics system [192]. A more realistic sensitivity in everyday use is 1 target cell in 10^4 [126,182].

Some immunophenotypes found on leukaemic cells are limited to certain normal tissues, and are not present in bone marrow, peripheral blood or cerebrospinal fluid (reviewed in ref. [182]). For example, in most cases of T-ALL, the lymphoblasts express nuclear TdT in combination with T-cell markers (e.g. CD3, CD5 or CD1). Although normal in developing T cells, such phenotypes are confined to the thymus. Thus, detection of individual TdT+ cells expressing such markers in the blood or marrow of T-ALL patients indicates residual disease.

In a proportion of B-lineage ALL and AML cases, the blast cells express immunophenotypes that are extremely rare or absent among normal haemopoietic cells [189,193] (reviewed in ref. [182]). Reading *et al.* [194] reported unusual coexpression of antigens in 85% of 272 cases of AML studied with a panel of 22 antibodies. Among the various phenotypic combinations suitable for study of residual disease in AML, the phe-

notype CD34/CD56, found in approximately 20% of cases of childhood AML, has proved to be one of the most informative [126]. Among normal CD34+ cells, CD56 is either undetectable or expressed at much lower levels than in blast cells [126,195].

Table 4.5 summarizes the phenotypic combinations that can be used for productive study of residual ALL. While the vast majority of T-ALLs are amenable to immunophenotypic analysis, only approximately 45% of B-lineage ALL cases express a phenotype suitable for sensitive analysis of residual disease. In most cases, intensity of antigen expression can also help in distinguishing leukaemic cells from the rare normal progenitors expressing these phenotypes. False-positive immunological results can derive from the use of antibodies that have nonspecific reactivities, such as cell binding through their Fc portion—a common feature of murine antibodies of IgG2 isotype [196]. The problem can be prevented by careful selection of optimal reagents and by saturation of Fc receptors with human or rabbit Ig. Phenotypic switches that occur at the time of relapse may result in false-negative monitoring of residual disease if they affect the 'leukaemia-associated' markers studied [197,198]. The investigation of multiple phenotypes in each case may help in reducing the problem.

Clinical studies

Among 18 patients with T-ALL, Bradstock *et al.* [188] identified six whose remission marrow samples contained 0.5–5% nucleated cells with T-cell marker plus nuclear TdT which indicated the presence of residual disease. Van Dongen *et al.* [199] used double-colour combinations including a T-cell marker (CD5) and TdT to monitor 26 T-ALL patients. Of the 12 relapses that developed in 10 patients, 11 were detected immunologically 4–21 weeks earlier than by routine morphological examination. None of the remaining 16 patients without detectable CD5/TdT double-labelled cells relapsed during a median follow-up of 43 months. Drach *et al.* [200] studied four patients with T-ALL by flow cytometry. None had detectable leukaemic cells and all remained in continuous complete remission with a median follow-up of 30 weeks after the last negative assay. Suspicious cells were seen in two of four evaluable cases of B-ALL. One of these patients subsequently relapsed, while in the other, phenotypically abnormal cells progressively disappeared during continued remission. The remaining two patients remained in continuous complete remission with no detectable leukaemic cells immunologically (follow-up time, 20 and 24 weeks after the negative finding). In one of our earlier studies, minimal residual disease (MRD) detection preceded overt relapse by 1–6 months in all 15 ALL patients; 22 patients were considered to be in clinical and immunological remission, although seven subsequently relapsed, two of these in the central nervous system [189]. The results of our recently conducted prospective study in childhood ALL indicate that MRD investigations are clinically useful [201].

Adriaansen *et al.* [123] studied 12 TdT+ AML cases during morphological remission, seven of which subsequently relapse once or twice (total of ten relapses); nine relapses were preceded by a gradual increase in phenotypically abnormal cells. The remaining five patients stayed in complete remission with a follow-up of 32–46 months. Although small proportions of phenotypically abnormal cells (<0.1% in the marrow) could be detected in these patients, they did not increase with serial sampling. Drach *et al.* [200] studied five AML patients in morphological remission; three showed the persistence or increase of phenotypically abnormal cells, followed by overt relapse. In our earlier study, immunological evidence of MRD was found in four of seven patients with AML, all of whom subsequently relapsed [189].

Detection of residual disease in cerebrospinal fluid

Approximately 5–10% of patients with ALL who enter remission will have an isolated CNS relapse [147]. Some of these patients may also have residual leukaemia in the bone marrow [202,203].

The first sign of CNS involvement is often the presence of malignant cells in the cerebrospinal fluid (CSF) [204], although it may be difficult to discriminate between leukaemic lymphoblasts and normal activated lymphocytes by routine morphological examination. Immunological methods can resolve this ambiguity. While B- and T-lymphocytes and monocytes are normally found in the CSF, cells expressing

nuclear TdT should be absent [205–207]. Thus, detection of even a single TdT+ cell would indicate CNS leukaemia. Hooijkaas *et al.* [206] reported the results of a 5-year follow-up study in which anti-TdT staining was used to analyse CSF from 113 children with TdT+ acute leukaemia or T-cell non-Hodgkin's lymphoma. In approximately 8% of the samples there was discordance between the results of morphological and immunological evaluation. In discordant cases, the results of immunological investigations appeared to be more informative than morphological examination in predicting clinical outcome. In our own study of over 1200 samples, the frequency of disagreement between morphology and immunology was only 1.9% (E. Coustan-Smith, D. Campana, C-H. Pui *et al.*, unpublished results). Thus, although routine examination of CSF samples by immunological methods would probably not be cost-effective, this approach can help in diagnosis when morphological findings are equivocal.

Acknowledgements

This work was supported by grants U01-CA60419, P01-CA20180 and P30-CA21765 from the National Cancer Institute and by the American Lebanese Syrian Associated Charities (ALSAC).

References

1 Catovsky D. (1981) *The Leukemic Cell*. Churchill Livingstone, Edinburgh.

2 Bernard A., Boumsell L., Dausset J., Milstein C. & Schlossman S.F. (1984) *Leucocyte Typing I*. Springer Verlag, Berlin.

3 Reinherz E.L., Haynes B.F., Nadler L.M. & Bernstein I.D. (1986) *Leukocyte Typing II*. Springer Verlag, Berlin.

4 McMichael A.J. (1987) *Leucocyte Typing III*. Oxford University Press, Oxford.

5 Knapp W., Dorken B., Gilks W.R. *et al.* (1989) *Leucocyte Typing IV*. Oxford University Press, Oxford.

6 Schlossman S.F., Boumsell L., Gilks W. *et al.* (1995) *Leucocyte Typing V*. Oxford University Press, Oxford.

7 Kishimoto T., Goyet S., Kikutani H. *et al.* (1997) *Leucocyte Typing VI*. Garland, New York.

8 Janossy G., Bollum F., Bradstock K.F. & Ashley J. (1980) Cellular phenotypes of normal and leukaemic hemopoietic cells determined by analysis with selected antibody combinations. *Blood*, **56**, 430–441.

9 Bradstock K.F., Janossy G., Pizzolo G. *et al.* (1980) Subpopulations of normal and leukemic human thymocytes: an analysis using monoclonal antibodies. *Journal of the National Cancer Institute*, **65**, 33–42.

10 Van Dongen J.J.M., Hooijkaas H., Comans-Bitter W.M., Benne W.M., Van Os T.M. & De Jong J.D.J. (1985) Triple immunological staining with colloidal gold, fluorescein and rhodamine as labels. *Journal of Immunological Methods*, **80**, 1–6.

11 Terstappen L.W.M.M. & Loken M.R. (1988) Five dimensional flow cytometry as a new approach for blood and bone marrow differentials. *Cytometry*, **9**, 548–553.

12 Mason D.Y., Erber W.N., Falini B., Stein H. & Gatter K.C. (1986) Immuno-enzymatic labelling of haematological samples with monoclonal antibodies. In: *Monoclonal Antibodies — methods in hematology*, (ed. P.C.L. Beverley), pp. 145–181. Churchill Livingstone, Edinburgh.

13 Erber W.M., Mynheer L.C. & Mason D.Y. (1986) APAAP labelling of blood and bone marrow samples for phenotyping leukaemia. *Lancet*, **i**, 761–765.

14 De Mey J., Hacker G.W., De Waele M. & Springall D.R. (1985) Gold probes in light microscopy. In: *Immunocytochemistry* (eds S. Van Noorden & J. Polak), pp. 71–88. John Wright, Oxford.

15 Greaves M.F. (1986) Differentiation-linked leukemogenesis in lymphocytes. *Science* **234**, 697–704.

16 Janossy G., Bollum F.J., Bradstock K.F., McMichael A., Rapson N. & Greaves M.F. (1979) Terminal transferase positive human bone marrow cells exhibit the antigenic phenotype of common acute lymphoblastic leukemia. *Journal of Immunology*, **123**, 1525–1529.

17 Desiderio S.V., Yancopoulos G.D., Paskind M. *et al.* (1984) Insertions of N regions into heavy chain genes is correlated with expression of terminal deoxycotransferase in B cells. *Nature*, **311**, 752–755.

18 Blackwell T.K. & Alt F.W. (1989) Molecular characterization of the lymphoid V(D)J recombination activity. *Journal of Biological Chemistry*, **264**, 10327–10330.

19 Oettinger M.A., Schatz D.G., Gorka C. & Baltimore D. (1990) RAG-1 and RAG-2 adjacent genes that synergistically activate VDJ recombination. *Science*, **248**, 1517–1520.

20 Campana D., Janossy G., Bofill M. *et al.* (1985) Human B cell development. I. Phenotypic differences of B lymphocytes in the bone marrow and peripheral lymphoid tissue. *Journal of Immunology*, **134**, 1524–1530.

21 Nadler L.M., Anderson K.C., Marti G. *et al.* (1983) B4, a human B lymphocyte-associated antigen expressed on normal, mitogen-activated, and malignant B lymphocytes. *Journal of Immunology*, **131**, 244–250.

22 Loken M.R., Shah V.O., Dattilio K.L. & Civin C.I. (1987) Flow cytometric analysis of human bone marrow. II. Normal B lymphocyte development. *Blood*, **70**, 1316–1324.

23 Mason D.Y., Cordell J.L., Tse A.G.D. *et al.* (1991) The IgM-associated protein mb-1 as a marker of normal and neoplastic B cells. *Journal of Immunology*, **147**, 2474–2482.

24 Ritz J., Pesando J.M., Notis-McConarty J. *et al.* (1980) A monoclonal antibody to human acute lymphoblastic leukaemia antigen. *Nature*, **284**, 583–585.

25 Pearl E.R., Vogler L.B., Okos A.J., Crist W.M., Lawton A.R. & Cooper M.D. (1978) B lymphocyte precursors in human bone marrow: an analysis of normal individuals and patients with antibody-deficiency states. *Journal of Immunology*, **120**, 1169–1175.

26 Takemori T., Mizuguchi J., Miyazoe I. *et al.* (1990) Two types of μ chain complexes are expressed during differentiation from pre-B to mature B cells. *EMBO Journal*, **9**, 2493–2501.

27 Schiff C., Milili M., Bossy D. *et al.* (1991) Lambda-like and V pre-B genes expression: an early B lineage marker of human leukemias. *Blood*, **7**, 1516–1525.

28 Benner R., Rijnbeek A-M., Schreier M.H. & Coutinho A. (1981) Frequency analysis of immunoglobulin V-gene expression and functional reactivities in bone marrow B cells. *Journal of Immunology*, **126**, 887–890.

29 Campana D. & Janossy G. (1988) Proliferation of normal and malignant human immature lymphoid cells. *Blood*, **71**, 1201–1210.

30 Osmond D.G. (1986) Population dynamics of bone marrow B lymphocytes. *Immunological Reviews*, **93**, 103–118.

31 Clevers H., Alarcon B., Wileman T. & Terhorst C. (1988) The T cell receptor/CD3 complex: a dynamic protein ensemble. *Annual Review of Immunology*, **6**, 629–662.

32 Lanier L.L., Allison J.P. & Phillips J.H. (1986) Correlation of cell surface antigen expression of human thymocytes by multi-color flow cytometric analysis: implications for differentiation. *Journal of Immunology*, **137**, 2501–2507.

33 Campana D., Coustan-Smith E., Wong L. & Janossy G. (1989) Expression of T cell receptor associated proteins during human T cell development. In: *Progress in Immunology* (ed. F. Melchers), pp. 1276–1279. Springer-Verlag, Berlin.

34 Reinherz E.L., Kung P.V., Goldstein G., Levey K.H. & Schlossman S.F. (1980) Discrete stages of human intrathymic differentiation. Analysis of normal thymocytes and leukemic lymphoblasts of T lineage. *Proceeding of the National Academy of Sciences*, **77**, 1588–1592.

35 Tidman N., Janossy G., Bodger M., Granger S., Kung P.C. & Goldstein G. (1981) Delineation of human thymocyte differentiation pathways utilizing double staining techniques with monoclonal antibodies. *Clinical and Experimental Immunology*, **45**, 457–462.

36 Lobach D.F., Hensley L.L., Ho W. & Haynes B. (1985) Human T cell antigen expression during early stages of fetal thymic maturation. *Journal of Immunology*, **135**, 1752–1759.

37 Furley A.J., Mizutani S., Weilbaecher K. *et al.* (1986) Developmentally regulated rearrangement and expression of genes encoding the T cell receptor–T3 complex. *Cell*, **46**, 75–87.

38 Campana D., Thompson J.S., Amlot P., Brown S. & Janossy G. (1987) The cytoplasmic expression of CD3 antigens in normal and malignant cells of the T lymphoid lineage. *Journal of Immunology*, **138**, 648–655.

39 Campana D., Janossy G., Coustan-Smith E. *et al.* (1989) The expression of T cell receptor-associated proteins during T cell ontogeny in man. *Journal of Immunology*, **142**, 57–66.

40 Haynes B.F., Denning S.M., Singer K.H. & Kurtzberg J. (1989) Ontogeny of T-cell precursors: a model for the initial stages of human T cell development. *Immunology Today*, **10**, 87–90.

41 Borst J., Van Dongen J.J.M., Bolhuis R.L.H. *et al.* (1988) Distinct molecular forms of human T cell receptor γ/δ detected on viable T cells by a monoclonal antibody. *Journal of Experimental Medicine*, **167**, 1625–1633.

42 Penit C. & Vasseur F. (1988) Sequential events in thymocyte differentiation and thymus regeneration revealed by a combination of bromodeoxyuridine DNA labelling and antimitotic drug treatment. *Journal of Immunology*, **140**, 3315–3323.

43 Brenner M.B., Strominger J.L. & Krangel M.S. (1988) The γδ T cell receptor. *Advances in Immunology*, **43**, 133–192.

44 Groh V., Porcelli S., Fabbi M. *et al.* (1989) Human lymphocytes bearing T cell receptor γ/δ are phenotypically diverse and evenly distributed throughout the lymphoid system. *Journal of Experimental Medicine*, **169**, 1277–1286.

45 Van Dongen J.J.M., Comans-Bitter W.M., Wolvers-Tettero I.L.M. & Borst J. (1990) Development of human T lymphocytes and their thymus-dependency. *Thymus*, **16**, 207–234.

46 Griffin J.D., Mayer R.J., Weinstein H.J. *et al.* (1983) Surface marker analysis of acute myeloblastic leukaemia: identification of differentiation associated phenotypes. *Blood*, **62**, 557–563.

47 Campana D. & Janossy G. (1987) Analysis of myeloid antigens on the cell surface and in the cytoplasm. In: *Leucocyte Typing III*.

(ed. A.J. McMichael), pp. 661–666. Oxford University Press, Oxford.

48 Favaloro E.J., Bradstock K.F., Kabral A., Grimsley P., Zowtyj H. & Zola H. (1988) Further characterization of human myeloid antigens (gp 160,95; gp 150; gp67): investigation of epitopic heterogeneity and non-hemopoietic distribution using panels of monoclonal antibodies belonging to CD11b, CD13 and CD33. *British Journal of Haematology*, **69**, 163–171.

49 Janossy G., Francis G.E., Capellaro D., Goldstone A.H. & Greaves M.F. (1978) Cell sorter analysis of the expression of two leukaemia associated antigens on human myeloid precursors. *Nature*, **276**, 176–178.

50 Civin C.I., Strauss L.C., Brovall C., Feckler M.J., Schwartz J.F. & Shaper J.H. (1984) Antigenic analysis of hematopoiesis. II. A hematopoietic progenitor cell surface antigen defined by a monoclonal antibody raised against KG-Ia cells. *Journal of Immunology*, **133**, 1–10.

51 Tindle R.W., Nichols R.A.B., Chan L., Campana D., Catovsky D. & Birnie G.D. (1985) A novel monoclonal antibody BI-3C5 recognizes myeloblasts and non-B non-T lymphoblasts in acute leukaemias and CGL blast crisis, and reacts with immature cells in normal bone marrow. *Leukemia Research*, **9**, 1–9.

52 Linch D.C., Allen C., Beverley P.C.L., Bynoe A.G., Scott C.S. & Hogg N. (1984) Monoclonal antibodies differentiating between monocytic and non-monocytic variants of AML. *Blood*, **63**, 566–573.

53 MacDonald S.M., Pulford K., Falini B., Micklen K. & Mason D.Y. (1986) A monoclonal antibody recognizing the p150/95 leucocyte differentiation antigen. *Immunology*, **59**, 427–431.

54 Knapp W., Strobl H. & Majdic O. (1994) Flow cytometric analysis of cell-surface and intracellular antigens in leukemia diagnosis. *Cytometry*, **18**, 187–198.

55 Andersson L.C., Gahmberg C.G., Teerenhovi L. & Vuopio P. (1979) Glycophorin A as a cell surface marker of early erythroid differentiation in acute leukemia. *International Journal of Cancer*, **23**, 717–722.

56 Greaves M.F., Sieff C. & Edwards P.A.W. (1983) Monoclonal anti-glycophorin as a probe for erythroleukemias. *Blood*, **61**, 645–650.

57 Vom dem Borne A.E.G.Kr., Modderman P.W., Admiraal L.G. & Nieuwenhuis H.K. (1989) Platelet antibodies, the overall results. In: *Leucocyte Typing IV* (eds W. Knapp, B. Dorken, W.R. Gilks *et al.*), pp. 951–966. Oxford University Press, Oxford.

58 Parravicini C.L. Soligo D., Berti E., Cattoretti G., Gaiera G. & Vago L. (1989) Immunohistochemical reactivity of anti-platelet mAb in normal human tissues and bone marrow. In: *Leucocyte Typing IV*, (eds W. Knapp, B. Dorken, W.R. Gilks *et al.*), pp. 981–985. Oxford University Press, Oxford.

59 McMichael A.J., Rust N.A., Pilch J.R. *et al.* (1981) Monoclonal antibody to human platelet glycoprotein I. Immunological studies. *British Journal of Haematology*, **49**, 501–509.

60 Gatter K.C., Cordell J.L., Turley H. *et al.* (1988) The immunohistological detection of platelets, megakaryocytes and thrombi in routinely processed specimens. *Histopathology*, **13**, 257–267.

61 Erber W.N., Breton-Gorius J., Villeval J.L., Oscier D.G., Bai Y. & Mason D.Y. (1987) Detection of cells of megakaryocytic lineage in haematological malignancies by immuno-alkaline phosphatase labelling of cell smears with a panel of monoclonal antibodies. *British Journal of Haematology*, **65**, 87–94.

62 Huang S. & Terstappen L.W.M.M. (1994) Lymphoid and myeloid differentiation of single human CD34+, HLA-DR+, CD38– hematopoietic stem cells. *Blood*, **83**, 1515–1526.

63 Craig W., Kay R., Cutler R.L. & Lansdorp P.M. (1993) Expression of Thy-1 on human hematopoietic progenitor cells. *Journal of Experimental Medicine*, **177**, 1331–1342.

64 Verfaillie C., Blakolmer K. & McGlave P. (1990) Purified primitive human hematopoietic progenitor cells with long-term *in vitro* repopulating capacity adhere selectively to irradiated bone marrow stroma. *Journal of Experimental Medicine*, **172**, 509–520.

65 Brand J., Srour E.F., van Besien K., Briddell R.A. & Hoffman R. (1990) Cytokine-dependent long-term culture of highly enriched precursors of hematopoietic progenitor cells form human bone marrow. *Journal of Clinical Investigation*, **86**, 932–941.

66 Baum C.M., Weissman I.L., Tsukamoto A.S., Bucle A.M. & Peault B. (1992) Isolation of a candidate human hematopoietic stem-cell population. *Proceedings of the National Academy of Sciences, USA*, **89**, 2804–2808.

67 Campana D., Coustan-Smith E. & Janossy G. (1985) Immunophenotyping in haematological diagnosis. In: *Clinical Haematology*. Vol. 3. *Advancing haematological techniques*, (ed. I. Cavill), pp. 889–920. Baillière Tindall, London.

68 Engel P., Wagner N. & Tedder T. (1995) CD79 Workshop Report. In: *Leucocyte Typing V*. (eds S.F. Schlossman, L. Boumsell, W. Gilks *et al.*), pp. 667–670. Oxford University Press, Oxford.

69 Dorken B., Moldenhauer G., Pezzutto A. *et al.* (1986) HD39 (B3), a B lineage restricted antigen whose cell surface expression is limited to resting and activated human B lymphocytes. *Journal of Immunology*, **136**, 4470–4478.

70 Chen Z., Sigaux F., Miglierina R. *et al.* (1986) Immunological typing of acute lymphoblastic leukemia: concurrent analysis by flow cytofluorometry and immunocytology. *Leukemia Research*, **10**, 1411–1416.

71 Mason D.Y., Stein H., Gerdes J. *et al.* (1987) Value of monoclonal anti-CD22 (p135) antibodies for the detection of normal and neoplastic B lymphoid cells. *Blood*, **69**, 836–843.

72 Boue D.R. & LeBien T.W. (1988) Expression and structure of CD22 in acute leukemia. *Blood*, **71**, 1480–1485.

73 Campana D., Patel M., Coustan-Smith E. & Janossy G. (1989) The expression of B cell associated antigens during B cell ontogeny. In: *Leucocyte Typing IV* (eds W. Knapp, B. Dorken, W.R. Gilks *et al.*), pp. 193–195. Oxford University Press, Oxford.

74 Link M.P., Stewart S.J., Warnke R.A. & Levy R. (1985) Discordance between surface and cytoplasmic expression of Leu 4 (T3) antigen in thymocytes and in blast cells from childhood T lymphoblastic malignancies. *Journal of Clinical Investigation*, **76**, 248–255.

75 Furley A.J., Chan L.C., Mizutani S. *et al.* (1987) Lineage specificity of rearrangement and expression of genes encoding the T cell receptor–T3 complex and Ig heavy chain in leukemia. *Leukemia*, **1**, 644–652.

76 Van Dongen J.J.M., Krissansen G.W., Wolvers-Tettero I.L.M. *et al.* (1988) Cytoplasmic expression of the CD3 antigen as a diagnostic marker for immature T-cell malignancies. *Blood*, **71**, 603–612.

77 Vogler L.B., Crist W.M., Bockman D.E., Pearl E.R., Lawton A.R. & Cooper M.D. (1978) Pre-B leukaemia: a new phenotype of childhood lymphoblastic leukaemia. *New England Journal of Medicine*, **298**, 872–877.

78 Campana D., Van Dongen J.J.M., Mehta A. *et al.* (1991) The stages of T cell receptor protein expression in T cell acute lymphoblastic leukemia. *Blood*, **77**, 1546–1554.

79 Pizzolo G., Vincenzi C., Nadali G. *et al.* (1994) Detection of membrane and intracellular antigens by flow cytometry following ORTHO PermeaFix TM fixation. *Leukemia*, **8**, 772–773.

80 Buccheri V., Mihaljevic B., Matutes E., Dyer M.J.S., Mason D.Y. & Catovsky D. (1993) mb-1: a new marker for B-lineage lymphoblastic leukemia. *Blood*, **82**, 853–857.

81 Janossy G., Coustan-Smith E. & Campana D. (1989) The reliability of cytoplasmic CD3 and CD22 antigen expression in the immunodiagnosis of acute leukaemia — a study of 500 cases. *Leukemia*, **3**, 170–181.

82 Korsmeyer S.J., Arnold A. & Bakhshi A. (1983) Immunoglobulin gene rearrangement and cell surface expression in acute lymphocytic leukemia of T cell and B cell precursor origins. *Journal of Clinical Investigation*, **71**, 301–311.

83 Greaves M.F., Hariri G., Newman R.A., Sutherland D.R., Ritter M.A. & Ritz J. (1983) Selective expression of the common acute lymphoblastic leukaemia (gp 100) antigen on immature lymphoid cells and their malignant counterparts. *Blood*, **61**, 628–639.

84 Greaves M.F., Janossy G., Peto J. & Kay H. (1981) Immunologically defined subclasses of acute lymphoblastic leukaemia in children: their relationship to presentation features and prognosis. *British Journal of Haematology*, **48**, 179–197.

85 Nadler L.M., Korsmeyer S.J., Anderson K.C. *et al.* (1984) B cell origin of non-T cell acute lymphoblastic leukemia. A model for discrete stages of neoplastic and normal pre-B cell differentiation. *Journal of Clinical Investigation*, **74**, 332–340.

86 Mirro J., Kitchingman G., Williams D. *et al.* (1986) Clinical and laboratory characteristics of acute leukemia with the 4;11 translocation. *Blood*, **67**, 689–697.

87 Pui C-H., Frankel L.S., Carroll A.J. *et al.* (1991) Clinical characteristics and treatment outcome of childhood acute lymphoblastic leukemia with the t(4;11)(q21;q23): a collaborative study of 40 cases. *Blood*, **77**, 440–447.

88 Ludwig W-D., Bartam C.R., Harbott J. *et al.* (1989) Phenotypic and genotypic heterogeneity in infant acute leukemia. I. Acute lymphoblastic leukemia. *Leukemia*, **3**, 431–439.

89 Behm F.G., Raimondi S.C., Schell M.J., Look A.T., Rivera G.K. & Pui C-H. (1992) Lack of CD45 antigen on blast cells in childhood acute lymphoblastic leukemia is associated with chromosomal hyperdiploidy and other favorable prognostic features. *Blood*, **79**, 1011–1016.

90 Carroll A.J., Crist W.M., Parmley R.T., Roper M., Cooper M.D. & Finley W.H. (1984) Pre-B cell leukemia associated with chromosome translocation 1;19. *Blood*, **63**, 721–728.

91 Borowitz M.J., Hunger S.P., Carroll A.J. *et al.* (1993) Predictability of the t(1;19)(q23;p13) from surface antigen phenotype: implications for screening cases of childhood acute lymphoblastic leukemia for molecular analysis: a Pediatric Oncology Group study. *Blood*, **82**, 1086–1091.

92 Koehler M., Behm F.G., Shuster J. *et al.* (1993) Transitional pre-B-cell acute lymphoblastic leukemia of childhood is associated with favorable prognostic clinical features and an excellent outcome: a Pediatric Oncology Group study. *Leukemia*, **7**, 2064–2068.

93 Flandrin G., Brouet J.C., Daniel M.T. & Preud'homme J. (1975) Acute leukemia with Burkitt's tumor cells. A study of six cases with special reference to lymphocytoid surface markers. *Blood*, **45**, 183–188.

94 First M.I.C. Cooperative Study Group (1985) Morphologic, immunologic, and cytogenetic working classification of acute lymphoblastic leukemias. *Cancer Genetics and Cytogenetics*, **23**, 189–197.

95 Finlay J.L. & Borcherding W. (1988) Acute B-lymphocytic leukemia with L1 morphology: a report of two pediatric cases. *Leukemia*, **2**, 60–62.

96 Michiels J., Adriaansen H.J., Hagemeijer A., Hooijkaas H., Van Dongen J.J. & Abels J. (1988) TdT positive B-cell acute lymphoblastic leukemia (B-ALL) without Burkitt characteristics. *British Journal of Haematology*, **68**, 423–426.

97 Goorha R., Bunin N., Mirro J. *et al.* (1987) Provocative pattern of rearrangements of the genes for the gamma and beta chains of the T-cell receptor in human leukemias. *Proceedings of the National Academy of Sciences, USA*, **84**, 4547–4551.

98 Tawa A., Benedict S.H., Hara J., Hozumi N. & Gelfand E.W. (1987) Rearrangement of the T cell receptor gamma-chain gene in childhood acute lymphoblastic leukemia. *Blood*, **70**, 1933–1939.

99 Van Dongen J.J.M., Wolvers-Tetteroo I.L.M., Wassenaar F., Borst J. & Van der Elsen P. (1989) Rearrangement and expression of T-cell receptor delta genes in T-cell acute lymphoblastic leukemias. *Blood*, **74**, 334–342.

100 Campana D., Coustan-Smith E., Behm F.G. & Goorha R. (1993) Normal and aberrant T-cell receptor protein expression in T-cell acute lymphoblastic leukemia. *Recent Results in Cancer Research*, **131**, 19–30.

101 Gouttefangeas C., Bensussan A. & Boumsell L. (1990) Study of the CD3-associated T-cell receptors reveals further differences between T-cell acute lymphoblastic lymphoma and leukemia. *Blood*, **75**, 931–938.

102 Drexler H.G. (1987) Classification of acute myeloid leukemias. A comparison of FAB and immunophenotyping. *Leukemia*, **1**, 697–705.

103 San Miguel J.F., Gonzales M., Canizo M.C., Anta J.P., Zola H. & Lopez Borrasca A. (1986) Surface marker analysis in acute myeloid leukaemia and correlation with FAB classification. *British Journal of Haematology*, **64**, 547–552.

104 Neame P.B., Soamboonsrup P., Browman G.P. *et al.* (1986) Classifying acute leukemia by immunophenotyping: a combined FAB-immunologic classification of AML. *Blood*, **68**, 1355–1361.

105 Van der Schoot C.E., Daams G.M., Pinkster J., Ver R. & von dem Borne A.E. (1990) Monoclonal antibodies against myeloperoxidase are valuable immunological reagents for the diagnosis of acute myeloid leukaemia. *British Journal of Haematology*, **74**, 173–179.

106 Drexler H.G., Thiel E. & Ludwig W.D. (1993) Acute myeloid leukemias expressing lymphoid-associated antigens: diagnostic incidence and prognostic significance. *Leukemia*, **7**, 489–498.

107 Chan L.C., Pegram S.M. & Greaves M.F. (1985) Contribution of immunophenotype to the classification and differential diagnosis of acute leukaemia. *Lancet*, **i**, 475–479.

108 Buccheri V., Shetty V., Yoshida N., Morilla R., Matutes E. & Catovsky D. (1992) The role of anti-myeloperoxidase antibody in the diagnosis and classification of acute leukemia: a comparison with light and electron microscopy cytochemistry. *British Journal of Haematology*, **80**, 62–68.

109 Ashman L.K., Roberts M.M., Gadd S.J., Cooper S.J. & Juttner C.A. (1988) Expression of a 150 kDa cell surface antigen identified with monoclonal antibody YB5.B8 is associated with poor prognosis in acute lymphoblastic leukemia. *Leukemia Research*, **12**, 923–929.

110 Buccheri V., Matutes E., Dyer M.J. & Catovsky D. (1993) Lineage commitment in biphenotypic acute leukemia. *Leukemia*, **7**, 919–927.

111 Pui C.H., Behm F.G. & Crist W.M. (1993) Clinical and biologic

relevance of immunologic marker studies in childhood acute lymphoblastic leukemia. *Blood*, **82**, 343–353.

112 Boucheix C., David B., Sebban C. *et al.* for the French Group on Therapy for Adult Acute Lymphoblastic Leukemia. (1994) Immunophenotype of adult acute lymphoblastic leukemia, clinical parameters, and outcome: an analysis of a prospective trial including 562 tested patients (LALA87). *Blood*, **84**, 1603–1612.

113 Sobol R.E., Mick R., Royston I. *et al.* (1987) Clinical importance of myeloid antigen expression in adult acute lymphoblastic leukemia. *New England Journal of Medicine*, **316**, 1111–1117.

114 Urbano-Ispizua A., Matutes E., Villamor N. *et al.* (1990) Clinical significance of the presence of myeloid associated antigens in acute lymphoblastic leukaemia. *British Journal of Haematology*, **75**, 202–207.

115 Wiersma S.R., Ortega J., Sobel E. & Weinberg K.I. (1991) Clinical importance of myeloid-antigen expression in acute lymphoblastic leukemia of childhood. *New England Journal of Medicine*, **324**, 800–808.

116 Childs C.C., Hirsch-Ginsberg C., Walters R.S. *et al.* (1989) Myeloid surface antigen-positive acute lymphoblastic leukemia (MY+ ALL): immunophenotypic, ultrastructural, cytogenetic, and molecular characteristics. *Leukemia*, **3**, 777–783.

117 Guyotat D., Campos L., Shi Z-H. *et al.* (1990) Myeloid surface antigen expression in adult acute lymphoblastic leukemia. *Leukemia*, **4**, 664–666.

118 Ferrara F., De Rosa C., Fasanaro A. *et al.* (1990) Myeloid antigen expression in adult acute lymphoblastic leukemia: clinicohematological correlations and prognostic relevance. *Human Pathology*, **4**, 93–98.

119 Pui C-H., Behm F.G., Singh B. *et al.* (1990) Myeloid-associated antigen expression lacks prognostic value in childhood acute lymphoblastic leukemia treated with intensive multiagent chemotherapy. *Blood*, **75**, 198–202.

120 Bradstock K.F., Hoffbrand A.V., Ganeshaguru K. *et al.* (1981) Terminal deoxynucleotidyl transferase expression in acute non-lymphoid leukaemia — an analysis by immunofluorescence. *British Journal of Haematology*, **47**, 133–143.

121 Vodilenich L., Tax W., Bai Y., Pegram S., Capel P. & Greaves M.F. (1983) A monoclonal antibody WT1 for detecting leukemias of T cell precursors. *Blood*, **62**, 1108–1013.

122 Lo Coco F., De Rossi G., Pasqualetti D. *et al.* (1989) CD7 positive acute myeloid leukaemia: a subtype associated with cell immaturity. *British Journal of Haematology*, **73**, 480–485.

123 Adriaansen H.J., Van Dongen J.J.M., Kappers-Klune C. *et al.* (1990) Terminal deoxynucleotidyl transferase positive subpopulations occur in the majority of ANLL: implications for the detection of minimal residual disease. *Leukemia*, **4**, 404–410.

124 Solary E., Casasnovas R.O., Campos L. *et al.* and the Groupe d'Etude Immunologique des Leucemies (GEIL) (1992) Surface markers in adult acute myeloblastic leukemia: correlation of CD19+, CD34+ and CD14+/DR– phenotypes with shorter survival. *Leukemia*, **6**, 393–399.

125 Griffin J.D., Hercend T., Beveridge R. & Schlossman S.F. (1983) Characterization of an antigen expressed by human natural killer cells. *Journal of Immunology*, **130**, 2947–2951.

126 Coustan-Smith E., Behm F.G., Hurwitz C.A., Rivera G.K. & Campana D. (1993) N-CAM (CD56) expression by CD34+ malignant myeloblasts has implications for minimal residual disease detection in acute myeloid leukemia. *Leukemia*, **7**, 853–858.

127 Hurwitz C.A., Raimondi S.C., Head D. *et al.* (1992) Distinctive immunophenotypic features of t(8;21)(q22;q22) acute myeloblastic leukemia in children. *Blood*, **80**, 3182–3188.

128 Greaves M.F., Chan L.C., Furley A.J.W., Watt S.M. & Molgaard H.V. (1986) Lineage promiscuity in hemopoietic differentiation and leukemia. *Blood*, **67**, 1–11.

129 Smith L.J., Curtis J.E., Messner H.A., Senn J.S., Furthmayr H. & McCulloch E.A. (1983) Lineage infidelity in acute leukemia. *Blood*, **61**, 1138–1145.

130 Saito M., Kumagai M., Okazaki T. *et al.* (1995) Stromal cell-mediated transcriptional regulation of the CD13/aminopeptidase N gene in leukemic cells. *Leukemia*, **9**, 1508–1516.

131 Shkolnik T., Schlossman S.F. & Griffin J.D. (1985) Acute undifferentiated leukemia: induction of partial differentiation by phorbol ester. *Leukemia Research*, **9**, 11–17.

132 Ragavachar A., Bartram C.R., Ganser A., Heil G., Kleihauer E. & Kubanek B. (1986) Acute undifferentiated leukemia: implications for cellular origin and clonality suggested by analysis of surface markers and immunoglobulin gene rearrangement. *Blood*, **68**, 658–663.

133 Hara J., Yumura-Yagi K., Tawa A. *et al.* (1989) Molecular analysis of acute undifferentiated leukemia: two distinct subgroups at the DNA and RNA levels. *Blood*, **74**, 1738–1746.

134 Campana D., Hansen-Hagge T.E., Matutes E. *et al.* (1990) Phenotypic, genotypic cytochemical and ultrastructural characterization of acute undifferentiated leukemia. *Leukemia*, **4**, 620–624.

135 Chessels J.M., Hurdisty R.M., Rapson N.Y. & Greaves M.F (1977) Acute lymphoblastic leukemia in children: classification and prognosis. *Lancet*, **ii**, 1307–1309.

136 Sen L. & Borella L. (1975) Clinical importance of lymphoblasts with T markers in childhood leukemia. *New England Journal of Medicine*, **292**, 828–832.

137 Patte C., Michon J., Frappaz D. *et al.* (1994) Therapy of Burkitt and other B-cell acute lymphoblastic leukaemia and lymphoma: experience with the LMB protocols of the SFOP in children and adults. *Baillières Clinical Haematology*, **7**, 339–348.

138 Crist W.M., Grossi C.E., Pullen J. & Cooper M.D. (1985) Immunologic markers in childhood acute lymphocytic leukemia. *Seminars in Oncology*, **12**, 105–121.

139 Greaves M.F., Janossy G., Peto J. & Kay H.E.M. (1981) Immunologically defined subclasses of acute lymphoblastic leukaemia in children: their relationship to presentation features and prognosis. *British Journal of Haematology*, **48**, 179–197.

140 Morgan E. & Hsu C.C.S. (1980) Prognostic significance of the acute lymphoblastic leukemia (ALL) cell-associated antigen in children with null cell ALL. *American Journal of Pediatric Hematology/Oncology*, **2**, 99–103.

141 Pui C.H. (1995) Childhood leukemias. *New England Journal of Medicine*, **332**, 1618–1630.

142 Pui C.H., Hancock M.L., Head D.R. *et al.* (1993) Clinical significance of CD34 expression in childhood acute lymphoblastic leukemia. *Blood*, **82**, 889–894.

143 Crist W.M., Boyett J., Roper M. *et al.* (1984) Pre-B-cell leukemia responds poorly to treatment: a Pediatric Oncology Group study. *Blood*, **63**, 407–414.

144 Crist W., Boyett J., Jackson J. *et al.* (1989) Prognostic importance of the pre-B-cell immunophenotype and other presenting features in B-lineage childhood acute lymphoblastic leukemia: a Pediatric Oncology Group study. *Blood*, **74**, 1252–1259.

145 Crist W.M., Carroll A.J., Shuster J.J. *et al.* (1990) Poor prognosis of children with pre-B acute lymphoblastic leukemia is associated with the t(1;19)(q23;p13): a Pediatric Oncology Group study. *Blood*, **76**, 117–122.

146 Raimondi S.C., Behm F.G., Roberson P.K. *et al.* (1990) Cytogenetics of pre-B-cell acute lymphoblastic leukemia with emphasis on

prognostic implications of the t(1;19). *Journal of Clinical Oncology*, **8**, 1380–1388.

147 Rivera G.K., Raimondi S.C., Hancock M.J. *et al.* (1991) Improved outcome in childhood acute lymphoblastic leukaemia with reinforced early treatment and rotational combination chemotherapy. *Lancet*, **i**, 61–63.

148 Dow L.W., Borella L., Sen L. *et al.* (1977) Initial prognostic factors and lymphoblast-erythrocyte rosette formation in 109 children with acute lymphoblastic leukemia. *Blood*, **50**, 671–682.

149 Tsukimoto I., Wong K.Y. & Lampkin B.C. (1976) Surface markers and prognostic factors in acute lymphoblastic leukemia. *New England Journal of Medicine*, **294**, 245–248.

150 Hammond D., Sather H., Nesbit M. *et al.* (1986) Analysis of prognostic factors in acute lymphoblastic leukemia. *Medical and Pediatric Oncology*, **14**, 124–127.

151 Nadler L.M., Reinherz E.L., Weinstein H.J., D'Orsi C.J. & Schlossman S.F. (1980) Heterogeneity of T-cell lymphoblastic malignancies. *Blood*, **55**, 806–810.

152 Crist W.M., Shuster J.J., Falletta J. *et al.* (1988) Clinical features and outcome in childhood T-cell leukemia-lymphoma according to stage of thymocyte differentiation: a Pediatric Oncology Group study. *Blood*, **72**, 1891–1897.

153 Pui C-H., Behm F.G., Singh B. *et al.* (1990) Heterogeneity of presenting features and their relation to treatment outcome in 120 children with T-cell acute lymphoblastic leukemia. *Blood*, **75**, 198–202.

154 Borowitz M.J., Dowell B.L., Boyett J.M. *et al.* (1985) Monoclonal antibody definition of T cell leukemia: a Pediatric Oncology Group study. *Blood*, **65**, 785–788.

155 Shuster J.J., Falletta J.M., Pullen D.J. *et al.* (1990) Prognostic factors in childhood T-cell acute lymphoblastic leukemia: a Pediatric Oncology Group Study. *Blood*, **75**, 166–173.

156 Thiel E., Kranz B.R., Raghavachar A. *et al.* (1989) Prethymic phenotype and genotype of pre-T (CD7+/ER-)-cell leukemia and its clinical significance within adult acute lymphoblastic leukemia. *Blood*, **73**, 1247–1258.

157 Digel W., Schultze J., Kunzmann R., Mertelsmann R. & Lindemann A. (1994) Poor prognosis of prethymic phenotype acute lymphoblastic leukemia (pre-T-ALL). *Leukemia*, **8**, 1406–1408.

158 Griffin J.D., Davis R., Nelson D.A. *et al.* (1986) Use of surface marker analysis to predict outcome of adult myeloblastic leukemia. *Blood*, **68**, 1232–1241.

159 Schwarzinger I., Valent P., Köller U. *et al.* (1990) Prognostic significance of surface marker expression on blasts of patients with *de novo* acute myeloblastic leukemia. *Journal of Clinical Oncology*, **8**, 423–430.

160 Merle-Beral H., Duc L.N.C., Leblond V. *et al.* (1989) Diagnostic and prognostic significance of myelomonocytic cell surface antigens in acute myeloid leukemia. *British Journal of Haematology*, **73**, 323–330.

161 San Miguel J.F., Ojeda E., Gonzalez M. *et al.* (1989) Prognostic value of immunological markers in acute myeloblastic leukemia. *Leukemia*, **3**, 108–111.

162 Bradstock K., Matthews J., Benson E., Page F., Bishop J. and the Australian Leukaemia Study Group (1994) Prognostic value of immunophenotyping in acute myeloid leukemia. *Blood*, **84**, 1220–1225.

163 Holowiecki J., Lutz D., Krzemien S. *et al.* (1986) CD-15 antigen detected by the VIM-D5 monoclonal antibody for prediction of ability to achieve complete remission in acute nonlymphocytic leukemia. *Acta Haematologica*, **76**, 16–19.

164 Borowitz M.J., Gockerman J.P., Moore J.D. *et al.* (1989)

Clinopathological and cytogenetic features of CD34 (MY10)-positive acute nonlymphocytic leukemia. *American Journal of Clinical Pathology*, **91**, 265–270.

165 Creutzig U., Harbott J., Sperling C. *et al.* (1995) Clinical significance of surface antigen expression in children with acute myeloid leukemia: results of study AML-BFM-87. *Blood*, **86**, 3097–3108.

166 Ball E.D., Davis R.B., Griffin J.D. *et al.* (1991) Prognostic value of lymphocyte surface markers in acute myeloid leukemia. *Blood*, **77**, 2242–2250.

167 Pui C-H., Raimondi S.C., Head D.R. *et al.* (1991) Characterization of childhood acute mixed-lineage leukemia at diagnosis and at relapse. *Blood*, **78**, 1327–1337.

168 Davey F.R., Mick R., Nelson D.A. *et al.* (1988) Morphologic and cytochemical characterization of adult lymphoid leukemias which express myeloid antigen. *Leukemia*, **2**, 420–426.

169 Pui C-H., Dahl G.V., Melvin S. *et al.* (1984) Acute leukaemias with mixed lymphoid and myeloid phenotype. *British Journal of Haematology*, **56**, 121–130.

170 Cross A.H., Goorha R.M., Nuss R. *et al.* (1988) Acute myeloid leukemia with T-lymphoid features: a distinct biologic and clinical entity. *Blood*, **72**, 579–587.

171 Jani P., Verbi W., Greaves M.F., Bevan D. & Bollum F. (1983) Terminal deoxynucleotidyl transferase in acute myeloid leukemia. *Leukemia Research*, **7**, 17–29.

172 Benedetto P., Mertelsmann R., Szatrowski T.H. *et al.* (1986) Prognostic significance of terminal deoxynucleotidyl transferase activity in acute non-lymphoblastic leukemia. *Journal of Clinical Oncology*, **4**, 489–495.

173 Swirsky D.M., Greaves M.F., Gray R.G. & Rees J.K.H. (1988) Terminal deoxynucleotidyl transferase and HLA-DR expression appear unrelated to prognosis of acute myeloid leukaemia. *British Journal of Haematology*, **70**, 193–198.

174 Caligaris-Cappio F. & Janossy G. (1985) Surface markers in chronic lymphoid leukaemias of B cell type. *Seminars in Hematology*, **22**, 1–12.

175 Matutes E. & Catovsky D. (1991) The classification of lymphoid leukemias. *Leukemia and Lymphoma*, **6** (Suppl.), 153–155.

176 Matutes E., Owusu-Ankomah K., Morilla R. *et al.* (1994) The immunological profile of B-cell disorders and proposal of a scoring system for the diagnosis of CLL. *Leukemia*, **8**, 1640–1645.

177 Matutes E., Morilla R., Owusu-Ankomah K., Houlihan A., Meeus P. & Catovsky D. (1994) The immunophenotype of hairy cell leukemia (HCL). Proposal for a scoring system to distinguish HCL from B-cell disorders with hairy or villous lymphocytes. *Leukemia and Lymphoma*, **14**(Suppl. 1), 57–61.

178 Matutes E., Morilla R., Owusu-Ankomah K., Houlihan A. & Catovsky D. (1994) The immunophenotype of splenic lymphoma with villous lymphocytes and its relevance to the differential diagnosis with other B-cell disorders. *Blood*, **83**, 1558–1562.

179 Matutes E. & Catovsky D. (1991) Mature T-cell leukemias and leukemia/lymphoma syndromes. Review of our experience in 175 cases. *Leukemia and Lymphoma*, **4**, 81–91.

180 Matutes E., Brito-Bapapulle V., Swansbury J. *et al.* (1991) Clinical and laboratory features of 78 cases of T-prolymphocytic leukemia. *Blood*, **78**, 3269–3274.

181 Hutchison R.E., Berard C.W., Shuster J.J., Link M.P., Pick T.E. & Murphy S.B. (1995) B-cell lineage confers a favorable outcome among children and adolescent with large-cell lymphoma: a Pediatric Oncology Group study. *Journal of Clinical Oncology*, **13**, 2023–2032.

182 Campana D. & Pui C.H. (1995) Detection of minimal residual

disease in acute leukemia: methodologic advances and clinical significance. *Blood*, **85**, 1416–1434.

183 Greaves M.F., Delia D., Janossy G. *et al.* (1980) Acute lymphoblastic leukaemia associated antigen. IV. Expression on non-leukaemic lymphoid cells. *Leukemia Research*, **4**, 15–21.

184 Sang B.C., Dias P., Shi L. *et al.* (1996) Monoclonal antibodies specific to the fusion region of E2A-pbx1 chimeric protein in t(1;19) ALL; characterization and diagnostic utility. *Blood*, **88**(Suppl. 1), 74a.

185 Ryan D.H. & Van Dongen J.J.M. (1988) Detection of residual disease in acute leukemia using immunological markers. In: *Immunologic Approaches to the Classification and Management of Lymphomas and Leukemias* (eds J.M. Bennett & K.A. Foon), pp. 173–203. Kluwer Academic Publishers, Norwell, MA.

186 Froelich T., Buchanan G., Cornet J., Sartain P. & Smith R. (1981) Terminal deoxynucleotidyl transferase-containing cells in peripheral blood: implications for the surveillance of patients with lymphoblastic leukemia or lymphoma in remission. *Blood*, **58**, 214–221.

187 Smith R., Hetherington M., Huntsman P. & Buchanan G. (1986) Surveillance of terminal deoxynucleotidyl transferase-positive cells in peripheral blood of patients with acute lymphoblastic leukemia (ALL). In: *Minimal Residual Disease in Acute Leukemia* (eds A. Hagenbeek & B. Lowenberg), pp. 134–140. M. Nijhoff Publishers, Dordrecht.

188 Bradstock K.F., Janossy G., Tidman N. *et al.* (1981) Immunological monitoring of residual disease in treated thymic acute lymphoblastic leukaemia. *Leukemia Research*, **5**, 301–306.

189 Campana D., Coustan-Smith E. & Janossy G. (1990) The immunological detection of minimal residual disease in acute leukemia. *Blood*, **76**, 163–171.

190 Van Dongen J.J.M., Hooijkaas H., Adriaansen H.J., Hahlen K. & Van Zanen G.E. (1986) Detection of minimal residual acute lymphoblastic leukemia by immunological marker analysis: possibilities and limitations. In: *Minimal Residual Disease in Acute Leukemia* (eds A. Hagenbeek & B. Lowenberg), pp. 113–120. M. Nijhoff Publishers, Dordrecht.

191 Janossy G., Campana D., Burnett A. *et al.* (1988) Autologous bone marrow transplantation in acute lymphoblastic leukaemia—preclinical immunologic studies. *Leukemia*, **2**, 485–495.

192 Gross H.J., Verwer B., Houck D. & Recktenwald D. (1993) Detection of rare cells at a frequency of one per million by flow cytometry. *Cytometry*, **14**, 519–524.

193 Hurwitz C.A., Gore S.D., Stone K.D. & Civin C.I. (1992) Flow cytometric detection of rare normal human marrow cells with immunophenotypes characteristic of acute lymphoblastic leukemia cells. *Leukemia*, **6**, 233–238.

194 Reading C.L., Estey E.H., Huh Y.O. *et al.* (1993) Expression of unusual immunophenotype combinations in acute myelogenous leukemia. *Blood*, **81**, 3083–3087.

195 Lanza F., Bi S., Castoldi G. & Goldman J.M. (1993) Abnormal expression of N-CAM (CD56) adhesion molecule on myeloid and progenitor cells from chronic myeloid leukemia. *Leukemia*, **7**, 1570–1575.

196 Anderson C. & Looney J. (1986) Human leukocyte IgG Fc receptors. *Immunology Today*, **7**, 264–269.

197 Greaves M.F., Paxton A., Janossy G., Pain C., Johnson S. & Lister T.A. (1980) Acute lymphoblastic leukaemia associated antigen. III. Alterations in expression during treatment and in relapse. *Leukemia Research*, **4**, 1–6.

198 Stass S., Mirro J., Melvin S., Pui C.H., Murphy S.B. & Williams D. (1984) Lineage switch in acute leukemia. *Blood*, **64**, 701–707.

199 Van Dongen J.J.M., Breit T.M., Adriaansen H.J., Beishizen A. & Hooijkaas H. (1992) Detection of minimal residual disease in acute leukemia by immunological marker analysis and polymerase chain reaction. *Leukemia*, **6**, 47–53.

200 Drach J., Drach D., Glassl H., Gattringer C. & Huber H. (1992) Flow cytometric determination of atypical antigen expression in acute leukemia for the study of minimal residual disease. *Cytometry*, **13**, 893–898.

201 Coustan-Smith E., Behm F.G., Sanchez J. *et al.* (1998) Immunologic detection of minimal residual disease in children with acute lymphoblastic leukemia. *Lancet.* (In press.)

202 Neale G.A.M., Pui C-H, Mahmoud H.H. *et al.* (1994) Molecular evidence for minimal residual bone marrow disease in children with isolated extramedullary relapse of T-cell acute lymphoblastic leukemia. *Leukemia*, **8**, 768–773.

203 Goulden N., Langlands K., Steward C. *et al.* (1994) PCR assessment of bone marrow status in 'isolated' extramedullary relapse of childhood B-precursor acute lymphoblastic leukaemia. *British Journal of Haematology*, **87**, 282–287.

204 Mahmoud H.H., Rivera G.K., Hancock M.L. *et al.* (1993) Low leukocyte counts with blast cells in cerebrospinal fluid of children with newly diagnosed acute lymphoblastic leukemia. *New England Journal of Medicine*, **329**, 314–318.

205 Bradstock K.F., Papageorgiou E.S. & Janossy G. (1981) Diagnosis of meningeal involvement in patients with acute lymphoblastic leukaemia using immunofluorescence for terminal transferase. *Cancer*, **47**, 2478–2483.

206 Hooijkaas H., Hahlen K., Adriaansen H.J., Dekker I., Van Zanen G.E. & Van Dongen J.J.M. (1989) Terminal deoxynucleotidyl transferase positive cells in cerebrospinal fluid and development of overt CNS leukemia: a 5-year follow-up study in 113 children with TdT positive leukemia or non-Hodgkin's lymphoma. *Blood*, **74**, 416–423.

207 Kranz B.R., Thiel E. & Thierfelder S. (1989) Immunocytochemical identification of meningeal leukemia and lymphoma: poly-L-lysine-coated slides permit multimarker analysis even with minute cerebrospinal fluid cell specimens. *Blood*, **73**, 1942–1947.

Acute Lymphoblastic Leukaemias

C.C. Bailey and S.E. Kinsey

Clinical features and diagnosis

Acute lymphoblastic leukaemia (ALL) commonly presents with a clinical history which extends over a period of 4–6 weeks. The first symptoms may be nonspecific infection, often in the upper respiratory tract, which either persists despite antibiotic therapy or, after initially improving, relapses. It may be noticed that the patient looks increasingly pale and has increasing lethargy and anorexia. During the same period the patient may start to complain of aching pains in the back and in the limbs. This bone pain may occasionally be more acute and localized and will then resemble the presentation of acute osteomyelitis. The pain may appear to be localized to the joints where it may mimic the onset of juvenile rheumatoid arthritis (Fig. 5.1). The symptom which usually precipitates the referral of the patient for a blood count is the appearance of either a purpuric rash or the onset of spontaneous or excessive bruising.

Examination of the patient will usually reveal signs of anaemia, cutaneous or mucous membrane haemorrhage, generalized lymphadenopathy and moderate enlargement of the liver and spleen. Careful examination of the retinae should be made for signs of retinal haemorrhage. All of these signs are, however, variable in their expression, and in some patients anaemia may be the only presenting feature.

Unusual presentations include dyspnoea or upper mediastinal obstruction associated with the presence of a large anterior or superior mediastinal mass. (Occasionally these symptoms may initially lead to the erroneous diagnosis of asthma associated with initial improvement in symptoms on commencing bronchodilators or oral steroids.) Pleural effusion may also be present in this syndrome which is most commonly seen in older children, has a strong male predominance and is associated with T-cell leukaemia (Fig. 5.2). Presentation with acute renal failure can occur in patients who have high white cell counts or who have extensive leukaemic infiltration of the kidney. Central nervous system (CNS) infiltration may present with signs of raised intracranial pressure and/or

with cranial nerve palsies, particularly of cranial nerves VI and VII. An exceedingly high presenting white cell count ($>200 \times 10^9$/l) may be associated with hyperviscosity syndrome and leukostasis, particularly in the coronary and cerebral vasculature.

Essential investigations

Full blood count. This usually reveals a normochromic normocytic anaemia, the mean haemoglobin level being 5 g/dl. The total white blood cell count is often within the normal range, but may be low, slightly elevated or occasionally greatly elevated. The differential count most commonly shows an absolute neutropenia and monocytopenia, with the majority of the cells being lymphocytes and leukaemic blast cells. The percentage of blast cells within the total varies from zero in some cases to 100% in others. The platelet count is usually decreased.

Bone marrow examination. This is essential even if the blood contains circulating leukaemic cells. On occasions the marrow may be difficult to aspirate, a so-called 'dry tap', and in these cases a trephine biopsy should be obtained. Bone marrow investigations must include light microscopy, cytochemistry, immunophenotyping, 'conventional' cytogenetics, DNA index and molecular techniques for identification of chromosomal abnormalities which may not be detectable by routine karyotyping. Light microscopy is required for FAB classification of leukaemic blasts, the scheme for this is outlined in Table 5.1.

Bone marrow should also be examined using a panel of monoclonal antibodies, to establish the cell marker characteristics of the leukaemic cells for that particular patient. Immunophenotyping is performed either by fluorescent activated cell sorting (FACS) analysis or alkaline phosphatase/anti-alkaline phosphatase (APAAP) techniques, cellular suspensions or smears respectively. Immunophenotypic classification of leukaemic cells has shown that these exist in several distinct subcategories, and that these are of clinical and prognostic importance. Table 5.2 shows the most common immunophenotyping patterns that have been described.

Cytogenetic evaluation of leukaemic blasts is a necessity. Certain abnormalities are recognized to relate to prognosis and others are described which relate to some leukaemic subtypes (Table 5.3).

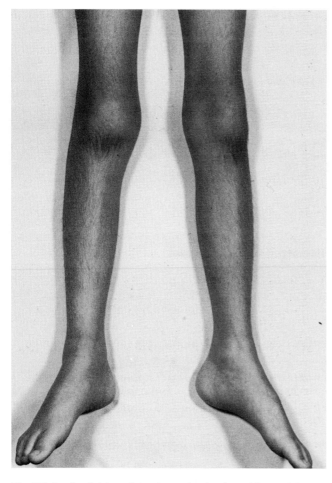

Fig. 5.1 Swollen joints and muscle wasting in a boy with ALL and a 3-month history of joint pain.

Conventional cytogenetic analysis by karyotype analysis is a routine investigation and remains important to identify emerging patterns of cytogenetic abnormality which may indicate association/prognosis in the future. However, it is well recognized that the molecular analysis of translocations and breakpoints is more likely to identify a specific abnormality than karyotype analysis alone, for example for t(9,22) BCR/abl and 11q23 abnormalities. Recently it has been identified that up to 30% of children with B-lineage ALL have translocation t(12;21) detectable by molecular techniques only and that this may be of prognostic significance [2]. Therefore it is recommended that molecular techniques are used to completely exclude the presence of Philadelphia chromosome positivity t(9,22) and 11q23 abnormalities and to identify the presence of t(12;21).

The role of numerical and structural karyotypic and molecular cytogenetics in the evaluation and elucidation of the pathogenesis of ALL cannot be understated. Up to this time, cytogenetics, cell morphology and immunophenotyping have only provided a clue to the likely treatment outcome. Numerical cytogenetic evaluation (ploidy) is known to be of value in prognosis for the treatment outcome and therefore may contribute to the assessment of overall risk and use of appropriate risk-stratified treatment. Laboratory techniques for the assessment of ploidy involve conventional karyotypic cytogenetic evaluation or flow-cytometric analysis of leukaemic cell DNA content; however, the latter will not provide information of any structural chromosome abnormality which may also be present [3].

Ploidy may be described as:

1 diploid (normal), DNA index 1.0;

2 pseudodiploid, 46 chromosomes, but with structural abnormalities present, DNA index 1.0;

3 hyperdiploid, 47–50 chromosomes, DNA index 1.01–1.15;

4 high hyperdiploid >50 chromosomes, DNA index >1.16;

5 hypodiploid/near haploid, <46 chromosomes, DNA index <1.0;

6 tetraploid, 92 chromosomes, DNA index 2.0.

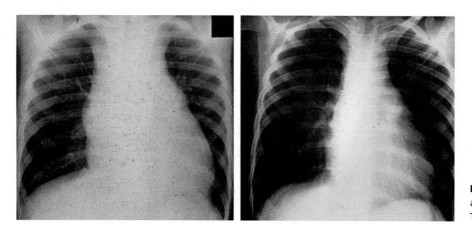

Fig. 5.2 Mediastinal widening (a) before and (b) 48 hours after therapy in a boy with T-ALL.

Table 5.1 The French–American–British (FAB) Morphological Classification Scheme for ALL. (From Bennett *et al.*, 1976 [1], with permission.)

Cytological features	L1	L2	L3
Cell size	Small cells predominate	Large, heterogeneous in size	Large and homogeneous
Nuclear chromatin	Homogeneous in any one case	Variable, heterogeneous in any one case	Finely stippled and homogeneous
Nuclear shape	Regular, occasional clefting or indentation	Irregular, clefting and indentation common	Regular, oval to round
Nucleoli	Not visible or small and inconspicuous	One or more present often large	Prominent; one or more vesicular
Amount of cytoplasm	Scanty	Variable often moderately abundant	Moderately abundant
Basophilia of cytoplasm	Slight or moderate rarely intense	Variable deep in some	Very deep
Cytoplasmic vacuolation	Variable	Variable	

Table 5.2 Immunophenotypic classification of ALL.

Leukaemic subtype	Null-ALL	C-ALL	Early Pre-B ALL	Pre-B-ALL	B-ALL	T-ALL
Nuclear TdT	+	+	+	+	–	+
HLA-DR(la)	+	+	+	+	+	–
CD10	–	+	+	+	– > +	–
CD19	+ > –	+	+	+	+	–
CD20	–	– > +	+	+	+	–
CD22	–	–	+	+	+	–
cCD22	+	+	+	NA	NA	–
CIg	–	–	–	+	NA	–
SIg	–	–	–	–	+	–
CD2	–	–	–	–	–	+

+ = typically positive; – = typically negative; + > – = majority of cases positive; – > + = majority of cases negative; NA = not applicable.

Table 5.3 Chromosomal abnormalities in ALL.

Abnormality	Likely leukaemic subtype
t(1;19)(q23;p13)	Pre-B, common
t(2;8)(p12;q24)	B
t(4;11)(q21;q23)	Null
del(6)(q21–25)	Common, B, T (+ other abnormalities)
t(8;14)(q24;q32)	B
t(8;22)(q34;q11)	B
t(9;22)(q43;q11)	Pre-B, common, null and rarely T
–9 and 9p t/del	Early T precursor
t(11;14)(q13;q32)	T
12p t/del	Common

With the increasing efficiency of cytogenetic techniques, subtle cytogenetic changes are more frequently found, leading to an increase in the number that are pseudodiploid compared with diploid [4].

Molecular markers, for example immunoglobulin heavy-chain (IgH) gene rearrangements in B-precursor ALL and T-cell receptor gene rearrangements (TCR$_\gamma$), are increasing in importance as a potential handle for assessment during (and following) treatment of minimal residual disease.

Cerebrospinal fluid examination. This examination should always be undertaken. The fluid should be examined microscopically and a cell count carried out. A cytocentrifuge preparation should then be made and examined for cell morphology. Counts of more than 5 per high-power field with recognizable blast cells on cytocentrifuge preparation are diagnostic of leukaemic infiltration. In the event of cells being present but with a cell count of less than 5 per high-power field being obtained, the cerebrospinal fluid (CSF) should be examined at weekly intervals until it is clear that the cells represent true CNS disease and not contamination of the specimen with peripheral blood. High peripheral blast count associated with traumatic CSF sampling may lead to incorrect diagnosis of CNS involvement, as a result of the contamination of the CSF specimen with peripheral blood. In difficult cases, immunophenotyping of CSF cells is invaluable.

Biochemical analyses. These should be undertaken for serum urate, urea and creatinine. Serum potassium, calcium and phosphate should also be measured. The presence of an elevated serum urate should alert the clinician to the presence of impending tumour lysis syndrome, which must be treated before the therapy for the leukaemia is commenced. In this context an ultrasound examination of the abdomen will sometimes reveal enlarged kidneys which, together with biochemical abnormality, is highly predictive of tumour lysis syndrome.

Immunoglobulins. The level of immunoglobulins should be measured. Some patients will have markedly decreased levels and this may be associated with poor ultimate outcome, even in the presence of other good risk features. [5].

Microbiological cultures. Cultures of blood, urine and faeces should be carried out, and appropriate swabs from the throat and the nose should be taken, to establish whether fever is associated with infection, and to determine the patient's resident flora. Identification of any pathogen will subsequently aid in antibiotic choices. Viral antibody titres should be measured to establish the level of immunity of the patient to viruses such as measles, varicella zoster, cytomegalovirus, Epstein–Barr and herpes simplex.

Radiology. A chest radiograph is the only X-ray which is routinely required. In patients with T-cell leukaemia, mediastinal enlargement is a frequent finding and may be so large that there is superior mediastinal obstruction. A variety of skeletal lesions may be seen, including lytic areas, periosteal elevation and metaphyseal bands, but these are of no prognostic significance and require no specific therapy. In patients with B-cell disease abdominal imaging is recommended.

Indicators of prognosis

Clinical features

The prognosis of ALL is most strongly influenced by the achievement of initial remission of the disease and by the duration of that initial remission. The ability to achieve remission is influenced by the therapy received by the patient. By considering various clinical and laboratory parameters present at diagnosis, attempts have been made to tailor therapy to risk features of the disease. The aim is to give more intensive therapy to those with adverse features and less intensive therapy to those with good prognostic features.

Data from the American Children's Cancer Group (CCG) and the British Medical Research Council acute lymphoblastic leukaemia studies (MRC UKALL) have been subjected to multivariate analysis in order to assess the influence of features measured at diagnosis on disease-free interval [6]. More recently, in addition to these initial features, the speed of response to therapy, dynamic staging, is being used to predict ultimate prognosis [7–11].

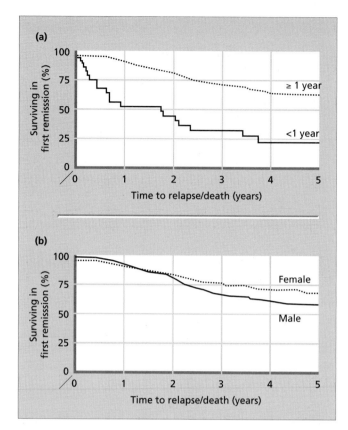

Fig. 5.3 Clinical outcome in the MRC UKALL X trial in children: (a) subdivided by age; (b) subdivided by sex.

While it is compelling to draw comparison between outcomes from different therapeutic approaches for different risk groups of patients with ALL, it has to be emphasized that response to therapy is of great importance, and that the influence of presenting features is interactive with the therapy received. Thus outcome for different risk groups cannot be extrapolated to potential response to differing therapy.

Age

Age at diagnosis has been shown to be an important indicator of prognosis (Fig. 5.3a), with children less than 1 year of age having a particularly poor outcome when treated with standard therapeutic protocols [12–14]. The CCG and MRC UKALL groups now both single out these infants for specifically designed therapeutic studies in an attempt to improve this outcome. Infants less than 1 year of age at presentation tend to have a high incidence of 11q23 cytogenetic abnormality, which is emerging as an important prognostic indicator of poor risk and is also seen in treatment-related acute myeloid leukaemia (AML). Age greater than 10 years predicts for a poor outcome [15,16], with a trend for this to worsen as age increases into the adult range.

Table 5.4 Features of the leukaemia/lymphoma syndrome.

Clinical features	Laboratory features
1. Lymphadenopathy >3 cm diameter	1. WBC > 5 × 10⁹/l
2. Splenomegaly > umbilicus or more	2. Hb > 10 g/dl
3. Mediastinal mass > one-third transthoracic diameter	3. T-ell positive

Sex

Both the CCG [17] and MRC UKALL [18–20] groups have shown male sex (Fig. 5.3b) to be a poor prognostic factor. The influence of male sex is interesting, because it does not appear to influence the ability to obtain an initial remission, nor to maintain this remission; it exerts its influence mainly after cessation of therapy. Boys then experience a greater incidence of bone marrow relapse than girls.

The incidence of testicular relapse is 12% [19,21–25], while ovarian relapse as an isolated event is rare. In the recent MRC trial UKALL VIII, the incidence of isolated testicular relapse appears to have been reduced to 5% and was significantly correlated with the presence of mediastinal mass and T-cell disease [25]. The majority of these testicular relapses occur within 1 year of the cessation of therapy, and unless further systemic therapy is given they will frequently be followed by bone marrow relapse. This raises the question whether the testicle acts as a sanctuary site from which reseeding of the marrow takes place or whether the testis is the early palpable tip of an iceberg of relapse taking place at multiple sites.

Bulky disease

Steinherz *et al.* [26] reported that analysis of the clinical course of 1537 children with ALL showed that there was a subgroup of 11.5% who had a poor outcome. This was associated with the presence of massive organomegaly or mass disease, defined as the presence of lymph nodes greater than 3 cm in diameter, the presence of a mediastinal mass greater than one-third of the transthoracic diameter or the presence of splenomegaly extending to or below the umbilicus.

Additionally, these patients tended to have a high peripheral white cell count at presentation greater than 50 × 10⁹/l, T-cell disease by immunophenotyping, preserved haemoglobin levels (>10 g/dl), male sex and age greater than 10 years compared with other children with ALL [16,26].

When bulky disease such as mediastinal mass is analysed as a single factor, it has a less strong prognostic influence [26,27] than when it occurs in the presence of abnormal laboratory features [28].

Steinherz also pointed out that the inverse was true — laboratory features alone are not such a strong prognostic indicator as when they are combined with a clinical feature [26]. Thus, the leukaemia/lymphoma syndrome, as this bulky presentation has been called, will be defined as the presence of at least one clinical and one laboratory feature from Table 5.4 and would be expected to predict a poor outcome.

Race

Black children with ALL in the USA have a significantly worse outcome than white children. They have a higher incidence of other poor prognostic features, such as a high white cell count, mediastinal mass and L2 morphology, and less frequently have favourable features, such as common ALL phenotype and hyperdiploid chromosomes [29].

In analysis, it has been suggested that if these differences are balanced for, then race, as such, may be irrelevant. The difference in prognosis may be accounted for in differences in socioeconomic status or in decreased access to medical care [30,31]. Similarly, it has been suggested that Asian children resident in the UK have a poorer outlook than similar white children. This is accounted for by socioeconomic status and language difficulties, leading to failure of compliance with therapy [32,33].

Hazard scoring systems

With increasing data on larger numbers of patients, statistical tests can be used to analyse the interaction of clinical and laboratory features felt to be influential with actual outcome. Following much statistical scrutiny, the largest investigations, MRC, Rome and St Jude, have developed mathematical models for hazard risks. Following analysis of the MRC UKALL X data, hazard ratio as a function of age, sex and white count determined by Cox regression analysis predicts those with a score greater than 0.8 as poor risk and those with a score less than 0.8 as standard risk [20,34,35]. More intensive treatment in the form of bone marrow transplantation from a matched sibling donor is recommended for the high-risk patients.

Indicators of prognosis—laboratory features

Full blood count

At any age and presentation the most important single prognostic indicator in ALL is the highest pretreatment white cell count. The higher this is, the less good the prognosis, with patients who have initial white cell counts at less than 100 × 10⁹/l doing particularly badly (Fig. 5.4). [6,20,27,34–36].

Preserved haemoglobin and decreased platelet levels are much less strong variables when assessed independently, but may be of prognostic significance when associated with other features [28]. Preservation of haemoglobin implies a higher pretreatment proliferative rate of marrow blast cells, with the leukaemia presenting before the haemoglobin has had time to fall.

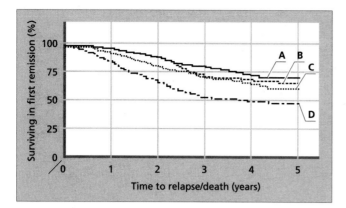

Fig. 5.4 Clinical outcome in the MRC UKALL X trial in children subdivided by white blood cell count at presentation. (A) <10 × 10⁹/l; (B) 10–19 × 10⁹/l; (C) 20–50 × 10⁹/l; (D) +50 × 10⁹/l.

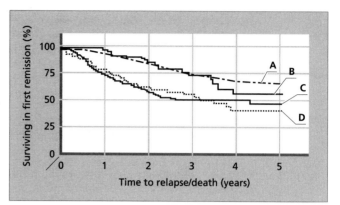

Fig. 5.5 Clinical outcome in the MRC UKALL X trial in children subdivided by cell type at presentation. (A) Common ALL; (B) pre-B-ALL; (C) T cell; (D) null cell.

Cell morphology

The cell morphology of the leukaemic cells has been related to prognosis. The French–American–British (FAB) Classification is now widely used; the majority of childhood leukaemias are of L1 morphology, while adults more frequently show L2 morphology.

In the CCG analysis of 3500 patients, the presence of more than 10% of cells with L2 morphology was shown to be associated with poor outcome. This worsened as the percentage of L2 cells increased. L3 morphology is associated with B-cell disease and carries a particularly poor outlook [37]. Similar results have also been reported from the FAB typing panel of the MRC UKALL group [38]. The periodic acid schiff (PAS) reaction in lymphoblasts also has prognostic bearing in relation to morphological and immunophenotypic features [39].

Cell marker studies

The use of panels of monoclonal antibodies has enabled ALL to be divided into well-defined subcategories. Common ALL, early pre-B-ALL, pre-B-ALL, B-ALL and T-ALL, and these are of prognostic significance (Fig. 5.5). Eighty-five per cent of childhood ALL is of B-lineage. Eighty per cent of patients will have C-ALL and will have the best outlook. Crist *et al.* [40] reported that 20–30% of patients will have cells which have positive reactions to cytoplasmic immunoglobulin but not to surface immunoglobulin—pre-B-ALL. This subset has a poorer prognosis than children with C-ALL [40–42].

Between 1 and 2% of patients present with cells with the characteristics of mature B cells identical to those seen in Burkitt's lymphoma. This group responds poorly to standard antileukaemic therapy and has a high incidence of early relapse. They respond better when treated with chemotherapy protocols designed for lymphoma therapy [43]. Between 10 and 15% of patients present with T-cell disease. They are more

frequently male, often present with a total white cell count of >50 × 10⁹/l and often have mass disease in the mediastinum and, as such, have a poor prognosis. However, it would appear that the T-cell characteristic is not in itself an independent prognostic indicator, and the patient presenting with T-cell lymphoblasts, but without the other adverse prognostic indicators, will have a prognosis equal to that of a patient with C-ALL [44].

Null-ALL occurs in a small percentage of children with ALL but more frequently in adults with the disease. This subgroup has an inferior prognosis to either C-ALL or T-ALL [45].

Biphenotypic leukaemia is said to occur when the leukaemic cell line expresses reactivity to antibodies specific to different lineages; for example, the spontaneous expression of both lymphoid and myeloid markers. This phenomena has been reported in up to 13% of childhood leukaemias and may occur more frequently than this in adult leukaemias [46,47]. The clinical significance of this phenomena is not at present clear and these patients should be treated as for ALL. Recent studies in infants in whom this phenomena is more often seen, and who, as a group, have a poor prognosis, have included the use of drugs active against the myeloid cell line.

Cytogenetics

Cytogenetic analysis of leukaemic blast cells is an essential investigation for the determination of prognosis. Analysis includes determination of the modal number of chromosomes and banding techniques to determine structural abnormalities within the chromosomes.

Children with a hyperdiploid leukaemia clone (>50 chromosomes) seem to have a favourable prognosis [48], while children who have hypodiploid or near haploid clones have a poorer outcome (Fig. 5.6) [49]. Children with a pseudodiploid clone (46 XX or XY but with intrinsic structural abnormalities) also fare poorly. It is now possible, by analysis of cellular DNA

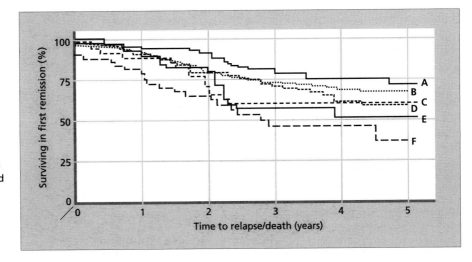

Fig. 5.6 Early analysis of clinical outcome in the MRC UKALL X trial in children subdivided by ploidy group at presentation. (A) 51+ chromosomes; (B) normal chromosome number; (C) pseudodiploid; (D) Ph,t(4;11), t(1;19); (E) <46 chromosomes; (F) 47–50 chromosomes.

flow cytometry, to determine the DNA ploidy of cells (see above).

Translocations are the commonest structural abnormality seen and seem to be associated with particular subtypes of ALL. t4;11(q21q23) is associated with null-ALL, particularly in infants, and carries a very poor prognosis [50]. t8;14(q24q23) occurs in B-cell leukaemia with its poor outcome [51]. t1;19(q23p13.3) is associated with pre-B-ALL, another poor outcome group [52], and t11;14(p13q13) occurs in T-cell leukaemia [53].

t9;22(q34q11) occurs in childhood ALL but is increasingly more common in adults with the condition. Patients with this translocation have a higher incidence of failure to achieve remission and a high early relapse rate [54–56].

Dynamic staging

This phrase has been coined to indicate the prognostic factors determined after the commencement of therapy and relating to the disease response to therapy over the first days or weeks of treatment to ultimate outcome.

Early studies by Jacquillat [7] in children and by Keating [8] in adults showed that bone marrow blast clearance by day 14 indicated a more favourable outcome in those patients who achieved clearance than in those who failed to do so. Miller *et al.* [9] showed that the clearance of blasts from the marrow by day 14 of therapy was an independent prognostic indicator of great significance. Rheim *et al.* [10], in the BFM 87 studies, showed that persistence of blasts after 1 week of treatment with corticosteroid alone indicated a poor prognosis. Data from the MRC UKALL VIII trial reported by Eden *et al.* [25] showed a highly significant disease-free survival for those clearing blasts to less than 5% to day 14 (*P* = 0.0002). Most recent studies are now investigating the significance of blast clearance from the bone marrow by day 7 of therapy [11].

Treatment

Modern therapy for ALL can be expected to be accompanied by a good success rate for remission induction, both in children and adults. In children there is also a good expectation of long-term disease-free survival, while in adults this may be achieved, but in fewer cases than in childhood. The treatment, however, is complex and intensive. A considerable amount of supportive care is necessary, particularly during remission induction. If the optimal results are to be achieved, this therapy should be undertaken in specialist units, using recognized treatment protocols. The maintenance or continuing therapy, while no less important, can more realistically be delivered nearer to the patient's home, allowing the concept of shared care to be pursued at this stage of therapy. Patient compliance during continuing therapy is exceedingly important. Noncompliance may significantly contribute to relapse rates. There is also evidence that a genetic variation exists in 6-mercaptopurine metabolism, with some patients being able to break down and excrete the drug more rapidly than others. This implies that rapid metabolizers have less therapeutic exposure to the drug than slow metabolizers.

Slow metabolizers, in their turn, experience more undesirable side effects such as major bone marrow suppression when they are treated with 6-mercaptopurine [57–59].

The newly diagnosed patient with acute lymphoblastic leukaemia will be anaemic, neutropenic and thrombocytopenic and may have hyperuricaemia and electrolyte disturbances. The first therapy offered, therefore, must be to improve the patient's overall condition, in order to prepare him or her for definitive antileukaemic therapy.

Anaemia should be corrected with transfusion of packed red blood cells. The only exception to this would be the rare patient who, because of an exceedingly elevated white cell count, has the hyperviscosity syndrome. However, in these patients, it is possible to overestimate the level of haemoglobin because of interference in the method of estimation and rehydration of these patients may unmask a severe anaemia. In these cases, anaemia can be corrected using whole blood as part of either an exchange transfusion procedure or leukopheresis to reduce the white cell count.

Patients with absolute neutrophil counts of less than $0.5 \times 10^9/l$ will frequently be pyrexial and often no obvious focus of infection can be found. This fever may sometimes therefore be a function of the disease process. However, after bacterial culture specimens have been obtained, therapy should be commenced empirically using an aminoglycoside antibiotic in combination with a ureidopenicillin or third- or fourth-generation cephalosporin or with one of the imipenem group of antibiotics.

Significant haemorrhage is unusual unless the platelet count is less than $20 \times 10^9/l$. Patients who are at particular risk are those in whom platelet levels as above are found in the presence of fever and infection. Such patients and patients with fundal haemorrhage or distressing mucous membrane haemorrhage should receive transfusions of platelets in order to raise the platelet count above $20 \times 10^9/l$.

Patients at particular risk for hyperuricaemia are those with large leukaemic cell mass, particularly those with B-cell leukaemia or T-cell leukaemia. There is also an increased risk in those patients who have enlarged kidneys as a result of leukaemic infiltration. Patients with the above risk factors may have normal uric acid levels at diagnosis, but develop raised levels after the commencement of antileukaemic therapy. Hyperuricaemia may be quickly followed by acute renal failure with rapid onset of hyperkalaemia, hyperphosphataemia, hypermagnesaemia and hypocalacaemia. This constellation of biochemical abnormalities, the tumour lysis syndrome, can then be accompanied by cardiac arrhythmia and death. It is important to note that dehydration and hypoxia contribute to tumour lysis. It is therefore extremely important that, if diagnostic procedures are to be performed under general anaesthetic, care is taken to correct any dehydration and to not allow any degree of hypoxia to occur.

Patients should commence intraveneous hydration therapy using twice the calculated maintenance fluid requirement. Allupurinol in a dose of $300–600\,mg/m^2$ per 24 hours should be commenced in order to block further formation of uric acid. Antileukaemic therapy should not be commenced until a diuresis has been obtained and any elevation of the serum uric acid has been corrected. In patients in whom a degree of renal failure already exists, or in whom it develops despite the above measures, dialysis or haemofiltration may be required in order to safely commence antileukaemic therapy [60].

Antileukaemic therapy is usually divided into three phases, remission induction, CNS-directed therapy, and maintenance or continuing therapy. In recent years various studies have explored the addition of intensification or consolidation blocks of treatment to the above pattern. These are an attempt to achieve further leukaemic cytoreductions in order to exploit the hypothesis of Goldie *et al.* [61].

The use of prognostic indicators and/or hazard score now identifies approximately 10% of patients who have a very high risk of treatment failure and who may be more appropriately treated with more intensive therapies such as bone marrow transplantation in first remission. Patients with B-cell leukaemia are more appropriately treated with lymphoma protocols. In the future, it may be possible to identify good-risk patients, for whom less intensive treatment will produce long-term survival with fewer late effects. However, at the present time no group of patients can be said to have better than an 85% chance of cure of their disease. Recent studies, such as those performed in Germany by Professor Reihm and his colleagues [62,63], have shown that low-risk patients have benefited less from intensification of therapy than have high-risk patients. Nevertheless, it is important that the 85% cure rate for the low-risk group is not accepted as satisfactory and that studies continue to include these patients in intensified protocols in order to improve their outcome further. It is also important to appreciate that the various phases of antileukaemic therapy, induction, consolidation, CNS therapy and continuing therapy are interactive, and that alterations in the treatment protocol to one phase of therapy may be reflected in altered outcomes in other areas. Examples might be that some patients may have received sufficient therapy for their underlying disease following intensive induction and consolidation and hence need less continuation therapy, while others may have profound myelotoxicity, reducing their ability to tolerate what may be essential consolidation therapy. Thus there may be advantageous or disadvantageous effects of early intensive therapy. Recent work has focused on the detection of minimal residual disease. This relies on identification of arrangements and rearrangements in the junctional regions generated by the immunoglobulin heavy-chain (IgH) gene, or the TCR gene, and then the amplification of these areas using the polymerase chain reaction (PCR). By identifying a specific 'finger-print' for the patient's leukaemia, PCR can then be used to detect minimal residual leukaemia in 90% or more of ALL. The value in assessing the completeness of remission and suitability for more intensive treatment of patients found to have residual disease is only just beginning to be fully evaluated [64–66].

The use of high doses of systemic agents such as methotrexate or cytosine arabinoside as CNS-directed therapy will inevitably have an effect on the disease in other areas of the body, and will interact with drugs given in consolidation or continuing therapy. Results of therapeutic studies comparing one therapy with another must therefore be interpreted in this light.

Remission induction

Remission induction in ALL is achieved using three drugs. Vincristine is given intravenously at weekly intervals for 4 weeks. Prednisolone is given orally daily over the same time period, and L-asparaginase is given either intravenously, intramuscularly or subcutaneously. The dose and route of administration of L-asparaginase varies in different treatment schedules.

The intravenous route is preferred in some schedules because of the undesirability of giving intramuscular or subcutaneous injections to individuals, who at this stage of their disease will almost certainly be thrombocytopenic. One of the major side effects of L-asparaginase is anaphylactic reaction. This is not uncommon when the intravenous route is used and is very rare when the drug is given either intramuscularly or subcutaneously [67].

The use of a three-drug schedule will be expected to achieve a remission rate of up to 90% in children with ALL, and up to 80% in adults with the disease. The addition of further drugs to induction therapy has not, to date, improved the remission induction rate in children, but appears to do so in adults. The most commonly used fourth drug is daunorubicin [68]. The addition of daunorubicin to the standard three-drug regimen was a randomized variable in the MRC UKALL VIII protocol in a dose of 45 mg/m^2 on days 1 and 2. The addition of daunorubicin induction therapy in the MRC UKALL VIII trial was associated with increased failed induction (nonremitters plus death in induction) compared with those not having daunorubicin—6 vs 3% [25]. However, there was a substantial reduction in the relapse rate (30 vs 38%) ($P = 0.06$) and disease-free survival at 5 years in remitters ($P = 0.08$). Deaths during induction were predominantly related to infection, particularly Gram negative, in those receiving daunorubicin. Even though there was an improvement in relapse-free survival, this does not translate into an improvement in overall disease-free survival, which results from a balance between increased toxicity and better disease control. However, the more intensive anthracycline therapy may confer better benefit in those presenting with white cell counts of greater than 50×10^9/l [25]. Other randomized studies have thus far failed to demonstrate any benefit in children [69].

In adult studies by the Cancer and Leukaemia Group B, however, the addition of daunorubicin to the induction regimen resulted in an improvement in remission induction from 47 to 83%. The length of the subsequent remission was, however, not increased [68].

It is important that, during remission induction, the antileukaemic therapy is continued in full dose, despite the inevitable cytopenias and fevers. The only reasons for dosage reduction would be the development of severe neuropathy secondary to vincristine therapy, pancreatitis due to asparaginase therapy, or diabetes which may be due to either or both of prednisolone and asparaginase.

Asparaginase can be continued in the face of an allergic reaction by changing to asparaginase obtained from a different source. Two sources are at present available, *E. coli*-derived asparaginase and *Erwinia* sp. asparaginase [70].

Intensification/consolidation therapy

The Goldie–Coldman hypothesis [61] suggests that an increase in the number of drug-resistant cells takes place as the mutation rate increases, and that the fraction of drug-resistant cells in a tumour population depends on whether the drug-resistant mutant occurs early or late in the treatment course.

Early aggressive chemotherapy to reduce the tumour cell population quickly should therefore decrease the likelihood of emergence of drug resistance. In the treatment of leukaemia, attempts to deliver intensive cytoreductive therapy in the first days of treatment have been accompanied in pilot studies for the MRC UKALL X study by unacceptable toxicity, the addition of daunorubicin in the standard three-drug induction regimen being probably the maximum tolerable increase in therapeutic aggressiveness at this stage.

The first major clinical studies to demonstrate the success of this approach were the BFM 76/79 regimens reported by Reihm *et al.* [62,63]. These regimens used a four-drug remission induction regimen (vincristine, prednisolone, L-asparaginase, daunorubicin), followed by an early intensification using cyclophosphamide, cytosine arabinoside and 6-thioguanine with cranial radiation therapy and intrathecal methotrexate. This was followed by a second intensification course and then maintenance chemotherapy using 6-mercaptopurine and methotrexate.

The regimen produced a 75% relapse-free survival rate at 4.5 years for high-risk patients. The German group has now gone on to modify the intensification pulses in terms of dosage of the drugs and timing of the second pulse, and has included standard-risk patients in the studies to explore the benefit which they may obtain from intensification. Early results suggest, however, that standard-risk patients have not shown the same benefit as that shown by the high-risk patients.

The American CCG conducted CCG106 for high-risk patients in which the BFM regimen was compared with a 'standard' regimen, without intensification, and a regimen from New York with intensification. The study showed that the two intensive regimens gave similar results but that both were superior to the standard regimen, in terms of remission induction and event-free survival [71].

The Medical Research Council in the UK conducted a trial from 1985 to 1990 in which the question of intensification was explored. UKALL X was designed to explore the optimal timing for the delivery of intensification. A standard regimen of four-drug induction, followed by cranial radiation therapy, plus intrathecal methotrexate and then continuing therapy using 6-mercaptopurine plus methotrexate, with monthly vincristine and prednisolone pulses (regimen (group) A), was compared with three regimens into which intensification blocks had been added (groups B–D). The intensification consisted of daunorubicin, cytosine arabinoside, etopside and 6-thioguanine given over 5 days.

In group B this pulse was given at week 5, in group C at

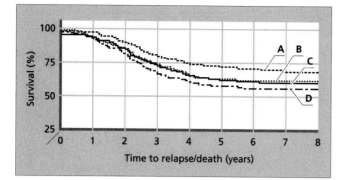

Fig. 5.7 Comparison of disease-free survival (DFS) in four randomized treatment arms in the MRC UKALL X trial (1993). Group A: *n* = 293, DFS = 71%; group B: *n* = 293, DFS = 62%; group C: *n* = 294, DFS = 61%; group D: *n* = 291, DFS = 57%.

Table 5.5 Age-related intrathecal methotrexate dosage for CNS prophylaxis.

Age (years)	Methotrexate rate (mg)
<1	7.5
<3	10
>3	12.5

week 20 and in group D at both weeks 5 and 20. The study showed that the regimen containing early and late intensification blocks was more effective than either no intensification or one intensification block (Fig. 5.7) [72].

Central nervous system-directed therapy

Chemotherapy for ALL improved through the 1960s such that the majority of children achieved remission of their disease, but as these remissions became longer, so 60–70% of them were terminated by the onset of CNS relapse. Studies from St Jude Hospital, Memphis, showed that radiation therapy to the craniospinal access could dramatically reduce this problem. Subsequent studies in the USA showed that the optimal therapy consisted of cranial radiation therapy with concurrent intrathecal injections of methotrexate [73,74].

The optimal dose of cranial radiation is 18 Gy for patients with standard-risk disease and 24 Gy for patients at high risk of CNS relapse (presenting white cell count >100 × 10⁹/l). Methotrexate is given concurrent with the cranial radiation therapy in an age-determined dose (Table 5.5). It is important to use such a dosage method, because of the relatively large size of the CNS space compared to the body size in the young infant.

Many children have received such therapy in the treatment of their leukaemia and have become long-term survivors. Follow-up of these children has shown that some of them have major problems with learning [75,76] and a small number have difficulties with growth and sexual development [77]. They appear to be worse the younger the child was at the time of therapy [78]. These late effects have been attributed to the cranial radiation therapy.

In order to avoid these late complications, the American CCG showed that for children aged 3–6 years, with presenting white cell count <10 × 10⁹/L cranial irradiation could be omitted so long as intrathecal methotrexate injections were continued throughout therapy [79].

Borsi and colleagues showed that methotrexate given intravenously in doses of 6–8 g/m² was able to create CSF methotrexate levels greater than the leukaemocidal level of 1 × 10⁻⁶ M [80,81]. Groups in the USA and the UK are now studying, in randomized trials, whether the addition of high-dose intraveneous methotrexate with folinic acid rescue at 24 hours to continued intrathecal methotrexate will have an additional benefit in terms of control of CNS disease. This approach also has the advantages that the high-dose therapy may confer increased therapeutic benefit over the systemic disease with longer event-free survival and may also be accompanied by fewer late sequelae than cranial radiation.

Children entered into these studies will need careful psychometric testing over the next few years, in order to ensure that high concentrations of methotrexate in the CNS are not accompanied by as yet unsuspected chemotherapy induced cerebral damage.

Continuing therapy

At the present time, maintenance or continuing therapy continues to be an essential part of therapy for ALL.

Very intensive induction and consolidation therapies may make the delivery of continuing therapy difficult because of reduced bone marrow tolerance, or even unnecessary, as exemplified by bone marrow transplantation. Present nontransplant, induction and consolidation therapies need to be followed by 2–3 years of continuing therapy. 6-Mercaptopurine and methotrexate taken orally form the backbone of continuing therapy, usually with the addition of monthly vincristine and prednisolone pulses.

Studies have been conducted in which the methotrexate has been given parenterally, rather than orally, but no significant survival advantage has been demonstrated [82]. Other studies have delivered the drugs in a pulsed form [83] or have sought to substitute the drugs given in pulses [84]. These studies also have failed to demonstrate advantage over simple, daily oral 6-mercaptopurine plus weekly oral methotrexate. The CCG 161 study in the USA experimented with the omission of the vincristine and the prednisolone pulses, but the study was altered when this omission was shown to be disadvantageous [85].

The manner in which the daily doses of 6-mercaptopurine are adjusted may be very important. Hale & Lilleyman [57] have recently shown that in MRC studies conducted since

1980, when clear guidelines for dose adjustment were issued, children have been prescribed 22% more 6-mercaptopurine than in similar studies before 1980. They postulate that this increased intensity of dose schedule may have been responsible for the marked survival in improvement seen over that time. They also showed that boys tolerated greater doses of 6-mercaptopurine for longer periods than did girls. They hypothesize that this greater tolerance to 6-mercaptopurine may underline the sex difference in survival seen in most studies of ALL. Koren and colleagues calculated the area under the concentration–time curve for patients, taking 1 mg of 6-mercaptopurine per m² of body area. They demonstrated differences in bioavailability of the mercaptopurine and showed that patients with a low bioavailability had a higher risk of relapse. They recommended the use of such a pharmocokinetic study early in continuing therapy in order to appropriately adjust the mercaptopurine dose [86].

The length of continuing therapy has progressively been reduced. The Children's Cancer Study Group showed that there was no advantage conferred by receiving 5 years' treatment, rather than 3 years [87], while the Medical Research Council showed that 3 years' therapy conferred no advantage when compared to 2 years for girls, but there was a slight advantage for boys [88]. With newer, more intensive induction and consolidation regimens, and a better understanding of the concept of minimal residual disease, further reductions in the level of continuing therapy may be able to be made, particularly if the 6-mercaptopurine dose is maintained at optimal levels.

Infants

Children of less than 12 months of age have a particularly poor outlook (Fig. 5.8) [6,36,89,90], they tend to have an increased incidence of poor prognostic features, such as high white cell count at presentation, CNS leukaemia at presentation, Null-cell disease and 4;11 translocation [13]. There is evidence that the disease in infants occurs at a more primitive stage of B-cell differentiation than occurs in older children [91].

There is frequently a myeloid element included in the leukaemic process, indicating that this may represent a biphenotypic process or true stem cell leukaemia. Molecular techniques have identified the presence of rearrangement of the MLL gene (11q23) in a high proportion of infants.

Recently, treatment protocols have been developed specifically for the therapy of infants and they have been excluded from the trials of therapy for older children. Remission induction is usually achieved using the three- or four-drug regimens of vincristine, prednisolone, asparaginase and daunorubicin. Consolidation with drugs conventionally used in the therapy of myeloid leukaemia, etoposide, cytosine arabinoside and 6-thioguanine, may help to control the myeloid element in the disease.

Central nervous system therapy must be achieved

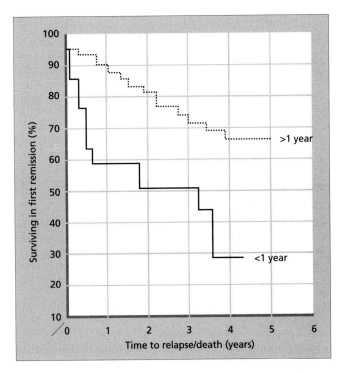

Fig. 5.8 Disease-free survival in the MRC UKALL VII clinical trial for patients under 1 year old at diagnosis versus the rest. <1 year old, *n* = 21; >1 year old, *n* = 810; *P* < 0.005.

chemotherapeutically, rather than with the use of radiotherapy, because of the vulnerability of the developing CNS. Intrathecal methotrexate given throughout maintenance, may be supplemented by intravenous infusions of methotrexate given in high-dose, or 'triple' intrathecal therapy with methotrexate, cytosine arabinoside and hydrocortisone may be preferred. These studies are, however, still investigational, and should only be administered from large treatment centres with considerable expertise in supportive care available.

Relapse

Bone marrow relapse

Bone marrow relapse is the site of failure in the majority of patients in whom disease recurs. The prognosis for further event-free survival is, in general, poor [92], but is influenced by various factors, among which the most important are the time at which the relapse takes place in relation to the initial therapy, the type of initial therapy given and the type of therapy employed to treat the relapse. The prognosis is best for those patients whose bone marrow relapse occurs more than 6 months after the completion of their initial therapy, and is worst for those patients in whom the relapse occurred while they are still receiving their initial course of therapy [93–95].

The prognosis worsens the shorter the length of the initial remission [95,96]. Patients who experience two or more bone marrow relapses are highly unlikely to be cured of their disease, while a small number may still be cured after a first bone marrow relapse [95,97]. The intensity of the initial therapy is related to the likelihood of sustained second remission, in that those patients relapsing after nonintensive initial therapy are more likely to have sustained second remissions than those in whom the relapse occurs following an intensive initial therapy.

Remission induction can be undertaken using a four-drug regimen including vincristine, a steroid, an anthracycline and asparaginase, and this will be successful in achieving a second remission in 90% of children [95,97,98]. This must be followed by further CNS-directed therapy because of the high risk of CNS re-seeding if this is not undertaken. The choice of CNS-directed therapy will depend upon the type of treatment given in the initial protocol, and on the plans for further treatment. An example would be a child who had not previously had cranial radiation therapy who might now be best treated using this option. However, if the plan is to proceed to bone marrow transplantation, this would not be the treatment of choice because of the need for total body irradiation in the transplant-conditioning regimen.

Similarly, the choice of consolidation/intensification therapy and continuing therapy is also influenced by the treatment given originally, the time at which the relapse takes place, and whether or not a transplant is planned. It is the policy in the UK at the present time to use the four-drug induction regimen as above, and to follow this with consolidated therapy utilizing cytosine arabinoside, cyclophosphamide, etoposide, epirubicin, asparaginase and dexamethasone, given over an 8-week period. Central nervous system preventative therapy is given using intrathecal and high-dose intravenous methotrexate therapy. Following this treatment, children with matched sibling donors proceed to bone marrow transplantation, whilst those without donors continue on a chemotherapy regimen for 100 weeks, in which a 6-week pulse of 6-mercaptopurine, methotrexate, vincristine and prednisolone is alternated with a 2-week pulse of cyclophosphamide, cytosine arabinoside, etoposide and thioguanine.

The previous study with randomization to autologous bone marrow transplantation has been discontinued due to lack of recruitment to the randomization, with physicians preferring to opt either for allogenic bone marrow transplants or continuing chemotherapy alone. Autografting in adult treatment is still being pursued. Some centres may feel that in some circumstances the use of unrelated bone marrow transplant should be considered. The long-term benefits of this form of therapy, with high treatment-related morbidity and mortality, remain unclear at present.

This therapy is appropriate for children whose disease relapses while on therapy or within 2 years of completing initial therapy. The very small percentage of children who experience very late relapse are more appropriately treated as if they had newly developed the disease.

Recent reports using similar therapeutic strategies have shown 90% remission rates, but still poor long-term survival rates [92,99].

Central nervous system relapse

Central nervous system relapse is the initial site of relapse, either as an isolated relapse or in combination with simultaneous bone marrow relapse in 10% of children. The most common presentation of CNS relapse is with symptoms of raised intracranial pressure, headache and vomiting. Occasionally a child will present with the onset of cranial nerve palsy, most commonly affecting cranial nerves VI or VII. A rare presentation of CNS relapse is increased appetite accompanied by excessive weight gain.

The prognosis following CNS relapse is poor [100]. Remission can be induced in the majority of patients with the use of six intrathecal injections of methotrexate, given at weekly intervals. Unless this is followed by further therapy to the CNS, however, further relapse is inevitable. The use of triple intrathecal therapy, using cytosine arabinoside and hydrocortisone, in addition to methotrexate, has been advocated in some studies, but there is little evidence to suggest any additional effectiveness over methotrexate alone [101].

Central nervous system relapse, if treated in isolation, will be followed in the majority of cases by bone marrow relapse. It is necessary, therefore, for patients to receive a further course of systemic induction therapy at the same time as the CNS-directed therapy.

If the child has relapsed following initial treatment which did not include cranial radiation therapy, the definitive CNS therapy of choice is either craniospinal irradiation [102] or total body irradiation given as part of the conditioning regimen for bone marrow transplantation. If neither of these options is possible then monthly intrathecal methotrexate injections for at least 1 year following the achievement of clearance of the blast cells from the cerebrospinal fluid should be given, along with systemic continuation therapy, which is usually given for 2 years from the date of the CNS relapse.

Testicular relapse

Testicular relapse usually presents as uni- or bilateral painless testicular enlargement. The testicle is the initial site of relapse in between 10 and 13% of boys [20,103]. It may occur during the initial therapy when the outlook is very poor or, more commonly, within 1 year after the cessation of therapy when the outlook is better [104]. It may occur as an isolated site of relapse, or in combination with either bone marrow or CNS relapse. Isolated testicular relapse will be followed by bone marrow relapse in a high percentage of cases, unless concurrent systemic therapy is given while the testicle is treated [104].

Testicular relapse may present as unilateral testicular

swelling, but studies have shown that it is frequently also present in the apparently unaffected testicle. Treatment must therefore be given to both testes. The usual prescription is to give four-drug induction therapy, with intrathecal methotrexate for CNS prophylaxis and to treat the testicle with radiation therapy to a dose of 24 Gy. This should be followed by continuing therapy for 2 years [105]. Those boys whose testicular relapse occurs during therapy, or within 6 months of its cessation, may be treated with more intensive consolidation/intensification therapy, or, if a bone marrow donor is available, with bone marrow transplantation. In this case the total body irradiation should be supplemented with a booster dose to the testis.

Boys treated with 24 Gy testicular radiation will inevitably be sterile, but may also suffer Leydig cell failure and require androgen replacement therapy subsequently [106].

Ocular relapse

Ocular relapse is a rare site of isolated relapse in acute lymphoblastic leukaemia. It usually presents as a red, painful eye and slit lamp examination reveals leukaemic infiltrates in the anterior chamber, the iris or the hypopyon. Ocular relapse is usually treated with local radiation therapy but, once again, because of the incidence of associated bone marrow relapse, systemic reinduction and continuing therapy should be given.

Bone marrow transplantation

In ALL allogenic bone marrow transplantation has been most commonly used as a rescue therapy following reinduction of remission, after relapse occurring either during therapy or within 1 year of completion of therapy. In these circumstances, further event-free survival rates of the order of 40% have been reported [107]. It is possible that for patients with particularly poor prognostic features at diagnosis, such as white cell count $>100 \times 10^9/l$, presence of t(4;11) or t(9;22) translocation or near haploid chromosome number, or for adult patients, bone marrow transplantation from a fully HLA-matched sibling donor, in first remission, may be the treatment of choice.

There are, however, no randomized studies to support this course of action, and the studies which have been reported have been criticized as being conducted on a highly selected group of patients who have been able to (i) achieve a remission and (ii) survive disease free until a transplant could be carried out.

Modern intensive regimens, such as the BFM and New York regimens, may give as good results. This question, at the present time, remains unanswered.

The role of autologous bone marrow transplantation is also unclear in ALL. The UK Medical Research Council attempted to clarify this by conducting a randomized control trial in patients during second remission, but this was discontinued due to nonrandomization because of physician choice of bone marrow transplant from either sibling or unrelated donors, or election to continue with chemotherapeutic regimens.

Supportive care

The field of supportive care for patients with ALL is very wide. It ranges from the resuscitation and preparation which is necessary before therapy begins (see above), through therapeutic and prophylactic treatment of infection to extensive psychosocial support.

While on therapy for acute leukaemia, patients are immune suppressed and, in addition, may have periods of profound neutropenia. They are therefore at risk from bacterial, viral and fungal infections and other opportunistic infections, particularly *Pneumocystis carinii* pneumonia.

Febrile illness occurring during periods of neutropenia should be treated empirically with broad-spectrum intravenous antibiotics. The combination of antibiotics chosen will depend upon local circumstances, taking into account the local microbiological epidemiology, and resistance patterns. A review of infections in the Medical Research Council UKALL X trial showed that the most common isolates were *Staph. aureus*, *Staph. epidermidis*, *E. coli*, *Pseudomonas* species and *Klebsiella* species. Until results of cultures are known, it is advisable to choose an antibiotic combination with a spectrum that cover these organisms. More recently there has been a re-emergence of Gram-positive organisms, in particular coagulase-negative staphylococci, streptococci and enterococci, are more frequently isolated.

The use of broad-spectrum antibiotic combinations has been very successful in the therapy of bacterial infection [108–110], but fungal infections are being reported with increasing frequency. In the neutropenic patient who remains febrile after 72 hours of appropriate antibiotic therapy, the empirical addition of amphotericin B should be considered [111]. Lipid-bound amphotericin B preparations are now available which are better tolerated by patients, and are associated with less nephrotoxicity, thus allowing the dose to be escalated for clinically suspected or microbiologically proven invasive fungal disease [112].

Mouth care is also of great importance during periods of neutropenia. As soon as possible after diagnosis, the patient should be seen by a dental hygienist and treatment should be given for any dental caries or infection. When the platelet count has recovered, full oral toilet should be carried out. In the meantime the mouth should be kept clean and moist by the frequent use of bacteriostatic mouth washes and by tooth cleaning using dental sponges, because ulceration and haemorrhage is frequent. Viral culture will reveal many of the mucosal ulcers to be infected with herpes simplex virus, which may become secondarily infected with *Candida albicans*. Herpes simplex should be treated with acyclovir and candidiasis with nystatin, or oral fluconazole for those who cannot tolerate nystatin.

When remission has been induced, the major dangers to the patient are viral infections, particularly measles, chickenpox and the protozoal infection pneumocystis carinii. Measles may pursue a particularly aggressive course in the immune suppressed, with the major dangers being the development of giant cell pneumonia, or measles encephalopathy [113]. Previous history of infection or immunization may not confer protection as it does in the normal individual, and all patients should therefore be considered at risk.

The patient cannot be immunized once leukaemia has been diagnosed because of the danger of dissemination of the live attenuated virus. However, it is common experience that the most usual source of contact is with the patient's siblings. Therefore, it is recommended that any nonimmunized siblings should receive immunization. If close contact occurs — 20 minutes in the same room as an individual who has measles or who develops it within 4 days—the patient should be given a dose of human immune globulin as soon as possible, in the hope that this will confer passive immunity. Despite these measures, measles remains a major cause of death in children in the UK, where large numbers of children in the population remain nonimmunized. The issue of poor herd immunity to measles has recently been addressed in the UK by an aggressive policy of immunization of school-age children.

Chickenpox can also pursue an aggressive course in the immune suppressed, with the development of widespread, sometimes haemorrhagic, skin lesions, hepatitis and pneumonitis. As with measles, a previous history of infection does not imply immunity, and all patients on therapy should be considered at risk. If close contact occurs—20 minutes in the same room as an individual with active chickenpox, or who develops chickenpox within 4 days—or close physical contact with an individual with open shingles, an intramuscular dose of zoster immune globulin should be given [114]. Should chickenpox develop despite these precautions, the patient should be treated with high-dose intravenous acyclovir.

Pneumocystis carinii pneumonia used to occur in patients during remission and was associated with a significant mortality. It can be prevented by the prophylactic use of trimethoprim-sulphamethoxazole given orally [115]. This therapy should now be included in all continuing therapy protocols. Patients who cannot tolerate oral trimethoprim-sulphamethoxazole may alternatively be treated with nebulized pentamidine.

Patients may develop other common viral infections, but generally these will not cause life-threatening illness; it is therefore important that this risk is not overemphasized, and it is our practice to encourage return to school or work as soon as possible after the neutrophil and platelet counts have recovered. This rehabilitation into a more normal lifestyle is essential. The aim of modern therapy is to reintroduce into society a patient who is not only disease free, but who is emotionally, socially and educationally intact and capable of playing a full role in that society.

In order to achieve this, it is essential to recognize the profound impact the diagnosis of leukaemia has on the patient and the family, and on the community in which the patient lives and works. The patient needs age-appropriate explanation of the diagnosis and the proposed treatment, and should be given opportunities to discuss any fear and apprehensions regarding the treatment and outlook.

The relatives' fears will vary according to the stage of illness and, in addition, they may be faced with additional stresses related to employment, finance or pre-existing marital problems. All of these areas need to be explored with them, and appropriate counselling and support should be provided.

Local community-based medical services will have little experience of the care of a leukaemic patient, and yet their help and support is essential to the patient. They may feel deskilled by the expertise of the major centre and should be given support and advice about what care needs to be provided for the patient, and when referral back to the major centre is needed.

Educational establishments need advice on the re-entry of the patient into the establishment. They may have fears regarding the courses of action to be taken should the child become ill in school and how to recognize problems, and they may need advice on what to expect of the patients' scholastic achievement. In order to achieve all of this, a multidisciplinary team is essential, consisting of the primary care physician, nurses and social workers. Access to psychology, dietetic advice, pharmacy and physiotherapy services should be available.

Late effects of treatment

The greatest concern regarding the late effects of treatment in leukaemia are the neuroendocrine effects of CNS therapy. It has been shown that children treated with 24 Gy cranial irradiation have, in some cases, suffered intellectual damage with progressive decline in verbal IQ, loss of attention span and academic failure. In addition, some children have been shown to have growth failure which may or may not be associated with loss of growth hormone secretion [77]. More recent treatment protocols have concentrated on the avoidance of radiation therapy for all except those at highest risk of CNS disease.

Reports on the neuroendocrine function of children treated with methotrexate, either intrathecally or intrathecally plus intravenously, suggest that these forms of therapy are not accompanied by the same sequelae as cranial irradiation. It is however known that methotrexate can be associated with the development of leucoencephalopathy and, therefore, children treated with CNS therapy protocols other than cranial irradiation need careful prolonged follow-up to assess any damage which may occur [116,117].

Other effects on growth are less serious. It is common for a degree of growth failure to occur during treatment, but this is often caught up once therapy stops. Children treated for leukaemia tend to have a higher incidence of obesity than their peers. Whether this is a direct effect associated with the treatment, or whether it reflects bad dietary habits cultivated during the inevitable family stress associated with diagnosis and therapy, is not clear.

Children treated prepubertally for their leukaemia usually enter puberty normally and have normal secondary sexual development. Some reports suggested that the ovaries of girls treated for leukaemia are smaller than normal [118]. Girls treated with cranial irradiation have been observed to have a higher than expected incidence of early onset of puberty. Despite this, many girls have now had pregnancies and have delivered normal offspring. Whether or not these girls will experience early menopause remains to be seen. Although boys experience a normal puberty, there are fewer reports of fatherhood among them than there are of motherhood for the girls, and it is likely that there is an incidence of subfertility [119].

Second primary tumours are a rare event in leukaemia survivors. The most common are new neoplasms of the haematological system or the development of glioma. Whether these are treatment-induced neoplasms or whether they represent a genetic predisposition to neoplasia is not clear.

The use of anthracyclines in induction and consolidation therapy has been associated with alterations in myocardial function. In most cases this has been detectable on echocardiography but has not, as yet, been of clinical significance except in those patients proceeding to further intensive, and potentially cardiomyopathic, therapies, such as bone marrow transplantation. However, there remains a worry regarding the long-term outlook for those with demonstrable myocardial changes.

Conclusion

Between 60 and 70% of children and between 20 and 40% of adults can now be expected to be long-term survivors of their leukaemia. It is possible that with an improved ability to stratify patients for their prognosis at the beginning of therapy, and to deliver more intensive therapies to those with less good outlooks, this could be improved in the future. Equally, as minimum residual disease technology is expanded, and the significance of small numbers of leukaemic cells detectable during remission becomes known, it may be possible to select patients for further treatments to prevent subsequent relapse.

Long-term follow-up has shown that relapse is rare once the patient has remained disease free for 3 years after the completion of therapy. Such patients will, however, need to be carefully followed up in the long-term follow-up clinics in order to further ascertain the true incidence of late effects of treatment, such as the development of second malignancies, the true incidence of fertility and infertility, the prognosis for long-term reproductive life in females and the degree of socioeconomic success achieved by the survivors. Increasing numbers of off-

spring are now being born to parents who survived childhood leukaemia, and these infants will need to be registered and monitored carefully for possible teratogenic effects of therapy or for the development of genetically determined malignant disease. This constitutes a logistic problem for the treatment centres which could only have been dreamed of three decades ago.

References

1 Bennett J.M., Catovsky K., Daniel M.T. *et al.* (1976) Proposals for the classification of the acute leukaemias (FAB Co-operative Group). *British Journal of Haematology*, **33**, 451–458.

2 Hiebert S.W., Ward D.C., Bray-Ward P. *et al.* (1995) Fusion of the TEL gene on 12p13 to the AML1 gene on 21q22 in acute lymphoblastic leukaemia. *Proceedings of National Academic Society*, **92**, 4917–4921.

3 Raimondi S.C. (1993) Current status of cytogenetic research in childhood acute lymphoblastic leukaemia. *Blood*, **81**, 2237–2251.

4 Pui C.J., Williams D.L., Roberson P.K. *et al.* (1988) Correlation of karyotype and immunophenotype in childhood acute lymphoblastic leukaemia. *Journal of Clinical Oncology*, **6**, 56.

5 Welch J.C. & Lilleyman J.S. (1995) Immunoglobulin concentrations in untreated lymphoblastic leukaemia. *Journal of Paediatric Haematology and Oncology*, **12**, 545–549.

6 Hammond G.D., Sather H.N., Nesbit M.E. *et al.* (1986) Analysis of prognostic factors in acute lymphoblastic leukaemia. *Medical and Paediatric Oncology*, **14**, 124–134.

7 Jacqillat C., Weil M., Gemon M.F. *et al.* (1973) Combination therapy in 130 patients with acute lymphoblastic leukaemia (protocol 06 LA 66-Paris). *Cancer Research*, **33**, 3278–3284.

8 Keating M.J., Smith T.C., Gehan E.A. *et al.* (1980) Factors related to length of complete remission in adult leukaemia. *Cancer*, **45**, 2017–2029.

9 Miller D.R., Coccia P.F., Bleyer A. *et al.* (1989) Early response to induction therapy as a prediction of disease free survival and late recurrence of childhood acute lymphoblastic leukaemia. A report from the Children's Cancer Study Group. *Journal of Clinical Oncology*, **7**, 1807–1815.

10 Reihm H., Feickert H.J., Schrappe M. *et al.* (1987) Therapy results in five ALL-BFM studies since 1970. Implications of risk factors for prognosis. *Haematology and Blood Transfusions*, **30**, 139–146.

11 Gaynon P.S., Bleyer W.A., Steinherz P.G. *et al.* (1990) Day 7 marrow response and outcome for children with acute lymphoblastic leukaemia and unfavourable presenting features. *Medical and Paediatric Oncology*, **18**, 273–279.

12 Blayer W.A. (1983) Acute lymphoid leukaemias. *Pediatric Annals*, **12**, 1–16.

13 Reaman G., Zeltzer P., Blayer W.A. *et al.* (1985) Acute lymphoblastic leukaemia in infants less than one year of age. A cumulative experience of the Children's Cancer Study Group. *Journal of Clinical Oncology*, **3**, 1513–1521.

14 Harousseau J.L., Tobelem G., Schaison G. *et al.* (1980) High risk acute lymphoblastic leukaemia. A study of 141 cases with initial white blood cell counts over 100 000/cu mm. *Cancer*, **46**, 1996–2003.

15 Crist W., Pullen J., Boyett J. *et al.* (1987) Acute lymphoblastic leukaemia in adolescents. Clinical and biologic features predict a poor prognosis. A Paediatric Oncology Group study. *Journal of Clinical Oncology*, **6**, 34–43.

16 Santana V.M., Dodge R.K. & Crist W.M. (1990) Presenting features and treatment outcome of adolescents with acute lymphoblastic leukaemia. *Leukemia*, **4**, 87–90.

17 Sather H., Miller D., Nesbitt M. *et al.* (1981) Differences in prognosis for boys and girls with acute lymphoblastic leukaemia. *Lancet*, **i**, 739–743.

18 Medical Research Council (1978) Effects of varying radiation schedule cyclophosphamide treatment and duration of treatment in acute lymphoblastic leukaemia. *British Medical Journal*, **11**, 787–791.

19 Medical Research Council (1982) Duration of therapy in childhood ALL. *Medical and Paediatric Oncology*, **10**, 511–520.

20 Chessells M.J., Richards S.M., Bailey C.C., Lilleyman J.S. & Eden O.B. (1995) Gender and treatment outcome in childhood lymphoblastic leukaemia: report from the Medical Research Council UKALL trials. *British Journal of Haematology*, **89**, 364–372.

21 Medical Research Council (1978) Testicular disease in acute lymphoblastic leukaemia in childhood. *British Medical Journal*, **1**, 334–338.

22 Nesbit M.E., Robinson L.C., Ortega J.A. *et al.* (1980) Testicular relapse in childhood acute lymphoblastic leukaemia associated with pre-treatment patient characteristics and treatment. *Cancer*, **45**, 2009–2016.

23 Land V.J., Berry D.H. & Herson J. (1979) Long term survival in childhood acute lymphoblastic leukaemia 'late' relapses. *Medical and Paediatric Oncology*, **7**, 19–24.

24 Wong K.J., Ballard E.T., Strayer F.H. *et al.* (1980) Clinical and occult testicular leukaemia in long term survivors of acute lymphoblastic leukaemia. *Journal of Paediatrics*, **96**, 567–574.

25 Eden O.B., Lilleyman J.S., Richards S., Shaw M.P. & Peto J. (1991) Results of Medical Research Council Leukaemia Trial UKALL VIII (Report on the Medical Research Council on behalf of the Working Party on Leukaemia in Childhood). *British Journal of Haematology*, **78**, 187–196.

26 Steinherz P., Siegel S. & Bleyer A. (1986) Lymphomatous presentation of acute lymphoblastic leukaemia. *Proceedings of the American Society of Clinical Oncology*, **5**, 153.

27 Chilcote R.R., Coccia P., Sather H.N. *et al.* (1984) Mediastinal mass in acute lymphoblastic leukaemia. *Medical and Paediatric Oncology*, **12**, 9–16.

28 Hann I.M., Scarffe J.H, Palmer M.K., Evans D.I.K. & Morris Jones P.H. (1981) Haemoglobin and prognosis in childhood acute lymphoblastic leukaemia. *Archives of Disease in Childhood*, **56**, 684–686.

29 Kalwinsky D.K., Rivera G., Dahl G.U. *et al.* (1985) Variation by race in presenting clinical and biological features of childhood acute lymphoblastic leukaemia. Implications for treatment outcome. *Leukaemia Research*, **9**, 817–823.

30 Walters T.R., Bushmore M. & Simone J. (1972) Poor prognosis in Negro children with acute lymphoblastic leukaemia. *Cancer*, **29**, 210–214.

31 Pendergrass T.W., Hoover R. & Godwin J.D. (1975) Prognosis of black children with acute lymphoblastic leukaemia. *Medical and Paediatric Oncology*, **1**, 143–148.

32 Mann J.R. & Oakhill A. (1983) Poor prognosis of ALL in Asian children. *British Medical Journal*, **286**, 839–841.

33 Varghese C., Barrett J.H., Johnston C., Shires M., Rider L. & Forman D. (1996) High risk of lymphomas in children of Asian origin: ethnicity of confounding by socioeconomic status. *British Journal of Cancer*, **74**, 1503–1505.

34 Mastrangelo R., Poplack D.G., Bleyer W.A. *et al.* (1986) Report and recommendations of the Rome Workshop concerning poor prognosis acute lymphoblastic leukaemia in children: biologic bases for staging, stratification and treatment. *Medical and Paediatric Oncology*, **14**, 191–194.

35 Rivera G.K., Pui C.H., Santana V.M. *et al.* (1993) Progress in the treatment of adolescents with acute lymphoblastic leukaemia. *Cancer*, **71**, 3400–3405.

36 Lilleyman J.S. & Eden O.B. (1986) United Kingdom Medical Research Council. Acute lymphoblastic leukaemia (UKALL) Trials I–VIII. Clinical features and results of treatment in four groups of children with adverse prognostic features. *Medical and Paediatric Oncology*, **14**, 182–186.

37 Miller D.R., Krailo M., Blayer W.A. *et al.* (1985) Prognostic implications of blast cell morphology in childhood acute lymphoblastic leukaemia. A report from the Children's Cancer Study Group. *Cancer Treatment Reports*, **69**, 1211–1221.

38 Lilleyman J.S., Hann I.M. & Stevens R.F. (1986) The clinical significance of blast cell morphology in childhood acute lymphoblastic leukaemia. *Medical and Paediatric Oncology*, **14**, 144–147.

39 Lilleyman J.S., Britton J.A., Anderson L.M., Richards S.M., Bailey C.C. & Chessells J.M. (1994) Periodic acid Schiff reaction in childhood lymphoblastic leukaemia. *Journal of Clinical Pathology*, **47**, 689–692.

40 Crist W.M., Grosse C.E., Pullen J. *et al.* (1985) Immunological markers in childhood acute lymphoblastic leukaemia. *Seminars in Oncology*, **12**, 105–121.

41 Brouet J.C., Preud'Homme J.L., Pen T.C. *et al.* (1979) Acute lymphoblastic leukaemia with pre-B cell characteristics. *Blood*, **54**, 269–273.

42 Pullen D.J., Falletta M.J., Crist W.M. *et al.* (1981) South-West Oncology Group experience with immunological phenotyping in acute lymphocytic leukaemia of childhood. *Cancer Research*, **41**, 4802–4809.

43 Hann I.M., Eden O.B., Barnes J. *et al.* (1990) 'Macho' chemotherapy for stage IV B cell lymphoma and B cell acute lymphoblastic leukaemia of childhood. United Kingdom Children's Cancer Study Group (UKCCSG). *British Journal of Haematology*, **76**, 359–364.

44 Poplack D.G. (1989) Acute lymphoblastic leukaemia. In: *Principles and Practice of Pediatric Oncology* (eds P.A. Pizzo & D.G. Poplack), p. 329. Lippincott, Philadelphia.

45 Greaves M.F. & Lister T.A. (1981) Prognostic importance of immunologic markers in adult acute lymphoblastic leukaemia. *New England Journal of Medicine*, **394**, 119–120.

46 Miro J., Zipf T.F., Pui C. *et al.* (1985) Acute mixed lineage leukaemia. Cytopathologic correlations and prognostic significance. *Blood*, **65**, 1115–1123.

47 Sobel R.E., Mick R., Royston I. *et al.* (1987) Clinical importance of myeloid antigen expression in adult acute lymphoblastic leukaemia. *New England Journal of Medicine*, **316**, 1111–1117.

48 Williams D.L., Tsiatis A., Brodeur G.M. *et al.* (1982) Prognostic significance of chromosome number in 136 untreated children with acute lymphoblastic leukaemia. *Blood*, **60**, 864–871.

49 Look A.T. (1985) The emerging of genetics of acute lymphoblastic leukaemia. Clinical and biological. *Seminars in Oncology*, **12**, 92–104.

50 Secker-Walker L.M., Steward E.C., Chan L. *et al.* (1985) The [4;11] translocation in acute leukaemia of childhood. The importance of additional chromosomal aberrations. *British Journal of Haematology*, **61**, 101–111.

51 Third International Workshop on Chromosomes in Leukaemia

(1983) Chromosome abnormalities and their clinical significance in acute lymphoblastic leukaemia. *Cancer Research*, **43**, 868–873.

52 Carroll A.J., Cris W.M., Parmley R. *et al.* (1984) Pre B cell leukaemia associated with chromosome translocation. *Blood*, **1**, 721–724.

53 Williams D.C., Look A.T., Melvin S.L. *et al.* (1984) New chromosomal translocations correlate with specific immunophenotypes of childhood acute lymphoblastic leukaemia. *Cell*, **36**, 101–109.

54 Ribero R.C., Abromowitch M., Raimond S.C. *et al.* (1987) Clinical and biological hallmarks of the Philadelphia chromosome in childhood acute lymphoblastic leukaemia. *Blood*, **70**, 948–953.

55 Secker-Walker L.M. (1990) Prognostic and biological importance of chromosome findings in acute lymphoblastic leukaemia. *Cancer Genetics and Cytogenetics*, **49**, 1–13.

56 Secker-Walker L.M. & Craig J.M. (1993) Prognostic implications of breakpoint and lineage heterogeneity in Philadelphia positive acute lymphoblastic leukaemia—a review. *Leukemia*, **7**, 147–151.

57 Hale J. & Lilleyman J.S. (1991) Importance of 6-mercaptopurine dose in lymphoblastic leukaemia. *Archives of Disease in Childhood*, **4**, 462–466.

58 Lennard M. & Lilleyman J.S. (1989) Importance of 6-mercaptopurine dose in acute lymphoblastic leukaemia. *Journal of Clinical Oncology*, **7**, 1815–1823.

59 Lennard L., Lilleyman J.S., Van Loor J. *et al.* (1990) Genetic variation in response to 6-mercaptopurine for childhood acute lymphoblastic leukaemia. *Lancet*, **366**, 225–229.

60 Heney D., Essex-Cater A., Brocklebank J.T. *et al.* (1990) Continuous arteriovenous haemofiltration in the treatment of lysis syndrome. *Pediatric Nephrology*, **4**, 245–247.

61 Goldie J.H., Coldman A.J. & Gudauskas G.A. (1982) Rationale for the use of alternating non cross resistant chemotherapy. *Cancer Treatment Reports*, **66**, 439–449 (abstract).

62 Henze G., Langerman H.J., Bramswig J. *et al.* (1981) Ergebrisse der studie BFM 76/79 zur behandlung der akute lymphoblastischen Leukaemie bei kindern und jugendlichen. *Klinische Padriatrie*, **193**, 145–154.

63 Riehm H., Gadner H., Henze G. *et al.* (1983) Acute lymphoblastic leukaemia. Treatment results in three BFM studies (1970–1981). In: *Leukaemic Research: advances in cell biology and treatment* (eds S.E. Murphy & J.R. Gilbert), pp. 251–260. Elsevier, New York.

64 Potter M.N., Cross N.C.P., Van Danzen J.J.M. *et al.* (1993) Molecular evidence of minimal residual disease after treatment for leukaemia and lymphoma — an updated meeting report and review. *Leukaemia*, **7**, 1302–1314.

65 Brisco M.J., Condon J., Hughes E. *et al.* (1994) Outcome prediction in childhood acute lymphoblastic leukaemia by molecular quantification of residual disease at the end of induction. *Lancet*, **343**, 196–200.

66 Steward C.G., Goulden N.J., Katz F. *et al.* (1994) A polymerase chain reaction study of the stability of Ig heavy chain and T cell receptor-gene rearrangements between presentation and relapse of childhood B lineage acute lymphoblastic leukaemia. *Blood*, **83**, 1355–1362.

67 Evans W.E., Tsiatis A. & Rivera G. (1982) Anaphylactoid reaction to *Escherichia coli* and *Erwinia asparaginase* in children with leukaemia. *Cancer*, **49**, 1378–1383.

68 Gottlieb A.J., Weinberg V., Ellison R.R. *et al.* (1984) Efficiency of daunorubicin in the therapy of adult acute lymphoblastic leukaemia. A prospective randomised trial by cancer and leukaemia group B. *Blood*, **64**, 267–274.

69 Schaison G., Lemerle S., Leverger G. *et al.* (1987) Usefulness of induction anthracycline in the treatment of acute lymphoblastic leukaemia in children. *SIOP Trondheim*, 193 (abstract).

70 King O.Y., Wilbur J.R., Mumford D.M. *et al.* (1974) Therapy with *Erwinia* L-asparaginase in children with acute leukaemia after anaphylaxis to *E. coli* L-asparaginase. *Cancer*, **33**, 611–614.

71 Gaynon P.S., Steinherz P.G., Blayer W.A. *et al.* (1988) Intensive therapy for children with acute lymphoblastic leukaemic and unfavourable presenting features: early conclusions of study CCG 106 by the Children's Cancer Study Group. *Lancet*, **i**, 921–924.

72 Chessells J.M., Bailey C.C., Richards S.M. *et al.* (1995) Intensification of treatment and survival in all children with lymphoblastic leukaemia: results of UK Medical Research Council trial UKALL X. *Lancet*, **345**, 143–148.

73 Aur R.J.A., Simone J.V., Husto H.O. *et al.* (1972) A comparative study of central nervous system irradiation and intensive chemotherapy early in remission in childhood acute lymphoblastic leukaemia. *Cancer*, **29**, 381–391.

74 Aur R.J.A., Simone J.V., Husto H.O. *et al.* (1971) Central nervous system therapy and combination chemotherapy of childhood acute lymphoblastic leukaemia. *Blood*, **37**, 272–281.

75 Eiser C. & Landsdowne R. (1978) Retrospective study of intellectual development in children treated for acute lymphoblastic leukaemia. *Archives of Disease in Childhood*, **52**, 525–529.

76 Meadows A.T., Massari D., Ferguson J. *et al.* (1981) Decline in IQ scores and cognitive dysfunction in children with acute lymphoblastic leukaemia treated with cranial irradiation. *Lancet*, **i**, 1015–1018.

77 Shalet S.M., Price D.A., Beardwell G.G. *et al.* (1979) Normal growth despite abnormalities of growth hormone secretion in children treated for acute leukaemia. *Journal of Pediatrics*, **94**, 719–722.

78 Blayer W.A., Fallvolita J., Robison L. *et al.* (1990) Influence of age, sex and concurrent methotrexate therapy and intellectual function after cranial irradiation during childhood. A report from the Children's Cancer Study Group. *Paediatric Haematology and Oncology*, **7**, 329–338.

79 Littman P., Coccia P., Blayer W.A. *et al.* (1987) Central nervous system (CNS) prophylaxis in children with low risk acute lymphoblastic leukaemia (ALL). *International Journal of Radiation Oncology, Biology and Physics*, **13**, 1443–1449.

80 Borsi J.D. & Moe P.J. (1987) Comparative study of the pharmacokinetics of methotrexate in a dose range of 0.5 g to 33.6 g/m² in children with acute lymphoblastic leukaemia. *Cancer*, **60**, 5–13.

81 Slordal L., Kolmannskog S., Moe P. *et al.* (1987) High dose methotrexate (6–8 g/m²) in childhood malignancies: clinical tolerability and pharmacokinetics. *Paediatric Haematology and Oncology*, **4**, 33–42.

82 Chessells J.M., Lieper A.D., Tiedemann K. *et al.* (1987) Oral methotrexate is as effective as intramuscular in maintenance therapy of acute lymphoblastic leukaemia. *Archives of Disease in Childhood*, **62**, 172–176.

83 Medical Research Council Leukaemia Trial UKALL V (1996) An attempt to reduce the immunosuppressive effects of therapy in childhood acute lymphoblastic leukaemia. Report to the council by the Working Party on Leukaemia in Childhood. *Journal of Clinical Oncology*, **4**, 1758–1764.

84 Spiers A.S.D., Roberts P.D., Marsh G.W. *et al.* (1975) Acute lymphoblastic leukaemia: cyclical chemotherapy with three combinations of four drugs (COAP-POMP-CART) regimen. *British Medical Journal*, **4**, 614–617.

85 Blayer W.A., Nickerson J., Coccia P.F. *et al.* (1985) Monthly pulses

of vincristine and prednisone prevent marrow and testicular relapse in childhood acute lymphoblastic leukaemia: one conclusion of the CCG 161 study of good prognosis ALL. *Proceedings of the American Society of Clinical Oncology*, **4**, 160.

86 Koren G., Ferrazini G. & Sulh H. (1990) Exposure to mercaptopurine as a prognostic factor in acute lymphocytic leukaemia in children. *New England Journal of Medicine*, **1**, 17–21.

87 Nesbitt M.E., Sather H.N., Robison L.L. *et al.* (1983) Randomised study of 3 years and 5 years of chemotherapy in childhood acute lymphoblastic leukaemia. *Journal of Clinical Oncology*, **1**, 308–316.

88 Medical Research Council (1982) Duration of chemotherapy in childhood acute lymphoblastic leukaemia. *Medical and Paediatric Oncology*, **10**, 511–520.

89 Sather H.N. (1986) Age at diagnosis in childhood acute lymphoblastic leukaemia. *Medical and Paediatric Oncology*, **14**, 166–172.

90 Pui C.H., Ribeiro R.C., Campana D. *et al.* (1996) Prognostic factors in the acute lymphoid and myeloid leukaemia of infants. *Leukaemia*, **10**, 952–956.

91 Dinndorf P.A. & Reaman G.H. (1986) Acute lymphoblastic leukaemia in infants. Evidence for B cell origin of disease by use on monoclonal antibody phenotyping. *Blood*, **68**, 975–978.

92 Culbert S.J., Shuster I.J., Land V.J. *et al.* (1991) Remission induction and continuation therapy in children in their first relapse of acute lymphoid leukaemia. A Pediatric Oncology Group study. *Cancer*, **67**, 37–42.

93 Nachman J., Baum E., Ramsay N. *et al.* (1986) Prognostic factors for reinduction and duration of second remission in children with acute lymphoblastic leukaemia. *Proceedings of the American Society of Clinical Oncology*, **5**, 200.

94 Blayer W.A., Sather H. & Hammond G.D. (1986) Prognosis and treatment after relapse of acute lymphoblastic leukaemia and non Hodgkin's lymphoma. *Cancer*, **58**, 590–594.

95 Behrendt H., Van Leeuwen E.F., Schuwirth C. *et al.* (1990) Bone marrow relapse occurring as first relapse in children with acute lymphoblastic leukaemia. *Medical and Paediatric Oncology*, **18**, 190–196.

96 Butturine A., Rivera G.K., Bortin M.M. *et al.* (1987) Which treatment for childhood acute lymphoblastic leukaemia in second remission? *Lancet*, **i**, 429–432.

97 Rivera G.K., Buchanan G., Boyett J.M. *et al.* (1986) Intensive retreatment of childhood acute lymphoblastic leukaemia in first bone marrow relapse. *New England Journal of Medicine*, **325**, 273–278.

98 Buchanan G.R., Rivera G.K., Boyett J.M. *et al.* (1988) Reinduction therapy in 297 children with acute lymphoblastic leukaemia in first bone marrow relapse. A Paediatric Oncology Group Study. *Blood*, **72**, 1286–1292.

99 Henze G., Fengler R., Hartmann R. *et al.* (1989) Chemotherapy for bone marrow relapse of childhood acute lymphoblastic leukaemia. *Cancer Chemotherapy and Pharmacology*, **24**, S19–26.

100 George S.L., Ochs J.M., Mauer A.A. *et al.* (1985) The importance of an isolated central nervous system relapse in children with acute lymphoblastic leukaemia. *Journal of Clinical Oncology*, **3**, 776–781.

101 Bleyer W.A. & Poplack D.G. (1985) Prophylaxis and treatment in the central nervous system and other sanctuaries. *Seminars in Oncology*, **12**, 131–148.

102 Land V.J., Thomas P.R.M. & Boyett J.M. (1985) Comparison of maintenance treatment for first central nervous system relapse in children with acute lymphoblastic leukaemia. A Paediatric Oncology Group Study. *Cancer*, **56**, 81–87.

103 Nesbitt M.E., Robison L.L., Ortega J.A. *et al.* (1980) Testicular relapse in childhood acute lymphoblastic leukaemia associated with pre-treatment patient characteristics and treatment. *Cancer*, **45**, 2009–2016.

104 Medical Research Council (1978) Testicular disease in acute lymphoblastic leukaemia in childhood. *British Medical Journal*, **i**, 334–338.

105 Uderzo C., Grazia Zurlo M., Adayoli L. *et al.* (1990) Treatment of isolated testicular relapse in childhood acute lymphoblastic leukaemia, in Italian multicentre study. Associazione Italiana Ematologia ed Oncologia Pediatrica. *Journal of Clinical Oncology*, **8**, 672–677.

106 Shalet S.M., Horver A., Ahmed S.R. *et al.* (1985) Leydig cell damage after testicular radiation for lymphoblastic leukaemia. *Medical and Paediatric Oncology*, **13**, 65–68.

107 Sanders J.E., Thomas E.D., Buckner C.D. *et al.* (1987) Marrow transplant for patients with acute lymphoblastic leukaemia in second remission. *Blood*, **70**, 324–326.

108 Hathorn J.W. (1989) Empirical antibiotics for febrile neutropenic cancer patients. *European Journal of Cancer and Clinical Oncology*, **25**, 543–551.

109 Wade J.C. (1989) Antibiotic therapy for the febrile granulocytopenic cancer patient: combination therapy versus monotherapy. *Reviews of Infectious Diseases*, **II**, S1572–S1581.

110 Lieschke G.J., Bell D., Rawlinson W. *et al.* (1989) Empiric single agent or combination antibiotic therapy for febrile episodes in neutropenic patients: an overview. *European Journal of Cancer and Clinical Oncology*, **25**, 537–542.

111 Hughes W.T., Armstrong D. & Bodey G.P. (1990) Guidelines for the use of antimicrobial agents in neutropenic patients with unexplained fever. *Journal of Infectious Diseases*, **161**, 381–396.

112 Chopra R., Blair S., Strong J. *et al.* (1991) Liposomal amphotericin B (Ambisome) in the treatment of fungal infections in neutropenic patients. *Journal of Antimicrobial Chemotherapy*, **28**, 93–104.

113 Murphy J.V. & Yunis E.J. (1976) Encephalopathy following measles infection in children with chronic illness. *Journal of Pediatrics*, **88**, 937–942.

114 Anonymous (1996) Human Varicella-Zoster Immunoglobulin (VZIG). In: *Immunisation Against Infectious Disease* (eds D.M. Salisbury & N.T. Begg), pp. 252–253. Her Majesty's Stationery Office, London.

115 Hughes W.T. (1977) *Pneumocystis carinii* pneumonia. *New England Journal of Medicine*, **297**, 1381–1383.

116 Ochs J.J. (1996) Neurotoxicity due to central nervous system therapy for childhood leukaemia. *American Journal of Pediatric Haematology and Oncology*, **11**, 93–105.

117 Ochs J.J., Mulhern R., Fairclough D. *et al.* (1991) Comparison of neuropsychologic functioning and clinical indicators of neurotoxicity in long term survivors of childhood leukaemia given cranial radiation or parenteral methotrexate a prospective study. *Journal of Clinical Oncology*, **9**, 145–151.

118 Himelstein-Braw R., Peters H. & Faber M. (1978) Morphological study of the ovaries of leukaemic children. *British Journal of Cancer*, **38**, 82–86.

119 Shalet G.M., Hann I.M. & Lendon M. (1981) Testicular function after combination chemotherapy in childhood for acute lymphoblastic leukaemia. *Archives of Disease in Childhood*, **56**, 275–278.

6 Chronic Lymphocytic Leukaemias

T.J. Hamblin and D.G. Oscier

History

John Menteith, a 28-year-old slater from Edinburgh, had been aware of a mass in the left side of his abdomen for 8 months before he died. John Hughes Bennett, the Englishman later to become Professor of Medicine in Edinburgh, reported in October 1845 [1] that at post-mortem he had massive enlargement of his liver, spleen and lymph nodes. Examination of his blood revealed 'the existence of true pus'. Six weeks later Rudolph Virchow in Berlin reported the case of Marie Straide, a 50-year-old cook, who died with a huge spleen and in her blood the reversal of the ratio of pigmented to colourless corpuscles [2]. These two early examples of 'lymphatic' and 'splenic' leukaemia began the unravelling of the complex puzzle that is the nature of the chronic leukaemias. Virchow was the first to recognize that splenic leukaemias had granular leucocytes with trefoil-like nuclei, in contrast to the lymphatic leukaemias with agranular leucocytes with smooth round nuclei [3], and in the same publication described lymphosarcoma as a malignant tumour of lymph nodes.

Ehrlich's histochemical stains confirmed the distinction between chronic lymphocytic leukaemia (CLL) and chronic myeloid leukaemia (CML) [4], but they also enabled Turk to draw attention to the resemblance between CLL and lymphosarcoma [5]. For the next 60 years the relationship between CLL and lymphosarcoma was controversial, although CLL was thought in the main to be a relatively benign tumour. Damashek called it 'an accumulation of incompetent lymphocytes' [6].

In the early 1970s, when B cells were identified as expressing surface immunoglobulin [7], it became apparent that most cases of CLL are tumours of B cells. Subsequent careful study of cellular morphology and lymphocyte markers has separated from true CLL a number of types of lymphoid tumours that are not CLL, among them prolymphocytic leukaemia (PLL), hairy cell leukaemia (HCL), hairy cell variants, splenic lymphoma with villous lymphocytes (SLVL) and mantle cell lymphoma (MCL).

Epidemiology

CLL is the commonest leukaemia in Europe and North America. The annual incidence varies with the age and sex structure of the population. Figures between 0.6 and 3.7 per 100 000 have been quoted for various areas of the USA [8]. The Leukaemia Research Fund Data Collection Study found an incidence in the UK of 6.15 per 100 000, although this concealed a variation between 1.3 and 13.7 per 100 000 in different health districts [9]. Since in our series more than three-quarters of patients were discovered because of an incidental blood count performed for irrelevant reasons, the exact prevalence must clearly depend on how assiduous is the case finding [10].

CLL is very rare below the age of 50 but after this there is a relatively rapid rise in incidence. It is unknown in children and patients below the age of 40 should be suspected of having a different type of lymphoma. Most authors suggest that the disease is approximately twice as common in men as in women [11,12]. However, the disease occurs approximately 6 years later in women than in men (Fig. 6.1) [8], so that although at any given age it is twice as common in men, the greater longevity of women means that this sex difference will be obscured in any series that includes large numbers of the old and very old.

There are no differences in the age-specific incidences between black and white Americans, but among Chinese, Japanese, Filipinos and American Indians the incidence is about five times less [13]. Among Jews the rate is twice that of non-Jewish North Americans [14].

CLL does occur in families, although rarely. First-degree relatives are three times more likely also to have CLL or another lymphoid neoplasm than the general population [15]. Autoimmune diseases are also reported to be more common in relatives of patients with CLL [16]. One study reported a high level of consanguinity in familial cases of CLL [17]. Concordance in several sets of identical twins has been reported [18]. In some familial cases the same immunoglobulin heavy-chain

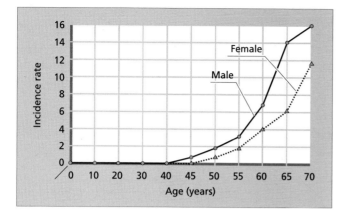

Fig. 6.1 Age-specific incidence rates for males (○) and females (△) of CLL, 1973–77, SEER Program areas. (Adapted from Young *et al.*, 1981 [8].)

variable-region gene has been used by both tumours, but even when this has been found in identical twins, different immunoglobulin gene rearrangements have been found, indicating that the tumours arose separately and postzygotically [19]. There is no association with HLA haplotype [20].

Aetiology

The cause of CLL is unknown. Exposure to ionizing radiation, drugs or chemicals has not been implicated [21–23]. No viral cause has been suggested. A single study among many negative studies has suggested that low-frequency electromagnetic fields might be an aetiological factor [24]. Although other lymphoid neoplasms are common among patients with immunodeficiency syndromes, this is not true for CLL.

Clinical features

Textbooks routinely tell us that about a quarter of patients are asymptomatic [25,26]. This is an underestimate due to selective nonreferral of patients with a lymphocytosis only and contamination of many of the older series with cases of MCL and SLVL. In our experience over 70% of patients present as a result of a blood test performed for an incidental reason [27]. Although patients usually present at age 60 years or over, when blood tests begin to be performed more commonly because of other illnesses, careful scrutiny of the case-notes will often reveal that a slight lymphocytosis had been disregarded several years previously.

Other presenting symptoms include those of anaemia and noticing enlarged lymph nodes or abdominal masses. Bruising and purpura are rare, as are systemic B symptoms. In some cases the appearance of shingles is the trigger for the blood test that makes the diagnosis [10].

The commonest clinical finding is lymphadenopathy which is present in 50% of patients, usually involving the cervical,

axillary or inguinal nodes [10]. The nodes are generally small (<2 cm in diameter), discrete and nontender. Epitrochlear nodes are occasionally found. Mediastinal glands are rare. Abdominal glands are rarely looked for, but in one series where lymphograms were performed they were found in more than 50% of patients [28]. Massive enlargement of lymph nodes, particularly abdominal nodes, should give rise to suspicion of Richter's syndrome, a rare transformation of CLL into a high-grade lymphoma (see below). Obstruction to airways or vascular or lymphatic channels by enlarged lymph nodes is very rare.

Splenic enlargement is found in up to a quarter of patients at presentation and may eventually be found in a half [10]. This sometimes causes symptoms of early satiety after meals and may result in hypersplenism, contributing to the anaemia and thrombocytopenia. Hepatomegaly is less frequent. Jaundice is usually a feature of complicating autoimmune haemolytic anaemia or, rarely, enlarged lymph nodes in the porta hepatis.

Extranodal involvement may be detected histologically but is seldom symptomatic. Most commonly we have seen prostatic infiltration giving rise to urinary symptoms. Infiltration of the kidney is well described [29], but is unrelated to the nephrotic syndrome which is occasionally seen [30]. Reports of gastrointestinal involvement [31] date from a period before MCL was clearly distinguished. Leukaemia cutis is rare [32] and more likely to be unsightly than dangerous. Occasional patients suffer an unexplained exfoliative dermatitis [10] (Fig. 6.2). Respiratory involvement is very rare [33]. Neurological involvement because of leukaemic infiltration of cranial or peripheral nerves has been reported, especially in the earlier literature [10,32]. The retro-orbital space, where deposits may cause proptosis and threaten sight, is among the commoner extranodal sites.

Infections are the major cause of death in between a quarter and a half of patients [10]. Bacterial infection of the respiratory tract, skin or urinary tract is the commonest problem and the usual organisms are *Strept. pneumoniae*, *Staph. aureus*, *Strept. pyogenes* and *E. coli*. They usually respond to conventional antibiotics. Until the advent of treatment with purine analogues opportunistic infections were rare, but there have been recent reports of infection with *Listeria monocytogenes* [34] and *Pneumocystis carinii* [35]. On the other hand, herpes zoster infections are extremely common. Nearly 30% of our patients developed shingles at some time in their illness, a fifth of these attacks occurring shortly before or at the time of diagnosis [10]. Some cases are very severe; recurrent attacks occur and postherpetic neuralgia is quite common. Rarely, the motor neurone is involved [10].

The principle autoimmune phenomenon in CLL is autoimmune haemolytic anaemia. Various series record the prevalence of autoimmune haemolytic anaemia to be between 2 and 35% [36,37]. Although there have been case reports of the association of CLL and systemic lupus erythematosus, rheumatoid arthritis, Sjögren's syndrome, ulcerative colitis,

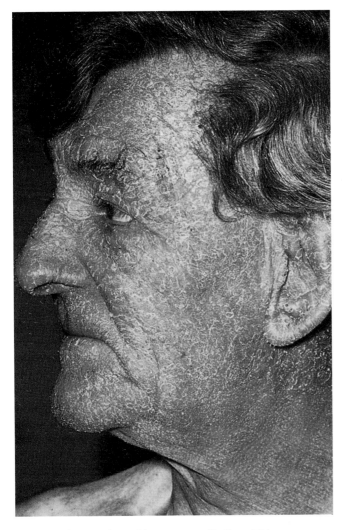

Fig. 6.2 Exfoliative dermatitis, a rare complication of CLL.

allergic vasculitis, pernicious anaemia and bullous pemphigoid [6,38–40], there is no reason to believe that these are other than chance occurrences.

Laboratory findings

White blood count

CLL is characterized by a persistent lymphocytosis in blood and bone marrow. Defining lymphocyte counts have been set at >5 × 10⁹/l [32], >10 × 10⁹/l [41] and >15 × 10⁹/l [42]. More important is evidence of monoclonality of the lymphocytes associated with the characteristic lymphocyte morphology. Monoclonality has been recognized by the finding of a single glucose-6-phosphate dehydrogenase isotype [43], a unique immunoglobulin (Ig) idiotype [44], clonal chromosomal abnormalities [45] and a single Ig gene rearrangement [46]. However, it is usually sufficient to demonstrate the expression of a single Ig light-chain type on the cell surface.

In many cases the lymphocyte count is very stable. In some it remains below 30 × 10⁹/l for the lifetime of the patient. Often there is a slowly progressive rise in lymphocyte count, usually taking more than a year to double. Counts that rise more rapidly than this are usually associated with an adverse prognosis. In some patients lymphocyte counts fluctuate without obvious cause, although they will often rise acutely in response to infection or if corticosteroids are given. Very high lymphocyte counts are occasionally seen. Counts over 500 × 10⁹/l may be associated with the hyperviscosity syndrome [47].

The leukaemic lymphocytes are small, round, monomorphic cells (see Plate 6.1 between pp. 292 and 293). The nucleus contains heavily clumped basophilic chromatin, and sometimes an indistinct nucleolus can be discerned. The cytoplasm is scanty, agranular, pale blue, and apparently fragile, since 'smudge' or 'smear' cells are usually plentiful in blood films. A small percentage of the CLL cells are larger with a prominent nucleolus (prolymphocytes). In some patients a small percentage of cells have a cleaved nucleus (see Plate 6.2) and in others small numbers of lymphoplasmacytoid cells (see Plate 6.3) are seen.

Immunophenotype

The lymphocytes of patients with CLL express surface Ig of a single light-chain type at about one-tenth the density of normal B cells; an estimated 9000 molecules per cell [48]. Most series include a few cases in which the expression is below the level of detectability [49]. Even in these, however, cytoplasmic monoclonal Ig may be detectable, sometimes in the form of crystals [50] (see Plate 6.4 between pp. 292 and 293). Most cases express IgM or co-express IgM and IgD on the surface of their cells. Early work showing the presence of IgG in a large number of cases was demonstrated to be the effect of binding of serum IgG to Fcγ II receptors [51]. However, a small percentage of patients whose disease may be classified as CLL by every other criterion undoubtedly express surface IgG or IgA [52]. Whatever the class of surface Ig, it caps and pinocytoses poorly in response to cross-linking [53].

MHC Class II is universally expressed. DR and DP are always present but DQ expression is more heterogeneous [54]. Other pan B-cell markers including CD19, CD20, CD24, CD37, CD40 and CD45RA are also ever present [55]. CD10, expressed during normal pre-B-cell ontogeny and during follicular development, is not found [56], nor is CD34, the antigen present on pluripotent stem cells [57]. The CD9 antigen, present on normal pre-B cells and a subpopulation of activated B cells, is found on less than 20% of CLLs [57]. Plasma cell antigens such as CD38 and PCA-1 (BB4) are not expressed by CLL cells [56].

The markers on CLL cells are distinct from those on normal B cells and most other B-cell tumours (Table 6.1). Apart from their low density of surface immunoglobulin, it was early

Table 6.1 Immunophenotype of various B-cell tumours.

	CLL	PLL	HCL	SLVL	MCL	FCCL
SIg	+	++	++	++	++	++
CD19, CD20, CD37, CD40	+	+	+	+	+	+
CD5	+	–	–	–	+	–
CD10	–	–	–	–	–	+
CD23	+	–	–	–	–	–
CD22	–	+	+	+	+	+
CD25	+	–	+	–	–	–
FMC7	–	++	++	+	+	+
CD11c	–	–	+	+	–	–
Mouse rosettes	+	–	–	–	–	–
CD35	–	+	+	+	+	+

FCCL = follicle centre cell lymphoma.

Table 6.2 Diagnostic scoring system for CLL.*

CD5	Pos.	1 point
CD22	Neg.	1 point
CD23	Pos.	1 point
Surface Ig	Dim	1 point
FMC7	Neg.	1 point

* Eighty-seven per cent scored 4 or 5, with scores of 0 or 1 in only 0.4%. Other B-cell leukaemias and lymphomas had scores of 0 or 1 in 89% and 72% of cases, respectively [61].

recognized that CLL cells formed rosettes with mouse erythrocytes [58]. Because the technology required is incompatible with flow cytometry, this test has largely been abandoned.

CD5, a 67-kDa antigen present on mature T cells and stage III thymocytes [59], is also present on virtually all CLL cells. Although it was originally thought that the CD5+ B cell was pathognomic for CLL, it should be noted that such cells are also found in MCL, a quite distinct and more malignant disease [60]. CD23, the low-affinity Fcε receptor, is present on most CLL cells but seldom on other B-cell malignancies [61]. Although cytoplasmic CD22 is expressed by CLL cells, this molecule is absent from or only weakly expressed on the surface of the cells. In other B-cell malignancies CD22 is found both on the surface of the cells and intracytoplasmically [62]. The antibody FMC7 has not been assigned a CD number but it is still very useful in CLL. It is present on only a very small percentage of CLL cells (usually <4%). Larger numbers indicate an adverse prognosis [63]. It is present on 30–60% of normal B cells, and is particularly strongly expressed on HCL and PLL cells.

About 50% of normal B cells express CD1c [64]. Rather fewer CLL cells do so, even though CD1c expression is commonly increased in most other B-cell tumours [65]. CD21 is the receptor for C3d and the Epstein–Barr virus (EBV). It is represented on CLL cells at reduced intensity and does not functionally support EBV transformation [66]. The complement receptor C3bR (CD35) is usually absent from CLL cells but it is present on normal B cells [66].

Matutes *et al.* [61] have proposed a scoring system which differentiates CLL from other B-cell leukaemias and lymphomas, based on the presence and density of staining of the following five markers: CD5, CD22, CD23, surface Ig and FMC7 (Table 6.2).

Anaemia and thrombocytopenia

A normochromic, normocytic anaemia is present in about 15% of patients [10]. Although anaemia carries a relatively poor prognosis in CLL, it is important to remember that this is only so when caused by marrow infiltration. Other causes of anaemia in this age group (such as iron deficiency or megaloblastic anaemia) will certainly be found in association with CLL.

About 20% of CLL patients have a positive Coombs' test at some time in their illness but only about 8% develop an autoimmune haemolytic anaemia (see Plate 6.5 between pp. 292 and 293) [67]. The autoantibody is a warm reacting polyclonal IgG, unrelated to the monoclonal IgM produced by the tumour. Only 1.8% of patients studied by the French Co-operative Group had a positive direct antiglobulin test (DAT) at entry into their trial [36]. However, this study included many stage A patients (Table 6.5) in whom the prevalence is much lower than in stages B and C. Among 198 patients (138 with stage A) studied by Hamblin *et al.* [67] for between 6 months and 22 years after presentation, there were 14 (7%) with a positive DAT of whom 10 (5%) had active haemolysis at some stage in their illness. The prevalence of positive DATs in stable stage A disease was 3%, in stages B and C 10%, and in progressive Stage A disease 18%.

Thrombocytopenia occurs in about 20% of patients [10]. In the majority it is caused by marrow infiltration suppressing normal haemopoiesis. Autoimmune thrombocytopenia is rare (<2% of patients) [68]. Mild thrombocytopenia can sometimes be caused by hypersplenism. Autoimmune neutropenia occurs in about one patient in 100 [69], and autoimmune red cell aplasia is even rarer [70]. Autoantibodies to other tissue-specific or nonspecific antigens are no commoner than in age-matched controls [67].

Immunology

Hypogammaglobulinaemia is extremely common. Only 15% of CLLs have normal serum immunoglobulins [10], and even these are likely to have a defect of antibody production when immunized with a new antigen [71]. Serum IgA is the first to be reduced, followed by IgM and IgG [10]. Levels of serum immunoglobulins are suppressed to a much greater extent than in any other B-cell tumour, apart from myeloma.

Contrary to the view that the CLL cell is an inert nonsecretory cell, it secretes both whole immunoglobulin and free light chains [72]. Light-chain secretion is invariably in excess of heavy-chain secretion [73]. Conventional cellulose acetate serum electrophoresis detects a monoclonal protein in 5–10% of patients [74]. However, more sensitive detection methods such as isoelectric focusing with immunofixation demonstrate monoclonal proteins in the serum or urine of the majority of patients [75]. Using a radioimmunoassay, Stevenson *et al.* [72] were able to show that in patients with very low immunoglobulins, up to 95% of the IgM and 65% of the IgD in the serum were idiotypic. Furthermore, the IgM was in the secreted pentomeric form and therefore not the result of membrane dissociation.

Surprisingly, T-cell numbers are increased in CLL, especially in early cases [76]. The greatest increase is in the CD8+ cells, so that the CD4 : CD8 ratio is often reversed. This is explained, at least in part, by a redirection of CD4+ cells to the bone marrow [77]. However, circulating T cells are functionally impaired, showing a reduced proliferative response to mitogens and antigens [78], reduced stimulation in the mixed lymphocyte reaction [79] and poor T-cell colony formation [80]. They also show diminished helper activity for B cells [81]. All of these functions deteriorate with increased stage of the disease.

Patients with CLL also show diminished NK activity [82], antibody-dependent cellular cytotoxicity (ADCC) [83] and lymphokine-activated killer (LAK) cell activity [84]. CLL cells secrete TGFβ which is a potent inhibitor of B-cell proliferation [85,86]. Patients have high levels of this cytokine which may be implicated in the hypogammaglobulinaemia [85]. The expression of CD25 on some CLL cells and the high levels of circulating soluble IL-2R may act as a sponge for endogenous IL-2 and thus down-regulate T-helper function [87].

Bone marrow

The bone marrow is inevitably infiltrated by small lymphocytes identical to those found in the blood. A defining level of at least 30% infiltration is useful but arbitrary [88]. Occasional patients have fewer lymphocytes, particularly early in their disease. In bone marrow trephine biopsies four histological patterns are described: interstitial, nodular, nodular and interstitial, and diffuse [89] (see Plate 6.6 between pp. 292 and 293). Interstitial involvement preserves the marrow architecture and is seen in more than a third of patients, depending on case selection. These are generally those with stage A disease. A pure nodular pattern is seen in only 10% of patients but a mixed nodular and interstitial pattern in about 30%. Extensive marrow replacement with diffuse involvement is found in less than 20%.

Lymph node histology

Normal lymph node architecture is effaced by a diffuse infiltration of small lymphocytes identical to those seen in the bone marrow. Also within the node are foci of larger cells containing nucleoli which are referred to as proliferation centres (see Plate 6.7 between pp. 292 and 293). Similar infiltrates can be seen in the spleen and bone marrow. The histology is indistinguishable from that of low-grade small lymphocytic lymphoma [42].

Chromosome studies

The first consistent chromosomal abnormality (trisomy 12) in CLL was not reported until 1979 [90]. The reason for this late discovery, compared to the other common leukaemias, was partly because the spontaneous mitotic rate in CLL is extremely low and partly because the standard mitogen used in the 1960s and 1970s was phytohaemagglutinin, a T-cell but not a B-cell stimulator. With the advent of a number of polyclonal B-cell activators such as lipopolysaccharide (LPS), pokeweed mitogen (PWM), EBV and 12-0 tetradecanoyl phorbol 13 acetate (TPA) [91], which are also mitogenic for leukaemic B-lymphocytes, many studies have shown that metaphases can be obtained in most cases of CLL [92–95]. An abnormal karyotype is found in about 50% of cases and of these approximately half have a single abnormality, one-quarter have two abnormalities while the remainder have a complex karyotype (Fig. 6.3) [96].

The most consistent abnormalities found are trisomy 12 [93,94,97,98], deletions or translocations of chromosome 13q [95,99,100] and deletions of chromosomes 11q and 6q (Fig. 6.4) [101,102]. In patients with a normal karyotype, metaphases may derive from either normal T cells or the clonal B-cell population. The use of fluorescent *in situ* hybridization (FISH) and molecular studies have demonstrated a higher prevalence of genetic abnormalities than are detectable by chromosomal analysis alone [103]. The identification of genes

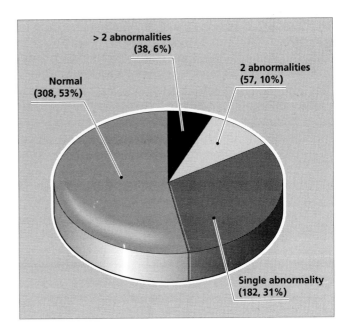

Fig. 6.3 Distribution of karyotypic abnormalities in CLL in the Bournemouth series (*n* = 585).

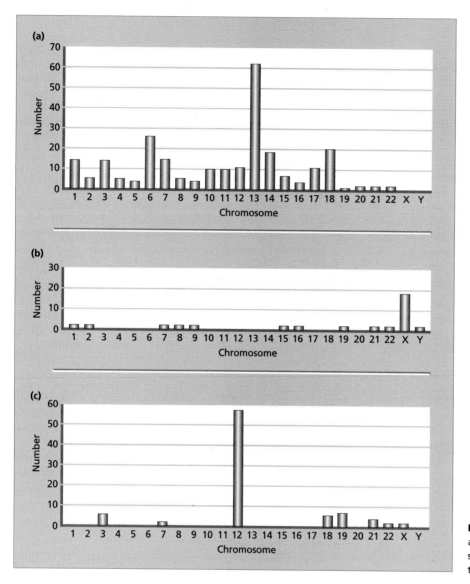

Fig. 6.4 Types of chromosomal abnormalities seen in the Bournemouth series: (a) structural; (b) monosomy; (c) trisomy.

important in the pathogenesis of leukaemia has largely resulted from the analysis of chromosomal translocations. In CLL most cytogenetic abnormalities result either in chromosomal loss or gain, and this largely accounts for the dearth of information on the genetic consequences of chromosomal abnormalities in CLL.

Karyotypic evolution occurs in approximately 15% of patients with CLL and may occur in the absence of clinical or morphological evolution [104].

Nature of the leukaemic cell

CLL is characterized by the accumulation of monoclonal lymphocytes. Although most leukaemic cells are apparently sequestered in G_0 [105], these bland, inactive, small lymphocytes nevertheless express antigens which in other situations,

would indicate cellular activation. It is not clear, therefore, whether CLL derives from a discrete and specialized B-cell lineage or represents a normal B cell frozen at a specific phase of maturation. Are its special characteristics related to its lineage or its stage of development, or are they a product of its neoplastic nature? Consequently, a whole range of reported biochemical properties of CLL cells, such as low catecholamine and cortisol receptors [106], altered lectin receptors [107], decreased dehydroascorbic acid uptake [108] and altered ect-ATPase kinetics [109], are of uncertain significance, since there is no valid population of control cells with which to compare them.

Cell-cycle status

CLL is considered to result from the gradual accumulation of long-lived noncycling lymphocytes. There are a small number of 'proliferating' cells denoted by positive Ki67 staining [110], but ethidium bromide staining shows these to be in G_1 and not in S phase [110]. This has been confirmed by Delmer *et al.* [111], who have demonstrated that in most cases of CLL there is an overexpression of cyclin D2 mRNA compared to normal resting B-lymphocytes. D-type cyclins are synthesized in early G_1. However, this block in differentiation is not irreversible, because it has been known for many years that *in vitro*, mitogens such as TPA and cytokines can induce CLL cells to increase immunoglobulin secretion and divide [112]. It has recently been shown that SIgM+ CLL cells express IgG and IgA transcripts, and that CD40-stimulated cells will secrete IgG and IgA in the presence of IL-10 [113]. Conversely, IgM-producing precursors have been found in the rare cases of SIgG+ CLL [114].

The factors responsible for the prolonged survival and failure of differentiation in CLL are poorly understood but are of practical importance, because the ability to induce apoptosis or terminal differentiation would have therapeutic implications. Many studies have attempted to analyse the ability of CLL cells to secrete and respond to cytokines, but their interpretation has been hindered by a number of technical factors. For example, the response to a particular cytokine may depend on the dose and duration of exposure, whether the cytokine is used singly or in combination and whether the leukaemic lymphocytes are activated or depleted of T and NK cells [115].

CLL cells express mRNA for IL-1β, IL-6, IL-7 (in some studies only), IL-8, IL-10, TNFα, TGFβ and BCL2 [115,116]. They respond to exogenous IL-2, IL-4, IL-5, IL-6, IL-7, IL-10, TNFα, TGFβ, IFNα and IFNγ. TNFα and IL-6 are possible autocrine growth factors [115], whereas TGFβ may be an autocrine growth inhibitor [85].

CLL cells consistently express BCL2 protein although at a lower level than follicular lymphoma cells bearing the t(14;18) translocation. Leukaemic cells die rapidly *in vitro* by apoptosis associated with a fall in BCL2 levels. Apoptosis may be prevented by co-culture with purified bone marrow-derived stromal cells [117] or the addition of IL-2, IFNα or IFNγ. IL-5 induces apoptosis by a mechanism which is independent of BCL2 expression [118].

The culture of CLL cells in the presence of cross-linked anti CD40 and IL-4 results in prolonged *in vitro* growth, but the *in vivo* significance of this finding is unclear [119].

CD5 positivity

CD5 is a 67-kD polypeptide with two N-linked carbohydrate sites [120]. The gene has been located to chromosome 11q13 [121]. The extracellular domain consists of three scavenger receptor cysteine-rich domains. Domain 1 is separated from domain 2 by a connecting peptide rich in threonine and proline residues. The cytoplasmic domain contains multiple potential sites for phosphorylation of serine/threonine or tyro-

sine [122]. The B-cell-specific molecule CD72 appears to be its natural ligand [123].

Caligaris-Cappio *et al.* [124] were the first to recognize a normal counterpart of the CD5+ B cell, located in the mantle zone of germinal centres in human lymph nodes. These cells share some of the characteristics of CLL cells but are not phenotypically identical [125]. They do not express the minimal levels of surface immunoglobulin characteristic of CLL cells, and do not overexpress Bcl-2. Moreover, in contrast to CLL cells, they do express C-*MYC* and are easily transformed by EBV [125].

The matter is confused by the fact that a quite distinct lymphoma arises from the mantle zone of lymph nodes [126]. While this is a tumour of CD5+ B cells it too is immunophenotypically distinguishable from CLL.

It has been recognized that substantial numbers of B cells in 20-week human fetal spleens and lymph nodes also express CD5 [127]. These cells are not present in liver or bone marrow [128]. Like the cells in CLL, they also express weak surface IgM plus IgD and their surface immunoglobulin caps poorly following cross-linking [129]. Again, like CLL, they do not express CD35 [57]. In the adult small numbers of CD5+ B cells are present in the blood and tonsil although, again, not in bone marrow [66]. In patients with rheumatoid arthritis and systemic lupus erythematosus, and after allogenetic bone marrow transplantation, CD5+ B cells are increased in number [130,131].

In mice, CD5+ B cells arising in fetal life comprise about 5% of circulating B-lymphocytes [132]. Strikingly, in certain strains of mice such as New Zealand Blacks (NZB) and Motheaten Viables (MeV), which are subject to autoimmune diseases, higher proportions (20–80%) of circulating B cells are CD5+ [133]. CD5+ B cells are particularly well represented in the murine peritoneum where they comprise 40–80% of B cells, but, as in humans, they are absent from the bone marrow [134]. Nor can this population be reconstituted by marrow transplantation into lethally irradiated animals [135]. In early life, there is a skewed usage by these cells of certain immunoglobulin heavy-chain variable-region genes, apparently driven by exposure to thymus-independent self antigens such as phosphatidyl choline [136].

The fact that there is a high prevalence of autoimmune phenomena in CLL has given support to those who consider it to be a tumour of a separate lineage of CD5+ B cells mainly involved in the production of autoantibodies [125]. This hypothesis is supported by the fact some CLL cells secrete polyreactive autoantibodies when stimulated *in vitro* [137], but some facts weigh against it. CD5+ B cells are not augmented in other strains of mice prone to autoimmunity [138], while Xid mice, which do not express the CD5 marker at all on B cells, have an incidence of autoimmunity that is similar to that in other strains [139]. Furthermore, it is now clear that in both mice and humans the germline configuration of many V_H gene products tends to favour weak reactions with autoantigens, irrespective of whether they are carried by CD5+ or CD5– B cells [140]. It has also become clear that CD5– B cells can be induced to express the antigen on stimulation with TPA [141]. Finally, the autoantibodies produced in CLL are not the product of the leukaemic clone but of the residual 'normal' B cells [67].

Adhesion molecules and activation markers

The homing and recirculation pattern of lymphocytes is determined by the presence of particular adhesion molecules on the surface of the cell. Unlike normal peripheral blood B cells, in CLL there is a low or absent expression of LFA-1 (CD11a/CD18) and ICAM-1 (CD54) [142,143]. On the other hand CD11b or CD11c, normally confined to the myeloid lineage, are sometimes found in CLL cells [144]. The lymphocyte homing receptors CD44 and L-selectin (CD62L) are expressed in the same way as in normal B cells [145,146].

Integrins are heterodimers of one of 15 alpha and one of eight beta subunits [147]. Of all the possible heterodimers, 21 are found in life and 13 on lymphocytes [148]. In CLL $\beta1$ forms heterodimers with $\alpha3$, $\alpha4$, $\alpha5$ and $\alpha6$; $\beta2$ with αL and $\beta7$ with $\alpha4$ [149–151]. It is not clear how expression of these molecules might affect the presentation of CLL, or what implications they hold for determining where in lymphocyte ontogeny the malignant cell arises. $\alpha4\beta7$ has been associated with nodal lymphomas [152], but no study in CLL has demonstrated whether this is true for this disease.

Part of the difficulty in correlating the integrin expression with cellular behaviour is in knowing whether or not the molecule is functional. Cellular activation is required for functional activity [151]. Virtually all B-cell malignancies express activation antigens [55]. The status of CLL as a tumour of resting B cells is challenged by the fact that it does so too. Virtually all cases express the B5 antigen [66] and CD39 [151]. Blast-1, CD71 and CD25 are each expressed on 50% of cases [153–155] and CD80 on 30% [151]. The low-affinity Fcϵ receptor, CD23, which is upregulated by IL-4, is present on most CLLs but seldom on other lymphoid tumours [61]. Other activation markers, B7/BB1, B8.7, CD54, CD71, CD77 and 4F2, are seldom expressed [153–155]. The significance of the presence of activation markers on CLL cells and of the contrast with cell-cycle status remains uncertain.

Immunoglobulin V genes

Immunoglobulin variable (V) domains are the products of combinatorial joining of V(D)J-gene segments. Each V domain has three hypervariable sequences, termed complementarity determining regions (CDRs). CDR1 and CDR2 are determined by the choice of V gene, and CDR3 by the V(D)J recombination. Sequence diversity in CDR3 is enhanced by the addition of nonencoded nucleotides at the splice sites, a process catalysed by terminal deoxynucleotidyl transferase (TdT). Further

diversity is produced by somatic mutations at or near the antibody combining site by hypothetical mutases, activated only within the germinal centre. Class switching of immunoglobulin heavy-chain constant-domain genes to epsilon, gamma or alpha occurs separately but at the same time and place.

There are now known to be 51 functional V_H genes, divided into seven families [156]. Early studies suggested that the rearrangement and expression of Ig gene segments in CLL might be nonrandom [157]. However, in a review of 75 cases of CLL for whom Ig gene sequences had been published, Schroeder & Dighiero found that 27 V_H genes had been used [158]. There was some suggestion of overuse of the V_H1 gene 51p1 [157] and of the V_H5 gene V251 [159], and, for the very few cases of CLL expressing class-switched Ig, the V_H4 gene V4–34 [52]. A similar overuse of the $V_\kappa III$ gene Humkv325 has been reported [160]. These results should be treated with caution, because close scrutiny of the individual case reports indicates that many of the patients did not have classical CLL. Our own experience confirms the biased usage of V4–34 in cases whose Ig has undergone class switching and, paradoxically, its underuse in cases that have not.

V4–34 is used by all anti-Ii cold agglutinins [161], while both 51p1 and Humkv325 are frequently used by monoclonal rheumatoid factors [162]. V251 and 51p1 are preferentially expressed in fetal life [163,164]. These facts have been marshalled to support a hypothesis that CLL is a tumour of a CD5+ B cell that arises early in fetal life and is committed to producing weak-acting autoreactive antibodies [137]. The case, however, is not strong. Fetal cells generally have short CDR3s whereas in CLL the reverse is true [158]. Furthermore, the V_H genes most well represented in the fetus, 31p1, 56p1 and 20p1, have not been described in CLL [158]. Clearly, this database needs to be expanded before any clear conclusions can be drawn.

Determination of whether the Ig genes of a leukaemic B cell have undergone somatic mutation would place its stage of maturation at either pre- or post-germinal centre. Although early reports suggested that Ig genes in CLL were in germline configuration [157], subsequent studies have disputed this [158]. Despite considerable doubt about the accuracy of diagnosis in many of the published cases, there appear to be two distinct patterns. Early reports have suggested corresponding clinical heterogeneity, although the evidence is not yet sufficient to point to two separate diseases [165].

Where somatic mutation has taken place there is no evidence of heterogeneity within the clone. This is quite unlike what is seen in low-grade follicular lymphoma where a pattern of evolving mutations is usually evident [166].

Low levels of surface immunoglobulin

Among normal B cells only anergic cells have such low levels of surface Ig as are seen in CLL [125]. In B cells anergy is the functionally silent state induced by the interaction of surface Ig with self antigen. Normal B cells anergized by exposure to soluble antigen respond by downregulating surface Ig [167]. Such cells respond poorly to ligation of the B-cell-receptor complex [168], although this block can be overcome by stimulation with CD40 and cytokines [169]. The resemblence to CLL cells is striking. Failure to respond to EBV stimulation [66], low levels of antiporter activity [170], poor response to mitogens [91], with poor signal transduction [171], high levels of Bcl-2 [172] and low levels of Fas [173], could all be the consequence of anergy and lead to the accumulation of functionally inert cells in G_0.

Cytogenetics and molecular genetics

Trisomy 12

Between 10 and 20% of patients with CLL have trisomy 12 detected by chromosomal analysis [91]. While it is clear that trisomy 12 can be detected by fluorescence *in situ* hybridization (FISH) using a centromeric probe for chromosome 12 in patients with an apparently normal karyotype, the overall prevalence of trisomy 12 detected by FISH varies from 10 to 30% of cases [103,174]. It is not known whether this variation reflects geographical differences or patient selection. Studies using Southern blotting have suggested that trisomy 12 involves the whole of the neoplastic clone [174], but more recently the combined use of FISH and immunophenotyping with a surface light-chain marker has shown that only 30–40% of the neoplastic clone have the extra chromosome [175]. This indicates that trisomy 12 must be a secondary event in leukaemogenesis. A recent study looking at prognostic factors in stage A CLL has confirmed that both atypical morphology and trisomy 12 are associated with disease progression, but in a multivariate analysis the effect of trisomy 12 was largely accounted for by its association with atypical morphology [176].

Chromosome 13

Although the original cytogenetic reports did not identify chromosome 13 abnormalities, subsequent studies have shown deletions or translocations of chromosome 13, mainly affecting band q14, to be common in CLL, occurring in between 15 and 25% of cases [91]. Of over 400 cases of CLL karyotyped in Bournemouth (Figs 6.3 & 6.4), 80 have had structural abnormalities of chromosome 13; of these two-thirds were deletions and one-third translocations [91]. The most frequently deleted segments were q12 to q14 and q14 to q22. The translocations all involved q14 but no consistent partner chromosome. In one-third of cases the translocations were complex, involving three or more chromosomes.

Since the retinoblastoma gene (*RB1*), a known tumour suppressor gene, is located at 13q14 it was an obvious candidate gene. Molecular and FISH studies using RB1 probes have

shown that many but not all patients with 13q14 deletions and translocations, as well as some patients with a normal karyotype, have *RB1* loss [177–179]. However, this loss is almost invariably heterozygous, and RNA and protein studies show that the retinoblastoma protein is expressed in CLL cells, suggesting that *RB1* loss is not an important event in the pathogenesis of CLL.

More recent studies using a panel of microsatellite markers have shown that genetic loss is found more frequently in a 1-megabase region telomeric to the *RB1* gene and homozygous loss of two anonymous probes, D13S19 and D13S25, is a frequent occurrence [180,181]. Investigation of patients with 13q14 translocations by FISH using a series of yeast artificial chromosome (YAC) probes consistently shows genetic loss with variable proximal and distal breakpoints, suggesting that the genetic consequence of 13q14 translocations is loss of genetic material rather than the creation of a fusion gene or the overexpression of an oncogene such as is typical for chromosomal translocations in haematological malignancies [182].

As with trisomy 12, combined immunophenotyping and FISH using 13q14 probes show that structural abnormalities of chromosome 13 may not involve the whole of the neoplastic clone [183]. However, it remains possible that a point mutation or a microdeletion of a critical gene could be an initiating or early event in at least some cases of CLL.

Despite being the commonest cytogenetic abnormalities in CLL with a combined incidence of 40–50% of all abnormalities, trisomy 12 and structural abnormalities of 13q rarely coexist. In a cytogenetic analysis of 400 cases, only eight patients were found to have both abnormalities occurring in the same clone [184]. In a separate study using FISH for trisomy 12 and *RB1* loss, 12 of 195 patients (6%) had both abnormalities (see Plate 6.8 between pp. 292 and 293) [183]. In both studies cells were identified with trisomy 12 alone, 13q loss alone and with both trisomy 12 and partial deletion of 13q. The low frequency of combined abnormalities raises the possibility that two independent molecular pathways may exist, both of which are important in the pathogenesis of CLL.

Support for this concept comes from analysis of immunoglobulin heavy-chain variable region (V_H) genes. Previous studies have suggested that in most cases of typical CLL the immunoglobulin V_H genes do not undergo somatic hypermutation. In a study of 16 cases of CLL with single chromosomal abnormalities, it has been found that none of nine cases with trisomy 12 showed somatic hypermutation, while all seven cases with structural abnormalities of 13q showed mutations without intraclonal heterogeneity [165]. These distinct mutational patterns suggest that cells harbouring the 13q14 abnormality appear to encounter the mutator mechanism of germinal centres, while those with trisomy 12 do not.

Chromosome 11q

Structural abnormalities of chromosome 11q in 5% of patients with CLL have been found by us. The majority of these abnormalities comprise large deletions, of which almost all involve band 11q23. One study using FISH with a YAC probe map to 11q23 found evidence of 11q deletions in 17% of cases of CLL [185]. In this series 11q deletions were associated with more advanced disease and extensive lymphadenopathy, but there was no significant difference in survival between patients with and without 11q deletions.

Chromosome 14q

The t(11;14)(q13;q32) translocation and the resultant overexpression of cyclin D1 is rarely reported in CLL. Cases in which the translocation has been found were usually atypical both in immunophenotype and morphology and there is some doubt about whether these cases are truly CLL, rather than a leukaemic phase of a MCL [186].

The t(14;18)(q32;q21) translocation and the light-chain variants t(2;28) and t(18;22) translocations, all of which result in the rearrangement of the *BCL2* gene, are rare in CLL — they are found in only 1–2% of cases [187,188]. Analysis of the *BCL2* breakpoints show that these are usually 5′ and distinct from the breakpoints associated with follicle centre cell lymphoma. The expression of BCL 2 protein is usually higher than that found in typical CLL but patients with *BCL2* rearrangements have no distinct clinical or morphological features.

The t(14;19)(q32;q13) translocation is another rare finding in CLL [189], occurring in 0.5% of cases. Lymphocyte morphology is frequently atypical and most patients have progressive disease. The breakpoint on chromosome 19 involves the *BCL3* gene which encodes an I-kB-like protein.

p53 gene

The p53 tumour suppressor gene is located on chromosome 17p13 and inactivation of p53, either by mutation or deletion, is the commonest genetic abnormality in malignant disease. p53 abnormalities may be detected by a single-strand conformation polymorphism analysis, immunochemistry or FISH. They are found in 10–15% of cases of CLL [190,191]. Where chromosome and molecular analyses have been performed concurrently, patients with deletions or mutations involving 17p13 almost invariably have a p53 mutation of the remaining allele. Clinically, there is a strong correlation between p53 mutations and advanced stage, resistance to chemotherapy (including to purine analogues) and short survival [192]. Amplification of the murine double minute 2 (*MDM2*) gene on chromosome 12 leads to overexpression of a protein which inactivates p53. No evidence of *MDM2* gene amplification has been found in CLL, but overexpression of *MDM2* RNA has been detected, although the clinical significance of this remains uncertain [193].

Table 6.3 Causes of reactive lymphocytosis.

Infectious mononucleosis
Cytomegalovirus
Toxoplasma gondii
Human immunodeficiency virus
Pertussis
Brucellosis
Congenital syphilis
Infectious hepatitis
Mumps
Varicella
Rubella
Adenovirus
Acute infectious lymphocytosis

Differential diagnosis

Reactive lymphocytoses (Table 6.3)

These usually occur in a younger age group than CLL. In some cases, such as infectious mononucleosis, the cells are clearly morphologically distinct, but in others the Romanowsky appearance is similar to CLL and the distinction must be made by immunophenotype.

Other B-cell tumours

Several other B-cell lymphomas characteristically have a leukaemic phase. Most of these are easily distinguished from CLL by the practised eye, but cell marker profiles are distinct (Table 6.1).

Prolymphocytic leukaemia

In PLL more than half the cells are prolymphocytes. Prolymphocytes are larger than CLL cells with less condensed chromatin, a single prominent nucleolus and more abundant pale agranular cytoplasm (see Plate 6.9 between pp. 292 and 239). They have high levels of surface immunoglobulin. Other details are discussed later in this chapter.

Hairy cell leukaemia

The neoplastic cells are larger than CLL cells with abundant sky-blue agranular cytoplasm with a serrated border. The nucleus has 'spongy' chromatin and a single nucleus. Characteristic markers are CD11c, CD25 and tartrate-resistant acid phosphatase positivity. HCL is discussed in detail in Chapter 8.

Splenic lymphoma with villous lymphocytes

The circulating lymphocytes have fine villous projections,

usually confined to one pole. The nucleus has condensed chromatin, though a single nucleolus may be distinguished. Cytoplasm may be slightly basophilic (see Plate 6.10). Further details are given later in the chapter.

Mantle cell lymphoma

The REAL Classification recognizes MCL as a specific entity, whereas it was lost in Group E of the Working Formulation and included within centrocytic lymphoma in the Kiel classification. The leukaemic cells are pleomorphic, medium to large in size, with slight nuclear irregularity and moderate indentation (see Plate 6.11). Small cells are very scanty. It bears most resemblance to CLL/PLL, and its CD5 positivity tends to confirm that mistaken diagnosis. Since many workers do not realize that CLL/PLL retains the low-intensity surface immunoglobulin intensity of CLL rather than gaining the high-intensity staining of PLL, they naturally assume that the bright SIg of MCL is what should be expected in CLL/PLL. The karyotype t(11;14) involving Bcl-1 (or cyclin-D) is characteristic but not pathognomonic, because it is also found in some cases of SLVL. Further details are found in Chapter 18.

Follicular lymphoma

About one-third of follicular lymphomas have a leukaemic phase. The cleaved cells of follicular lymphoma are very small, have little or no visible cytoplasm, have a smooth rather than clumped nuclear chromatin pattern and have an irregular or angular nuclear outline with characteristic nuclear clefts or their indentations (see Plate 6.12). The membrane phenotype is distinctive (Table 6.1). Follicular lymphoma is considered in detail in Chapter 18.

CD5– chronic lymphocytic leukaemia

Although CD5 positivity is regarded as a defining feature of CLL, many series include a minority of cases which are CD5–. Since many other types of B-cell lymphoma can resemble CLL clinically, and predominately involve blood and bone marrow, it is difficult to decide whether these are true cases of CLL. Scrutiny of individual cases in the literature frequently exposes them as atypical in other features, but often insufficient detail is given. A review of 12 cases of CD5– CLL showed them to be CD23– with bright surface Ig [194]. They were of advanced stage with splenomegaly. An unbiased observer might wonder how they differed from PLL. Further study is clearly warranted.

T-cell leukaemias

The T-cell leukaemias are included within the differential diagnosis for completeness. The existance of a T-cell leukaemia which is morphologically indistinguishable from B-CLL is controversial. A form of T-PLL with a predominance of small prolymphocytes could be confused with CLL, but the nucleolus is distinct and the membrane phenotype very different. Recently, Hoyer *et al.* have described 25 cases of T-CLL in which the lymphocytes were small with absent or inconspicuous nucleoli, round or irregular nuclei and minimal agranular cytoplasm [195]. Twenty-two were CD4+ and three CD8+. Recurring cytogenetic abnormalities involved bands 14q11 and 14q32. The median age at presentation was 57 years with a male preponderance (1.5:1, male:female). Shotty lymphadenopathy was present in 56%, slight or moderate splenomegaly in 40% and skin involvement in 4%. The clinical course was aggressive and refractory to alkylating agents and intensive chemotherapy. Two similar patients have been described by Wong *et al.* [196]. The resemblance of all these cases to T-PLL is striking, and Matutes & Catovsky [197] have designated them a small cell variant of T-PLL.

T hairy cell leukaemia is very rare and not really to be confused. ATLL has a very characteristic cell morphology and membrane phenotype (see Chapter 7). In some cases of cutaneous T-cell lymphoma the Sézary cells are very small and condensed so that the nuclear convolutions are overlooked. Again the phenotype is distinctive.

In large granular lymphocytic (LGL) leukaemia the lymphocytes are larger than in CLL with more abundant cytoplasm with azurophil granules (See Plate 6.13). The difficult differential is not from CLL but from a reactive T-cell lymphocytosis and must usually be made by examining T-cell receptor gene rearrangement.

Natural history, staging and prognosis

The natural history of CLL is extremely variable. For a large proportion of patients, long survival without symptoms, signs or progression is the rule. The longest reported survivor is 36 years [198]. On the other hand other patients may present with a barely raised white cell count and a single enlarged lymph node, yet within months develop bone marrow failure and massive lymphadenopathy and hepatosplenomegaly. Thankfully, such cases are rare and the usual pattern of progression is for a slow increase in white cell count, degree of marrow infiltration, and size of lymph nodes and spleen. More than half will die from an unrelated cause [10].

There are three factors which affect the prognosis in CLL: (i) the tumour mass; (ii) the rate of progression; (iii) the sensitivity of the tumour to chemotherapy. Two commonly used staging systems are thought to be good indices of tumour mass but state nothing about the rate of progression of the disease nor about the sensitivity to chemotherapy.

The Rai Staging System [199] (Table 6.4) correlates well with survival. However, stages I and II do not differ significantly and neither do stages III and IV, so that three

Table 6.4 Rai Clinical Staging System.

Stage 0	Lymphocytosis in blood and marrow only
Stage I	Lymphocytosis plus lymphadenopathy
Stage II	Lymphocytosis plus splenomegaly or hepatomegaly
Stage III	Lymphocytosis plus anaemia (Hb < 110 g/l)
Stage IV	Lymphocytosis plus thrombocytopenia (platelets < 100 × 10^9/l)

Table 6.5 Binet Clinical Staging System.

Stage A	<3 involved sites, Hb > 100 g/l, platelets > 100 × 10^9/l
Stage B	>3 involved sites, Hb > 100 g/l, platelets > 100 × 10^9/l
Stage C	Hb < 100 g/l or platelets < 100 × 10^9/l

Involved sites are liver, spleen and lymph nodes in inguinal, axilliary and cervical regions.

groups are sufficient. Median survivals for stage 0 is 12 years, for stages I or II is 7 years and for stages III and IV is less than 12 months.

The Binet Staging System [200] (Table 6.5) has only three groups and takes a different level of haemoglobin to signify anaemia but is otherwise similar with similar results. The median survival for group A is 9 years, for group B 8 years and group C 2 years.

Neither system specifies that anaemia or thrombocytopenia should be the result of marrow failure, but this is an important stipulation. Anaemia or thrombocytopenia with an autoimmune, or other, cause does not carry the same grave prognosis. It is difficult to see why neither staging system makes no allowance for the sex difference in the normal range for haemoglobin.

It is sometimes useful to adopt the International Workshop on CLLs recommendation to combine the Binet and Rai stages in the following manner: A(0), A(I), A(II), B(I), B(II), C(III), C(IV) [201].

There have been several other staging systems suggested (reviewed by Montserrat & Rozman [202]), but none has found wide acceptance.

Other prognostic measurements

A decision on whether to treat and how to do so is generally made on the basis of stage (see below). It is usual practice to delay treatment in stage A disease. Nevertheless, about a quarter of stage A patients will eventually progress [10] and other prognostic markers would be of value for the early recognition of this group.

The absolute number of circulating lymphocytes can be regarded as a rough and ready measure of tumour mass, but a high lymphocyte count alone is not a good indication of the need for treatment. However, patients whose lymphocyte counts remain below 30 × 10^9/l are usually best left without chemotherapy [203].

It should be noted that both the Rai and Binet Scoring Systems set the haemoglobin required for advanced stage disease much lower than the lower limit of the normal range. Several groups have noted that any fall in haemoglobin is an adverse prognostic factor [204,205]. The French Co-operative Group demonstrated that a subset of stage A patients that they

designated A, and defined as having a haemoglobin less than 120 g/l or a white cell count greater than 30 × 10^9/l, had a worse prognosis and would benefit from early treatment [206]. This observation has not yet been confirmed in other studies and suffers from the hazards of retrospective subset analysis.

A large multicentre European study has shown karyotype to be an independent prognostic factor in CLL [96]. The median survival in patients with a normal karyotype was more than 15 years, compared to 7.7 years for patients with a clonal abnormality. Patients with a complex karyotype have the worse prognosis. Abnormalities of chromosomes 12 and 14q conferred a poorer prognosis than did 13q abnormalities.

Lymphocyte doubling time (LDT) is a further independent variable. LDTs of less than 12 months are associated with a poor prognosis [207]. This is the simplest measurement of the progressive nature of the disease. There have been several attempts to find an *in vitro* correlate with this progressive nature, including tritiated thymidine incorporation [208], mitogenic activity after polyclonal lymphocyte stimulation [209], the percentage of lymphocytes in S phase by flow cytometry [109] and the percentage of cells positive for Ki67 or PCNA [210,211]. All are beyond the reach of the general haematologist.

A diffuse bone marrow histological pattern confers a worse prognosis than nondiffuse [89], but diffuse infiltration is very rare in stage A disease. A collaborative group from the Royal Marsden, Bournemouth and Plymouth has defined a set of criteria for atypical lymphocyte morphology in CLL [176]. The presence of either more than 10% circulating prolymphocytes or more than 15% of cells with a cleaved nucleus and/or lymphoplasmacytic features correlated well with the presence of trisomy 12 and with progression in stage A disease.

Montserrat & Rozman [202] proposed criteria which included a nondiffuse bone marrow histology, haemoglobin greater than 130 g/l and white cell count less than 30 × 10^9/l, to identify 'smouldering' CLL akin to benign monoclonal gammopathy. Such a form of CLL would be unlikely to progress and have a survival probability no worse than age- and sex-matched controls (Table 6.6). Nevertheless, even with these criteria, 20% of smouldering CLL will eventually progress to a stage requiring treatment.

Table 6.6 Criteria for smouldering CLL.

Stage A
Nondiffuse bone marrow histopathology
Hb > 130 g/l
Lymphocyte count < 30×10^9/l
Lymphocyte doubling time > 12 months

The third criterion upon which survival depends, namely the sensitivity of tumour cells to chemotherapy, is not easy to assess *in vitro*. Bosanquet *et al.* [212] have had some success with the DISC assay but this remains to be fully evaluated in a large study.

Complications

Autoimmunity

Autoimmune haemolytic anaemia is a strikingly common complication of CLL, occurring in between 10 and 20% of patients depending on stage [67]. Autoimmune thrombocytopenia, neutropenia and pure red cell aplasia all occur, but less frequently [68–70]. Other autoimmune phenomena are no commoner than in age-matched controls [67]. Any explanation of autoimmunity in CLL must address the question why the range of activity is so restricted.

The hypothesis that is currently in favour draws on the suggestion that CLL is a tumour of B1-B-cells destined to produce weak-reacting IgM 'autoantibodies' [125]. It is suggested that such autoreactive B cells might act as antigen-presenting cells (APC) presenting restricted haematopoietic self antigens to residual normal B cells. One difficulty with this idea is the inertness of the CLL cells. They bear a close resemblance to anergic B cells, and such cells are poor at processing and presenting antigen [213]. Thus a further extension of the hypothesis has to locate the APC function within the microenvironment of the spleen where it is supposed that interaction with activated T cells, particularly via the CD40–CD40 ligand connection, is able to upregulate the expression of CD80 and CD86 which are necessary for antigen presentation [214].

A further factor to accommodate within the hypothesis is the relationship of autoimmunity to treatment. Damashek suggested that haemolysis might be triggered by treatment with X-rays or alkylating agents [215]. Two such case reports have subsequently appeared in the literature [216,217], but among 37 haemolytic episodes in his series, Hansen found only five where treatment with X-rays or alkylating agents had been given in the previous 2 months [218]. Recently, it has become apparent that haemolysis after treatment with fludarabine or cladribine is much commoner than after other forms of treatment [219,220]. Since these drugs produce a

much more profound T-cell suppression than alkylating agents or X-rays, the hypothesis that breakdown in T-cell regulation by the combined effect of the tumour, old age and treatment is supported [221].

Transformation

Transformation in CLL is a rare event. Three forms have been recognized.

Prolymphocytic transformation

The existence of variable proportions of atypical large cells with prominent nucleoli has long been recognized as a feature of CLL. The accumulation of such cells accompanied by progressive clinical deterioration and refractiveness to treatment was described by Enno *et al.* [222] as a prolymphocytoid transformation of CLL (see Plate 6.14 between pp. 292 and 293). Melo *et al.* [223] examined the relationship between CLL and PLL by studying 164 cases of typical CLL submitted to the first MRC trial on CLL, together with 146 cases sent in as atypical CLL or PLL. They were separated on the basis of the percentage of prolymphocytes on the blood film. One hundred and seventy-four cases with less than 10% prolymphocytes were designated CLL, 84 with 11–55% prolymphocytes were called CLL/PLL and 42 with more than 55% were recognized as PLL.

In many respects the CLL/PLL group were intermediate between CLL and PLL. They resembled the CLL groups in having more lymphadenopathy and an older age at presentation, but were more like the PLL group in having large spleens and a worse prognosis.

Cell markers, in general, resemble those of CLL rather than PLL, although the prolymphocytes tend to be positive for FMC7 and membrane CD22. More than half the group had stable numbers of prolymphocytes and could not be thought of as progressing at all. However, in a minority there was a gradual progression to a PLL-like blood picture. In only two did the cell markers change to those of PLL. Patients with greater than 15% prolymphocytes in their blood have a poor prognosis. They tend to respond poorly to single-agent chemotherapy.

Richter's syndrome

In 1928 Richter described an aggressive lymphoma occurring in a patient with CLL and gave his name to a phenomenon which occurs in up to 3% of patients [224]. The patients with previously indolent disease experience a sudden clinical deterioration with rapidly enlarging lymph node or nodes, often with hepatosplenomegaly in the face of an unchanging or even falling white cell count. B symptoms are often present. Other signs that Richter's transformation is occurring include a sudden rise in LDH, the appearance of a paraprotein, fever or weight loss, evidence of extranodal disease, hypercalcaemia and bony destruction [225]. Histologically, the tumour is a diffuse large cell lymphoma [226].

Whether Richter's syndrome is the transformation of CLL into a high-grade lymphoma or the development of an independent aggressive tumour has been disputed. Molecular studies have made it clear that both can occur with equal frequency [227–231].

Acute lymphoblastic leukaemia

Transformation of CLL to acute lymphoblastic leukaemia (ALL) is controversial. The first convincing report demonstrated blast cells with surface immunoglobulin which would be uncharacteristic for classical ALL [232]. One of the two cases had surface IgMκ with rheumatoid factor activity on both lymphocytes and lymphoblasts, and it now seems more likely that this and subsequent cases represent either a Richter-like transformation of CLL with peripheral blood spillover of the high-grade lymphoma cells, or a similar high-grade transformation of a different B-cell lymphoma with a superficial resemblance to CLL. In at least one of the reported cases the CD5 antigen was retained during the blastic phase [233]. However, in another case the blasts were shown to be TdT positive [234], and in this and other cases the blast cells had the characteristics of ALL [235]. In such cases, however, it has not been established that the ALL belongs to the same clone as the CLL. As techniques for determining this have grown more sophisticated, it is notable that case reports of ALL transformation of CLL have ceased appearing. At present a sceptical viewpoint is warranted.

Second malignancies

Because of the age of the population nonhaematological causes are common in patients with CLL. Several studies have reported greater numbers than might have been expected [236–239], but such studies are inconclusive because in the elderly both CLL and other malignancies may be clinically silent, and the finding of one might bias the physician and prevent the other being found. A role for impaired immune surveillance has been postulated.

Haematological malignancies

It might be expected that haematologists would be assiduous in reporting cases of CLL and other haematological malignancies. Myeloma [240], myelodysplastic syndrome [241], chronic myeloid leukaemia and acute myeloblastic leukaemia [10] have all been seen in our unit in association with CLL. Apart from two cases of myeloma [242,243], none of these tumours have been shown to be clonally related to the CLL. Given the massive underdiagnosis of CLL in the community, it is very likely that these are chance associations.

Management

CLL is probably incurable. Fortunately, a large proportion of patients do not require treatment. Several trials of early vs deferred treatment of stage A CLL have indicated no benefit for early treatment [244–247]. Indeed there may be a slight disadvantage in treating this group. There is an argument that some patients with stage B might also benefit from deferring treatment. Unfortunately, no prospective trial has examined this.

Indications for treatment are a falling haemoglobin or platelet count, progression to a later stage of disease, unsightly or painful lymphadenopathy or organomegaly, other disease-related symptoms, a lymphocyte doubling time of less than 12 months or transformation of disease [176].

Response criteria

A National Cancer Institute sponsored Working Group recommended criteria of response in CLL in 1988 [248]. Complete response (CR) was defined as freedom from clinical disease for at least 2 months with a 'normal' blood count (haemoglobin >110 g/l, neutrophils >1.5 × 10^9/l, lymphocytes <4 × 10^9/l, platelets >100 × 10^9/l) without transfusion; no constitutional symptoms, no lymphadenopathy or hepatosplenomegaly and fewer than 30% small lymphocytes in the bone marrow.

A partial response (PR) was defined as at least a 50% reduction in the numbers of lymphocytes in the blood, together with at least a 50% reduction in lymphadenopathy and/or hepatosplenomegaly. At least one of the following should be maintained for at least 2 months: haemoglobin greater than 110 g/l; platelets greater than 100 × 10^9/l; or a 50% improvement in platelet or red cell count over pretreatment values without transfusions.

The MD Anderson Cancer Treatment Center introduced a further type of response, a nodular complete response [249]. These patients fulfilled the criteria for a CR except for the presence of lymphoid nodules on trephine biopsy.

In all of these responses it is usual to find that the disease remains easily detectable by more sensitive methods. A population of CD5/CD19+ cells can be detected by dual-colour immunofluorescence, while molecular techniques will detect a single immunoglobulin heavy-chain gene rearrangement.

Corticosteroids

Corticosteroids are effective agents in many cases of CLL. They are generally reserved as first-line agents in patients presenting with autoimmune haemolytic anaemia or thrombocytopenia or as salvage therapy in patients with refractory disease. The dose for autoimmune disease is prednisolone 40 mg/m^2 daily for 14 days, tapering over another 2 weeks. Prednisolone alone will control CLL in about 10% of cases, but because of steroid-induced side effects it should not be used as a treatment of choice. Characteristically patients on corticosteroids have an initial rise in lymphocyte count. This is due to redistribution of lymphocytes among compartments and does not carry a sinister significance.

In end-stage refractory CLL high-dose methyl prednisolone has a place [250]. Dosages of 250 mg/m² daily for 5 days can restore normal haemoglobin and platelet counts, although the risk of infection is high.

Alkylating agents

Chlorambucil is long established as the treatment of choice in CLL. Given orally it is well tolerated, and avoids the usual alkylating agent side effects of alopecia and gastrointestinal intolerance. A number of different regimens have been used, ranging from 0.1 mg/kg daily given indefinitely to 0.7 mg/kg daily for 4 days every month [244]. No randomized study has compared the efficacy of continuous vs intermittent chlorambucil in CLL, although many doctors feel that continuous chlorambucil would be more likely to induce secondary myelodysplastic syndrome [251].

A Yugoslavian trial compared a continuous high daily dose of chlorambucil (15 mg/day) with a single dose (75 mg) given intermittently every 4 weeks together with prednisolone (50 mg/day tapered to 15 mg/day over 6 weeks) followed by 30 mg/day for 7 days with each subsequent course of chlorambucil [252]. The high daily dose was associated with greater toxicity and diminished compliance but gave a higher CR rate (70 vs 30%) and a significantly longer survival (median survival 6 years vs 3 years *P* < 0.01.)

There is conflicting evidence as to whether adding prednisolone to chlorambucil improves response or survival [244,253]. Current practice in the UK is to use prednisolone if there is evidence of autoimmune disease, and during the first course of treatment if the patient presents with significant thrombocytopenia. Cyclophosphamide (50–100 mg/day) is an acceptable alternative to chlorambucil in the few patients who have allergic rashes on the latter. Cyclophosphamide causes more alopecia but less marrow toxicity than chlorambucil.

Combination chemotherapy

The combination of cyclophosphamide, vincristine and prednisolone (COP) is no better than chlorambucil alone in inducing CR or prolonging survival in Rai stage II or Binet stage B or C CLL [244,254,255]. The neurotoxicity of vincristine, especially in elderly patients, makes it an unacceptable drug in CLL.

An anthracycline-containing combination may have an advantage over chlorambucil alone in advanced stage disease. In the French Co-operative Trial, CHOP (cyclophosphamide, vincristine, doxorubicin and prednisolone) gave a higher response rate than chlorambucil and prednisolone (77 vs 53%) for stage B disease, and a survival advantage over COP (median survival 57 months vs 25 months) for stage C disease

[256]. This trial was criticized because of small numbers (only 59 patients with stage C disease), because of the low dose of doxorubicin (25 mg/m²), and because of the poor results achieved with COP compared to other trials [244]. A subsequent French study again showed a higher response rate for CHOP compared with chlorambucil and prednisolone in stage B disease, but no improvement in survival [257]. A Danish trial [258] and a Swedish trial [259] both confirmed higher response rates for CHOP in conventional doses compared with chlorambucil, but neither showed a survival advantage.

Intensive regimens such as M2 (cyclophosphamide, BCNU, melphalan and prednisolone) [260] and POACH (prednisolone, vincristine, cytarabine, cyclophosphamide and doxorubicin) [261] have proved to be no better than chlorambucil and prednisolone in phase III trials. The place of anthracyclines in CLL therefore remains controversial, and is currently being investigated in the MRC CLL III trial which compares chlorambucil and epirubicin with chlorambucil alone [244].

Purine analogues

The purine analogue cytosine arabinoside is one of the most active single agents in the treatment of acute leukaemias and high-grade lymphomas, yet it only has modest activity in CLL [262]. Attempts to devise more effective purine analogues for the treatment of CLL have independently yielded three promising agents, fludarabine, cladribine and pentostatin.

Fludarabine

This purine analogue was developed as a water-soluble and adenosine deaminase-resistant derivative of vidarabine [263]. 9-β Arabinofuranosyl-2-fluoroadenine-5'-monophosphate (Fig. 6.5), was first introduced at high dose for the treatment of acute leukaemia but had unacceptable neurotoxicity [264]. However, at dosages of 25 mg/m²/day by 30-minute intravenous infusion for 5 days every 28 days, it is the most effective single agent known in CLL.

In 12 phase I and phase II studies among 1298 patients with relapsed or refractory disease, a 41% response rate (CR + PR) was seen [265]. Among previously untreated patients the response rate was almost twice as high (79%), with the majority being complete or nodular responses [266].

In phase III studies fludarabine has been compared with CAP (chlorambucil, doxorubicin and prednisolone) in a multicentre European study [267]. In previously untreated patients the response rates were greater in the fludarabine arm (71 vs 60%). The same was true for previously treated patients (48 vs 27%). The difference was only significant for the previously treated group. In this group median remission duration was 324 days for the fludarabine group and 179 days for the CAP group. This difference was not statistically significant, and

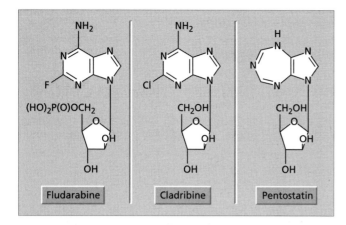

Fig. 6.5 Comparative structures of fludarabine, cladribine and pentostatin.

neither was the difference between median survivals at 728 and 731 days respectively. On the other hand in the previously untreated group fludarabine induced significantly longer remissions and significantly longer survivals. Alopecia and nausea and vomiting were significantly more frequent in the CAP arm, but infections were commoner in the fludarabine arm.

In a similar French study fludarabine gave a significantly higher response rate in stage B CLL compared with either CAP or CHOP, but for stage C patients there was no difference between the treatment groups [268]. In an American study of previously untreated patients the incidence of CR and overall responses was significantly greater for patients treated with fludarabine than for those treated with chlorambucil [269]. Neither of these trials is sufficiently mature to give survival data.

Complete remissions obtained with fludarabine are long lasting. Mean time to progression was 33 months for previously untreated patients and 21 months for previously treated patients [270]. Occasionally, although not usually, all molecular evidence of the CLL is abolished [271]. Second remissions are obtainable in those patients who received fludarabine as first-line therapy, but may not be the case in those who are already refractory to alkylating agents [270]. In a study of 91 young patients from the failure of fludarabine therapy, Seymour *et al.* [272] found that 83% of those relapsing after receiving fludarabine as a first-line therapy responded to a second round of fludarabine-containing therapy, whereas only 7% of those relapsing after responding to fludarabine salvage therapy responded to any subsequent treatment.

Fludarabine has also been used in combination with other agents. Neither combination with chlorambucil [273] nor with doxorubicin [274] gave higher response rates than have been recorded with fludarabine alone. In a direct comparison with single-agent fludarabine in 264 patients, the combination of fludarabine with prednisolone did not influence response rate

or survival; however, there was a higher incidence of opportunistic infections [275].

Fludarabine potentiates the metabolism of cytosine arabinoside (ara-C) [276] and, by making use of this fact, the combination of fludarabine, ara-C and cisplatin was given to 17 patients with CLL who were refractory to fludarabine. Six responded, including two CRs [277].

Cladribine

2-Chlorodeoxyadenosine (Fig. 6.5) is converted to its active triphosphate in cells with high levels of deoxycytidine kinase and low 5′-nucleotidase activity [278]. It was originally developed as an immunosuppressive agent but was shown to have antiproliferative activity against a variety of leukaemic cell lines [279]. In phase I studies it was found to be both immunosuppressive and myelosuppressive [280]. Phase II studies demonstrated a very high response rate in hairy cell leukaemia [281].

Cladribine may be given as a 7-day continuous infusion in a dose of 0.1 mg/kg/day or as a daily 2-hour infusion of 0.12 mg/kg/day for 5 days. In each case the dose is repeated every 28 days. In CLL six studies showed overall responses (CR + PR) of 43% in relapsed and refractory patients [265,282]. In three trials of 71 untreated patients the response rate was 83%, with 32% CR [283–285]. Remissions in patients achieving CR lasted for a median of 42 months and those achieving PR lasted for a median of 18 months [286]. It is usual for retreated patients to respond [287]. Juliusson *et al.* [288] reported a lack of cross-resistance in patients refractory to fludarabine, but this was not confirmed by a larger series of patients [289].

A phase I study of cladribine with chlorambucil demonstrated that it was feasible to combine two courses of half-dose cladribine with standard doses of chlorambucil without unacceptable toxicity [290].

Pentostatin

2-Deoxycoformycin (Fig. 6.5) is a purine analogue harvested from fermentation cultures of the soil organism *Streptomyces antibioticus* [291]. It is a potent inhibitor of the enzyme adenosine deaminase. This leads to the accumulation of 2-deoxyadenosine and its nucleotides within the cell. 2-Deoxyadenosine is phosphorylated to dATP, which accumulates in cells and downregulates ribonucleoside reductase so that DNA replication and repair is impaired [265].

Although pentostatin was originally introduced for the treatment of hairy cell leukaemia, it is also effective in the treatment of CLL, but apparently less so than fludarabine or cladribine. In four separate studies involving 121 previously treated patients, there were three CRs and 26 PRs (overall response rate 24%) [292–295]. The usual dose is 4 mg/m² weekly intravenously. It is well tolerated.

Side effects of purine analogues

Myelotoxicity is a feature of all three purine analogues, and has been well reviewed by Cheson [280]. With the doses used to treat CLL, neutropenia occurs in between 30 and 80% of patients, and it is worse in previously treated and unresponsive patients. Neutrophil counts seldom fall below $0.5 \times 10^9/l$. Thrombocytopenia also occurs with all three drugs. With fludarabine, platelet counts seldom fall below $75 \times 10^9/l$, with cladribine grade IV thrombocytopenia (platelets $<25 \times 10^9/l$) occurs in about 30% of patients. There is less experience with pentostatin, but its effect seems intermediate between the other two. Myelotoxicity usually recovers within 3 weeks of treatment.

Immunosuppression is a more important side effect and it is cumulative. Lymphocytopenia develops rapidly, mainly affecting the CD4+ T cells. O'Brien *et al.* [275] tested 217 patients with CLL treated with fludarabine. Median CD4 counts declined from $1.015 \times 10^9/l$ pretreatment to $0.169 \times 10^9/l$ after three treatments to $0.148 \times 10^9/l$ after six treatments. Similar falls have been reported with cladribine and pentostatin. Lymphocytopenia is prolonged with all three drugs and may barely have recovered after 2 years.

The immunosuppression has important consequences. Opportunist infections, especially *Pneumocystis carinii* [35], *Listeria monocytogenes* [34], disseminated candidiasis [296], *Aspergillus niger* [296], atypical mycobacteria [296], *Cytomegalovirus* [297] and *Cryptococcus* [298], are a serious hazard to be guarded against. Some authors recommend prophylactic cotrimoxazole and antifungals [296]. The combination of corticosteroids with purine analogues makes such infections more likely [275]. Transfusion-related graft-versus-host (GVH) disease has been observed [299] and it is recommended that all patients treated with purine analogues should receive irradiated blood products [299].

Autoimmune phenomena are also commoner in patients with CLL treated with purine analogues. Myint *et al.* [219] reported the development of autoimmune haemolytic anaemia (AIHA) in 12 out of 52 patients treated with fludarabine. The anaemia tends to be severe, with an abrupt onset after as few as one or as many as 12 courses. It is usually possible to control the anaemia with corticosteroids. Re-exposure to fludarabine or cladribine is likely to re-ignite the haemolytic process unless accompanied by corticosteroids. Second attacks are often difficult to control. Autoimmune thrombocytopenia [300] and pure red cell aplasia [301] also occur. The phenomen may be seen with all three drugs [302,303].

It is not clear whether patients with a history of AIHA or a positive antiglobulin test should be treated with purine analogues. Although such a history was found in patients who haemolysed with fludarabine, the majority of patients had no such history. Furthermore, some patients with such a history have been successfully treated with no special precautions.

Less well-established treatments

Monoclonal antibodies

There have been several reports of treatment of CLL with monoclonal antibodies directed against cell surface molecules [304–309]. These studies have attempted to invoke natural effectors such as complement [305], natural killer cells [304] or cytotoxic T cells [309], or have attempted to direct ribosomal inactivating proteins (RIP) [306,307] or radioisotopes [308] to the cell surface. Of the targets chosen, only idiotypic immunoglobulin is truly tumour specific [304], but differentiation antigens such as CD5, CD19, CD20, CD25 and CDw52 are present on most CLL cells and on such normal lymphocytes that the patient could afford to lose for a limited period. Among the RIP, blocked ricin A-chain [307], saporin [310] and modified diphtheria toxin [311] have been the most popular. Despite huge investment in these approaches they have not fulfilled their promise. In most cases transitory falls in lymphocyte counts have been the limits of their success.

Other biological agents

Interferon alpha effectively reduces the white cell count in stage A CLL [312]. Unfortunately it has no effect in those patients who actually need treatment. When used after fludarabine in patients who obtain near complete remission, it does not eliminate minimal residual disease nor does it delay relapse [313]

Two phase II trials of IL-2 in refractory stage C CLL showed minor responses only [314,315]. The usual extreme toxicity was evident.

Splenectomy and splenic irradiation

Splenic irradiation was evaluated in the first two MRC trials. It was found to be as effective as chlorambucil for both response and survival [244]. An Italian trial reported an overall response rate (CR and PR) of 83%. However, the response duration was only 9 months and second responses were rare [316]. Splenectomy is a valuable adjunct to treatment in selected patients [317]

Bone marrow transplantation

Theoretically, allogeneic bone marrow transplantation offers the best chance for cure of CLL, but is only applicable to a small minority of young patients. The combined registries of the European Group for Bone Marrow Transplantation (EBMT) and the International Bone Marrow Transplant Registry (IBMR) reported 70 allogeneic bone marrow transplants in CLL between 1984 and 1995 [318]. The conditioning regimen was usually cyclophosphamide and total body irradiation and GVH prophylaxis was methotrexate and cyclosporin. Only 3%

were in CR prior to transplantation. Engraftment occurred in all bar two patients and complete remission was achieved in 75%. GVH disease occurred in 47% and relapse within 54 months in 15%. Five patients have died of progressive leukaemia and 35 of treatment-related complications. Actuarial survival was 48% at 3 years.

The same registries reported autologous transplants in 29 patients [318]. Nine have received peripheral blood stem cells (PBSC), 19 bone marrow (15 purged) and one combined bone marrow and peripheral blood. At the time of the transplant 69% were in CR. Although 83% of the total group achieved CR post transplant, only 27% of those not in CR before the transplant did so. Only two patients have died of treatment-related complications, but another four have died from progressive disease. Actuarial survival was 40% at 3 years.

A group at Boston has treated 41 patients with CLL, who following conventional chemotherapy reached a state of minimal disease, with high-dose chemoradiotherapy followed by either a T-cell-depleted matched sibling allogeneic bone marrow transplant (13 patients) or a monoclonal antibody purged marrow autograft (28 patients) [319]. Four patients died of infection-related GVH disease and two died of autologous transplant-related complications. Thirty-one patients were tested by polymerase chain reaction (PCR) amplification of IgH rearrangements for minimal residual disease at the time of transplant and all were positive. However, all bar five eventually became PCR negative; only these five have relapsed. The actuarial disease-free survival for the whole group was 77% at 19 months.

The Houston group have reported 22 patients with advanced CLL treated with high-dose cyclophosphamide and total body irradiation by bone marrow transplantation. Eleven received syngeneic or matched sibling allogeneic bone marrow, and 11 autologous bone marrow harvested during a previous fludarabine-induced CR [320]. Of the 11 who received syngeneic or allogeneic marrow, seven achieved CR, two a nodular CR and one a PR. Ten patients were alive 2–36 months after the transplantation. Of those receiving autologous marrow, six patients achieved CR, four a nodular CR and one a PR. However, two patients relapsed with CLL and three with a Richter's transformation. Two developed immune cytopenias while in morphological remission and one of these died of cytomegalovirus pneumonia. Six of the 11 remained in CR 2–29 months following transplantation.

Only small numbers of patients have been treated with PBSC transplants. However, it has been demonstrated that patients with CLL have resting mean peripheral blood myeloid progenitor cell (CFU-GM) counts 30 times higher than controls [321]. Although this finding is encouraging, it is not yet clear whether it will be routinely possible to generate PBSCs in patients who have been previously treated with purine analogues. Thus transplantation remains an experimental technique which is not yet ready for phase III evaluation.

Treatment of complications

Infections in CLL are frequently associated with profound hypogammaglobulinaemia. Consideration has been given to the use of prophylactic intravenous immunoglobulin in patients at high risk of infection. In a phase III placebo-controlled double-blind study, intravenous Ig at a dose of 400 mg/kg every 3 weeks for 1 year significantly reduced the number of bacterial infections and increased the infection-free intervals in patients with CLL with a serum IgG of less than 3 g/l [322]. However, the numbers of severe bacterial infections and viral infections were not reduced and there was no survival benefit. Intavenous immunoglobulin is expensive, and its use has not been evaluated in cost-benefit terms, nor in comparison with prophylactic oral antibiotics.

Immune cytopenias usually respond to treatment with prednisolone 40–60 mg/m^2 daily. Unresponsive disease may require splenectomy, intravenous Ig or treatment with cyclosporin. The latter is usually recommended for patients with pure red cell aplasia [323].

Treatment of transformation of CLL is difficult. Prolymphocytoid transformation of CLL often responds to treatment. Alkylating agents, anthracyclines and purine analogues may all have a place [324]. Richter's syndrome remains a problem. In a study of 39 patients, Robertson et al. [226] found a median survival of 5 months despite multiagent chemotherapy. Usually CHOP-based regimens are used but only partial responses are likely.

Strategy for treatment

At present there is no indication to treat patients with stage A disease unless it is progressive. Such patients should be observed at a frequency determined by the presence or absence of adverse prognostic factors. Patients who require treatment should preferably be entered into clinical trials. Whether or not an anthracycline should be incorporated into first-line therapy remains to be determined. Similarly, although the purine analogues undoubtedly produce a higher CR rate than any other regimen, this has yet to be translated into a survival advantage. Furthermore, there is no evidence that patients treated with fludarabine or cladribine as a first-line agent survive any better than those for whom it is reserved for chlorambucil-resistant disease. For patients not entered into trials intermittent chlorambucil remains the treatment of choice, and fludarabine or cladribine is reserved for unresponsive disease.

Patients under the age of 60 should be considered for entry into trials with curative intent. These will usually entail treatment with purine analogues followed by high-dose chemoradiotherapy and stem cell rescue. At present it is not possible to give a preference for autografts or allografts, and this should remain the subject of further study. Although PBSC transplants carry less associated morbidity than bone marrow autografts, it is not yet possible to give an assurance that PBSC can be regularly generated after purine analogue treatment. Most workers have preferred high-dose cyclophosphamide and total body irradiation as a conditioning regimen, but less intensive regimens such as BEAM (BCNU, etoposide, ara-C and melphalan), which are regularly used for non-Hodgkin's lymphoma, have not been properly evaluated in CLL.

Disease that is resistant to alkylating agents, anthracyclines and purine analogues is still a major problem. Possible strategies in such patients include local radiotherapy for symptomatic relief (including splenic irradiation for hypersplenism), splenectomy, regular leucaphereses, high-dose methylprednisolone, experimental chemotherapeutic protocols (including fludarabine, ara-C and cisplatin) and monoclonal antibodies.

Prolymphocytic leukaemia

PLL was first recognized as a separate entity by Galton *et al.* [325] in 1974. It occurs in the same age group as CLL with a similar male preponderance. It is, however, much rarer. One large series from a tertiary referral centre found it to represent about 10% of all lymphocytic leukaemias [41]; in our experience it represents about 1% [10], being rarer than MCL in leukaemic phase, SLVL and HCL. The cause is unknown, but since some cases clearly evolve from CLL, it is likely to be of similar aetiology. Familial cases have not been reported. Because it is a much more aggressive disease than CLL, it is unlikely that large numbers of patients remain symptomless and undiagnosed.

Cell-marker studies have made it clear that while 80% of cases of PLL are derived from B cells, the remainder, although the cell morphology is usually indistinguishable, are tumours of T cells [326].

The characteristic clinical feature of both types of PLL is splenomegaly, usually in the absence of palpable lymphadenopathy in B-PLL, although in T-PLL lymph-node enlargement is seen in about half of patients and skin infiltration in one-third of patients [327]. The rash, which occurs on the torso, face and arms, is papular, nonscaling and not itchy. Skin biopsy shows dense cellular infiltrates around blood vessels and skin appendages in the dermis, but no Pautrier microabscesses characteristic of cutaneous T-cell lymphoma.

The lymphocyte count is most often greater than 100 × 10⁹/l at presentation, and the lymphocyte doubling time is short, usually a matter of a few months only. Anaemia and thrombocytopenia are found in over 50% of cases at presentation. In a third of cases of B-PLL a monoclonal Ig band is found in the serum, but profound hypogammaglobulinaemia, as seen in CLL, is not common.

The prolymphocyte is larger than the characteristic CLL cell. The round nucleus has moderately condensed chromatin and a prominent central nucleolus. Cytoplasm is relatively abundant, pale and agranular (see Plate 6.9 between pp. 292 and

293). In T-PLL the large granular pattern of staining with acid phosphatase and alpha-naphthyl acetate esterase is seen [328]. Smear cells are not usually seen. By definition more than 55% of lymphocytes must be prolymphocytes [223]. It is important to examine the cells at the thin end of the film, as their distinctive morphology is not apparent at the thick end, and the unwary are prone to misdiagnose the disease as CLL.

The bone marrow and spleen show diffuse infiltration with prolymphocytes. If the lymph nodes are involved they show effacement of architecture with diffuse infiltration. The liver shows dense infiltration of portal tracts and sinusoids [326].

The lymphocyte markers of B-PLL are characteristic. The surface Ig is usually IgM or IgM plus IgD, although both IgG and IgA have been seen. It is much denser than in CLL, indeed perhaps denser than with any other B-cell tumour [223]. Other pan-B-cell markers, CD19, CD20, CD24 and CD37, are positive. The cells do not form mouse rosettes and are CD23– [223]. In most cases they are CD5–, although cases with clear evidence of having transformed from CLL may show some CD5 positivity. The cells are surface CD22+ and FMC7+ [223].

In T-PLL the predominant phenotype is CD3+, CD4+, CD7+ and, CD8–, but in about a third of cases the cells coexpress CD4m and CD8 or are CD8+ and CD4– [327]. These phenotypic differences have no effect on the behaviour of the disease.

A karyotypic abnormality is seen in about 60% of cases of B-PLL. No consistent abnormality has been found, but prominent among them have been translocations or deletions at 14q32, a t(6;12)(q15;p13) translocation, a t(2;3)(q35;q14) translocation and trisomy 12 [329]. T-PLL almost invariably demonstrates inv(14)(q11;q32) or other 14q abnormalities [330]. The 14q11 breakpoint involves the T-cell receptor alpha and beta chain genes [331]. The breakpoints at 14q32 are not homogeneous and span a region of at least 300 kilobases not involving the Ig heavy-chain gene [332].

B-PLL pursues an aggressive clinical course with a median survival of less than 3 years [333]. Less than 20% of patients respond to treatment with chlorambucil or COP [334]. Low-dose splenic irradiation has proved an effective treatment in some patients [335]. About 50% respond to combination chemotherapy with CHOP, but remissions are usually short lived. Treatment with purine analogues remains experimental, but responses to fludarabine, pentostatin and cladrabine have been reported [324,336,337].

The outlook in T-PLL is even grimmer, with a reported median survival of 7 months [338]. CHOP chemotherapy has been reported to produce CR in 6% and PR in 27% [339]. Similar responses (10% CR and 38% PR) have been reported with pentostatin [340]. Promising responses to CAMPATH-1H have been described [341].

Splenic lymphoma with villous lymphocytes

A combination of splenomegaly, circulating atypical hairy cells and a paraprotein was first described in 1979 [342]. A variety of different names has been used to describe this disorder and the term 'splenic lymphoma with villous lymphocytes' (SLVL) was introduced by the group at the Royal Marsden Hospital in 1987 [343]. The median age at diagnosis is approximately 70 years with few cases reported below the age of 50. Among 50 cases investigated at the Royal Marsden [344], there were 32 men and 18 women, whereas the 33 cases seen in Bournemouth included 14 men and 19 women. There is little data on the incidence on SLVL compared to other chronic B-cell lymphoproliferative disorders. Since 1984 we have seen 33 cases of SLVL, 12 cases of PLL, 15 cases of HCL and 583 patients with CLL.

The most frequent presenting features are fatigue, abdominal discomfort or an incidental finding based on a routine blood count. On examination most patients have splenomegaly which frequently extends below the umbilicus. Between 20 and 40% present with hepatomegaly, whereas lymphadenopathy is usually absent. The lymphocyte count varies between 10 and $50 \times 10^9/l$ with a median of $30 \times 10^9/l$. Approximately 30% of patients are anaemic at presentation while 10% are thrombocytopenic.

The diagnostic feature of SLVL is the presence of circulating lymphocytes which are usually larger than those found in CLL. The cytoplasm is irregular with short villi localized to one pole of the cell. The nucleus is central with clumped chromatin and a single prominent nucleolus in 50% of cases (see Plate 6.10 between pp. 292 and 293). There is usually an associated population of cells with plasmacytoid features and cytoplasmic basophilia. Between 50 and 70% of patients have a low-level paraprotein which is usually IgM but sometimes IgG. The Royal Marsden Group have determined the immunophenotype of 100 cases of SLVL [345]. Cells from all cases express moderate or strong surface immunoglobulin usually IgM+D or IgM alone, CD19, CD37 and HLA DR. Eighty per cent express CD22, CD24 and FMC7. CD5, CD10, CD11c, CD23, CD25, CD38, HC2 and B-LY-7 are expressed in a minority of cases. The immunophenotype is distinct from CLL and typical HCL but there is overlap with PLL and hairy cell variant.

The marrow in SLVL is easily aspirable and villous lymphocytes are found in over 50% of cases. The trephine biopsy usually shows a nodular infiltrate. Splenic histology shows infiltration primarily of the white pulp but sometimes with extension to the red pulp.

An abnormal karyotype is found in the majority of cases and is frequently complex [346]. Recurring abnormalities include deletions or translocations of 7q, particularly involving bands 7q22 and 7q34–36. Another recurring abnormality is the t(11;14) translocation found in 15% of cases. BCR1 rearrangements have been found in patients with a normal karyotype and novel breakpoints distinct from the major translocation cluster associated with MCL have been identified [347].

Little is known about the aetiology or pathogenesis of SLVL. The splenic histology in SLVL is identical to that found in mar-ginal cell lymphoma of the spleen [348] and analysis of the Ig heavy-chain variable-region genes shows somatic hypermutation with evidence of antigen selection in some cases but no clonal heterogeneity consistent with derivation from a hypermutated antigen responsive IgM+ memory cell [349].

SLVL is frequently a benign disorder with a median survival of 7–10 years [350]. The usual indication for treatment is hypersplenism but a minority of patients undergo transformation to an aggressive large cell lymphoma. Alkylating agents with or without steroids produce a partial response characterized by a reduction in spleen size, a fall in lymphocyte count and improvement in haemoglobin and platelet count in 50–70% of patients. The median duration of response is 3 years and sequential courses of treatment may be necessary. Where splenectomy has been performed either as initial treatment or in patients failing chemotherapy, the results have been excellent and durable and splenectomy is currently considered the treatment of choice for symptomatic patients with no contraindications to surgery [344]. In older less fit patients splenic irradiation can lead to objective responses. There are recent anecdotal reports of good responses with fludarabine.

Large granular lymphocytosis

Large lymphocytes with abundant pale cytoplasm containing fine or coarse azurophilic granules comprise 10–15% of normal peripheral blood lymphocytes (see Plate 6.13 between pp. 292 and 293). They may be subdivided into a CD3+ population, which are thought to represent activated cytotoxic T-lymphocytes, and CD3– natural killer (NK) cells.

An increase in large granular lymphocytes (LGLs) may be transient or persistent. Transient increases occur following viral infections, myocardial infarction and bone marrow transplantation and comprise CD3+ or CD3– lineages or a combination of the two. Persistent increases may also involve either lineage and can frequently, but not invariably, be shown to be clonal disorders. The incidence of large granular lymphocytosis is unknown. The Yorkshire Leukaemia Study Group investigated blood samples from 748 adults with either an absolute lymphocyte count of more than $4.5 \times 10^9/l$ or with more than 25% LGLs [351]. There was an expansion of LGLs in 269 cases and of 112 cases which were re-analysed at least 6 months later, 92 (82%) had a persisting large granular lymphocytosis. The clinical and laboratory features of CD3+ and CD3– LGLs will be discussed separately.

CD3+ large granular lymphocytes

In clonal proliferations of CD3+ LGLs the median age of presentation is 55–60 years and there is an equal sex distribution [352]. The most frequent presenting features are fatigue, constitutional symptoms and infection. In the largest single centre series from the Mayo Clinic, 28% of patients were asymptomatic at diagnosis [353]. On examination, 20–50% of patients have slight or moderate splenomegaly. Hepatomegaly is less common and lymphadenopathy is rare. There is a strong association with rheumatoid arthritis which coexists in 20–30% of cases. Eighty per cent of patients are neutropenic at presentation and 40% have a neutrophil count of less than 0.5 × 10⁹/l. Also 50% of patients are anaemic and 20% are thrombocytopenic. Only 70% of patients have a lymphocyte count of more than 4 × 10⁹/l but most have less than 25% LGLs and the median LGL count is 1.5 × 10⁹/l with a range of 0.1–10 × 10⁹/l. The typical immunophenotype is CD2+, CD3+, CD4–, CD8+, CD16+, CD57+. Southern analysis reveals clonal rearrangements of the TCRαβ genes in the majority of cases and of the TCRγδ genes in a minority. There is a high incidence of serological abnormalities including rheumatoid factor, antinuclear antibody and antineutrophil antibodies.

The mechanism of neutropenia is poorly understood but in some cases may be autoimmune. CD3+ LGLs should be considered to be a possible cause of chronic neutropenia, particularly in the context of rheumatoid arthritis and also of adult-onset cyclical neutropenia. Severe anaemia as a result of pure red cell aplasia may be due to a direct inhibitory effect of the leukaemic LGLs. The natural history of this disorder is uncertain but in the Mayo Clinic series the actuarial mean survival was 161 months. Sixty-nine per cent of patients required treatment and the main indications were symptomatic anaemia, B symptoms and recurrent neutropenic infections. There are a number of treatment options and 70% of patients respond to prednisolone, oral cyclophosphamide or a combination of the two. In the Mayo Clinic series the median duration of initial therapy was 12 months and the use of cyclophosphamide with or without prednisolone gave a median duration of response of 34 months compared to 12 months with prednisolone alone. Low-dose oral methotrexate may be effective as initial treatment or in patients who have failed a trial of steroids [354]. There are case reports of successful responses to fludarabine [355], and to granulocyte colony-stimulating factor(G-CSF) and cyclosporin-A [356] in patients with severe neutropenia. Splenectomy has been of benefit in a minority of patients with severe neutropenia and moderate splenomegaly [357].

CD3– large granular lymphocytes

Patients with CD3– LGLs may also pursue a chronic course characterized by mild or moderate neutropenia. The incidence of rheumatoid arthritis is much lower than with CD3+ cases. By definition all cases lack TCR rearrangements and the percentage of cases with clonal CD3– LGL populations is uncertain. Using X-inactivation studies one group showed that two of six women had a clonal LGL population whereas another study found no evidence of clonality in seven women with CD3– LGLs [358].

In contrast, there is a true CD3– LGL leukaemia which is rare in Europe and America but more common in Asia [352,359]. The median age of presentation is 39 years and most patients present with constitutional symptoms and massive hepatosplenomegaly. Thirty per cent have lymphadenopathy and gastrointestinal and CNS involvement is common. The lymphocyte count is higher than in CD3+ LGL leukaemia and most patients are anaemic and thrombocytopenic, although only 20% have severe neutropenia. The usual immunophenotype is CD3–, CD4–, CD8–, CD16+, CD56+, CD57–. Clonality may be confirmed by the finding of cytogenetic abnormalities and a proportion of patients have clonal integration of EBV, although this appears to be more common in Japanese cases than in European or American patients. Most patients pursue a rapidly progressive course, although in some there is a preceding chronic phase. The response to intensive chemotherapy is poor.

References

1 Bennett J.H. (1845) Two cases of disease and enlargement of the spleen in which death took place from the presence of purulent matter in the blood. *Edinburgh Medical and Surgical Journal*, **64**, 413–423.

2 Virchow R. (1845) Weisses Blut. *Neue Notizen Gebiete Natur-Heilkunde*, **36**, 151–156.

3 Virchow R. (1847) Weisses Blut und Milztumoren. *Med Z*, **16**, 9–15.

4 Ehrlich P. (1891) *Farbenanalytische Untersuchungen zur Histologie und Klinik des Blutes*. Hirschwald, Berlin.

5 Turk W. (1903) Ein System der Lymphomatosen. *Wiener Klinische Wochenschrift*, **16**, 1073–1085.

6 Damashek W. (1967) Chronic lymphocytic leukemia—an accumulative disease of immunologically incompetent lymphocytes. *Blood*, **29**, 566–584.

7 Aisenberg A.C. & Bloch K.J. (1972) Immunoglobulins on the surface of neoplastic lymphocytes. *New England Journal of Medicine*, **287**, 272–276.

8 Young J.L., Percy C.L. & Asire A.J. (eds) (1981) *SEER: incidence and mortality data: 1973–1977. NCI Monographs*, 57. NIH Publication No. 81-2330. National Institutes of Health, Bethesda.

9 Cartwright R.A., Alexander F.E., McKinney P.A. & Ricketts T.J. (1990) *Leukaemia and Lymphoma. An atlas of distribution within areas of England and Wales 1984–8*. Leukaemia Research Fund, London.

10 Hamblin T.J. (1987) Chronic lymphocytic leukaemia. *Baillière's Clinical Haematology*, **1**, 449–491.

11 Court-Brown W.M. & Doll R. (1959) Adult leukaemia: trends in mortality in relation to aetiology. *British Medical Journal*, **1**, 1063–1069.

12 Fraumeni J.R. & Miller R.W. (1967) Epidemiology of human leukaemia: recent observations. *Journal of the National Cancer Institute*, **38**, 593–605.

13 Weiss N.S. (1978) *Geographical Variation in the Incidence of the Leukemias and the Lymphomas. NCI Monographs*, 53 (ed. B.E. Henderson), p. 139. NIH publication No. 79-1864. National Institutes of Health, Bethesda.

14 MacMahon B. & Koller E.K. (1957) Ethnic differences in the incidences of leukemia. *Blood*, **12**, 1–10.

15 Cuttner J. (1992) Increased incidence of hematologic malignan-

cies in first degree relatives of patients with chronic lymphocytic leukemia. *Cancer Investigation*, **10**, 103–109.

16 Gunz F.W. & Veale A.M.O. (1969) Leukemia in close relatives, accident or predisposition? *Journal of the National Cancer Institute*, **42**, 517–524.

17 Kunita S., Kamer Y. & Ota K. (1974) Genetic studies on familial leukemia. *Cancer*, **34**, 1098–1101.

18 Conley C.L., Misiti J. & Laster A.J. (1980) Genetic factors predisposing to chronic lymphocytic leukemia and to auto-immune disease. *Medicine*, **59**, 323–334.

19 Brok-Simoni F., Rechavi G., Katzir N. & Ben-Bassat I. (1987) Chronic lymphocytic leukaemia in twin sisters. Monozygous but not identical. *Lancet*, **i**, 329.

20 Jones H.P. & Whittaker J.A. (1991) Chronic lymphatic leukaemia: an investigation of HLA antigen frequencies and white cell differential counts in patients, relatives and controls. *Leukemia Research*, **15**, 543–549.

21 Bizzozero O.J., Johnson K.G., Ciocco A. *et al.* (1967) Radiation related leukemia in Hiroshima and Nagasaki 1946–1964. II. Observations on type specific leukemia, survivorship and clinical behaviour. *Annals of Internal Medicine*, **66**, 522–530.

22 Zahm S.H., Weisenburger D.D., Babbitt P.A. *et al.* (1992) Use of hair coloring products and the risk of lymphoma, multiple myeloma and chronic lymphocytic leukemia. *American Journal of Public Health*, **82**, 990–997.

23 Cronkite E.P. (1987) An historical account of clinical investigations on chronic lymphocytic leukemia in the Medical Research Center, Brookhaven National Laboratory. *Blood Cells*, **12**, 285–295.

24 Floderus B., Persson T., Stenlind C. *et al.* (1993) Occupational exposure to electromagnetic fields in relation to leukemia and brain tumours: a case-control study in Sweden. *Cancer Causes Control*, **4**, 465–476.

25 Kipps T.J. (1995) Chronic lymphocytic leukemia and related disease. In: *Williams Hematology* (eds E. Beutler, M.A. Lichtman, B.S. Coller & T.J. Kipps), 5th edn, pp. 1017–1039. McGraw-Hill, New York.

26 Foerster J. (1993) Chronic lymphocytic leukemia. In: *Wintrobe's Clinical Hematology* (eds G.R. Lee, T.C. Bithell, J. Foerster, J.W. Athens & J.N. Lukens), 9th edn, pp. 2034–2053. Lea & Febiger, Philadelphia.

27 Hamblin T.J., Oscier D.G., Stevens J.R. & Smith J.L. (1987) Long survival in B-CLL correlates with surface IgMK phenotype. *British Journal of Haematology*, **66**, 21–26.

28 Auclerc M.F., Desprez-Cyrely J.P., Maral J. *et al.* (1984) Prognostic value of lymphograms in chronic lymphocytic leukemia. *Cancer*, **53**, 888–895.

29 Norris H.J. & Weiner M. (1961) The renal lesion in leukemia. *American Journal of the Medical Sciences*, **241**, 512–524.

30 Dathan J.R.E., Heyworth M.F. & MacIver A.G. (1974) Nephrotic syndrome in chronic lymphocytic leukaemia. *British Medical Journal*, **3**, 655–657.

31 Cornes J.S. & Jones T.G. (1962) Leukaemic lesions of the gastrointestinal tract. *Journal of Clinical Pathology*, **15**, 305–313.

32 Sweet D.L. Jr, Golomb H.M. & Altmann J.E. (1977) The clinical features of chronic lymphocytic leukaemia. *Clinical Haematology*, **6**, 185–202.

33 Green R.A. & Nichols N.J. (1959) Pulmonary involvement in leukemia. *American Review of Respiratory Disease*, **80**, 833–840.

34 Spielberger R.T., Stock W. & Larson R.A. (1993) Listeriosis after 2-chlorodeoxyadenosine treatment. *New England Journal of Medicine*, **328**, 813–814.

35 Byrd J.C., Hargis J.B., Kester K.E., Hospental D.R., Knutson S.W. & Diehl L.F. (1995) Opportunistic infections with fludaribine in previously treated patients with low grade lymphoid malignancies: a role for *Pneumocystis carinii* pneumonia prophylaxis. *American Journal of Hematology*, **49**, 135–142.

36 Dighiero G., Travade P., Chevret S., Fenaux P., Chastang C. and the French Co-operative Group on CLL. (1991) B cell chronic lymphocytic leukemia: present status and future directions. *Blood*, **78**, 1901–1914.

37 Bergsagel D.E. (1967) The chronic leukemias: a review of disease manifestations and the aims of therapy. *Canadian Medical Association Journal*, **96**, 1615–1620.

38 Miller D.G. (1992) Patterns of immunological deficiency in lymphomas and leukemias. *Annals of Internal Medicine*, **57**, 703–715.

39 Parker A.C. & Bennett M. (1976) Pernicious anaemia and lymphoproliferative disease. *Scandinavian Journal of Haematology*, **17**, 395–397.

40 Goodnough L.T. & Muir A. (1980) Bullous pemphigoid as a manifestation of chronic lymphocytic leukemia. *Archives of Internal Medicine*, **140**, 1526–1527.

41 Catovsky D. (1984) Chronic lymphocytic, prolymphocytic and hairy cell leukaemias. In: *Haematology. 1 Leukaemias* (eds J.M. Goldman & H.D. Preisler), pp. 266–268. Butterworths, London.

42 Skarin A.T. (1985) Pathology and morphology of chronic leukemias and related disorders. In: *Neoplastic Diseases of the Blood* (eds P.H. Wiernik, G.P. Cancellos, R.A. Kyle & C.A. Schiffer), pp. 19–50. Churchill Livingstone, New York.

43 Fialkow P.J., Najfeld V., Reddy A., Singer J. & Steinmann L. (1978) Chronic lymphocytic leukaemia: clonal origin in a committed B lymphocyte progenitor. *Lancet*, **ii**, 444–446.

44 Hamblin T.J., Abdul-Ahad A.K., Gordon J., Stevenson F.K. & Stevenson G.T. (1980) Preliminary evidence in treating lymphocytic leukaemia with antibody to immunoglobulin idiotypes on the cell surface. *British Journal of Cancer*, **42**, 495–502.

45 Gahrton G., Robert K.-H., Friberg K., Zech L. & Bird A.G. (1980) Non-random chromosomal aberrations in chronic lymphocytic leukemia revealed by polyclonal B-cell mitogen stimulation. *Blood*, **56**, 640–647.

46 Korsmeyer S.J., Hieter P.A., Ravetch J.V. *et al.* (1981) Developmental hierarchy of immunoglobulin gene rearrangements in human leukemic pre-B cells. *Proceedings of the National Academy of Sciences, USA*, **78**, 7096–8100.

47 Baer M.R., Stein R.S. & Dessypris E.N. (1985) Chronic lymphocytic leukemia with hyperleukocytosis: the hyperviscosity syndrome. *Cancer*, **56**, 2865–2869.

48 Ternynck T., Diaghiero G., Fallezou J. & Binet J.L. (1974) Comparison of normal and CLL lymphocyte surface Ig determinants using peroxidase-labelled antibodies. I. Detection and quantitation of light chain determinants. *Blood*, **43**, 789–795.

49 Hamblin T.J. & Hough D. (1977) Chronic lymphatic leukaemia: correlation of immunofluorescent characteristic with clinical features. *British Journal of Haematology*, **36**, 359–365.

50 Cawley J.C., Smith J.L., Goldstone A.H. *et al.* (1976) IgA and IgM cytoplasmic inclusions in a series of cases with chronic lymphocytic leukaemia. *Clinical and Experimental Immunology*, **23**, 78–80.

51 Stevenson F.K., Hamblin T.J. & Stevenson G.T. (1981) The nature of IgG on the surface of B lymphocytes in chronic lymphocytic leukemia. *Journal of Experimental Medicine*, **154**, 1965–1969.

52 Hashimoto S., Dono M., Watai M. *et al.* (1995) Somatic diversification and selection of IgH and L chains variable region

genes in IgG+, CD5+ chronic lymphocytic leukemia B cells. *Journal of Experimental Medicine*, **181**, 1507–1517.

53 Slease R.B., Wistar R. Jr & Scher I. (1979) Surface immunoglobulin density in human peripheral blood mononuclear cells. *Blood*, **54**, 72–87.

54 Fermand J.P., Schmitt C. & Brouet J.C. (1985) Distribution of class II DC antigens on normal and leukaemic lymphoid cells. *European Journal of Immunology*, **15**, 1183–1187.

55 Freedman A.S., Boyd A.W., Berrebi A. *et al.* (1987) Expression of B cell activation antigens on normal and malignant B cells. *Leukemia*, **1**, 9–15.

56 Anderson K.C., Bates M.P., Slaughenhaupt B.L. *et al.* (1984) Expression of human B cell associated antigens on leukaemias and lymphomas: a model of B cell differentiation. *Blood*, **63**, 1424–1431.

57 Freedman A.S. & Nadler L.M. (1993) Immunologic markers in B-cell chronic lymphocytic leukemia. In: *Chronic Lymphocytic Leukemia: scientific advances and clinical developments* (ed. B.D. Cheson), pp. 1–32. Marcel Dekker, New York.

58 Catovsky D., Cherchi M., Okos A., Hegde V. & Galton D.A.G. (1976) Mouse red cell rosettes in B lymphoproliferative disorders. *British Journal of Haematology*, **33**, 173–177.

59 Foon K.A., Schroff R.W. & Gale R.P. (1982) Surface markers on leukaemia and lymphoma cells. *Blood*, **60**, 1–19.

60 Bain B.J. & Catovsky D. (1995) The leukaemic phase of non-Hodgkin's lymphoma. *Journal of Clinical Pathology*, **48**, 189–193.

61 Matutes E., Owusu-Ankomah K., Morilla R. *et al.* (1994) The immunological profile of B-cell disorders and proposal of a scoring system for the diagnosis of CLL. *Leukemia*, **8**, 1640–1645.

62 Caligaris-Cappio F., Gobbi M., Bergui L. *et al.* (1984) B chronic lymphocytic leukemia patients with stable benign disease show a distinctive membrane phenotype. *British Journal of Haematology*, **56**, 655–660.

63 Catovsky D., Cherchi M., Brooks J., Bradley J. & Zola H. (1981) Heterogeneity of B cell leukemias demonstrated by the monoclonal antibody FMC7. *Blood*, **33**, 173–177.

64 Delia D., Cattoretti G., Polli N. *et al.* (1988) CD1c but neither CD1a nor CD1b molecules are expressed on normal, activated, and malignant B cells. Identification of a new B cell subset. *Blood*, **72**, 241–247.

65 Orazi A., Cattoretti G., Polli N. & Rilke F. (1991) Distinct morphophenotypic features of chronic B lymphocytic leukemia identified with CD1c and CD23 antibodies. *European Journal of Haematology*, **47**, 28–35.

66 Freedman A.S., Boyd A.W., Bieber F. *et al.* (1987) Normal cellular counterparts of B cell chronic lymphocytic leukemia. *Blood*, **70**, 418–427.

67 Hamblin T.J., Oscier D.G. & Young B.J. (1986) Autoimmunity in chronic lymphocytic leukaemia. *Journal of Clinical Pathology*, **39**, 713–716.

68 Ebbe S., Wittels B. & Damashek W. (1962) Autoimmune thrombocytopenic purpura ('ITP type') with chronic lymphocytic leukemia. *Blood*, **19**, 23–27.

69 Rustagi P., Han T., Ziolkowski L., Currie M. & Logue G. (1983) Antigranulocyte antibodies in chronic lymphocytic leukemia and other chronic lymphoproliferative disorders. *Blood*, **62**(Suppl. 1), 106.

70 Abeloff M.D. & Waterbury M.D. (1974) Pure red cell aplasia and chronic lymphocytic leukemia. *Archives of Internal Medicine*, **134**, 721–724.

71 Hamblin T.J., Verrier Jones J. & Peacock D.B. (1975) The immune response to φx174 in man: (i) primary and secondary antibody production in patients with chronic lymphocytic leukaemia. *Clinical and Experimental Immunology*, **21**, 101–108.

72 Stevenson F.K., Hamblin T.J., Stevenson G.T. & Tutt A.C. (1980) Extracellular idiotypic immunoglobulin arising from human leukaemic B lymphocytes. *Journal of Experimental Medicine*, **152**, 1484–1496.

73 Hannam-Harris A.C., Gordon J. & Smith J.L. (1980) Immunoglobulin synthesis by neoplastic B lymphocytes; free light chain synthesis as a marker of B cell differentiation. *Journal of Immunology*, **125**, 2177–2181.

74 Alexanian R. (1975) Monoclonal gammapathy in lymphoma. *Archives of Internal Medicine*, **135**, 62–66.

75 Sinclair D., Dagg J.H., Mowat A.M., Parrott D.M.V. & Stott D.I. (1984) Serum paraproteins in chronic lymphocytic leukaemia. *Journal of Clinical Pathology*, **37**, 463–466.

76 Kay N.E. (1981) Abnormal T cell subpopulation function in CLL: excessive suppressor and deficient helper activity with respect to B cell proliferation. *Blood*, **57**, 418–420.

77 Pizzolo G., Chilosi M., Ambrozetti A., Semenzato A., Fiore-Donati L. & Peron A.G. (1983) Immunohistologic study of bone marrow involvement in B chronic lymphocytic leukemia. *Blood*, **62**, 1289–1296.

78 Bouroncle B.A., Klausen K.P. & Aschenbrand J.R. (1969) Studies of the delayed response to phytohaemagglutinin (PHA) stimulated lymphocytes in 25 chronic lymphocytic leukemias before and after therapy. *Blood*, **34**, 166–178.

79 Han T., Bloom M.L., Dadey B. *et al.* (1982) Lack of autologous mixed lymphocyte reaction in patients with chronic lymphocytic leukemia: evidence for autoreactive T cell dysfunction not correlated with phenotype, karyotype or clinical status. *Blood*, **60**, 1075–1081.

80 Foa R. & Catovsky D. (1979) T lymphocyte colonies in normal blood, bone marrow and lymphoproliferative disorders. *Clinical and Experimental Immunology*, **36**, 488–495.

81 Chiorazzi N., Fu S., Ghodrat M., Kunkel H.G., Rai K. & Gee T. (1979) T cell helper defect in patients with chronic lymphocytic leukemia. *Journal of Immunology*, **122**, 1087–1090.

82 Foa R., Lauria F., Lusso P. *et al.* (1984) Discrepancy between phenotypic and functional features of natural killer T lymphocytes in B cell chronic lymphocytic leukaemia. *British Journal of Haematology*, **58**, 509–516.

83 Platsoucas C.D., Fernandes G., Gupta S.L. *et al.* (1980) Defective spontaneous and antibody-dependent cytotoxicity mediated by E-rosette positive and E-rosette negative cells in untreated patients with chronic lymphocytic leukemia. Augmentation by *in vitro* treatment with interferon. *Journal of Immunology*, **125**, 1216–1223.

84 Foa R., Fierro M.T., Raspadori D. *et al.* (1990) Lymphokine-activated killer (LAK) cell activity in B and T chronic lymphoid leukemia: defective LAK generation and reduced susceptibility of the leukemic cells to allogeneic and autologous LAK effectors. *Blood*, **76**, 1349–1354.

85 Lotz M., Ranheim E. & Kipps T.J. (1994) Transforming growth factor beta as endogenous growth inhibitor of chronic lymphocytic leukemia B cells. *Journal of Experimental Medicine*, **179**, 999–1004.

86 Kehrl J.H., Taylor A., Kim S.J. & Fauci A.S. (1991) Transforming growth factor-beta is a potent negative regulator of human lymphocytes. *Annals of the New York Academy of Sciences*, **628**, 345–353.

87 Semenzato G., Foa R., Agostini C. *et al.* (1987) High serum levels

of soluble interleukin 2 receptor in patients with B chronic lymphocytic leukemia. *Blood*, **70**, 396–400.

88 International Workshop on Chronic Lymphocytic Leukemia (1989) Chronic lymphocytic leukemia: recommendations for diagnosis, staging and response criteria. *Annals of Internal Medicine*, **110**, 236–238.

89 Rozman C., Hernandez-Nieto L., Montserrat E. & Brugues R. (1981) Prognostic significance of bone marrow patterns in chronic lymphocytic leukaemia. *British Journal of Haematology*, **47**, 529–537.

90 Gahrton G., Zech L., Robert K-H. & Bird A.G. (1979) Mitogenic stimulation of leukemic cells by Epstein–Barr virus. *New England Journal of Medicine*, **301**, 438.

91 Oscier D.G. (1994) Cytogenetic and molecular abnormalities in chronic lymphocytic leukaemia. *Blood Reviews*, **8**, 88–97.

92 Gahrton G., Robert K-H., Friberg K., Zech L. & Bird A.G. (1980) Non-random chromosomal aberrations in chronic lymphocytic leukemia revealed by polyclonal B-cell stimulation. *Blood*, **56**, 640–647.

93 Han T., Ozer H., Sadamori N. *et al.* (1984) Prognostic importance of cytogenetic abnormalities in patients with chronic lymphocytic leukemia. *New England Journal of Medicine*, **310**, 288–292.

94 Pittman S. & Catovsky D. (1984) Prognostic significance of chromosomal abnormalities in chronic lymphocytic leukaemia. *British Journal of Haematology*, **58**, 649–660.

95 Fitchett M., Griffiths M.J., Oscier D.G., Johnson S. & Seabright M. (1987) Chromosome abnormalities involving band 13q14 in hematologic malignancies. *Cancer Genetics and Cytogenetics*, **24**, 143–150.

96 Juliusson G., Oscier D.G., Fitchett M. *et al.* (1990) Prognostic subgroups in B-cell chronic lymphocytic leukemia defined by specific chromosomal abnormalities. *New England Journal of Medicine*, **323**, 720–724.

97 Geisler G.H., Philip P. & Hansen M.M. (1989) B-cell chronic lymphocytic leukaemia: clonal chromosomal abnormalities and prognosis in 89 cases. *European Journal of Haematology*, **43**, 397–403.

98 Bird M.L., Ueshima Y., Rowley J.D., Haren J.M. & Vardiman J.W. (1989) Chromosomal abnormalities in B cell chronic lymphocytic leukemia and their clinical correlations. *Leukemia*, **3**, 182–191.

99 Oscier D.G., Fitchett M. & Hamblin T.J. (1988) Chromosomal abnormalities in B-CLL. *Nouvelle Revue Française d'Hematologie*, **30**, 397–398.

100 Petersen L.C., Lindquist L., Church S. & Kay N.E. (1992) Frequent clonal abnormalities of chromosome band 13q14 in B cell chronic lymphocytic leukemia. Multiple clones, subclones and nonclonal alterations in 82 mid-western patients. *Genes Chromosomes Cancer*, **4**, 273–280.

101 Döhner H., Stilgenbauer S., Liebisch P. *et al.* (1995) 11q deletions are the second most common chromosome aberration in B-cell chronic lymphocytic leukemia and are associated with advanced stages and marked lymphadenopathy. *Blood*, **86** (Suppl. 1), 1369a.

102 Offit K., Parsa N.L., Gaidano G. *et al.* (1993) 6q deletions define distinct clinico-pathologic subsets of non-Hodgkin's lymphoma. *Blood*, **82**, 2157–2162.

103 Que T.H., Marco G., Ellis J. *et al.* (1993) Trisomy 12 in chronic lymphocytic leukemia detected by fluorescence *in situ* hybridisation: analysis by stage, immunophenotype and morphology. *Blood*, **82**, 571–575.

104 Oscier D., Fitchett M., Herbert T. & Lambert R. (1991) Karyotypic evolution in B-cell chronic lymphocytic leukaemia. *Genes Chromosomes Cancer*, **3**, 16–20.

105 Andreeff M., Danzyrkiewicz Z., Sharpless T.K., Clarkson B.D. & Melamed M.R. (1980) Discrimination of human leukemia subtypes by flow cytometric analysis of cellular DNA and RNA. *Blood*, **55**, 282–293.

106 Sheppard J.R., Gommus R. & Moldow C.F. (1977) Catecholamine hormone receptors are reduced on chronic lymphocytic leukaemic lymphocytes. *Nature*, **269**, 693–695.

107 Speckart S.F., Boldt D.H. & MacDermott R.P. (1978) Chronic lymphatic leukemia (CLL): cell surface changes detected by lectin binding and their relation to altered glycosyltransferase activity. *Blood*, **52**, 681–695.

108 Stahl R.L., Farber C.M., Liebes L.F. *et al.* (1985) Relationship of dehydroascorbic acid transport to cell lineages in lymphocytes from normal subjects and patients with CLL. *Cancer Research*, **45**, 6507–6512.

109 Gutmann H.R., Chow Y.M., Vesella R.L. *et al.* (1983) The kinetic properties of ecto-ATPase of human peripheral blood lymphocytes and of chronic lymphatic leukemia cells. *Blood*, **62**, 1041–1046.

110 Orchard J.A. & Oscier D.G. (1996) Prognostic value of Ki 67 and cell cycle analysis in chronic lymphocytic leukaemia. *British Journal of Haematology*, **93**(Suppl. 2), 116.

111 Delmer A., Ajchenbaum-Cymbalista F., Tang R. *et al.* (1995) Overexpression of Cyclin D2 in chronic B-cell malignancies. *Blood*, **85**, 2870–2876.

112 Okamura J., Gelfand E.W. & Letarte M. (1982) Heterogeneity of the response of chronic lymphocytic leukemia cells to phorbol ester. *Blood*, **60**, 1082–1088.

113 Malisan F., Fluckiger A-C., Ho S., Guret C., Banchereau J. & Martinez-Valdez H. (1996) B-chronic lymphocytic leukemias can undergo isotype switching *in vivo* and can be induced to differentiate and switch *in vitro*. *Blood*, **87**, 717–724.

114 Dono M., Hashimoto S., Fais F. *et al.* (1996) Evidence for progenitors of chronic lymphocytic leukemia B cells that undergo intraclonal differentiation and diversification. *Blood*, **87**, 1586–1594.

115 Hoffbrand A.V., Panayiotidis P., Reittie J. & Ganeshaguru K. (1993) Autocrine and paracrine growth loops in chronic lymphocytic leukemia. *Seminars in Hematology*, **30**, 306–317.

116 di Celle P.F., Carbone A., Marchis D. *et al.* (1994) Cytokine gene expression in B-cell chronic lymphocytic leukemia: evidence of constitutive Interleukin-8 (IL-8) mRNA expression and secretion of biologically active IL-8 protein. *Blood*, **84**, 220–228.

117 Panayiotidis P., Jones D., Ganeshaguru K., Foroni L. & Hoffbrand A.V. (1996) Human bone marrow stromal cells prevent apoptosis and support the survival or chronic lymphocytic leukaemia cells *in vitro*. *British Journal of Haematology*, **92**, 97–103.

118 Mainou-Fowler T., Craig V.A., Copplestone J.A., Hamon M.D. & Prentice A.G. (1994) Interleukin-5 (IL-5) increases spontaneous apoptosis of B-cell chronic lymphocytic leukemia cells *in vitro* independently of bcl-2 expression, and is inhibited by IL-4. *Blood*, **84**, 2297–2304.

119 Fluckiger A.C., Rossi J.F., Bussel A., Bryon P., Banchereau J. & Defrance T. (1992) Responsiveness of chronic lymphocytic leukemia B cells activated via surface Igs or CD40 to B-cell tropic factors. *Blood*, **80**, 3173–3181.

120 Bournsell L., Coppin H., Pham D. *et al.* (1980) An antigen shared by a human T cell subset and B cell chronic lymphocytic leukemia cells. *Journal of Experimental Medicine*, **152**, 229–234.

121 Barclay A.N., Binkeland M.L., Brown M.H. *et al.* (1993) *The Leuco-cyte Antigen Facts Book.* Academic, London.

122 Freeman M. (1990) An ancient highly conserved family of cysteine-rich protein domains revealed by cloning type I and type II murine macrophage scavenger receptors. *Proceedings of the National Academy of Sciences,* USA, **87**, 8810–8814.

123 Van de Velde H., von Hoegen I., Luo W., Parnes J. & Thielemans K. (1991) The B cell surface protein CD72/Lyb-2 is the ligand for CD5. *Nature,* **351**, 662–665.

124 Caligaris-Cappio F., Gobbi M., Bofill M. & Janossy G. (1982) Infrequent normal B lymphocytes express features of B chronic lymphocytic leukaemia. *Journal of Experimental Medicine,* **155**, 623–627.

125 Caligaris-Cappio F. (1996) B-chronic lymphocytic leukaemia: a malignancy of anti-self B cells. *Blood,* **87**, 2615–2620.

126 Vandenberghe E. (1994) Mantle cell lymphoma. *Blood Reviews,* **8**, 79–87.

127 Antin J.H., Emerson S.P., Martin P., Gaddol N. & Ault K.A. (1986) Leu 1 (CD5) B cells, a major lymphoid sub-population in human fetal spleen: phenotypic and functional studies. *Journal of Immunology,* **136**, 505–510.

128 Kipps T.J. (1989) The CD5 B cell. *Advances in Immunology,* **47**, 117–185.

129 Caligaris-Cappio F. & Janossy G. (1985) Surface markers on chronic lymphoid leukemias of B cell type. *Seminars in Hematology,* **22**, 1–12.

130 Antin J.H., Ault K.A., Rappeport J.M. & Smith B.R. (1987) B lymphocyte reconstitution after human bone marrow transplantation. *Journal of Clinical Investigation,* **80**, 325–332.

131 Plater-Zyberk C., Maini R.N., Lam K., Kennedy D. & Janossy G. (1985) A rheumatoid arthritis B cell subset expresses a phenotype similar to that in chronic lymphocytic leukemia. *Arthritis and Rheumatism,* **28**, 971–976.

132 Manohar V., Brown E., Leiserson W.M. & Chused T.M. (1982) Expression of Ly-1 by a subset of B lymphocytes. *Journal of Immunology,* **129**, 532–538.

133 Herzenberg L.A., Stall A.M., Lalor P.A., Sidman C., Moore W.A. & Pards D.R. (1986) The Lyl-B cell lineage. *Immunological Reviews,* **93**, 81–102.

134 Hayakawa K., Hardy R.R. & Herzenberg L.A. (1986) Peritoneal Ly1-B cells: genetic control, autoantibody production, increased lambda light chain expression. *European Journal of Immunology,* **16**, 450–456.

135 Hayakawa K., Hardy R.R. & Herzenberg L.A. (1985) Progenitors for Lyl-B cells are distinct from progenitors for other B cells. *Journal of Experimental Medicine,* **161**, 1554–1568.

136 Mercolino T.J., Locke A.L., Afshari A. *et al.* (1989) Restricted immunoglobulin variable gene usage by normal Ly-1 (CD5+) B cells that recognise phosphatidyl choline. *Journal of Experimental Medicine,* **169**, 1869–1877.

137 Broker B.M., Klajman A., Youinan P. *et al.* (1988) Chronic lymphocytic leukemic (CLL) cells secrete multispecific autoantibodies. *Journal of Autoimmunity,* **1**, 469–481.

138 Dighiero G. (1987) Relevance of murine models in elucidating the origin of B-CLL lymphocytes and related immune associated phenomena. *Seminars in Hematology,* **24**, 240–251.

139 Dighireo G., Poncet P., Rouyre S. & Mazie J.C. (1986) Newborn Xia mice carry the genetic information for the production of natural autoantibodies. *Journal of Immunology,* **136**, 4000–4005.

140 Kaushik A., Meyer R., Fidanza V., Lim A., Bona C. & Dighiero G. (1991) Ly1 and V gene expression among hybridomas secreting natural autoantibody. *Journal of Autoimmunity,* **3**, 687–700.

141 Miller R.A. & Gralow J. (1984) The induction of Leu-1 antigen expression in human malignant and normal B cells by phorbolmyristic acetate (PMA). *Journal of Immunology,* **133**, 3408–3412.

142 Inghirami G., Wieczorek R., Zhu B., Silber R., Della-Favera R. & Knowles D.M. (1988) Differential expression of LFA-1 molecules in non-Hodgkin's lymphoma and lymphoid leukemias. *Blood,* **72**, 1431–1434.

143 Maio M., Pinto A., Carbone A. *et al.* (1990) Differential expression of CD54/intercellular adhesion molecule-1 in myeloid leukemias and in lymproliferative disorders. *Blood,* **76**, 783–790.

144 Wormsley S., Baird S., Gadol N., Rai K. & Sobal R. (1990) Characteristics of CD11c+ CD5+ chronic B-cell leukemias and the identification of normal peripheral blood B-cell subsets with chronic lymphoid leukemia immunophenotypes. *Blood,* **76**, 123–130.

145 Csanaky G., Vass J.A., Miloserits J., Ocsovszki I., Szornor A. & Schirelczerm M. (1994) Expression and function of L selectin molecules (Lecam-1) in B-cell chronic lymphocytic leukemia. *Haematologica,* **79**, 132–136.

146 Picker L.J., Medeiros L.J., Weiss L.M., Warnke R.A. & Butcher E.C. (1988) Expression of lymphocyte having receptor antigen in non-Hodgkin's lymphoma. *American Journal of Pathology,* **130**, 496–504.

147 Hynes R.O. (1992) Integrins: versatility, modulation and signalling in cell adhesion. *Cell,* **68**, 11–25.

148 Hemler M.E. (1990) VLA proteins in the integrin family: structures, functions and their role on leukocytes. *Annual Review of Immunology,* **8**, 365–400.

149 Moller P., Eichelman A., Konetz K. & Mechtersheimer G. (1992) Adhesion molecules VLA-1 to VLA-6 define discrete stages of peripheral B lymphocyte development and characterize different types of B cell neoplasia. *Leukemia,* **6**, 256–264.

150 Vincent A.M. (1996) *Adhesion mechanisms in CLL and HCL.* PhD thesis, University of Liverpool.

151 Baldini L.G.M. & Cro L.M. (1994) Structure and function of VLA integrins: differential expression in B cell leukemia/lymphoma. *Leukemia and Lymphoma,* **12**, 197–203.

152 Andrew D.P., Berlin C., Honda J. *et al.* (1994) Distinct but overlapping epitopes are involved in $\alpha 4\beta 7$ mediated adhesion to vascular cell adhesion molecule-1 mucosal adhesion-1, fibronectin and lymphocyte aggregation. *Journal of Immunology,* **153**, 3847–3861.

153 Gordon J., Mellstedt H., Arman P., Biberefield P., Bjorkholm M. & Klein G. (1983) Phenotypes in chronic B-lymphocytic leukemia probed by monoclonal antibodies and immunoglobulin secretion studies: identification of stages of maturation arrest and the relation to clinical findings. *Blood,* **62**, 910–917.

154 Lewandrowski K., Medeiros L. & Harris N. (1990) Expression of the activation antigen, 4F2, by non-Hodgkin's lymphomas of B-cell phenotype. *Cancer,* **66**, 1158–1164.

155 Karrag S., Leprence C., Merle-Beral H., Debre P., Richard Y. & Galanaud P. (1990) B8.7 antigen expression on B-CLL cells and its relationship to the LMW-BCGF responsiveness. *Leukemia Research,* **14**, 809–814.

156 Cook G.P. & Tomlinson T.M. (1995) The human immunoglobulin VH repertoire. *Immunology Today,* **16**, 237–242.

157 Kipps T.J., Tomhave E., Pratt L.F., Duffy S., Chen P.P. & Carson D.A. (1989) Developmentally restricted VH gene expressed at

high frequency in chronic lymphocytic leukemia. *Proceedings of the National Academy of Sciences, USA*, **86**, 5913–5917.

158 Schroeder H.W. Jr & Dighiero G. (1994) The pathogenesis of chronic lymphocytic leukemia: analysis of the antibody repertoire. *Immunology Today*, **15**, 288–294.

159 Cai J., Humphries C., Richardson A & Tucker P.W. (1992) Extensive and selective mutation of a rearranged VH5 gene in human B cell chronic lymphocytic leukemia. *Journal of Experimental Medicine*, **176**, 1073–1081.

160 Kipps T.J., Tomhave E., Chen P.P. & Carson D.A. (1988) Autoantibody associated kappa light chain variable region gene expressed in chronic lymphocytic leukemia with little or no somatic mutation. Implications for etiology and immunotherapy. *Journal of Experimental Medicine*, **167**, 840–852.

161 Pascual V.K., Victor K., Spellerberg M., Hamblin T.J., Stevenson F.K. & Capra D. (1992) VH restriction among human cold agglutinins: the VH4-21 gene segment is required to encode anti-I and anti-i specificities. *Journal of Immunology*, **149**, 2337–2344.

162 Kipps T.J. (1993) Implications of anti-idiotype antibodies. In: *Chronic Lymphocytic Leukaemia—scientific advances and clinical developments* (ed. B.D. Cheson), pp. 123–146. Marcel Dekker, New York.

163 Schroeder H.W. Jr, Hillson J.L. & Perlmutter R.M. (1987) Early restriction of the human antibody repertoire. *Science*, **238**, 791–793.

164 Kipps T.J., Robbins B.A. & Carson D.A. (1990) Uniform high frequency expression of autoantibody associated cross reactive idiotypes in the primary B cell follicles in human fetal spleen. *Journal of Experimental Medicine*, **171**, 189–196.

165 Oscier D.G., Thomset A., Zhu D. & Stevenson F.K. (1995) Different roles of somatic hypermutation in VH genes among subsets of chronic lymphocytic leukaemia defined by chromosome abnormalities. *Blood*, **86**(Suppl. 1), 840a.

166 Zhu D., Hawkins R., Hamblin T.J. & Stevenson F.K. (1994) Clonal history of a human follicular lymphoma revealed in the immunoglobulin variable region genes. *British Journal of Haematology*, **86**, 505–512.

167 Goodnow C.C., Crosbie J., Adelstein S. *et al.* (1988) Altered immunoglobulin expression and functional silencing of self reactive B lymphocytes in transgenic mice. *Nature*, **334**, 676–682.

168 Cooke M.D., Heath A.W., Shokat A.M. *et al.* (1994) Immunoglobulin signal transduction guides the specificity of B cell–T cell interactions and is blocked in tolerant self reactive B cells. *Journal of Experimental Medicine*, **179**, 425–438.

169 Eris J.M., Basten A., Brink R. *et al.* (1994) Anergic self reactive B-cells present self antigens and respond normally to CD40-dependent T-cell signals but are defective in antigen-receptor mediated functions. *Proceedings of the National Academy of Sciences*, **91**, 4392–4396.

170 Ghigo D., Gaidano G.L., Treves S. *et al.* (1991) Na+/H+ antiporter has different properties in human B lymphocytes according to CD5 expression and malignant phenotype. *European Journal of Immunology*, **21**, 583–588.

171 Michel F., Merle Beral H., Legac E., Michel A., Debre P. & Bismuth G. (1993) Defective calcium response in B chronic lymphocytic leukemia cells. *Journal of Immunology*, **150**, 3624–3633.

172 Schena M., Larrsson L.G., Gottardi D. *et al.* (1992) Growth and differentiation associated expression of Bcl-2 in B chronic lymphocytic leukemia cells. *Blood*, **79**, 2981–2989.

173 Mapara M.Y., Bargon R., Zugck C. *et al.* (1993) APO-1 mediated apoptosis or proliferation in chronic B lymphocytic leukemia:

correlation with Bcl-2 oncogene expression. *European Journal of Immunology*, **23**, 702–708.

174 Einhorn S., Burvall K., Juliusson G., Gahrton G. & Meeker T. (1989) Molecular analyses of chromosome 12 in chronic lymphocytic leukemia. *Leukemia*, **3**, 871–874.

175 Garcia-Marco J., Matutes E., Morilla R. *et al.* (1994) Trisomy 12 in B-cell chronic lymphocytic leukaemia: assessment of lineage restriction by simultaneous analysis of immunophenotype and genotype in interphase cells by fluorescence *in situ* hybridization. *British Journal of Haematology*, **83**, 44–50.

176 Oscier D.G., Copplestone J.A., Chapman R. *et al.* (1994) Atypical lymphocyte morphology and abnormal karyotype predict disease progression in stage A and A0 chronic lymphocytic leukaemia. *Blood*, **84**(Suppl. 1), 452a.

177 Oscier D.G., Chapman R. & Cowell J. (1990) Deletion of a retinoblastoma gene in B cell chronic lymphocytic leukaemia. *Blood*, **76**, 241a.

178 Liu Y., Szekely L., Grander D. *et al.* (1993) Chronic lymphocytic leukemia cells with allelic deletions at 13q14 commonly have one intact RB1 gene: evidence for a role of an adjacent locus. *Proceedings of the National Academy of Sciences USA*, **90**, 8697–8701.

179 Stilgenbauer S., Döhner H., Bulgay-Mörschel M., Weitz S., Bentz M. & Lichter P. (1993) High frequency of monoallelic retinoblastoma gene deletion in B-cell chronic lymphoid leukemia shown by interphase cytogenetics. *Blood*, **81**, 2118–2124.

180 Hawthorn L.A., Chapman R., Oscier D. & Cowell J.K. (1993) The consistent 13q14 translocation breakpoint seen in chronic B-cell leukaemia (B-CLL) involves deletion of the D13S25 locus which lies distal to the retinoblastoma predisposition gene. *Oncogene*, **8**, 1415–1419.

181 Liu Y., Hermanson M., Grandér D. *et al.* (1995) 13q deletions in lymphoid malignancies. *Blood*, **86**, 1911–1915.

182 Gardiner A.C., Corcoran M.M. & Oscier D.G. (1996) Different region of loss from chromosome 13q14 translocations in B CLL determined by FISH using Yac probes. *British Journal of Haematology*, **92**(Suppl. 1), 80.

183 Garcia-Marco J., Jones D., Coman S. *et al.* (1995) Lineage restriction of trisomy 12 and Rb1 deletions in chronic lymphocytic leukemia (CLL) by combined immunophenotyping and dual color interphase FISH. *Blood*, **86**(Suppl. 1), 344a.

184 Mould S., Gardiner A., Corcoran M. & Oscier D.G. (1996) Trisomy 12 and structural abnormalities of 13q14 occurring in the same clone in chronic lymphocytic leukaemia. *British Journal of Haematology*, **92**, 389–392.

185 Dohner H., Stilgenbauer P., Liebisch A. *et al.* (1995) 11q deletions are the second most common chromosome aberration in B-cell chronic lymphocytic leukemia and are associated with advanced stage and marked lymphadenopathy. *Blood*, **86**(Suppl. 1), 345a.

186 Cuneo A., Balboni M., Piva N. *et al.* (1995) Atypical chronic lymphocytic leukaemia with t(11;14)(q13;q32): karyotype evolution and prolymphocytic transformation. *British Journal of Haematology*, **90**, 409–416.

187 Dyer M.J.S., Zani V.J., Lu W.Z. *et al.* (1994) BCL2 translocations in leukemias of mature B cells. *Blood*, **83**, 3682–3688.

188 Merup M., Spasokoukotskaja T., Einhorn S., Smith C.I.E., Gahrton G. & Juliusson G. (1996) Bcl-2 rearrangements with breakpoints in both vcr and mbr in non-Hodgkin's lymphomas and chronic lymphocytic leukaemia. *British Journal of Haematology*, **92**, 647–652.

189 Michaux L., Mecucci C., Stul M. *et al.* (1996) BCL3 rearrange-

ment and t(14;19)(q32;q13) in lymphoproliferative disorders. *Genes, Chromosomes and Cancer*, **15**, 38–47.

190 Fenaux P., Preudhomme C., Luc J. *et al.* (1992) Mutations of the p53 gene in B-cell chronic lymphocytic leukemia: a report on 39 cases with cytogenetic analysis. *Leukemia*, **6**, 246–250.

191 El Roulby S., Thomas A., Costin D. *et al.* (1993) p53 gene mutation in B-cell chronic lymphocytic leukemia is associated with drug resistance and is independent of MDR1/MDR3 gene expression. *Blood*, **82**, 3452–3459.

192 Döhner H., Fischer K., Bentz M. *et al.* (1995) p53 gene deletion predicts for poor survival and non-response to therapy with purine analogs in chronic B-cell leukemias. *Blood*, **85**, 1580–1589.

193 Watanabe T., Hotta T., Ichikawa A. *et al.* (1994) The MDM2 oncogene overexpression in chronic lymphocytic leukemia and low-grade lymphoma of B-cell origin. *Blood*, **84**, 3158–3165.

194 Salomon-Nguyeu F., Valensi F. & Merle-Beral-H. (1995) A scoring system for the classification of CD5– B CLL versus CD5+ B CLL and B PLL. *Leukemia and Lymphoma*, **4**, 45–50.

195 Hoyer J.D., Ross C.W., Li C.Y. *et al.* (1995) True T cell chronic lymphocytic leukemia: a morphologic and immunophenotypic study of 25 cases. *Blood*, **86**, 1163–1169.

196 Wong K.F., Chan J.K.C. & Sin V.C. (1996) T-cell form of chronic lymphocytic leukaemia: a reaffirmation of its existence. *British Journal of Haematology*, **93**, 157–159.

197 Matutes E. & Catovsky D. (1996) Similarities between T-cell chronic lymphocytic leukemia and the small cell variant of T-prolymphocytic leukemia. *Blood*, **87**, 3520–3521.

198 Marlow A.A. & Evans E.R. (1977) Chronic lymphocytic leukemia: first physical sign after 22 years. *Western Journal of Medicine*, **77**, 408–409.

199 Rai K.R., Sawitsky A., Cronkite E.R. *et al.* (1977) Clinical staging of chronic lymphocytic leukemia. *Blood*, **46**, 219–234.

200 Binet J-L., Leprier M., Dighiero G. *et al.* (1977) A clinical staging system for chronic lymphocytic leukemia. *Cancer*, **40**, 855–864.

201 Binet J-L., Catovsky D., Chandra P. *et al.* (1981) Chronic lymphocytic leukaemia: proposals for a revised prognostic staging system. *British Journal of Haematology*, **48**, 365–367.

202 Montserrat E. & Rozman C. (1993) Chronic lymphocytic leukaemia: prognostic factors and natural history. *Baillière's Clinical Haematology*, **4**, 849–866.

203 Montserrat E., Vinolas E., Reverter J.C. & Rozman C. (1988) Natural history of chronic lymphocytic leukemia; on the progression and prognosis of early clinical stages. *Nouvelle Revue Française d'Hematologie*, **30**, 359–361.

204 French Co-operative Group on Chronic Lymphocytic Leukemia (1990) Natural history of stage A chronic lymphocytic leukaemia untreated patients. *British Journal of Haematology*, **76**, 45–57.

205 Molica S. (1991) Progression and survival studies in early chronic lymphocytic leukemia. *Blood*, **78**, 895–899.

206 International Workshop on CLL. (1989) Prognostic factors in early chronic lymphocytic leukaemia. *Lancet*, **ii**, 968–969.

207 Montserrat E., Sanchez-Bisono J., Vinolus N. *et al.* (1986) Lymphocyte doubling time in chronic lymphocytic leukaemia: analysis of prognostic significance. *British Journal of Haematology*, **62**, 567–575.

208 Moayeri H. & Sokal J.E. (1979) *In vitro* leukocyte thymidine uptake and prognosis in chronic lymphocytic leukemia. *American Journal of Medicine*, **66**, 773–778.

209 Juliusson G., Robert K-H., Nilsson B. *et al.* (1985) Prognostic value of B-cell mitogen-induced and spontaneous thymidine

uptake *in vitro* in chronic lymphocytic leukaemia cells. *British Journal of Haematology*, **66**, 429–436.

210 Skoog L., Tani E., Svedmgv E. & Johansson B. (1995) Growth fractions in non-Hodgkin's lymphoma and reactive lymphadenitis determined by Ki67 monoclonal antibody in fine needle aspirates. *Diagnostic Cytopathology*, **12**, 234–238.

211 Czader M., Porwit A., Tani E., Ost A., Mazar J. & Auer G. (1995) DNA image cytometry and the expression of proliferative markers (proliferating cell nuclear antigen and Ki67) in non-Hodgkin's lymphomas. *Modern Pathology*, **8**, 51–58.

212 Bosanquet A.G. & Bell P.B. (1996) Novel *ex vivo* analysis of non-classical pleiotropic drug resistance and collateral sensitivity induced by therapy provides a rationale for treatment strategies in chronic lymphocytic leukaemia. *Blood*, **87**, 1692–1671.

213 Hodgkins P.D. & Basten A. (1995) B cell activation, tolerance and antigen presenting function. *Current Opinions in Immunology*, **7**, 121–129.

214 Ranheim E.A. & Kipps T.J. (1993) Activated T cells induce expression of B7/BB1 on normal or leukemic B cells through a CD40 dependent signal. *Journal of Experimental Medicine*, **177**, 925–929.

215 Lewis F.B., Schwarz R.S. & Damashek W. (1996) X-irradiation and alkylating agents as possible trigger mechanisms in autoimmune complications of malignant lymphoproliferative diseases. *Clinical and Experimental Immunology*, **1**, 3–11.

216 Catovsky D. & Foa R. (1990) B-cell chronic lymphocytic leukaemia. In: *The Lymphoid Leukaemias* (eds D. Catovsky & R. Foa), pp. 73–112. Butterworths, London.

217 Thompson-Moya L., Martin T., Heuft H.G., Neubaur A. & Herrmann R. (1989) Allergic reaction with immune hemolytic anemia arising from chlorambucil. *American Journal of Hematology*, **32**, 230–231.

218 Hansen M.M. (1973) Chronic lymphocytic leukaemia: clinical studies based on 189 cases followed for a long time. *Scandinavian Journal of Haematology*, **18**(Suppl. 1), 1–282.

219 Myint H., Copplestone J.A., Orchard J. *et al.* (1995) Fludarabine related autoimmune haemolytic anaemia in patients with chronic lymphocytic leukaemia. *British Journal of Haematology*, **91**, 341–344.

220 Chasty R.C., Myint H., Oscier D.G. *et al.* (1996) Autoimmune haemolysis in patients with B-CLL treated with chlorodeoxyadenosine (CDA). *British Journal of Haematology*, **92**(Suppl. 1), 71.

221 Weinberg K. & Parkman R. (1995) Age, the thymus and T lymphocytes. *New England Journal of Medicine*, **332**, 182–183.

222 Enno A., Catovsky D., O'Brien M. *et al.* (1979) Prolymphocytoid transformation of chronic lymphocytic leukemia. *British Journal of Haematology*, **41**, 9–18.

223 Melo J.V., Catovsky D. & Galton D.A.G. (1986) The relationship between chronic lymphocytic leukaemia and prolymphocytic leukaemia. I Clinical and laboratory features of 300 patients and characterisation of an intermediate group. *British Journal of Haematology*, **63**, 377–387.

224 Richter N. (1928) Generalised reticular sarcoma of lymph nodes associated with lymphatic leukemia. *American Journal of Pathology*, **4**, 285–299.

225 Robertson L.E., Pugh W., O'Brien S. *et al.* (1993) Richter's syndrome: a report on 39 cases. *Journal of Clinical Oncology*, **11**, 1985–1989.

226 Trump D.L., Mann R.B., Phelps R., Roberts H. & Conley C.L. (1980) Richter's syndrome: diffuse histiocytic lymphoma in patients with chronic lymphocytic leukemia. A report of five

cases and review of the literature. *American Journal of Medicine*, **68**, 539–547.

227 Kruger A., Sadullah S., Chapman R. *et al.* (1993) Use of a retinoblastoma gene probe to investigate clonality in Richter's syndrome. *Leukemia*, **7**, 1891–1895.

228 Baylis K.M., Kueck B.D., Hanson C.A., Matthaeus W.G. & Almayno V.A. (1990) Richter's syndrome presenting as primary central nervous system lymphoma. Transformation of an identical clone. *American Journal of Clinical Pathology*, **93**, 117–123.

229 Bentoli L.F., Kubagawa H., Borzillo G.V. *et al.* (1987) Analysis with anti-idiotype antibody of a patient with chronic lymphocytic leukemia and a large cell lymphoma (Richter's syndrome). *Blood*, **70**, 45–50.

230 Miyamura K., Osada H., Yamaguchi T. *et al.* (1990) Single clonal origin of neoplastic B cells with different immunoglobulin light chains in a patient with Richter's syndrome. *Cancer*, **86**, 140–144.

231 Tohda S., Morio T., Suzuki T. *et al.* (1990) Richter's syndrome with two B cell clones possessing different surface immunoglobulins and immunoglobulin gene rearrangements. *American Journal of Hematology*, **35**, 32–36.

232 Brouet J.C., Preud'homme J.L., Seligman M. & Bernard J. (1973) Blast cells with surface immunoglobulin in two cases of acute blast crisis supervening on chronic lymphocytic leukaemia. *British Medical Journal*, **4**, 23–24.

233 Miller A.L.C., Habershaw J.A., Dhaliwhal H.S. & Lister T.A. (1984) Chronic lymphocytic leukaemia presenting as a blast cell crisis. *Leukemia Research*, **8**, 905–912.

234 Januszewicz E., Cooper I.A., Pilkington G. & Jose D. (1983) Blastic transformation of chronic lymphocytic leukemia. *American Journal of Hematology*, **15**, 399–402.

235 Frenkel E.P., Ligler F.S., Graham M.S. *et al.* (1981) Acute lymphocytic leukemia transformation of chronic lymphatic leukemia: substantiation by flow cytometry. *American Journal Hematology*, **10**, 391–398.

236 Beresford O.D. (1952) Chronic lymphatic leukaemia associated with malignant disease. *British Journal of Cancer*, **5**, 339–344.

237 Mannusow D., Weineman B.H. (1975) Subsequent neoplasia in chronic lymphocytic leukemia. *Journal of the American Medical Association*, **232**, 267–269.

238 Davis J.W., Weiss W.S. & Armstrong B.K. (1987) Second cancers in patients with chronic lymphocytic leukemia. *Journal of the National Cancer Institute*, **78**, 91–94.

239 Mellemgaard A., Geisler C.H. & Storm H.H. (1994) Risk of kidney cancer and other second solid malignancies in patients with chronic lymphocytic leukemia. *European Journal of Haematology*, **53**, 218–222.

240 Jeha T., Hamblin T.J. & Smith J.L. (1981) Coincident chronic lymphocytic leukemia and osteosclerotic multiple myeloma. *Blood*, **57**, 617–619.

241 Copplestone J.A., Mufti G.J., Hamblin T.J. & Oscier D.G. (1986) Immunological abnormalities in myelodysplastic syndromes. II Co-existent lymphoid or plasma cell neoplasms. A report of 20 cases unrelated to chemotherapy. *British Journal of Haematology*, **63**, 149–159.

242 Fermand J.P., James J.M., Hevait P. & Brouet J.C. (1985) Associated chronic lymphocytic leukemia and multiple myeloma: origin from a single clone. *Blood*, **66**, 291–293.

243 Saltman D.L., Ross J.A., Banks R.E., Ford A.M. & Mackie M.J. (1989) Molecular evidence for a single clone origin in diphenotypic concomitant chronic lymphocytic leukemia and multiple myeloma. *Blood*, **74**, 2062–2065.

244 Catovsky D., Richards S., Fooks J. & Hamblin T.J. (1991) CLL trials in the United Kingdom. The Medical Research Council CLL Trials 1, 2 and 3. In: *Advances in Chronic Lymphocytic Leukemia* (eds A. Polliak & E. Montserrat), pp. 105–111. Harwood, Chur.

245 French Co-operative Group on Chronic Lymphocytic Leukemia (1990) Effects of chlorambucil and therapeutic decision in initial forms of chronic lymphocytic leukemia (stage A). Results of a randomised clinical trial on 612 patients. *Blood*, **75**, 1414–1421.

246 Shustik C., Mick R., Silver R., Sawitsky A., Rai K.R. & Shapiro I. (1988) Treatment of early chronic lymphocytic leukemia: intermittent chlorambucil versus observation. *Haematology and Oncology*, **6**, 7–12.

247 Spanish Co-operative Group (PETHEMA) (1991) Treatment of chronic lymphocytic leukemia: a preliminary report of Spanish (PETHEMA) trials. In: *Advances in Chronic Lymphocytic Leukemia* (eds A. Polliak & E. Montserrat), pp. 105–111. Harwood, Chur.

248 Cheson B.D., Bennett J.M., Rai K.R. *et al.* (1988) Guidelines for clinical protocols for chronic lymphocytic leukemia: recommendations of the National Cancer Institute — sponsored working group. *American Journal of Hematology*, **29**, 152–163.

249 Keating M.J., Kantarjian H., O'Brien S. *et al.* (1991) Fludarabine: a new agent with marked cytoreductive activity in untreated chronic lymphocytic leukemia. *Journal of Clinical Oncology*, **9**, 44–49.

250 Bosanquet A.G., McCann S.R., Crotty G.M., Mills M.J. & Catovsky D. (1995) Methylprednisolone in advanced chronic lymphocytic leukaemia: rationale for, and effectiveness of treatment suggested by DiSC assay. *Acta Haematologica*, **93**, 73–79.

251 Robertson L.E., Estey E., Kantarjian H. *et al.* (1994) Therapy related leukemia and myelodysplastic syndrome in chronic lymphocytic leukemia. *Leukemia*, **8**, 2047–2051.

252 Jacksic B. & Brugiatelli H. (1988) High dose continuous chlorambucil vs intermittent chlorambucil plus prednisolone for treatment of B CLL: IGCI CLL–01 trial. *Nouvelle Revue Française d'Hematologie*, **30**, 437–442.

253 Han T., Ezdinli E.Z., Shimoaka K. & Desai D.V. (1973) Chlorambucil vs combined chlorambucil-corticosteroid therapy in chronic lymphocytic leukemia. *Cancer*, **31**, 502–508.

254 Montserrat E., Alcala A., Parody R. *et al.* (1985) Treatment of chronic lymphocytic leukemia in advanced stages: a randomised trial comparing chlorambucil plus prednisolone versus cyclophosphamide, vincristine and prednisolone. *Cancer*, **56**, 2369–2375.

255 French Co-operative Group on Chronic Lymphocytic Leukemia (1990) A randomized clinical trial of chlorambucil versus COP in stage B chronic lymphocytic leukemia. *Blood*, **75**, 1422–1425.

256 French Co-operative Group on Chronic Lymphocytic Leukemia (1986) Benefit of the CHOP regimen in advanced untreated chronic lymphocytic leukemia. Results of a randomized clinical trial. *Lancet*, **i**, 1346–1349.

257 French Co-operative Group on Chronic Lymphocytic Leukemia (1994) Is the CHOP regimen a good treatment for advanced CLL? Results from two randomized clinical trials. *Leukemia and Lymphoma*, **13**, 449–456.

258 Hansen M.M., Andersen E., Christensen B.E. *et al.* (1988) CHOP versus prednisolone and chlorambucil in chronic lymphocytic leukemia (CLL): preliminary results of a randomized multicenter study. *Nouvelle Revue Française d'Hematologie*, **30**, 433–436.

259 Kimby E., Bjorkholm M., Gahrton G. *et al.* (1994) Chlorambucil/prednisolone vs CHOP in symptomatic low grade non-

Hodgkin's lymphomas: a randomized trial from the Lymphoma Group of Central Sweden. *Annals of Oncology*, **5**(Suppl. 1), 67–71.

260 Case D.C.J., Porensky R.S. & Fanning J.P. (1985) Combination chemotherapy with M2 protocol (BCNU, Cyclophosphamide, Vincristine, Melphalan and Prednisolone) for chronic lymphocytic leukemia (stages III and I). *Oncology*, **42**, 350–353.

261 Keating M.J. (1988) Multiple agent chemotherapy (POACH) in previously treated and untreated patients with chronic lymphocytic leukemia. *Leukemia*, **2**, 157–164.

262 Robertson L.E., Hall R., Keating M.J. *et al.* (1993) High dose cytosine arabinoside in chronic lymphocytic leukemia: a clinical and pharmacological analysis. *Leukemia and Lymphoma*, **10**, 43–48.

263 Brockman R.M., Schabel F.M. & Montgomery J.A. (1977) Biological activity of 9-β-D-arabinofuranosyl-2-fluoroadenine, a metabolically stable analogue of 9-β-D-arabinofuranosyladenine. *Biochemical Pharmacology*, **26**, 2193–2196.

264 Cheson B.D., Vena D.A., Foss F.M. & Sorensen J.M. (1994) Neurotoxicity of purine analogues: a review. *Journal of Clinical Oncology*, **12**, 2216–2228.

265 Pott-Hoeck C. & Hidderman W. (1995) Purine analogues in the treatment of low grade lymphomas and chronic lymphocytic leukemia. *Annals of Oncology*, **6**, 421–433.

266 Keating M.R., Kantarjian H., O'Brien S. *et al.* (1991) Fludarabine: a new agent with marked cytoreductive activity in untreated CLL. *Journal of Clinical Oncology*, **9**, 44–49.

267 French Co-operative Group on CLL, Johnson S., Smith A.G. *et al.* (1996) Multicentre prospective randomised trial of fludarabine versus cyclophosphamide, doxorubicin, and prednisolone (CAP) for treatment of advanced stage chronic lymphocytic leukaemia. *Lancet*, **347**, 1432–1438.

268 French Co-operative Group on CLL (1994) Comparison of fludarabine (FDR), CAP and CHOP in previously untreated stage B and C chronic lymphocytic leukemia (CLL). First interim results of a randomized clinical trial in 247 patients. *Blood*, **84**(Suppl. 1), 461a.

269 Rai K.R., Peterson B., Keating M.J. *et al.* (1995) Fludarabine induces a high complete remission rate in previously untreated patients with active chronic lymphocytic leukemia (CLL). A randomized inter-group study. *Blood*, **86**(Suppl. 1), 607a.

270 Keating M.R., O'Brien S., Kantarjian H. *et al.* (1993) Long term follow up of patients with chronic lymphocytic leukemia treated with fludarabine as a single agent. *Blood*, **81**, 2878–2884.

271 Cull G., Richardson D.S., Howe D.J., Hopkins J.A., Johnson S.A. & Phillips M.J. (1995) Molecular complete response in a patient with chronic lymphocytic leukaemia treated with 2-chlorodeoxyadenosine. *Acta Oncologica*, **34**, 536–537.

272 Seymour J.F., Robertson L.E., O'Brien S., Lerner S. & Keating M.J. (1995) Survival of young patients with chronic lymphocytic leukemia failing fludarabine therapy: a basis for the use of myeloablative therapies. *Leukemia and Lymphoma*, **18**, 493–496.

273 Robertson L.E., O'Brien S., Kantarjian H. *et al.* (1995) Fludarabine plus doxorubicin in previously treated chronic lymphocytic leukemia. *Leukemia*, **9**, 934–935.

274 Elias L., Stock-Novock D., Head D.R. *et al.* (1996) A phase I trial of the combination of fludarabine monophosphate and chlorambucil in CLL: a South West Oncology Group study. *Leukemia*, **7**, 361–365.

275 O'Brien S., Kantarjian H., Beran M. *et al.* (1993) Results of fludarabine and prednisolone therapy in 264 patients with chronic lymphocytic leukemia with multivariate analysis-derived prognostic model for response to treatment. *Blood*, **82**, 1695–1700.

276 Gandhi V., Kemena A, Keating M.J. & Plunkett W. (1992) Fludarabine infusion potentiates arabinosylcytosine metabolism in lymphocytes of patients with chronic lymphocytic leukemia. *Cancer Research*, **52**, 897–903.

277 Robertson L.E., Kantarjian H., O'Brien S. *et al.* (1993) Cisplatin, fludarabine and ara-C (PFA): a regimen for advanced refractory CLL. *Proceedings of the American Society of Clinical Oncology*, **12**, 1014a.

278 Kawasaki H., Camera C.J., Piro I.D. *et al.* (1993) Relationship of deoxycytidine kinase and cytoplasmic 5' nucleotidase to the chemotherapeutic efficacy of 2-chlorodeoxyadenosine. *Blood*, **81**, 597–601.

279 Carson D.A., Wasson D.B., Taetle R. *et al.* (1983) Specific toxicity of 2-chlorodeoxyadenosine towards resting and proliferating human lymphocytes. *Blood*, **62**, 737–743.

280 Cheson B.D. (1995) Infectious and immunosuppressive complications of purine analogue therapy. *Journal of Clinical Oncology*, **13**, 2431–2448.

281 Piro L.D., Carneva C.J., Carson D.A. *et al.* (1990) Lasting remissions in hairy cell leukemia induced by a single infusion of 2-chlorodeoxyadenosine. *New England Journal of Medicine*, **322**, 1117–1121.

282 Tallman M.S., Hakiman D., Zanzig C. *et al.* (1995) Cladribine in the treatment of relapsing or refractory chronic lymphocytic leukemia. *Journal of Clinical Oncology*, **13**, 983–988.

283 Saven A., Leven R.H., Kosty M., Beutler E. & Piro L.D. (1995) 2-Chlorodeoxyadenosine activity in patients with untreated chronic lymphocytic leukemia. *Journal of Clinical Oncology*, **13**, 570–574.

284 Delannoy A., Martiat P., Gala S.L. *et al.* (1995) 2-Chlorodeoxyadenosine for patients with previously untreated chronic lymphocytic leukemia (CLL). *Leukemia*, **9**, 1130–1135.

285 Mulligan S.P., Eliadis P., Dall B. *et al.* (1995) 2-Chlorodeoxyadenosine (2-CdA) in previously untreated chronic lymphocytic leukemia (CLL). Preliminary analysis from the Australian Leukemia Study Group Trial. *Blood*, **86**(Suppl. 1), 349a.

286 Juliusson G. & Liliemark J. (1995) Long term survival following cladribine (2-chlorodeoxyadenosine) in 117 patients with chronic lymphocytic leukemia (CLL). *Blood*, **86**(Suppl. 1), 350a.

287 Juliusson G. & Liliemark J. (1994) Retreatment of chronic lymphocytic leukemia with 2-chlorodeoxyadenosine (2-CdA) at relapse following 2-CdA-induced remission: no acquired resistance. *Leukemia and Lymphoma*, **13**, 75–88.

288 Juliusson G., Elmhorn-Rosenberg A. & Liliemark J. (1992) Response to 2-chlorodeoxyadenosine in patients with chronic lymphocytic leukemia resistant to fludarabine. *New England Journal of Medicine*, **327**, 1056–1061.

289 O'Brien S., Kantarjian H., Estey E. *et al.* (1994) Lack of effect of 2-chlorodeoxyadenosine in patients with chronic lymphocytic leukemia refractory to fludarabine. *New England Journal of Medicine*, **330**, 319–322.

290 Tefferi A., Witzig T.E., Reid J.M., Li C.Y. & Ames M.M. (1994) Phase I study of combined 2-chlorodeoxyadenosine and chlorambucil in chronic lymphocytic leukemia and low grade lymphoma. *Journal of Clinical Oncology*, **12**, 569–574.

291 Kane B.J., Kuhn J.G. & Roush M.K. (1992) Pentostatin: an adenosine deaminase inhibitor for the treatment of hairy cell leukemia. *Annals of Pharmacotherapy*, **26**, 939–947.

292 Grever M.R., Leiby J.M. & Kraut E.H. (1985) Low dose deoxyco-

formycin in lymphoid malignancy. *Journal of Clinical Oncology*, **3**, 1196–1201.

293 O'Dwyer P., Wagner B., Leyland-Jones B. *et al.* (1988) 2-Deoxycoformycin (Pentostatin) for lymphoid malignancies. *Annals of Internal Medicine*, **108**, 733–743.

294 Dillman R.O., Mick R. & McIntyre O.R. (1989) Pentostatin in chronic lymphocytic leukemia. A phase II trial of Cancer and Leukemia group B. *Journal of Clinical Oncology*, **7**, 433–438.

295 Ho A.D., Thaler J., Strykmans P. *et al.* (1990) Pentostatin in refractory CLL: a phase II trial of the EORTC. *Journal of the National Cancer Institute*, **82**, 1416–1420.

296 Byrd J.C., Hargis J.B., Kester K.E., Hospenthal D.R., Knutson S.W. & Diehl L.F. (1995) Opportunistic pulmonary infections with fludarabine in previously treated patients with low grade lymphoid malignancies: a role for *Pneumocystis carinnii* pneumonia prophylaxis. *American Journal of Hematology*, **49**, 135–142.

297 Schilling P.J. & Vadham-Raj S. (1990) Concurrent cytomegalovirus and pneumocystis pneumonia after fludarabine therapy for chronic lymphocytic leukemia. *New England Journal of Medicine*, **323**, 833–834.

298 Leenders A., Sonnenveld P. & de Marie S. (1995) Cryptococcal meningitis following fludarabine treatment for chronic lymphocytic leukemia. *European Journal of Microbiology and Infectious Diseases*, **14**, 826–828.

299 Maung Z.T., Wood A.C., Jackson G.H., Turner G.E., Appleton A.C. & Hamilton P.J. (1994) Transfusion associated graft versus host disease in fludarabine treated B chronic lymphocytic leukemia. *British Journal of Haematology*, **88**, 649–652.

300 Montillo M., Tedeschi A. & Leoni P. (1994) Recurrence of autoimmune thrombocytopenia after treatment with fludarabine in a patient with chronic lymphocytic leukemia. *Leukemia and Lymphoma*, **15**, 187–188.

301 Leporier M., Reman O. & Troussard X. (1993) Pure red cell aplasia with fludarabine for chronic lymphocytic leukemia. *Lancet*, **342**, 555.

302 Byrd J.C., Hertler A.A., Weiss R.B., Freuman J., Kwender S.L. & Diehl L.F. (1995) Fatal recurrence of autoimmune hemolytic anemia following pentostatin therapy in a patient with a history of fludarabine associated hemolytic anemia. *Annals of Oncology*, **6**, 300–301.

303 Fleischman R.A. & Croy D. (1995) Acute onset of severe autoimmune hemolytic anemia after treatment with 2-chlorodeoxyadenosine for chronic lymphocytic leukemia. *American Journal of Hematology*, **48**, 293.

304 Hamblin T.J., Abdul-Ahad A.K., Gordon J., Stevenson F.K. & Stevenson G.T. (1980) Preliminary evidence in treating lymphocytic leukaemia with antibody to immunoglobulin idiotypes on the cell surfaces. *British Journal of Cancer*, **42**, 495–502.

305 Dyer M.J., Hale G., Hayhoe F.G. & Waldmann H. (1989) Effects of CAMPATH-1 antibodies *in vivo* in patients with lymphoid malignancies: influence of antibody isotype. *Blood*, **73**, 1431–1439.

306 Hertler A.A., Schlossman D.M., Borowitz M.J., Blythman H.E., Cassellas P. & Frankel A.E. (1989) An anti CD% immunotoxin for chronic lymphocytic leukemia: enhancement of cytotoxicity with human serum albumin-monensin. *International Journal of Cancer*, **43**, 215–219.

307 Grossbard M.L., Lambert J.M., Goldmacher V.S. *et al.* (1993) Anti-B4 blocked ricin: a phase I trial of 7 day continuous infusion in patients with B cell neoplasms. *Journal of Clinical Oncology*, **11**, 726–737.

308 DeNardo G.L., Lewis J.P., DeNardo S.J. & O'Grady L.F. (1994)

Effect of Lym-1 radioimmunoconjugate on refractory chronic lymphocytic leukemia. *Cancer*, **73**, 1425–1432.

309 De Gast G.C., Van Hauten A.A., Haagen I.A. *et al.* (1995) Clinical experience with CD5 × CD19 bispecific antibodies in patients with B cell malignancies. *Journal of Hemotherapy*, **4**, 433–437.

310 Bregni M., Sienna S., Formosa A. *et al.* (1989) B cell restricted saporin immunotoxins: activity against B-cell lines and chronic lymphocytic leukemia cells. *Blood*, **73**, 753–762.

311 Kreitman R.J., Chaudhary V.K., Kozak R.W., Fitzgerald D.J., Waldman T.A. & Pastan I. (1992) Recombinant toxins containing the variable domains of the anti-Tac monoclonal antibody to the interleukin-2 receptor kill malignant cells from patients with chronic lymphocytic leukemia. *Blood*, **80**, 2344–2352.

312 Zeigler-Heitbrock H.W., Schlag R., Flieger D. & Thiele E. (1989) Favorable response of early stage B CLL patients to treatment with IFN alpha 2. *Blood*, **73**, 1426–1430.

313 O'Brien S., Kantarjian H., Beran M. *et al.* (1995) Interferon maintenance therapy for patients with chronic lymphocytic leukemia in remission after fludarabine therapy. *Blood*, **86**, 1298–1300.

314 Allison M.A., Jones S.E. & McGaffey P. (1989) Phase II trial of outpatient interleukin-2 in malignant lymphoma, chronic lymphocytic leukemia and selected solid tumours. *Journal of Clinical Oncology*, **7**, 75–80.

315 Kay N.E., Oken M.M., Mazza J.J. & Bradley E.C. (1988) Evidence for tumour reduction in refractory or relapsed B-CLL patients with infusional interleukin-2. *Nouvelle Revue Française d'Hematologie*, **30**, 475–478.

316 Chisise T., Caprist G. & Dal Fior S. (1991) Splenic irradiation in chronic lymphocytic leukemia. *European Journal of Haematology*, **46**, 202–204.

317 Delpero J.R., Gastart J.A., Letreut G.P. *et al.* (1987) The value of splenectomy in chronic lymphocytic leukemia. *Cancer*, **59**, 340–345.

318 Michallet M., Archimbaud E., Rowlings P.A., Horowitz Z.M., Gratwohl A. & Gale R.P. (1995) Hematopoietic stem cell transplant for chronic lymphocytic leukemia. *Blood*, **86**(Suppl. 1), 457a.

319 Gribben J.G., Barlett-Pandite L., Provan A. *et al.* (1995) Disease free status and absence of PCR detectable minimal residual disease suggests eradication of B-CLL following autologous and allogeneic BMT. *Blood*, **86**(Suppl. 1), 457a.

320 Khouri I.F., Keating M.J., Vriesendorp H.M. *et al.* (1994) Autologous and allogeneic bone marrow transplantation for chronic lymphocytic leukemia: preliminary results. *Journal of Clinical Oncology*, **12**, 748–758.

321 Tsatalas C., Chalkia P., Athanasiadis G. *et al.* (1995) Increased peripheral blood normal myeloid progenitor cells (CFU-GM) in chronic lymphocytic leukemia: a perspective for autologous peripheral stem cell transplantation. *European Journal of Haematology*, **54**, 235–240.

322 Co-operative Group for the Study of Immunoglobulin in CLL (1988) Intravenous immunoglobulin for the prevention of infection in chronic lymphocytic leukemia. *New England Journal of Medicine*, **319**, 902–970.

323 Tura S., Finelli C., Bandini G. *et al.* (1988) Cyclosporin A in the treatment of CLL associated pure red cell aplasia and bone marrow hypoplasia. *Nouvelle Revue Française d'Hematologie*, **30**, 479–481.

324 Kantarjian H.M., Childs C., O'Brien S. *et al.* (1991) Efficiency of fludarabine, a new adenine nucleoside analogue in patients with prolymphocytic leukemia and the prolymphocytoid variant of

chronic lymphocytic leukemia. *American Journal of Medicine*, **90**, 223–228.

325 Galton D.A.G., Goldman J.M., Wiltshaw E. *et al.* (1974) Prolymphocytic leukaemia. *British Journal of Haematology*, **27**, 7–23.

326 Matutes E. & Catovsky D. (1991) Mature T cell leukaemias and leukaemia/lymphoma syndromes. Review of our experience in 175 cases. *Leukemia and Lymphoma*, **4**, 81–91.

327 Matutes E., Brito-Bapapulle V., Swansbury J. *et al.* (1991) Clinical and laboratory features of 78 cases of prolymphocytic leukemia. *Blood*, **78**, 3269–3274.

328 Catovsky D. & Foa R. (1990) *The Lymphoid Leukaemias*. Butterworths, London.

329 Brito-Bapapulle V., Pittman S., Melo J.V. *et al.* (1987) Cytogenetic studies on prolymphocytic leukaemia. 1 B cell prolymphocytic leukaemia. *Hematologic Pathology*, **1**, 27–33.

330 Matutes E., Brito-Bapapulle V., Swansbury J. *et al.* (1991) Clinical and laboratory features of T-prolymphocytic leukaemia. *Blood*, **78**, 3269–3274.

331 Croce C.M., Isobe M., Polumbo A. *et al.* (1985) Gene for alpha chain of human T cell receptor: location on chromosome 14 region involved in T cell neoplasms. *Science*, **227**, 1044–1047.

332 Brito-Bapapulle V. & Catovsky D. (1991) Inversions and tandem translocations involving chromosome 14q11 and 14q32 in T prolymphocytic leukemia and T cell leukemias in patients with ataxia telangectasia. *Cancer, Genetics and Cytogenetics*, **55**, 1–9.

333 Melo J.V., Catovsky D., Gregory W.M. & Galton D.A.G. (1987) The relationship between chronic lymphocytic leukemia and prolymphocytic leukemia. (i) Analysis of survival and prognostic features. *British Journal of Haematology*, **65**, 23–29.

334 Melo J.V., Catovsky D. & Galton D.A.G. (1986) The relationship between chronic lymphocytic leukemia and prolymphocytic leukaemia. (ii) Patterns of evolution of 'prolymphocytoid transformation'. *British Journal of Haematology*, **64**, 77–86.

335 Oscier D.G., Catovsky D., Errington R.D. *et al.* (1981) Splenic irradiation in B prolymphocytic leukaemia. *British Journal of Haematology*, **48**, 577–584.

336 Dearden C. & Catovsky D. (1990) Deoxycoformycin in the treatment of mature B cell malignancies. *British Journal of Cancer*, **62**, 4–5.

337 Barton K., Larson R.A., O'Brien S. & Rabin M.J. (1992) Rapid response of B-cell prolymphocytic leukemia to 2-chlorodeoxyadenosine. *Journal of Clinical Oncology*, **10**, 1821.

338 Tsai L.M., Tsai C.C., Hyde T.P. *et al.* (1984) T cell prolymphocytic leukemia with helper cell phenotype and a review of the literature. *Cancer*, **54**, 463–470.

339 Catovsky D. (1993) Diagnosis and treatment of CLL variants. In: *Chronic Lymphocytic Leukemia: scientific advances and clinical developments* (ed. B. Cheson), pp. 369–397. Marcel Dekker, New York.

340 Witzig T.E., Weitz J.J., Lundberg T.H. & Tefferi A. (1994) Treatment of refractory T cell chronic lymphocytic leukemia with purine nucleoside analogues. *Leukemia and Lymphoma*, **14**, 137–139.

341 Catovsky D. (1995) Chronic lymphoproliferative disorders. *Current Opinion in Oncology*, **7**, 3–11.

342 Neiman R.S., Sullivan A.L. & Jaffe R. (1979) Malignant lymphoma simulating leukaemic reticuloendotheliosis. A clinicopathologic study of ten cases. *Cancer*, **43**, 329–342.

343 Melo J.V., Robinson D.S.F., Gregory C. & Catovsky D. (1987) Splenic B cell lymphoma with 'villous' lymphocytes in the peripheral blood: a disorder distinct from hairy cell leukemia. *Leukemia*, **1**, 294–299.

344 Mulligan S.P. & Catovsky D. (1992) Splenic lymphoma with villous lymphocytes. *Leukemia and Lymphoma*, **6**, 97–105.

345 Matutes E., Morilla R., Owusu-Ankomah K., Houlihan A. & Catovsky D. (1994) The immunophenotype of splenic lymphoma with villous lymphocytes and its relevance to the differential diagnosis with other B-cell disorders. *Blood*, **83**, 1558–1562.

346 Oscier D.G., Matutes E., Gardiner E. *et al.* (1993) Cytogenetic studies in splenic lymphoma with villous lymphocytes. *British Journal of Haematology*, **85**, 487–491.

347 Jadayel D., Matutes E., Dyer M.J.S. *et al.* (1994) Splenic lymphoma with villous lymphocytes: analysis of BCL-1 rearrangements and expression of the cyclin D1 gene. *Blood*, **83**, 3664–3671.

348 Isaacson P.G., Matutes E., Burke M. & Catovsky D. (1994) The histopathology of splenic lymphoma with villous lymphocytes. *Blood*, **84**, 3828–3834.

349 Zhu D., Oscier D.G. & Stevenson F.K. (1995) Splenic lymphoma with villous lymphocytes involves B cells with extensively mutated Ig heavy chain variable region genes. *Blood*, **85**, 1603–1607.

350 Mulligan S.P., Matutes E., Dearden C. & Catovsky D. (1991) Splenic lymphoma with villous lymphocytes: natural history and response to therapy in 50 cases. *British Journal of Haematology*, **78**, 206–209.

351 Scott C.S., Richards S.J., Sivakumaran M. *et al.* (1993) Transient and persistent expansions of large granular lymphocytes (LGL) and NK-associated (NKa) cells: the Yorkshire Leukemia Group study. *British Journal of Haematology*, **83**, 504–515.

352 Loughran T.P. Jr (1993) Clonal diseases of large granular lymphocytes. *Blood*, **82**, 1–14.

353 Dhodapkar M.V., Li C-Y., Lust J.A., Tefferi A. & Phyliky R.L. (1994) Clinical spectrum of clonal proliferations of T-large granular lymphocytes: a T-cell clonopathy of undetermined significance? *Blood*, **84**, 1602–1627.

354 Loughran T.P. Jr, Kidd P.G. & Starkebaum G. (1994) Treatment of large granular lymphocyte leukemia with oral low-dose methotrexate. *Blood*, **84**, 2164–2170.

355 Cooper D.L., Henderson-Bakas M. & Berliner N. (1993) Lymphoproliferative disorder of granular lymphocytes associated with severe neutropenia. Response to therapy with granulocyte colony stimulating factor. *Cancer*, **72**, 1607–1611.

356 Jakubowski A., Winton E.F., Gencarelli A. & Gabrilove J. (1995) Treatment of chronic neutropenia associated with granular lymphocytosis with cyclosporin A and filgrastim. *American Journal of Hematology*, **50**, 288–291.

357 Loughran T.P., Starkelbaum G., Clark E., Wallace P. & Kadin M.E. (1987) Evaluation of splenectomy in large granular lymphocyte leukemia. *British Journal of Haematology*, **67**, 135–140.

358 Kelly A., Richards S.J., Sivakumaran M. *et al.* (1994) Clonality of CD3 negative large granular lymphocyte proliferations determined by PCR based X-inactivation studies. *Journal of Clinical Pathology*, **47**, 399–404.

359 Jaffe E.S. (1996) Classification of natural killer (NK) cell and NK-like T-cell malignancies. *Blood.* **87**, 1207–1210.

7   Adult T-cell Leukaemia/ Lymphoma

E. Matutes and D. Catovsky

Introduction

Within the spectrum of post-thymic (mature) T-cell malignancies, adult T-cell leukaemia/lymphoma (ATLL) is a distinct clinicopathological entity. The disease was first described by Takatsuki and colleagues in 1977 [1] and later its full heterogeneous nature recognized. The main interest in ATLL lies in its aetiological relationship with the human T-cell leukaemia virus type 1 or HTLV-I [2]. Although ATLL and HTLV-I were initially considered to be clustered mainly in two geographical areas, Japan and the Caribbean, seroepidemiological surveys worldwide and routine screening of lymphoid malignancies have led to the recognition that the disease and its retrovirus are more widespread than originally thought. This chapter will describe the main clinical and biological features of ATLL and discuss epidemiological and virological aspects of its relationship with HTLV-I.

Clinical features

ATLL often presents with a leukaemic picture and, less commonly, as a lymphoma with little or no peripheral blood involvement. The leukaemic manifestations of ATLL are variable and include smouldering, chronic and acute forms [3–5]. Our experience is based on 52 ATLL patients studied over the past 10 years and includes 46 black patients of Caribbean origin, two born in Africa, one Japanese, two of Iranian descent and one from Chile.

The clinical and laboratory features are summarized in Table 7.1. ATLL affects adults (median age: 47 years) and, exceptionally, infants. Material has been reviewed from an 18-month-old baby with HTLV-I + ATLL included in a series of Brazilian cases [6]; few other paediatric cases have been reported [7,8]. These rare cases suggest that there is not always a long period of latency between the infection with HTLV-I and the development of ATLL. The clinical and laboratory features of our series of ATLL patients studied in the UK (mostly of Caribbean descent) have been compared with a larger series of Japanese

and Brazilian patients. The only difference encountered was the age of onset, which was a decade younger in the Caribbean and Brazilian patients [9,10] compared to the Japanese patients. This probably reflects the influence of different environmental cofactors which are responsible for the development of ATLL in HTLV-I carriers in these two distinct geographical regions.

Males and females are equally affected, which contrasts with the female prevalence in tropical spastic paraparesis which is another disease associated with HTLV-I. Lymphadenopathy is the most common physical finding, whereas the liver and spleen are less often enlarged (Table 7.1). Skin lesions are frequent and seen as a maculopapular rash or nodules but generalized erythrodermia is rare. Hypercalcaemia is a characteristic manifestation of ATLL and is seen in half of the cases at presentation and up to two-thirds during the course of the disease. Despite this, osteolytic lesions are relatively rare [11]. In the series reported there was only one case in whom the disease manifested almost exclusively with bone tumours, lytic lesions and hypercalcaemia, with no evidence of organomegaly or blood and bone marrow involvement.

Central nervous system (CNS) involvement by the leukaemia, either manifested by cranial nerve palsies or peripheral neuropathy with the presence of atypical lymphocytes in the cerebral spinal fluid (CSF), is also infrequent but was seen in six patients. Pulmonary involvement has been documented in a high proportion of Japanese patients and this has been seen in all clinical subtypes including chronic and smouldering ATLL [12]. In some cases the infiltrates correspond to opportunistic infections such as pneumocystis, fungal and cryptococcal, infections which are common in ATLL and underline the immunodeficiency associated with HTLV-I.

In rare cases, the disease presents as a lymphoma of the gastrointestinal tract [13]. In our experience, and also in Japanese reports, there seems to be an association between HTLV-I and infestation by *Strongyloides stercoralis*. Strongyloidiasis preceded or complicated the leukaemia in 4 of our patients. This finding and the observation that up to 40% of patients with *Strongy-*

Table 7.1 Clinical and laboratory features of ATLL*.

Feature	Incidence
Lymphadenopathy	70%
Splenomegaly	31%
Hepatomegaly	27%
Skin lesions	41%
Hypercalcaemia†	74%
Anaemia (<10 g/dl)	14%
Thrombocytopenia (< 100 × 10⁹/l)	17%
WBC (× 10⁹/l)	
Median	31
Range	4–263

* Series of 52 cases studied in the UK. Forty had leukaemic ATLL: acute (33), smouldering (five) and chronic (two), and 12 patients had lymphoma type ATLL.
† Observed at presentation in 51% and in 23% during the evolution of the disease. In only 10% was associated with osteolytic lesions.

Table 7.2 Clinical forms of ATLL.

Leukaemia (75% of cases)

Acute	Acute or subacute onset; leucocytosis with atypical lymphoid cells; hypercalcaemia, lymphadenopathy and other organ involvement
Chronic	Slowly progressive or stable leucocytosis with atypical lymphoid cells; rarely skin lesions or lymphadenopathy and LDH below twice the upper normal level
Smouldering	Skin rash with or without transient lymphadenopathy; normal WBC; T-cell clonality and clonal integration of HTLV-I

Lymphoma (25% of cases)
Lymphadenopathy/organomegaly with no blood involvement

loides infestation and HTLV-I⁺ serology have a monoclonal pattern of integration of the retrovirus, a feature not seen in healthy carriers [14], has lead to the hypothesis that this parasite may play a secondary role in the development or progression to ATLL [9].

Clinical forms of acute T-cell leukaemia/lymphoma

The acute form of ATLL is the most frequent, accounting for 65% of the cases. The cases of lymphoma may be indistinguishable on clinical and histopathological grounds from other types of T-cell non-Hodgkin's lymphoma (NHL). The remaining 10% of patients present as chronic or smouldering ATLL (Table 7.2).

Chronic ATLL is rare in our experience but it may represent up to 15% of cases in Japan. This form is characterized by persistent T-cell lymphocytosis with little or no organ involvement and with lactic dehydrogenase (LDH) values up to twice the upper normal level. Within a period of months to several years the disease may become acute. Shirono *et al.* [15] suggested that a high proliferative rate of the blood lymphocytes in chronic ATLL, as measured by staining with the monoclonal antibody Ki-67, correlates with rapid progression of the disease.

Smouldering ATLL [3], designated also as 'pre-leukaemic' form [5], is characterized by skin lesions responsive to topical steroids, transient minor or no lymph-node enlargement and pulmonary infiltrates. The patients are otherwise asymptomatic and the leucocyte count is normal with less than 3% atypical lymphoid cells, which is similar to the findings in normal HTLV-I carriers. Unlike normal carriers, smouldering ATLL has, by definition, an abnormal T-cell clone which needs to be documented by chromosomal abnormalities and/or DNA

analysis showing the monoclonal integration of proviral DNA in the blood lymphocytes [16,17].

Familial acute T-cell leukaemia/lymphoma

Familial ATLL has been documented in endemic regions such as Japan [18,19], but it is less common in countries with a lower HTLV-I seroprevalence such as the USA where it has been reported in Caribbean immigrants [20]. The first familial cluster of ATLL has been reported in the UK in two siblings of Afro-Caribbean descent, one of whom was born in the UK and found to be an HTLV-I carrier 4 years prior to the development of ATLL [21]. Serological studies in this family, in which the mother was HTLV-I antibody positive, support the vertical transmission of HTLV-I. The fact that in most of the familial clusters, the patients did not have contact for a number of years, as in ours, suggests that environmental factors have little influence in the predisposition to develop ATLL.

Laboratory investigations

A number of tests are necessary to make the diagnosis of ATLL and distinguish this disease from other mature T-cell malignancies. These include.
1 Blood counts, bone marrow aspirate and trephine biopsy with particular attention to the morphology of the lymphocytes.
2 Immunophenotype of the blood lymphocytes and/or of any other tissue involved (e.g. lymph node).
3 Biochemistry profile to detect hypercalcaemia and the degree of liver and renal involvement.
4 Tissue biopsies for histological classification.
5 HTLV-I status assessed by serology and/or DNA analysis by Southern blots with specific probes for HTLV-I.

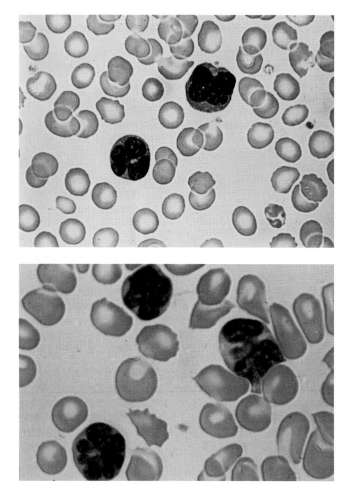

Fig. 7.1 ATLL cells in peripheral blood films showing marked nuclear irregularities characteristic of flower-like cells.

Morphological diagnosis

Leucocytosis with very atypical lymphoid cells is a consistent finding in the leukaemic forms of ATLL. The white blood cell count tends to rise over a short period of time, except in the chronic cases in which it may be stable for months or years.

Examination of peripheral blood films is one of the most important diagnostic procedures in ATLL. The lymphocytes are characterized by marked pleomorphism with respect to size, nuclear irregularities and degree of chromatin condensation. The most typical cell is a medium-sized lymphocyte with a highly irregular nucleus, often polylobed, which gives the designation 'flower-like' (Fig. 7.1). The nuclear indentations in ATLL cells are readily visible by light microscopy. This is not the case in the hyperchromatic cerebriform cells of Sézary's syndrome; these have very narrow indentations which often require ultrastructural analysis for their visualization. In some cases, however, a minor proportion of lymphocytes in ATLL may resemble Sézary cells. The cytoplasm of ATLL cells is often scanty and agranular and nucleoli are inconspicuous. Large

immunoblast-like cells with loose nuclear chromatin, prominent nucleoli and basophilic cytoplasm are occasionally identified in the peripheral blood, but usually they represent less than 5% of the lymphoid cells. These cells are often more abundant in lymph nodes, which thus resemble a large cell NHL of immunoblastic type.

The blood picture tends to be less pleomorphic in chronic ATLL, although cells with an irregular nuclear outline still predominate and, in smouldering ATLL, only a minority (<3%) of lymphocytes are polylobated; a picture seen in healthy HTLV-I carriers.

The bone marrow is not heavily involved in ATLL. Atypical lymphocytes with the same morphology as those in the peripheral blood are admixed with normal haemopoietic cells. Although bone marrow trephines and aspirates are informative, they are not essential for diagnosis.

Hypercalcaemia

This is the most characteristic and distinct biochemical abnormality of ATLL. Hypercalcaemia is extremely rare in NHL [22] and in other types of T-cell malignancy. Half of the cases in the study reported here had elevated serum calcium levels at presentation which developed in several others during the course of the disease (Table 7.1). Hypercalcaemia is more frequent in patients with high white blood cell counts; it is only associated with osteolytic lesions, documented either by X-ray and/or bone scan, in 15%.

The mechanism of hypercalcaemia is thought to be related to the release of cytokines by the malignant cells, particularly parathyroid-related protein (PTH-rP), IL-1 and tumour necrosis factor beta (TNFβ), as serum levels of PTH and 1,25 hydroxyvitamin D_3 are not increased. ATLL cells in culture and HTLV-I+ cell lines have been shown to produce and release PTH-rP to the media and to express PTH-rP messenger RNA [23]. Furthermore, the gene coding for PTH-rP has been shown to be highly expressed in ATLL cells and in lymphocytes from HTLV-I carriers, correlating with the proportion of HTLV-I infected cells [24]. These findings suggest that infection with HTLV-I induces the expression of the PTH-rP gene. This is supported by evidence that HTLV-I tax causes transactivation of the PTH-rP promoters on these cells [24].

Other biochemical tests

Serum lactic dehydrogenase (LDH), albumin levels, and estimation of the liver and renal function may help in the patient's management, to distinguish acute from chronic ATLL and assess the extent of the disease. There is evidence that serum levels of beta-2-microglobulin have prognostic significance, with those patients with high levels having poor outcome and shorter survival [25]. The prognostic significance of mutations of the p53 gene has also recently been reported. These are frequently found in the acute type, either presenting *d'amblee* or

Table 7.3 Immunological markers in ATLL*: I.

Marker	% of positive cases†
TdT/CD1a (thymic marker)	0
Er/CD2 (E-rosette receptor)	86
CD3 (membrane expression)	76‡
CD5	92
CD7	15
CD4+ CD8–	93
CD4+ CD8+	6
CD4– CD8–	2
CD25 (alpha-chain IL-2 receptor)	88
HLA-DR (Class II MHC)	47
CD38	66

* Based on our series of ATLL cases.
† More than 20% of cells positive with a given antibody.
‡ Cells from two cases were membrane CD3– but cytoplasmic CD3+.

Table 7.4 Immunological markers in ATLL*: II.

Functional phenotype	MAb		% of positive cases
	CD45RA	CD29/CD45RO	
'Hybrid'	++	++	50
'Helper-inducer'	–	++	50

* Ten cases studied.

Immunological markers

ATLL cells display a mature/post-thymic T-cell phenotype, being always negative with CD1a, a marker of cortical thymocytes, and the nuclear enzyme terminal deoxynucleotidyl transferase (TdT). The cells are positive with most T-cell markers, CD2 or E-rosette receptor, CD3 and CD5 (Table 7.3). CD3 is always positive in the cytoplasm of these cells but may be weakly expressed or even negative when tested on the membrane in a minority of cases [27]. It has been suggested that the defective membrane expression of CD3 and of the T-cell receptor complex results from cell activation, and that this plays a pathogenetic role in the development and/or progression of ATLL [28]. A novel serum factor designated CD3 down-regulatory factor has been recently documented in ATLL [29]. CD7 is often negative in ATLL and this contrasts with findings in T-prolymphocytic leukaemia (T-PLL), in which this monoclonal antibody (MAb) is always positive [30].

ATLL cells characteristically express in their membrane the p55 alpha chain of the IL-2 receptor detected by anti-Tac (CD25). Other T-cell activation antigens—Class II MHC determinants and CD38—are less often positive.

Reactivity with MAbs which identify the two major T-cell subsets, CD4 and CD8–, indicates that ATLL cells from most cases have a CD4+, CD8– phenotype. This is similar to findings in other T-cell malignancies [30,31]. The coexpression or lack of expression of CD4 and CD8 is rare and is more commonly seen in lymph nodes than in the circulating cells. It has been suggested that the rare cases of acute ATLL with CD4+, CD8+ cells have a more aggressive clinical course [32] than those with the more common CD4+, CD8– phenotype.

Despite their phenotype, ATLL cells suppress *in vitro* B-cell differentiation as measured by the B-cell immunoglobulin (Ig) synthesis on a pokeweed mitogen-driven system [33,34]. It is still controversial whether the leukaemic cells suppress directly the synthesis of Ig or act instead as inducers of suppression, whose function is thought to be mediated by CD4–, CD8+ lymphocytes. Immunophenotypic studies with MAbs that identify two functional subpopulations of normal blood CD4+ lymphocytes, the suppressor-inducer/naive cells (CD45RA+) and the helper-inducer/primed cells (CD29+/CD45R0+), have not clarified this issue either. In fact, in 50% of cases ATLL cells coexpress all these antigens; this is a 'hybrid phenotype' (Table 7.4), a pattern which is rarely found in normal CD4+ lymphocytes. In the other 50% of cases, ATLL cells have a 'helper-inducer' phenotype [35,36]. These findings are supported by observations in healthy HTLV-I+ carriers in whom all the CD4+ lymphocytes infected with HTLV-I have the CD45R0+ helper-inducer phenotype [37], which is found in normal individuals in 50% of CD4+ cells.

Interleukin-2 receptors

A special feature of ATLL cells is the expression of a high number of IL-2 receptors [38–40]. Normal resting T-lymphocytes only acquire these receptors upon activation. IL-2 receptors can be detected in the patients' sera by an enzyme-linked immunosorbent assay (ELISA). The serum levels correlate with tumour load, and they are significantly higher in the acute and lymphoma forms than in the chronic and smouldering types and in HTLV-I+ carriers [41,42].

Early work suggested that the expression of the IL-2 receptors played a key role in the development of ATLL. The bases of this hypothesis were.

1 The higher number of IL-2 receptors displayed by ATLL cells compared to normal activated T-lymphocytes. This was later shown to result from the continuous transcription of the IL-2 receptor gene with increased levels of IL-2 receptor mRNA [43].

2 The infection of normal cells with HTLV-I results on IL-2 receptor expression (cells become anti-Tac positive) [44,45]. It has been shown that, in contrast to normal controls, HTLV-I+ healthy carriers have Tac+ lymphocytes in the circulation [46].

3 The growth of some HTLV-I+ ATLL cell lines becomes independent of exogenous IL-2 some time after culture. Again this is different from findings with normal T cells.

These arguments have supported the view that the leukaemia is maintained by an autocrine mechanism of growth, firstly requiring IL-2 and subsequently becoming independent of it. This theory was weakened when it was shown that ATLL cells do not secrete IL-2 to promote growth, do not have increased levels of mRNA for IL-2 and do not respond with proliferation to exogenous IL-2 despite the abundance of this receptor. Still, a possible role for IL-2 receptors in leukaemogenesis has not been ruled out. In healthy carriers, HTLV-I infection turns on the IL-2 receptor gene, resulting in lymphocytes in a permanent state of 'activation' and thus highly susceptible to other factors which may promote the emergence of a malignant clone.

Histology of affected tissues

Histological analysis is always necessary in the lymphoma form of ATLL and less systematically in cases presenting as leukaemia. The tissues most frequently examined are lymph nodes, skin and bone marrow. Although there is no unique histological pattern for ATLL and there is a degree of overlap with findings in other T-cell malignancies, some features have emerged as characteristic.

Lymph nodes

There is always a diffuse pattern of infiltration and a marked degree of pleomorphism (Fig. 7.2). Analysis of 56 T-NHL, including HTLV-I+ and HTLV-I- cases by Lennert *et al.* [47], showed that 70% of cases with the pleomorphic type of NHL, particularly those with large- and medium-sized cells, corresponded to HTLV-I+ cases. However, pleomorphism by itself does not allow for a case to be classified as HTLV-I+. In addition, a minority of cases may have a diffuse pattern of infiltration by small cells. Similarly, immunohistochemical findings are not unique to ATLL. For instance, reactivity with anti-Tac and lack of expression of CD7 are the most frequent patterns in ATLL but are not exclusive of this disease [47,48].

Some difficulties exist in applying the NCI Working Formulation or the Kiel Classification [49,50] to classify HTLV-I+ lymphomas, because ATLL does not fit into a single disease category. Some cases may be classified as high grade whereas others may fit into the intermediate grade and, rarely, they appear as low grade based on the histological and cytological characteristics. For instance, large cells and/or immunoblasts may be the predominant population in some cases, whereas in others there is an admixture of small, medium and large cells. In the recently reported proposals for the classification of lymphomas by the International Lymphoma Study Group, ATLL is placed as a separate entity within the peripheral T-cell lymphomas but without a specific histological pattern [51].

ATLL cells show marked nuclear irregularities in lymph

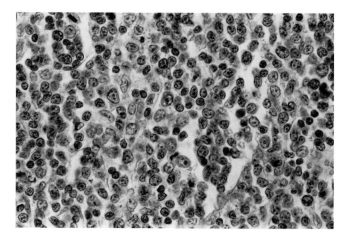

Fig. 7.2 Lymph-node biopsy from an ATLL case showing infiltration by lymphoid cells of variable size and degree of chromatin condensation.

nodes as seen in the peripheral blood. Immunoblasts are large, have a regular or oval nucleus with open chromatin, one or several nucleoli and a deeply basophilic cytoplasm [52]. No major differences in lymph-node histology have been reported between Japanese and Caribbean cases. Only rare cases will display patterns suggestive of angioimmunoblastic lymphadenopathy or Hodgkin's disease, including the presence of atypical giant cells resembling Reed–Sternberg cells in a lymphocytic background [53,54].

Skin lesions

Cutaneous lesions in ATLL are seen in 30–40% of patients [55]. They often constitute the first clinical manifestation in smouldering ATLL preceding by months or years a florid leukaemic phase. The skin infiltration usually involves the dermis (Fig. 7.3). Epidermotropism and even Pautrier's microabcesses resembling the lesions seen in mycosis fungoides and Sézary's syndrome have been documented in some Japanese, Caribbean and Brazilian patients with ATLL [6,50,55]. The lymphocytes infiltrating the skin are pleomorphic and convoluted and have features similar to those of circulating ATLL cells. Typical Sézary-like cells with serpentine/cerebriform nucleus are rare. The presence of epidermotropism and Sézary-like cells in the skin infiltrates may still be compatible with a diagnosis of HTLV-I+ ATLL if other features of the disease are present.

Serological surveys in patients with cutaneous T-cell lymphoma in nonendemic areas have shown that HTLV-I is not associated with this group of disorders [56]. Unusual cases of HTLV-I+ mycosis fungoides have nevertheless been documented in Japan [57] and a case of HTLV-I+ positive Sézary cell leukaemia has been studied in a Caucasian patient born in Greece [58]. It is uncertain whether some of these cases should be reclassified as ATLL based on the HTLV-I findings. If the clin-

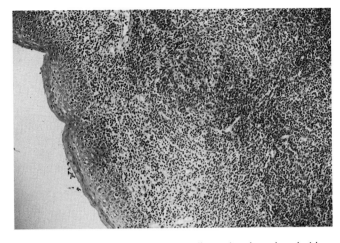

Fig. 7.3 Skin biopsy from a case of ATLL illustrating dense lymphoid infiltration but confined to the dermis.

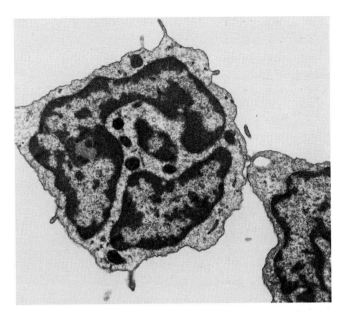

Fig. 7.4 Electron photomicrograph from a patient with ATLL showing a typical circulating cell with an irregular nucleus divided into three nuclear lobes.

icopathological features are typical of one of the known T-cell disorders, then a diagnosis of ATLL should not be made based only on HTLV-I serology. On the other hand, if a T-cell malignancy does not fit into any of the well-defined disease entities, the threshold for diagnosing ATLL should be low, as it is apparent that this disease is quite variable in its clinical and laboratory manifestations.

Bone marrow

This is usually moderately involved in ATLL, both in the leukaemia and lymphoma forms, suggesting that the disease originates in peripheral lymphoid tissues rather than in the bone marrow. The marrow aspirates may show 5–20% of convoluted lymphocytes. The most characteristic feature in the trephine biopsies is a marked proliferation of osteoclasts which are responsible for and correlate with the hypercalcaemia of ATLL [59].

Electron microscopy of acute T-cell leukaemia/lymphoma cells

Although ultrastructural analysis is not required for a diagnosis of ATLL, it is helpful in difficult cases, particularly when considering the alternative diagnoses of small cell variant of Sézary's syndrome or T-PLL. Electron microscopy allows a more precise assessment of the morphology and nuclear irregularities. A range of small to large cells, as seen by light microscopy, is also recognized by electron microscopy. The most characteristic cell type is a medium size lymphocyte with a highly irregular nucleus, often comprising two or more independent nuclear lobes (Fig. 7.4). Rarely the nucleus of these cells adopts the cerebriform or serpentine configuration of Sézary cells. In the latter condition, the nuclear indentations are narrow and the number of nuclear segments is two or less.

The ratio between the length of the longest indentation and the maximal nuclear diameter (I/N) is greater than 0.66 in at least 22% of cells from Sézary's syndrome, whereas in ATLL this ratio is seen only in 10% of cells. Several studies have suggested that ATLL can be distinguished from Sézary cells by ultrastructural analysis but there is some degree of overlap [60,61]. Nucleoli are usually small except in immunoblasts which often display one to three nucleoli. The amount and type of cytoplasmic organelles varies from case to case but deposits of glycogen, as seen in Sézary cells, and lysosomal granules are common in ATLL [61]. Cells in two cases that we studied had parallel tubular arrays, a structure characteristic of normal and leukaemic large granular lymphocytes.

Evidence of HTLV-I infection can be demonstrated by electron microscopy after ATLL cells are cultured for 5–7 days in the presence of mitogens and IL-2 by the budding and release of type-C retrovirus particles from the cell membrane [46,62] (Fig. 7.5).

Detection of HTLV-I

This represents one of the most important tests for the diagnosis of ATLL. Serum antibodies (IgM, IgG) to HTLV-I can be detected by serological assays or by demonstrating viral or proviral proteins in the infected cells. The serological assays commercially available are of variable sensitivity and specificity. ELISA and radioimmunoassay are the most commonly used. Both are highly sensitive but not specific enough. For example, ELISA may have 1–2% false positives, mainly in patients with autoimmune disorders and/or hypergamma-

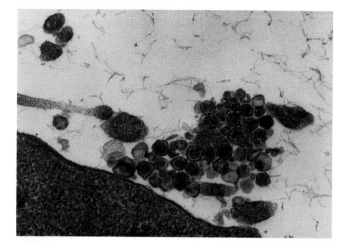

Fig. 7.5 Electron photomicrograph of a cell from a healthy HTLV-I carrier after 25-day culture showing release of type-C retrovirus particles.

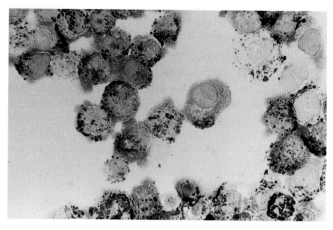

Fig. 7.6 HTLV-I-infected cells showing strong reactivity with a MAb against the HTLV-I core protein p19 (immunoperoxidase technique).

globulinaemia. The gelatin particle agglutination test is widely used in Japan as first-line screening because of its simplicity and low cost; its specificity is similar to that of ELISA. The indirect immunofluorescence test introduced by Hinuma *et al.* [63] and its modification, indirect immunoperoxidase, applied by us [64] uses acetone-fixed HTLV-I+ cells on cytocentrifuge slides. The most specific assay for antibody analysis is Western blotting that uses purified HTLV-I proteins extracted from infected cells. Sera with antibodies to HTLV-I are revealed as discrete specific bands into a nitrocellulose paper corresponding to the major core proteins p19, p24-, envelope protein gp46-, transmembrane protein gp21 and tax protein. Confirmation of HTLV-I infection requires positivity for at least two viral gene protein products [65]. Western blotting also allows, to some extent, to distinguish HTLV-I from the closely related virus HTLV-II. The nucleotide sequence homology between these two retroviruses (65%) does not allow a distinction by standard serological tests, whereas a differential pattern of bands by Western blotting, strong p19 and negative or weak p24, indicates HTLV-I and the reverse pattern suggests HTLV-II. When results are not clear cut, molecular analysis by the polymerase chain reaction (PCR) is required to identify type-specific viral sequences [66].

A number of new assays useful for the serological discrimination between HTLV-I and HTLV-II have recently become available. These are Western blotting using recombinant proteins which contain amino-acid sequences for the envelope proteins, gp46 for HTLV-I and gp52 for HTLV-II [67], and ELISA methods using synthetic peptides derived from gp46 and gp21 [68]. The use of these assays will reduce the need for more laborious and costly investigations.

HTLV-I can also be detected by investigating the expression of the retroviral core proteins p19 and p24 by indirect immunofluorescence or immunoperoxidase methods with MAbs specific to p19 and p24 (Fig. 7.6) [46]. This assay requires *in vitro* culture, as the leukaemic or normal HTLV-I infected cells do not express these core proteins on the resting state. Molecular analysis allows the detection of proviral DNA integrated in the host DNA by Southern blotting using specific probes for HTLV-I [69] and PCR, which is very sensitive when using primers for the gag, env and tax HTLV-I proteins [66]. Southern blotting can demonstrate a monoclonal pattern of integration of HTLV-I proviral DNA in ATLL cells. HTLV-I integration is not detectable by this method in seropositive carriers but, if detected, shows a polyclonal pattern.

Relationship of HTLV-I with acute T-cell leukaemia/lymphoma and other diseases

The role of retroviruses as aetiological agents in animal leukaemias has been known for many years [70]. Major advances took place in the 1970s with the discovery of reverse transcriptase, which is essential for the replication and DNA integration of retroviruses, and of T-cell growth factor (IL-2) which allowed the long-term culture of T-lymphocytes. These discoveries led to the first isolation of HTLV-I by Gallo *et al.* [2,56] from cultured cells from a black patient, diagnosed first as mycosis fungoides and later revised as ATLL [71]. Almost at the same time, Hinuma *et al.* [63] discovered, in a cell line established by Miyoshi from a patient with ATLL, a retrovirus, then designated ATLV. The identity between HTLV-I and ATLV was later established [72]. Serological surveys in the early 1980s in Japan established the link between the disease and the virus by showing that the majority of patients with ATLL have antibodies to HTLV-I. The association of HTLV-I with ATLL was later established in black Caribbeans resident in the UK [73]. Subsequent seroepidemiological surveys in the Caribbean [74] identified this region together with Japan as the main endemic areas for the retrovirus. Definitive evidence for the aetiological role of HTLV-I came from the demonstration of monoclonal integration of proviral DNA in the leukaemic cells [69], confirming that ATLL arises from the malignant transformation of a cell previously infected with HTLV-I.

It has become apparent in the last few years that HTLV-I is linked to a spectrum of diseases other than ATLL. Although their intimate pathogenic mechanism is unknown, it is suspected that they result from an immunological imbalance, immunosuppression or hyperimmune response resulting from the infection with HTLV-I.

The best documented of these disorders is HTLV-I associated myelopathy, also known as tropical spastic paraparesis (TSP) [75,76]. This is a progressive spastic myelopathy which affects primarily the spinal cord. The disease clusters in the same areas as HTLV-I and ATLL and can be distinguished from other chronic myelopathies, for example multiple sclerosis. Unlike ATLL, TSP affects predominantly females and in the UK is seen among the black population immigrant from the Caribbean [77]. Patients with TSP have a high titre of antibodies to HTLV-I in the serum and in the CSF. The blood from TSP patients has lymphocytes which undergo spontaneous proliferation and a subpopulation of cytotoxic CD8+ T cells which recognize HTLV-I proteins and are able to kill HTLV-I infected cells [68]. These cytotoxic cells may play a role in the aetiopathogenesis of TSP. Post-mortem findings demonstrate infiltration of the damaged CNS by CD8+ lymphocytes and macrophages. TSP and ATLL have been found rarely associated in the same patients in Japan and in the Caribbean [78–81] and recently in three Chilean patients [82]. Usually, the leukaemia has a protractive clinical course corresponding to that of smouldering and chronic ATLL or presents as lymphoma. The low occurrence of ATLL (1/1500) and TSP (1/2500) among HTLV-I carriers explains the low incidence of both diseases occurring simultaneously.

Polymyositis is another manifestation of HTLV-I infection. Clinically and pathologically it is indistinguishable from the disease seen in HTLV-I⁻ individuals, but its incidence is higher in those infected with the retrovirus [83].

HTLV-I associated arthropathy is a recently described disorder also linked to HTLV-I. It may be seen in TSP or, rarely, in ATLL patients [84,85] and it is characterized by synovial proliferation and lymphocytic infiltration with atypical convoluted cells. It has been postulated that HTLV-I infected cells stimulate directly or through the release of cytokines, in particular IL-1, the proliferation of synovial cells leading to the arthropathy.

Other manifestations seen in adult carriers of HTLV-I include pulmonary infiltrates, peripheral neuropathy, uveitis, etc. Of interest, too, are the clinical manifestations in HTLV-I+ children and infants born from seropositive mothers, chiefly a syndrome of persistent lymphadenopathy and a form of eczema or chronic dermatitis.

Epidemiology

Two main geographical areas, southwest of Japan and the Caribbean islands, were recognized in the 1980s to be endemic for HTLV-I and ATLL. It also became apparent that both were prevalent among Japanese and Caribbean populations immigrant to the USA and Europe respectively [11,73,86]. Evidence for HTLV-I infection was reported subsequently from West and Central Africa [2]. Although some of the latter findings have been conflicting, possibly as a result of cross-reactivity with HIV proteins in some of the serological assays, some studies were confirmed by Western blotting [87]. Although HTLV-I associated diseases have not been reported with high frequency in Africa, some cases of ATLL have been documented [88] and two such patients are included in our series.

In Japan, HTLV-I is prevalent in Kyushu, Shikoku and Okinawa. The most recent nationwide study estimated an annual incidence of about 700 cases of ATLL. Half of them originated in Kyushu and the remainder in metropolitan areas. The risk for developing ATLL appears to be 1.5 times higher in males [89]. Clusters of ATLL and seropositivity for HTLV-I have been also observed in northern regions such as Hokkaido and Tohaku [90].

ATLL is prevalent in most islands of the Caribbean, Jamaica, Trinidad and Martinique, etc., where over two-thirds of lymphomas are of the T-cell type and most have the features of ATLL [74,91,92]. The majority of patients in our series originated from these and other islands, including St Vincent, Guyana and Dominique. HTLV-I is not prevalent in Cuba despite its vicinity to Jamaica [93]. This difference may relate to racial rather than geographical factors after these islands were colonized. For example, Jamaica was colonized in the seventeenth century by the British, who took African slaves which became the main black population [91]. Cuba was colonized by the Spanish and although slaves were brought from Africa, there was a high degree of intermarriage between the races and, as a result, the black African population never became predominant. They now represent 15% of the population, with the remainder being mulattos and white Europeans.

Seroepidemiological studies, and a detailed investigation of T-lymphoid malignancies, have lead to the discovery of new geographical clusters for ATLL. Thus, HTLV-I infection has now been shown to occur in some South American countries, in particular, Colombia and Chile where TSP has also been documented [94,95] as well as ATLL [96–98]. Fourteen Brazilian patients have been reported with ATLL in a series which included five whites of Portuguese descent [6] and, more recently, it has been shown that ATLL is one of the commonest diseases within the spectrum of T-cell malignancies [10], correlating with a high rate of seroprevalence in this country which in blood donors is 0.5% [99].

A high prevalence of HTLV-I antibodies among the Mashadi Jews who originated from northeastern Iran has been reported [100]. Few patients with ATLL have been documented in Iran

[101] and two patients in our series were born there. A HTLV-I+ cluster has been recognized in an Iraqi family with two members suffering from lymphoma and TSP respectively [102]. More recently, a high seroprevalence for HTLV-I has been reported in Melanesia, particularly in Papua New Guinea and the Solomon Islands and in Australian aborigines [103,104]. Data on the molecular characterization of HTLV-I in some of the Melanesian and Australian variants differ in nucleotide sequence up to 9% from the Japanese and Caribbean isolates and share some homology with the simian T-lymphotropic viruses (STLV) [105]. These data would support the old origin of HTLV-I with an independent evolution in these areas or its origin in nonhuman primates.

Modes of transmission of HTLV-I

HTLV-I is an exogenous retrovirus which is transmitted by viable infected cells. The major route of transmission is horizontal from mother to child. The prevalence of HTLV-I carriers in children born from seropositive mothers in Japan is about 22% [106]. The intrauterine or vertical route of transmission is rare (1–4% of HTLV-I infection in infants), although HTLV-I infected T-lymphocytes have been demonstrated in cord blood [107]. The transmission during the postnatal period is by breastfeeding [106]. There is evidence for both HTLV-I infected cells in mother's milk and oral infection through human milk in animal models. An active prophylactic programme is currently in progress in Japan aimed at refraining HTLV-I positive mothers from breastfeeding. Preliminary results show a significant decline in mother to child transmission [106].

Another major route of HTLV-I transmission is through cellular blood products. This was initially suspected because of a relative high frequency of HTLV-I antibodies in the sera from patients with haematological malignancies, other than ATLL, who had received multiple transfusions. The rate of transmission is as high as 32–53% in some studies [68,108]. The risk for seroconversion is greater when the blood is stored for less than 6 days, suggesting that infected viable cells are required for the successful transmission of HTLV-I. Kataoka *et al.* [109] demonstrated the transmission in rabbits with as little as 0.01 ml of HTLV-I infected blood. This raises the issue of the risk for HTLV-I infection by accidental inoculation among laboratory workers. Screening for HTLV-I on blood products started in Japan in 1986 and this is currently taking place also in other endemic areas including the USA. These policies seem to be having a positive effect, as shown by the decrease in HTLV-I infection in recipients of blood products [110,111]. In the UK, a recent survey from the North London Blood Transfusion Centre has shown a low frequency (1/20 000) of true, confirmed HTLV-I antibody-positive individuals among the blood donors [112] and therefore these data probably do not justify the costs of universal blood donation screening in this country.

Although TSP may develop in patients who have acquired the retroviral infection by blood transfusion, ATLL has not been reported or seems extremely rare. On the other hand, there has been a recent report of a case of ATLL following allogeneic bone marrow transplantation; the donor lymphocytes became infected by HTLV-I [113].

The sexual route of transmission, from male to female, has been suggested by seroepidemiological data and by the presence of HTLV-I infected cells in the seminal fluid of carriers. Unlike HIV, the transmission of HTLV-I by this route requires many years of sexual relation and therefore it is likely that it does not represent the major route of spread of this virus [106].

Pathogenesis of HTLV-I induced malignancy

The mechanisms by which HTLV-I causes ATLL are still unknown. HTLV-I does not carry an oncogene and, without exception, the tumour cells are monoclonal with respect to the site of proviral integration [69]. In contrast with retroviruses involved in animal malignancies, HTLV-I is nonrandomly integrated into the DNA [114]. Animal viruses, for example avian leukaemia virus, either carry an oncogene or integrate in a specific site near to a proto-oncogene [115].

HTLV-I has the basic genes of retroviruses: *gag, pol* and *env*, which code, respectively, for the internal core proteins, the enzyme reverse transcriptase and the envelope proteins. In common with HTLV-II, HIV and the simian and bovine leukaemia viruses, the nucleotide sequence of HTLV-I has revealed a novel region known as the long open reading (lor) frame [66]. In this region a protein of 40 KDa which codes for the *tax* (transactivator) gene and previously designated *px* [66,115,116], has been considered responsible for the cellular transformation and immortalization of the infected cells by inducing the continuous expression of IL-2 and IL-2 receptor genes. The tax protein appears to be involved in the post-transcriptional activation of cellular genes which bind to the provirus long terminal repeat (LTR) and upregulate its transcription [117,118]. Another gene designated *rex* [119] seems to regulate the expression of the *tax* gene and facilitate the transport of the virus from the nucleus to the cytoplasm. Thus, HTLV-I viral replication and gene expression is controlled by these two viral regulators, tax and rex.

Because only 1 in 1500 HTLV-I carriers develops ATLL, and there is a long period of latency between HTLV-I infection and the development of the disease (usually over 20 years), a mechanism of leukaemogenesis through multiple steps has been suggested [118,120]. The initial oncogenic step is HTLV-I infection and additional events, for example chromosome aberrations, are likely to be involved in the evolution of the T-cell clone and the development of ATLL. There is a minority of patients who are HTLV-I⁻ and this suggests that the role of HTLV-I may be substituted by other factors in rare cases. Detailed studies on HTLV-I carriers and cases of smouldering

ATLL may elucidate the late steps of oncogenesis and the critical factors involved in the development of ATLL.

Chromosome abnormalities

Cytogenetic abnormalities are found in up to 90% of ATLL cases, particularly in the lymphoma and acute types [121]. Most of the reports come from Japan [122–124], but findings in Caribbean patients [125,126] show similar abnormalities. Unlike other malignancies such as Burkitt's lymphoma, the chromosome changes are not specific to ATLL. The most frequent numerical changes are trisomies of chromosomes 3,7 and in females, monosomy X. Structural abnormalities are often complex; they frequently involve 6q, 14q, 3q, 1q and 10p. Deletion of chromosome 6 occurs often at bands q15 and/or q21; this is also found in cutaneous T-cell lymphoma and in T-PLL [126]. Abnormalities of chromosome 14, seen in about 17% of cases, involve bands q32 or q11. The rearrangement inv(14) (q11q32), which is characteristic of T-PLL [127], is rare in ATLL [121]. Chromosome changes are less frequent and not as complex in smouldering ATLL as in the other clinical forms. This implies that chromosome aberrations correlate with disease progression. In this context, Sanada *et al.* [16] reported a case of smouldering ATLL with monoclonal integration of HTLV-I but in whom four different clones were documented by cytogenetic analysis. This suggests that all the abnormal clones were derived from a cell with a normal karyotype infected by HTLV-I.

Diagnostic criteria and differential diagnosis

Because of overlapping features between the mature T-cell malignancies, the diagnosis of ATLL should always be based on a multiparameter approach which takes into account clinical and laboratory features, HTLV-I status and geographical factors. A constellation of findings which are highly characteristic, if not unique, to ATLL are hypercalcaemia, a pleomorphic blood picture with convoluted or 'flower' cells displaying a CD4+ CD25+ phenotype and clustering of the disease in regions endemic for HTLV-I. Demonstration of HTLV-I antibodies in the patient's sera is an essential confirmatory test. The serological documentation of HTLV-I may not in itself be diagnostic in endemic areas, because of the prevalence of HTLV-I in patients with other types of malignancies. DNA analysis demonstrating the clonal integration of the HTLV-I proviral DNA in the tumour cells is required to confirm the diagnosis and it is essential when the overall picture is not characteristic of ATLL.

The differential diagnosis of ATLL always arises with two mature T-cell disorders, T-PLL and Sézary's syndrome, in which the cells have a CD4+ phenotype and may also express CD25. Hypercalcaemia is not seen in these diseases and the patients have other features, for example splenomegaly and an elevated white blood cell count greater than $100 \times 10^9/l$ in T-PLL, and diffuse erythroderma in Sézary's syndrome. The morphology of the leukaemic T cells is also distinct, although difficult cases require the use of electron microscopy to analyse in detail the cell morphology. HTLV-I is, with few exceptions [57,58,128], negative in Sézary's syndrome and cutaneous T-cell lymphoma [56]. Although recent reports have suggested that a subgroup of cutaneous T-cell lymphomas may be associated with HTLV-I or to a close related retrovirus by the presence of retroviral sequences in the cell DNA and/or release of retrovirus particles after cell culture [129,130], our preliminary findings do not confirm this. In addition, these data should be taken with caution as a clonal integration of the virus into the neoplastic cells has not been demonstrated and all these cases of bona fide cutaneous T-cell lymphomas are, unlike ATLL, HTLV-I antibody negative. A link has not been established either between HTLV-I and T-PLL, as all our cases were HTLV-I negative including two black patients born in the Caribbean [131]. In addition, no link was found in an unusual case of Sézary's syndrome with immunoblastic transformation in a black Caribbean, whose cells had a CD4+ CD25+ phenotype, and the lymph-node histology may well be consistent with the diagnosis of ATLL [132].

A different problem is caused by the few cases of HTLV-I-ATLL documented in a Brazilian series [6,10] and others reported from Japan [133,134]. In none of these was there any serological or molecular evidence of HTLV-I involvement, whereas the clinical and laboratory features were otherwise consistent with ATLL. An analogy can be drawn with Burkitt's lymphoma in which there is a clear association with Epstein–Barr virus (EBV) in the majority of African patients but which is lacking in the sporadic disease with the same features in nonendemic areas. In order to improve the diagnostic criteria for ATLL, a scoring system has recently been proposed which integrates a number of clinical and laboratory features (Table 7.5). By applying this proposal, all ATLL studied scored 5 or over, with more than half scoring between 8 and 10, and this included the five Brazilian patients who were HTLV-I- by serology and PCR [10]. In contrast, the score in T-cell malignancies, other than ATLL, is always less than 5. This system may be helpful to distinguish HTLV-I- ATLL from non-ATLL disorders.

Prognosis and treatment

ATLL is an aggressive malignancy with poor prognosis; the median survival ranges from 5 to 13 months [135–137; our own data] in Caribbean and Japanese patients. Acute ATLL responds poorly to therapeutic modalities used in high-grade NHL such as CHOP (cyclophosphamide, vincristine, doxorubicin, prednisolone) or M-BACOP (Table 7.6). The lymphoma form of ATLL, although also often resistant to therapy, has a slightly better prognosis. It has been suggested that the resistance to chemotherapy in ATLL is related to the overexpression of the p-glycoprotein encoded by the multidrug resistant

Table 7.5 Scoring system for the diagnosis of ATLL.

Feature	Score 2	Score 1	Score 0
T-markers positive	CD4+ CD25+	CD4+ only	CD4−
Morphology (LM, TEM)	Typical ATLL cells	Not typical of ATLL, T-PLL or Sézary's syndrome	Typical Sézary's syndrome and T-PLL cells

Histology
  Lymph node
  Skin (infiltration area)
		Pleomorphic T cell
		Dermis
			Epidermis

HTLV-I (serology, DNA)	Positive		Negative
Clinical features Hypercalcaemia	Present		Absent
Geographical clustering		Endemic area	Sporadic

LM = light microscopy; TEM = transmission electron microscopy.

Table 7.6 Response to treatment in ATLL*.

Therapy	Number of patients	Partial	Complete
CHOP/M-BACOP	27	6	5
Deoxycoformycin	25	1	2
Etoposide (oral)	4	0	2
ALL-type regimen	3	3	0

* Results in our series. Includes patients who have received more than one treatment modality.

gene [138]. Patients with the chronic and smouldering forms of ATLL run a protracted clinical course until progression occurs and then the disease becomes acute. Extracorporeal photochemotherapy has been used in a few chronic and smouldering ATLL patients with some benefit for the skin lesions [139]. Transient spontaneous remissions have been documented in few cases [140–142].

The majority of ATLL patients have been treated with CHOP or similar combinations and some good partial or complete responses have been obtained, particularly when higher doses and more frequent injections are given, as with the combination VEPA (vincristine, doxorubicin, prednisolone, cyclophosphamide) used in Japan [137]. Other treatments employed include the adenosine deaminase inhibitor 2′ deoxycoformycin and the MAb anti-Tac [143–145]. When deoxycoformycin was used in 25 cases of ATLL, responses were documented in only three, one partial and two complete [146]. One of the two complete remitters relapsed 3 years later and was then resistant to deoxycoformycin; the other patient died when in complete remission from an opportunistic infec-

tion [147]. The results of chemotherapy in our series is given in Table 7.6. Of interest is the complete response in two patients with etoposide used as a single agent, lasting 3 and 12 months.

ATLL patients have a high incidence of opportunistic infections, particularly lung infiltrates [12]. These are often not related to the degree of neutropenia and can be seen in both treated and untreated patients and may occur during remission. It is likely that they result from the immunodeficiency state caused by HTLV-I. This is supported by the high frequency of infections seen also in healthy HTLV-I+ carriers.

It is apparent that more effective therapeutical modalities are needed to treat ATLL. One new approach which appears to be attractive, and with potential for responses, is a conjugate of recombinant IL-2 with diphtheria toxin which was shown *in vitro* to be highly cytotoxic to ATLL cells [148]. Another strategy has recently been delineated with the use of a combination of interferon alpha and zidovudine. Preliminary results in few ATLL patients are encouraging, with half of them achieving complete or partial responses [149,150]. A larger number of patients needs to be evaluated and also long-term follow-up is needed to see whether such responses are long-lasting.

References

1 Takatsuki K., Uchiyama J., Sagawa K. *et al.* (1977) Adult T-cell leukaemia in Japan. In: *Topics in Hematology* (eds S. Seno, F. Takaku & S. Irino), pp. 73–77. Excerpta Medica, Amsterdam.
2 Gallo R.C., Essex M.E. & Gross L. (eds) (1984) *Human T-cell Leukemia/Lymphoma Virus.* Cold Spring Harbor Laboratory, New York.
3 Yamaguchi K., Nishimura H., Kohrogi H. *et al.* (1983) A proposal for smoldering adult T-cell leukemia: a clinicopathologic study of five cases. *Blood,* **62**, 758–766.
4 Takatsuki K., Yamaguchi K., Kawano F. *et al.* (1985) Clinical

diversity in adult T-cell leukemia-lymphoma. *Cancer Research*, **45**, 4644–4645.

5 Kinoshita K., Amagasaki T., Ikeda S. *et al.* (1985) Preleukemic state of adult T cell leukemia: abnormal T lymphocytosis induced by human adult T cell leukemia-lymphoma virus. *Blood*, **66**, 120–127.

6 Pombo de Oliveira M.S., Matutes E., Famadas L.C. *et al.* (1990) Adult T-cell leukaemia/lymphoma in Brazil and its relation to HTLV-I. *Lancet*, **336**, 987–990.

7 Vilmer E., le Deist F., Fisher A. *et al.* (1985) Smouldering T lymphoma related to HTLV-I in a Sicilian child. *Lancet*, **ii**, 1301–1302.

8 Brindle R.J., Eglin R.P., Parsons A.I. *et al.* (1988) HTLV-I, HIV, hepatitis B and hepatitis delta in the Pacific and Southeast Asia. A serological survey. *Epidemiology and Infection*, **100**, 153–156.

9 Yamaguchi K., Matutes E., Catovsky D. *et al.* (1987) *Strongyloides stercoralis* as candidate cofactor for HTLV-I induced malignancies. *Lancet*, **ii**, 94–95.

10 Pombo de Oliveira M.S., Matutes E., Schulz T. *et al.* (1995) T-cell malignancies in Brazil. Clinico-pathological and molecular studies of HTLV-I-positive and -negative cases. *International Journal of Cancer*, **60**, 823–827.

11 Bunn P.A. Jr, Schechter G.P., Jaffe E. *et al.* (1983) Clinical course of retrovirus-associated adult T-cell lymphoma in the United States. *New England Journal of Medicine*, **309**, 257–264.

12 Yoshioka R., Yamaguchi K., Yoshinaga T. *et al.* (1985) Pulmonary complications in patients with adult T-cell leukemia. *Cancer*, **55**, 2491–2494.

13 Hattori T., Asou N., Suzushima H. *et al.* (1991) Leukaemia of novel gastrointestinal T-lymphocyte population infected with HTLV-I. *Lancet*, **337**, 76–77.

14 Nakada K., Yamaguchi K., Furugen S. *et al.* (1987) Monoclonal integration of HTLV-I proviral DNA in patients with strongyloidiasis. *International Journal of Cancer*, **40**, 145–148.

15 Shirono K., Hattori T. & Takatsuki K. (1989) Prognostic usefulness of Ki-67 antigen expression of adult T-cell leukaemia. *Lancet*, **ii**, 1044.

16 Sanada I., Nakada K. & Furugen S. (1986) Chromosomal abnormalities in a patient with smoldering adult T-cell leukemia: evidence for a multistep pathogenesis. *Leukemia Research*, **10**, 1377–1382.

17 Yamaguchi K., Seiki M. & Yoshida M. (1984) The detection of human T cell leukemia virus proviral DNA and its application for classification and diagnosis of T cell malignancy. *Blood*, **63**, 1235–1240.

18 Ichimaru M., Kinoshita K., Kamihira S. *et al.* (1982) Familial disposition of adult T-cell leukemia and lymphoma. *GANN Monograph on Cancer Research*, **28**, 185–193.

19 Yamaguchi K., Sung Yul L., Shimizu T. *et al.* (1985) Concurrence of lymphoma type adult T-cell leukemia in three sisters. *Cancer*, **56**, 1688–1690.

20 Ratner L. & Poiesz B.J. (1988) Leukemias associated with human T-cell lymphotropic virus type I in a non-endemic region. *Medicine*, **67**, 401–421.

21 Matutes E., Spittle M.F., Smith N.P. *et al.* (1995) The first report of familial adult T-cell leukaemia lymphoma in the United Kingdom. *British Journal of Haematology*, **89**, 615–619.

22 Canellos G.P. (1974) Hypercalcemia in malignant lymphoma and leukemia. *Annals of the New York Academy of Science*, **230**, 240–246.

23 Honda S., Yamaguchi K., Miyake Y. *et al.* (1988) Production of parathyroid hormone-related protein in adult T-cell leukemia cells. *Japanese Journal of Cancer Research*, **79**, 1264–1268.

24 Watanabe T., Yamaguchi K., Takatsuki K. *et al.* (1990) Constitutive expression of parathyroid hormone-related protein gene in human T cell leukemia virus type 1 (HTLV-I) carriers and adult T cell leukemia patients that can be trans-activated by HTLV-I tax gene. *Journal of Experimental Medicine*, **172**, 759–765.

25 Sadamori N., Mine M., Hakariya S. *et al.* (1995) Clinical significance of B2-microglobulin in serum of adult T cell leukemia. *Leukemia*, **9**, 594–597.

26 Nishimura S., Asou N., Suzushima H. *et al.* (1995) p53 gene mutation and loss of heterozygosity are associated with increased risk of disease progression in adult T cell leukemia. *Leukemia*, **9**, 598–604.

27 Tsuda H. & Takatsuki K. (1984) Specific decrease in T3 antigen density in adult T-cell leukaemia cells: I. Flow microfluorometric analysis. *British Journal of Cancer*, **50**, 843–845.

28 Shirono K., Hattori T., Matsuoka M. *et al.* (1988) Adult T cell leukemia cell lines that originated from primary leukemic clones also had a defect of expression of CD3-T cell receptor complex. *Leukemia*, **2**, 728–733.

29 Maeda Y., Matsuda M., Irimajiri K. & Horiuchi A. (1994) Downregulation of CD3 antigen on adult T cell leukemia cells. *Leukemia and Lymphoma*, **13**, 249–256.

30 Matutes E., Brito-Babapulle V., Worner I. *et al.* (1988) T-cell chronic lymphocytic leukaemia: the spectrum of mature T-cell disorders. *Nouvelle Revue Française d'Hematologie*, **30**, 347–351.

31 Matutes E. & Catovsky D. (1991) Mature T-cell leukemias and leukemia/lymphoma syndromes. Review of our experience in 175 cases. *Leukemia and Lymphoma*, **4**, 81–91.

32 Tamura K., Unoki T., Sagawa K. *et al.* (1985) Clinical features of OKT4+/OKT8+ adult T-cell leukemia. *Leukemia Research*, **9**, 1353–1359.

33 Yamada Y. (1983) Phenotypic and functional analysis of leukemic cells from 16 patients with adult T-cell leukemia/lymphoma. *Blood*, **61**, 192–199.

34 Miedema F., Terpstra F.G., Smit J.W. *et al.* (1984) Functional properties of neoplastic T cells in adult T-cell lymphoma/leukemia patients from the Caribbean. *Blood*, **63**, 477–481.

35 Worner I., Matutes E., Beverley P.C.L. *et al.* (1990) The distribution of CD45R, CD29 and CD45RO (UCHL1) antigens in mature CD4 positive T-cell leukaemias. *British Journal of Haematology*, **74**, 439–444.

36 Imamura N., Inada T., Mtasiwa D.M. *et al.* (1989) Phenotype and function of Japanese adult T-cell leukaemia cells. *Lancet*, **ii**, 214.

37 Richardson J.H., Edwards A.J., Cruickshank J.K. *et al.* (1990). *In vivo* cellular tropism of human T-cell leukemia virus type 1. *Journal of Virology*, **64**, 5682–5687.

38 Waldmann T.A., Greene W.C., Sarin P.S. *et al.* (1984) Functional and phenotypic comparison of human T cell leukemia/lymphoma virus positive adult T cell leukemia with human T cell leukemia/lymphoma virus negative Sezary leukemia, and their distinction using anti-Tac monoclonal antibody identifying the human receptor for T cell growth factor. *Journal of Clinical Investigation*, **73**, 1711–1718.

39 Tsudo M., Uchiyama T., Uchino H. *et al.* (1983) Failure of regulation of Tac antigen/TCGF receptor on adult T-cell leukemia cells by anti-TAC monoclonal antibody. *Blood*, **61**, 1014–1016.

40 Lando Z., Sarin P., Megson M. *et al.* (1983) Association of human T-cell leukaemia/lymphoma virus with the Tac antigen marker for the human T-cell growth factor receptor. *Nature*, **305**, 733–736.

41 Yasuda N., Lai P.K., Ip S.H. *et al.* (1988) Soluble interleukin 2

receptors in sera of Japanese patients with adult T cell leukemia mark activity of disease. *Blood*, **71**, 1021–1026.

42 Yamaguchi K., Nishimura Y., Kiyokawa T. *et al.* (1989) Elevated serum levels of soluble interleukin-2 receptors in HTLV-I-associated myelopathy. *Journal of Laboratory and Clinical Medicine*, **114**, 407–410.

43 Yodoi J. & Uchiyama T. (1986) IL-2 receptor dysfunction and adult T-cell leukemia. *Immunological Reviews*, **92**, 135–156.

44 Mann D.L., Popovic M., Murray C. *et al.* (1983) Cell surface antigen expression in newborn cord blood lymphocytes infected with HTLV. *Journal of Immunology*, **131**, 2021–2024.

45 Hoxie J.A., Matthews D.M. & Cines D.B. (1984) Infection of human endothelial cells by human T-cell leukemia virus type I. *Proceedings of the National Academy of Science, USA*, **81**, 7591–7595.

46 Matutes E., Dalgleish A.G., Weiss R.A. *et al.* (1986) Studies in healthy human T-cell leukemia-lymphoma virus (HTLV-I) carriers from the Caribbean. *International Journal of Cancer*, **38**, 41–45.

47 Lennert K., Kikuchi M., Sato E. *et al.* (1984) HTLV-positive and -negative T-cell lymphomas. Morphological and immunohistochemical differences between European and HTLV-positive Japanese T-cell lymphomas. *International Journal of Cancer*, **35**, 65–72.

48 Su I-J., Wang C-H., Cheng A-L. *et al.* (1988) Characterization of the spectrum of postthymic T-cell malignancies in Taiwan. *Cancer*, **61**, 2060–2070.

49 Suchi T., Lennert K., Tu L-Y. *et al.* (1987) Histopathology and immunohistochemistry of peripheral T cell lymphomas: a proposal for their classification. *Journal of Clinical Pathology*, **40**, 995–1015.

50 National Cancer Institute Sponsored Study of Classifications of Non-Hodgkin's Lymphomas (1982) Summary and description of a working formulation for clinical use. *Cancer*, **49**, 2112–2135.

51 Harris N.L., Jaffe E.S., Stein H. *et al.* (1994) A revised European–American classification of lymphoid neoplasms: a proposal from the International Lymphoma Study Group. *Blood*, **84**, 1361–1392.

52 O'Brien C.J., Lampert I.A. & Catovsky D. (1983) The histopathology of adult T-cell lymphoma leukaemia in blacks from the Caribbean. *Histopathology*, **7**, 349–364.

53 Duggan D.B., Ehrlich G.D., Davey F.P. *et al.* (1988) HTLV-I-induced lymphoma mimicking Hodgkin's disease. Diagnosis by polymerase chain reaction amplification of specific HTLV-I sequences in tumour DNA. *Blood*, **71**, 1027–1032.

54 Ohshima K., Kikuchi M., Yoshida T. *et al.* (1990) Lymph nodes in incipient adult T-cell leukemia-lymphoma with Hodgkin's disease-like histologic features. *Cancer*, **67**, 1622–1628.

55 Mitsui T., Suchi T. & Kikuchi M. (1982) Macroscopical and histopathological analyses on cutaneous lymphomatous lesions of peripheral T cell nature. *GANN Monograph on Cancer Research*, **28**, 135–145.

56 Gallo R.C., Kalyanaraman V.S., Sarngadharan M.G. *et al.* (1983) Association of the human type C retrovirus with a subset of adult T-cell cancers. *Cancer Research*, **43**, 3892–3899.

57 Kinoshita K., Tatsuhiko A., Momita S. *et al.* (1985) Association of adult human T-cell leukemia virus (ATLV/HTLV) with mycosis fungoides and extranodal cutaneous T-cell malignant lymphoma. *Journal of Kyushu Hematological Society*, **33**, 31–36.

58 Matutes E., Keeling D.M., Newland A.C. *et al.* (1990) Sezary cell-like leukemia: a distinct type of mature T cell malignancy. *Leukemia*, **4**, 262–266.

59 Grossman B., Schechter G.P., Horton J.E. *et al.* (1981) Hypercalcemia associated with T-cell lymphoma-leukemia. *American Journal of Clinical Pathology*, **75**, 149–155.

60 Shimoyama M., Minato K., Saito H. *et al.* (1979) Comparison of clinical, morphologic and immunologic characteristics of adult T-cell leukemia-lymphoma and cutaneous T-cell lymphoma. *Japanese Journal of Clinical Oncology*, **9**, 357–372.

61 Eimoto T., Mitsui T. & Kikuchi M. (1981) Ultrastructure of adult T-cell leukemia/lymphoma. *Virchows Archives (Cell Pathology)*, **38**, 189–208.

62 Matutes E., Brito-Babapulle V. & Catovsky D. (1985) Clinical, immunological, ultrastructural and cytogenetic studies in black patients with adult T cell leukemia/lymphoma. In: *Retroviruses in Human Lymphoma/Leukemia* (ed. M. Miwa), pp. 59–70 Japan Scientific Society Press, Tokyo.

63 Hinuma Y., Nagata K., Hanaoka M. *et al.* (1981) Adult T-cell leukemia antigen in an ATL cell line and detection of antibodies to the antigen in human sera. *Proceedings of the National Academy of Science, USA*, **78**, 6476–6480.

64 Yamaguchi K., Matutes E., Kiyokawa Y. *et al.* (1988) Comparison of immunoperoxidase staining with indirect immunofluorescence, ELISA and Western blotting assays for detecting anti-HTLV-I antibodies in systemic lupus erythematosus. *Journal of Clinical Pathology*, **41**, 57–61.

65 Anderson D.W., Epstein J.S., Lee T-H. *et al.* (1989) Serological confirmation of human T-lymphotropic virus type I infection in healthy blood plasma donors. *Blood*, **74**, 2581–2589.

66 Seiki M., Hattori S., Hirayama Y. *et al.* (1983) Human adult T-cell leukemia virus: complete nucleotide sequence of the provirus genome integrated in leukemia cell DNA. *Proceedings of the National Academy of Science, USA*, **79**, 3618–3622.

67 Chen Y-M.A., Lee T-H., Wiktor S.Z. *et al.* (1990) Type-specific antigens for serological discrimination of HTLV-I and HTLV-II infection. *Lancet*, **336**, 1153–1155.

68 *International Retrovirus Conference. Current Issue in Human Retrovirology: HTLV.* Montego Bay, Jamaica, February 1991.

69 Yoshida M., Seiki M., Yamaguchi K. *et al.* (1984) Monoclonal integration of human T-cell leukemia provirus in all primary tumors of adult T-cell leukemia suggests causative role of human T-cell virus in the disease. *Proceedings of the National Academy of Science, USA*, **81**, 2534–2537.

70 Gross L. (1983) *Oncogenic Viruses*, 3rd edn. Pergamon, Oxford.

71 Poiesz B.J., Ruscetti F.W., Gazdar A.F. *et al.* (1980) Detection and isolation of type C retrovirus particles from fresh and cultured lymphocytes of a patient with cutaneous T cell lymphoma. *Proceedings of the National Academy of Science, USA*, **77**, 7415–7419.

72 Popovic M., Reitz M.S., Sarngadharam M.G. *et al.* (1982) The virus of Japanese adult T-cell leukaemia is a member of the human T-cell leukaemia group. *Nature*, **300**, 63–66.

73 Catovsky D., Greaves M.F., Rose M. *et al.* (1982) Adult T-cell lymphoma-leukaemia in blacks from the West Indies. *Lancet*, **i**, 639–643.

74 Blattner W.A., Gibbs W.N., Saxinger C. *et al.* (1983) Human T-cell leukaemia/lymphoma virus-associated lymphoreticular neoplasia in Jamaica. *Lancet*, **ii**, 61–64.

75 Gessain A., Barin F., Vernant J.C. *et al.* (1985) Antibodies to human T-lymphotropic virus type 1 in patients with tropical spastic paraparesis. *Lancet*, **ii**, 407–410.

76 Osame M., Matsumoto M., Usuku K. *et al.* (1987) Chronic progressive myelopathy associated with elevated antibodies to human T-lymphotropic virus type 1 and adult T-cell leukemia-like cells. *Annals of Neurology*, **21**, 117–122.

77 Dalgleish A., Richardson J., Matutes E. *et al.* (1988) HTLV-I infection in tropical spastic paraparesis: lymphocyte culture and serologic response. *AIDS Research and Human Retroviruses*, **4**, 475–485.

78 Scully R.E., Mark E.J., McNeely W.F. *et al.* (1989) Case records of the Massachusetts General Hospital. *New England Journal of Medicine*, **321**, 663–675.

79 Veyssier-Belot C., Couderc L.J., Desgranges C.L. *et al.* (1990) Kaposi's sarcoma and HTLV-I infection. *Lancet*, **336**, 575.

80 Kawano F., Tsukamoto A., Satoh M. *et al.* (1982) HTLV-I associated myelopathy/tropical spastic paraparesis with adult T-cell leukemia. *Leukemia*, **6**, 66–67.

81 Bartholomew C., Cleghorn F., Charles W. *et al.* (1986) HTLV-I and tropical spastic paraparesis. *Lancet*, **ii**, 99–100.

82 Cartier L., Castillo J.L., Cabrera M.E. *et al.* (1995) HTLV-I positive progressive spastic paraparesis (TSP) associated with a lymphoid disorder in three Chilean patients. *Leukemia and Lymphoma*, **17**, 459–464.

83 Morgan O. StC., Rodgers-Johnson P., Mora C. *et al.* (1989) HTLV-I and polymyositis in Jamaica. *Lancet*, **ii**, 1182–1184.

84 Nishioka K., Maruyama I., Sato K. *et al.* (1989) Chronic inflammatory arthropathy associated with HTLV-I. *Lancet*, **i**, 441.

85 Kitajima I., Maruyama I, Maruyama Y *et al.* (1989) Polyarthritis in human T lymphotropic virus type I-associated myelopathy. *Arthritis and Rheumatism*, **32**, 1342–1344.

86 Robert-Guroff M., Coutinho R.A., Zadelhoff A.W. *et al.* (1984) Prevalence of HTLV-specific antibodies in Surinam emigrants to the Netherlands. *Leukaemia Research*, **8**, 501–504.

87 Delaporte E., Peeters M., Simoni M. *et al.* (1989) HTLV-I infection in Western Equatorial Africa. *Lancet*, **ii**, 1226.

88 Hahn B.H., Shaw G.M., Popovic M. *et al.* (1984) Molecular cloning and analysis of a new variant of human T-cell leukemia virus (HTLV-Ib) from an African patient with adult T-cell leukemia-lymphoma. *International Journal of Cancer*, **34**, 613–618.

89 Tajima K., the T- and B-cell Malignancy Study Group and Co-authors (1990) The 4th nation-wide study of adult T-cell leukaemia/lymphoma (ATL) in Japan: estimates of risk of ATL and its geographical and clinical features. *International Journal of Cancer*, **45**, 237–243.

90 The T- and B-cell Malignancy Study Group (1988) The third nation-wide study on adult T-cell leukaemia/lymphoma (ATL) in Japan: characteristic patterns of HLA antigen and HTLV-I infection in ATL patients and their relatives. *International Journal of Cancer*, **41**, 505–512.

91 Bartholomew C., Charles W., Saxinger C. *et al.* (1985) Racial and other characteristics of human T cell leukaemia/lymphoma (HTLV-I) and AIDS (HTLV-III) in Trinidad. *British Medical Journal*, **290**, 1243–1246.

92 Gessain A., Jouannelle A., Escarmant P. *et al.* (1984) HTLV antibodies in patients with non-Hodgkin lymphomas in Martinique. *Lancet*, **i**, 1183–1184.

93 Hernandez Ramirez P., Rivero Jimenez R., Ballester Santovenia M. *et al.* (1991) Very low seroprevalance of HTLV-I/II in Cuba: antibodies in blood donors and in hematological and nonhematological patients. *Vox Sanguinis*, **61**, 277–278.

94 Roman G.C., Roman L.N., Spencer P.S. *et al.* (1985) Tropical spastic paraparesis: a neuroepidemiological study in Colombia. *Annals of Neurology*, **17**, 361–365.

95 Cartier-Rovirosa L., Mora C., Araya F. *et al.* (1989) HTLV-I positive spastic paraparesis in a temperate zone. *Lancet*, **i**, 556–557.

96 Montserrat E., Lozano M., Urbano-Ispizua A. *et al.* (1989) Adult T-cell leukemia in a Chilean resident in Spain: long lasting remission after 2-deoxycoformycin treatment. *Leukemia and Lymphoma*, **1**, 47–49.

97 Cabrera M.E., Gray A.M., Cartier L. *et al.* (1991) Simultaneous adult T-cell leukemia/lymphoma and sub-acute polyneuropathy in a patient from Chile. *Leukemia*, **5**, 350–353.

98 Cabrera M.E., Labra S., Catovsky D. *et al.* (1994) HTLV-I positive adult T-cell leukaemia/lymphoma (ATLL) in Chile. *Leukemia*, **8**, 1763–1767.

99 Matutes E., Schulz T., Andrada Serpa M.J. *et al.* (1994) Report of the Second International Symposium on HTLV in Brazil. *Leukemia*, **8**, 1092–1094.

100 Meytes D., Schochat B., Lee H. *et al.* (1990) Serological and molecular survey for HTLV-I infection in a high-risk Middle Eastern group. *Lancet*, **336**, 1533–1535.

101 Sidi Y., Meytes D., Shohat B. *et al.* (1990) Adult T-cell lymphoma in Israeli patients of Iranian origin. *Cancer*, **65**, 590–593.

102 Denic S., Nolan P., Doherty J. *et al.* (1990) HTLV-I infection in Iraq. *Lancet*, **336**, 1135–1136.

103 Yanagihara R., Jenkins C.L., Alexander S.S. *et al.* (1990) Human T lymphotropic virus type I infection in Papua New Guinea: high prevalence among the Hagahai confirmed by western analysis. *Journal of Infectious Diseases*, **162**, 649–654.

104 Gessain A., Yanigahira R., Franchini G. *et al.* (1991) Highly divergent molecular variants of human T-lymphotropic virus type 1 from isolated populations in Papua New Guinea and the Solomon Islands. *Proceedings of the National Academy of Science, USA*, **88**, 7694–7698.

105 Blattner W.A. & Gallo R.C. (1994) Epidemiology of HTLV-I and HTLV-II infection. In: *Adult T-cell Leukaemia* (ed. K. Takatsuki), pp. 45–90. Oxford University Press, Oxford.

106 Hino S. (1990) Milk-borne transmission of HTLV-I from carrier mothers and its prevention. *Haematology Reviews*, **3**, 223–233.

107 Komuro A., Hayami M., Fujii H. *et al.* (1983) Vertical transmission of adult T-cell leukaemia virus. *Lancet*, **i**, 240.

108 Sato H. & Okochi K. (1990) Transmission of HTLV-I through blood transfusion and its prevention. *Haematology Reviews*, **3**, 235–245.

109 Kataoka R., Takehara N., Iwahara Y. *et al.* (1990) Transmission of HTLV-I by blood transfusion and its prevention by passive immunization in rabbits. *Blood*, **76**, 1657–1661.

110 Nishimura Y., Yamaguchi K., Kiyokawa T. *et al.* (1989) Prevention of transmission of human T-cell lymphotropic virus type-I by blood transfusion by screening of donors. *Transfusion*, **29**, 372.

111 Yamaguchi K., Nishimura Y., Fukuyoshi Y. *et al.* (1990) Decrease of HTLV-I infection in haemodialysis patients after donor screening. *Lancet*, **336**, 1070.

112 Brennan M., Runganga J., Barbara J.A.J. *et al.* (1993) Prevalence of antibodies to human T cell leukaemia/lymphoma virus in blood donors in north London. *British Medical Journal*, **307**, 1235–1239.

113 Ljungman P., Lawler M., Asjo B. *et al.* (1994) Infection of donor lymphocytes with human T lymphotropic virus type I (HTLV-I) following allogeneic bone marrow transplantation for HTLV-I positive adult T-cell leukaemia. *British Journal of Haematology*, **88**, 403–405.

114 Seiki M., Eddy R., Shows T.B. *et al.* (1984) Nonspecific integration of the HTLV provirus genome into adult T-cell leukaemia cells. *Nature*, **309**, 640–642.

115 Gallo R.C. (1986) The first human retrovirus. *Scientific American*, **255**, 78–88.

116 Wong-Staal F. & Gallo R.C. (1985) Human T-lymphotropic retroviruses. *Nature*, **317**, 395–403.

117 Seiki M., Inoue J., Takeda T. *et al.* (1985) The p40 of human T-cell leukemia virus type I is a trans-acting activator of viral gene transcription. *Japanese Journal of Cancer Research (Gann)*, **76**, 1127–1131.

118 Miwa M. (1990) Mechanism of oncogenesis of adult T-cell leukemia/lymphoma. *Hematology Reviews*, **3**, 247–255.

119 Kiyokawa T., Seiki M., Iwashita S. *et al.* (1985) p27 and p21 proteins encoded by the Px sequence of human T-cell leukemia virus type I. *Proceedings of the National Academy of Science, USA*, **82**, 8359–8363.

120 Okamoto T., Ohno Y., Tsugane S. *et al.* (1989) Multi-step carcinogenesis model for adult T-cell leukemia. *Japanese Journal of Cancer Research*, **80**, 191–195.

121 Kamada N., Tanaka K., Takechi M. *et al.* (1989) Chromosome aberrations in adult T cell leukemia. *Hematology Reviews*, **3**, 257–270.

122 Ueshima Y., Fukuhara S., Hattori T. *et al.* (1981) Chromosome studies in adult T cell leukaemia in Japan. Significance of trisomy 7. *Blood*, **58**, 420–425.

123 Miyamoto K., Tomita N., Ishii A. *et al.* (1984) Chromosome abnormalities of leukemia cells in adult patients with T-cell leukemia. *Journal of the National Cancer Institute*, **73**, 353–362.

124 Sanada I., Tanaka R., Kumagai E. *et al.* (1985) Chromosomal aberrations in adult T cell leukemia: relationship to the clinical severity. *Blood*, **65**, 649–654.

125 Brito-Babapulle V., Matutes E., Hegde U. *et al.* (1984) Adult T-cell lymphoma/leukemia in a Caribbean patient: cytogenetic, immunologic and ultrastructural findings. *Cancer, Genetics and Cytogenetics*, **12**, 343–357.

126 Brito-Babapulle V., Matutes E., Parreira L. *et al.* (1986) Abnormalities of chromosome 7q and Tac expression in T-cell leukemias. *Blood*, **67**, 516–521.

127 Brito-Babapulle V., Pomfret M., Matutes E. *et al.* (1987) Cytogenetic studies on prolymphocytic leukemia. II. T-cell prolymphocytic leukemia. *Blood*, **70**, 926–931.

128 Kaplanski S., Wong-Staal F., Farnarier-Seidel C. *et al.* (1986) Detection of HTLV-I (human T-cell lymphotropic virus, Type I) proviral DNA in leukemic cells from a French patient with Sezary syndrome. *Leukemia Research*, **10**, 375–380.

129 Hall W.W., Liu C.R., Schneewind O. *et al.* (1991) A deleted HTLV-I provirus in blood and cutaneous lesions of patients with mycosis fungoides. *Science*, **253**, 317–320.

130 Zucker-Franklin D., Coutavas E.E., Rush M.G. & Zouzias D.C. (1991) Detection of human T-lymphotropic-virus-like particles in cultures of peripheral-blood lymphocytes from patients with mycosis fungoides. *Proceedings of the National Academy of Science (Washington)*, **88**, 7630–7634.

131 Matutes E., Brito-Babapulle V., Swansbury J. *et al.* (1991) Clinical and laboratory features of 78 cases of T-prolymphocytic leukemia. *Blood*, **78**, 3269–3274.

132 Matutes E., Schulz T., Dyer M. *et al.* (1995) Immunoblastic transformation of a Sezary syndrome in a Black Caribbean patient without evidence of HTLV-I. *Leukemia and Lymphoma*, **18**, 521–527.

133 Shimoyama M., Kagami Y., Shimotohno K. *et al.* (1986) Adult T-cell leukemia/lymphoma not associated with human T-cell leukemia virus type I. *Proceedings of the National Academy of Science, USA*, **83**, 4524–4528.

134 Shimoyama M., Abe T., Miyamoto K. *et al.* (1987) Chromosome aberrations and clinical features of adult T cell leukemia-lymphoma not associated with human T cell leukemia virus type I. *Blood*, **69**, 984–989.

135 Yamaguchi K., Yoshioka R., Kiyokawa T. *et al.* (1986) Lymphoma type adult T-cell leukemia — a clinicopathologic study of HTLV related T-cell type malignant lymphoma. *Hematological Oncology*, **4**, 59–65.

136 Shimamoto Y., Yamaguchi M., Miyamoto Y. *et al.* (1990) The differences between lymphoma and leukemia type of adult T-cell leukemia. *Leukemia and Lymphoma*, **1**, 101–112.

137 Shimamoto Y., Suga K., Shimojo M. *et al.* (1990) Comparison of CHOP versus VEPA therapy in patients with lymphoma type of adult T-cell leukemia. *Leukemia and Lymphoma*, **2**, 335–340.

138 Kato S., Nishimura J., Muta K. *et al.* (1990) Overexpression of P-glycoprotein in adult T-cell leukaemia. *Lancet*, **336**, 573.

139 Futami G., Kiyokawa T., Yamaguchi K. *et al.* (1990) Treatment of adult T cell leukaemia by extracorporeal photochemotherapy. *Leukemia and Lymphoma*, **2**, 195–200.

140 Kimura I., Tsubota T., Hayashi K. *et al.* (1983) Spontaneous, complete remission in adult T-cell leukemia: a case report. *Japanese Journal of Clinical Oncology* **13**(Suppl 2), 231–236.

141 Schnitzer B., Lovett E.J. & Kahn L.E. (1983) Adult T-cell leukaemia with spontaneous remission. *Lancet*, **ii**, 1030.

142 Murakawa M., Shibuya T., Teshima T. *et al.* (1990) Spontaneous remission from acute exacerbation of chronic adult T-cell leukemia. *Blut*, **61**, 346–349.

143 Yamaguchi K., Takatsuki K., Dearden C. *et al.* (1988) Chemotherapy with deoxycoformycin in mature T-cell malignancies. In: *Cancer Chemotherapy: Challenges for the future* (ed. K. Kimura), Vol. 3, pp. 216–220. Excerpta Medica, Tokyo.

144 Dearden C.E., Matutes E. & Catovsky D. (1991) Deoxycoformycin in the treatment of mature T-cell leukaemias. *British Journal of Cancer*, **64**, 903–906.

145 Waldmann T.A., Goldman C.K., Bongiovanni K.F. *et al.* (1988) Therapy of patients with human T-cell lymphotropic virus I-induced adult T-cell leukemia with anti-Tac, a monoclonal antibody to the receptor for Interleukin-2. *Blood*, **72**, 1805–1816.

146 Mercieca J., Matutes E., Dearden C. *et al.* (1994) The role of pentostatin in the treatment of T-cell malignancies: analysis of response rate in 145 patients according to disease subtype. *Journal of Clinical Oncology*, **12**, 2588–2593.

147 Mattock C., Anderson N.A.B., Sheldon C.E. *et al.* (1986) Spontaneous remission and relapse in adult T cell lymphoma/leukaemia associated with HTLV-I. *British Medical Journal*, **292**, 1171–1172.

148 Kiyokawa T., Shirono K., Hattori T. *et al.* (1989) Cytotoxicity of Interleukin 2-toxin toward lymphocytes from patients with adult T-cell leukemia. *Cancer Research*, **49**, 4042–4046.

149 Gill P.S., Harrington W., Kaplan M.H. *et al.* (1995) Treatment of adult T-cell leukemia-lymphoma with a combination of interferon alfa and zidovudine. *New England Journal of Medicine*, **332**, 1744–1748.

150 Hermine O., Bouscary D., Gessain A. *et al.* (1995) Brief report: treatment of adult T-cell leukemia-lymphoma with zidovudine and interferon alfa. *New England Journal of Medicine*, **332**, 1749–1751.

8 Hairy Cell Leukaemia

J. Burthem and J.C. Cawley

Introduction

Although the first description of what is now understood as hairy cell leukaemia (HCL) was probably given by Rosenthal & Lee in 1951 [1], it was the detailed report in 1958 from Bouroncle *et al.* [2] of Columbus, Ohio that led to the disease being widely regarded as a distinct entity. These latter authors clearly identified 'reticulum cells' with a serrated border in a group of 26 patients presenting a well-defined clinicopathological picture which they chose to call leukaemic reticuloendotheliosis. In much of the earlier literature this was the preferred term, but since the late 1970s the disease has been increasingly referred to as hairy cell leukaemia. Symmers' statement in 1978 [3] that 'it is difficult to conceive how a disease that has become so widely known as "hairy-cell leukaemia" can ever be referred to by any more mundane name' has been completely justified and the disease is now almost exclusively referred to by its descriptive name.

Clincal and laboratory aspects

Aetiology and epidemiology

The factors underlying the development of HCL are not understood. Several studies have emphasized an unexpectedly high occurrence in certain groups [4], suggesting the possibility of an occupation-related incidence. In particular, exposure to benzene, solvents and related compounds has been implicated, but such risk factors have not been confirmed in all studies [4–7]. There have been isolated reports of familial occurrence [8,9].

The possibility of a viral aetiology for HCL was suggested after the discovery of an HTLV-II genome integrated in the abnormal cells of cases of 'T-cell HCL' [10]. However, subsequent studies suggest that this is not a generalized phenomenon [11,12], and does not extend to the B-cell form of the disease. Similarly, although Epstein–Barr virus (EBV) has been implicated in certain cases of HCL [13], later serological and molecular studies have not confirmed a widespread role for the virus [14,15].

Clinical presentation

HCL is typically a disease of middle-aged males (males : females ratio approximately 4 : 1). It is not a disease of childhood, but it is by no means exceptional either in patients under 40 or in those over 70 [16]. The incidence of HCL is 3 per million in a year [4]. The disease has a worldwide distribution, although it is relatively rare in certain geographical areas, notably in Japan [17].

Most (approximately 75%) patients present with non-specific symptoms, perhaps at least partially attributable to anaemia. Symptoms probably due to infection are among the presenting complaints of about 30%, while a haemorrhagic tendency is noted in some 20% [16].

Splenomegaly is by far the most constant physical finding, being present in about 85% of patients at presentation and in a higher proportion at some stage of the illness [16]. Discomfort caused by splenomegaly is usually slight and the severe pain of splenic infarction is rare.

Hepatomegaly is much less common, being detectable in only some 50% of patients; marked hepatomegaly is rare. Lymphadenopathy is minimal and when present (<20% of cases) is minor and limited to one node site [16]. Moderate intra-abdominal adenopathy, which can be demonstrated by lymphangiography or CT scanning, is less rare, but substantial peripheral lymphadenopathy attributable to the disease is exceptional [18]. Massive abdominal adenopathy is a recognized late complication of the disorder (see below).

Laboratory findings

Peripheral blood

Anaemia, leucopenia and thrombocytopenia are characteristic

of HCL, and pancytopenia is present in 70% of patients [16]. The anaemia is typically of moderate degree (mean Hb approximately 10 g/dl) and is usually associated with a high-normal or definitely elevated MCV [16]. Slight anisocytosis, piokilocytosis and occasional circulating nucleated red cells are frequently seen, and in a few patients normoblasts may be numerous. A number of factors contribute to the anaemia of HCL. Splenic red cell pooling and haemodilution consequent upon raised plasma volume increase in proportion to spleen size [19,20]. Red cell survival is often moderately reduced [20]; HC-derived marrow-suppressive factors (principally TNFα) have been repeatedly described [21,22].

Although the majority of patients with HCL are leucopenic at presentation, the leucocyte count is the most variable of the standard haematological parameters, being normal or elevated in about 30% of patients. The percentage of circulating morphological hairy cells (HCs) (see below) varies from 0 to 100% but, in general, increases with the leucocyte count. Nearly all patients (>95%) are neutropenic (<2.5 × 10⁹/l) at presentation. The neutrophils are also often qualitatively abnormal with an increased alkaline phosphatase content [23] and defective microbicidal properties [24]. There is no corresponding deficiency of eosinophils or basophils, but profound monocytopenia is nearly always present [25].

Thrombocytopenia is found at presentation in more than 80% of patients [16]. Splenic sequestration [20] is a major factor in patients who have not been splenectomized, but defective production may also be important. Platelets may show a storage pool defect, but this is not usually a major cause of clinical bleeding [26].

Bone marrow

The bone marrow is inaspirable or yields hypocellular non-diagnostic material in 50% of cases, perhaps because of the moderate or marked increases in stromal reticulin fibres that characterize the disease.

The number of infiltrating HCs is very variable and precise quantitation is often difficult since they are frequently less hairy than in the blood. Granulocyte and monocyte precursors are profoundly reduced and may show dysplastic features [27], while cells of the erythroid and megakaryocytic series are often relatively spared [16].

Biochemistry

Despite the microscopic hepatic infiltration consistently present in the disease, liver function tests are usually normal. Serum immunoglobulins are usually normal or raised (40% of cases). Significant paraproteinaemia is rare [28], but a low level of paraprotein can be identified in around 10% of cases when sensitive techniques are used [29].

Complications

Infection

Improvements in therapy of HCL have meant that significant prolonged neutropenia is now unusual. Consequently, the importance of infection as a cause of morbidity and mortality has been significantly reduced. In general, the infections resemble those occurring in patients with marrow suppression. There does, however, appear to be a particular susceptibility to atypical mycobacterial infections [30]; such infection is usually widely disseminated and associated with pulmonary involvement. Most patients will respond to antituberculous drugs or to therapy of the underlying HCL.

This peculiar susceptibility to mycobacterial infection has been related to the severe peripheral monocytopenia of the disease and to impaired granuloma formation with scanty macrophages [31]. However, tissue macrophages are in general not particularly reduced in HCL [16], and it seems likely that the immune defect has a more complex basis. For example, not only neutrophils and monocytes, but also T cells, are functionally defective [16]. The marked susceptibility to infection means that all pyrexias of unknown origin in the disease must be thoroughly investigated for occult infection. However, fevers may sometimes have an immunological basis (see below). If all attempts to find an infective organism are unsuccessful, and there is no evidence of excess immunological activity, an empirical trial of antituberculous therapy is justified [16].

Autoimmune disorders

A range of autoimmune disorders have now been described in HCL, the most common is a systemic vasculitic syndrome with persistent fever, malaise, weight loss and arthralgia, and with potential involvement of a number of organs especially the skin [32]. Less commonly, the disease may present with classical features of polyarteritis nodosa, or other autoimmune phenomena [32–34]. A raised erythrocyte sedimentation rate (ESR), immune complexes, rheumatoid factor or antinuclear antibodies may be found. The cause of the immunological disturbance remains obscure, but such complications are usually associated with active disease and resolve when HCL is effectively treated. Steroids may be helpful.

Bone

Osteolytic lesions (most commonly at the femoral neck) attributable to HCs may occur with or without paraproteinaemia, and may result in fracture [35] Persistent localized pain is the usual symptom, and MRI or technetium scanning may be helpful where plain X-ray fails to reveal the lesion [36]. Bone involvement probably indicates a high tumour burden and, although local radiation therapy is effective, systemic treatment is usually also required [35].

Second malignancy in hairy cell leukaemia

An increased risk of a second malignancy has been long recognized, and there is a twofold risk of a second primary cancer within 1 year of diagnosis [37]. It is now clear, however, that this risk also extends to treated patients. Death from second malignancy is now a major cause of mortality in interferon-treated patients [38]. Whether the risk of second malignancy also extends to nucleoside-treated patients is unclear at present.

Abdominal lymph node enlargement

Substantial abdominal adenopathy may be seen in up to 15% of patients, generally appearing late in the disease and involving the upper aortic and retropancreatic regions (Fig. 8.1) [39]. The abnormal cells found in the lymph glands are larger than typical HCs and do not circulate [40]. Patients with abdominal adenopathy respond much less well to treatment than does typical disease, and it seems appropriate to regard this complication as a form of 'transformation' of HCL [40].

Other complications

Haemorrhage is frequently associated with infection, but is rarely a major cause of death. Skin purpura and ecchymoses are the most common bleeding manifestations. Thrombocytopenia is an important aetiological factor in its own right but may also contribute to rashes with an infiltrative [16] or vasculitic basis [41].

In those rare cases where significant paraproteinaemia is present it is usually of the same light-chain type as the immunoglobulin produced by the HCs [42]. However, this is not always so, and the paraprotein may then be the product of coexisting myeloma [43]. Chylous and serous ascitic and pleural effusions have been recorded [20] and splenic rupture is another uncommon complication of the disease [44].

Pathology

Bone marrow

The bone marrow is probably always, or almost always, involved and its histology is diagnostic [45]. Splenic involvement may occasionally be prominent in patients with inconspicuous infiltration of the marrow. The mononuclear cell infiltrate may be partial or complete, but is always diffuse [45]. The mononuclear cells, although they do not display obvious cytoplasmic hairs, nevertheless present a distinctive appearance in which the well-defined nuclei are separated from one

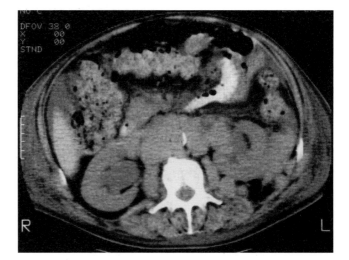

Fig. 8.1 CT scan illustrating extensive enlargement of prevertebral abdominal lymph nodes in a case of HCL.

another by a clear zone of cytoplasm or by clear spaces, imparting what has been described as a 'halo' appearance [45].

A second distinctive feature of the bone marrow is the consistent finding of fine reticulin fibrosis. The precise composition of this reticulin is unclear. However, infiltrating fibroblasts are uncommon, and the fibrosis seems to result, at least in part, from the production and assembly of a fibronectin matrix by the HCs themselves [46].

Spleen

The cut surface of the spleen presents a homogeneous dark-red appearance with no evidence of circumscribed tumour, and malphigian bodies are atrophic or absent. Histological examination shows diffuse infiltration of the red pulp by mononuclear cells containing slightly irregular nuclei with fine stippled chromatin. The red pulp is so heavily infiltrated by HCs that it is frequently difficult to distinguish cords and sinuses. In certain areas there are variable size blood-filled spaces, lined by HCs rather than endothelial cells. These structures—pseudosinuses—are pathognomonic of HCL [47].

In addition to HCs, the splenic cords contain readily identifiable macrophages and plasma cells; the latter do not show light-chain restriction of their intracytoplasmic immunoglobulin and are therefore presumably reactive in nature [16].

Liver

Despite the frequent absence of clinical hepatomegaly, evidence of HC infiltration is nearly always found [48]. There is infiltration of both the sinusoids and portal tracts, but the general architecture of the liver remains intact. Sinusoidal involvement is distinctive, the HCs attaching to the sinusoidal wall in a manner analogous to Kupffer cells [49]. Portal tract involvement may be relatively inconspicuous or take the form of pseudosinus-like lesions encircled by reticulin fibres.

Lymph nodes

Enlargement of peripheral lymph nodes is rarely a feature of HCL. However, when node material has been examined histologically it has usually been found to be involved. Despite this, and even when the HC infiltration is conspicuous, there is usually some preservation of node architecture, with recognizable residual follicles [48]. In those cases with major abdominal adenopathy (see earlier), the nodes are considerably expanded, with a diffuse infiltration consisting of typical HCs and atypical HCs of larger and more primitive appearance [40].

Diagnosis

The features of typical HCL have become so well known that the great majority of cases are now readily diagnosed by simple morphological examination of blood and marrow films against a background of isolated splenomegaly and/or peripheral pancytopenia. In such cases immunological markers and cytochemistry are merely confirmatory.

Of the various cytochemical techniques that have been used in the past, tartrate-resistant acid phosphatase staining (TRAP) remains of considerable value. TRAP is reviewed in the section 'Cytology and cytochemistry' below; other cytochemical reactivities are no longer of diagnostic importance.

The immunophenotypic features of typical HCL have now been well established, and a useful diagnostic panel is given in Table 8.1.

Occasionally, diagnostic difficulties arise. This is generally when HCs are so scanty that doubt is raised about the diagnosis, or when there are significant clinical or pathological atypia.

When the patient is very leucopenic, HCs may be inconspicuous in the blood, but they are then usually readily identified in buffy-coat preparations and in the marrow. A range of monoclonal antibodies (MAbs) are now available that react with HCs in fixed paraffin-embedded tissues, but in general these MAbs are not very specific (e.g. CD20 [50], CD45RA [50] or DBA.44 [51]) and their principle value lies in recognizing residual disease after treatment.

When atypia are present, the question arises whether the patient has one of the two recognized HCL-like conditions. These disorders (HCL variant and splenic lymphoma with villous lymphocytes) generally have different therapeutic requirements or respond differently to therapy, and must therefore be accurately discriminated from typical HCL.

Hairy cell leukaemia variant

The closely related disorder HCL variant (HCL-V) presents with a picture similar to that of typical HCL, but the white cell

Table 8.1 A panel of monoclonal antibodies (MAbs) useful in the confirmation of typical HCL.

Marker	Reactivity
CD5	–
CD11c	+++
CD20	+++
CD22	+++
CD25	++
B-ly7*	++
HC2*	++

* These MAbs are principally used to distinguish HCL from SLVL or HCL-V and may be omitted in otherwise typical disease.

count is higher (generally $50–100 \times 10^9$/l) and monocytes are typically present in the peripheral blood [52,53]. The abnormal cells are smaller than typical HCs, with less cytoplasm and less conspicuous hairs. The round, centrally placed nucleus has more clumped chromatin and a nucleolus is usually present. Bone marrow is generally aspirable and not fibrotic. Immunophenotypically, the cells mark as mature B cells expressing CD19, CD20, CD22 and FMC7. They may frequently express the hairy cell markers CD11c and B-Ly7, but CD25 and HC2 are not usually expressed and TRAP reactivity is weak or absent [54,55]. Although relatively benign, the disorder responds less well to treatment than does typical HCL [53].

Splenic lymphoma with villous lymphocytes

Splenic lymphoma with villous lymphocytes (SLVL) is less commonly confused with HCL, but circulating 'hairy cells' are present and its clinical features may lead to diagnostic confusion. The principle clinical feature is splenic enlargement which may be considerable. Lymph gland enlargement is more common than in HCL, but is not always seen. Monocytopenia is not a feature, and a monoclonal IgM may be present [56–58].

Like HCL-V, the malignant cells are smaller than HCs, but they generally circulate in smaller numbers than in HCL-V. The nucleus is round/ovoid and centrally placed with condensed chromatin; a small nucleolus is often present. Short villi may be present, but these are often confined to the poles of the cell. Bone marrow involvement is usually nodular or patchy but may occasionally show a paratrabecular pattern [58,59]. The abnormal cells express typical mature B-cell markers and TRAP reactivity is generally present, but is usually weaker than in typical HCL. One or two HCL markers (CD11c, B-Ly7, HC2 and CD25) may be present, whereas in typical HCL three or four of these markers are expressed together [55].

Treatment

It is now clear that almost all newly diagnosed cases of HCL will respond to treatment with nucleoside analogues, and that the majority of patients can expect prolonged remission and perhaps cure. The sensitivity of HCL to nucleosides means that this class of drugs is now the treatment of first choice for most patients.

Alternative treatments, principally interferon alpha or splenectomy, retain a role in limited clinical circumstances. Similarly, colony-stimulating factors may be useful in some, but not all, patients.

The current treatment options are reviewed below, and an overall treatment strategy is presented. The possible mechanisms of action of the drugs are then discussed.

The nucleosides: chlorodeoxyadenosine, deoxycoformycin and fludarabine

Chlorodeoxyadenosine

When given as a continuous intravenous infusion for 7 days at a dose of 0.1 mg/kg daily, around 95% of patients will respond to chlorodeoxyadenosine (CDA) and over 80% will enter a complete remission [60]. Residual HCs are detectable by sensitive methods in the bone marrow of some patients, and prolonged follow-up has not yet been possible. However, early relapse rates are very low [61]. Those patients who respond incompletely to CDA, or who relapse after an initial remission, may respond to retreatment with CDA or to other nucleosides [62].

The principle toxicity of CDA is a dose-related neutropenia with a mean nadir of 0.4×10^9/l. Fever is common, and occurs in up to half of patients. This fever is often culture negative, but infections are seen in up to 40% and may occasionally be fatal [61,63]. Opportunistic infections may occur early after treatment, but do not appear to be a long-term problem despite the prolonged CD4 lymphopenia induced by the drug [62].

Deoxycoformycin

The most usual treatment regimen for deoxycoformycin (DCF) is to give 4 mg/m² as an intravenous bolus once every 14 days until maximum response is obtained; if remission occurs, two more doses are then given (median treatment time 4–7 months). Response rates are very similar to those obtained with CDA, around 90% responding and up to 80% achieving a complete remission [64,65]. Again, residual HCs can often be identified in the bone marrow of DCF-treated patients, but after follow up of 3–4 years around 80% remain in remission [65]. Relapsed patients may respond to further DCF; resistant disease may be successfully treated with other nucleosides [66].

The severe bone marrow, CNS or renal side effects historically associated with DCF are not a feature of current regimens [67]. Nevertheless, significant neutropenia occurs in 45% of patients, and infections (which are occasionally fatal) are seen in 30% [67]. The prolonged CD4 lymphopenia of DCF does not appear to cause problems [68]. Nausea and vomiting are the most frequent adverse reactions, but respond to prophylactic antiemetics. A skin rash (often photosensitive) is seen in 70% but is rarely severe [67].

Fludarabine

Fludarabine is structurally and functionally similar to CDA and DCF, and has been successfully employed in HCL patients resistant to other treatments [69,70]. However there is as yet no widespread experience with its use; at present, therefore, fludarabine cannot be recommended as a first-choice treatment in HCL.

Interferon

In HCL, interferon alpha (IFNα) prolongs survival, improves quality of life, and provides cost-effective therapy [71]. The optimal dose remains unclear, but a common regimen is to give 2×10^6 U/m² day for 4–6 months, followed by the same dose three times each week until 1 year. This regimen will induce normal blood counts in 80% of patients, although few achieve complete bone marrow remission [72,73]. Lower doses may be better tolerated and give an equal, but slower, response. Long-term 'maintenance' treatment prolongs remission, but is not always well tolerated by patients [72]. Remission may be lengthy, but in most patients HCs reappear 6–10 months after treatment is stopped, and re-treatment is generally required after around 30 months [73]. Relapsed patients may respond to reinduction with IFNα, and IFNα does not appear to reduce sensitivity to subsequent treatment with nucleosides [65].

The side effects of IFNα are well known and are usually restricted to 'flu-like' symptoms that resolve after a few weeks' treatment [74]. A more major problem, however, is that of IFNα resistance [75,76]. Primary resistance is seen in 10–15% of patients, and may be the result of IFNα receptor absence or dysfunction [77]. Some acquired resistance may arise by a similar mechanism, but in other cases it is mediated by neutralizing anti-IFNα antibodies. The frequency of such antibodies is greatest for IFNα2a (20%) and least for natural interferon (1–2%) [78]. When neutralizing antibodies are associated with loss of responsiveness, dose adjustment or substitution of an alternative IFNα preparation is usually effective [79].

Splenectomy

Removal of the spleen was recognized to be effective treatment for HCL when the disorder was first described [2], and until recently splenectomy was often performed. Although it has now largely been supplanted by nucleoside therapy, removal of the spleen does not reduce the response to other therapies and may still occasionally be indicated.

Splenectomy improves survival in patients with substantial splenomegaly (>4 cm). The extent of HC infiltration of the marrow and platelet count are the best indicators of the likely response to surgery. Within the best prognostic group (platelet count >60 × 10⁹/l and marrow HCs <85%), a sustained improvement for over 4 years may be expected [80]. In contrast, the presence of significant marrow failure greatly reduces response duration, and the removal of impalpable spleens does not improve survival [81].

Following splenectomy, 40–60% of patients show an almost complete response in terms of return of platelets, haemoglobin and neutrophils to satisfactory levels. A further 30–40% of patients will show a partial response (platelet response >Hb >neutrophils), while some 10–20% will derive no benefit. The response to surgery is usually obvious within 2 weeks and, as might be expected, prognosis is best in complete responders.

Colony-stimulating factors

Granulocyte colony-stimulating factor (G-CSF) administration corrects neutropenia and leads to the resolution of infection in most cases of untreated HCL. However, the effect is not sustained, and counts fall rapidly when treatment is withdrawn [82,83]. G-CSF also maintains neutrophil counts during IFNα therapy [83].

Granulocyte-macrophage colony-stimulating factor (GM-CSF) has been less well studied, but has been reported to support neutrophil counts in untreated patients [84].

Combination treatment

Several groups have investigated the use of combinations of treatments in HCL. Splenectomy does not significantly prolong the remission of IFN-treated patients [85], and combining IFN with nucleosides does not improve the effectiveness of the latter agents [86]. In very neutropenic patients, initial treatment with IFN (and perhaps G-CSF) to improve the patient's general condition and reduce disease activity, may reduce the risk of infection during subsequent nucleoside treatment [87]. This latter strategy has not, however, been widely used.

Treatment strategy

When marrow function is well maintained, patients with HCL generally remain well. Moreover, such patients may remain in this stable state for some time. Thus, although there have been great advances in therapy, it seems reasonable to withhold treatment until there is risk of debility. In this regard, the criteria for commencing treatment proposed at the Second International Workshop on HCL (1986) remain useful [88]. Thus, treatment is indicated in the presence of recurrent/serious infections or of a significant bleeding tendency, or when marrow suppression is manifest by haemoglobin less than 12

g/dl, platelets less than 100 × 10⁹/l or neutrophils less than 1.5 × 10⁹/l.

When treatment is required, the choice for most patients will be to use either CDA or DCF. There are no clear direct comparative data concerning the two agents, but there is a perception [89] that CDA may have a superior side-effect profile and perhaps efficacy. CDA and DCF are also the treatment of choice in those patients who have relapsed following IFNα.

IFNα may be preferred in patients intolerant of nucleosides or in those patients who have previously responded well to the cytokine. In such patients, maintenance therapy may be justified. There are no published data regarding the effectiveness of IFNα in nucleoside-resistant patients.

Splenectomy may retain a role for those patients wishing to avoid drug treatment, or in those patients with the rare 'pure splenic HCL'.

Mechanism of action of the anti-HCL drugs

Nucleoside drugs are analogues of 2'-deoxyadenosine and either inhibit the enzyme adenosine deaminase (in the case of DCF) or are resistant to its effects (CDA and fludarabine) [90]. As a result, in nucleoside-treated cells, purine nucleosides enter an alternative metabolic pathway in which they are phosphorylated rather than deaminated. This phosphorylation pathway is a particular feature of lymphoid cells and the net effect of the drugs is to cause an accumulation of purine nucleotide triphosphates in lymphocytes (either deoxyadenosine triphosphate—DCF, or the triphosphate form of the drug—CDA/fludarabine) [90].

Such an accumulation is clearly toxic. The drugs cause fairly rapid apoptosis of sensitive cells *in vitro*, and it has been suggested that the accumulated nucleoside triphosphates may cause cell death by inhibiting normal DNA repair [91], disrupting RNA metabolism [92] or interfering with the related metabolic pathways that control transmethylation [91]. However, all these factors also operate in other lymphoid cells, and the precise mechanism(s) that underlie the particular sensitivity of HCL to these drugs remains unclear.

Similarly, the precise action of IFNα in HCL has not been clearly determined. In general, IFN effects can be mediated either directly by an influence on cell division and growth, or indirectly by modulation of the immune response.

In HCL, a range of effects of IFNα on other immune cells have been described, but HCs appear relatively resistant to killing by such cells and it is generally believed that IFNα mediates its effects directly against the malignant HC [93].

Many such direct effects have been described. IFNα modifies intracellular signals in many cells [94], and in HCs may specifically alter intracellular free calcium and protein phosphorylation [95]; the cytokine also alters proto-oncogene expression in HC-derived cell-lines [96]. IFNα also inhibits the proliferation of HCs induced by B-cell growth factor (BCGF) or by TFNα, and may therefore interfere with the autocrine growth of HCs [97,98]. Finally, IFNα causes changes in HC morphology, surface antigen expression and cytoskeletal structure (e.g. refs [97,99]).

No clear, single effect of IFNα has yet emerged to explain the particular sensitivity of HCs to IFNα. However, all these IFNα-induced changes may indicate an alteration in the state of activation/differentiation of the malignant cell, the net effect of which is to reduce the ability of the HC to proliferate or survive.

Biology of the malignant cell

Cytology and cytochemistry

Although HCs derive their name from the numerous tiny cytoplasmic projections which extend for variable distances from the periphery of the cells, it is in fact a combination of characteristics that identifies the HC in Romanowsky preparations. The eccentric nucleus with its distinctive fine chromatin condensation and inconspicuous nucleoli, the pale slate-blue cytoplasm, as well as the surface hairs, all form part of the initial diagnostic impression.

Seven isoenzymes of acid phosphatase are demonstrable by gel electrophoresis in normal and pathological leucocytes. Isoenzyme 5 is largely restricted to the HCs of HCL and, unlike the other isoenzymes of acid phosphatase, is resistant to tartaric acid [100]. TRAP can be readily detected cytochemically and its demonstration has become an important confirmatory diagnostic test in the disease. Provided certain technical points [101] are observed, moderate or strong TRAP can probably be demonstrated in all genuine examples of HCL (Fig. 8.2). The converse, however, is not true and at least moderate TRAP activity may occasionally be observed in other cell types [102].

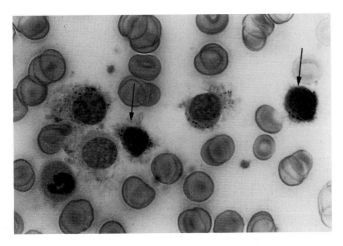

Fig. 8.2 Five hairy cells and a neutrophil. The cells demonstrate variable positivity: two of the hairy cells show a strong reaction (arrowed), while the neutrophil has not stained, demonstrating the effectiveness of the tartrate inhibition (TRAP).

Ultrastructure

The fine structural features of the HC are those of a metabolically active cell deriving much of its energy from oxidative mitochondrial metabolism [16] (Fig. 8.3). The nucleus displays slight to moderate peripheral chromatin condensation and nucleoli are inconspicuous. The surface hairs of HCs are readily seen as fine microvilli and less frequent, broadly based structures; these form the distinctive combination of finger-like projections and ridge-like ruffles seen by scanning electron microscopy (Fig. 8.4). Modest numbers of free ribosomes and a few short strands of rough endoplasmic reticulum account for the distinctive slate-blue cytoplasm of Romanowsky preparations. The Golgi apparatus is only moderately developed, but numerous vacuoles and vesicles are often seen scattered throughout the cytoplasm.

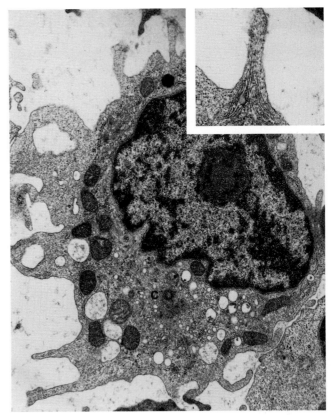

Fig. 8.3 Hairy cell. In order to minimize preparative artefact, this specimen was obtained by dextran sedimentation and fixation in suspension. Fine microvilli and more broadly based surface projections are present. The inset shows how, in favourable planes of section, microfibrils are seen entering the microvilli. Vacuoles and vesicles of varying size are particularly prominent in this cell. A centriole (c) is present in transverse section and microtubules are seen converging on the nearby pericentriolar satellites. The eccentric nuclear profile with its moderate peripheral chromatin condensation is typical; the nucleolus contains a distinct pars amorpha and a poorly defined nucleolonema. (× 13 000, inset × 21 500.)

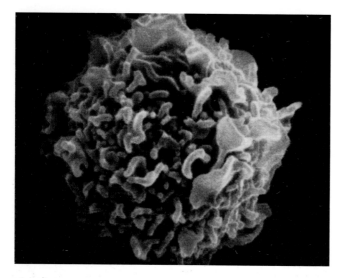

Fig. 8.4 Hairy cell displaying the typical hybrid surface morphology of monocytoid ruffles and lymphoid microvilli. (SEM, × 12 000.)

TRAP is demonstrable at the ultrastructural level in at least some of the cytoplasmic granules [16]. In addition, an endogenous peroxidase distinct from myeloperoxidase can be seen in strands of endoplasmic reticulum, but not in cytoplasmic granules. The exact nature of this HC peroxidase is unknown, but it resembles that seen in cells of the megakaryocyte series.

Distinctive cylindrical structures known as ribosome–lamella (R–L) complexes are found in approximately 50% of cases. In a given patient they may be very infrequent, or they may occur in many of the HCs. Although these structures may occasionally occur in a variety of other haematological and nonhaematological cell types, they are more common in HCL than in other haematological malignancies. As their name suggests, R–L complexes are composed of ribosomal granules associated with an elaborate system of fibrils — the lamella component (Fig. 8.5). The function of R–L complexes is unknown, but they are not involved in immunoglobulin synthesis because nearby endoplasmic reticulum can be shown to contain immunoglobulin by peroxidase immuno-electron microscopy, while the R–L complexes themselves are unreactive.

The diagnostic importance of electron microscopy has probably been overstated, because the usual reasons for diagnostic difficulty — paucity or atypia of HCs — are not overcome by ultrastructural examination.

Karyotype

The closely defined nature of HCL, and the homogeneity in the behaviour of the malignant cells, suggests that a consistent genetic lesion may underlie the disorder. Karyotypic studies have not, however, found any consistent abnormality. The incidence of karyotypic abnormality identified in recent studies has varied between 19 and 67% [103,104], and a wide range of common B-cell abnormalities, including 14q+, have been identified [105]; the most HC-specific abnormalities involve chromosome 5, but these are not seen in all patients [104]. It is also interesting to note that HCs show high rates of nonclonal chromosomal change, suggesting some chromosomal instability [103,104].

Differentiation and activation

It is now recognized that HCL represents a clonal proliferation of B cells at a late stage of differentiation and that the abnormal cells have features of cell activation. A wide body of evidence supports this and is reviewed below.

Immunoglobulin studies

HCs show typical features of late B-cell differentiation. The abnormal cells have rearranged both heavy- and light-chain Ig loci [106]. They synthesize Ig, express the molecule strongly at their surface, and show a limited capacity for Ig secretion. Ig heavy-chain switching has, at least partly, occurred since all Ig types other than IgE have reported on the malignant cells. IgG is most frequently expressed (approx. 50%) [28,103,107]. The Ig genes in HCL, unlike those in plasma cells, have not undergone somatic mutation [108].

Certain features of Ig expression by HCs are not, however, completely understood. Surface Ig is most often the relatively uncommon IgG3 subtype [109]. Furthermore, and in contrast to other B cells, many cases of HCL express multiple heavy-chain isotypes on the surface of the malignant clone [28,103,107]. This unusual feature is difficult to explain, because the simultaneous expression of Ig heavy chains other than M and D is not compatible with current models of Ig class switching [110].

Surface antigen expression

The immunological surface markers of HCs confirm the late-B-cell nature of the malignant cell. CD19, CD20, CD22, CD40 and FMC7 are expressed, while early B-cell markers such as CD10 are not usually present [111]. Plasma cell markers such as PCA-1 are expressed [112], but the cells show no other features of plasmacytoid differentiation. In other regards the surface antigens expressed by HCs are typical of an activated B cell. Markers such as CD21 and CD24, which are normally lost after activation, are only weakly expressed [111], while activation antigens such as CD25 and CD72 are strongly represented [111].

However, not all B-cell activation antigens are present on HCs; for example, both CD38 and CD23 are weakly expressed or are absent [111]. Furthermore, HCs express a group of antigens not generally found on B cells. For example, markers

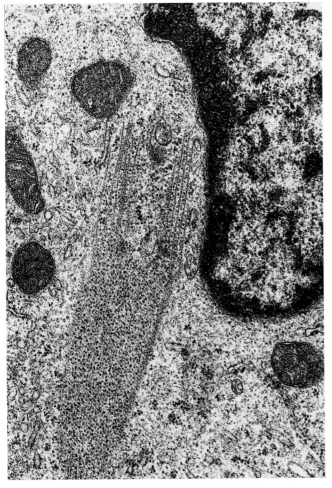

(a)

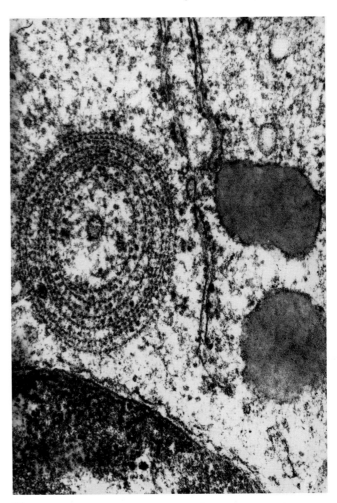

(b)

Fig. 8.5 (a) Ribosome–lamella (R–L) complex. In its upper part, the complex is cut obliquely. Careful examination of the obliquely sectioned area reveals the two-dimensional net-like structure described in the text. (× 72 000.) (b) R–L complex in transverse section. The coils of the lamella component of the complex are seen to be composed of distinct subunits which sometimes appear to be separated, but are often joined. The ribosomes, which are concentrically arranged approximately midway between the coils, sometimes appear to be connected with the subunits of the lamella component. Two prominent lipid droplets are present. (× 66 000.)

such as CD11c and B-Ly7 are not generally represented on B cells; rather they are regarded to be activation markers on monocytes and T cells respectively.

Thus, the surface antigen expression confirms the late B, but pre-plasma cell, differentiation of the HC. Surface antigens also indicate that the HC is an activated cell. However the HC should not be regarded as a typical 'activated B cell' because although some markers of B-cell activation are expressed, others are not. Furthermore, other HC antigens, although clearly associated with activation, are generally a feature of non-B-cell lineages.

Cytoskeleton

The most characteristic feature of the HC is its cytoplasmic hairs; these too are likely to be a reflection of the activated nature of the malignant cell. Microtubules and the intermediate filament vimentin are both well represented in the malignant cell but do not appear to be essential to the 'hairy' phenotype [113]. The actin cytoskeleton is, however, important; actin filaments extend into the fine hairs of the malignant cell and are responsible for the pleats and ruffles that characterize the HC phenotype [16,114]. Similar appearances can be induced in other normal and malignant lymphocytes by phorbol ester treatment [115,116], further supporting the concept that the cytoskeletal structure is also a reflection of the activated nature of the HC.

Despite the distinctive appearance of HCs, their cytoskeleton is not 'fixed' and its organization is altered in response to environmental stimuli such as adhesion or cytokines [117,118].

Interaction with the environment

In tissues, normal and malignant lymphoid cells receive specific signals that influence adhesion, migration and, ultimately, their proliferation and survival. Such signals derive from the interaction of the cell with adhesive and soluble factors in the tissue microenvironment. It is these interactions that underlie the unique tissue distribution and behaviour of the different lymphoid malignancies.

In HCL, the malignant cell interacts with, and responds to, a range of cytokines and adhesive elements.

Adhesion

HCs are strongly adhesive cells *in vitro*, and their distinctive adhesive responses are reflected *in vivo* in the unusual tissue distribution that characterizes HCL.

All classes of adhesion receptor are represented. Lymphocyte selectin is variably expressed, as are certain members of the immunoglobulin superfamily (CD32 (FcγRII receptor) and CD22) [111]. Other Ig superfamily molecules such as ICAM-1 are more variably represented [119]. The integrin family has been more intensively studied, and it has been shown that a unique profile of receptors is expressed [120]. Several of the HC integrins are markers of B-cell activation (αXβ2 and α5β1), while others reflect activation in other cell types (αHβ7 and αvβ3).

Particular integrin receptors have now been linked to HC behaviour (reviewed in ref [120]). Thus, the integrin α4β1 is strongly expressed on HCs and has been implicated in the initial cell–cell adhesion that governs HC entry into tissues, particularly bone marrow and spleen. α5β1 is very strongly expressed, and is essential to fibronectin synthesis/assembly by HCs (discussed above in relation to HCL bone marrow fibrosis). Finally, the integrin αvβ3 induces HC's motility on substrata such as vitronectin, and may be important in invasion of splenic red pulp by HCs. No role in HC behaviour has yet been identified for the other highly expressed integrin receptors, namely, αHβ7 (B-Ly7) and αXβ2 (CD11c/CD18).

Cytokines

HCs express receptors for a range of cytokines. Two of these, TNFα and LMW-BCGF, induce low-level proliferation of HCs. Moreover, both these cytokines may be secreted by the malignant cell, providing a potential autocrine growth loop [121,122]. TNFα may also have wider effects on the behaviour and survival of the HC [122].

Two 'myeloid growth factor' receptors, namely, the M-CSF (macrophage colony stimulating factor) [123] and GM-CSF receptors [124], are expressed. Neither mediates proliferation, but both influence the interaction of HCs with their environment. M-CSF enhances HC motility on a range of substrata [118], while GM-CSF has antiadhesive properties and reduces HC adhesion [124].

When considering the interleukins, receptors are expressed for IL-2, IL-6 and IL-15. Of these, the strong CD25 (IL-2α) expression by HCs has lead to extensive study of IL-2 and its receptor. It is now established that HCs possess all three components (alpha, beta and gamma) of the IL-2R, but that only the alpha chain is strongly expressed. As a result, the malignant cell can assemble relatively few functional high-affinity receptors at their surface [125,126]. The alpha chain is secreted from the cell surface into the serum [127], but its function there is not clear. The functional responses induced in HCs by other interleukins are poorly defined at present.

Signalling

There is an accumulating body of evidence suggesting pronounced signalling activity in HCs. Protein tyrosine kinases of the *src* family are very active [128,129], as are serine/threonine kinases such as calcium/calmodulin-dependent kinase II [130]. Furthermore, free intracellular calcium levels in HCs are higher than in related cell types such as CLL and normal B cells [130], while in such cells pharmacological stimulation of PKC can induce HC-like features [115,116]. Finally, tyrosine phosphatases such as CD45 [131] are strongly represented.

Since the oncogenic event underlying HCL remains obscure, it is difficult to assess the significance of these various signalling phenomena. However it is clear that, despite the activated nature of the HC, most if not all the signalling processes outlined above can be both downregulated or stimulated further. Thus, the elevated free intracellular calcium levels of HCs can be reduced by IFN and increased by BCGF [130]. Similarly, tyrosine phosphorylation signals are responsive to both cytokines and adhesion [120].

The future

Current treatment for HCL is so effective it is unlikely that major therapeutic advances will now be made. What does the future now hold? Of course no one knows, but it is clear that at least one major question remains, namely, what is the basic cellular abnormality resulting in the fascinating phenotype of the HC? Enough is now known to predict that the oncogenic event involves specific, but incomplete, cell activation. Rapid progress in the relevant areas of cell/molecular biology suggests that elucidation of the precise nature of this oncogenic event, and its consequences, is now within reach.

References

1 Rosenthal N. & Lee S.L. (1951) Reticulum cell leukemia: a clinical and morphological entity. Report of 16 cases. In: *Thirtieth Annual*

Meeting of the American Society of Clinical Pathologists (Chicago), 16–19 October.

2 Bouroncle B.A., Wiseman B.K. & Doan C.A. (1958) Leukemic reticuloendotheliosis. *Blood*, **13**, 609–630.

3 Symmers W. St C. (ed.) (1978) *Systemic Pathology*. Churchill Livingstone, Edinburgh.

4 Staines A. & Cartwright R.A. (1993) Hairy-cell leukaemia; descriptive epidemiology and a case-control study. *British Journal of Haematology*, **85**, 714–717.

5 Oleske D., Golomb H.M., Farber M.D. & Levy P.S. (1985) A case-control inquiry into the etiology of hairy-cell leukemia. *American Journal of Epidemiology*, **121**, 675–683.

6 Aksoy M. (1987) Chronic lymphoid leukemia and hairy-cell leukemia due to chronic exposure to benzene—report of 3 cases. *British Journal of Haematology*, **66**, 209–211.

7 Flandrin G. & Collado S. (1987) Is male predominance (4/1) in hairy-cell leukemia related to occupational exposure to ionizing-radiation, benzene and other solvents. *British Journal of Haematology*, **67**, 119–120.

8 Gramatovici M., Bennett J.M., Hiscock J.G. & Grewal K.S. (1993) Three cases of familial hairy cell leukemia. *American Journal of Hematology*, **42**, 337–339.

9 Ward F.T., Baker J., Krishnan J., Dow N. & Kjobech C.H. (1990) Hairy cell leukemia in two siblings. A human leukocyte antigen-linked disease? *Cancer*, **65**, 319–321.

10 Kalyanaraman V.S., Sarngadharan M.G., Robertguroff M. *et al.* (1982) A new subtype of human t-cell leukemia-virus (htlv-II) associated with a T-cell variant of hairy-cell leukemia. *Science*, **218**, 571–573.

11 Lion T., Razvi N., Golomb H.M. & Brownstein R.H. (1988) B-lymphocytic hairy cells contain no HTLV-II DNA sequences. *Blood*, **72**, 1428–1430.

12 Hjelle B., Mills R., Swenson S., Mertz G., Key C. & Allen S. (1991) Incidence of hairy cell leukemia, mycosis fungoides, and chronic lymphocytic leukemia in first known HTLV-II-endemic population. *Journal of Infectious Diseases*, **163**, 435–440.

13 Wolf B.C., Martin A.W., Neiman R.S. *et al.* (1990) The detection of Epstein–Barr virus in hairy cell leukemia cells by in situ hybridization. *American Journal of Pathology*, **136**, 717–723.

14 Chang K.L., Chen Y.Y. & Weiss L.M. (1993) Lack of evidence of Epstein–Barr virus in hairy cell leukemia and monocytoid B-cell lymphoma. *Human Pathology*, **24**, 58–61.

15 Hamilton-Dutoit S.J. & Pallesen G. (1992) A survey of Epstein–Barr virus gene expression in sporadic non-Hodgkin's lymphomas. Detection of Epstein–Barr virus in a subset of peripheral T-cell lymphomas. *American Journal of Pathology*, **140**, 1315–1325.

16 Cawley J.C., Burns G.F., Hayhoe F.G.H. (eds) (1980) *Hairy-cell Leukaemia*. Springer, Heidelberg.

17 Katayama I., Hirashima K., Maruyama K. *et al.* (1987) Hairy-cell leukemia in Japanese patients — a study with monoclonal-antibodies. *Leukemia*, **1**, 301–305.

18 Budman D.R., Koziner B., Arlin A. *et al.* (1979) Massive adenopathy mimicking lymphoma in leukemic reticuloendotheliosis. *American Journal of Medicine*, **66**, 160–162.

19 Lewis S.M., Catovsky D., Hows J.M. & Ardalan B. (1977) Splenic red cell pooling in hairy cell leukaemia. *British Journal of Haematology*, **35**, 351–357.

20 Castro-Malaspina H., Najean Y. & Flandrin G. (1979) Erythro-

kinetic studies in hairy cell leukaemia. *British Journal of Haematology*, **42**, 189–197.

21 Taniguchi N., Kuratsune H., Kanamaru A. *et al.* (1989) Inhibition against CFU-C and CFU-E colony formation by soluble factor(s) derived from hairy cells. *Blood*, **73**, 907–913.

22 Foa R., Guarini A., Francia-di-Celle P. *et al.* (1992) Constitutive production of tumor necrosis factor-alpha in hairy cell leukemia: possible role in the pathogenesis of the cytopenia(s) and effect of treatment with interferon-alpha. *Journal of Clinical Oncology*, **10**, 954–959.

23 Hayhoe F.G., Flemens R.J., Burns G.F. *et al.* (1977) Leukocyte alkaline phosphatase scores in hairy cell leukaemia. *British Journal of Haematology*, **37**, 158–159.

24 Child J.A., Cawley J.C., Martin S. & Ghoneim A.T.M. (1978) Microbiocidal function of the neutrophils in hairy-cell leukaemia. *Acta Haematologica*, **62**, 191–198.

25 Seshadri R.S., Brown E.J. & Zipursky A. (1976) Leukemic reticuloendotheliosis. A failure of monocyte production. *New England Journal of Medicine*, **295**, 181–184.

26 Zuzel M., Cawley J.C., Paton R.C., Burn G.F. & McNichol G.P. (1979) Platelet function in hairy-cell leukaemia. *Journal of Clinical Pathology*, **32**, 814–821.

27 Pittaluga S., Verhoef G., Maes A., Boogaerts M.A. & De-Wolf-Peeters C. (1994) Bone marrow trephines. Findings in patients with hairy cell leukaemia before and after treatment. *Histopathology*, **25**, 129–135.

28 Burns G.F., Cawley J.C., Worman C.P. *et al.* (1978) Multiple heavy chain isotypes on the surface of the cells of hairy-cell leukaemia. *Blood*, **52**, 1132–1136.

29 Hansen D.A., Robbins B.A., Bylund D.J. Piro L.D., Saven A. & Ellison D.J. (1994) Identification of monoclonal immunoglobulins and quantitative immunoglobulin abnormalities in hairy cell leukemia and chronic lymphocytic leukemia. *American Journal of Clinical Pathology*, **102**, 580–585.

30 Marie J.P., Degos L. & Flandrin G. (1977) Hairy cell leukaemia and tuberculosis. *New England Journal of Medicine*, **297**, 1354.

31 Rice L., Shenkenberg T., Lynch E.C. & Wheeler T.M. (1982) Granulomatous infections complicating hairy-cell leukaemia. *Cancer*, **49**, 1924–1928.

32 Westbrook C.A. & Golde D.W. (1985) Autoimmune-disease in hairy-cell leukaemia — clinical syndromes and treatment. *British Journal of Haematology*, **61**, 349–356.

33 Domingo A., Crespo N., Fernandez-de-Sevilla A., Domenech P., Jordan C. & Callis M. (1992) Hairy cell leukemia and autoimmune hemolytic anemia. *Leukemia*, **6**, 606–607.

34 Salvarani C., Capozzoli N., Baricchi R. *et al.* (1989) Autoimmune disease in hairy-cell leukemia: systemic vasculitis and anticardiolipin syndrome [letter]. *Clinical and Experimental Rheumatology*, **7**, 329–330.

35 Lembersky B.C., Ratain M.J. & Golomb H.M. (1988) Skeletal complications in hairy cell leukemia: diagnosis and therapy. *Journal of Clinical Oncology*, **6**, 1280–1284.

36 Herold C.J., Wittich G.R., Schwarzinger I. *et al.* (1988) Skeletal involvement in hairy cell leukemia. *Skeletal Radiology*, **17**, 171–175.

37 Bernstein L., Newton P. & Ross R.K. (1990) Epidemiology of hairy cell leukemia in Los Angeles County. *Cancer Research*, **50**, 3605–3609.

38 Kampmeier P., Spielberger R., Dickstein J., Mick R., Golomb H. & Vardiman J.W. (1994) Increased incidence of second neoplasms

in patients treated with interferon alpha 2b for hairy cell leukemia: a clinicopathologic assessment. *Blood*, **83**, 2931–2938.

39 Mercieca J., Puga M., Matutes E., Moskovic E., Salim S. & Catovsky D. (1994) Incidence and significance of abdominal lymphadenopathy in hairy cell leukaemia. *Leukemia and Lymphoma*, **14**(Suppl. 1), 79–83.

40 Mercieca J., Matutes E., Moskovic E. *et al.* (1992) Massive abdominal lymphadenopathy in hairy cell leukaemia: a report of 12 cases. *British Journal of Haematology*, **82**, 547–554.

41 Elkan K.B., Hughes G.R.V., Catovsky D. *et al.* (1979) Hairy-cell leukaemia and polyarteritis nodosa. *Lancet*, **ii**, 280–282.

42 Jansen J., Bolhuis R.L.H., Vanieuwkoop J.A., Schuit H.R.E. & Kroese W.F.S. (1983) Paraproteinemia plus osteolytic lesions in typical hairy-cell leukaemia. *British Journal of Haematology*, **54**, 531–541.

43 Catovsky D., Costello C. & Loukopoulus D. (1981) Hairy cell leukaemia and myelomatosis: chance association or clinical manifestations of the same B-cell disease spectrum. *Blood*, **57**, 758–763.

44 Keidan A.J., Lin Yin J.A. & Gordon Smith E.C. (1984) Uncommon complications of hairy cell leukaemia. *British Journal of Haematology*, **57**, 176–177.

45 Burke J.S. (1978) The value of the bone-marrow in the diagnosis of hairy cell leukemia. *American Journal of Clinical Pathology*, **70**, 876–884.

46 Burthem J. & Cawley J.C. (1994) The bone marrow fibrosis of hairy-cell leukaemia is caused by the synthesis and assembly of a fibronectin matrix by the hairy cells. *Blood*, **83**, 497–504.

47 Nanba K., Soban E.J., Bowling M.C. & Berad C.W. (1977) Splenic pseudosinuses and hepatic angiomatous lesions. Distinctive features of hairy cell leukemia. *American Journal of Clinical Pathology*, **67**, 415–426.

48 Burke J.S., Byrne G.E. & Rappaport H. (1974) Hairy cell leukemia (leukemic reticuloendotheliosis). A clinical pathologic study of 21 patients. *Cancer*, **33**, 2267–2274.

49 Delsol G., Pelligrin M., Corberand J., Guiu M., Pris J. & Fabre J. (1977) *Kupffer Cells and Other Liver Sinusoidal Cells*. Elsevier, Amsterdam.

50 Falini B., Pileri S.A., Flenghi L. *et al.* (1990) Selection of a panel of monoclonal antibodies for monitoring residual disease in peripheral blood and bone marrow of interferon-treated hairy cell leukaemia patients. *British Journal of Haematology*, **76**, 460–468.

51 Ellison D.J., Sharpe R.W., Robbins B.A. *et al.* (1994) Immunomorphologic analysis of bone marrow biopsies after treatment with 2-chlorodeoxyadenosine for hairy cell leukemia. *Blood*, **84**, 4310–4315.

52 Cawley J.C., Burns G.F. & Hayhoe F.G.J. (1980) A chronic lymphoproliferative disorder with distinctive features — a distinct variant of hairy-cell leukemia. *Leukemia Research*, **4**, 547.

53 Sainati L., Matutes E., Mulligan S. *et al.* (1990) A variant form of hairy cell leukemia resistant to alpha-interferon: clinical and phenotypic characteristics of 17 patients. *Blood*, **76**, 157–162.

54 Catovsky D., Obrien M., Melo J.V., Wardle J. & Brozovic M. (1984) Hairy-cell leukemia (hcl) variant — an intermediate disease between hcl and b prolymphocytic leukemia. *Seminars in Oncology*, **11**, 362–369.

55 Matutes E., Morilla R., Owusu-Ankomah K., Houlihan A. & Catovsky D. (1994) The immunophenotype of splenic lymphoma with villous lymphocytes and its relevance to the differential diagnosis with other B-cell disorders. *Blood*, **83**, 1558–1562.

56 Melo J.V., Robinson D.S.F., Gregory C. & Catovsky D. (1987) Splenic b-cell lymphoma with villous lymphocytes in the peripheral-blood — a disorder distinct from hairy-cell leukaemia. *Leukemia*, **1**, 294–298.

57 Catovsky D. & Foa R. (eds) (1990) *The Lymphoid Leukaemias: the leukaemic phase of non-Hodgkins lymphoma*. Butterworths, London.

58 Neiman R.S., Sullivan A.L. & Jaffe R. (1979) Malignant lymphoma simulating leukemic reticuloendotheliosis: a clinicopathologic study of 10 cases. *Cancer*, **43**, 329–343.

59 Isaacson P.G., Matutes E., Burke M. & Catovsky D. (1994) The histopathology of splenic lymphoma with villous lymphocytes. *Blood*, **84**, 3828–3834.

60 Saven A. & Piro L. (1994) Newer purine analogues for the treatment of hairy-cell leukemia. *New England Journal of Medicine*, **330**, 691–697.

61 Piro L.D., Ellison D.J. & Saven A. (1994) The Scripps Clinic experience with 2-chlorodeoxyadenosine in the treatment of hairy cell leukemia. *Leukemia and Lymphoma*, **14**(Suppl. 1), 121–125.

62 Lauria F., Benfenati D., Raspadori D. *et al.* (1994) Retreatment with 2-CdA of progressed HCL patients. *Leukemia and Lymphoma*, **14**(Suppl. 1), 143–145.

63 Bryson H.M. & Sorkin E.M. (1993) Cladribine. A review of its pharmacodynamic and pharmacokinetic properties and therapeutic potential in haematological malignancies. *Drugs*, **46**, 872–894.

64 Annino L., Ferrari A., Giona F. *et al.* (1994) Deoxycoformycin induces long-lasting remissions in hairy cell leukemia: clinical and biological results of two different regimens. *Leukemia and Lymphoma*, **14**(Suppl. 1):115–119.

65 Catovsky D., Matutes E., Talavera J.G. *et al.* (1994) Long term results with 2'deoxycoformycin in hairy cell leukemia. *Leukemia and Lymphoma*, **14**(Suppl. 1), 109–113.

66 Kraut E.H., Grever M.R. & Bouroncle B.A. (1994) Long-term follow-up of patients with hairy cell leukemia after treatment with 2'-deoxycoformycin. *Blood*, **84**, 4061–4063.

67 Brogden R.N. & Sorkin E.M. (1993) Pentostatin. A review of its pharmacodynamic and pharmacokinetic properties, and therapeutic potential in lymphoproliferative disorders. *Drugs*, **46**, 652–677.

68 Urba W.J., Baseler M.W., Kopp W.C. *et al.* (1989) Deoxycoformycin-induced immunosuppression in patients with hairy cell leukemia. *Blood*, **73**, 38–46.

69 Kraut E.H. & Chun H.G. (1991) Fludarabine phosphate in refractory hairy cell leukemia. *American Journal of Hematology*, **37**, 59–60.

70 Kantarjian H.M., Schachner J. & Keating M.J. (1991) Fludarabine therapy in hairy cell leukemia. *Cancer*, **67**, 1291–1293.

71 Ozer H., Golomb H.M., Zimmerman H. & Spiegel R.J. (1989) Cost-benefit analysis of interferon alfa-2b in treatment of hairy cell leukemia. *Journal of the National Cancer Institute*, **81**, 594–602.

72 Golomb H.M., Ratain M.J., Fefer A. *et al.* (1988) Randomized study of the duration of treatment with interferon alfa-2B in patients with hairy cell leukemia. *Journal of the National Cancer Institute*, **80**, 369–373.

73 Berman E., Heller G., Kempin S., Gee T., Tran L.L. & Clarkson B. (1990) Incidence of response and long-term follow-up in patients with hairy cell leukemia treated with recombinant interferon alfa-2a [see comments]. *Blood*, **75**, 839–845.

74 Galvani D.W. & Cawley J.C. (1990) The current status of interferon alpha in haemic malignancy. *Blood Reviews*, **4**, 175–180.

75 Ratain M.J., Golomb H.M., Vardiman J.W. *et al.* (1988)

Relapse after interferon alfa-2b therapy for hairy-cell leukemia: analysis of prognostic variables. *Journal of Clinical Oncology*, **6**, 1714–1721.

76 Zinzani P.L., Lauria F., Raspadori D. *et al.* (1992) Results in hairy-cell leukemia patients treated with alpha-interferon: predictive prognostic factors. *European Journal of Haematology*, **49**, 133–137.

77 Platanias L.C., Pfeffer L.M., Barton K.P., Vardiman J.W., Golomb H.M. & Colamonici O.R. (1992) Expression of the IFN alpha receptor in hairy cell leukaemia. *British Journal of Haematology*, **82**, 541–546.

78 Antonelli G. & Dianzani F. (1993) Antibodies to interferon in patients. *Archives of Virology*, **8**(Suppl.), 271–277.

79 von-Wussow P., Pralle H., Hochkeppel H.K. *et al.* (1991) Effective natural interferon-alpha therapy in recombinant interferon-alpha-resistant patients with hairy cell leukemia. *Blood*, **78**, 38–43.

80 Ratain M.J., Vardiman J.W., Barker C.M. & Golomb H.M. (1988) Prognostic variables in hairy cell leukemia after splenectomy as initial therapy. *Cancer*, **62**, 2420–2424.

81 Jansen J. & Hermans J. (1981) Splenectomy in hairy-cell leukemia — a retrospective multi-center analysis. *Cancer*, **47**, 2066–2076.

82 Lorber C., Willfort A., Ohler L. *et al.* (1993) Granulocyte colony-stimulating factor (rh G-CSF) as an adjunct to interferon alpha therapy of neutropenic patients with hairy cell leukemia. *Annals of Hematology*, **67**, 13–16.

83 Glaspy J.A., Souza L., Scates S. *et al.* (1992) Treatment of hairy cell leukemia with granulocyte colony-stimulating factor and recombinant consensus interferon or recombinant interferon-alpha-2b. *Journal of Immunotherapy*, **11**, 198–208.

84 Lindemann A., Herrmann F., Mertelsmann R., Gamm H. & Rumpelt H.J. (1990) Splenic hematopoiesis following GM-CSF therapy in a patient with hairy cell leukemia [letter]. *Leukemia*, **4**, 606–607.

85 Damasio E.E. & Frassoldati A. (1994) Splenectomy following complete response to alpha interferon (IFN) therapy in patients with hairy cell leukemia (HCL): results of the HCL88 protocol. Italian Cooperative Group for the Study of Hairy Cell Leukemia (ICGHCL). *Leukemia and Lymphoma*, **14**(Suppl. 1), 95–98.

86 Martin A., Nerenstone S., Urba W.J. *et al.* (1990) Treatment of hairy cell leukemia with alternating cycles of pentostatin and recombinant leukocyte A interferon: results of a phase II study. *Journal of Clinical Oncology*, **8**, 721–730.

87 Habermann T.M., Andersen J.W., Cassileth P.A., Bennett J.M. & Oken M.M. (1992) Sequential administration of recombinant interferon alpha and deoxycoformycin in the treatment of hairy cell leukaemia. *British Journal of Haemotology*, **80**, 466.

88 Catovsky D., Golomb H.M. & Golde D.W. (1987) General Commentary on the Second International Workshop. *Leukemia*, **1**, 407–409.

89 Arena F.P. (1994) Treatment of hairy-cell leukaemia in a decade of change. Appraisal of community based oncologists' opinions. *Leukemia and Lymphoma*, **14**(Suppl. 1), 85–88.

90 Carrera M.D., Saven A. & Piro L.D. (1994) Purine metabolism of lymphocytes. Targets for chemotherapy drug development. *New Drug Therapy*, **8**, 357–380.

91 Ganeshaguru K., de-Mel W.C., Sissolak G. *et al.* (1991) Increase in 2′,5′-oligoadenylate synthetase caused by deoxycoformycin in hairy cell leukaemia. *Advances in Experimental Medicine and Biology*, **309A**, 65–68.

92 Ho A.D., Ganeshaguru K., Knauf W. *et al.* (1989) Enzyme activities of leukemic cells and biochemical changes induced by deoxycoformycin *in vitro* — lack of correlation with clinical response. *Leukemia Research*, **13**, 269–278.

93 Vedantham S., Gamliel H. & Golomb H.M. (1992) Mechanism of interferon action in hairy cell leukemia: a model of effective cancer biotherapy. *Cancer Research*, **52**, 1056–1066.

94 Pellegrini S. & Schindler C. (1993) Early events in signalling by interferons. *Trends in Biochemical Science*, **18**, 338–342.

95 Genot E., Bismuth G., Degos L., Sigaux F. & Wietzerbin J. (1992) Interferon-alpha downregulates the abnormal intracytoplasmic free calcium concentration of tumor cells in hairy cell leukemia. *Blood*, **80**, 2060–2065.

96 Harvey W.H., Harb O.S., Kosak S.T., Sheaffer J.C., Lowe L.R. & Heerema N.A. (1994) Interferon-alpha-2b downregulation of oncogenes H-*ras*, c-*raf-2*, c-*kit*, c-*myc*, c-*myb* and c-*fos* in ESKOL, a hairy cell leukemic line, results in temporal perturbation of signal transduction cascade. *Leukemia Research*, **18**, 577–585.

97 Gamliel H., Brownstein B.H., Gurfel D., Wu S.H., Rosner M.C. & Golomb H.M. (1990) B-cell growth factor-induced and alpha-interferon-inhibited proliferation of hairy cells coincides with modulation of cell surface antigens. *Cancer Research*, **50**, 4111–4120.

98 Heslop H.E., Brenner M.K., Ganeshaguru K. & Hoffbrand A.V. (1991) Possible mechanism of action of interferon alpha in chronic B-cell malignancies. *British Journal of Haematology*, **79**(Suppl. 1), 14–16.

99 Hassan I.B., Lantz M. & Sundstrom C. (1991) Effect of alpha-IFN on cytokine-induced antigen expression and secretion of TNF, LT and IgM in HCL. *Leukemia Research*, **15**, 903–910.

100 Li C.Y., Yam L.T. & Lam K.W. (1970) Studies of acid phosphatase isoenzymes in human leukocytes. Demonstration of isoenzyme cell specificity. *Journal of Histochemistry and Cytochemistry*, **18**, 901–910.

101 Janckila A.J., Li C.Y., Lam K.W. & Yam L.T. (1978) The cytochemistry of tartrate-resistant acid phosphatase. Technical considerations. *American Journal of Clinical Pathology*, **70**, 45–55.

102 Drexler H.G. & Gignac S.M. (1994) Characterization and expression of tartrate-resistant acid phosphatase (TRAP) in hematopoietic cells. *Leukemia*, **8**, 359–368.

103 Kluin-Nelemans H.C., Beverstock G.C., Mollevanger P. *et al.* (1994) Proliferation and cytogenetic analysis of hairy cell leukemia upon stimulation via the CD40 antigen. *Blood*, **84**, 3134–3141.

104 Haglund U., Juliusson G., Stellan B. & Gahrton G. (1994) Hairy cell leukemia is characterized by clonal chromosome abnormalities clustered to specific regions. *Blood*, **83**, 2637–2645.

105 Juliusson G. & Gahrton G. (1993) Cytogenetics in CLL and related disorders. *Baillière's Clinical Haematology*, **6**, 821–848.

106 Korsmeyer S.J., Greene W.C. & Cossman J. (1983) Rearrangement and expression of immunoglobulin genes and expression of Tac antigen in hairy cell leukemia. *Proceedings of the National Academy of Sciences, USA*, **80**, 4522–4526.

107 Jansen J., Schuit H.R.E., Meijer C.J.L.M., Vannieuwkoop J.A. & Hijmans W. (1982) Cell markers in hairy-cell leukemia studied in cells from 51 patients. *Blood*, **59**, 52–60.

108 Wagner S.D., Martinelli V. & Luzzatto L. (1994) Similar patterns of V kappa gene usage but different degrees of somatic mutation in hairy cell leukemia, prolymphocytic leukemia, Waldenstrom's macroglobulinemia, and myeloma. *Blood*, **83**, 3647–3653.

109 Kluin-Nelemans H.C., Krouwels M.M., Jansen J.H. *et al.* (1990)

Hairy cell leukemia preferentially expresses the IgG3-subclass. *Blood*, **75**, 972–975.

110 Snapper C.M. & Finkelman F.D. (1993) Immunoglobulin class switching. In: *Fundamental Immunology* (ed. W.E. Paul), 3rd edn, pp. 337–364. Raven, New York.

111 Knapp W., Dorken B., Gilks W.R. *et al.* (eds) (1989) Leukocyte typing IV. In: *White Cell Differentiation Antigens*. Oxford, Oxford University Press.

112 Anderson K.C., Boyd A.W., Fisher D.C., Leslie D., Schlossman S.F. & Nadler L.M. (1985) Hairy-cell leukemia—a tumor of pre-plasma cells. *Blood*, **65**, 620–629.

113 Zauli D., Gobbi M., Crespi C., Tazzari P.L., Miserocchi F. & Tassinari A. (1988) Cytoskeleton organization of normal and neoplastic lymphocytes and lymphoid cell lines of T and B origin. *British Journal of Haematology*, **68**, 405–409.

114 Caligaris-Cappio F.G., Bergui L., Corbascio G., Tousco F. & Marchisio P.C. (1986) Cytoskeletal organisation is aberrantly rearranged in the cells of B chronic lymphocytic leukemia. *Blood*, **67**, 233–239.

115 Gazitt Y., Leizerowitz R. & Polliack A. (1988) Induction of plasmacytoid and hairy cell features by phorbol esters (TPA) in B-lymphoma cells: attempted correlation with disease activity. *Hematological Oncology*, **6**, 307–318.

116 Al-Katib A., Mohammad R.M., Dan M. *et al.* (1993) Bryostatin 1-induced hairy cell features on chronic lymphocytic leukemia cells *in vitro*. *Experimental Hematology*, **21**, 61–65.

117 Burthem J., Baker P.K., Hunt J.A. & Cawley J.C. (1994) The function of c-*fms* in hairy-cell leukemia: macrophage colony-stimulating factor stimulates hairy-cell movement. *Blood*, **83**, 1381–1389.

118 Burthem J., Baker P.K., Hunt J.A. & Cawley J.C. (1994) Hairy cell interactions with extracellular matrix: expression of specific integrin receptors and their role in the cell's response to specific adhesive proteins. *Blood*, **84**, 873–882.

119 Jansen J.H., van-der-Harst D., Wientjens G.J. *et al.* (1992) Induction of CD11a/leukocyte function antigen-1 and CD54/intercellular adhesion molecule-1 on hairy cell leukemia cells is accompanied by enhanced susceptibility to T-cell but not lymphokine-activated killer-cell cytotoxicity [see comments]. *Blood*, **80**, 478–483.

120 Burthem J. & Cawley J.C. (1994) Specific tissue invasion, localisation and matrix modification in hairy-cell leukemia. *Leukemia and Lymphoma*, **14**(Suppl. 1), 19–22.

121 Ford R.J., Yoshimura J., Morgan J., Quesada J., Montagna R. & Maizel A. (1985) Growth factor-mediated tumour cell proliferation in hairy-cell leukemia. *Journal of Experimental Medicine*, **162**, 1093–1098.

122 Cordingley F.T., Bianchi A., Hoffbrand A.V. *et al.* (1988) Tumour necrosis factor as an autocrine tumour growth factor for chronic B-cell malignancies. *Lancet*, **1**, 969–971.

123 Till K.J., Lopez A., Slupsky J. & Cawley J.C. (1993) C-*fms* protein expression by B-cells, with particular reference to the hairy cells of hairy-cell leukaemia. *British Journal of Haematology*, **83**, 223–231.

124 Till K.J., Burthem J., Lopez A. & Cawley J.C. (1996) Expression and function of the granulocyte–macrophage colony-stimulating factor (GM-CSF) receptor on mature B-cells: GM-CSF inhibits the chemotaxis, adhesion and motility of these cells. *Blood*, **88**, 479–486.

125 Trentin L., Zambello R., Benati C. *et al.* (1992) Expression and functional role of the p75 interleukin 2 receptor chain on leukemic hairy cells. *Cancer Research*, **52**, 5223–5228.

126 de-Totero D., Carbone A., Tazzari P.L. *et al.* (1994) Expression of the IL2 receptor alpha, beta and gamma chains in hairy cell leukemia. *Leukemia and Lymphoma*, **14**(Suppl. 1), 27–32.

127 Burton J. & Kay N.E. (1994) Does IL-2 receptor expression and secretion in chronic B-cell leukemia have a role in down-regulation of the immune system? *Leukemia*, **8**, 92–96.

128 Lower E.E., Franco R.S. & Martelo O.J. (1992) Increased tyrosine protein kinase activity in hairy cell and monocytic leukemias. *American Journal of the Medical Sciences*, **303**, 387–391.

129 Lynch S.A., Bruggs J.S., Fromowitz F. *et al.* (1993) Increased expression of the src proto-oncogene in hairy cell leukemia and a subgroup of B-cell lymphomas. *Leukemia*, **7**, 1416–1422.

130 Genot E. & Wietzerbin J. (1994) Investigating hairy cell leukemia dysregulations. Looking for interferon alpha site of action in hairy cells. *Leukemia and Lymphoma*, **14**(Suppl. 1), 23–26.

131 Martin J.M., Boras V.F., Houwen B. & Francovich N. (1988) Hairy cell leukemia and anti-leukocyte common antigen. *American Journal of Clinical Pathology*, **90**, 412–420.

9 Acute Myeloid Leukaemia: Clinical Features and Management

J.A. Whittaker

Clinical features

The presenting features of acute myeloid leukaemia (AML) are often directly related to bone marrow failure which may have been present from a few days to several months. This results in varying degrees of anaemia, granulocytopenia and thrombocytopenia, which are the direct or indirect causes of many of the symptoms and signs at presentation. In a minority of AML patients, the presenting clinical features may also be due to infiltration of tissues with leukaemic cells.

The clinical features of leukaemia are well reviewed in the older literature [1–3].

Clinical features related to bone marrow failure

Anaemia

Pallor and tiredness are the commonest symptoms of anaemia and occur in the majority of adult patients, of whom 80% have an initial haemoglobin concentration below 11 g/dl. The median haemoglobin concentration is 9 g/dl and, in the elderly or when anaemia has been present for some time, this may result in cardiorespiratory symptoms, particularly dyspnoea, tachycardia, syncope and angina. Apart from tachycardia, signs of anaemia are uncommon except in severely anaemic patients where pulmonary oedema and congestive cardiac failure can occur. Marrow failure is almost certainly mainly due to a direct reduction in stem cells and may be associated with ineffective erythropoiesis, especially in erythroleukaemia. Simple 'crowding-out' of erythroid tissue by leukaemic cells is unlikely to occur.

Anaemia due to marrow failure may be made worse by accelerated destruction of red cells and by blood loss. Marked haemolytic anaemia is rare, although a shortened red cell survival can be demonstrated in some patients. Reticulocytosis may occur, occasionally with circulating nucleated red cells seen in the blood of patients with erythroleukaemia, but these changes are unusual in other AML subtypes.

Granulocytopenia

Fever occurs commonly in AML patients at presentation and throughout the induction period. Infection, especially septicaemia, is the commonest cause of fever and must always be considered as a likely cause of fever, particularly in patients with granulocyte counts below 1.0×10^9/l. Although the median white cell count in AML patients [1] is $15-20 \times 10^9$/l, one third of patients are neutropenic at diagnosis with granulocyte counts of $0.5-1.9 \times 10^9$/l.

Fever without clinical or laboratory confirmation of infection occurs in about one-third of febrile episodes and in a small proportion of patients may be related to widespread disease. In patients who have started treatment, infection is even more likely as a cause of fever, but in a few patients fever is due to reactions to drugs or to transfusion of blood products.

The causes of infection in leukaemia patients are discussed in Chapter 25.

Thrombocytopenia

Bleeding occurs in 60% of AML patients at presentation [1] and throughout the induction period and is almost always secondary to severe thrombocytopenia caused by marrow failure. There is a complex, poorly understood relationship between thrombocytopenia and bleeding, but the highest risk of bleeding is in patients with platelet counts less than 20×10^9/l, although many patients will not bleed at these and lower counts. Most patients do not bleed spontaenously at higher platelet counts, although bleeding is more frequent in patients with systemic infections or severe anaemia. Defects of platelet function, so frequently seen in myeloproliferative disorders, rarely occur in AML [4].

The skin is the commonest site of bleeding with small petechial haemorrhages seen especially over the lower legs and feet (Fig. 9.1). Bleeding from the gums is common, particularly in patients with poor dental hygiene, and bleeding into the mucous membranes of the buccal cavity, tonsillar bed and

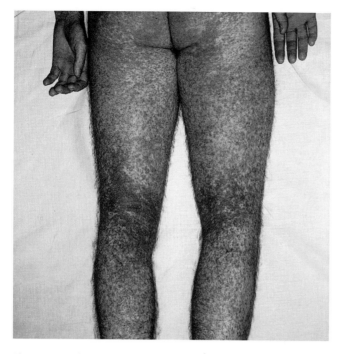

Fig. 9.1 Petechial rash over the lower extremities in a 33-year-old man with AML (M2) and a platelet count of 10 × 10⁹/l.

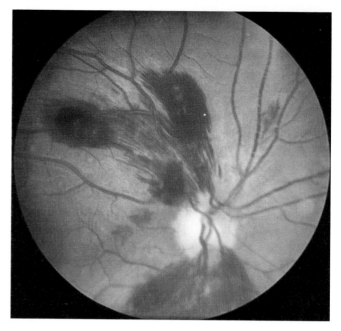

Fig. 9.2 Retinal bleeding in AML (same patient as shown in Fig. 9.1).

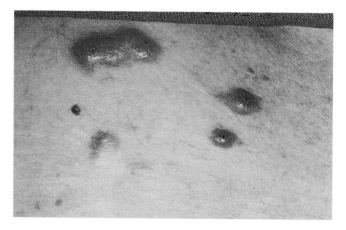

Fig. 9.3 Leukaemic skin deposits in a 35-year-old woman with AML (M5).

pharynx is frequent. Epistaxis is less usual, although potentially much more troublesome, and frank haematuria is rare, although microscopic haematuria is common and often undetected. Usually, blood loss from the gastrointestinal tract is microscopic, but may be severe and even life threatening in patients with active peptic ulceration. In women, menorrhagia is common and it is probably wisest to suppress menstruation until remission is achieved.

Haemorrhage in the eye is most often seen in the retina (Fig. 9.2), where it may occasionally cause visual disturbances, especially blind spots. Haemorrhage into the vitreous is even more serious, but fortunately rarely seen. Subconjunctival haemorrhage is not usually serious, although it will inevitably cause considerable concern to the patient.

Intracranial bleeding is extremely serious and often results in death. Fortunately, the general availability of platelet concentrates has reduced dramatically the number of deaths from this cause.

Clinical features due to leukaemic infiltration

Skin

Leukaemic skin deposits (Fig. 9.3) can occur occasionally in patients with any of the subtypes of AML, but are most frequently seen in acute monocytic leukaemia (FAB M5) and acute myelomonocytic leukaemia (FAB M4). They usually occur as small, rose-coloured or purple papular lesions which may be multiple and generalized or, less commonly, few in number [5]. The ability of leukaemic monocytes to migrate to the skin has been demonstrated in skin windows [6–8] and skin abrasions result in the migration of leukaemic cells in M5 patients, whereas only normal inflammatory cells migrate in other subtypes of AML [8]. These findings may explain the high incidence of skin infiltration in M4 and M5 disease.

Mouth and gums

Gingival hypertrophy due to infiltration with leukaemic cells (Fig. 9.4) occurs in 25% of patients with M5a, 50% with M5b and 50% with M4 disease [5], but in only 5–8% of other AML subtypes [1]. Infiltration of the tongue, producing macroglossia and tonsillar infiltration, is seen rarely in M4 and M5 disease.

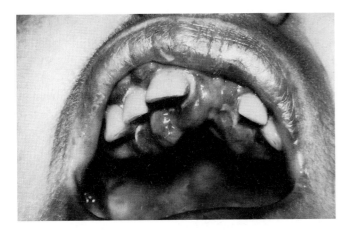

Fig. 9.4 Gum hypertrophy in a patient with AML (M4).

Eyes

All the parts of the eye have occasionally been affected by leukaemic deposits, but these disorders are less frequently seen in AML than in acute lymphoblastic leukaemia (ALL), where choroidal and neural infiltrates frequently coexist with meningeal leukaemia. However, retinal infiltrates probably occur with the same frequency in AML and ALL in childhood [9].

Liver, spleen and lymph nodes

Lymphadenopathy and hepatosplenomegaly occur in about 40% of patients, but are usually minimal and often clinically undetectable. Significant enlargement of the liver, spleen and lymph nodes occurs in about 10% of patients and may indicate an underlying alternative diagnosis, for example, AML transformation secondary to chronic myeloid leukaemia.

Bone

Bone and joint pain is rare at presentation, but not uncommon terminally in patients with a rapidly increasing number of leukaemia cells. It may be caused by bone infarcts [10], by periosteal elevation due to leukaemic tissue, or by increased blood flow with raised marrow pressure [11,12]. Bone pain is often associated with tenderness at major sites of marrow production, especially the sternum. Pain and tenderness over long bones, seen not infrequently in children with ALL [13], is rare in adults, but when present may be due to periosteal elevation, in which case the abnormality may be seen on X-ray.

The rapid disappearance of bone pain following successful cytoreduction indicates a possible relationship to leukaemic deposits.

Other organs

Infiltration occurs in other organs, but rarely causes clinical

symptoms at presentation. The kidneys, lung and pleura, heart and pericardium, and gastrointestinal tract may be involved. Leukaemia in the lung and pleura have been associated with bleeding into the lung parenchyma and pleura, and deposits in the heart with pericardial bleeding and tamponade, but these syndromes are rare.

Other clinical features

Nonspecific skin lesions apparently unrelated to leukaemic infiltration include pruritus, urticaria, papules, vesicles and erythema multiforme. Painful indurated erythematous plaques have been reported [14].

Herpes simplex, although rare at diagnosis, is seen frequently during treatment. Herpes zoster is occasionally encountered, but is much less common than in patients with ALL, chronic lymphatic leukaemia and other lymphoid neoplasms. Varicella is rarely seen, but can be rapidly fatal in association with the severe immunosuppression usually found in AML patients. These and other viral infections are discussed in Chapter 25.

Bleeding from deficiency of clotting factors

This type of bleeding episode (Fig. 9.5) usually presents a different clinical picture from that due to thrombocytopenia, although both may be present in the same patient. Ecchymoses and haematomas, particularly at sites of venepuncture and marrow aspiration, are frequent, and major internal haemorrhage into the gastrointestinal tract, liver, spleen or genitourinary tract may occur. The commonest cause is disseminated intravascular coagulation (DIC) associated particularly with acute promyelocytic leukaemia [FAB M3].

Many AML patients show mild alterations in other coagulation factors, especially those factors manufactured in the liver, although these disturbances do not usually give rise to clinical disorders. Prothrombin (factor II) is decreased in up to 23% of patients [4], factor V in about 20% [15], but in up to 90% of patients with acute promyelocytic leukaemia [16], combined factor VII and factor X deficiency or factor X deficiency alone occur in about one-quarter of patients.

Increases in fibrinogen, factor VIII and occasionally other coagulation factors have been reported [4], and it has been suggested that these indicate a hypercoagulable state, perhaps with an increased risk of thromboembolic disease and possibly as an overshoot following DIC. However, many alterations in coagulation relate to multiple deficiencies, for which there is no convincing explanation.

Blood in acute myeloid leukaemia

The appearances of the blood film directly relate to marrow failure and to infiltration with leukaemic cells. Red cell changes are unusual unless haemolysis or DIC is a feature. The

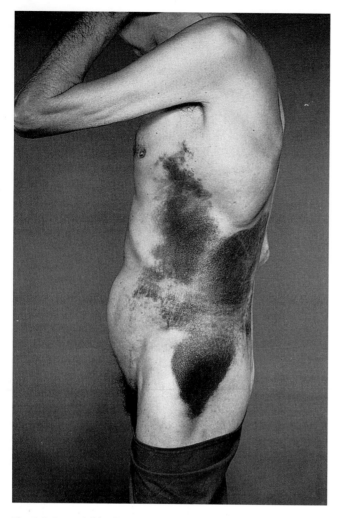

Fig. 9.5 Purpuric bleeding in a patient with AML (M2) and multiple clotting factor deficiencies (factors II, V, VII, X).

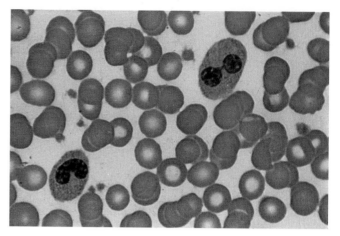

Fig. 9.6 Pelger–Hüet anomaly in the blood of a patient with AML (M1).

total leucocyte count may be increased, normal or decreased, but most often reflects the number of blasts present. Most patients show some degree of neutropenia at presentation, which may be severe. Neutrophils are often abnormal with few or absent granules and occasionally a Pelger-like abnormality of the nucleus (Fig. 9.6). These abnormal neutrophils are usually functionally and metabolically abnormal with poor mobilization and phagocytic properties [17,18], decreased bactericidal activity [19], decreased peroxidase and decreased terminal deoxynucleotide transferase [20].

Leukaemic blasts are present in varying numbers from zero to counts exceeding $200 \times 10^9/l$, with a median count of 15–20 $\times 10^9/l$. There is a direct relationship between blast counts in blood and bone marrow and patients with high blood blast counts usually have almost complete replacement of the bone marrow by leukaemic cells. However, quite frequently, the blasts seen in the blood differ in morphological characteristics from those in the marrow, particularly in leukaemia with a monocytoid component. Consequently, attempts to classify

leukaemia from the characteristics of blood blasts should not be made.

Auer rods in leukaemic blasts, due to the coalescence of primary granules, are pathognomic of AML, but are seen in less than 20% of patients. They are usually more easily seen in marrow aspirates, but are often detectable in blood blasts and rarely in neutrophil granulocytes.

The morphological features of AML, including bone marrow appearances, are fully described in Chapter 2.

Special clinical problems

Acute monocytic leukaemia (FAB M5)

Acute monocytic leukaemia is associated with a high frequency of extramedullary disease [5,21,22], particularly hepatosplenomegaly (50%), lymphadenopathy (42%), skin deposits (33%) and gum infiltration (25%). Less frequently, perianal deposits, gastrointestinal tract infiltration, bladder disease and deposits in lung and pleura are present [5]. Patients have a poor prognosis, largely due to a high incidence of central nervous system (CNS) disease [21,22] with a risk of leukaemic meningitis five times greater than for other subtypes of AML [23]. Renal failure and hypokalaemia occur frequently in association with increased levels of serum lysozyme, often in patients with high blood blast cell counts. The presence of excessive lysozyme in the glomerular filtrate in M5 disease produces renal tubular dysfunction resulting in the excretion of lysozyme in the urine [24]. Disseminated intravascular coagulation is an occasional problem [22,25].

Patients with M5 disease need careful clinical assessment, including examination of cerebrospinal fluid (CSF) and assessment of renal function before treatment starts. Potentially nephrotoxic antibiotics, for example aminoglycosides, if required, should be used with care, as they can cause a marked increase in the excretion of urinary lysozyme. Assessment of

Table 9.1 Laboratory findings in patients with DIC.

Laboratory test	Severe DIC (with clinical disease)	Moderate DIC (often without clinical problems)	Mild DIC (often without clinical problems)
Primary changes			
Plasma fibrinogen	< 1 g/l	Usually normal	Usually normal
FDP	Raised	Raised	Raised
Platelet count*	< 50 × 10⁹/l	Variable	Variable
Thrombin time	Very long†	Variable	Often normal
Secondary changes			
Prothrombin time	Very long†	Variable	Normal
Partial thromboplastin time	Very long†	Variable	Normal
Clotting time	Very long†	Variable	Normal
Factors II, V, VII, IX, X, XI, XII	Low	Variable	Normal
Plasminogen	Low	Low or normal	Variable
Plasminogen activator	Variable	Variable	Variable

* Low platelet count may be related to marrow failure and in isolation does not give reliable evidence of DIC in acute promyelocytic leukaemia.

† Blood often incoagulable.

renal function before treatment is also worthwhile in patients with M4 disease, where many of the clinical features of M5 disease have been described. Asymptomatic leukaemic infiltration has been observed in CSF in more than half the patients in one small series [26] and there is some evidence for an association between the eosinophilic variant of M4, the chromosome abnormality, inv(16)(p13;q22), and CNS disease [27].

Acute promyelocytic leukaemia (FAB M3)

About 10–15% of adult AML patients have acute promyelocytic leukaemia (M3) characterized by abnormal promyelocytes which constitute more than 50% of marrow cells [28] containing distinctive large granules and multiple Auer rods and frequently showing a bilobed nucleus. A rarer atypical hypogranular variant has been described [29,30], in which cells often show a bilobed or multilobed nucleus. The white cell count is usually much higher than in the hypergranular form, sometimes exceeding 200 × 10⁹/l. Almost all cases are characterized by an abnormal karyotype with a 15;17 chromosomal translocation [31,32]. Patients with hypergranular M3 and those with the hypogranular variant may present with potentially fatal excessive bleeding [33–39], which is often inappropriate to the degree of thrombocytopenia. Bleeding is due to DIC which occurs in 75% of M3 patients [40–42] accompanied by secondary fibrinolysis and is thought to be related to the release of procoagulants from the azurophilic granules in the leukaemic promyelocytes [43–47]. These procoagulants are antigenically related to brain tissue factor [46]. Occasionally, DIC can complicate other subtypes of AML [48], including acute monocytic leukaemia. Somewhat surprisingly, there is no evidence to link the severity of DIC with the number of circulating promyelocytes, although often DIC appears to be precipitated by treatment, presumably by the release of large amounts of procoagulant, when disruption of promyelocytes is maximal.

The laboratory features of DIC (Table 9.1) include a prolonged prothrombin time, a prolonged partial thromboplastin time, some reduction in platelet count, which is often severe, and reduction in plasma fibrinogen level. Depending on the severity of the DIC process, various combinations of these abnormalities are seen (see Chapter 26 for full discussion).

Associated with DIC, there is a high frequency of renal [49] and respiratory [49,50] failure which carry a poor prognosis and are probably related to deposition of microthrombi in the kidney and lungs. The acute respiratory distress syndrome (ARDS) is characterized by pulmonary platelet sequestration with frequent pulmonary haemorrhage and thrombosis [51–53]. ARDS is unusual at presentation and is more commonly precipitated by cytotoxic treatment. In one large series, no patient with ARDS requiring artificial ventilation survived [49]. Renal failure is associated with renal cortical necrosis, but many patients may survive with renal dialysis.

Leucostasis and hyperviscosity

Between 10 and 15% of AML patients have a leucocyte count above 100 × 10⁹/l at presentation [54,55] and these patients have a poor prognosis due to vascular infiltration of the CNS and lungs [56,57]. A high incidence of fatal bleeding at presentation and during induction treatment is characteristic [56–59]. Half of all patients with AML and hyperleucocytosis have clinical or other evidence of leucostasis in the CNS or lungs, with pulmonary leucostasis the single worst prognostic factor. Three-quarters of these patients have M4 or M5 disease.

Patients with hyperleucocytosis are usually protected from hyperviscosity by anaemia [60], but inappropriate transfusion may result in a clinical hyperviscosity syndrome with lethargy, unsteadiness of gait, visual disturbances and coma.

In patients with AML and hyperleucocytosis, large, relatively undeformable myeloblasts impede the microcirculation [61], causing plugging of the vessel lumen with leucocyte aggregates and thrombi [62,63]. The vessels become distended and leaky, leading to tissue infiltration by myeloblasts, occasionally associated with vascular rupture. The process is exacerbated by subsequent release of vasoactive peptides and nucleotides, which enhance stasis and cell aggregation [63]. It is not clear whether vessels in the brain and lung are uniquely susceptible to leucostasis, or merely supply vital organs whose function is crucial to survival.

Success in reducing the white cell count is an important predictor of survival in AML patients with hyperleucocytosis [57]. Consequently, treatment must include early, intensive leukapheresis to reduce the leucocyte count significantly below 100 × 10⁹/l before anaemia is corrected.

Leukaemia in the central nervous system

Leukaemia in the CNS, which carries a very poor prognosis with early death for most patients, appears to be increasing in incidence as AML patients survive for longer periods, although a large post-mortem study has suggested a decrease [64]. The older literature describes an incidence for clinical disease of 5% [1], with most reports suggesting 10% [65–67] as the true incidence. Leukaemic pleocytosis without overt clinical disease may be even more frequent, especially in patients with M4 and M5 disease [26,68,69]. Additionally, there is a particularly high risk of CNS disease in children, with several studies reporting an incidence of 20% [70–73].

Unlike ALL [74], most series have not described prognostic indicators for CNS disease in AML patients, although Meyer *et al.* [26] showed that patients with CNS disease were younger and had more hepatosplenomegaly.

There is a greater frequency of focal neurological lesions in AML patients with CNS disease [75] than in ALL patients, where focal disease is unusual. The incidence varies from 30 to 66% and lesions are often multiple [27].

The clinical features of CNS leukaemia are those of increased intracranial pressure, especially headaches, vomiting, neck stiffness, papilloedema and VIth nerve paresis. Other cranial nerve palsies may occur, especially when focal disease is present. The diagnosis should be established by examination of a cytocentrifuge preparation of CSF in which leukaemic cells can be identified. Computerized tomography of the brain is useful in adults where focal lesions are suspected, especially where CSF examination is negative.

CNS disease probably occurs at presentation when there may be large numbers of leukaemic blasts circulating. As most cytotoxic drugs do not cross the blood–brain barrier in appreciable amounts, leukaemic cells are able to proliferate slowly, eventually producing the clinical picture of CNS infiltration [76]. In childhood ALL, patients with CNS disease have a higher incidence of thrombocytopenia than those patients who remain free of disease and it seems likely that this leads to a higher risk of microscopic bleeding into the CNS, which then allows seeding of leukaemic cells.

Metabolic problems

Renal function

Renal function is often abnormal at presentation as a consequence of the disease (hyperuricaemia, hypokalaemia, renal infiltration), or of infection or its treatment. It is essential that uric acid production and electrolyte levels are corrected before treatment is started. Uric acid levels should be monitored throughout the induction period. Prophylactic treatment with allopurinol is advisable, as the initial white cell count may not reflect the total body mass of leukaemic cells.

Hepatic function

Many cytotoxic drugs, especially the anthracycline antibiotics, are metabolized in the liver and are more toxic in the presence of liver cell damage. Consequently, it is essential that liver function should be assessed before treatment commences and again before subsequent treatments are given. An otherwise unexplained rise in serum bilirubin or an increase in levels of liver cell enzymes are indications to reduce or delay the administration of anthracyclines.

Cardiac function

The anthracycline antibiotics, used widely in remission induction treatments, show a cumulative cardiotoxicity [77] which may be potentiated by hypokalaemia [78,79]. The clinical features are those of congestive heart failure, the most striking characteristic being the rapidly progressive course [80,81]. The condition may be controlled if diagnosed early and treated intensively, but the ECG, chest X-ray and measurement of cardiac enzymes are unhelpful in predicting its onset [81,82]. However, monitoring of changes in echocardiograph [83] and radionuclide scintiangiography [84,85] allow early diagnosis, but cardiac biopsy, which has proved useful for patients with solid tumours [86], is inappropriate for AML patients, most of whom are thrombocytopenic. If none of these methods is available, the total dose of anthracyclines should be limited to about 500 mg/m².

Purine metabolism

The lysis of leukaemic cells, which occurs spontaneously, or more usually in association with cytoreduction, liberates purines which are converted first to hypoxanthine and then to xanthine and uric acid by the enzyme xanthine oxidase. Uric acid may be deposited in various body tissues, but its clinical effects are seen almost exclusively in the kidneys and joints. Deposits of uric acid in the renal parenchyma, renal pelvis and ureters can result in acute renal failure. In most cases, serum uric acid is raised and urinary urate excretion is two to three times that seen in normal subjects.

Gouty arthropathy caused by deposits of uric acid crystals in large joints is rare prior to treatment, but not uncommon thereafter, especially in patients with high leucocyte counts. The pattern of joint involvement is 'secondary', nearly always single and most often affects the ankle or knee joints and less frequently the hip, wrist, elbow and shoulder. The small joints of the foot, most frequently involved in primary gout, are seldom affected.

The introduction of the xanthine oxidase inhibitor allopurinol [87] has dramatically decreased the frequency of both urate nephropathy and arthropathy. The block in the conversion of hypoxanthine and xanthine to uric acid results in an increase in the serum levels of these substances and, although neither is appreciably more soluble than uric acid, their excretion occurs by a different mechanism so that they do not damage the kidneys, even if present in large quantities. However, large joint arthropathy caused by accumulation of xanthine crystals has been described, but is very rare.

Allopurinol, 300 mg daily, should be administered to all AML patients during remission induction. The breakdown of 6-mercaptopurine to thiouric acid is catalysed by xanthine oxidase, therefore when this drug is used in AML treatment, its dosage should be reduced to 25%. However, 6-thioguanine does not depend on xanthine oxidase for its breakdown, and it can be given in normal dosage together with allopurinol.

Calcium metabolism

Disturbance of calcium metabolism is very much less frequently seen in AML than in patients with disseminated malignancy, chronic myeloid leukaemia (CML) or adult T-cell leukaemia/lymphoma. However, both hypercalcaemia or hypocalcaemia may occur in AML. The cause of hypercalcaemia is uncertain, but has been attributed to direct production by leukaemia cells of a parathormone-like substance with the ability to activate osteoclasts [88,89]. Initial treatment should be with rehydration using 2–3 l/day of 0.9% saline.

Calcitonine or diphosphonates may be used if hypercalcaemia is protracted. Diphosphonates act by inhibiting cell-mediated bone resorption [90] and, although they probably act more slowly than calcitonin, their effects are longer lasting [91]. However, the achievement of complete remission is the only certain way of restoring normal calcium metabolism.

Hypocalcaemia is unusual in AML [92], but may be seen as a response to treatment [93] in patients with initial large tumour masses. In addition, it has also been noted in relapse. As with hypercalcaemia, remission of AML restores hypocalcaemia to normal. Other methods of treatment, such as the administration of calcium chloride or magnesium salts, are less successful.

Prognostic factors

For many years, haematologists have searched for features of AML which might allow treatment to be tailored specifically to different types of disease. However, unlike ALL, there are no clear good prognostic factors for patients with AML, although there are features which predict a poor outcome. Certain factors can help predict the achievement and maintenance of complete remission in AML and the best known of these are described below.

Cytogenetics. Good responses to treatment can be predicted by the presence of t(8;21)(q22;q22), which is associated with M2 morphology, and inv(16)(q13;q22), which is closely linked with M4 eosinophilic morphology. The t(15;17) abnormality associated with M3 disease also predicts a better outlook [94,95].

Certain features are associated with a poorer outlook, including absence of chromosome 5 and the 5q– anomaly. Similarly, absence of chromosome 7 or 7q– is a disadvantage. An additional 8 chromosome, abnormalities of chromosome 11, especially 11q–, and abnormalities of chromosome 3, are unfavourable [94,95].

Immunophenotype. The presence of CD13, CD14, CD34, CD11b, CD11c and HLA DR all indicate a poorer outlook, while conversely, low levels or the absence of these markers may confer a better outlook [96].

Morphology. Patients with M3 disease have a better outlook, as do patients with M4 eosinophilic morphology, while patients with M0, M6 and M7 disease appear to have a poorer outlook. However, morphological subtype is generally less important than cytogenetics and immunophenotype.

Multidrug resistance. The multidrug resistance (MDR) phenotype, as indicated by the presence of the glycoprotein p170, is associated with resistance to various drugs which it seems to exclude from leukaemia cells by an efflux mechanism. MDR expression is associated with a poorer outcome, but its presence can be modulated by cyclosporin A and other cyclosporin analogues. The place of these modulators in AML treatment is currently under investigation [97].

Other laboratory studies. The proliferation of leukaemic blasts in culture and a low tritiated thymidine labelling index appear to relate to a poor outlook [98–100].

Patients treated (no.)	Anthracycline	Median age (years)	CR (%)	MRD (months)	Reference
226	DNR	47	58	12	Yates *et al.* [110]
117	DNR	43	72	NA	Sauter *et al.* [111]
58	DNR	36	56	8–18	Rai *et al.* [108]
40	DNR/DXR	NA	60	12.5	Preisler *et al.* [107]
508	DNR	53	66	17	Vogler *et al.* [133]
211	DNR	NA	53	12	Preisler *et al.* [114]

Table 9.2 Some remission induction regimens using an anthracycline and ara-C (3 + 7) in the treatment of adult AML.

CR = complete remission; DNR = daunorubicin; DXR = doxorubicin; MRD = mean remission duration; NA = not available.

Clinical features. The patient's age at diagnosis is perhaps the most important prognostic determinant, with children and teenagers having the best outlook. Remission rates and survival durations decrease with each decade of life, with the elderly having a poor prognosis [101,102].

Other clinical features indicating a poor prognosis are a white cell count greater than 100×10^9/l, the detection of leukaemic blasts in the CSF and the presence of extra-medullary leukaemia. Secondary leukaemia, whether as a transformation of another haematological process (e.g. MDS, polycythaemia) or following the use of drugs or X-ray therapy, also confers a poor outlook [101,102].

Treatment

Since the introduction of useful cytotoxic agents, such as the anthracyclines and cytosine arabinoside (ara-C), 30 or more years ago, the induction treatment of AML has developed rapidly. The addition of newer treatment agents, for example etoposide, idarubicin and mitoxantrone, has complemented these advances, so that high remission rates can now be achieved using various drug combinations. While comparisons of these regimens in induction and maintenance treatment continue, further advances in chemotherapy are likely to be slower.

Induction chemotherapy

Single-agent chemotherapy

There is no longer any place for the use of single agents in induction chemotherapy, as remission rates are low and the duration of these remissions is short. The older literature indicates that anthracyclines and ara-C used alone at standard dosage can produce remission rates of 50% and above [103–105]. However, cytosine arabinoside used as a high-dose intravenous infusion has a definite place in the management of relapsed and resistant AML and its use is considered separately.

Combination chemotherapy

The chief aims of combination chemotherapy are the rapid production of early complete remission (CR) and the reduction of the risk of the emergence of disease resistance. Modern treatments result in rapid marrow hypoplasia requiring a period of haematological support until marrow recovery occurs.

Cytosine arabinoside with an anthracycline

Combinations of an anthracycline antibiotic and ara-C with or without 6-thioguanine are now standard AML induction regimens and can be expected to give CR rates of 60–80% in patients under 60 years. Perhaps the most frequent method of administering these drugs is a combination of 3 days of anthracycline and 7 days of ara-C (Table 9.2), the so-called 'three plus seven' regimen [106–115]. The addition to anthracycline/ara-C combinations of 6-thioguanine (DAT) does not improve the CR rate or the remission duration [116–122], but many regimens still include this agent.

Anthracycline dosages have varied, but doxorubicin, 30–45 mg/m²/day, or daunorubicin, 45–60 mg/m²/day, are usual and seem equally effective. The timing of the anthracycline, at the beginning or the end of the ara-C infusion, does not produce any difference in remission rate [123]. Ara-C at a dose of 100–200 mg/m²/day is given by continuous intravenous or subcutaneous infusion and both routes are probably more effective than total-dose injection [124]. Treatment with ara-C for 7 days appears to be better than 5 [108], but equal to 10 days [106,125], which has been associated with a higher rate of gastrointestinal toxicity. However, others have claimed a greater antileukaemic effectiveness for a 10-day infusion without increased haematological toxicity.

Recently, efforts have been made to improve the effectiveness of these standard induction regimens by substituting alternative anthracycline drugs. One such anthracycline is idarubicin (4'-demethoxydaunorubin) which is more rapidly taken into leukaemic blasts than daunorubicin and has a longer plasma half-life. Several comparative studies [126–128] suggest that idarubicin may produce higher remission rates earlier in the induction phase of treatment and is at least as effective overall as daunorubicin. The use of alternative anthracyclines is more fully discussed in Chapter 10.

Cytosine arabinoside combined with other agents

Mitoxantrone in combinations with ara-C gives good remission rates which some consider to be better than those obtained with daunorubicin [129].

Etoposide used in combination with ara-C and daunorubicin has given similar remission rates to combinations of an anthracycline with ara-C [130], with a probable increase in the length of remission [131,132].

Combinations of vincristine and prednisolone with ara-C for 5 or 10 days [133–135] give slightly lower remission rates than those for ara-C and anthracyclines and, as a consequence, these regimens have fallen out of favour.

Induction combinations including amsacrine

Amsacrine (AMSA), an acridine derivative which has proved useful as a single agent, when combined with other drugs has given encouraging results in the treatment of relapsed or resistant AML. Results of drug combinations containing ara-C with [136] or without [137] 6-thioguanine or with etoposide [138] have given CR rates of 32–70%. AMSA combined with 5-azacytidine has shown similar promise [139].

In a randomized trial of DAT (3 + 5) versus AMSA, ara-C and 6-thioguanine, Berman *et al.* [140] showed a CR rate of 70% for AMSA-treated patients which was statistically significantly different in age-stratified groupings. While there remain some doubts about the cardiotoxicity of AMSA, in combination with ara-C it can be regarded as a very useful agent for AML treatment in both *de novo* and relapsed or resistant patients.

Consolidation and maintenance of remission

A further major objective in leukaemia treatment is the prevention of disease recurrence once remission has been established. Many patients subsequently relapse, presumably because their induction treatment did not completely abolish the leukaemia, but although methods for detecting minimal residual disease are improving, they cannot yet be reliably used in AML.

Consequently, some form of maintenance or consolidation treatment is required to eliminate residual disease. Even low doses of the agents used to induce remission when given in the postremission phase are probably more effective than nothing and it is probable that, as in the case of ALL, more intensive postremission treatment will achieve a longer disease-free survival and an increase in cure rates.

Traditionally, maintenance treatment consists of doses of drugs lower than those given in induction chemotherapy, whereas consolidation treatment involves either repeating the induction chemotherapy or intensifying treatment with chemotherapy using additional drugs. It appears that prolonged maintenance treatment does not confer any benefit over shorter more intensive consolidation treatments [142,143], which have now become standard in treatment protocols.

Several approaches to intensive consolidation treatment are currently under investigation, but to date most experience has been gained with high-dose ara-C (HDAC). Several studies have reported 5-year survival rates above 30% using either HDAC alone [143,144] or in combination with an anthracycline [145–147] and these results appear to give superior

Table 9.3 Results of intensification treatment in AML.

Intensification treatment	No. of patients	Median age (years)	Median follow-up (years)	Actuarial probability of CR at 5 years (%)	Reference
DXR; ara-C; 5 Aza; POMP	30	NA (range 18–50)	3.5	40	Weinstein *et al.* [70]
ara-C	94	NA (range 18–74)	NA	30	Mayer *et al.* [141]
HD ara-C; AMSA	123	46	2	30	Cassileth *et al.* [149]
HD ara-C; DXR; ara-C; AMSA	123	55	1.8	47	Preisler *et al.* [114]
HD ara-C; AMSA, Etop; L-asp	74	48	3	34	Tallman *et al.* [148]
HD ara-C; DNR; ara-C	118	44	3.5	37	Rohatiner *et al.* [122]
HD ara-C; DNR	87	38	3.5	49	Wolff *et al.* [147]

AMSA = amsacrine; ara-C = cytosine arabinoside; 5 Aza = 5-azacytidine; DNR = daunorubicin; DXR = doxorubicin; Etop = etoposide; HD ara-C = high-dose cytosine arabinoside; L-asp = L-asparaginase; NA = not available; POMP = prednisone, vincristine, methotrexate, pruinethol.

remission durations to those obtained with less intensive maintenance therapies.

Not all patients with AML in remission will tolerate the toxicity associated with intensive consolidation regimens and selection, often on the grounds of age, will need to be carefully made. A further question is just how many courses of consolidation treatment give optimum results and exactly how these should be timed. These problems are more fully discussed in Chapter 10 and the results of some intensive consolidation treatments are shown in Table 9.3.

Treatment of patients with relapsed or resistant disease

About 15% of AML patients are primarily resistant to chemotherapy and up to 70% of those achieving remission can be expected to relapse. A second CR can be obtained for about half of these patients with treatment with conventional induction chemotherapy [120] and, as for first remissions, these CR rates are age related. The CR rate is related also to the length of the first remission, patients with short first remissions being unlikely to obtain further remissions. Second remissions are disappointingly short and almost always shorter than first remissions. The incidence of drug-resistant disease is much higher in relapsed patients and death due to the inability to tolerate repeated intensive treatments is common [150].

The causes of induction failure are shown in Table 9.4, patients with drug-resistant disease (type I and type II failure) having a particularly poor outlook. For these patients, HDAC alone or in combination has given encouraging results. Usually, HDAC is given by intravenous infusion in doses up to 3 g/m² every 12 h on 8–12 occasions either alone [151–153] or with amsacrine [154] or etoposide, but recently a randomized trial in refractory or relapsed leukaemia has shown no differ-

ence in outcome for HDAC alone compared with HDAC and etoposide [155].

Complete remission rates in studies using HDAC alone or in combination with other agents are 50–60% for relapsed AML and 20–40% for patients with resistant disease.

Etoposide has achieved remission rates higher than 30% in refractory AML in combination with mitoxantrone [156,157] or with aclacinomycin [158]. One of these studies [156] gave a median remission duration of 15 months.

A variety of other agents alone or in combination have been tried in refractory and relapsed AML, generally with less promising results often attributed to the toxicity of the treatment. Drugs which have shown promise as single agents, and are therefore worth further study, include 2-chlorodeoxyadenosine [159], 5-azacytidine [160] and carboplatin [161].

Reasons for failure of induction chemotherapy

In spite of recent improvements in remission rates, a significant number of AML patients still fail to reach CR. It has long been obvious that some patients die from septicaemia and other infections associated with severe neutropenia resulting from intensive chemotherapy and, although improvements in supportive care have reduced the number of these deaths, they continue to be a problem. Estey *et al.* [162] found that two-thirds of those dying after the third week of induction treatment, before which CR is unusual, had marrow hypoplasia and these patients might have entered remission with better supportive care. Infection accounted for 73% of deaths during the first four courses of treatment. Of these, 34% were bacterial alone, 15% fungal alone and 11% resulted from a combination of bacterial and fungal infection. Surprisingly, a high proportion of deaths were caused by haemorrhage (33%).

I	Major drug resistance	Failure to produce significant marrow hypoplasia; patient surviving for >7 days after chemotherapy finishes
II	Relative drug resistance	(i) Chemotherapy produces hypoplasia; leukaemic cells repopulate marrow in >40 days (ii) As for (i), but with repopulation by some normal cells
III	Regeneration failure	Marrow severely hypoplastic for >40 days after chemotherapy finishes
IV	Hypoplastic death	Patient dies during severe marrow hypoplasia†
V	Inadequate trial	Patient dies <7 days after chemotherapy with a cellular bone marrow
VI	Extramedullary persistence	Patient enters complete haematological remission, but leukaemic cells persist in extramedullary sites (principally CSF, liver or spleen)

Table 9.4 Causes of induction failure in AML*.

* Modified from Preisler *et al.* [106].
† Classified as regeneration failure if death occurs >40 days after chemotherapy.

However, it is important to distinguish these deaths from those related to failure to eradicate leukaemia after an adequate trial of chemotherapy. The majority of treatment failures are a result of drug resistance (types I and II) or early death of the patient with type IV or V failure.

Special problems of treatment

Treatment in the elderly

The incidence of AML increases with each decade of life and, with increasing life expectancy, the majority of newly presenting patients are now over 50 years with a peak incidence in the elderly. However, remission rates and survival duration for AML patients is closely related to age [163–165], with elderly patients faring badly. Intensive modern induction treatments produce high remission rates, which are often achievable only in patients under 60 years, possibly because the elderly are less well able to tolerate the septicaemia frequently associated with severe neutropenia, but also related to the high incidence of preceding myelodysplastic syndromes (MDS) in older patients. Differences in the length of disease-free survival between younger and older patient groups have been further accentuated in recent years by intensive postinduction chemotherapy and bone marrow transplantation, treatments not usually applicable to the elderly.

Consequently, any less intensive treatment likely to produce reasonable CR rates is worthy of consideration for older patients. Several recently reported alternatives are shown in Table 9.5. Induction treatment with an anthracycline antibiotic and ara-C is best tolerated at lower than normal dosages. Results are related to age, with satisfactory CR rates for patients aged 60–70 years, but lower rates for those over 70 years.

The intensity of the induction regimens used in Table 9.5 varies somewhat and some authors have shown that a lower daunorubicin dose achieves more favourable results in the elderly [110]. However, several studies have used more intensive treatment regimens; for example, Tilly *et al.* [170] used a DAT 'four plus seven' regimen with a 52% CR rate. Löwenberg *et al.* [169] randomized patients to DAT 'three plus seven' or to palliative treatment and supportive care only. Overall survival, although short, was significantly longer for the DAT-treated group. These authors suggest that conservative treatments should be reserved for selected patients who are unlikely to tolerate DAT treatment.

Yin *et al.* [171], using mitozantrone and ara-C, reported CR rates of 64% in *de novo* AML and 28% in patients who had preceding MDS or secondary AML, while Arlin *et al.* [172] achieved similar results with the same drug combination. However, neither study suggests a convincing advantage for the use of mitozantrone over daunorubicin.

Patients who are very elderly (over 75 years) or who have a preceding history of significant medical illness can be effectively treated with low-dose ara-C. There are reports of several hundred patients with AML receiving low-dose ara-C treatment [175–181]. Treatment is well tolerated, with response rates of 30–50% in *de novo* AML and 8–22% in secondary AML. Toxicity is low, with few treatment-related deaths, although some reports stress profound neutropenia and thrombocytopenia requiring intensive support. Low-dose ara-C treatment seems to be most beneficial in patients with a low to moderate leukaemic cell mass, that is, those with early AML, hypoplastic myeloid leukaemia or refractory anaemia with excess of myeloblasts in transformation. The bone marrow blast cell count may be helpful in predicting response with little or no effect when blast cell counts exceed 85%.

Postinduction chemotherapy for elderly patients in remission is needed if remission duration is to be usefully prolonged. Few of the remission induction studies in Table 9.5 give details of survival. Available data [120,143,171] show that disease-free survival is only 15% at 44 months [171] and only 5% at 5 years [120]. A randomized trial using three escalating doses of ara-C as postinduction chemotherapy [143] showed a

Table 9.5 Results of induction treatment of AML in elderly patients.

Induction treatment	No. of patients	CR (%)	Age (years)	Reference
RBZ, ara-C, VCR, Pred	59	48	>60	Keating *et al.* [166]
DNR, ara-C, 6TG	40	28	>70	Kahn *et al.* [167]
DNR, ara-C, 6TG	315	48	>60	Rees *et al.* [120]
DNR, ara-C, 6TG	176	43	>60	Rees & Gray [168]
DNR, ara-C, VCR	31	58	>65	Löwenberg *et al.* [169]
DNR, ara-C	46	52	>65	Tilly *et al.* [170]
MTX, ara-C	104	64	>60	Yin *et al.* [171]
DNR, ara-C/MTX, ara-C	99	41	>60	Arlin *et al.* [172]
MTX, ara-C	104	58	>60	Liu Yin [165]
DNR, ara-C	388	53	>60	Stone *et al.* [174]
DNR, ara-C	173	59	>65	Dombret *et al.* [173]

ara-C = cytosine arabinoside; CR = complete remission; DNR = daunorubicin; MTX = mitozantrone; Pred = prednisone; RBZ = rubidazone; 6TG = 6-thioguanine; VCR = vincristine.

dose–effect relationship in patients less than 60 years, but no clear relationship in the elderly. High-dose postinduction chemotherapy is unlikely to be tolerated by elderly patients and further studies of consolidation and maintenance chemotherapy are needed.

Treatment in childhood

Until recently, treatment results in childhood AML differed little from those in adults and the infrequent occurrence of the disease made for slow progress. However, the use of intensive induction and postremission treatments has resulted in high remission rates and in the prolongation of survival [70,182–194]. Some modern protocols and their results are summarized in Table 9.6. These treatments are possibly even more intensive than those described above for adults and require the full range of support facilities.

Induction treatment using a combination of ara-C and an anthracycline, with or without the addition of vincristine and prednisone, gives CR rates of approximately 80% [70,189–192], but as in adult trials, the addition of etoposide does not seem to improve remission rates [186]. However, CR rates are generally higher than in most adult trials, possibly because of the lower incidence of toxicity-related deaths and leukaemia drug resistance.

In children under 3 years, the anthracycline used for induc-

tion treatment should be chosen with care in view of the finding of high toxicity related mortality with doxorubicin (29%), but not with daunorubicin (1%) [184].

There is a clear need for postremission chemotherapy, although the most effective treatment is not clear.

Creutzig *et al.* [183], using an intensive sequential 57-day induction including vincristine, doxorubicin, prednisone and ara-C, followed by 2-monthly cycles of doxorubicin, ara-C and 6-thioguanine, obtained a 51% disease-free survival at 3 years. The same authors, using a more conventional induction treatment with daunorubicin and ara-C, have subsequently reported a 52% 5-year disease-free survival following two courses of high-dose ara-C and etoposide as postremission treatment [186].

Although postremission therapy, summarized in Table 9.6, remains complex, inclusion of at least two courses of high-dose cytosine arabinoside is now standard and one study [190] has shown a better disease-free survival in a group receiving a six-dose HDAC treatment compared with a group receiving four doses.

Both induction and postremission treatment of childhood AML continues to intensify, but some authors have questioned the need for intensive treatment for all patients [185] following their identification of low-risk patient groups with a particularly good outlook. These low-risk groups included patients who had FAB M1 with Auer rods, FAB M2 with a

Table 9.6 Induction and postremission treatment of AML in childhood.

Induction treatment	Postremission treatment	CR (%)	DFS at 3 years (%)	No. of patients	Reference
DXR, ara-C (3 + 7) VCR, Pred (3 + 7) × 2	Complex multidrug	70	56	83	Weinstein *et al.* [182] Weinstein *et al.* [70]
DNR, ara-C, 6TG (3 + 7) × 2	Complex multidrug + maintenance to 2 years	85	35	207	Steuber *et al.* [189]
DNR, ara-C, Etop (3 + 10) × 1 (2 + 5) × 1	HDAC/Etop × 2 + maintenance to 18 months	80	52*	210 (1993)	Creutzig *et al.* [185] Creutzig *et al.* [186]
DNR, ara-C, 6TG (3 + 7) × 1 (2 + 5) × 1	HDAC × 4 Etop, Aza × 4 POMP × 4 DNR, Ara-C × 4	85	34	140	Ravindranath *et al.* [190]
DNR, ara-C (3 + 7) × 2	HDAC/L-asp × 2 + 3 maintenance courses + ABMT or allo BMT	76	37	142	Woods *et al.* [187,188]
DXR, ara-C (3 + 7) × 1 (2 + 5) × 1	Complex multidrug	78	36*	490	Nesbit *et al.* [192]
DNR, ara-C, 6TG (3 + 7) × 1 DNR, ara-C (2 + 5) × 1	Complex multidrug *or* Allo BMT/ABMT	79	31*	161	Amadori *et al.* [191]

ABMT = autologous bone marrow transplantation; allo = allogeneic; ara-C = cytosine arabinoside; L-asp = L-asparaginase; Aza = 5-azacytidine; DFS = disease-free survival; DNR = daunorubicin; DXR = doxorubicin; Etop = etoposide; HDAC = high-dose ara-C; POMP = prednisolone, vincristine, methotrexate, 6-mercaptopurine; Pred = prednisone; 6TG = 6-thioguanine; VCR = vincristine.
* 5-year survival.

white cell count below 20 × 10⁹/l, FAB M3 or FAB M4 with eosinophilia. Hyperleucocytosis, especially with FAB M5 morphology, carried a poor prognosis. It seems likely that, as with ALL in children, it may soon be possible to incorporate prognostic factors into treatment protocols as our understanding of the disease increases.

Central nervous system disease

Compared with adult AML, the relapse rate is lower in children, but CNS relapses, which are unusual in adults, occur more frequently with an incidence of about 20% in children [70,71]. As with adults, children with myelomonocytic (M4) or monocytic (M5) disease have the highest risk of CNS leukaemia [26,70]. In a series of 111 adult AML relapses, only six were in the CNS [132], but in a large study [70,182] including both children and adults not given CNS prophylaxis, CNS relapse was uncommon in adults, but relatively frequent in the children.

As a result of these observtions, the need for CNS prophylaxis in childhood AML is now generally accepted. The most effective treatment is not clear, but both cranial radiotherapy and intrathecal cytosine arabinoside have been used successfully. However, the exact value of these treatments is unknown, as none have included a true control group. Additionally, one group [186] found the beneficial effect of cranial radiotherapy confined to 'good risk' patients.

Treatment of acute promyelocytic leukaemia

Acute promyelocytic leukaemia (FAB M3), characterized by specific morphology (see Chapter 2), the t(15;17) translocation and often by a coagulopathy, was until relatively recently treated similarly to other forms of adult AML. Thus treated, it had a poor prognosis with an early high death rate related to bleeding from DIC, often precipitated by induction treatment [48,195,196]. Early death from intracerebral haemorrhage was particularly frequent in patients over 30 years [49] and could be anticipated by the appearance of large retinal haemorrhages. However, better management of DIC-related bleeding improved remission rates to 60–80% [28,33,197], leading to a generally longer survival than for patients with other subtypes of AML [198,199]. Induction chemotherapy was similar to that used for other AML subtypes using ara-C and an anthracycline with or without 6TG.

The observation that all-*trans* retinoic acid (ATRA) can stimulate the differentiation of M3 blasts, both *in vitro* and *in vivo*, has changed patient management and ATRA is now a part of standard treatment. Initially, ATRA used alone in newly diagnosed patients gave remission rates of about 90% [200–204]. These authors and others confirmed the action of ATRA as a differentiating agent leading to normal haematopoiesis. In addition, they reported swift improvement in the associated coagulopathy, but they also noted two

specific problems. Up to 50% of patients treated with ATRA alone developed 'ATRA syndrome' characterized by a rapid rise in circulating polymorphonuclear leucocytes associated with weight gain, fever, occasional renal failure and cardiopulmonary failure and responsible for the deaths of some patients [202,205,206]. However, induction treatment with an anthracycline and ara-C at this stage was associated with the lowering of white cell counts and complete remission [207]. A second problem in patients treated with ATRA alone was the development of drug resistance, with almost all the patients relapsing within a few months [201,202,208].

Because of these problems, induction treatment of M3 AML now usually incorporates combined treatment with ATRA and intensive chemotherapy and this approach has been compared with the use of intensive chemotherapy alone in several clinical trials.

Several nonrandomized trials have shown high remission rates (85–96%) and high rates of disease-free survival when remission is induced using ATRA alone, followed immediately by up to three courses of induction chemotherapy with ara-C and an anthracycline [207,209–211]. Using this approach, the best long-term disease-free survival is 70% at 4 years [207].

In addition, in an especially large, but uncontrolled study, 481 patients achieved CR using ATRA and then received intensive consolidation treatment with an anthracycline and ara-C. There was a low risk of relapse, 81% of patients being alive at 2 years [212].

Fewer randomized studies are available, but a large European cooperative study [213,214] compared induction chemotherapy of daunorubicin and ara-C used alone or preceded by ATRA. Event-free survival was significantly better in the ATRA-treated group, so much so that the trial was discontinued at 18 months and further analysis has confirmed better survival with higher event-free survival in ATRA-treated patients [209].

Patients with FAB M3 who relapse after achieving CR with chemotherapy alone can be expected to achieve a second remission with ATRA treatment in 85–90% of cases [201,210,215,216], although most of these patients will relapse again within 12 months. When patients relapse after reaching a first remission with ATRA, most will not respond again, even using higher doses, although second remissions have been reported in late relapsing patients [210,214].

All-trans retinoic acid syndrome

A progressive rise in white cell count is seen in most patients treated with ATRA and occasionally this may be associated with an 'ATRA syndrome' of fever, weight gain, oedema, pleural effusion, respiratory distress and occasionally hypotension and renal failure. Rarely, the syndrome occurs in patients with a normal white cell count, although its severity seems to parallel the count in most patients and rapid rises in the count seem more likely to be associated with cardiopulmonary and renal failure [202–207]. The syndrome seems less likely to occur where ATRA is used with early induction chemotherapy and some authors suggest an association with CD13 expression on the leukaemic blast cells [206–210].

The ATRA syndrome, initially thought to relate to leukostasis and thrombosis, seems more like a variant of ARDS. It has been postulated that ATRA may stimulate cytokine expression by leukaemic blasts, with secretion of G-CSF and IL-IB stimulating leukocytosis.

The early introduction of chemotherapy appears to reduce the incidence of the ATRA syndrome to about 5% or less [211,213]. Others have treated the ATRA syndrome successfully using oral prednisolone [217] or intravenous dexamethasone [206,210,215] and avoiding the early introduction of leukaemia chemotherapy. However, there is general agreement that patients who present with a white cell count greater than $15 \times 10^9/l$ require immediate treatment with chemotherapy and intravenous steroids.

Management of coagulopathy

The use of ATRA in the induction treatment of FAB M3 has resulted in a significant reduction in the number of patients exhibiting clinical signs of bleeding or thrombosis associated with the laboratory changes of a coagulopathy. This improvement comes from the slow cell death seen with ATRA treatment which results in a median time to the disappearance of coagulopathy of about 3 days, compared with 6 days for chemotherapy [213]. Primary fibrinolysis disappears after 5 days of ATRA treatment, although DIC persists for 2–3 weeks [218,219], probably resulting in very occasional examples of thromboembolic disease during this period [220].

Prior to the use of ATRA, some authorities recommended the use of heparin by continuous intravenous infusion to treat DIC [197,198], but this approach is now seldom used. The coagulopathy associated with acute promyelocytic leukaemia is fully discussed in Chapter 26.

Allogeneic bone marrow transplantation

All patients aged 50 years or less with newly diagnosed AML should be tissue typed and attempts made to identify a potential sibling bone marrow donor. The decision on when to perform bone marrow transplantation (BMT) from a matched donor is fully discussed in Chapter 22. However, it is important to identify potential BMT donors early, as more than 50% of adults in first remission following chemotherapy can be expected to relapse. Up to 30% of these patients will be cured by allogeneic BMT carried out during a second CR [221–223]. In addition, 15–20% of patients who are resistant to attempts to induce a first CR can be cured by BMT, providing that they have minimal disease at the time of transplantation.

There are now many prospective studies comparing BMT from matched siblings with chemotherapy alone [224] showing cure rates of 40–64% for BMT and 19–24% for chemotherapy. However, many of the chemotherapy-only arms of these trials would be considered inadequate compared with today's protocols, so that firm conclusions probably cannot be drawn from these studies when making a decision whether or not to use BMT in first CR.

The place of unrelated donor transplants in AML is discussed in Chapter 22.

Autologous transplantation

Patients with newly diagnosed AML who do not have a sibling donor should be considered for autologous bone marrow transplantation (ABMT) or peripheral blood stem cell transplant (PBSCT). The place of these treatments in the management of AML in first CR is still not clear and few randomized clinical trials of autologous transplantation vs chemotherapy alone are available. A detailed discussion of ABMT and PBSCT in AML is to be found in Chapter 23.

Most trials of ABMT in first remission AML show disease-free survival rates of 40–50%, with rates of 25–30% in second remission or early first relapse [225,226]. A number of patients achieving long disease-free survival after first relapse have been transplanted using cells collected in first CR.

A randomized trial comparing allogeneic BMT, ABMT and chemotherapy alone for AML patients in first CR has shown a 4-year disease-free survival of 55% for allogeneic BMT, 48% for the autologous group and 30% for the group receiving chemotherapy alone [227].

Thus it seems relevant to collect cells for either ABMT or PBSCT on all AML patients reaching first CR who do not have an allogeneic BMT donor. These stored cells can then be made available for transplantation in second or subsequent CR.

References

1 Boggs D.R., Wintrobe M.M. & Cartwright G.E. (1962) The acute leukaemias. Analysis of 322 cases and review of the literature. *Medicine*, **41**, 163–225.

2 Roath S., Israels M.C.G. & Wilkinson J.F. (1964) The acute leukaemias: a study of 580 patients. *Quarterly Journal of Medicine*, **33**, 256–283.

3 Wiernik P.H. (1982) Acute leukemias of adults. In: *Cancer: principles and practice of oncology* (eds V.T. Devita, S. Hellman & S.A. Rosenberg), pp. 1402–1426. J.B. Lippincott, Philadelphia.

4 Rosner F., Dobbs J.V., Ritz N.D. *et al.* (1970) Disturbances of hemostasis in acute myeloblastic leukemia. *Acta Haematologica*, **43**, 65–72.

5 Straus D.J., Mertelsmann R., Koziner B. *et al.* (1980) The acute monocytic leukemias: multidisciplinary studies in 45 patients. *Medicine*, **59**, 409–425.

6 Schiffer C.A. & Wiernik P.H. (1977) Functional evaluation of circulating leukemic cells in acute non-lymphocytic leukemia. *Leukemia Research*, **1**, 271–277.

7 Ohta H. & Hatsuda T. (1973) Ready release of intracellular

muramidase (lysozyme) from mononuclear cells in skin window exudates. *Acta Haematologica*, **49**, 159–165.

8 Schmalzl F., Huber H., Asamer M. *et al.* (1969) Cytochemical and immunohistologic investigations on the source and the functional changes of mononuclear cells in skin window exudates. *Blood*, **34**, 129–140.

9 Robb R.M., Ervin L.D. & Shallan S.E. (1979) An autopsy study of eye involvement in acute leukaemia of childhood. *Medical and Pediatric Oncology*, **6**, 171–177.

10 Kundel D.W., Brecher G., Bodey G.P. *et al.* (1964) Reticulin fibrosis and bone infarction in acute leukaemia. Implications for prognosis. *Blood*, **23**, 526–544.

11 Petrakis N.L. (1954) Bone marrow pressure in leukemic and non-leukemic patients. *Journal of Clinical Investigation*, **33**, 27–34.

12 Petrakis N.L., Masouredis S.P. & Miller P. (1953) The local blood flow in human bone marrow in leukemia and neoplastic diseases as determined by the clearance rate of radionuclide (^{131}I). *Journal of Clinical Investigation*, **32**, 952–963.

13 Hann I.M., Gupta S., Palmer M.K. *et al.* (1979) The prognostic significance of radiological and symptomatic bone involvement in childhood acute lymphoblastic leukemia. *Medical and Pediatric Oncology*, **6**, 51–55.

14 Klock J.C. & Oken R.L. (1976) Febrile neutrophilic dermatosis in acute myelogenous leukaemia. *Cancer*, **37**, 922–927.

15 Brakman P., Snyder J., Henderson E.S. *et al.* (1970) Blood coagulation and fibrinolysis in acute leukaemia. *British Journal of Haematology*, **18**, 135–145.

16 Didisheim P., Thrombold J.S., Vandervoort R.L.E. *et al.* (1964) Acute promyelocytic leukemia with fibrinogen and factor V deficiencies. *Blood*, **23**, 717–728.

17 Boggs D.R. (1960) The cellular composition of the inflammatory exudates in human leukemias. *Blood*, **15**, 466–475.

18 Holland J.F., Senn H. & Banerjee T. (1971) Quantitative studies of localized leukocyte mobilization in acute leukaemia. *Blood*, **37**, 499–511.

19 Solberg C.O., Schreiner A.S., Hellum K.B. *et al.* (1975) Neutrophil granulocyte function in the early diagnosis of acute myelomonocytic and myeloblastic leukemia. *Acta Medica Scandinavica*, **197**, 147–151.

20 Srivastava D.I.S., Kahn S.A. & Henderson E.S. (1976) High terminal deoxynucleotidyl transferase activity in acute myelogenous leukemia. *Cancer Research*, **36**, 3847–3850.

21 Sultan C., Imbert M., Richard M-F. *et al.* (1977) Pure acute monocytic leukemia. *American Journal of Clinical Pathology*, **68**, 752–757.

22 Tobelem G., Jacquillat C., Chastang C. *et al.* (1980) Acute monoblastic leukemia: a clinical and biologic study of 74 cases. *Blood*, **55**, 71–76.

23 Boros L. & Bennett J.M. (1984) The acute myeloid leukemias. In: Goldman J.M. & Priesler H.D. (eds) *Leukemias*, pp. 104–135. Butterworths, London.

24 Osserman E.T. & Lawlor D.P. (1966) Serum and urinary lysozyme (muramidase) in monocytic and myelomonocytic leukaemia. *Journal of Experimental Medicine*, **124**, 921–951.

25 Shaw M.T. (1978) The distinctive features of acute monocytic leukaemia. *American Journal of Haematology*, **4**, 97–103.

26 Meyer R.I., Ferreira P.P.C., Cuttner J. *et al.* (1980) Central nervous system involvement and presentation in acute granulocytic leukemia. *American Journal of Medicine*, **68**, 691–694.

27 Holmes R., Keating M.J., Cork A. *et al.* (1985) A unique pattern of central nervous system leukemia in acute myelomonocytic leukemia associated with inv (16) (p13, q22). *Blood*, **65**, 1071–1078.

28 Bernard J., Weil M., Boiron M. *et al.* (1973) Acute promyelocytic leukemia. Results of treatment by daunorubicin. *Blood*, **41**, 489–496.

29 Bennett J.M., Catovsky D., Daniel M.T. *et al.* (1980) A variant form of hypergranular promyelocytic leukemia (M3). *British Journal of Haematology*, **44**, 169–170.

30 Golomb H.M., Rowley J.D., Vardiman J.W. *et al.* (1980) 'Microgranular' acute promyelocytic leukemia: a distinct clinical, ultrastructural and cytogenetic entity. *Blood*, **55**, 253–259.

31 Kaneko Y. & Sakurai M. (1977) 15;17 translocation in acute promyelocytic leukaemia. *Lancet*, **i**, 961.

32 Van den Berghe H., Louwagie A., Broeckaert-van Orshoven A. *et al.* (1979) Chromosome abnormalities in acute promyelocytic leukemia (APL). *Cancer*, **43**, 558–562.

33 Gralnick H.R. & Sultan C. (1975) Acute promyelocytic leukaemia, haemorrhagic manifestations and morphologic criteria. (Annotation.) *British Journal of Haematology*, **29**, 373–376.

34 Rosenthal R.L. (1963) Acute promyelocytic leukemia associated with hypofibrinogenemia. *Blood*, **21**, 495–508.

35 Bernard J., Lasneret J., Chome J. *et al.* (1963) A cytological and histological study of acute promyelocytic leukemia. *Journal of Clinical Pathology*, **16**, 319–325.

36 Polliack A. (1971) Acute promyelocytic leukemia with disseminated intravascular coagulation. *American Journal of Clinical Pathology*, **56**, 155–161.

37 Goldman J.M. (1974) Acute promyelocytic leukaemia. *British Medical Journal*, **1**, 380–382.

38 Valdivieso M., Rodriguez V. & Drewinko B. (1975) Clinical and morphological correlations in acute promyelocytic leukemia. *Medical and Pediatric Oncology*, **1**, 37–50.

39 Jones M.E. & Saleem A. (1978) Acute promyelocytic leukemia. A review of the literature. *American Journal of Medicine*, **65**, 673–677.

40 Hillstead L.K. (1957) Acute promyelocytic leukemia. *Acta Medica Scandinavica*, **159**, 189–194.

41 Randj J., Moloney W.C. & Sise H.S. (1969) Coagulation defects in acute promyelocytic leukemia. *Archives of Internal Medicine*, **123**, 39–48.

42 Albarracin N.S. & Haust N.D. (1971) Intravascular coagulation in promyelocytic leukemia. *American Journal of Clinical Pathology*, **55**, 677–685.

43 Groopman J. & Ellman L. (1979) Acute promyelocytic leukemia. *American Journal of Hematology*, **7**, 395–408.

44 Gralnick H.R. & Abrell E. (1973) Studies of the procoagulant and fibrinolytic activity of promyelocytes in acute promyelocytic leukaemia. *British Journal of Haematology*, **24**, 89–99.

45 Sultan C., Gouault-Heilmann M. & Tulliez M. (1973) Relationship between blast-cell morphology and occurrence of a syndrome of disseminated intravascular coagulation. *British Journal of Haematology*, **24**, 255–259.

46 Gouault-Heilmann M., Chardon E., Sultan C. *et al.* (1975) The procoagulant factor of leukaemic promyelocytes. Demonstration of immunologic cross reactivity with human brain tissue factor. *British Journal of Haematology*, **30**, 151–158.

47 Sakuragawa N., Takahashi K., Hoshiyama M. *et al.* (1976) Pathologic cells as procoagulant substance of disseminated intravascular coagulation syndrome in acute promyelocytic leukemia. *Thrombosis Research*, **8**, 263–273.

48 Gralnick H.R., Marchesi S. & Givelber H. (1972) Intravascular

coagulation in acute leukemia. Clinical and subclinical abnormalities. *Blood*, **40**, 709–718.

49 Cordonnier C., Vernant J.P., Brun B. *et al.* (1985) Acute promyelocytic leukemia in 57 previously untreated patients. *Cancer*, **55**, 18–25.

50 Blaisdell F.W. (1974) Pathophysiology of the respiratory distress syndrome. *Archives of Surgery*, **108**, 44–49.

51 Bone R.C., Francis P.B. & Pierce A.K. (1976) Intravascular coagulation associated with the adult respiratory distress syndrome. *American Journal of Medicine*, **61**, 585–589.

52 Schneider R.C., Zapol W.M. & Carvalho A.C. (1980) Platelet consumption and sequestration in severe acute respiratory failure. *American Review of Respiratory Diseases*, **122**, 445–451.

53 Mainwaring D. & Curreri P.W. (1982) Platelet and neutrophil sequestration after fragment D induced respiratory disease. *Circulatory Shock*, **9**, 75–80.

54 Wiernik P.H. & Serpick A.A. (1970) Factors affecting remission and survival in adult acute nonlymphocytic leukemia. *Medicine*, **49**, 505–513.

55 Crowther D., Beard M.E.J., Bateman C.J.T. *et al.* (1975) Factors influencing prognosis in adults with acute myelogenous leukaemia. *British Journal of Cancer*, **32**, 456–464.

56 Hug V., Keating M., McCredie K. *et al.* (1983) Clinical course and response to treatment of patients with acute myelogenous leukemia presenting with a high leukocyte count. *Cancer*, **52**, 773–779.

57 Lester T.J., Johnson J.W. & Cuttner J. (1985) Pulmonary leukostasis as the single worst prognostic factor in patients with acute myelocytic leukemia and hyperleukocytosis. *American Journal of Medicine*, **79**, 43–48.

58 Vernant J.P., Brun B., Mannoni P. *et al.* (1979) Respiratory distress of hyperleukocytic granulocytic leukemias. *Cancer*, **44**, 264–268.

59 Prakash U.B., Divertie M.B. & Banks P.M. (1979) Aggressive therapy in acute respiratory failure from leukemic pulmonary infiltrates. *Chest*, **75**, 345–350.

60 Berg J., Vincent P.C. & Gunz F.W. (1979) Extreme leukocytosis and prognosis of newly diagnosed patients with acute nonlymphocytic leukemia. *Medical Journal of Australia*, **i**, 480–482.

61 Lichtman M.A. (1973) Rheology of leukocytes, leukocyte suspension and blood in leukemia. Possible relationship to clinical manifestations. *Journal of Clinical Investigation*, **52**, 350–358.

62 Freireich E.J., Thomas L.B., Frei E. *et al.* (1960) A distinctive type of intracerebral hemorrhage associated with 'blastic crisis' in patients with leukemia. *Cancer*, **13**, 146–154.

63 McKee L.C. & Collins R.D. (1974) Intravascular leukocyte thrombi and aggregates as a cause of morbidity and mortality in leukemia. *Medicine*, **53**, 463–478.

64 Barcos M., Lane W., Gomez G.A. *et al.* (1987) An autopsy study of 1206 acute and chronic leukemias (1958–1982). *Cancer*, **60**, 827–837.

65 Dawson D.W., Rosenthal D.S. & Moloney W.C. (1979) Neurological complications of acute leukemia in adults: changing rate. *Annals of Internal Medicine*, **79**, 541–544.

66 Law I.P. & Blom J. (1977) Adult acute leukemia: frequency of central nervous system involvement in long term survivors. *Cancer*, **40**, 1304–1306.

67 Steward D.J., Keating M.J., McCredie K.B. *et al.* (1981) Natural history of central nervous system acute leukemia in adults. *Cancer*, **47**, 184–196.

68 Cuttner J., Conjalka M.S., Reilly M. *et al.* (1980) Association of monocytic leukemia in patients with extreme leucocytosis. *American Journal of Medicine*, **69**, 555–558.

69 Ruggero D., Baccarani M., Zaccaria A. *et al.* (1977) Nervous system involvement in adult myeloid leukemia. *Hematologica*, **62**, 312–317.

70 Weinstein H.J., Mayer R.J., Rosenthal D.S. *et al.* (1983) Chemotherapy for acute myelogenous leukemia in children and adults: VAPA update. *Blood*, **62**, 315–319.

71 Dahl G.V., Simone J.V., Hustu H.O. *et al.* (1978) Preventive central nervous system irradiation in children with acute nonlymphocytic leukemia. *Cancer*, **42**, 2187–2192.

72 Choi S. & Simone J.V. (1976) Acute non-lymphocytic leukemia in 171 children. *Medical and Pediatric Oncology*, **2**, 119–146.

73 Kay H.E.M. (1976) Development of CNS leukaemia in acute myeloid leukaemia in children. *Archives of Diseases of Childhood*, **51**, 73–74.

74 West R.J., Graham-Pole J., Hardisty R.M. *et al.* (1972) Factors in pathogenesis of central nervous system leukaemia. *British Medical Journal*, **3**, 311–314.

75 Pippard M.J., Callender S.T. & Sheldon P.W.E. (1979) Infiltration of central nervous system in adult acute myeloid leukaemia. *British Medical Journal*, **1**, 227–229.

76 Kuo A.H-M., Yataganas X., Galicich J.H. *et al.* (1975) Proliferative kinetics of central nervous system leukaemia. *Cancer*, **36**, 232–239.

77 Lefrak E.A., Pitha J., Rosenheim S.K. *et al.* (1973) A clinicopathological analysis of adriamycin cardiotoxicity. *Cancer*, **32**, 302–314.

78 Legha S.S., Keating M.J., McCredie K.B. *et al.* (1982) Evaluation of AMSA in previously treated patients with acute leukemia: results of therapy in 109 adults. *Blood*, **60**, 484–490.

79 Minow R.A., Benjamin R.S. & Gottlieb J.A. (1975) Adriamycin (NSC-123127) cardiomyopathy — an overview with determination of risk factors. *Cancer Chemotherapy Reports*, **6**, 195–199.

80 Al-Ismail S.A.D. & Whittaker J.A. (1979) Systolic time interval as index of schedule dependent doxorubicin cardiotoxicity in patients with acute myelogenous leukaemia. *British Medical Journal*, **1**, 1392–1395.

81 Al-Ismail S.A.D., Parry D.H. & Whittaker J.A. (1977) Anthracycline cardiotoxicity and acute myelogenous leukaemia. *British Medical Journal*, **1**, 815–817.

82 Rinehart J.J., Lewis R.P. & Balcerzak S.P. (1974) Adriamycin cardiotoxicity in man. *Annals of Internal Medicine*, **81**, 475–478.

83 Bloom K.R., Bini R.M., Williams C.M. *et al.* (1978) Echocardiography in adriamycin cardiotoxicity. *Cancer*, **41**, 1265–1269.

84 Alexander J., Dainiak N., Berger H.J. *et al.* (1979) Serial assessment of doxorubicin cardiotoxicity with quantitative radionuclide angiocardiography. *New England Journal of Medicine*, **300**, 278–283.

85 Singer J.W., Narahara K.A., Ritchie J.L. *et al.* (1978) Time and dose-dependent changes in ejection fraction determined by radionuclide angiography after anthracycline therapy. *Cancer Treatment Reports*, **62**, 945–948.

86 Mortensen S.A., Olsen H.S. & Baandrup U. (1986) Chronic anthracycline cardiotoxicity: haemodynamic and histopathological manifestations suggesting a restrictive endomyocardial disease. *British Heart Journal*, **55**, 274–282.

87 De Conti R.C. & Calabresi P. (1960) Use of allopurinol for prevention and control of hyperuricemia in patients with neoplastic disease. *New England Journal of Medicine*, **274**, 481–486.

88 Mundy G.R., Ibbotson K.J. & D'Souza S.M. (1985) Tumor products and the calcemia of malignancy. *Journal of Clinical Investigation*, **76**, 391–394.

89 Hasselbalch H., Birgens H.S. & Geisler C. (1985) Hypercalcaemia in the accelerated phase of chronic myelogenous leukaemia: no

relationship to the phenotype of the blast cells. *Scandinavian Journal of Haematology*, **35**, 333–338.

90 Body J.J., Borkowski A., Cleeren A. *et al.* (1986) Treatment of malignancy-associated hypercalcaemia with intravenous amino-hydroxypropylidene diphosphonate. *Journal of Clinical Oncology*, **4**, 1177–1183.

91 Ralston S.H., Gardner M.D., Dryburgh F.J. *et al.* (1985) Compari-son of aminohydroxypropylidine disphosphonate, mithramycin and corticosteroids/calcitonin on treatment of cancer associated hypercalcemia. *Lancet*, **ii**, 907.

92 Mir M.A. & Delamore I.W. (1978) Metabolic disorders in acute myeloid leukaemia. *British Journal of Haematology*, **40**, 79–92.

93 Freedman D.R., Shannon M., Dandova P. *et al.* (1982) Hypo-parathyroidism and hypocalcaemia during treatment for acute leukaemia. *British Medical Journal*, **84**, 700–702.

94 Schiffer C.A., Lee E.J., Romiyasu T. *et al.* (1989) Prognostic impact of cytogenetic abnormalities in patients with *de novo* acute non-lymphocytic leukemia. *Blood*, **73**, 263–270.

95 Bloomfield C.D., Lawrence D., Arthur D.C. *et al.* (1994) Curative impact of intensification with high dose cytarabine (HiDAC) in acute myeloid leukemia (AML) varies by cytogenetic group. *Blood*, **84**(Suppl.), 111.

96 Solary E., Cassanovas R.O., Campos L. *et al.* (1992) Surface markers in adult acute myeloblastic leukemia: correlation of CD19+, CD23+ and CD14+/DR phenotypes with shorter survival. *Leukemia*, **6**, 393–399.

97 Campos L., Gyotat D., Archimbaud D. *et al.* (1992) Clinical significance of multidrug resistance P-glycoprotein expression on acute non lymphoblastic leukemia cells at diagnosis. *Blood*, **79**, 473–476.

98 Short T., Miller K.R. Desforges J.D. (1987) The predictive value of *in vitro* techniques in acute non lymphocytic leukemia. *Leukemia Research*, **11**, 687–691.

99 Raza A., Preisler H.D., Day I. *et al.* (1990) Direct relationship between remission duration in acute myeloid leukaemia and cell cycle kinetics. *Blood*, **76**, 2191–2197.

100 Löwenberg B., Van Putten W.W., Touw I.P. *et al.* (1993) Autonomous proliferation of leukemic cells *in vitro* as a determi-nant of prognosis in adult acute myeloid leukemia. *New England Journal of Medicine*, **328**, 614–619.

101 Wood R.B., Dallimore C.M., Smith S.A. & Whittaker J.A. (1984) Use of logistic regression analysis to improve prediction of prog-nosis in acute myeloid leukemia. *Leukemia Research*, **8**, 667–679.

102 Estey E., Smith I.L., Keating M.J. *et al.* (1989) Prediction of sur-vival during induction therapy in patients with newly diagnosed acute myeloblastic leukemia. *Leukemia*, **3**, 257–262.

103 Wiernik P.H. & Serpick A.A. (1972) A randomized clinical trial of daunorubicin and a combination of prednisone, vincristine, 6-mercaptopurine and methotrexate in adult acute nonlympho-cytic leukemia. *Cancer Research*, **32**, 2023–2026.

104 Jacquillat C., Weil M., Gemon-Auclere M.F. *et al.* (1976) Clinical study of rubidazone (22050 RP), a new daunorubicin derived compound, in 170 patients with acute leukemia and other malig-nancies. *Cancer*, **37**, 653–659.

105 Bodey G.P., Coltman C., Freireich E.J. *et al.* (1974) Chemotherapy of acute leukemia. Comparison of cytosine arabinoside alone and in combination with vincristine, prednisone and cyclophos-phamide. *Archives of Internal Medicine*, **133**, 260–266.

106 Preisler H.D., Rustum Y., Henderson E.S. *et al.* (1979) Treatment of acute nonlymphocytic leukemia: use of anthracycline-cytosine arabinoside induction therapy and comparison of two mainte-nance regimens. *Blood*, **53**, 455–464.

107 Preisler H.D., Bjornsson S., Henderson E.S. *et al.* (1979) Remis-sion induction in acute nonlymphocytic leukemia: comparison of a seven-day and ten-day infusion of cytosine arabinoside in com-bination with adriamycin. *Medical and Pediatric Oncology*, **7**, 269–275.

108 Rai K.R., Holland J.R., Glidewell O.J. *et al.* (1981) Treatment of acute myelocytic leukemia: a study by Cancer and Leukemia Group B. *Blood*, **58**, 1203–1212.

109 Link H., Frauer H.M., Ostendorf P. *et al.* (1985) Therapy for acute myeloid leukemia in 119 adults: a comparison of two treatment protocols. *Blut*, **51**, 49–57.

110 Yates J., Glidewell O., Wiernik P. *et al.* (1982) Cytosine arabi-noside with daunorubicin or adriamycin for therapy of acute myelocytic leukemia: a CALGB study. *Blood*, **60**, 454–462.

111 Sauter C., Berchtold W., Fopp M. *et al.* (1984) Acute myelogenous leukaemia: maintenance chemotherapy after early consolidation treatment does not prolong survival. *Lancet*, **i**, 379–382.

112 Omura G.A., Vogler W.R. & Lefante J. (1982) Treatment of acute myelogenous leukemia: influence of three induction regimens and maintenance with chemotherapy or BCG immunotherapy. *Cancer*, **49**, 1530–1536.

113 Mayer R.J., Schiffer C.A., Peterson B.A. *et al.* (1987) Intensive postremission therapy in adults with acute nonlymphocytic leukemia using various dose schedules of ara-C. A progress report from the CALGB. *Seminars in Oncology*, **14**(Suppl.), 25–31.

114 Preisler H.D., Davis R.B., Krishner J. *et al.* (1987) Comparison of three remission induction regimens and two postinduction strategies for the treatment of acute nonlymphocytic leukemia: Cancer and Leukemia Group B Study. *Blood*, **69**, 1441–1449.

115 Cassileth P.A. & Katz M.E. (1977) Chemotherapy for adult acute nonlymphocytic leukemia with daunorubicin and cytosine arabi-noside. *Cancer Treatment Reports*, **61**, 1441–1445.

116 Glucksberg H., Cheever M., Fefer A. *et al.* (1981) Intensification therapy in acute nonlymphocytic leukemia (ANL) in adults (Abstract) *Proceedings of the American Association for Cancer Research and the American Society of Clinical Oncology*, **22**, 232.

117 Cassileth P.A., Begg C.B., Bennett J.M. *et al.* (1984) A randomized study of the efficacy of consolidation therapy in adult acute non-lymphocytic leukemia. *Blood*, **63**, 843–847.

118 Büchner T., Urbanitz D., Hiddeman W. *et al.* (1985) Intensified induction and consolidation with or without maintenance chemotherapy for AML: two multicenter studies of the German AML Cooperative Group. *Journal of Clinical Oncology*, **3**, 1583–1589.

119 Clarkson B.D., Gee T., Mertelsmann R. *et al.* (1988) Current status of treatment of acute leukemia in adults: an overview of the memorial experience and review of the literature. *Critical Reviews in Oncology/Hematology*, **4**, 221–248.

120 Rees J.K.H., Gray R.G., Swirsky D. *et al.* (1986) Principle results of the Medical Research Council's 8th acute myeloid leukaemia trial. *Lancet*, **ii**, 1236–1241.

121 Rees J.K.H. & Gray R.G. (1990) Remission induction and post-remission therapy in acute myelogenous leukaemia. British MRC study. *Haematology and Blood Transfusion*, **33**, 243–248.

122 Rohatiner A.Z.S., Gregory W.M., Bassan R. *et al.* (1988) Short-term therapy for acute myelogenous leukaemia. *Journal of Clinical Oncology*, **6**, 218–226.

123 Archimbaud E., Fiere D., Treille-Ritouet D. *et al.* (1987) Influence of daunorubicin and cytarabine sequencing on the outcome of therapy in acute myelogenous leukaemia: a randomized trial. *Cancer Treatment Reports*, **71**, 571–574.

124 Gale R.P., Foon K.A., Cline M.J. *et al.* (1981) Intensive

chemotherapy for acute myelogenous leukemia. *Annals of Internal Medicine*, **94**, 753–757.

125 Dietman R.O., Davis R.B., Green M.R. *et al.* (1991) A comparative study of two different doses of cytarabine for acute myeloid leukemia: a phase III trial of Cancer and Leukemia Group B. *Blood*, **78**, 2520–2526.

126 Berman E., Heller G., Santorsa J. *et al.* (1991) Results of a randomised trial comparing idarubicin and cytosine arabinoside with daunorubicin and cytosine arabinoside in adult patients with newly diagnosed acute myelogenous leukemia. *Blood*, **77**, 1666–1674.

127 Vogler W.R., Velez-Garcia E., Weiner R.S. *et al.* (1992) A phase III trial comparing idarubicin and daunorubicin in acute myelogenous leukemia: a Southeastern Cancer Study Group study. *Journal of Clinical Oncology*, **10**, 1103–1111.

128 Wiernik P.H., Bands P.L.C., Case D.C. *et al.* (1992) Cytarabine plus idarubicin or daunorubicin as consolidation therapy for previously untreated adult patients with acute myeloid leukemia. *Blood*, **79**, 313–319.

129 Arlin Z., Case D.C., Moore J. *et al.* (1990) Randomized multicenter trial of cytosine arabinoside with mitoxantrone or daunorubicin in previously untreated adult patients with acute nonlymphocytic leukemia (ANNLL). *Leukemia*, **4**, 177–183.

130 Ho A.D., Bernadett B., Haas R. *et al.* (1991) Etoposide in acute leukemia: past experience and future perspectives. *Cancer*, **67**, 281–284.

131 Carella A.M., Martinengo M., Santini G. *et al.* (1987) Idarubicin in combination with etoposide and cytarabine in adult untreated nonlymphoblastic leukemia. *European Journal of Cancer and Clinical Oncology*, **12**, 1673–1678.

132 Bishop J.F., Löwenthal R.N., Joshua D. *et al.* (1990) Etoposide in acute nonlymphocytic leukemia. *Blood*, **75**, 27–32.

133 Vogler W.R., Winton E.F., Gordon D.S. *et al.* (1984) A randomized comparison of postremission therapy in acute myelogenous leukemia: a Southeastern Cancer Study Group trial. *Blood*, **63**, 1039–1045.

134 Hewlett J.S., Chen T., Balcerzak S.P. *et al.* (1985) High rate of long-term survival in adult acute leukemia following ten-day chemotherapy (OAP) induction. *Archives of Internal Medicine*, **145**, 1006–1012.

135 Keating M.J., Smith T.L., McCredie K.B. *et al.* (1981) A four year experience with anthracycline, cytosine arabinoside, vincristine and prednisone combination chemotherapy in 325 adults with acute leukemia. *Cancer*, **47**, 2779–2788.

136 Arlin Z.A., Flomenburg B., Gee T.S. *et al.* (1981) Treatment of acute leukemia in relapse with 4′ (9-acridinylamino) methanesulfon-m-anisidide (AMSA) in combination with cytosine arabinoside and thioguanine. *Cancer Clinical Trials*, **4**, 317–321.

137 Hines J.D., Oken M.M., Mazza J.J. *et al.* (1984) High dose cytosine arabinoside and m-AMSA is effective therapy in relapsed acute nonlymphocytic leukemia. *Journal of Clinical Oncology*, **2**, 545–549.

138 Tschopp L., von Fliedner V.E., Sauter C. *et al.* (1986) Efficacy and clinical cross-resistance of a new combination therapy (AMSA/VP16) in previously treated patients with acute nonlymphocytic leukemia. *Journal of Clinical Oncology*, **4**, 318–324.

139 Winton E.F., Hearn E.B., Martelo O. *et al.* (1985) Sequentially administered 5-azacitidine and amsacrine in refractory adult acute leukemia: a phase I–II trial of the Southeastern Cancer Study Group. *Cancer Treatment Reports*, **69**, 807–811.

140 Berman E., Zalmen A.A., Gaynor J. *et al.* (1988) Comparative trial of cytarabine and thioguanine in combination with amsacrine or daunorubicin in patients with untreated acute nonlymphocytic leukemia: results of the L-16M protocol. *Leukemia*, **3**, 115–121.

141 Mayer R.J., Weinstein H.J., Coral F.S. *et al.* (1982) The role of intensive postinduction chemotherapy in the management of patients with acute myelogenous leukemia. *Cancer Treatment Reports*, **66**, 1455–1462.

142 Preisler H.D., Anderson K. & Rai K. (1989) The frequency of long term remission in patients with acute myelogenous leukaemia treated with conventional maintenance chemotherapy: a study of 760 patients with a minimal follow-up time of six years. *British Journal of Haematology*, **71**, 189–194.

143 Haronsseau J.L., Milpied N., Briere J. *et al.* (1991) Double intensive consolidation chemotherapy in adult acute myeloid leukemia. *Journal of Clinical Oncology*, **9**, 1432–1437.

144 Mayer R.J., Davis R.B., Schiffer C.A. *et al.* (1994) Intensive postremission chemotherapy in adults with acute myeloid leukemia. *New England Journal of Medicine*, **331**, 896–903.

145 Champlin P.A., Gajewski J., Nimer S. *et al.* (1990) Post remission chemotherapy for adults with daunorubicin consolidation treatment. *Journal of Clinical Oncology*, **8**, 1199–1206.

146 Schiller G.J., Gajewski J., Nimer S. *et al.* (1992) Long term outcome of high dose cytarabine-based consolidation chemotherapy for adults with acute myelogenous leukemia. *Blood*, **80**, 2977–2982.

147 Wolff S.N., Herzig R.H., Fay J.W. *et al.* (1989) High dose cytarabine and daunorubicin as consolidation therapy for acute myeloid leukemia in first remission — long term follow up and results. *Journal of Clinical Oncology*, **7**, 1260–1267.

148 Tallman M.S., Appelbaum F.R., Amos D. *et al.* (1987) Evaluation of intensive postremission chemotherapy for adults with acute nonlymphocytic leukemia using high-dose cytosine arabinoside with L-asparaginase and amsacrine with etoposide. *Journal of Clinical Oncology*, **5**, 918–926.

149 Cassileth P.A., Begg C.B., Silber R. *et al.* (1987) Prolonged unmaintained remission after intensive consolidation therapy in adult acute nonlymphocytic leukemia. *Cancer Treatment Reports*, **71**, 137–140.

150 Goldberg J., Grunwald H., Vogler W.R. *et al.* (1985) Treatment of patients with nonlymphocytic leukemia in relapse: a leukemia intergroup study. *American Journal of Hematology*, **19**, 167–176.

151 Herzig R.H., Wolff S.N., Lazarus H.M. *et al.* (1983) High-dose cytosine arabinoside therapy for refractory leukemia. *Blood*, **62**, 361–369.

152 Cantin G. & Brennan J.K. (1984) High-dose cytosine arabinoside for acute nonlymphocytic leukemia. *American Journal of Hematology*, **16**, 59–66.

153 Herzig R.H., Lazarus H.M., Wolff S.N. *et al.* (1985) High-dose cytosine arabinoside therapy with and without anthracycline antibiotics for remission and reinduction of acute nonlymphoblastic leukemia. *Journal of Clinical Oncology*, **3**, 992–997.

154 Zittoun R., Marie J.P., Zittoun J. *et al.* (1985) Modulation of cytosine arabinoside (Ara-C) and high-dose Ara-C in acute leukemia. *Seminars in Oncology*, **12**(Suppl.), 139–143.

155 Vogler W.R., McCarley D.L., Stagg M. *et al.* (1994) A phase III trial of high dose cytosine arabinoside with or without etoposide in relapsed and refractory acute myelogenous leukemia. A Southeastern Cancer Study Group Trial. *Leukemia*, **8**, 1847–1853.

156 Daenen S., Lowenberg B., Sonneveld W.L. *et al.* (1994) Efficacy of etoposide and mitoxantrone in patients with acute myelogenous

leukemia refractory to standard induction therapy and intermediate-dose cytarabine and amsidine. *Leukemia*, **8**, 6–10.

157 Rowe J.M., Andersen J.W., Mazza J.J. *et al.* (1994) Treatment of relapsed and refractory AML with mitoxantrone and etoposide. In: *Acute Leukemias IV: prognostic factors* (eds T. Bücher, W. Hiddleman & B. Wormann), pp. 235–238. Springer-Verlag, Berlin.

158 Rowe J.M., Chang A.Y.C., Bennett J.M. (1988) Aclacinomycin A and etoposide (VP-16-213): an effective regimen in previously treated patients with refractory acute myelogenous leukemia. *Blood*, **71**, 992–996.

159 Santana V.M., Marrow J., Kearns C. *et al.* (1992) 2-Chlorodeoxyadenosine produces a high rate of hematologic remission in relapsed acute myeloid leukemia. *Journal of Clinical Oncology*, **10**, 364–370.

160 Petti M.C., Mandelli F., Zagonel V. *et al.* (1993) A pilot study of 5-aza-2'-deoxycytidine (Decitabine) in the treatment of poor prognosis acute myelogenous leukemia patients: preliminary results. *Leukemia*, **7**, 36–41.

161 Vogler W.R., Harrington D.P., Winton E.F. *et al.* (1992) Phase II clinical trial of carboplatin in relapsed and refractory leukemia. *Leukemia*, **6**, 1072–1073.

162 Estey E.H., Keating M.J., McCredie K.B. *et al.* (1982) Causes of initial remission induction failure in acute myelogenous leukemia. *Blood*, **60**, 309–315.

163 Curtis J.E., Till J.E., Messner H.A. *et al.* (1979) Comparison of outcomes and prognostic factors for two groups of patients with acute myeloblastic leukemia. *Leukemia Research*, **3**, 409–416.

164 Bernard P., Reiffers J., Lacombe F. *et al.* (1984) A stage classification for prognosis in adult acute myelogenous leukaemia based upon patients age, bone marrow karyotype and clinical features. *Scandinavian Journal of Haematology*, **32**, 429–440.

165 Liu Yin J.A. (1993) Acute myeloid leukaemia in the elderly: biology and treatment. *British Journal of Haematology*, **83**, 1–6.

166 Keating M.J., McCredie K.B., Benjamin R.S. *et al.* (1981) Treatment of patients over 50 years of age with acute myelogenous leukemia with a combination of rubidazone and cytosine arabinoside, vincristine and prednisone (ROAP). *Blood*, **58**, 584–591.

167 Kahn S.B., Begg C.B., Mazza J.J. *et al.* (1984) Full dose versus attenuated dose daunorubicin, cytosine arabinoside and 6-thioguanine in the treatment of acute nonlymphocytic leukemia in the elderly. *Journal of Clinical Oncology*, **2**, 865–870.

168 Rees J.K.H. & Gray R.G. (1987) Comparison of 1 + 5 DAT and 3 + 10 DAT followed by COAP or MAZE consolidation therapy in the treatment of acute myeloid leukemia. MRC Ninth AML trial. *Seminars in Oncology*, **4**, 32–36.

169 Löwenberg B., Zittoun R., Jehn K.U. *et al.* (1989) On the value of intensive remission-induction chemotherapy in elderly patients of 65+ years with acute myeloid leukemia: a randomised phase III study of the European Organisation for Research and Treatment of Cancer Leukaemia Group. *Journal of Clinical Oncology*, **7**, 1268–1274.

170 Tilly H., Castaigne S., Bordessoule D. *et al.* (1990) Low-dose cytosine versus intensive chemotherapy in the treatment of acute nonlymphocytic leukemia in the elderly. *Journal of Clinical Oncology*, **8**, 272–279.

171 Yin J.A.L., Johnson P.R.E., Davies J.M. *et al.* (1991) Mitozantrone and cytosine arabinoside as first line therapy in elderly patients with acute myeloid leukemia. *British Journal of Haematology*, **79**, 415–420.

172 Arlin Z., Case D.C., Moore J. *et al.* (1990) Randomised multi-center trial of cytosine arabinoside with mitoxantrone or daunorubicin in previously untreated adult patients with acute nonlymphocytic leukemia (ANLL). *Leukemia*, **4**, 177–183.

173 Dombret H., Chastang C., Fenaux P. *et al.* (1995) A controlled study of recombinant human granulocyte colony-stimulating factor in elderly patients after treatment for acute myelogenous leukemia. *New England Journal of Medicine*, **332**, 1678–1683.

174 Stone R.M., Berg D.J., George S.L. *et al.* (1995) Granulocyte-macrophage colony-stimulating factor after initial chemotherapy for elderly patients with primary acute myelogenous leukemia. *New England Journal of Medicine*, **332**, 1671–1677.

175 Manoharan A., Leyden M.J. & Sullivan J. (1984) Low-dose cytarabine in acute myeloid leukaemia. *Medical Journal of Australia*, **141**, 643–646.

176 Tilly H., Castaigne S., Bourdessoule D. *et al.* (1985) Low-dose cytosine arabinoside treatment for acute non-lymphocytic leukemia in elderly patients. *Cancer*, **55**, 1633–1636.

177 Jensen M.K. & Ahlbom G. (1985) Low dose cytosine arabinoside in the treatment of acute non-lymphocytic leukaemia. *Scandinavian Journal of Haematology*, **34**, 261–263.

178 Mufti G.J., Oscier D.G., Hamblin T.J. *et al.* (1983) Low doses of cytarbine in the treatment of myelodysplastic syndrome and acute myeloid leukaemia. *New England Journal of Medicine*, **309**, 1653–1654.

179 Pinkerton P.H., London B. & Cowan D.H. (1985) Low dose cytosine arabinoside in acute myeloid leukemia. *American Journal of Hematology*, **19**, 415–417.

180 Powell B.L., Capizzi R.L., Muss H.B. *et al.* (1989) Low-dose AraC therapy for acute myelogenous leukemia in elderly patients. *Leukemia*, **3**, 23–28.

181 Manoharan A. (1983) Low-dose cytarabine therapy in hypoplastic acute leukemia. *New England Journal of Medicine*, **309**, 1652–1653.

182 Weinstein H.J., Mayer R.J., Rosenthal D.S. *et al.* (1980) Treatment of acute myelogenous leukemia in children and adults. *New England Journal of Medicine*, **303**, 473–478.

183 Creutzig U., Ritter J., Riehm H. *et al.* (1985) Improved treatment results in childhood acute myelogenous leukemia: a report of the German cooperative study AML-BFM-78. *Blood*, **65**, 298–304.

184 Buckley J.D., Lampkin B.C., Nesbit M.E. *et al.* (1989) Remission induction in children with acute non-lymphocytic leukemia using cytosine arabinoside and doxorubicin or daunorubicin: a report from the Childrens' Cancer Study Group. *Medical and Pediatric Oncology*, **17**, 382–390.

185 Creutzig U., Ritter J. & Schellong G. (1990) Identification of two risk groups in childhood acute myelogenous leukemia after therapy intensification in study AML-BFM-83 as compared with study AML-BFM-78. *Blood*, **75**, 1932–1940.

186 Creutzig U., Ritter J., Zimmerman M. *et al.* (1993) Does cranial irradiation reduce the risk for bone marrow relapse in acute myelogenous leukemia? Unexpected results of the Childhood Actue Myelogenous Leukemia Study BFM-87. *Journal of Clinical Oncology*, **11**, 279–286.

187 Woods W.G., Raymann F.B., Lampkin B.C. *et al.* (1990) The role of timing of high dose cytosine arabinoside intensification and of maintenance therapy in the treatment of children with acute nonlymphocytic leukemia. *Cancer*, **66**, 1106–1113.

188 Woods W.G., Kobrinsky N., Buckley S. *et al.* (1993) Intensively timed induction therapy followed by autologous or allogeneic bone marrow transplantation for children with acute myeloid

leukemia or myelodysplastic syndrome: a Children's Cancer Group pilot study. *Journal of Clinical Oncology*, **11**, 1448–1457.

189 Steuber C.P., Civin C., Raymann F. *et al.* (1991) Therapy of childhood acute nonlymphocytic leukemia: a Pediatric Oncology Group Study (POG 8101). *Journal of Clinical Oncology*, **9**, 247–258.

190 Ravindranath Y., Steuber C.P., Krischer J.P. *et al.* (1991) High dose cytosine arabinoside for intensification of early therapy in childhood acute myeloid leukemia: a Pediatric Oncology Group Study. *Journal of Clinical Oncology*, **9**, 572–580.

191 Amadori S., Testi A.M., Arico M. *et al.* (1993) Prospective comparative study of bone marow transplantation and post-remission chemotherapy for childhood acute myelogenous leukemia. *Journal of Clinical Oncology*, **11**, 1046–1054.

192 Nesbit M.E., Buckley J.D., Feig S.A. *et al.* (1994) Chemotherapy for induction of remission of childhood acute myeloid leukemia followed by marrow transplantation or multiagent chemotherapy: a report from the Children's Cancer Group. *Journal of Clinical Oncology*, **12**, 127–135.

193 Ritter J., Creutzig U., Schellong G. *et al.* (1992) Treatment results of three consecutive German AML trials. *Leukemia*, **6**(Suppl. 2), 59–62.

194 Grier H.E., Gelber R.D., Link M.P. *et al.* (1992) Intensive sequential chemotherapy for children with acute myelogenous leukemia: VAPA 80-035 and HI-C-Daze. *Leukemia*, **6**(Suppl 2), 48–51.

195 Drapkin R.L., Gee T.S., Dowling M.D. *et al.* (1978) Prophylactic heparin therapy in acute promyelocytic leukemia. *Cancer*, **41**, 2484–2490.

196 Rodeghiero R., Arvisati G., Castaman G. *et al.* (1990) Early deaths and anti-hemorrhagic treatments in acute promyelocytic leukemia. A GIMEMA retrospective study in 268 consecutive patients. *Blood*, **75**, 2112–2117.

197 Arlin Z., Kempin S., Mertelsmann R. *et al.* (1984) Primary therapy of acute promyelocytic leukemia: results of amsacrine and daunorubicin-based therapy. *Blood*, **63**, 211–212.

198 Kantarjian H.M., Keating M.J., Walters R.S. *et al.* (1987) Acute promyelocytic leukemia: the M.D. Anderson Hospital experience. *American Journal of Medicine*, **80**, 879–884.

199 Kantarjian H.M., Keating M.J., Walters R.S. *et al.* (1987) Role of maintenance chemotherapy in acute promyelocytic leukemia. *Cancer*, **59**, 1258–1263.

200 Huang M., Yu-Chen Y., Shu-Rong C. *et al.* (1988) Use of all-*trans* retinoic acid in the treatment of acute promyelocytic leukemia. *Blood*, **72**, 567–572.

201 Degos L., Chomienne C., Daniel M.T. *et al.* (1990) Treatment of first relapse in acute promyelocytic leukaemia with all-*trans* retinoic acid. *Lancet*, **336**, 1440–1441.

202 Castaigne S., Chomienne C., Daniel M.T. *et al.* (1990) All-*trans* retinoic acid as a differentiating therapy for acute promyelocytic leukemias. 1. Clinical results. *Blood*, **76**, 1704–1717.

203 Warrell R.P., Frankel S.R., Miller W. *et al.* (1991) Differentiation therapy of acute promyelocytic leukemia with tretinoin (all-*trans* retinoic acid). *New England Journal of Medicine*, **324**, 1385–1393.

204 Chen Z.X., Xue Y.Q., Zhang R. *et al.* (1991) A clinical and experimental study on all-*trans* retinoic acid treatment acute promyelocytic leukemia patients. *Blood*, **78**, 1413–1419.

205 Fenaux P., Castaigne S., Chomienne C. *et al.* (1992) All-*trans* retinoic acid treatment for patients with acute promyelocytic leukemia. *Leukemia*, **6**, 64–66.

206 Frankel S.R., Eardley A., Lauwers G. *et al.* (1992) The 'retinoic acid syndrome' in acute promyelocytic leukemia. *Annals of Internal Medicine*, **117**, 292–296.

207 Fenaux P., Castaigne S., Dombret H. *et al.* (1992) All-*trans* retinoic acid followed by intensive chemotherapy gives a high complete remission rate and may prolong remissions in newly diagnosed acute promyelocytic leukemia. *Blood*, **80**, 2176–2181.

208 Ohashi H., Ichikawa A., Takagi N. *et al.* (1992) Remission induction of acute promyelocytic leukemia by all-*trans* retinoic acid: molecular evidence of restoration of normal hematopoiesis after differentiation and subsequent extinction of leukemic clone. *Leukemia*, **6**, 859–862.

209 Degos L., Dombret H., Chomienne C. *et al.* (1995) All-*trans* retinoic acid as a differentiating agent in the treatment of acute promyelocytic leukemia. *Blood*, **85**, 2643–2653.

210 Warrell R.P., Maslak P., Eardley A. *et al.* (1994) Treatment of acute promyelocytic leukemia with all-*trans* retinoic acid: an update of the New York experience. *Leukemia*, **8**, 926–933.

211 Kanamaru A., Takemoto Y., Tanimoto M. *et al.* (1995) All-*trans* retinoic acid for the treatment of newly diagnosed acute promyelocytic leukemia. *Blood*, **85**, 1202–1206.

212 Sun G., Ouyang R., Cher S. *et al.* (1994) Follow up of 481 patients with APL after CR using ATRA. *Chinese Journal of Hematology*, **15**, 411–413.

213 Fenaux P., Le Deley M.C., Castaigne S. *et al.* (1993) Effect of all-*trans* retinoic acid in newly diagnosed acute promyelocytic leukemia. Results of a multi center randomized trial. *Blood*, **82**, 3241–3249.

214 Fenaux P., Wattle E., Archimbaud E. *et al.* (1994) Prolonged follow-up confirms that all-*trans* retinoic acid (ATRA) followed by chemotherapy reduces the risk of relapse in newly diagnosed acute promyelocytic leukemia (APL). *Blood*, **84**, 666–667.

215 Frankel S.R., Eardley A., Heller G. *et al.* (1994) All-*trans* retinoic acid for acute promyelocytic leukemia. Results of the New York Study. *Annals of Internal Medicine*, **120**, 279–286.

216 Ohno R., Yoshida H. & Fukutani H. (1993) Multi institutional study of all-*trans* retinoic acid as a differentiation therapy of refractory acute promyelocytic leukemia. *Leukemia*, **7**, 1722–1727.

217 Wiley J.S. & Firkin F.C. (1995) Reduction of pulmonary toxicity by prednisolone prophylaxis during all-*trans* retinoic acid treatment of acute promyelocytic leukemia. *Leukemia*, **9**, 774–778.

218 Dombret H., Scrobohaci M.L., Ghorra P. *et al.* (1993) Coagulation disorders associated with acute promyelocytic leukemia: corrective effect of all-*trans* retinoic acid treatment. *Leukemia*, **7**, 2–9.

219 Tapiovaara H., Matikainen S., Hurme M. *et al.* (1994) Induction of differentiation of promyelocytic NB4 cells by retinoic acid is associated with rapid increase in urokinase activity subsequently down regulated by production of inhibitors. *Blood*, **83**, 1883–1891.

220 Hashimoto S., Koike T., Tatewaki W. *et al.* (1994) Fatal thromboembolism in acute promyelocytic leukemia during all-*trans* retinoic acid therapy combined with antifibrinolytic therapy for prophylaxis of hemorrhage. *Leukemia*, **8**, 1113–1115.

221 Clift R.A., Buckner C.D., Appelbaum F.R. *et al.* (1992) Allogenic marrow transplantation during untreated first relapse of acute myeloid leukemia. *Journal of Clinical Oncology*, **10**, 1723–1729.

222 Blume K.G., Kopecky K.J., Henslee-Downey J.P. *et al.* (1993) A prospective randomized comparison of total body irradiation/ etoposide versus busulfan-cyclophosphamide as preparatory

regimens for bone marrow transplantation in patients with leukemia who were not in first remission: a Southwest Oncology Group Study. *Blood*, **81**, 2187–2193.

223 Biggs J.C., Horowitz M.M., Gale R.P. *et al.* (1992) Bone marrow transplants may cure patients with acute leukemia never achieving remission with chemotherapy. *Blood*, **80**, 1090–1093.

224 Appelbaum F.R. (1997) The use of bone marrow and peripheral blood stem cell transplantation in the treatment of cancer. *Cancer Journal for Clinicians*. (In press.)

225 Yeager A.M., Kaizer H., Santos G.W. *et al.* (1986) Autologous bone marrow transplantation in patients with acute non-lymphocytic leukemia, using *ex vivo* marrow treatment with 4-hydroperoxycyclophosphamide. *New England Journal of Medicine*, **323**, 260–262.

226 Chopra R., Goldstone A.H., McMillan K.K. *et al.* (1991) Successful treatment of acute myeloid leukemia beyond first remission with autologous bone marrow transplantation using busulphan/cyclophosphamide and unpurged marrow. The British Autograft Group Experience. *Journal of Clinical Oncology*, **9**, 1840–1847.

227 Zittoun R.A., Mandelli F., Willeinze R. *et al.* (1995) Autologous or allogeneic bone marrow transplantation compared with intensive chemotherapy in acute myelogenous leukemia. *New England Journal of Medicine*, **332**, 217–223.

10 Acute Myeloid Leukaemia: Recent Clinical Trial Data and Future Prospects

L.G. Robinson and A.K. Burnett

Introduction

A number of factors over the past 20 years have contributed to an improved outcome for patients with acute myeloid leukaemia (AML). The linchpins of chemotherapy have always been an anthracycline and a cytosine arabinoside (ara-C), so any improvements which have been seen must be attributed to other aspects of care such as:

1 an improvement in blood product support;
2 better antibiotic, antifungal and antiviral agents;
3 an improved understanding of how and when to use antimicrobials;
4 improved technique of venous access;
5 the development of specialist teams for dealing with the different aspects of care.

Only some of these improvements have been validated in randomized trials, and adopted as a result; however, the evolution of improved antimicrobial agents has generally been a product of many large phase III studies.

It is now clearly recognized that AML is a heterogeneous disease with a variable response to chemotherapy, and while it is permissible to claim therapeutic progress as measured by increased remission rates and, in younger patients, a better chance of long-term survival, these improvements have only emphasized the variability of response between patients with this disease. This is most marked when age is considered, but there are several other robust prognostic indicators which may lead to future therapeutic progress based on individualization of treatment to suit particular prognostic subgroups.

In recent years considerable international effort has been devoted to a few questions related to the treatment of AML involving prospective randomized trials. The hope has been to clearly determine the benefit of a particular therapeutic option. Sometimes such large trials produce greater uncertainty, because once other variables are properly controlled for, the expected benefit becomes difficult to demonstrate with statistical confidence. Similarly when studies do show benefit,

it is because a control arm has done less well than would have been expected, or perhaps general progress in the field has been capable of producing equally as good results but by using a different approach.

This chapter examines some of the recent randomized trial activity which has addressed some key areas in AML treatment:

1 the role of growth factors;
2 whether there are better alternatives to daunorubicin in induction therapy;
3 the role of autologous bone marrow transplantation;
4 the role of high-dose ara-C in the consolidation phase.

Haemopoietic growth factors

The role of the myeloid haemopoietic growth factors (granulocyte colony-stimulating factor (G-CSF), granulocyte-macrophage CSF (GM-CSF) in the treatment of patients with AML remains controversial, despite several studies that have examined their safety and efficacy.

Although there seems to be clear evidence that they reduce the period of neutropenia in AML patients receiving cytotoxic chemotherapy and following bone marrow transplant, this has yet to be translated into a statistically significant reduction in infection rates, infection-related mortality, improved complete remission rates or overall survival. Indeed, some studies suggest the converse is true and have raised issues about their safety. However, despite *in vitro* data suggesting a distinct pharmacological action leading to potentiation of the action of conventional cytotoxic agents, there is little to suggest that growth factors promote leukaemic proliferation in the patient.

Interpretation of the results of these studies, however, is difficult because of multiple factors, including: the misleading reporting of probability values; a lack of use of appropriate confidence limits; the variation in supportive care practice; the heterogeneity of patients and treatment regimens, and the timing, duration and dose of the growth factor used.

Biology of growth factors

Haemopoietic growth factors are glycoprotein hormones that regulate the differentiation and proliferation of haemopoietic progenitor cells and the function of mature blood cells by actions at multiple levels [1–3]. Since their discovery in the 1960s, they have now been cloned and purified and are produced by recombinant DNA techniques, making them readily available for clinical use.

Each is encoded for by a different gene, with that for GM-CSF lying on chromosome 5 [4] and that for G-CSF on chromosome 17 [5]. The biological effects are mediated through specific binding to a low number of high-affinity receptors on the surface of target cells [6,7]. Disturbingly, receptors have been detected on myeloid leukaemic cells [8–10] in addition to normal haemopoietic cells and nonhaemopoietic cells [11–13].

The actions of these growth factors include:

1 The regulation of progenitor cell growth and differentiation.
2 The regulation of the function of mature blood cells.
3 The stimulation of the proliferation of leukaemic cells *in vitro* with terminal differentiation and growth arrest.
4 The stimulation of the growth of nonhaemopoietic cells, e.g. fibroblasts, endothelial cells.

Mechanisms of action of growth factors

Growth factors may play a role in both the treatment and supportive care of patients with AML. Numerous possible mechanisms of action have been described, and these may depend on not only the particular factor used but also the dose and timing of administration. These mechanisms of action include.

1 The recruitment of leukaemic cells from the G_0 to S phase, which gives a superior efficacy of cytotoxics, e.g. ara-C [14]. A higher proportion of cells in S phase has been confirmed in some studies following growth-factor priming. This mechanism is also the basis for time-sequential regimens such as

fludarabine, ara-C and G-CSF (FLAG), which show promising results in the treatment of relapsed or refractory disease. Other studies, however, have failed to confirm this finding [15], perhaps casting some doubt on this as the primary mechanism of action.

2 The ability to overcome the defective cellular maturation seen in AML aiming to decrease and deplete the self-renewal potential of the malignant clone (differentiation therapy).

3 The alteration of intracellular drug metabolism [16]. Increased incorporation of ara-C into DNA (1.5–8.5-fold) has been seen in patients studied due to an increased activation of DNA polymerase α. This leads to a mean threefold increase in ara-C toxicity over that of patients not treated with growth factors.

4 An effect on drug-induced damage and DNA repair mechanisms [17,18].

5 An alteration in the ara-cCTP/cCTP ratio.

It seems likely that multiple mechanisms are involved which may be synergistic.

Efficacy of growth factors

At least 10 randomized studies (Table 10.1) examining the efficacy of growth-factor use in AML have been published [19–28]. Many of these have been in elderly subjects, which is probably appropriate because the aim is to reduce deaths during induction, which is a substantially greater problem in older patients. These trials have used variable doses and dosing schedules, and both G-CSF and GM-CSF have been examined. The end points include: neutrophil recovery, infection rates, febrile episodes, complete remission (CR) rates, remission duration and overall survival.

All agree that, with growth-factor support with G-CSF or GM-CSF before, during or after chemotherapy, the period of neutropenia (recovery to counts >0.5–1.0 × 10⁹/l) is reduced by approximately 7 days with no significant effect on platelet recovery. Despite the well-known correlation between the

Table 10.1 Effect of use of growth factors (G-CSF/GM-CSF) in patients with AML undergoing chemotherapy.

Study	CSF	No. of patients	Effect on neutrophil recovery	Effect on infection rate	Effect on CR rate	Effect on remission duration	Effect on survival
Estey *et al.* 1990 [19]	GM	65	NS	NS	NS	—	—
Buchner *et al.* 1991 [20]	GM	92	Increased	NS	NS	NS	—
Rowe *et al.* 1993 [21]	GM	118	Increased	Decreased	NS	—	Increased
Estey *et al.* 1992 [22]	GM	232	Increased	—	Decreased	NS	Decreased
Archimbaud *et al.* 1993 [23]	GM	58	NS	—	NS	NS	NS
Bettellheim *et al.* 1991 [24]	GM	57	Increased	—	—	—	—
Buchner *et al.* 1993 [25]	GM	63	Increased	—	NS	Increased	—
Ohno *et al.* 1990 [26]	G	61	Increased	Decreased	NS	NS	—
Ohno *et al.* 1994 [27]	G	58	Increased	NS	NS	NS	NS
Estey *et al.* 1994 [28]	G	197	Increased	NS	NS	—	NS

NS = nonsignificant difference (*P* > 0.05).

duration of neutropenia and the risk of infection, this accelerated rate of neutrophil recovery has not consistently translated into statistically significant reductions in infection rates or incidence of fatal infections. Two studies do report this finding [21,26], one using G-CSF and the other GM-CSF, but the other studies do not confirm this. Again there is also no consistent pattern of reduction in antibiotic usage or hospital stay.

Despite the pharmacological synergism with ara-C, no studies have found an improved CR rate and only the ECOG study demonstrated improved survival [21]. One study, in which GM-CSF was administered before and during chemotherapy to newly diagnosed cases of AML, reported a reduction in CR and survival rate [22]. Alterations in CR rates and survival may reflect both effects on fatal infections, numbers of leukaemia blasts and their sensitivity to chemotherapy.

Perhaps the least ambiguous test of the sensitization strategy is remission duration. This has been infrequently studied, with only one study reporting an improvement [20], but notably with only a short follow-up period.

In spite of the fact that these studies have involved nearly 1000 randomized patients, no clear benefit has emerged. This, however, could reflect the heterogeneous study design and the probability that these studies have not been large enough.

Safety of growth factors

Although there has been concern over the safety of these agents because they have been shown to stimulate the growth of leukaemic cells *in vitro* [29–31], regrowth of leukaemia secondary to growth-factor administration has not emerged as a clinical problem. The nonhaematological toxicity is negligible. There has been a recent report associating use with AML/MDS in patients with aplastic anaemia [32], although as the numbers are small and this is a known complication of the disease process under treatment, the significance is questionable.

In conclusion, although myeloid growth factors offer a theoretical advantage in both the treatment and supportive care of patients with AML, the currently available literature does not support their routine use. Thrombocytopenia remains a significant clinical problem. A placebo-controlled trial of IL-6 has been completed but is not yet published and studies on the recently cloned thrombopoietic growth factors in AML are awaited with interest.

Anthracyclines in treatment

The anthracycline daunorubicin has formed the backbone of induction chemotherapy in AML. Over the years a number of studies have addressed the question what the most appropriate dose should be. Certainly for younger patients 45 mg/m² has been shown to be superior to 30 mg/m² [33].

There is probably no particular advantage in further dose escalation. In older patients the benefits of a higher dose may be less clear.

In recent years a newer anthracycline, idarubicin, and an anthracenedione, mitoxantrone, have both been directly compared with daunorubicin in induction schedules in a number of studies with some fairly clear answers.

Daunorubicin vs idarubicin

Six randomized trials have now compared two different anthracyclines, daunorubicin vs idarubicin, in otherwise standard protocols (Table 10.2) [34–39]. Idarubicin (4' demethoxydaunorubicin), by virtue of its more lipophilic properties, is taken up more rapidly into cells and indeed may be less susceptible to the effects of drug efflux—regulated by the product of the *MDR* gene. It induces more DNA single-strand breaks and has a more prolonged plasma half-life. Five of these studies have shown a significantly higher CR rate in the idarubicin arm with similar toxicity, providing a substantial body of evidence to support the superiority of the new agent. Some caution is still required, because in some studies the results of the control arm are inferior to what is regularly achieved in large multicentre contemporary trials using conventional schedules. There is also concern about the equivalence of dose between the arms.

Daunorubicin vs mitoxantrone

Mitoxantrone, an anthracenedione, has been proposed as an alternative agent to the anthracyclines with less toxicity, particularly cardiac. Four studies [40–43] have compared its efficacy and safety to that of daunorubicin, with only one

Table 10.2 Comparison of the use of idarubicin (I) and daunorubicin (D) in the treatment of AML.

Study	No. of patients	Effect on CR rate I vs D	Effect on survival	Effect on response duration
Gonzalez-Llaven et al. 1991 [34]	62	60 vs 42%, P value not given	—	—
Reiffers et al. 1988 [35]	64	70 vs 73%, NS	—	—
Vogler et al. 1992 [36]	230	71 vs 58%, P = 0.003	NS	NS
Mandelli et al. 1991 [38]	255	40 vs 39%, NS	NS	NS
Berman et al. 1992 [39]	130	80 vs 58%, P = 0.05	I > D	—
Wiernik et al. 1992 [37]	214	70 vs 59%, P = 0.035	I > D	I > D

Table 10.3 Comparison of the use of mitozantrone (M) and daunorubicin (D) in the treatment of AML.

Study	No. of patients	Effect on CR rate M vs D	Effect on survival	Effect on mortality
Johnson *et al.* 1990 [40]	88	64.4 vs 61.9%, NS	NS	NS
Arlin *et al.* 1990 [41]	216	63 vs 53%, NS (*P* = 0.15)	NS	—
Wahlin *et al.* 1991 [42]	44	67 vs 70%, NS	NS	NS
Lowenberg *et al.* 1991 [43]	488	52.5 vs 37.6%, *P* = 0.002	NS	NS

reporting a favourable advantage in terms of a significantly increased CR rate but with no improvement in overall survival rate (Table 10.3). Interestingly, toxicity profiles for the 2 days were comparable with no proven reduction in cardiac toxicity, which was expected.

Initially, there appears to be stronger evidence to substitute idarubicin for daunorubicin rather than mitoxantrone. The weight of evidence for mitoxantrone is less convincing, but there is certainly some evidence to suggest superiority. Studies to directly compare mitoxantrone and idarubicin are currently underway and from the studies presented, it should not be presumed, that one is superior to another. These trials were recently subjected to data overview analysis from a comprehensive dataset, which confirmed that there were advantages for both drugs over daunorubicin, but studies between idarubicin and mitoxantrone were not available [44].

Autologous bone marrow transplantation

Many patients have been treated with high-dose therapy and autologous bone marrow transplantation (ABMT) since the introduction of this approach for relapsed disease in the late 1970s by the Houston Group [45]. The several hundred cases recorded in the registries of the European Group for Bone Marrow Transplantation (EBMT) and Autologous Bone Marrow Transplant Registry (ABMTR) merely reflect a proportion of this activity. The initial single-institution studies were very encouraging at the time as a viable alternative for patients who lacked sibling donors and therefore could not be offered allogeneic BMT, which was then considered optimal for all patients in first remission. ABMT offered a relatively low procedural mortality and morbidity and therefore could be an option for patients up to 50 or 60 years of age, which represents a substantial proportion of patients with AML who enter remission [46–50]. Another feature of these early studies was that relapse after 2 years was a relatively unusual occurrence, and in that respect the pattern of relapse was more akin to that seen after allogeneic BMT than that seen with contemporary chemotherapy where plateaus of relapse-free survival were

not usually apparent. Protracted haemopoietic recovery, particularly thrombocytopenia, was common and seemed much more frequent in AML than in other diseases where more prior chemotherapy had often been given before the autograft [51].

It was clear that the development of ABMT as a 'last-ditch' effort to salvage patients who had relapsed and failed reinduction treatment was only of temporary benefit if any. Many studies were therefore undertaken in first remission and produced 5-year survivals of 45–55%, from which many patients are now in continued complete remission (CCR) 10–15 years later. For many this represented sufficient evidence to adopt ABMT as standard care, but there were some reservations which stimulated a number of major trial groups to conduct proper prospective randomized trials, some of which have now been reported.

These trials have only addressed a small proportion of the issues relevant to the role of ABMT in AML, but nevertheless have been a valuable experience from which to move on. Among the doubts raised about the single-arm studies was the degree of unconscious case selection which took place. In contemporary survival curves of the time a substantial proportion of (perhaps 25%) patients relapsed in the first 6 months. Such patients would often have been excluded from transplanted populations, who tended to receive the treatment at about 4–6 months into remission. This effect was well illustrated by time-censoring studies, which suggest that the outlook for patients who survived to 6 months was around 40%; this may not have been much less successful than transplant outcomes [52]. The proportion of patients who were not offered autologous BMT because, although in remission, were in some other respect not considered fit, was not known.

Prospective randomized trials

Nine prospective randomized trials have been reported [53–56], with the results of others pending. They have a broadly similar aim — to evaluate the role of ABMT in first remission — but there are important differences in design and therefore the nature of the question asked. In all cases, trial entrants who are found to have an HLA-compatible sibling are expected to receive allogeneic BMT. With careful statistical analysis these data can delineate the impact of allogeneic BMT in the context of contemporary alternatives. In most but not all studies the recipients of allografts appeared to have a better prospect of survival; however, in most cases this was based on a superficial analysis.

Two study groups (MRC and HOVON) compared the addition of autograft to no further treatment — all patients had received respectable consolidation treatment. The MRC Trial was unique in that more chemotherapy was given (four courses) before the ABMT [60]. These study protocols are depicted in schema A in Fig. 10.1. The results of the HOVON study have not been published. The majority of trials

Table 10.4 Randomized studies of autograft in AML.

Study group	No. of patients randomized	Purged marrow	Autograft vs chemotherapy	Autograft vs no further treatment	Adults (A) Children (C)	Effect of autograft Relapse risk	Effect of autograft Overall survival
BGMT-84 [53]	35	–	+		A	↓	↓
BGMT-87 [54]	77	–	+		A	↓	NS
EORCT/GIMEMA [55]	254	–	+		A	↓	NS
GOELAM [56]	151	–	+		A	↓	NS
AIEOP [57]	72		+		C	No	NS
POG [58]	232	+	+		C	↓	NS
CCSG [59]	412		+		C	No	NS
MRC 10 [60]	381	–		+	100C	↓	↑NS*
HOVON 4	124	–		+	A	NK	NK

* Significant in 2-year survivors.
NK = not known.

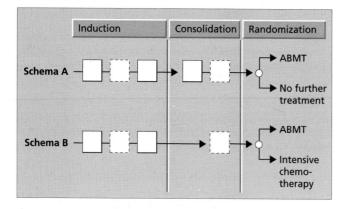

Fig. 10.1 Design of prospective studies of autograft in AML.

compared ABMT to some form of further chemotherapy, usually following only one consolidation chemotherapy course. These would follow schema B in Fig. 10.1. There are other important differences between protocols, the most important of which is the age profile of the study population. The MRC, CCSG, POG and AIEOP groups have all conducted studies in children (Table 10.4). This becomes a relevant factor when one tries to form an overall impression of effect from all trials, because of the 1728 patients involved in these nine trials, over 800 were children.

Other differences between study designs are probably less crucial. *In vitro* purging of the autograft was not attempted in the MRC, HOVON, EORTC, BGMT or GOELAM Trials. In general either cyclophosphamide and total body irradiation or busulphan/cyclophosphamide was used as myeloablative treatment. These studies were initiated before peripheral stem cell transplantation became the preferred source of haemopoietic stem cells.

In total these studies have randomized in excess of 1700 patients and uncovered some broadly similar experiences

about the logistics of trials of this design. Only 30–40% of patients in remission who could have been randomized were so, which was of considerable relevance to the original question. This was not, as might have been anticipated, exclusively a result of early relapse, but of failure of the patient or physician to accept randomization. This may often be because of the toxicity of the preceding chemotherapy. A smaller proportion of patients or physicians elected to have the ABMT. It is remarkable that there seems to be little correlation between the proportion of patients randomized and the amount of prior chemotherapy. This failure to randomize 60–70% of available patients is not only statistically inefficient but also modifies what question is actually being asked, and whether the data obtained from this selected group can be reasonably extrapolated to all patients with AML who enter remission.

A major consideration in interpretation is that it is now well established that there is considerable interpatient variation in risk of relapse, and therefore, if possible, account should be taken of the risk profile of patient groups when interpreting treatment effect. At present it is not possible to segregate patients in most of these trials in this way. However, patient age is one of these factors and it is possible to view these trials in the context of whether they have been conducted partially or exclusively in children (e.g. CCSG, POG, AEIOP, MRC). Given that the outcome of chemotherapy alone for children is better than for older patients, it is conceivable that it is more difficult to demonstrate a benefit for BMT in this age group than in older patients where the relapse risk is higher.

Despite these differences in detail a number of general observations can be made about these trials. Only a minority of patients who were eligible for randomization were randomized, and even then there was variable compliance with the allocated treatment. It is clear that the outcome for those who received an autograft did at least as well as patients in the original single-arm studies. The procedural mortality has varied between trials but was 15% in the POG trial in children compared with 6.5% in the GEOLAM Trial. It is noticeable that, with the possible exception of the BGMT 87 and the EORTC Trials, the chemotherapy arms have shown evidence of improvement compared with what was expected in the early and mid 1980s. Therefore, although it appears that ABMT has more than fulfilled the potential it demonstrated in the early 1980s, chemotherapy — particularly in children — has also improved. This makes it much more difficult to demonstrate benefit. In spite of this, and even in the MRC Trial where the chemotherapy arm was arguably the most intensive, it is still possible to clearly demonstrate a reduced risk of relapse in the ABMT arm of most trials. This has not yet converted to an overall survival advantage. Its potential is partly inhibited by procedural mortality, but also by a superior probability of survival from relapse in the chemotherapy arm — as most clearly demonstrated in the EORTC Trial. These effects may also be related to age. For example, the EORTC Study was limited to adults. The results of the chemotherapy were poorer than those normally seen even in that age group in contemporary studies; however, a proportion of such patients appeared to be salvageable when they relapsed. In contrast, the MRC trial in this age group resulted in a satisfactory survival in the chemotherapy patients but an unfortunately high procedural-related mortality in the autograft arm, and there was no difference in survival between those who relapsed from chemotherapy or ABMT. In the younger patients in the MRC Study the failure to demonstrate an overall difference was not because of an excess of deaths in the ABMT arm, but resulted from an increased salvage after relapse after chemotherapy even although the relapse risk was already 50%.

ABMT clearly offers a reduced risk of relapse on these intentions to treat analysis, even in subgroups considered to have favourable prognoses. It should be remembered that several patients in such analyses may not have received the ABMT (35% in the MRC Trial). It is associated with an important procedural mortality which requires to be substantially reduced before the superior antileukaemic effect produces clinical benefit. There are also subgroups of patients (e.g. children) who appear to be more amenable to salvage therapy after relapse and in whom the overall benefit is therefore not apparent. In such circumstances the immediate and late toxic effects become the dominant consideration and this has reduced the value of ABMT as part of first-line management in children.

Several other issues regarding ABMT could be resolved in randomized trials which to date have not been attempted. The most significant of these might be to establish what contribution the elective use of delaying the transplant either until second remission — as in the design of the MRC Trial — or as primary treatment of relapse. Both appear to be valid options which need to be formally tested, but it is not clear which treatment modality is best in second remission. Such studies will have a high level of patient fall-out, requiring major international collaboration and huge numbers of patients, and therefore may never be carried out. A second unresolved issue

is whether purging of the bone marrow (or stem cells) is helpful. Registry data might suggest that a viable trial could be mounted in patients either who entered initial remission late (e.g. requiring more than one course) or whose treatment plan deliberately uses ABMT early in remission [61], since these are the subgroups who appear to benefit most from purging.

Cytosine arabinoside treatment

Cytosine arabinoside (ara-C) has been a key drug in the treatment of AML for over 30 years, both in the induction and the consolidation phases. The dosing schedule has varied substantially and several randomized trials of different schedules were conducted a number of years ago. Higher dose treatments of up to $3.0\,g/m^2$ over 6 days have been used over the years but formal comparisons of higher dosing schedules have been infrequent. There has long been a view that high-dose [62] ara-C used as consolidation could achieve results equivalent to BMT.

The most important recent prospective trial has been carried out by the CALGB, where three ara-C doses were compared [63]. Doses of $100\,mg/m^2$/day by continuous infusion for 5 days or $400\,mg/m^2$/day for 5 days by continuous infusion or $3.0\,g/m^2$ b.d. by 3-hour infusion on days 1, 3 and 5 were allocated for a total of four courses. In practice it was difficult for all courses to be given as intended. However this study established that the highest dose was the most effective in younger patients (<60 years), but was too toxic in older patients.

Neurotoxicity occurred in older patients, for which an elevated serum creatinine and alkaline phosphatase were associated risk factors [64]. The direct comparison between the three dose schedules showed respective disease-free survivals of 21, 25 and 39% in the 100 mg, 400 mg and 3.0 g study arms; however, there was a higher relative proportion of younger patients in the 3.0 g arm, which may have slightly exaggerated the benefit. In patients under 60 who received the high-dose arm the prospect of disease-free survival was 44% and survival was 52%, suggesting that this approach may be an equivalent option to BMT. This poses the question what is the best consolidation in younger patients.

Major trial groups have invested considerable effort in recent years in attempting to answer this question. In patients under 60 years an overall conclusion can be drawn that more intensive treatment is better. In the case of transplantation, however, such a benefit is inhibited because of procedure-related mortality. It is also apparent that some patients — predominantly children with good risk disease — can be salvaged if they relapse. Interestingly, the trend over recent years to intensify treatment has not modified the longstanding observation that the major determinants of successful reinduction therapy are the duration of first remission and the age of the patient. It is generally assumed that transplantation is the best treatment of second remission, but this has not been formally tested in a prospective trial, and a retrospective comparison suggests that only younger patients with first-remission durations of more than 1 year, and older patients with first complete remission (CR) of less than 1 year, had significantly superior survivals following allogeneic BMT [65].

While it can reasonably be concluded that more initial treatment will reduce relapse risk, it is not clear by how much. The MRC Trial gave four intensive courses of chemotherapy, which produced a survival from diagnosis of 40% at 6 years. However, even in that context, autograft was able to reduce the relapse risk by a further 20%. The reduction in relapse risk was seen in patients of all risk groups. The issue now, therefore, is whether a fifth course can provide additional benefit without the additional toxicity associated with BMT.

Future clinical trials

Important improvements in the outcome for younger patients with AML have been achieved in the last decade. Remission rates are high and the risk of relapse has been reduced somewhat. Randomized trials have contributed much to this progress, although there are probably several effective remission induction schedules and a long follow-up is still required to ascertain if ABMT is beneficial. It is now very clear that the risk categorization of the patient based on a number of parameters—principally cytogenetics [66]—needs to be taken into account when deciding which is the best therapeutic option. Allocating treatment options to the different risk groups will become the norm.

The major therapeutic challenges are in the older patient groups, which comprise the majority of those with the disease. There are probably at least two categories of patients in this age group. The first category is those considered fit for conventional treatment and for whom information on clinical outcomes is available from clinical trials. However, a substantial additional proportion of patients, the second category, are not considered fit for intensive chemotherapy and receive nonprotocol, somewhat less toxic, treatment. Both approaches may be appropriate. For various reasons related to the biology of older patients and the disease in the elderly, primary drug resistance is a major problem. This may now be amenable to modulation. Of particular interest will be the imminent randomized trials of PSC-833 (Novartis), which is a cyclosporin analogue without the immunosuppressive or nephrotoxic effects [67]. *In vitro* evidence confirms that the concentrations required to modulate the *MDR* mechanism are achievable clinically without excessive toxicity. Whether such modulation should be limited only to remission induction treatment is a mute point. Prognostic factors may identify a small number of elderly (>60 years) patients who benefit from intensive chemotherapy—but it appears that for the majority there is a limited future for the strategy for dose escalation. A better understanding of the disease in this age group may lead to more effective treatment, such as facilitating differentiation or inducing cell death by activation of apoptotic mechanisms. In these patients improving survival will be more difficult and delivering treatment which is compatible with a good quality of life is the therapeutic goal.

References

1 Metcalf D. (1985) The granulocyte-macrophage colony stimulating factors. *Science*, **229**, 16–22.
2 Clark S.C. & Kamen R. (1987) The human haemopoietic colony-stimulating factors. *Science*, **236**, 1229–1237.
3 Sieff C.A. (1987) Haemopoietic growth factors. *Journal of Clinical Investigation*, **79**, 1549–1557.
4 Wong G.G., Witek J.S., Temple P.A. *et al.* (1985) Purified human granulocyte-macrophage colony stimulating factor: direct action on neutrophils. *Science*, **225**, 810–815.
5 Simmers R.N., Webber L.M., Shannon M.F. *et al.* (1987) Localisation of the G-CSF gene on chromosome 17 proximal to the breakpoint in the t(15:17) in acute promyelocytic leukaemia. *Blood*, **70**, 330–332.
6 Sherr C.J., Rettenmeir C.W., Sacca R. *et al.* (1985) The c-*fms* proto-oncogene product is related to the receptor for the mononuclear phagocyte growth factor CSF-1. *Cell*, **41**, 665–676.
7 Park L.S., Freid D., Gillis S. & Urdal D.L. (1986) Characterisation of the cell surface for human granulocyte/macrophage colony-stimulating factor. *Journal of Experimental Medicine*, **164**, 251–262.
8 Gasson J.C., Kaufman S.E., Weisbart R.H., Tomonaga M. & Golde P.W. (1986) High affinity binding of granulocyte-macrophage colony-stimulating factor to normal and leukaemia human myeloid cells. *Proceedings of the National Academy of Sciences, USA*, **83**, 669–673.
9 Nicola N.A., Beyley C.G. & Metcalf D. (1985) Identification of the human analogue of a regulator that induces differentiation in murine leukemic cells. *Nature*, **314**, 625–628.
10 Souza L.M., Boore T.C., Gabrilove J. *et al.* (1986) Recombinant human granulocyte colony stimulating factor: effects on normal and leukaemic myeloid cells. *Science* **232**, 61–65.
11 Rettemeir C.W., Sacca R., Furman W.L. *et al.* (1986) Expression of the human c-*fms* proto-oncogene product (colony stimulating factor-1 receptor) on peripheral blood mononuclear cells and choriocarcinoma cell line. *Journal of Clinical Investigation*, **77**, 1740–1746.
12 Pollard J.W., Bartocci A., Arecci R., Orlofsky A., Ladner M.B. & Stanley E.R. (1987) Apparent role of the macrophage growth factor CSF-1 in placental development. *Nature*, **330**, 484–486.
13 Baldwin G.C., Gasson J.C., Kaufman S.E. *et al.* (1989) Non haemopoietic tumor cells express functional GM-CSF receptors. *Blood*, **73**, 1033–1037.
14 Tafuri A. & Andreeff M. (1990) Kinetic rationale for cytokine induced recruitment of myeloblastic leukaemia followed by cycle-specific chemotherapy *in vitro*. *Leukemia*, **4**, 826–834.
15 Young G.S., Minden M.D. & McCulloch E.A. (1993) Influence of schedule on regulated sensitivity of AML blasts to cytosine arabinoside. *Leukemia*, **7**, 1012–1019.
16 Karp J.E., Burke P.J., Donehover R.C. & Ross C. (1990) Effects of rh-GM-CSF on intracellular Ara-C pharmacology *in vitro* in acute myeloblastic leukaemia: comparability with drug induced humoral stimulatory activity. *Leukemia*, **4**, 553–556.
17 Link C.J., Burt R.K. & Bohn V.A. (1991) Gene specific repair if DNA damage induced by UV irradiation and cancer chemotherapies. *Cancer Cells*, **3**, 427–436.

18 Mikita T. & Beardsley C.P. (1988) Functional consequences of ara-binosylcytosine structural in DNA. *Biochemistry*, **27**, 4698–4705.

19 Estey E.H., Dixon D., Kantarjian H.M. *et al.* (1990) Treatment of poor prognosis newly diagnosed acute myeloid leukemia with ara-C and recombinant human granulocyte-macrophage colony stimulating factor. *Blood*, **75**, 1766–1769.

20 Buchner T., Hiddemann W., Koenigsmann M. *et al.* (1991) Recombinant human granulocyte-macrophage colony stimulating factor after chemotherapy in patients with acute myeloid leukemia at higher age or after relapse. *Blood*, **78**, 1190–1197.

21 Rowe J.M., Andersen J., Mazza J.J. *et al.* (1993) Phase III randomised placebo controlled study of granulocyte-macrophage colony stimulating factor (GM-CSF) in adult patients (55–70 years) with acute myelogenous leukemia (AML). A study of the Eastern Cooperative Oncology Group (ECOG). *Blood*, **82**, 329a.

22 Estey E., Thall P.F., Kantarjian H. *et al.* (1992) Treatment of newly diagnosed acute myelogenous leukemia with granulocyte-macrophage colony stimulating factor (GM-CSF) before and during continuous infusion high-dose ara-C + daunorubicin: comparison to patients treated without GM-CSF. *Blood*, **79**, 2246–2255.

23 Archimbaud E., Fenaux P., Reiffers J. *et al.* (1993) Granulocyte-macrophage colony stimulating factor in association to timed-sequential chemotherapy with mitoxantrone, etoposide and cytarabine for refractory acute myelogenous leukemia. *Leukemia*, **7**, 372–377.

24 Bettelheim P., Valent P., Andreef M. *et al.* (1991) Recombinant human granulocyte-macrophage colony stimulating factor in combination with standard induction chemotherapy in *de novo* acute myeloid leukemia. *Blood*, **77**, 700–711.

25 Buchner T., Hiddemann W., Rottmann R. *et al.* (1993) Multiple course chemotherapy with or without GM-CSF priming and long term administration for newly diagnosed AML. *Proceedings of the American Society of Clinical Oncology*, **12**, 301.

26 Ohno R., Tomonaga M., Kobayashi T. *et al.* (1990) Effect of granulocyte colony stimulating factor after intensive induction therapy in relapsed refractory acute leukemia. *New England Journal of Medicine*, **323**, 871–877.

27 Ohno R., Naoe T., Kanamaru A. *et al.* (1994) Leukemia Study Group: a double-blind controlled study of granulocyte colony-stimulating factor started two days before induction chemotherapy in refractory acute myeloid leukemia. *Blood*, **83**, 2086–2092.

28 Estey E., Thall P., Andreeff M. *et al.* (1994) Use of G-CSF before, during and after Fludarabine and ara-C induction chemotherapy of newly diagnosed AML or MDS: comparison with Fludarabine + ara-C without G-CSF. *Journal of Clinical Oncology*, **12**(4), 671–678.

29 Griffin J.D., Young D., Herrmenn F. *et al.* (1986) Effects of recombinant human GM-CSF on proliferation of clonogenic cells in acute myeloblastic leukemia. *Blood*, **67**, 1448–1453.

30 Miyauchi J., Kelleher C.A., Yang Y.C. *et al.* (1987) The effects of three recombinant growth factors, IL-3, GM-CSF and G-CSF on the blast cells of acute myeloblastic leukemia maintained in short-term suspension culture. *Blood*, **70**, 657–663.

31 Vellenga E., Young D.C., Wagner K., Wiper D., Ostapovicz D. & Griffin J. (1987) The effects of GM-CSF and G-CSF in promoting growth of clonogenic cells in acute myeloblastic leukemia. *Blood*, **69**, 1771–1776.

32 Imashuku S., Hibi S., Katooka-Mormoto Y. *et al.* (1995) Myelodysplasia and acute myeloid leukaemia in cases of aplastic anaemia and congenital neutropenia following G-CSF administration. *British Journal of Haematology*, **89**, 188–190.

33 Yates J., Glidewell O., Wiernick P. *et al.* (1982) Cytosine arabinoside with daunorubicin or adriamycin for therapy of acute myelocytic leukemia: a CALGB Study. *Blood*, **60**, 454–462.

34 Gonzalez-Llaven J., Rubio-Borja K.E., Martinez O. & Multicentric group ICHAC (1991) Efficacy of idarubicin plus ara-C in induction remission of *de novo* adult acute nonlymphoblastic leukaemia. *Haematologica*, **76**(Suppl. 4), 128.

35 Reiffers J., Hurteloup P., Stoppa A.M. *et al.* (1988) A prospective controlled study comparing idarubicin and daunorubicin as induction treatment for acute non-lymphoblastic leukemia in the elderly. *Haematologica*, **73**(Suppl. 1), 126.

36 Vogler W.R., Velez-Garcia E., Weiner R.S. *et al.* (1992) A phase III trial comparing idarubicin and daunorubicin in combination with cytarabine in acute myelogenous leukemia: a Southeastern Cancer Study Group Study. *Journal of Clinical Oncology*, **10**, 1103–1111.

37 Wiernik P.H., Banks P.L.C., Case D.C. *et al.* (1992) Cytarabine plus idarubicin and daunorubicin as induction and consolidation therapy for previously untreated adult patients with acute myeloid leukaemia. *Blood*, **79**, 313–319.

38 Mandelli F., Petti M.C., Ardia A. *et al.* (1991) A multicentric study from the Italian Co-operative Group GIEMMA. *European Journal of Cancer*, **27**, 750–755.

39 Berman E., Heller G., Santorsa J. *et al.* (1992) Results of a randomised trial comparing idarubicin and cytosine arabinoside with daunorubicin and cytosine arabinoside in adult patients with newly diagnosed acute myelogenous leukemia. *Blood*, **77**, 1666–1674.

40 Johnson S.A., Prentice A.G., Copplestone J.A. & Phillips M.J. (1990) Randomised study of mitoxantrone/cytosine arabinoside (2 + 5) and daunorubicin/cytosine arabinoside (2 + 5) in the treatment of acute myelogenous leukaemia. In: *4th Proceedings of the UK Novantrone Symposium (London)*, pp. 87–94. Media Medica, Chichester.

41 Arlin Z., Case D.C., Moore J. *et al.* and the Lederle Cooperative Group (1990) Randomised multicenter trial of cytosine arabinoside with mitoxantrone or daunorubicin in previously untreated adult patients with acute nonlymphoblastic leukaemia (ANLL). *Leukemia*, **4**, 177–183.

42 Wahlin A., Hornsten P., Hedenus M. & Malm C. (1991) Mitoxantrone and cytarabine versus daunorubicin and cytarabine in previously treated patients with acute myeloid leukaemia. *Cancer, Chemotherapy and Pharmacology*, **28**(6), 480–483.

43 Lowenberg B., Fiere D., Zimoun R. *et al.* (1991) Mitoxantrone versus daunorubicin in induction of acute myelogenous leukemia in elderly patients and low dose ara-C vs control as maintenance. An EORTC phase III trial (AML9) *Haematologica*, **76**(Suppl. 4), 91.

44 Wheatley K. (1995) Meta-analysis of randomized trials of idarubicin (IDAR) or mitozantrone (MTO) versus daunorubicin (DNR) as induction therapy for acute myeloid leukemia. *Blood*, **86**, 434a.

45 Dicke A., Spitzer G., Peters L. *et al.* (1979) Autologous bone marrow transplantation in relapsed adult acute leukaemia. *Lancet*, **i**, 514–517.

46 Burnett A.K., Tansey P., Watkins R. *et al.* (1984) Transplantation of unpurged autologous bone marrow in acute myeloid leukaemia in first remission. *Lancet*, **ii**, 1068–1070.

47 Stewart R., Buckner C., Bensinger W. *et al.* (1985) Autologous marrow transplantation in patients with acute non-lymphocytic leukemia in first remission. *Experimental Hematology*, **13**, 267–272.

48 Goldstone A.H., Anderson C.C., Linch D.C. *et al.* (1986) Autologous bone marrow transplantation following high dose therapy for

the treatment of adult patients with acute myeloid leukaemia. *British Journal of Haematology*, **64**, 529–537.

49 Lowenberg B., Verdonk L.J., Dekker A.W. *et al.* (1990) Autologous bone marrow transplantation in acute myeloid leukaemia in first remission: results of a Dutch prospective study. *Journal of Clinical Oncology*, **8**, 287–294.

50 Yeager A.M., Kaiser H., Santos G.W. *et al.* (1986) Autologous bone marrow transplantation in patients with acute non-lymphocytic leukaemia using *ex vivo* marrow treatment with 4-hyroperoxycyclophosphamide. *New England Journal of Medicine*, **315**, 141–147.

51 Pendry K., Alcorn M.J. & Burnett A.K. (1993) Factors influencing haematological recovery in 53 patients with acute myeloid leukaemia in first remission after autologous bone marrow transplantation. *British Journal of Haematology*, 83, 45–52.

52 Butturini A. & Gale R.P. (1989) Chemotherapy versus transplantation in acute leukaemia. *British Journal of Haematology*, **72**, 1–8.

53 Reiffers J., Gaspard M.H., Maraninchi D. *et al.* (1989) Comparison of allogeneic or autologous bone marrow transplantation and chemotherapy in patients with acute myeloid leukaemia in first remission: a prospective controlled trial. *British Journal of Haematology*, **72**, 57–63.

54 Reiffers J., Stoppa A.M., Attal M. *et al.* (1993) Autologous stem cell transplantation versus chemotherapy for adult patients with acute myeloid leukaemia in first remission: the BGMT Group experience. *Nouvelle Revue Française d'Hematologie*, **35**, 17.

55 Zittoun R.A., Mandelli F., Willemze R. *et al.* (1995) Autologous or allogeneic bone marrow transplantation compared with intensive chemotherapy in acute myelogenous leukaemia. *New England Journal of Medicine*, **332**, 217–223.

56 Harousseau J.L., Cahn J.Y., Pignon B. *et al.* (1997) Comparisons of autologous marrow transplantation and intensive chemotherapy as post remission therapy in adult acute myeloid leukaemia. *Blood*, **90**, 2978–2986.

57 Amadori S., Testi A.M., Arico M. *et al.* (1993) Prospective comparative study bone marrow transplantation and post-remission chemotherapy for childhood acute myelogenous leukaemia. *Journal of Clinical Oncology*, **11**, 1046–1054.

58 Ravindranath Y., Yeager A.M., Chang M.N. *et al.* (1996) Autolo-gous bone marrow transplantation versus intensive consolidation chemotherapy for acute myeloid leukemia in childhood. *New England Journal of Medicine*, **334**, 1428–1434.

59 Woods W.G., Kobrinsky N., Buckley J. *et al.* (1994) Timing intensive induction therapy improves post-remission outcome in acute myeloid leukemia (AML) irrespective of the use of bone marrow transplantation (BMT). *Blood*, **84**(Suppl. 1), 232a (abstract 912).

60 Burnett A.K., Goldstone A.H., Stevens R.F. *et al.* (1998) The addition of autologous bone marrow transplantation to intensive chemotherapy for acute myeloid leukaemia in first remission significantly reduces the risk of relapse and prolongs survival. *Lancet* (in press).

61 Gorin N.C., Labopin M., Meloni G. *et al.* (1991) Autologous bone marrow transplantation for acute myeloid leukemia in Europe: further evidence of the role of marrow purging by masfosfamide. *Leukemia*, **5**, 896–904.

62 Wolff S.N., Herzig R.H., Fay J.W. *et al.* (1989) High-dose cytarabine and daunorubicin as consolidation therapy for acute myeloid leukemia in first remission: long-term follow-up and results. *Journal of Clinical Oncology*, **7**, 1260–1267.

63 Mayer R.J., Davies R.B., Schiffer C.A. *et al.* (1994) Intensive post-remission chemotherapy in adults with acute myeloid leukemia. *New England Journal of Medicine*, **331**, 896–903.

64 Rubin E.H., Anderson J.W., Berg D.T., Schiffer C.A., Mayer R.J. & Stone R.M. (1992) Risk factors for high-dose cytarabine neurotoxicity: an analysis of a cancer and leukemia group B trial in patients with acute myeloid leukemia. *Journal of Clinical Oncology*, **10**, 948–953.

65 Gale R.P., Horowitz M.M., Rees J.K.H. *et al.* (1996) Chemotherapy versus transplants for acute myelogenous leukemia in second remission. *Leukemia*, **10**, 13–19.

66 Gale R.P., Horowitz M.M., Weiner R.S. *et al.* (1995) Impact of cytogenetic abnormalities on outcome of bone marrow transplants in acute myelogenous leukemia in first remission. *Bone Marrow Transplantation*, **16**, 203–208.

67 Boote D.T., Dennis I.F., Twentyman P.R. *et al.* (1996) Phase I study of Etoposide with SDZ PSC 833 as a modulator of multidrug resistance in patients with cancer. *Journal of Clinical Oncology*, **14**, 610–618.

11 Myelodysplasia and Preleukaemia

C.G. Geary and A.T. Macheta

Introduction

The term preleukaemia has a number of different connotations, but is now customarily used to describe an acquired haematological abnormality preceding the onset of acute leukaemia (AL). Such cases had been recognized since the beginning of the century [1], but comprehensive descriptions did not appear until the late 1940s and the 1950s [2,3]. Galton [4] has pointed out that, in these early days, haematologists were more concerned with identifying specific nutritional deficiencies responsible for abnormal marrow morphology, particularly megaloblastosis, than in defining the potentially leukaemic evolution of certain refractory (or 'achrestic') anaemias [5], although such a possibility was recognized.

Following the classic paper reported by Block *et al.* [6], the broad clinical and morphological features of preleukaemia were defined. Thus, it was noted to anticipate acute myeloblastic leukaemia (AML) rather than acute lymphoblastic leukaemia (ALL). The morphological abnormalities were, by definition, not diagnostic of AL, but the blood picture was often characterized by multiple cytopenias in the presence of a hypercellular marrow. Clinically, the symptomatology reflected a degree of bone marrow failure rather than the toxic, metabolic and extramedullary features often seen in AL. The prognosis was poor; in Block's original series of 13 patients, the median survival was only 27 months.

Since this clinicopathological definition of the preleukaemic syndrome, detailed evaluation of the bone marrow picture has permitted the identification of clinically similar patients whose marrows show a modest increase in the number of blast cells, as well as other dysplastic features. Those in whom a diagnosis of haemopoietic neoplasia was made with more certainty, were labelled as cases of 'smouldering' leukaemia by Rheingold *et al.* [7], but were often, somewhat confusingly, included under the older title of preleukaemia. Although the latter term was originally used retrospectively, with increasing experience and the help of cytogenetic, cultural and, now, molecular biological techniques, it is often reasonable to use it prospectively, to define patients with an intrinsic marrow disorder in whom there is a high risk of AL developing at some stage.

Patients with congenital disorders such as Fanconi's anaemia, Bloom's syndrome, ataxia telangiectasia and Down's syndrome, in whom there is also an increased risk of AL, were traditionally excluded from consideration of preleukaemia, as were those with well-defined acquired haematological disease, such as chronic myeloproliferative disorders. However, Mayer & Cannellos [8] have suggested that the latter groups might be referred to as examples of 'secondary' preleukaemia, 'primary' disease referring to those patients in which a clonal disorder erupts in a previously normal marrow. Although the great majority of descriptions of preleukaemia refer to the early stages of AML, it is now recognized that syndromes anticipating the onset of ALL and lymphoma do occasionally occur. The best example of the former progression is, perhaps, the aplastic phase sometimes ushering in ALL in children [9,10], while idiopathic nontropical splenomegaly, mixed connective tissue disorders and phenylhydantoin-induced lymphadenopathy occasionally anticipate B-cell lymphomas [11]. Finally, rare cases of ALL or biphenotypic leukaemia following apparently typical myelodysplasia have also been reported.

Definitions

The term 'preleukaemia' was coined at a time when the morphological abnormalities present in various refractory marrow disorders were still being described and evaluated; thus there was considerable overlap in terminology, and in the clinical and morphological features defined in various groups of patients. Diagnostic labels ranged from those describing cases without identifiable leukaemic blast cells (aregenerative anaemia, haemopoietic dysplasia, refractory anaemia with hypercellular marrow, refractory sideroblastic anaemia), to those in which leukaemia was a more certain diagnosis ('atypical' leukaemia, oligoblastic, smouldering or subacute leukaemia, subacute or chronic myelomonocytic leukaemia,

196   *Chapter 11*

chronic erythraemic myelosis and refractory anaemia with excess of blasts) [12]. Recently, the term myelodysplastic syndrome (MDS) has been increasingly used. Although this descriptive term is perhaps preferable to preleukaemia, it must be emphasized that similar morphological abnormalities may be seen in situations other than those caused by intrinsic marrow disorder; for example, after cytotoxic chemotherapy, or immunological damage to the marrow [13], in endocrine disorders, or as a paraneoplastic phenomenon [14,15]. Many of the morphological abnormalities seen in myelodysplasia occur in untreated megaloblastic anaemia [16,17] and also in patients with AIDS [18–20]. Attempts at classification on purely morphological grounds had thus proved difficult, but in 1982 the FAB group proposed a comprehensive classification of the MDS which is of value in predicting the likely risk of leukaemia in each group [21].

Incidence

The incidence of preleukaemia is not known with certainty. Early reports, often based on retrospective clinical studies of patients with AL, implied that it was very low [22,23], but later surveys suggested an incidence of at least 10% of those adult patients, eventually diagnosed as suffering from acute non-lymphocytic leukaemia [24–26]. According to Saarni & Linman [27], as many as 30% of their patients with acute myelomonocytic leukaemia had a recognizable preleukaemic phase.

A careful study, performed on behalf of the Leukaemia Research Fund in the UK in 1984–88, showed considerable local geographical variation in the incidence of MDS, with an average figure of 3.6 new cases per 100 000 population per year [28]. Another study, of the Dusseldorf population, carried out by Aul and his colleagues [29], suggested a crude incidence rate of 4.1 per 100 000 per year in the 5 years preceding publication of the study in 1992; 20% of these cases came to light as a result of routine blood counts performed for incidental reasons rather than suspected haematological disease. Williamson and his colleagues [30] have recently published an epidemiological study of MDS at a clinic in Bournemouth, UK, which serves an area with a large elderly population. The crude incidence rate found by these workers was a much higher 12.6 per 100 000 per year. Age-specific incidence rates are shown in Fig. 11.1. All studies of this type have shown that the incidence of MDS, like that of AML, rises steeply with age; the latter disease is, of course, more likely to be preceded by a myelodysplastic phase in the elderly. With the exception of the 5q– syndrome, MDS is commoner in males than females, and this may be particularly true of paediatric cases. One of the difficulties in establishing true incidence rates for MDS in different populations reflects problems in defining minimal criteria for the diagnosis. Elderly patients may be overlooked, especially if asymptomatic; on the other hand, the use of electronic blood counters means that minor deviations from

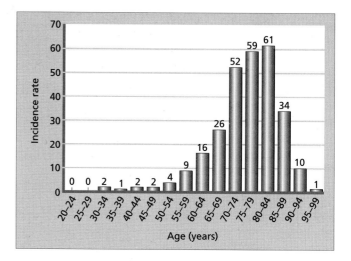

Fig. 11.1 Age distribution at diagnosis of MDS. (From Williamson *et al.*, 1994 [30], with permission.) Age-specific incidence rates (per 100 000 cases): <50 years = 0.5; 50–59 = 5.3; 60–69 = 15; 70–79 = 49; ≥80 years = 89.

normal are more readily detected, perhaps prompting bone marrow examination. These considerations are important in trying to decide whether there has been an absolute increase in the incidence of primary MDS, as some studies have suggested [31,32], or whether recent trends simply reflect an increasing awareness of the diagnosis. Some studies have found a higher incidence of exposure to chemical myelotoxins, such as benzene, in MDS patients than in control groups [33]. In a recent study of 400 newly diagnosed cases of MDS in the UK, using case controls, West and his colleagues [34] identified exposure to low-level radiation (such as in repeated dental X-rays), halogenated hydrocarbons and benzene-related compounds, as possible risk factors. An interesting feature of this study was that MDS sufferers seemed to be less fertile than the average; hypothalamic posterior hypophysis insufficiency has been reported in clinical evaluation of patients with the monosomy 7 syndrome. Other studies have suggested an increased risk of MDS in first-degree relatives of adults with the disease.

Preleukaemic syndromes analogous to those occurring in the elderly do occasionally occur in childhood or in young adults, sometimes on a familial basis, and those associated with secondary (therapy-linked) leukaemia can arise at any age. The increasing use of intensive chemotherapy for malignant disease is reflected in a rise in the incidence of this type of MDS as these patients are cured of, or remain in long-term remission from, the primary disease.

Pathogenesis of myelodysplasia

Studies with glucose 6-phosphate dehydrogenase (G6PD) isoenzyme markers [35], as well as cytogenetic markers, and the cultural behaviour of marrows from patients with MDS [36–39], suggested that these are clonal disorders, and that the clinical and morphological evolution of the disease reflects clonal expansion of an abnormal haematopoietic progenitor cell. Recent work using X-linked DNA analysis has confirmed the clonal nature of most cases of MDS, although occasional exceptions have been noted [40,41]. Some workers have suggested that there is no essential difference between 'preleukaemic' MDS and AL [42], but the usually slower tempo of clinical evolution in preleukaemia, as well as the morphology, justify distinction between the two groups. The biological differences reflect varying abnormalities involving cellular differentiation, regulation and expansion of the abnormal clone at the expense of normal cells. Evolution of MDS into AML may occur as a result of clonal evolution, sometimes with new chromosomal markers [43,44]. In other patients, there is a gradual rise in marrow and blood blast cell numbers over a period of weeks or months, until the patient fulfils the criteria for the diagnosis of AML, i.e. with more than 30% marrow blasts [45]. Koeffler & Golde [46] have suggested that this occurs as a result of increasing dislocation between proliferation and maturation of the neoplastic cell line, with more prominent arrest at the level of the blast cell. Thus, the preleukaemic disorders may not be distinct entities but represent stages in a multiphasic 'proliferative' disorder which has a high risk, eventually, of terminating in AL if the patient lives long enough. Several events or 'hits' occur during the evolution of MDS; one could cause proliferation of a genetically unstable clone of haemopoietic stem cells, while another could induce chromosomal abnormalities in a subclone, which then gains functional ascendancy [47], a further hit may then result in acute leukaemia. The morphological phenotype must depend on the gene localization of the change which the target cell sustains during somatic mutation [48].

Classification of the myelodysplastic syndrome

In 1976 the FAB cooperative group introduced semiquantitative methods of assessing morphological features in AL [49]. The group recognized the practical importance of assessing morphological features in AL and of separating from AML those borderline cases previously characterized as refractory anaemia with excess of blasts (RAEB) by Dreyfus [25]. Such cases were recognized as unsuitable for treatment by the intensive chemotherapy protocols used for *de novo* AML. In 1982 the FAB group attempted to analyse the spectrum of MDS in more detail, particularly the risk of evolution to acute leukaemia [16]. The group examined, in particular, the transitional zones between RAEB and AML on the one hand, and between RAEB and simple refractory anaemia with ring sideroblasts (RARS) and without ring sideroblasts (RA) on the other. They found that the dysplastic changes seen in RAEB (and in some cases of AML) were often also seen in the marrows of these latter patients; although blast cells were not present in the blood or increased in the marrow, they were considered to represent one end of a spectrum of neoplastic

Table 11.1 FAB types: quantitative features in MDS [4,50].

Type	Blood picture	Marrow
Refractory anaemia (RA)	<1% blasts	Dysplasia in one or more lineages. <5% blasts
RA with ring sideroblasts (RAS)	<1% blasts	As RA with ring sideroblasts representing at least 15% erythroblasts
RA with excess of blasts (RAEB)	<5% blasts	As RA with 5–20% blasts
RAEB in transformation (RAEB-t)	As RAEB but with 5% blasts, or with Auer rods	As RA with 20–30% blasts or as RAEB with Auer rods
Chronic myelomonocytic leukaemia (CMML)	As any of the above with >1 × 10^9/l monocytes	As any of the above + promonocytes

disorder in which five morphological variants might be identified. The chief distinguishing features of this classification are shown in Table 11.1. Arbitrary quantitative boundaries are set between the MDS and AML. A level of 30% marrow blasts is deemed to distinguish the two groups, while at the other end of the spectrum, patients with fewer than 5% blasts are allocated into the RA and RARS groups. Patients whose marrows showed 20–30% blast cells, or who had more than 5% blasts in the blood, were identified as refractory anaemia with excess of blasts in transformation (RAEB-t). If the blood monocyte count exceeded 1000/μl, the case was identified as chronic myelomonocytic leukaemia (CMML), provided the marrow appearances were consistent with a diagnosis of MDS. Although this purely morphological classification has been criticized on the grounds that it takes no account of other biological parameters, such as karyotype, or cultural patterns of granulocyte/macrophage colony-forming unit (GM-CFU) and erythroid burst-forming unit (E-BFU) production, or erythrokinetic patterns [51], subsequent attempts to classify large numbers of MDS patients have found it to be reproducible [52,53]. Moreover, this approach to classification has the merit of emphasizing that MDS results from a clonal proliferation; in this context, the precise number of blast cells seen in the marrow may not be crucial in making a diagnosis of leukaemia. Although the FAB group identify a marrow blast count of 5% as discriminating RAEB from RA and RARS, the normal marrow rarely shows more than 2% blasts, even when there is infection, so that a patient persistently showing 3–5% blasts must be regarded as having 'early' leukaemia; this can often be confirmed histologically (see below). The term preleukaemia would then logically apply only to patients with 2% or less blasts in their marrows [54].

Clinical findings

Patients with primary (*de novo*) MDS are usually middle aged or elderly, with a median age in excess of 60 years. Nevertheless, in an analysis of 554 patients with primary MDS, Fenaux *et al.* [55] found that 6.7% were aged 50 or less at diagnosis. Symptomatology reflects incipient bone marrow failure, so that patients commonly complain of weakness (though symptoms are often relatively mild, reflecting the gradual onset of marrow failure), epistaxes or easy bruising. Recurrent infections, usually bacterial, occasionally fungal, or mouth ulcers, reflect chronic neutropenia. Fever without overt infection is sometimes seen. Extramedullary evidence of leukaemia, such as organomegaly, is much less conspicuous than in acute or chronic leukaemias; slight splenomegaly may occur in up to 20% of cases, particularly in CMML, although autopsy studies have sometimes failed to demonstrate leukaemic infiltration of the spleen. Gum hypertrophy occurs only rarely in CMML [56]. Occasionally, these patients also present with pleural or pericardial effusions, skin infiltration or lymphadenopathy [57]. Dermatological changes in MDS have recently attracted attention. In addition to bacterial abscesses and leukaemia cutis, Sweet's syndrome (Fig. 11.2) (neutrophilic dermatosis) has recently been defined as a characteristic complication [58] and is often accompanied by fever and a blood neutrophilia.

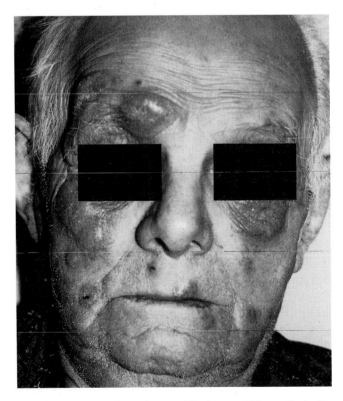

Fig. 11.2 Sweet's syndrome (neutrophilic dermatosis) in a patient with a chronic proliferative marrow disorder. (Courtesy of Dr D. Gorst, Royal Infirmary, Lancaster.)

Skin vasculitides have also been noted; these and other manifestations of vasculitis may be prodromes of the developing marrow disorder [59]. Rarely patients may present with more comprehensive evidence of autoimmune disease, such as haemolytic anaemia, or systemic lupus erythematosis [60,61], which may be responsive to immunosuppressants. Except for lysozymuria with accompanying hypokalaemia, found in CMML, metabolic and electrolyte disturbances—often present in acute leukaemia—seem to be rare in MDS.

Morphological abnormalities

A diagnosis of MDS can usually be suspected from inspection of the blood film and marrow aspirate (Table 11.2), and if appropriate, trephine biopsy. Characteristically, there are multiple cytopenias in the blood with a hypercellular marrow showing evidence of maturation arrest and dysplasia ('trilineage dysplasia'), but an isolated cytopenia, or bicytopenia, also occurs and the marrow may show significant dysplasia of only one cell line [62]. A proportion of patients (of the order of 25%) have hypoplastic marrows at diagnosis [63].

Erythropoiesis

Anaemia is usually, but not invariably, present; 5–10% of patients with MDS have normal haematocrits at diagnosis [64], but erythrokinetic studies have shown that ineffective erythropoiesis, manifest by macrocytosis and erythroid hyperplasia, is an early and characteristic feature [65]. Other cases show normochromic, normocytic blood pictures, usually with anisocytosis and poikilocytosis, while patients with refractory sideroblastic anaemia (RARS) often show red cell dimorphism. Ovalocytes are occasionally conspicuous, but not diagnostic of preleukaemia, although they are said to be particularly common in the 5q-syndrome (see below). Nucleated red cells may be present; reticulocytopenia is usual, but reticulocytosis occasionally occurs. Conversely, red cell aplasia may be the presenting feature of MDS, or develop during the course of the disease [66].

In addition to nonspecific signs of dyserythropoiesis, such as pyknosis, polyploidy, multinuclearity, nuclear budding and, rarely, internuclear bridging of erythroblasts, abnormal sideroblasts are frequently seen in the marrow. The FAB group defines 15% of the total erythroblast population as a significant number; such cases would be designated as refractory sideroblastic anaemia or, by the FAB group, refractory anaemia with ring sideroblasts (RARS). However, Hast & Reizenstein [67,68] claim that careful evaluation of the type of pathological sideroblast is important in establishing the risk of leukaemia. It may be higher in those patients who have a predominance of nonring or 'intermediate' sideroblasts, which must, nevertheless, be regarded as abnormal.

A variety of red cell glycolytic enzyme abnormalities have been described; no characteristic pattern which will permit the

Table 11.2 Morphological and functional abnormalities in MDS.

	Blood	Marrow
Erythropoiesis	Anisocytosis and poikilocytosis; macrocytes, ovalocytes, hypochromic or stippled cells, nucleated red cells	Nuclear budding, megaloblasts, multinucleate erythroblasts, sideroblasts, PAS positivity
	Enzyme defects; cell surface antigen changes; PNH-like lesions; HbF ↑, acquired HbH	
Myelopoiesis	Nuclear blebs, hyposegmentation ('Pelger' anomaly), giant lobes, hypersegmentation, nuclear clumping, atypical monocytes	Maturation arrest, atypical blast and mononuclear cells ('paramyeloid' cells),* abnormal or deficient granulation, vacuolation
	Reduced bacteriocidal, chemotactic and phagocytic activity	Reduced myeloperoxidase, chloracetate and alkaline phosphatase activity
Thrombopoiesis	Giant forms deficient in granules; membrane abnormalities	Giant or micromegakaryocytes
	Abnormal adhesion, aggregation; prolonged bleeding time	

PAS = periodic acid-Schiff stain.
* See text.

identification of preleukaemic from other dyserythropoietic states has emerged, although a decrease in pyruvate kinase activity is particularly common [69]. Folate deficiency may give very similar patterns of enzyme abnormality. Newman [70] and his colleagues found, in their series, that 80% of patients with preleukaemia had increased fetal haemoglobin levels; a few patients with preleukaemia have developed haemoglobin H disease, giving rise to the red cell morphological changes seen in thalassaemia. The intracellular precipitates of excess B-chain tetrameres, resembling 'golf-balls', can then be seen in reticulocyte or brilliant cresyl-blue preparations [71,72]. Alterations in erythrocyte membrane antigens have been documented in MDS, as in AL itself. A decrease in A_1 agglutinogen activity is the most usual, but modifications of the H antigen also occur [73,74]. Blood-group antigens may change with the onset of blast crisis [75].

One interesting antigenic change found in the erythrocytes is that involving the *I*/*i* locus. Expression of I antigen is decreased in several dyserythropoietic anaemias, as well as in aplastic anaemia and in AL, whereas i antigen is frequently increased in MDS, but only in some cases of AL. Moreover, a PNH clone may emerge in patients with MDS. There appear to be different patterns of red cell sensitivity to complement in the various types of dyserythropoietic anaemia. The paper by Ricard *et al.* [16] gives a full account of this subject.

Granulopoiesis

Neutropenia is the most commonly observed abnormality, but there may be a relative or absolute monocytosis, and even, occasionally, a neutrophil leucytosis. Neutrophils often show nuclear and cytoplasmic abnormalities, with defective or anomalous granules being particularly frequent (Table 11.2). The loss of primary granules is frequently paralleled by the loss of peroxidase activity. In occasional patients there may be a total absence of specific granules in apparently 'mature' neutrophils which contain azurophil granules [76–78]. A Pelger–Huet anomaly is often present; hypersegmentation is less common. A distinctive nuclear abnormality, affecting mainly mature granulocytes, has been described by Felman *et al.* [79]. Abnormal chromatin condensation gives the nucleus a fragmented or 'cog-wheel' appearance, lacking segmentation. These patients often have a leucocytosis and granulocytic hyperplasia in the marrow; the prognosis is usually poor. In some cases of CMML, cells intermediate between monocytes and myelocytes are conspicuous in the blood and marrow. These have been called 'paramyeloid' cells or 'mononuclear neutrophils'. Their identity may be clarified by the combined esterase preparation, which, however, often gives anomalous results in MDS [80]. Cytochemical abnormalities of this type are also sometimes seen in nonleukaemic disorders, such as megaloblastic anaemia [81]. The leucocyte alkaline phosphatase (LAP) score in preleukaemia is usually normal or low, but there is no distinctive pattern in MDS. Defects of neutrophil function occur in up to 50% of patients with MDS, and contribute to the high incidence of infection. The association between monosomy 7 syndromes and neutrophil functional defects is well established; these include defective chemotaxis, phagocytosis, superoxide generation and bacteriocidal activity [82].

A marrow blast cell count of 5% was used as an important discriminating feature by the FAB group in their classification. However, in a severely dysplastic and cellular marrow, a precise count may be difficult to achieve against a background of atypical promyelocytes, myelocytes, monocytes and erythroid hyperplasia. Heimpel [78] has emphasized the difficulties encountered in performing accurate myelograms in such patients. Some observers have taken myeloblasts and promyelocytes together and require a limit of 10% for the diagnosis of leukaemia. However, the FAB group [17] has suggested that promyelocytes should be disregarded and have also recognized two different types of blast cell, according to their nuclear:cytoplasmic ratio and the presence of cytoplasmic granules (types I and II blast cells). Goasguen and his group [83] have recently proposed recognition of a more 'mature' blast cell (type III). These cells have more than 6, and sometimes more than 20 granules, but lack a Golgi zone and should therefore not be counted as promyelocytes (although the nucleus may be eccentrically placed). Inclusion of these cells in the marrow blast count identifies patients with a worse prognosis. Abnormally small blast cells are sometimes seen in MDS, both in smears and histological sections of the marrow [84]. Auer rods are occasionally seen in patients with MDS, especially in RAEB-t; although evidence is somewhat conflicting, their presence usually heralds rapid progression of the disease [85,86] when seen in other morphological subtypes. There is some evidence that cases of RAEB-t displaying Auer rods respond more readily to therapy.

Lymphopoiesis

Lymphocyte morphology is not distinctively abnormal in MDS, but quantitative and qualitative changes in specific lymphocyte subsets have been described, and these may contribute to the propensity of certain patients to suffer infections, autoimmune disease and even second malignancies. When lymphopenia occurs in MDS this usually reflects reduction in T-cell numbers, particularly CD4+ cells [87–89]. Deficient NK (natural killer) cell function has also been described in various types of MDS [88]. A poor response to phytohaemagglutinin (PHA) and concanavalin A has been reported [89] and there is tentative evidence of a decreased ability to mediate DNA repair [90]. Results from these and other studies support the thesis that preleukaemic MDS often reflects a defect of the haemopoietic stem cell manifest in several, if not all, cell lines, but DNA studies of 11 patients with loss of part, or all of, chromosome 5 suggested that the lymphoid cell lines are not always involved [91]. Similar results accrued from studies of patients with monosomy 7 [92] or trisomy 8. However, it has also been suggested that a primary defect in T cells, or their factors, might result in defective haematopoiesis, or at least contribute to peripheral cytopenias [93]. Although B-cell lymphocyte populations usually seem to be normal in MDS, there is some evidence for aberrant function [94], resulting in both hypo- and hyper-gammaglobulinaemia [87]. Autoantibodies to red cells, resulting in a positive red cell antiglobulin test, and even sometimes autoimmune haemolytic anaemia, seem to be unusually common in MDS, while Copplestone *et al.* [95] found paraprotein bands in up to 15% of cases. Concomitant lymphoproliferative or immunoproliferative neoplastic disorders are well documented in MDS [96]; chronic lymphocytic leukaemia, lymphocytic lymphoma, hairy cell leukaemia, as well as rare entities such as large granular lymphocytic

leukaemia, have all been reported [87]. The association of sideroblastic anaemia with myeloma has been known for many years [97]; although originally depicted as an example of 'secondary' sideroblastic anaemia, it seems likely that some such cases represent simultaneous involvement of myeloid/erythroid cell lines, as well as B cells; in a proportion of myeloma patients the two diseases apparently occurred as part of the natural history, and not as a result of the treatment of the primary disorder [98], although the majority are a result of therapy with alkylating agents [99]. Copplestone and his colleagues [100] have reported 20 patients who were simultaneously diagnosed as having myeloma or lymphoproliferative disease and MDS: Hamblin [87] has suggested that the high incidence of concomitant immunoglobulin-secreting tumours in MDS, when compared with chronic myeloid leukaemia (CML), another 'stem cell' disease, might reflect chronic infection resulting from neutrophil dysfunction; B-cell proliferation might then lead to the accumulation of genetic 'errors'. Alternatively, production of abnormal cytokines by cells of the monocyte or macrophage lineage could result in the emergence of an abnormal clone. In summary, although there are variable immunological defects in many cases of MDS, it is uncertain whether these are primary or secondary events.

Megakaryocytes and platelets

At least 50% of patients with MDS are thrombocytopenic [101], but thrombocytosis sometimes occurs, particularly in RARS and in the 5q– syndrome (see p. 202). Occasionally an isolated thrombocytopenia is the only cytopenia observed. Ultrastructural examination shows vacuolation, defective or absent microtubules, dilated canalicular systems, and giant platelet granules, which do not participate in the release reaction during aggregation [102]. Abnormal platelet function can be demonstrated by the bleeding time, and by tests of adhesion and aggregation [103]; the bleeding time may be prolonged in the presence of a normal platelet count. A defect in thromboxane A_2 activity has been described in two patients with MDS who had a haemorrhagic tendency in spite of normal platelet counts [104]. In the marrow there may be decreased or increased numbers of megakaryocytes, but these are morphologically abnormal; often the nucleus is small and nonlobulated. These cells (micromegakaryocytes) may be capable of producing small numbers of dysplastic platelets, which, occasionally, are unusually large; they represent cytoplasmic maturation of a cell unable to duplicate DNA [76]. Micromegakaryocytes may be as small as 20 μm in diameter and are sometimes mistaken for primitive granulocytic cells, or even lymphocytes [78]. Nevertheless, they can be identified by immunocytochemistry (antibody to factor VIII or platelet-specific glycoprotein IBB/IIIA), or by electron microscopic demonstration of platelet peroxidase [105,106]. Thrombocytopenia in MDS is thus often due to ineffective thrombocytopoiesis. It has been suggested that more than 10% mono or bi-nucleated megakaryocytes are a useful diagnostic feature of the preleukaemic MDS, but they also occur in small numbers in chronic myeloproliferative disease, for example CML, and in some nonmalignant disorders.

Bone marrow histology

Recent studies have confirmed the observation, reported in the original paper by Block *et al.* [6], that bone marrow histology is an important investigation in preleukaemic dysplasia [107]: aspirates and trephine biopsies are complementary procedures. Marrow cellularity can be assessed more accurately and myelofibrosis identified. Apoptosis is a conspicuous feature in some cases of MDS. Lymphoid aggregates are occasionally seen in this disease: their significance is unknown [108]. Pronounced reticulin fibrosis is sometimes present. In hypocellular marrows this feature is useful in distinguishing MDS from idiopathic or drug-related aplastic anaemia in which the reticulin pattern is usually normal [109]. Collagen fibrosis is uncommon in this type of dysplasia, but it does occasionally occur and can lead to confusion with other types of fibrotic bone marrow disorder [110]; this subject is discussed below. In addition to assessing cellularity, bone marrow histology is useful in detecting disruption of the normal bone marrow architecture. One characteristic feature is displacement of granulopoiesis from its normal, paratrabecular, position. Tricot and his colleagues [84], using plastic-embedded trephine biopsies to study patients with MDS, have described abnormal histological patterns consisting of small aggregates of blast cells and promyelocytes. Small foci of these primitive cells (sometimes as few as three to five cells) were found clustering centrally in the intertrabecular marrow regions and the authors described this phenomenon as abnormal localization of immature precursors (ALIP) (Fig. 11.3). In addition, these aggregates of primitive cells are often accompanied by more differentiated elements, displaying monocytoid or granulocytic characteristics. The authors have reported that this is a more discriminating way of recognizing blast cell infiltration in MDS than by examining marrow aspirates. Moreover, they reported this phenomenon to be an adverse prognostic finding, in relation to patients with RA or RARS. However, Mangi and his colleagues [111] have emphasized the importance of immunohistochemical recognition of early progenitor cells in bone marrow biopsies: in conventional haematoxylin and eosin (H & E) preparations it may be impossible to distinguish between proerythroblasts and myeloblasts, and, because erythroid hyperplasia is often found in MDS marrows, this can be misleading. Although ALIP cannot now be regarded as pathognomonic for MDS (it is also seen after the use of haemopoietic growth factors and in the early stage of recovery after allogeneic marrow transplantation), it does, presumably, reflect abnormal growth patterns of granulopoiesis which are a feature of this syndrome [108]. Dyserythropoiesis, dysmegakaryopoiesis and dysgranulopoiesis may all be detected in well-prepared biopsy specimens; in particular the abnormal megakaryoblastic and megakaryocytic morphology character-

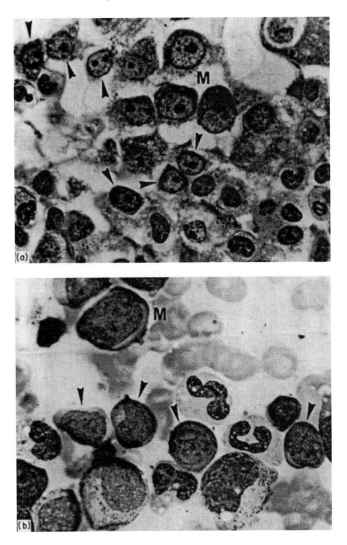

Fig. 11.3 (a) ALIP positivity. Proliferation of small blastic elements (arrows) distributed throughout the intertrabecular areas. These small blastic elements are accompanied by myeloblasts and promyelocytes (M). (b) Bone marrow smear, showing multiple small-sized blasts (arrows); the nucleus has a fine chromatin pattern and one or more nucleoli; these cells have a small rim of cytoplasm. Notice the typical myeloblast (M) with its larger size. The small-sized blasts may be the equivalent of the ALIP blasts, observed in trephine biopsies. (Reproduced by kind permission of Dr G.M. Tricot [84]).

istic of the 5q– syndrome can be distinguished histologically from the more pleomorphic changes seen in other forms of MDS, the cells being monolobar and characteristically larger, at 30–40 μm diameter, with a round, eccentrically placed nucleus [112].

Specific types of the myelodysplastic syndrome

Although there is considerable overlap between the various types of preleukaemic MDSs, and clinicopathological entities are harder to define than in AL or the chronic myeloproliferative syndrome, some discriminating features have emerged.

Refractory anaemia

Refractory anaemia (RA) is clearly a heterogeneous diagnosis, and not all cases are necessarily potentially preleukaemic. Some may have poorly defined biochemical lesions affecting erythropoiesis, and not clonal disorders [113,114]. It is particularly important to exclude alcoholism in this group and it must be remembered that thrombocytopenia may also occur in these patients. The FAB group described patients, usually over the age of 50, with anaemia, reticulocytopenia, erythroid hyperplasia and/or dyserythropoiesis, and, less frequently, dysgranulopoiesis, but with fewer than 5% blasts in the marrow. Subsumed into this group are some of the syndromes recognized by earlier authors, such as Vilter *et al.* [115], who classified the refractory anaemias into five different types.

Although blast cells are absent from the blood, the presence of minor changes in the granulocytic and megakaryocytic series are of particular importance in allotting the patient to the preleukaemic syndrome, but leukaemia may ensue in an occasional patient who presents only with macrocytosis without anaemia [116,117]. In one series [117], 48 out of 53 patients with RA had leucocyte counts of less than $3.9 \times 10^9/l$ and/or platelet counts of less than $130 \times 10^9/l$, suggesting that, even at diagnosis, there was evidence of involvement of the pluripotent haemopoietic stem cell. The term 'refractory pancytopenia' might be more appropriate for such cases. The incidence of acute leukaemia in this group may be higher than that in refractory sideroblastic anaemia, with figures ranging up to 30% [117].

Red cell aplasia

Red cell aplasia (RCA) is recognized as a preleukaemic syndrome, especially in the elderly; karyotopic analysis is important in such patients to distinguish those particularly at risk [118]. In these, response to immunosuppressants is less likely, although it has also been suggested that failure of immune surveillance might allow the emergence of both autoimmune abnormalities and neoplasia [13]. It is of interest that macrocytosis and dyserythropoiesis sometimes persist after remission of RCA in the adult with immunosuppressants. In one review, Fitchen found the incidence of AL in RCA to be only 7% (eight of 108 cases), although others have reported higher figures [119,120]. This disparity probably reflects differences in patient selection and diagnosis; in particular, patients with thymoma do not seem to be vulnerable to leukaemia. Lacombe *et al.* [121] found that patients with RCA resulting from stem cell defects usually exhibited poor autologous growth of BFU-E and CFU-E using a plasma clot technique. Patients with RCA resulting from an autoimmune process often exhibited at least some growth, and this correlated with the response to immunosuppressants. Amegakaryocytic thrombocytopenia is now also recognized as a preleukaemic picture.

The 5q− syndrome

This is a reasonably well defined entity, which is of particular interest because the deleted material often involves several genes concerned with the production of haemopoietic growth factors, such as GM-CSF, IL-3, IL-4 and IL-5, and the FMS gene, which encodes the receptor for CSF-1. Reduced leucocyte interferon production in patients with the 5q− syndrome has been described. Loss of a portion of the long arm of chromosome 5 is seen frequently in therapy-related myelodysplasia and acute leukaemias, often with other karyotypic abnormalities, but when it occurs alone it is characteristically associated with a relatively indolent form of RA, with only a small risk of acute leukaemia. The initial haematological correlation was with refractory macrocytic anaemia, occurring in elderly women, in which a distinctive deletion of the long arm of chromosome 5 was noted [122]. However, ovalocytic macrocytosis is now regarded as less specific than the presence of megakaryocytic abnormalities, particularly hyperplasia and hypolobulation: many of these patients also have increased platelet counts. Kerkhofs *et al.* [123] concluded that this syndrome can be discriminated from other types of MDS by the presence of megakaryocytic hypolobulation with three of the following features: (i) macrocytic anaemia, (ii) normal or low numbers of erythroid marrow precursor cells, (iii) absence of ring sideroblasts and (iv) normal or high platelet count. Nevertheless the cytogenetic abnormality has also been identified in other haematological syndromes, including pure red cell aplasia, essential thrombocythaemia, and even acute lymphoblastic leukaemia [124–127]. When patients present with the typical features of the 5q− syndrome described above, they are more likely to have a cytogenetically normal cell line in addition; in the nontypical cases, Kerkhofs *et al.* [123] found that 100% of cultured cells showed the abnormality. This might help to explain the higher incidence of acute leukaemia in nontypical cases. Abnormalities of chromosome 5 are more frequently found in patients with secondary MDS than in those with therapy-related AML and no previous preleukaemic phase [127]. In contrast to the usual preponderance of males with MDS in the classical 5q− syndrome, females outnumber males by a ratio of 2:1, and it is possible that this reflects different patterns of exposure to myelotoxins. Homozygous deletions of the FMS gene in a young woman with RA and the 5q− syndrome has recently been described [128], but the pathogenetic role of the genetic deletion in the heterozygote is not understood, especially as unaffected cells such as T-lymphocytes and fibroblasts continue to elaborate identical growth factors [54]. The association of specific interstitial deletions of the long arm of chromosome 5 with dysplastic haemopoiesis has prompted the question whether the deletion of the genetic material is critical to the process of transformation and clonal growth; the breakpoints in the damaged chromosome differ somewhat in different cases, although the proximal break is characteristically at

5q 13–15 and the distal break at 5q 31–33; (5)(q13 q33) is the most commonly encountered deletion, occurring in 40% of cases [129]. Whether minor differences in the breakpoints have morphological correlates, or influence the risk of progression, is currently being investigated [130]. The proximal breakpoint is closer to the centromere in elderly patients, whereas the distal breakpoint is independent of age. Abnormalities of the genes encoding FMS and its receptor CSF-1 might be implicated in the spectrum of functional morphological abnormalities seen in this syndrome, although red cell hypoplasia is less easily explained. Research is also currently directed at the possibility that the deletion involves tumour suppressor genes [129]. Thus, although a large number of genes related to haemopoietic cell growth and differentiation on the long arm of chromosome 5 have been identified, the significance of these deletions, at the molecular level, is not yet fully understood [54].

Refractory sideroblastic anaemia

One of the most difficult problems in the classification of the preleukaemic myelodysplasias is the question whether all cases of primary acquired sideroblastic anaemia should be included for consideration [131,132]. The exact genetic lesion in this disorder is unknown, but it produces defects in DNA synthesis [133] as well as disordered mitochondrial function [134]. Impairment of haem synthesis causes mitochondrial iron overload which may, secondarily, further inhibit mitochondrial function, although no consistent pattern of enzyme deficiency has been identified, at least in acquired disease. Mutations of mitochondrial DNA are currently being sought in this disease [135,136]. Some 20% of patients with preleukaemia have sideroblastic changes in their marrows, although the percentage of erythroblasts showing pathological sideroblasts varies widely [64,137]. The FAB group now define 15% of the total erythroblasts (not the total cell population) as a discriminating feature in making the diagnosis. That some cases of refractory sideroblastic anaemia (RARS) are, indeed, clonal disorders was suggested originally by the characteristic dual red cell populations seen in the blood, and has also been proved by cytogenetic (and in one instance) by isoenzyme segregation studies. Among the cytogenetic abnormalities encountered in RARS are deletions of chromosomes 5, 11 and 20; loss of the Y chromosome in males is also common but less significant. One interesting abnormality is inversion of the long arm of chromosome 3, which has been found in sideroblastic patients with thrombocytosis [138]. Acute leukaemia has been reported to follow, in the various series, in proportions ranging from 0 to 24%. AML is the typical progression in such cases, but other evolutions and associations have been reported, including ALL, CLL, and even hairy cell leukaemia [139–145]. Classic primary sideroblastic anaemia may evolve into a syndrome resembling agnogenic myeloid metaplasia, and polycythaemia vera following RARS has also been described [117,146]. The heterogeneity of the natural history of primary sideroblastic anaemia has recently been emphasized by a large French study [147], which identified a relationship to chronic myeloproliferative disease as well as acute leukaemia. In the study of younger patients with MDS previously cited [55], no cases of RARS were discovered.

Patients who present with, or subsequently develop, leucopenia or thrombocytopenia seem to be at greater risk of developing leukaemia than those with anaemia only [117,142,144]. Thrombocytosis occasionally seen in primary RAS, is a favourable prognostic factor [143], while male sex is associated with a higher incidence of leukaemia [144]. The risk of acute leukaemia is also increased in those with abnormal marrow karyotypes, especially monosomy 7 or deletion 20q, or with complex abnormalities.

Heimpel [114] has suggested that the haematologist should carefully discriminate between cases in which there is a panmyelosis, if not a pancytopenia, and those who present with 'pure' sideroblastic anaemia, i.e. in which the morphological abnormalities are strictly confined to the erythroid series; the risk of leukaemia seems to be much lower in the latter group. In a recent study, Gattermann and colleagues [148] found a lower incidence of AL in RARS patients who showed only dyserythropoiesis (1.9% at 5 years) compared with 48% in those who also showed dysplasias of other lineages at diagnosis. These latter patients had a much worse overall survival and were more likely to show poor growth in clonal assays. Nevertheless, bone marrow cytology is a relatively crude way of deciding whether these additional cell lines are involved in a clonal disorder, and others have suggested that the separation into two groups is artificial, all gradations being seen [149]. It is also possible that a series of genetic changes occur, even in the most indolent cases or RARS, affecting first erythropoiesis and, later, other cell lineages, as the clonal disorder evolves. The evolution to acute leukaemia could reflect a further genetic change—in the rare cases where leukaemia has entered remission, sideroblastic morphology has persisted [136,150].

Some observers have claimed that patients with erythroblast iron overload should be segregated into at least two groups, according to the proportion of 'complete' ring sideroblasts defined as erythroblasts containing at least six iron granules, covering one-third or more of the perimeter of the nucleus. Early evolution into leukaemia was noted by Hast & Reizenstein [67,68] to be associated with a preponderance of 'nonring', though pathological, sideroblasts. They noted that the typical features of cytopenic myelodysplasia are more likely to be associated with nonring forms. In their study, 50% of patients with this latter morphological abnormality eventually developed AL, a figure substantially higher than that cited above for RARS as a generic group; these former patients would now be classified as RA. Garand and his co-workers [147], in their study, defined a better prognosis for patients with 'pure' acquired idiopathic sideroblastic anaemia (AISA) than in patients classified as RA. Cazzola *et al.* [151] have also described distinctive erythrokinetic patterns for the two groups, although May *et al.* were unable to confirm this [152]. Marrow culture studies *in vitro* often show near normal patterns in chronic idiopathic sideroblastic anaemia, also suggesting a low propensity to leukaemic evolution [153,154].

Thus, it is valuable to distinguish between refractory anaemia with and without large numbers of ring sideroblasts, as they may present clinically as somewhat different entities, as regards chronicity, risk of AL and incidence of clinical iron overload. There is evidence that the latter complication is influenced by the HLA group of the patient. Cartwright *et al.* [155] found that the incidence of HLA-A3, at over 70% in a group of RARS patients with clinical evidence of iron overload, was comparable to that found in primary haemochromatosis; it was of interest that family members of the patients with sideroblastic anaemia sometimes also evinced evidence of mild iron overload. The haemochromatosis gene is widely distributed in the population, its presence may contribute to the severity of iron overload in certain patients with sideroblastic anaemia [156].

Paroxysmal nocturnal haemoglobinuria

Paroxysmal nocturnal haemoglobinuria (PNH) occupies a central position within the hierarchy of preleukaemic syndromes [157]. It is an acquired disorder of haemopoiesis, characterized by episodes of intravascular haemolysis, and a variable neutropenia and thrombocytopenia associated, in the typical case, with a fluctuating marrow hypoplasia, although others show erythroid hyperplasia [158,159]. Serological evidence of PNH, such as a positive sucrose-lysis or Ham test, reflecting abnormalities, or lack, of cell membrane proteins, is found not only in relation to hypoplastic anaemia, but also in various congenital dyserythropoietic disorders, in MDS, acute leukaemia and chronic myeloproliferative disorders [157,160–162]. There is good evidence that PNH is a clonal disorder [163], yet the incidence of AL in classical PNH is low; 18 cases have been described, of which four were examples of erythroleukaemia (for review see ref. [162]). It has been suggested that the propensity to evolve into leukaemia is low, unless there is another unstable clone also present in the marrow. Patients with PNH, whose marrows are cytogenetically normal, may have a low risk of leukaemia [164]. A recent case report suggests that the leukaemic clone does not necessarily emerge from that originally displaying the PNH abnormality [165], although in most cases it seems to do so [166,167]. Occasionally a PNH clone disappears [168].

Chronic erythraemic myelosis

This term is no longer included in the FAB classification of myelodysplasia, although it was encompassed by earlier classifications of refractory anaemia and smouldering leukaemia [115,169–170].

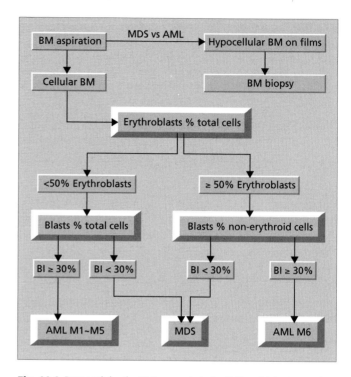

Fig. 11.4 Proposals by the FAB group to help distinguish between the spectrum seen in MDS from AML [172]. BI = blasts; BM = bone marrow.

Erythroid hyperplasia is a common feature in myelodysplasia, and it is likely that many cases would now be allocated the diagnosis of RA, RARS or RAEB. The FAB group suggested that in categorizing a new case, the erythroid component should be disregarded if the myeloid : erythroid ratio is less than 1, and a blast count performed only on the remaining myeloid cells [172]. In this way, a distinction between myelodysplasia and acute erythroleukaemia (FAB variant M6) is achieved, if the '30% rule' is followed (Fig. 11.4). There is evidence to suggest that the M6 variant usually evolves out of a previous myelodysplastic syndrome [4]. However, other criteria for classifying erythroleukaemia have been proposed, and, in particular, the tempo of clinical progression and type of karyotypic abnormality detected [173,174].

Refractory anaemia with excess of blast cells and in transformation

The FAB group define refractory anaemia with excess of blast cells (RAEB) as those patients who exhibit more than 5% but less than 20% blast cells in the marrow [21]; an occasional blast cell (less than 5%) may be present in the blood, which otherwise typically shows a pancytopenia. Erythroid hyperplasia may be conspicuous, although there is typically evidence of trilineage dysplasia. This group includes cases previously referred to as oligoblastic or smouldering leukaemia. However, the FAB group has introduced the useful term RAEB in transformation (RAEB-t) to identify patients who have more obvious infiltration of the marrow (20–30%), at which level the formal diagnosis of AL is established. The leukaemic cell mass is probably larger in such patients and splenomegaly, and even hepatomegaly, may be present; the presence of significant organomegaly is usually a poor prognostic sign [26,175]. Auer rods are more likely to be seen in the blast cells of this group. Nevertheless, some patients with RAEB-t have a relatively indolent course [176].

Subacute and chronic myelomonocytic leukaemia

Linman [177] first suggested the term chronic myelomonocytic leukaemia (CMML) for a group of patients with a 'myeloproliferative' disorder characterized by peripheral monocytosis and a marrow showing proliferation of immature myeloid cells; others noted that blast cells are less conspicuous than in acute myelomonocytic leukaemia (AMML). The clinical picture is not that of an acute leukaemia and the course sometimes surprisingly indolent, with relatively slight anaemia, although some cases, nevertheless, gradually progress to acute monocytic or myelomonocytic leukaemia. CMML is particularly commonly associated with RAS gene deletions.

The FAB group proposed inclusion of CMML in the spectrum of MDS. This was logical, because, despite a conspicuous peripheral monocytosis (and sometimes granulocytosis), the marrow 'picture' is usually similar to that of other patients with MDS, and, in particular, to that of patients with RAEB. Nevertheless, CMML can be regarded as a disease that shows features of both myelodysplasia and myeloproliferative disease, and either dysplasia or proliferation can dominate the picture in individual patients [178]. The distinguishing feature is a peripheral monocytosis greater than $1 \times 10^9/l$, and often in the range $5-10 \times 10^9/l$. The monocytes often show nuclear abnormalities, with bizarre convolution; paramyeloid cells are frequent, while granulocytes may be hypersegmented or show hypogranulation. Some patients also have small numbers of immature granulocytes in the blood. When considered in conjunction with the granulocytic hyperplasia sometimes seen in the marrow, these patients have, in the past, been confused with Philadelphia-negative (Ph-) CML, but discriminating features between classical Philadelphia-positive (Ph+) CML, atypical (aCML) and CMML have emerged following the publication of a number of morphological, cytogenetic and molecular biology studies [179,180]. This differential diagnosis is discussed in Chapter 13, but the distinguishing features between CMML and aCML (which is BCR-ABL as well as Philadelphia negative) are regarded as: more conspicuous monocytosis, but fewer immature granulocytes, including blasts, in the blood of patients with CMML as compared with aCML, and more granulocytic hyperplasia in the marrows of patients with the latter disease. In contrast to CML, basophilia is not usually seen in either aCML or CMML. The distinction between the three diseases is important, because the natural history and prognosis of each differs, as does response to chemotherapy and interferon.

The FAB group [181] have recently performed a statistical analysis on the morphological features of the blood and marrow pictures of these cases and have proposed a group of predictive parameters which should enable a discriminating diagnosis to be made. In addition to those previously identified, marrow erythroid hyperplasia was found to occur more frequently in CMML—as it does in other types of MDS—than in CML or aCML. This classification is shown in Table 11.3; interestingly, the Group found that dysplasia was more conspicuous in aCML than in CMML. The situation is further complicated by the observation that a characteristic karyotypic abnormality (5;12 translocation) has been described in both CMML and aCML [182]. Whether 'juvenile' CML should be regarded as a type of myelodysplastic syndrome, perhaps linked to CMML, remains a matter of dispute.

The picture of CMML may supervene in the accelerated phase of a chronic myeloproliferative disorder [183]. One interesting feature is the frequency with which a polyclonal hyperimmunoglobulinaemia is present; in one series two out of 35 patients also showed an M-protein, but it must be remembered that the latter finding is not uncommon in the elderly [184]. Many of these patients show increased lysozyme levels in serum and urine which show a rough correlation with the leucocyte count, and this may lead to nephropathy. Serum uric acid and vitamin B_{12} levels are frequently increased in patients with higher counts, again demonstrating some overlap with the chronic myeloproliferative disorders.

Although some very chronic cases have been reported, presenting sometimes with a solitary monocytosis [43,185,186], ('chronic monocytic leukaemia') and minimal cytopenia or dysplasia, it is doubtful whether the group as a whole has a survival that is significantly better than patients with RAEB (Table 11.4). Patients with a high risk of developing leukaemia often have more primitive cells in the blood at diagnosis, and this may be reflected in the marrow picture with blast counts of up to 20% or more, suggesting that some of these patients should be regarded as examples of RAEB-t. Sexauer *et al.* [188] had earlier suggested the term 'subacute myelomonocytic leukaemia' for these patients. The differential diagnosis of CMML includes leukaemoid blood pictures due to carcinoma, Hodgkin's disease and certain chronic infections, such as subacute bacterial endocarditis.

Table 11.3 Predictive parameters in CML, aCML and CMML. (From Bennett *et al.*, 1994 [181], with permission.)

Parameter	CML	aCML	CMML
1. Basophils	+	–	
2. Immature granulocytes	+	+	–
3. Granulocyte dysplasia	–	+	–
4. Monocytes	–	–	+
5. Bone marrow precursors	–	–	+

Table 11.4 Survival and leukaemic progression in 1081 patients with primary MDS. (From Mufti, 1990 [187], with permission.)

FAB subtype	Patients No.	Patients %	Survival (months)	Median survival (months)	Leukaemic progression (%)
RA	305	28	18–64	50	12
RAS	262	24	14–76+	51	8
RAEB	248	23	7–16	11	44
RAEB-t	91	9	2.5–11	5	60
CMML	175	16	9–60+	11	14

Morphological-immunological and Cytogenetic (MIC) Third Co-operative Study Group data, collected from 11 independent studies reported between 1982 and 1987.

Chronic neutrophilic leukaemia

The rare marrow disorder chronic neutrophilic leukaemia (CNL) is now customarily included within the spectrum of MDS, although it does not have special identification within the FAB classification. A particular point of interest is its association with monoclonal gammopathy or even myeloma. Its natural history is discussed further in Chapter 13.

The aplasia-leukaemia syndrome

A number of associations between marrow hypoplasia and leukaemia have been defined. Firstly, typical aplastic anaemia, irrespective of aetiology, may terminate, usually after a period of some years, as AL. Except in constitutional aplasia (e.g. Fanconi's anaemia), such cases are uncommon, although the hitherto poor prognosis in acquired aplastic anaemia may have concealed an association between the two diseases; however, a period of myelodysplasia usually intervenes (see below). In a few cases, the agent causing the initial aplastic phase is known to be leukaemogenic, and this has been best documented for benzene [189] and radiation [190]. In other cases, for example chloramphenicol- or phenylbutazone-induced aplasia, it is unlikely that the agent itself is leukaemogenic, but the persistence of an abnormal marrow permits the emergence of a leukaemic clone, perhaps as the result of a further insult: PNH might be regarded as evidence of this transformation. The possibility also arises that some cases of apparently idiopathic aplasia are in reality clonal disorders in which the abnormal clone is too small to be identified morphologically [191]. Such a situation might arise if, following an episode of severe bone marrow damage, a PNH or preleukaemic clone was relatively resistant to the agent causing the damage [159].

Secondly, AL may arise *de novo* as a hypoplastic marrow syndrome. Because of reduced marrow cellularity, the absolute number of blast cells can be difficult to quantify on aspirate, but trephine biopsy reveals the true nature of the disease. When over 30% of the total marrow cells are blasts, the criteria for the diagnosis of AL are fulfilled. Such cases may account

for up to 7.5% of patients with AML, although the majority are elderly. The condition has been called hypoplastic AL and hypocellular AL [192–194]. Splenomegaly is inconspicuous. There is always pancytopenia but an occasional blast cell is seen in the blood. The prognosis is poor: in one study of 15 cases the median survival was only 8 months [195]. In this series, 10 cases were classified as FAB M1, three as M2, one as M4 and one as lymphoblastic L2. Marrow cellularity may increase as the disease becomes more frankly blastic. Although the prognosis is poor, occasional remissions of hypoplastic AL have been reported.

Thirdly, MDS may present with a hypoplastic marrow, and the differential diagnosis can be difficult [63,195,196]. Most cases of this type fit the criteria for RA and RAEB; a few cases of hypoplastic CMML have been reported [63]. Again, this may evolve from previous aplasia, and some observers claim that a definite aplastic phase can be discerned as part of the natural history of MDS [197]. A sideroblastic phase may intervene between aplasia and AL [198]. The close association between aplastic anaemia and MDS has been emphasized by a number of recent clinical and morphological studies. Thus Applebaum *et al.* [199] found that some 4% of patients with morphologically 'typical' aplastic anaemia had acquired clonal abnormalities on cytogenetic analysis at diagnosis; these were often of the type seen in MDS. de Planque *et al.* [200], reporting on the European Co-operative Study, found that, 2 years after diagnosis of aplasia treated with antithymocyte globulin, 10% of patients demonstrated clonal cytogenetic abnormalities, while at 10 years 15% of cases showed clinical, cytogenetic or morphological evidence of clonal disorders [201,202]. In another study Tichelli *et al.* [203] found an incidence of clonal disorder of 42%, 15 years after an initial diagnosis of aplastic anaemia, in 117 patients. Comparable results were reported from a study in Manchester [204]. One cytogenetic abnormality characteristically found in hypoplastic MDS is trisomy 6; the morphological evidence of dysplasia is often rather inconspicuous, and the patients have sometimes responded to immunosuppressive therapy [205]. Whether the presence of a clonal abnormality in otherwise 'typical' aplastic anaemia confers a worse prognosis is at present unclear, but a patient with an abnormality characteristic of MDS, such as 5q–, monosomy 7 or trisomy 8, should probably be regarded as having preleukaemia and treated as such. However, Bacigalupo's group have shown that cytogenetic abnormalities in aplastic anaemia may disappear [206], so further studies of the natural history of these cases is required; they might be analogous to the spontaneous remissions occasionally occurring in MDS, PNH and even AL. Fohlmeister *et al.* [197,207] found that the presence of dysplastic micromegakaryocytes, a focal increase in megakaryocytes, or an increase in marrow reticulin were all particularly associated with later evolution to leukaemia and suggested that these cases were better classified as hypocellular MDS. These, and other, studies suggest that a proportion of patients classified at present as examples of acquired aplastic

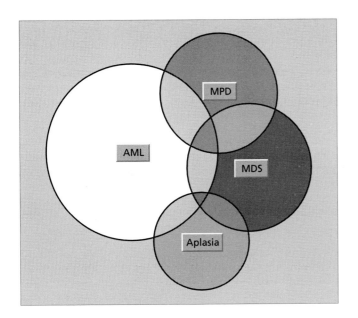

Fig. 11.5 Venn diagram showing the overlapping domains of AML, MDS, myeloproliferative syndromes (MPD) and some cases of aplastic anaemia (aplasia). Cases showing transitional features are increasingly recognized, but may be difficult to classify.

anaemia (AA) have a potentially preleukaemic disease, and that in some the marrow disorder is of a clonal nature *ab initio* (Fig. 11.5) [208], although it is also possible that the use of immunosuppressive therapy to treat aplasia is responsible. Analysis of clonality in such patients with DNA probes [208] may be of use in ascertaining whether attempts to distinguish between aplastic anaemia and hypocellular MDS are justifiable and meaningful. However, Young [210] has recently discussed the pitfalls in interpreting evidence of clonality in bone marrow cells from patients with AA.

Overlap between the myelodysplastic syndrome and myeloproliferative disorders

Whereas the morphological hallmark of MDS is abnormal maturation, with quantitative and functional deficiencies of the end cell, the myeloproliferative disorders (MPD) are characterized, for most of their course, by overproduction of one or more cell lines without, at least at first, conspicuous morphological or functional defects. Nevertheless, a number of recent studies have illustrated the overlap between these groups. CMML is an obvious example, as is the type of RARS associated with thrombocytosis. The monosomy 7 syndrome in children also occupies the borderline between (MPD) and MPS. Again, diagnostic difficulty may arise in the later stages of classic CML, dysplastic features becoming prominent as the disease enters an 'accelerated' phase [183]. The same is true of polycythaemia vera; although AL often seems to erupt explosively in this disease, in other cases it may be preceded by a

period of MDS [211], and in most cases this can be attributed to previous myelosuppressive therapy, although it has also been recorded in patients treated by venesection alone [212]. Of course, the previous history and, usually, conspicuous extramedullary haemopoiesis will distinguish such cases, but there are others in which classification is difficult. These cases are sometimes referred to as 'atypical' myeloproliferative disorders, and the clinical features, morphology and natural history share features of both MPD and MDS, although, in general, survival is less good than in classic MPD. A number of karyotypic abnormalities, such as monosomy 7, trisomy 8, 13q–, t(1;7) and 20q–, are seen in both MDS and MPD [182]. The inference must be that a particular genetic lesion in the haemopoietic cell may be expressed in different ways, giving rise to different haematological pictures. The morphological and clinical features of the disease, which emerge following this genetic insult, may be determined by humoral factors and cellular interactions in the marrow environment.

Myelofibrosis in the myelodysplastic syndrome

Significant marrow fibrosis, usually reticulin, rarely collagen, has been defined in a number of patients with MDS, and is especially common in secondary MDS. Reports are often confusing, referring to 'mild' or 'marked' fibrosis [110], and early reports probably included some cases which would now be classified as AML: this could be true of the patients described by Sultan *et al.* [213] under the label 'acute myelodysplasia with myelofibrosis'. These patients had a clinical course similar to that of those with AML, and had pancytopenia, or leucoerythroblastosis, fibrotic marrows with trilineage dysplasia and increased numbers of blasts, although their lineage was undecided.

It is not certain how this syndrome differs from 'malignant myelosclerosis', described by Lewis & Szur [214], some 18 years earlier, and by Bearman *et al.* [215] and Manohoran *et al.* [216]. The patients in these reported groups also had rapidly fatal diseases, often with severe systemic symptoms, such as fever, and the later studies emphasized the presence of megakaryocytic hyperplasia; some, at least, of these cases would now be classified as M7 on the FAB criteria, although progression from a pre-existing MPD cannot be excluded in others [110]. The diagnosis of AL may not be possible from poorly cellular aspirates, but trephine biopsy, when it reveals that 30% of the identifiable cells are blasts, confirms the diagnosis [108,217].

Another group of patients has a more chronic course and display, usually, multiple cytopenias, fibrotic marrows with trilineage MDS, and, sometimes, extramedullary haematopoiesis. Poikilocytosis is often marked, although the tear-drop cells characteristic of chronic myelofibrosis are not always seen. The usual features of MDS have been present, and ALIP may be demonstrated. The difficulties in assigning a diagnostic label to these cases have been emphasized by

Verhoel *et al.* [218], while Pagliuca and his colleagues [219] describe in detail the haematological and histological features of 10 such cases. The mean survival rate in this last group was 30 months, i.e. comparable to that in nonfibrotic MDS, but others have reported a less good prognosis. Occasionally these cases seem to respond to high-dose corticosteroids.

Therapy-related myelodysplasia

Therapy-related myelodysplasia (t-MDS) and leukaemia are now recognized as serious complications of chemotherapy and/or radiotherapy given for a variety of malignant and, occasionally, nonmalignant diseases [220]. These complications were initially reported in patients treated for Hodgkin's disease and myeloma; however, the more widespread and intensive use of alkylating agents and DNA–topoisomerase II inhibitors, which can damage haemopoietic cells, and the improved survival of the patients concerned, have resulted in leukaemia/MDS being seen more often in patients with solid tumours, including non-Hodgkin's lymphomas, breast, lung, ovarian and other cancers [99,221].

Such cases may account for as many as 10–15% of AML patients seen [222]. The clinical and pathological features of therapy-related leukaemias are discussed in greater detail in Chapter 12. Early studies (before the introduction of the FAB criteria) did not distinguish between leukaemia and MDS, although many of the reported patients had fewer than the definitive 30% bone marrow blasts. It was clear, however, that the majority of such patients evinced a preleukaemic phase, characterized by cytopenias and morphological abnormalities in blood and bone marrow [223,224]. This preleukaemic phase may be overlooked and falsely attributed to myelosuppression from chemotherapy, or to progression of the primary disease. More recently, reviews have distinguished between therapy-related leukaemia and t-MDS, and some have attempted to classify the latter according to FAB definitions [225,226]. Presentation as MDS may account for at least 50% of all cases of therapy-related leukaemia and t-MDS, and at least 50% of these will evolve, if the patient survives, into AL.

The poor prognosis of t-MDS has been repeatedly emphasized, with many patients succumbing to infections or bleeding caused by cytopenias, while showing no evidence of progression to AL or of the primary malignant disease [225,227]. Chemotherapy and/or radiotherapy probably cause an irreversible mutation in the haemopoietic stem cell, with its clonal proliferation subsequently leading to the evolution of AL; immune suppression is probably an important contributing factor [228]. The incidence of t-MDS in large, treated patient groups has not been defined accurately, but it is probably higher than that for AL itself, because some patients die from the primary disease before the latter becomes manifest. The haematological changes can be subtle, for example, macrocytosis or mild cytopenias, and may be overlooked. Biological and genetic abnormalities characteristic of MDS may be present in patients who appear clinically and morphologically

normal [229]. Factors influencing the risks of developing t-MDS include age (children are at less risk than adults), the primary disease, and the type, as well as the amount and duration of the treatment given. The leukaemogenic effects of different chemotherapeutic agents probably differ, but they have been best documented in relation to the alkylating agents, procarbazine and nitrosoureas [221,230], and more recently to etoposide and other DNA–topoisomerase II reactive drugs. This latter group often develop t-AML with no preleukaemic phase and are frequently associated with 11q23 abnormalities, whereas alkylating agents tend to be associated with whole or partial deletions of chromosomes 5 and/or 7 [231–235]. Pederson-Bjergaard *et al.* [232] suggest that there may be a synergistic leukaemogenic effect between the two classes of drug. Treatment with alkylator-based regimens and radiation, either concurrently or sequentially, does not appear to increase the risk of leukaemogenesis above that of drugs alone [236,237]. Recent reports have highlighted t-MDS/AML as a frequent and serious late complication of potentially curative transplant procedures (autologous marrow and peripheral blood stem cell transplants) for Hodgkin's and non-Hodgkin's lymphoma [238,239]; these patients are likely to have had particularly heavy treatment, and to exhibit residual immunosuppression.

The latency period from the start of treatment of the primary malignancy to the development of a therapy-related marrow disorder is usually about 4–5 years, but it may be many years. The risk peaks within the first decade after the chemotherapy for the primary disease, while the risks during the second decade are thought to be low [236]. As in primary MDS, the clinical manifestations are commonly related to cytopenias. Organomegaly and lymphadenopathy are uncommon. Anaemia and thrombocytopenia are the major features. Severe neutropenia at diagnosis (less than 0.5×10^9/l) is less common, but it may become more pronounced with time. There are few, if any, features in the blood which distinguish secondary from primary MDS, although oval macrocytes may be more conspicuous. However, the marrow is more commonly hypocellular than in *de novo* MDS and reticulin fibrosis is present in up to 50% of cases. Primary and secondary MDS with marrow fibrosis appear clinically and morphologically similar with a poor survival and megakaryocytic hyperplasia, although it has been suggested that there are some differences such as a higher number of megakaryoblasts in the primary form [240]. If obtainable, the marrow aspirate usually shows severe tri-lineage myelodysplasia [223].

Erythroid abnormalities are conspicuous from an early stage. Periodic acid-Schiff (PAS) stain often shows diffuse or granular positivity [223] and micro- and megakaryocytes are commonly conspicuous, especially with monosomy 7. All these features may be seen in *de novo* MDS, but it is our impression, as well as that of others [225,241], that the dysplasia is more pronounced than in *de novo* MDS, especially when fewer than 5% blasts (FAB types RA and RAS) are present. The presence of the primary disease may cause further confusion, for

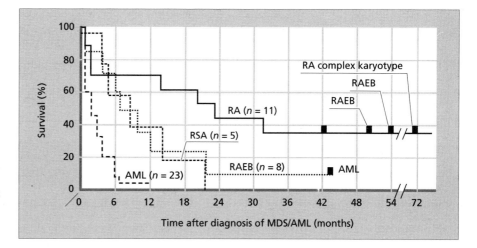

Fig. 11.6 Prognosis of secondary MDS/AML showing the poor prognosis in secondary MDS/AML of all morphological types seen at Manchester Royal Infirmary and Christie Hospital, Manchester over approximately 8 years.

example plasmablasts or residual lymphoma. Subclassification of t-MDS cases according to FAB criteria has been attempted in some reports [225,226], although this can prove difficult and some cases cannot readily be classified in this way [241]. The value of such attempts at classification remains debatable as, with the possible exception of those classed as RA, the prognosis is equally poor.

Several studies have emphasized the poor outlook of patients with t-MDS [225,227]. About half will evolve into an AL that is generally refractory to conventional therapy. Other patients succumb to the effects of cytopenias without progression to t-AML, but there is little difference in survival between the two groups. Figure 11.6 shows our experience of cases classified into FAB groups. Survival was somewhat better for patients with RA. Patients with therapy-related RSA fared badly, in contrast to the expected outcome in *de novo* disease. A similar, higher than expected rate of evolution to AML from therapy-related RARS was seen by Kantarjian *et al.* [227]. Pederson-Bjergaard & Preben [242] found that complete remission of the primary tumour, or a malignant lymphoma as the primary tumour, was the most significant independent prognostic factor for longer survival. Other factors included the platelet count, the number of chromosomal aberrations, the haemoglobin and the percentage of blasts in the marrow. However, even with the three most favourable prognostic factors, the predicted 5-year survival in their study was still depressingly low. The series of Kantarjian *et al.* included 57 cases of t-MDS whose median survival was only 45 weeks [227]. Age, cytogenetic pattern and marrow blast percentage emerged as important prognostic features for survival.

Paediatric myelodysplasia

Myelodysplasia appears to be a rare disorder in childhood, although it seems likely that such cases have been underdiagnosed. In the UK a National Registry for paediatric myelodysplasia has been set up and in the future, may yield more information about the incidence of these disorders, and lead to a widely accepted classification. A small number (about 17%) of childhood AML cases seem to be preceded by a preleukaemic phase [243]. Studies have suggested that MDS accounts for between 1.1 and 8.7% of haematological malignancies in childhood [244,245]. Congenital bone marrow disorders, such as Fanconi's anaemia and Schwachman's syndrome, may develop MDS as a prelude to AML, and these conditions should be considered in any child who presents with cytopenias and morphological evidence of myelodysplasia in blood and/or marrow. Other predisposing conditions for childhood MDS/AML include the constitutional chromosome disorders trisomy 21 (Down's syndrome) and trisomy 8, DNA repair deficiency syndromes such as ataxia telangiectasia, Bloom's syndrome, xeroderma pigmentosum and the Li–Fraumeni syndrome [246]. Children with neurofibromatosis show a higher than expected rate of both juvenile chronic myeloid leukaemia (JCML) and typical CML. MDS arising when a congenital bone marrow disorder is already present has been termed 'secondary' MDS. Therapy-related MDS in children has been described, especially after chemotherapy for Hodgkin's disease and ALL, although children may be at less risk than adults. Nevertheless, in view of the greater life expectancy of children, a higher proportion of cases might be expected to transform to AML and this appears to be the case. Bone marrow transplantation is the only curative treatment available at present.

There is little published literature dealing specifically with paediatric myelodysplasia and the FAB group have yet to develop a classification suitable for this disease in children. Chessells recently proposed a classification (Table 11.5) which included JCML and infantile monosomy 7 syndrome, both of which show morphological evidence of myelodysplasia and are the commonest forms of myelodysplasia seen in paediatric practice [247]. The classification includes some other conditions having myeloproliferative as well as myelodysplastic features, such as those seen in Down's syndrome. Others feel, however, that the conventional FAB criteria can be usefully applied to most cases of childhood MDS. In a recent review of

Table 11.5 Classification of paediatric myelodysplasia. (From Chessells, 1991 [246], with permission.)

Primary myelodysplasia
    Juvenile chronic myeloid leukaemia (JCML)
    Infantile monosomy 7 syndrome
    Refractory anaemia (RA)
    Refractory anaemia with ring sideroblasts (RARS)
    Refractory anaemia with excess blasts (RAEB)
    Refractory anaemia with excess blasts in transformation (RAEB-t)

Proliferative MDS
    Down's sydrome
    MDS with eosinophilia
    Atypical CML
    Familial MDS
    Miscellaneous

Secondary myelodysplasia
    Familial
    Therapy induced

110 cases, the more advanced forms of MDS (RAEB and RAEB-t) accounted for 64% of cases whereas CMML (18%) was less common [248,249].

Juvenile chronic myeloid leukaemia was distinguished from the adult type of CML some 30 years ago [249]. It is sometimes referred to as CMML of childhood in French and European literature, a name which Chessells feels may be more appropriate [247], although it has some distinctive features that set it apart from the typical adult form of CMML. The condition is commoner in boys and there is an association with neurofibromatosis [251,252]. It presents with pallor, splenomegaly, generalized lymphadenopathy and bleeding from thrombocytopenia. A facial rash, often with a butterfly distribution, may be present at diagnosis and this can also precede other features by many months. The rash can involve the trunk and, when biopsied, shows an infiltrative lesion consisting of lymphocytes and histiocytes. Cutaneous xanthomas may be present. Progression of the disease is accompanied by wasting, lymphadenopathy, often suppurative, and progressive splenomegaly. The blood count usually shows anaemia, thrombocytopenia and a raised white cell count but not usually greater than $50 \times 10^9/l$, while the blood film shows monocytes, eosinophils, abnormal neutrophils and occasional blast cells. The marrow shows monocytosis and blast cells, as well as trilineage myelodysplasia, with similarities to CMML described in adults. The appearances may resemble the infantile monosomy 7 syndrome [253], although the platelet count is lower and the HbF level is usually raised to more than 10% in JCML [254]. Erythrocytes may show a fetal red cell enzyme pattern. Cytogenetic analysis may be abnormal but there are no consistent abnormalities [252]. In culture there is spontaneous growth of macrophage colonies without the need for added GM-CSF. Chessells [247] reports a median age of diagnosis of 3 years and a poor median survival of only 6 months in

14 children seen in her clinic over a period of 20 years. Currently, allogeneic bone marrow transplantation would seem to be the treatment of choice and, in view of the poor prognosis, alternative donors should be looked for in the absence of a suitable sibling donor. A frank blast transformation, as seen in Ph+ CML, does not seem to occur, although there may be an increase in blast cells and normoblastaemia as the disease progresses.

The infantile myelodysplasia: syndrome with monosomy 7 was initially described by Teasedale *et al.* in 1970 [255]. The disease is commoner in boys, presenting with recurrent infections, cytopenias and splenomegaly. A rash similar to that in JCML may be seen occasionally [247]. The morphology of the blood and marrow may resemble RA, RAEB or JCML. Bleeding is a less prominent feature than in JCML and thrombocytopenia is milder. The fetal haemoglobin is rarely above 10%. Cytogenetic analysis shows metaphases lacking a chromosome 7 in a variable, but usually major, proportion of the cells. There is an autonomous growth of macrophage colonies in culture, as in JCML [253]. Neutrophils show defective chemotaxis and chemokinesis; this may account for the high susceptibility to bacterial infection which appears to be a prominent clinical feature of the syndrome. The median survival in infantile monosomy 7 appears better than in JCML, although there is a predilection for the subsequent development of AML. Some patients may experience a prolonged remission from intensive AML chemotherapy, but bone marrow transplantation appears to be the treatment of choice. Questions remain regarding the timing of the procedure and the precise role for intensive chemotherapy.

There is little information regarding the forms of primary MDS that are seen more commonly in adults. Refractory anaemia with ring sideroblasts appears to be very rare and must be distinguished from the congenital sideroblastic anaemias in which the mean corpuscular volume (MCV) is reduced and dysplastic changes are seen only in the erythron. The possibility of an underlying mitochondrial cytopathy should be considered. These patients may have metabolic acidosis, cortical neurological impairment or evidence of multiorgan dysfunction, but the haematological manifestations may be the sole clinical features over a long period of time. Haemopoiesis is neither clonal nor cytogenetically abnormal. The diagnosis is confirmed by the demonstration of a deletion in mitochondrial DNA [256]. Other studies have reported a predominance of the more aggressive forms of MDS, i.e. RAEB and RAEB-t, with a high rate of evolution to AML [257]. Intensive chemotherapy does not yield long remissions, and this, again, suggests that bone marrow transplantation prior to the development of AML is the best option.

A recent report summarized the clinical, morphological and cytogenetic features in 68 children with myelodysplasia presenting to a single institution—the largest group of cases published so far [258]. Using the conventional FAB system of classification, 50% of the cases were categorized as CMML, with RA and RAEB the next most common subtypes. The prognosis was very variable and the classification thus of limited use. The addition of features, such as HbF level and cytogenetics, to the FAB system allowed the incorporation of JCML and infantile monosomy 7 syndrome, resulting in patient groups with significant differences in survival. The proportion of blasts in the blood or marrow, or the presence of ALIP, were not significant variables, and the Bournemouth score was not a sufficient discriminant. A prognostic scoring index based on platelet count, HbF level and cytogenetic complexity did, however, identify groups with highly significant differences in survival. A HbF level of greater than 10%, a platelet count of less than $40 \times 10^9/l$ and a complex karyotype (i.e. two or more clonal or structural abnormalities) were each allowed one point. Patients with a score of zero had a 5-year survival of 61.6% (CI 33–84%), whereas those with a score of two or three all died within 4 years of diagnosis. This revised classification may, in the future, prove helpful in making treatment choices in paediatric MDS.

Children with Down's syndrome have a 27-fold increased risk of developing acute leukaemias, especially acute lymphoblastic and the otherwise uncommon M7 variant, but they can also develop a myeloproliferative syndrome in the neonatal period known as transient abnormal myelopoiesis (TAM), which may resemble an acute leukaemia but usually regresses spontaneously. Some children who develop TAM do go on to develop AL after 6 months to 3 years, but the precise relationship between the two is not fully established. The true incidence of TAM is not clear. Clinically affected babies have enlargement of the liver and the spleen and the blood count shows macrocytosis with many blast cells. Moderate anaemia is usually present and the platelet count is variable. Myelodysplastic features may be seen in the blood film. Progressive marrow failure does not occur and treatment is supportive. It has been suggested that the blast cells seen in TAM may be multipotent stem cells [259]. TAM has been seen in apparently normal children who are actually mosaics for trisomy 21; the proliferating cells are those with the trisomy 21 karyotype. Zipursky *et al.* [260] recently summarized their experience in 23 cases of MDS occurring in Down's syndrome. MDS was characterized by thrombocytopenia, dysmegakaryocytopoiesis and increased megakaryoblasts. The most common abnormal karyotype was trisomy 8, which was present in almost half the patients.

Diagnosis

In most cases, careful scrutiny of blood film and marrow appearances permits a confident diagnosis of MDS, but in some the haematologist has to rely on more sophisticated methods to confirm the diagnosis. The diagnosis of MDS is based on quantitative and qualitative changes in the blood and marrow, as described above, which cannot be attributed to any other cause. Among the differential diagnoses which must be

carefully excluded in this age group are nutritional deficiencies, drug-induced dyshaemopoiesis, metabolic disturbances such as hypothyroidism and liver failure, alcoholism, the anaemia of chronic dis-orders, immune cytopenias including those due to HTLV infection and nonhaematological malignancies. The presence of a clonal abnormality in marrow cells, and clonal abnormalities of the proliferative capacity of cultured marrow, provide supportive evidence. Greenberg and his colleagues have defined leukaemic growth patterns as microcluster or macrocluster formation with defective maturation and persistence of blast cells within the cell aggregates, or very low colony formation [261]. However, GM-CFU studies in MDS have given variable results and may be of greater value in following evolution than in making an initial diagnosis. Thus Rosenthal & Moloney [93] found normal patterns in some patients with refractory 'dysmyelopoietic' anaemia. Our own studies [37] suggested that, although proliferative defects were often more conspicuous in patients with preleukaemia than in cytopenia as a result of other forms of marrow disease, there was overlap between the two groups, so that in an individual patient this test might not be discriminating. The greatest difficulty arises in relation to patients who present with isolated cytopenias, or dysplasia of only one cell lineage, and in whom marrow cytogenetic analysis is normal. 'Minimal criteria' for the diagnosis of preleukaemic MDS have not been defined by the FAB group, but Linman & Bagby [262] and Saarni & Linman [27] proposed such criteria in a retrospective analysis of their patients. These did not include an increase in marrow blast cells. It is of interest that even when carefully defined criteria are used, mistakes may occur. For example, Todd & Pierre [263] used morphological criteria defined by Saarni & Linman prospectively to study 326 patients: 31 (10%) of these, who were labelled as preleukaemic, eventually recovered, achieving normal blood counts, and 5% progressed to agnogenic myeloid metaplasia. Tricot [264] has suggested that the diagnosis of MDS should be considered in the context of cytopenia only when other conditions known to produce dyshaematopoiesis are excluded, and the patient either (i) shows dysplasia of at least two cell lines on marrow aspirate and/or trephine, or (ii) if exhibiting an abnormality of only a single cell line, also shows an acquired clonal chromosome abnormality in the marrow. The presence of Pelger cells and micromegakaryocytes together seems to distinguish preleukaemia from other refractory cytopenias [265]. Culligan & Jacobs [266] have proposed a 'spectrum' of diagnostic certainty in MDS, ranging from those patients who have only minimal dysplasia, but normal karyotype and progenitor cell growth ('uncertain, possibly early MDS'), to those with overt trilineage dysplasia, or clonal cytogenetic abnormality, X-linked monoclonality, or abnormal progenitor cells in the peripheral blood ('MDS confirmed'). It is likely that the haematologist will make increasing use of X-linked DNA polymorphisms and *RAS* mutations to corroborate a morphological suspicion of MDS; for example, Anttila *et al.*

[267] have recently reported on the value of studies of DNA methylation of the calcitonin-5 gene to identify MDS amongst elderly patients who present only with solitary macrocytosis.

Cytogenetic abnormalities in primary and secondary myelodysplastic syndrome

Up to 70% of patients with MDS show cytogenetic abnormalities, of which 5q–, monosomy 7 and trisomy 8 are the commonest; in others the chromosomal abnormality may be 'submicroscopic'. Fluorescence *in situ* hybridization (FISH) is increasingly used to demonstrate cytogenetic abnormalities in these patients: the technique has improved the specificity of cytogenetic analysis, and the identification of cell lineages involved in suspected clonal proliferations [130]. These are discussed in more detail in Chapter 3. Despite the morphological association of the 5q– abnormality, there is no distinctive cytogenetic aberration in the preleukaemic syndrome that is not also found in AML. However, there are significant differences in the incidence of the various abnormalities. In preleukaemia t(8;21) and t(15;17) are rare, as is the Philadelphia chromosome t(9;22). On the other hand, 5q– and 20q– abnormalities are more common. Monosomy 7 is seen in a wide spectrum of myeloid disorders, especially in children, where it may be 'familial'. The precise role of deletion of one chromosome 7 in the pathogenesis of myeloid dysplasias is not understood, but Fenaux and his colleagues have suggested that –7 could be a cytogenetic marker for myeloid leukaemia that develops in the context of either a constitutional genetic instability, or acquired genotoxic damage, rather than the primary initiating event [129]. The 20q– deletion has been particularly associated with RARS, although in a review of 174 cases of MDS, Knapp [268] found that no chromosome abnormality was specifically associated with any preleukaemia or MDS classification. However, structural rearrangements of the short arm of chromosome 12 were found to occur in 15% of cases of CMML reported by Heim & Mitelman [269]. The t(5;12) breakpoint has recently been cloned; it results in fusion of a novel gene, *TEL*, to the platelet-3 derived growth factor receptor beta gene [270]. Chromosomal abnormalities are more frequently found in RAEB and RAEB-t than in other types of MDS, while in secondary MDS, complex abnormalities involving multiple chromosomes are characteristic [271]. Chromosomal loss or gain, or interstitial deletions, are much more characteristic of MDS than translocations, although these do occur in 5% of cases (Table 11.6), and are particularly associated with DNA–topoisomerase II reactive drugs. The prognostic value of the FAB subtypes is enhanced when combined with cytogenetic patterns, and Yunis *et al.* [272] have proposed a prognostic classification based on cytogenetic analysis. The presence of a cytogenetically abnormal clone in the marrow does not necessarily mean that the patient will develop leukaemia, and some studies have shown little difference in survival in patients with a single stable abnormality and those with normal karyotypes [273]. The worst prognosis is found in patients with multiple or complex lesions, but patients with hypodiploid karyotypes also fare badly [274]. The evolution of a new karyotypic abnormality can herald a change in the tempo of the disease and may be associated with a change in morphology, or increasing blast count [275]. The persistence of some normal metaphases, on the other hand, seems to correlate with a better prognosis [12]. Occasionally an abnormal clone may disappear from the marrow, and this has rarely accompanied spontaneous remission of the marrow disorder [276,277]. In one case, remission followed withdrawal of immunosuppressive therapy for a connective tissue disorder [228].

Cytogenetic findings in therapy-related myelodysplasia/acute myeloblastic leukaemia

Cytogenetic findings have been reported in several large series of t-MDS/AML [278–281]. Abnormalities, which are usually complex, are more commonly found than in primary MDS and the number of abnormalities seen per case tends to be greater [281], with chromosome numbers 5 and 7 being most often affected. These may take the form of monosomies, or partial deletions of the long arms of these chromsomes, sometimes as single changes but more commonly in association with other abnormalities. Le Beau *et al.* [282] found that 45 out of 47 t-MDS patients showed abnormalities of chromosomes 5 and/or

Chromosomal loss or gain	Deletions	Translocations	Others
–5	5(q13.3–33.1)	(1;3)(p36;q21)	
–7	(7q)x	(1;7)(p11;p11)	inv(3)(q21,q26)
–17	11(q14–23)	(2;11)(p21;q23)	i(17q)
–Y	12(p11–13)	(6;9)(p23;q34)	
+8	(13q)x	(11;21)(q24;q11 i.e. q11.2)	
+21	20(q11–13)		

Table 11.6 Single recurring karyotypic abnormalities in primary and therapy-related MDS. (From Mufti, 1990 [187], with permission.)

– = Monosomy; + = trisomy; p = short arm; q = long arm; bands deleted are shown in brackets; inv = inversion of chromosome bands; i = isochromosome; x = deletions are of variable size.

7. The frequent involvement of these chromosomes has been noted by others. The most common abnormalities seen are −7 (41%), del 5q− (28%), −5 (11%) and der(21q−)(9%). Other abnormalities sometimes seen include 7q−, +8, der(12p), t(1,7), −12, der(17p), der(3p), der(6p), der(3q), der(11q), −17, −18 and der(19q) [283]. The type of therapy may influence the type of cytogenetic abnormality which evolves. In the series of t-MDSs/AML of Kantarjian *et al.* [227], chromosomes 5 and/or 7 abnormalities were significantly more common in patients treated with alkylating agents, procarbazine and nitrosoureas, compared to patients receiving other drugs or irradiation alone. Similarly, Pederson-Bjergaard *et al.* [232] found a correlation between prior therapy with alkylating agents, a preceding myelodysplastic phase, and abnormalities of these chromosomes. The same authors, in an update of 91 cases of t-MDS/AML [242], analysed chromosomal aberrations to determine whether they were consistently present in all abnormal metaphases, or only in some. The inference is that the former could represent primary cytogenetic events during leukaemogenesis and be of crucial importance in the pathogenesis of the disease, although *RAS* mutations may occur before the appearance of monosomy 7. Consistently observed abnormalities, in addition to those involving chromosomes 5 and 7, included 11q23 rearrangements (particularly associated with DNA–topoisomerase II reactive drugs), monosomies 17 and 18 (17q aberrations, 3q rearrangements), trisomy 1q and rearrangement of 21q [232,242].

Clinical course and prognosis

Preleukaemic MDS is a serious diagnosis. Although there is some variation, and rare spontaneous remissions do occur [276,277], most studies have reported median survivals of less than 30 months: Tricot [284] found that only 8% of patients survived more than 5 years after the diagnosis. Most patients with MDS are elderly, and they frequently die of marrow insufficiency before AL develops, infection being particularly common; in one series of 86 patients, 64% died of infection [285]. It is not known whether all patients would progress to the stage of AL if they lived long enough. In some studies, patients who died of AL actually lived longer than those who did not, emphasizing the dangers of infection or haemorrhage in this phase of the disease. There is a wide variation in the incidence of AL in the various published series. Hoelzer *et al.* [12] reviewed the clinical findings and prognosis of 962 published cases of MDS and found that 297 patients (31%) developed leukaemia, Foucar *et al.* [139], analysing the natural history of 109 cases of MDS according to the FAB classification, found that the five morphological subtypes separate into only two disease groups when survival and cause of death are considered. Patients with RA or RARS are more likely to survive or die of unrelated disorders, while those classified as RAEB-t had a median survival of only 6 months.

In general, patients with an increase in marrow blasts have a poor prognosis; however, long survival does occasionally occur, even in the presence of conspicuous blastic infiltration of the marrow (Fig. 11.7). The great majority of patients transform to FAB types M2, M4 or M6, but ALL and even biphenotypic AL have been described [287–290]. Progression from MDS to ALL with the Ph chromosome has been described [291]. Most lymphoid transformations from previous MDS seem to display early B (CD10−, CD19+, TdT+) or hybrid myeloid–lymphoid phenotypes; unlike the situation in lymphoblastic transformation of classical CGL, the common ALL phenotype CD10+ CD19+ is unusual [292]. T-cell lymphoblastic transformation has also been defined in a case of MDS [293].

The features associated with a poor prognosis include: increasing age; severity of anaemia, granulocytopenia or thrombocytopenia at diagnosis; increasing blood or marrow blast count; abnormal localization of immature precursors (ALIP) in the bone marrow trephine; the presence of monosomy 7 or complex cytogenetic abnormalities, and organomegaly. A number of scoring systems have been devised to predict survival, using quantitative or qualitative features in MDS based on the FAB classification; these should reflect both the severity of marrow failure and the risk of acute leukaemia. The best known is the Bournemouth score which assesses the severity of pancytopenia and blastic infiltration of the marrow [294]. In CMML, patients with high leucocyte counts fared worse than those with neutrophil counts of less than 16×10^9/l or monocyte counts of less than 2.6×10^9/l, and the score has been modified in respect of this MDS subtype [295]. Other studies have confirmed that the severity of dysmegakaryocytopoiesis and dysgranulopoiesis has some correlation with survival [296], although patients with erythroid hyperplasia may fare better than those with erythroid depression. Aul's group [297] have defined an alternative prognostic profile. In their scale 1 'point' is allotted to each of the following: marrow blast count >5%, LDH >200, haemoglobin <9 g/dl and platelet count <100 × 10^9/l. Three groups were defined according to survival and risk of transformation. Low-risk patients (0 points) had a 91% 2-year survival and negligible risk of leukaemia. Corresponding figures for intermediate (1–2 points) or high-risk (3–4 points) patients were: 50% with 19% risk of AML, and 9% with 54% risk of AML. An international prognostic scoring system has recently been generated from a study of 816 patients with MDS. Age influenced survival but not risk of leukaemia [298].

A deterioration in GM-CFU proliferation, with micro- or macrocluster growth, often heralds the onset of AL. There is some correlation between the degree of marrow infiltration by blasts, plating efficiency and prognosis. Thus, Verma *et al.* [299] were able to identify five different growth patterns on culture; those patients whose marrows grew only clusters containing predominantly blast cells fared worse, and Spitzer *et al.* found similar correlations [300]. These results were often indistinguishable from those found in AL. In a recent review of

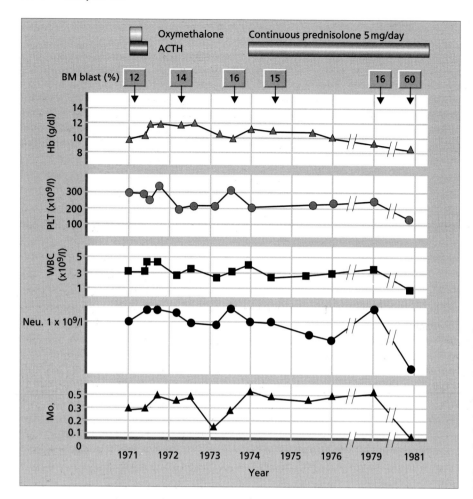

Fig. 11.7 Ten-year survival in a 52-year-old female patient with smouldering leukaemia. In spite of showing a significant increase in bone marrow (BM) blasts, the patient remained clinically well for much of this time, with only a slight peripheral blood cytopenia. Death followed shortly after an abrupt rise in BM blast count which coincided with the onset of more profound pancytopenia. The proliferative capacity of the marrow in respect of CFU-GM during the oligoblastic phase was drastically reduced. (From Geary, 1983 [285], with permission.) ACTH = adrenocorticotrophic hormone; Hb = haemoglobin; Mo. = monocytes; Neu. = neutrophils; PLT = platelets; WBC = white blood cells

marrow culture studies in 179 patients with various types of MDS, Greenberg was able to correlate clinical outcome with marrow growth *in vitro*. An interesting phenomenon was acquisition of resistance to the normal inhibitory action of prostaglandin E [261]. However, Francis *et al.* [301] demonstrated that perturbation of endogenous colony stimulating activity (CSA) may be a more discriminating prognostic indicator than colony growth per se. The rate of leukaemic transformation was greatest in those with raised CSA levels. Flow cytometry measurements of marrow DNA indicate a poor prognosis for patients with a high proportion of cells in G_0/G_1.

Treatment

Despite much effort and many clinical trials, no therapy, apart from allogeneic bone marrow transplantation, has been shown definitely to prolong survival in MDS patients [302]. The danger to life relates particularly to the consequences of marrow failure, and the risk of AL evolving at some time. There is wide variation in the clinical course of patients with these disorders, and any treatment recommended must be considered with the likely progress of a newly diagnosed case: the prognostic indices referred to previously are often useful.

Thus, many patients with RARS, and some with RA, lead an indolent course, and little treatment may be desirable, apart from correction of any underlying haematinic deficiency. Although high-dose pyridoxine is customarily given in sideroblastic anaemia, there is usually little response. Some patients in these groups, who have only mild thrombocytopenia and/or neutropenia, may suffer little disability, while others require occasional blood transfusions, although even elderly patients may tolerate surprisingly low haematocrits, in the absence of cardiovascular insufficiency. In these patients, the problems are similar to those in any patient with chronic marrow failure—in particular, intercurrent infection can seriously depress residual haemopoietic function. Androgenic steroids have been tried, but with little success, although Ruutu *et al.* have reported interesting results when androgens were used in combination with haemarginate [303]. The attenuated androgen danazol has been reported to be effective in improving thrombocytopenia, possibly by abrogating an associated immune-mediated mechanism rather than stimulating megakaryocyte production [304]. The role of corticosteroids is also rather controversial: although Bagby and his colleagues reported improvements in up to 15% of cases, which could be predicted by *in vitro* studies, other workers have not found them to be of sustained value, except in those cases where there is clear evidence of an associated autoimmune disease [61]. There have been few trials of immunotherapy in MDS; marrow GM-CFU growth improved after subcutaneous BCG inoculations, but this was not reflected in the peripheral blood counts [305]. Lithium salts are occasionally useful in profoundly neutropenic patients [306]. A recent report suggests that patients with RA and RAEB, as well as those with hypoplastic MDS, may respond to antithymocyte globulin [307].

Chemotherapy

Ablation of the dysplastic clonal proliferation is the logical radical treatment for MDS, but, except in those younger individuals who are candidates for allogeneic bone marrow transplantation (see Chapter 22), this is rarely achieved. Myelodysplasia, and AML evolving from it, are characterized by relative resistance to antileukaemic chemotherapy. The biological reasons for this are uncertain: one possibility is that, in MDS the residual normal stem cell pool is so much reduced that repopulation of the marrow, with remission, is rarely achieved; certainly the aplastic phase following chemotherapy is much longer in MDS than in AML patients. Nevertheless, studies of long-term bone marrow culture in MDS patients suggests that some patients at the less 'leukaemic' end of the spectrum do have identifiable normal haemopoietic precursors [308]; moreover, abrogation of a cytogenetically abnormal clone, with restoration of polyclonal haemopoiesis, has been described in occasional patients (see below). Alasano and his colleagues [309], using a PCR assay at the phosphoglycerate kinase locus on the X chromosome, analysed haemopoietic colonies cultured from five patients with MDS: three of the five had some polyclonal progenitors. The implication is that it may be possible to 'purify' these progenitors for autotransplantation. Interest is now focused, in particular, on acquisition of the multidrug-resistance gene (P-glycoprotein), which is commonly found in MDS patients and may reflect previous exposure to chemical mutagens, including cytotoxic drugs [310].

The advanced age of the majority of patients with MDS, who often have other diseases, renders intensive chemotherapy unsuitable in most cases. Nevertheless, recent experience has shown that complete remissions can be achieved in selected cases, although remission periods are substantially shorter than in AML patients [302,311]. Evaluation of the value of intensive chemotherapy in the various studies reported is difficult because of the small numbers involved, patient selection and different chemotherapy protocols [304]. Some of the best results reported have been from Michels *et al.* (61% CR in 31 patients with *de novo* RAEB-t) [312] and from de Witte's group, who observed CR rates of 57% in patients over the age of 45 and 71% for those under that age [313]. These figures are of particular interest, because they are similar to those obtained by the same team in patients with *de novo* AML; the corollary is that age is an important factor determining remission, whether the patient suffers from AML or MDS; nevertheless, the recent MRC trial has confirmed that evidence of a preceding myelodysplastic phase is an important adverse factor in determining outcome after chemotherapy. Estey and his colleagues, using intensive chemotherapy which included idarubicin, fludarabine and cytosine arabinoside, with or without G-CSF, has also reported remission rates in excess of 50% in patients over 60, including some with karyotypic abnormalities [311,314]. Nevertheless, most reports record short CR times, although remission is initially followed by complete haematological recovery. Thus, in a recent review, Loeffler *et al.* combined several series totalling more than 100 patients, and found the median duration of remission to be well below 12 months [315]. In the series reported by de Witte *et al.*, only 7% of patients were alive at 3 years; comparable results were reported from the Memorial Sloan Kettering Cancer Center. Estey's studies showed that, despite encouraging initial results, no patient over the age of 60 was in CR 2 years later. Apart from age, and previous cytotoxic chemotherapy, an abnormal karyotype is an important adverse factor in determining relapse-free survival rate [316]. So far, there is little information comparing the results of intensive chemotherapy in the various subgroups of MDS, as this has been attempted only rarely in RA and RARS, unless followed by allogeneic transplantation. However, RAEB-t at diagnosis and the presence of Auer rods were associated with better results in the series reported by Michels *et al.* [312]. Most, but not all, studies have suggested better results, in established MDS, if chemotherapy is started before evolution to frank AML, but most workers would not now attempt this therapy in patients over 65 who are still in a stable MDS phase. The chemotherapy of AML in elderly patients is discussed in Chapter 9.

Single-agent therapy

Patients with CMML, whose clinical and morphological features exhibit more conspicuously 'proliferative' features than other types of MDS, such as leucocytosis and splenomegaly, may respond to various types of cytotoxic therapy. Cytosine arabinoside, hydroxyurea, etoposide, mercaptopurine and busulphan have been used in these patients. The subject has been reviewed by Hamblin & Oscier [317]. Bagby [318] has suggested that in MDS patients in whom T-cell functional defects can be identified *in vitro*, azathioprine should be tried in small doses (e.g. 50 mg/day). Occasional successes have been reported in patients who have not responded to steroids.

Bone marrow transplantation

Experience with allogeneic marrow transplantation in MDS is accruing from a number of centres, and the international bone marrow transplant registries have now collected data on several hundred patients who have been transplanted for MDS. This has been summarized by de Witte & Gratwohl [319] and by Anderson *et al.* [320], and is discussed further in

Chapter 22. The disappointing results with intensive chemotherapy alone suggest that remission induction, when achieved, should be followed by transplantation, as a form of consolidation therapy. In the case of high-grade MDS this is best done earlier than later, and the evidence is that the eventual outcome is influenced by the proportion of residual blasts in the marrow at the time of transplantation, with those patients who are morphologically in complete remission faring best. Autologous transplants may be feasible if sufficient numbers of polyclonal stem cells can be identified in MDS patients.

One analysis of cases reported to the European Bone Marrow Transplant group showed a 3-year disease-free survival in 32% of patients transplanted for RAEB, and 27% of patients who had RAEB-t. The relapse rate is higher in patients with secondary MDS, whether transplanted in the MDS or frankly leukaemic stages. Experience from the Seattle group [320], where 50% of relapses occurred after the 12-month landmark, suggests that the outcome might be improved by more intensive conditioning. In low-grade MDS, there is as yet less experience, but a number of younger patients with RA and RARS have been transplanted with disease-free survival rates of 50% or more; conditioning regimens must include marrow ablative radiotherapy or chemotherapy [321]. Patients with the morphological and clinical features of severe aplastic anaemia, but with the cytogenetic abnormalities found in MDS, are probably best treated as cases of hypocellular MDS. Patients with RA and RARS under the age of 55 who have cytogenetic abnormalities, or cytopenias other than anaemia, or leukaemic *in vitro* growth characteristics, are best treated by chemotherapy and transplantation, if a donor is available, because the prognosis in this group is so poor. In younger patients without these characteristics, transplantation should still be considered; although few patients under the age of 50 with RARS have so far been reported, the inexorable progression of bone marrow failure in this disorder, as well as the risk of acute leukaemia, argues in favour of transplantation. Another consideration influencing early rather than late transplantation is that of sensitization to blood products if red cell or platelet transfusions become necessary, and iron overload, particularly in RARS.

Very few marrow transplants have so far been reported in CMML. O'Donnell *et al.* [321] reported on the progress of two cases: one died from transplant-related complications, but the other was alive 3 years later.

Differentiation therapy

The concept of differentiation therapy in the treatment of MDS is based on experimental maturation of leukaemic cell lines with simultaneous induction in self-renewal capacity. Theoretically, prolonged treatment could produce 'extinction' of the neoplastic clone and re-establishment of polyclonal haemopoiesis; indeed rare spontaneous remissions of MDS

have been reported [277]. A number of agents have been studied in clinical practice: these include cytosine arabinoside, vitamin D analogues, 13-*cis* retinoic acid, and interferons (IFN) alpha and gamma. Haemopoietic growth factors also fall into this category and are considered below. Cytosine arabinoside can induce differentiation of certain leukaemic cell lines cultured *in vitro*, and in 1979 Baccarani & Tura [322] reported that a patient with RAEB treated with small doses of this agent responded with clinical improvement and amelioration of the blood picture. There was also an improvement in marrow morphology without a complete remission. Many studies of the use of this agent have been reported. Although it was originally postulated that cytosine arabinoside was acting as a differentiating agent, improving maturation in the dysplastic cell line, clinical experience suggests that the beneficial effects, when they occur, reflect its cytotoxic action, following inhibition of DNA synthesis. Thus, responses do not usually occur unless at least 750 mg of the drug are given, and most patients who respond pass through a hypoplastic phase, reflected by a more profound thrombocytopenia in the blood [323]. The response is nevertheless of interest, because, as noted above, it confirms that some patients with MDS have a residue of normal (or at least, less dysplastic) haemopoietic stem cells. There is now a wide literature, but, unfortunately, a paucity of controlled trials, on the use of low-dose cytosine in MDS; some of the larger reports include AML as well as MDS patients [304]. A detailed analysis of 510 cases of AML and MDS treated with this agent concluded that although complete remissions of up to 17% were obtained in MDS patients, with a median response duration of about 15 months, the results were unpredictable and often involved episodes of potentially dangerous cytopenia, associated with periods of marrow hypoplasia [324]. Supportive therapy, particularly with platelet infusions, was often required and hospital admission necessary. Therefore, enthusiasm for low-dose cytosine use alone has waned, although it may be effective in selected patients [304], particularly as, in the only randomized trial reported so far, there was no important difference in the rate of progression to AML, or in the overall survival [325]. One recent trial has explored the combined use of cytosine arabinoside with retinioic acid (Medical Research Council), while there have also been small trials of cytosine arabinoside with cytokines (GM-CSF). So far, the clinical results have not been very impressive, although the rationale — haemopoietic growth factors induce proliferation of leukaemic cells and enhance the cytotoxicity of cytosine—is sound. A new cytarabine analogue, cytarabine ocfosfate, which can be given orally, has recently undergone trials in Japan, and may be suitable for outpatient administration: the results of this trial are awaited. The same group have described treatment of MDS patients using a new anthracycline (aclarubicin) in combination with very low dose cytosine, with some success [326].

A number of other cytotoxic agents have been tried as differentiating agents, including 6-mercaptopurine and etoposide

[327,328], which can both be given orally. There has recently been interest in 5-azacytidine as a cytotoxic differentiating agent [329,330]. This drug is a ring analogue of the pyrimidine nucleoside cytosine, and, like cytosine arabinoside, a cycle-specific agent with effects on DNA metabolism. Initial results were encouraging and the drug does enhance cellular differentiation, and subsequent evaluation suggested that it may be superior to low-dose cytosine arabinoside, although toxicity remains a problem [331]. Promising results were reported with a related analogue, 5 aza-2' deoxycytidine (Decitabine). Four of 10 patients, with previously resistant disease, achieved remissions [332].

Noncytotoxic differentiating agents

A number of other differentiating agents have been explored. 13-*cis*-retinoic acid has been used in MDS and acute promyelocytic leukaemia, and some early trials suggested improvements in up to 30% of patients with MDS [333]. Unfortunately, at the dosage required (up to 100mg/m² for several months) there was often unacceptable toxicity, with hyperkeratosis, stomatitis and hepatotoxicity being particularly troublesome [334]. Later in a double-blind randomized trial, MDS patients were treated with 13-*cis*-retinoic acid, or a placebo, and little benefit was discerned in the former group [335]. A number of later small trials also showed little benefit, including one in which alpha-tocopherol was used in order to reduce dermatological toxicity, and in which the patients were able to tolerate high doses of the retinoid. Other differentiating agents, such as 1:25 dihydroxyvitamin D_3, have only marginal effects in these patients, despite *in vitro* activity, although it has been suggested that dosage-limiting hypercalcaemia may prevent a response. New vitamin D analogues, which have less effects on calcium metabolism, are currently under investigation [336]. Yet another agent which has been investigated recently is hexamethylene bisacetamide (HEMBA), a compound related to dimethyl sulphoxide (DMSO), an agent very effective at producing differentiation in erythroleukaemia and HL-60 leukaemia cell lines. Improvement was usually transient, but it was of interest that one patient with MDS achieved a remission lasting some months [337].

Interferons

All three classes of interferons (leucocyte, fibroblast and immune) are able to suppress haemopoiesis, although there appears to be some difference in their mechanism of action. In the presence of IFNα, -β and -δ, colony formation by haemopoietic progenitor cells is reduced in culture. It was initially hoped that this effect might be more pronounced in relation to dysplastic haemopoiesis than normal progenitors, and anecdotal reports have suggested that isolated cases of MDS will respond to IFNα: in one case a karyotypic abnormality characteristic of MDS disappeared after treatment. However,

larger trials, sometimes using very large doses of interferon for prolonged periods, have shown only rather marginal improvements in blood counts [338], although sometimes marrow blasts have diminished. Moreover, the use of interferon does not seem to have delayed the onset of AL. Interferon has also been combined with other agents: for example, in one study a combination of IFNα, 1:25 dihydroxyvitamin D and retinoic acid in patients with MDS or AML gave results comparable to those obtained with cytarabine used alone, although marrow hypoplasia was less frequent than in the control group [339]. The effects of the different types of interferon can be augmented *in vitro* if combined with other biological agents such as tumour necrosis factor (TNFα), but there is little clinical information about the value of this combination so far. Future trials might combine the use of interferon with the various types of haemopoietic growth factor [340]. On present evidence, it may reasonably be concluded that interferon has much less predictable and beneficial effects in MDS than it does in patients with CML, but of course the side effects, particularly the flu-like syndrome encountered with large doses of interferon, are the same.

Haemopoietic growth factors

If the haematological defects in MDS are related to aberrations in the balance between self-renewal, proliferation and maturation, as has been demonstrated *in vitro*, these might be susceptible to the influence of recombinant haemopoietic growth factors (HGFs). There is now substantial experience in the use of these factors in MDS patients, although the important information about whether this therapy works by stimulating residual normal haemopoietic progenitor cells, or by inducing differentiation of leukaemic cells, is still inconclusive. As with differentiating agents, the latter mechanism could, theoretically, produce clonal extinction of the neoplastic cell line. Growth factors differ in their effects on different haemopoietic cell compartments. For instance, IL-3 and GM-CSF stimulate proliferation in early haemopoietic cell compartments, whereas G-CSF and M-CSF are able to provoke differentiation, as well as proliferation, in the 'committed' precursor cells by giving rise to granulocytes and monocytes.

Ganser & Hoelzer [341] and Greenberg [342] have recently reviewed the results using both GM-CSF and G-CSF in MDS patients. These authors recorded treatment of 232 patients with GM-CSF; about 80% showed a significant increase in their granulocyte counts. There was a reticulocytosis and rise in platelet count in, respectively, 20 and 6% of the patients, with a simultaneous increase in marrow cellularity. In a randomized trial using small doses of subcutaneous GM-CSF for periods of up to 90 days, the patients in the treatment arm had significant increases in neutrophils, monocytes and eosinophils and, importantly, a halving in the infection rate compared with the control arm. In another trial, involving 40 MDS patients, half of whom had RA, G-CSF was given for periods of 7 or 14 days [343]. Most of the patients showed significant increases in neutrophil counts, and, interestingly, some showed a decrease in marrow blast counts. Seven of the 11 patients who had infections before therapy was commenced experienced resolution of the infection. Most workers noted an improvement in neutrophil function, as shown by studies of *in vitro* chemotaxis and phagacytosis, and this was often sustained for some weeks or months after treatment. There are adverse effects of GM-CSF treatment, and some patients have found fever and bone pain to be troublesome; capillary leakage also occurs. There is some evidence that extramedullary haemopoiesis, reflected in increasing splenomegaly, may be influenced by GM-CSF treatment. Earlier fears that cytokines might cause acceleration of blast cell kinetics have not been realized, although it seems unwise to use them in RAEB-t.

Taken together, although there is less information on G-CSF in MDS, these studies suggest that both GM-CSF and G-CSF are useful in treating life-threatening neutropenia and/or infections in these patients, but there is still little information so far on their use as prophylactic long-term therapy. Greenberg has shown that G-CSF is more effective at promoting differentiation, compared with proliferation in MDS cells [261,342]. A number of multicentre control trials are currently in progress to elucidate their effect on infection rates and overall survival. One interesting combination is that of the synergistic effects of low-dose cytosine arabinoside with GM-CSF in myelodysplasia. The cytoxic drug has been given in both low and conventional doses. These protocols have been used in RAEB and RAEB-t patients, but so far the response rates do not seem to differ substantially from the use of low-dose cytosine arabinoside alone.

Interleukins 3 and 6

Both these cytokines have been used as treatments for patients with MDS, particularly in an attempt to increase the platelet count. Generally the results have been rather disappointing, although in one trial using IL-6, platelet counts in five of 16 thrombocytopenic patients did rise, with two patients achieving counts of over 50×10^9/l. Since IL-3 acts mainly on early progenitors, it is possible that combination with cytokines acting on later progenitors might have a synergystic effect. Some recent trials with IL-3 have been reviewed [302,331].

Erythropoietin

Several investigators have found that serum erythropoietin (EPO) levels are lower than might be expected for the severity of anaemia in patients with MDS, although there is considerable variation. Recombinant human (EPO) at pharmacological doses has been used by several groups in order to treat the hypoproliferative anaemia of MDS, by overcoming defective erthyroid maturation. Generally, results have been rather disappointing and it is now clear that 'inappropriately' low endogenous EPO levels do not always predict response to the treatment; usually the patients have required high doses of erythropoietin, presumably reflecting a decreased responsiveness of the dysplastic marrow cells to erythropoietins. One review of recent experience with r-EPO involving 308 patients in 15 different trials suggested that up to 20% of MDS patients showed some response, although those with substantial transfusion requirements often did not respond well [302]. Evidence is also conflicting as to whether patients with a specific class of MDS, such as RARS, are more likely to respond. Rose *et al.* found that RA patients with EPO levels less than 100 U/l had a response rate of 54% [344]. Ganser & Hoelzer have produced a meta-analysis of published reports on the efficacy of EPO in MDS patients — those responding had no transfusion needs, endogeneous EPO levels less than 200 U/l, absence of marrow ring sideroblasts, and, probably, absence of a cytogenetic abnormality [345]. Interest has now moved to the use of EPO with other growth factors such as G-CSF. As EPO acts mainly on committed erythroid progenitors, it is logical to combine treatment with a cytokine acting at an earlier stage, in the hope of enhancing E-BFU production, as has been demonstrated *in vitro*. Early information does indeed suggest that a combination of G-CSF with EPO is more effective than the use of recombinant EPO alone. Further details of these studies are awaited, but it is of interest that patients with refractory sideroblastic anaemia, who usually show a poor response to erythropoietin alone, have been reported to show a response rate of up to 60% [346].

Conclusions

Only ablation of the neoplastic haemopoietic clone, with parallel reconstitution of normal haemopoiesis, can cure a patient with MDS. Relatively few patients are suitable candidates for allogeneic bone marrow transplantation at present, and for the rest manipulation of the haemopoietic defect, with a veiw to improving peripheral cytopenias, and supportive therapy, must suffice. Differentiation therapy has so far been rather disappointing, but it is still in its infancy; the fact that a few patients do respond, occasionally dramatically, but unpredictably, indicates the heterogeneity of the underlying disease and its biological defect. It is possible that the use of differentiating agents, in combination with newer HGFs, might prove more effective. A better understanding of the genetic and molecular abnormalities underlying the bone marrow defect is needed; this might permit the identification of particular patient groups that are not necessarily recognizable solely by morphology, who might respond to different agents, perhaps combined with appropriate chemotherapy [304,340].

Relationship of myelodysplasia to acute myeloid leukaemia and other clonal marrow disorders

Morphological features suggest that certain cases of apparently *de novo* AML arise, in reality, out of pre-existing MDS that had not been recognized clinically [347]. These include a relatively low marrow blast cell count, erythroid hyperplasia with megaloblastic features, dysplastic megakaryocytes, or the presence of the 5q– lesion. However, in a recent study of 332 patients with AML, 11.7% of whom showed trilineage MDS, no excess of abnormalities of chromosomes 5, 7 or 8 were noted, although evidence of MDS was seen particularly in patients with erythroleukaemia [348]. AML associated with inversion of chromosome 3 is commonly preceded by a phase of MDS. If trilineage myelodysplasia is identified, it may recur after chemotherapy-induced remission is obtained, and has been labelled 'post-leukaemic' myelodysplasia by Foucar *et al.* [349]. As previously noted, ring sideroblasts may reappear after successful therapy of AML with a previous, sideroblastic phase. Generally, the prognosis in such cases is worse than in AML without dysplastic features, although 'postleukaemic' phases may be extended [349,350]. Jowitt *et al.* have shown that 'clonal' remissions of AML are often characterized by residual morphological evidence of dysplasia [351]. Fialkow *et al.* [352] have suggested that AML in children and young adults is a different disease to that occurring in the elderly, where a preleukaemic phase is more likely to be detected clinically and morphologically. These differences may reflect different target cells within the hirearchy of haemopoietic stem cells, with the disease in older people arising at a more primitive level. Distinctive biological features characterizing the two groups have been identified [353].

The morphological spectrum seen in MDS overlaps with that of the chronic myeloproliferative disorders as well as with AL. This is best seen in relation to CMML, but some cases described as atypical myeloproliferative disease, with or without myeloid metaplasia, often show dysplastic features. Indeed, some features seen in MDS do occur in the later stages of polycythaemia vera, and in agnogenic myeloid metaplasia. RARS may evolve into myelofibrosis, agnogenic myeloid metaplasia or even polycythaemia, while marrow fibrosis is encountered in MDS. Moreover, as noted previously, there now seems to be a close relationship between some cases of congenital and acquired aplastic anaemia and MDS, so it may be legitimate to identify a spectrum of marrow morphology which includes AML, MDS, MPD and aplastic anaemia. Such a scheme will accommodate the transitional cases noted above which are often difficult to classify by existing rules (see Fig. 11.4).

References

1 Von Leube W. (1990) Uber einen fall von rapid verlaufender schwerer Anaemie mit gleichzeitiger leukamischer Beschaffenheit des Blutes. *Berliner Klinische Wochenschrift*, **37**, 851–1900.

2 Hamilton-Paterson J.L. (1949) Pre-leukaemic anaemia. *Acta Haematologica (Basel)*, **2**, 309–316.

3 Bjorkman S.E. (1956) Chronic refractory anaemia with sideroblastic bone marrow: a study of four cases. *Blood*, **11**, 250–259.

4 Galton D.A.G. (1984) The myelodysplastic syndromes. *Clinical and Laboratory Haematology*, **6**, 99–112.

5 Wilkinson J.F. & Israels M.C.G. (1935) Achrestic anaemia. *British Medical Journal*, **1**, 139–143, 194–197.

6 Block M., Jacobson L.O. & Bethard W.F. (1953) Preleukemic acute human leukaemia. *Journal of the American Medical Association*, **152**, 1018–1028.

7 Rheingold J.J., Kaufmann R., Adelson E. *et al.* (1963) Smouldering acute leukemia. *New England Journal of Medicine*, **268**, 812–815.

8 Mayer R.J. & Cannellos G.P. (1990) Pre-leukaemic syndromes and other myeloproliferative disorders. In: *Leukaemia* (eds E.S. Henderson & T.A. Lister), 5th edn, pp. 613–637. Saunders, London.

9 Melhorn D.K., Gross S. & Newman A.S. (1970) Acute childhood leukaemia presenting as aplastic anaemia: the response to corticosteroids. *Journal of Paediatrics*, **77**, 647–652.

10 Breatnack F., Chessels J.M. & Greaves M.F. (1981) The aplastic presentation of childhood leukaemia: a feature of common ALL. *British Journal of Haematology*, **49**, 387–393.

11 Kay H.E.M. (1983) The leukaemias: pathogenesis and treatment. In: *Diseases of the Blood* (eds R.M. Hardisty & D.J. Weatherall), p. 797–828. Blackwell Scientific Publications, Oxford.

12 Hoelzer D., Ganser A. & Heimpel H. (1984) 'Atypical' leukaemias: pre-leukaemia, smouldering leukaemia and hypoplastic leukaemia. In: *Leukaemia* (eds E. Thiel & S. Thierfelder), pp. 69–101. Springer Verlag, Berlin.

13 Miescher P.A., Favre H. & Beris P. (1991) Autoimmune myelodysplasias. *Seminars in Haematology*, **28**, 322–329.

14 Raz I., Shinar E. & Polliack A. (1984) Pancytopenia with hypercellular bone marrow — a possible paraneoplastic syndrome in carcinoma of the lung: a report of 3 cases. *American Journal of Haematology*, **16**, 403–408.

15 Barry R.E. & Salmon P.R. (1969) Recurrent leukaemoid reaction in pernicious anaemia complicated by gastric carcinoma. *British Medical Journal*, **2**, 612–613.

16 Ricard M.F., Sigaux F., Imbert M. *et al.* (1979) Complementary investigations in myelodysplastic syndromes. In: *Pre-leukaemia* (eds F. Schmalzl & K.P. Hellriegel), pp. 56–66. Springer Verlag, Berlin.

17 Dokal I.S., Cox T.M. & Galton D.A.G. (1990) Vitamin B_{12} and folate deficiency presenting as leukaemia. *British Medical Journal*, **300**, 1263–1264.

18 Costello C. (1988) Haematological abnormalities in human immunodeficiency virus (HIV) disease. *Journal of Clinical Pathology*, **41**, 71–715.

19 Zon L., Arlein C. & Groopman J.E. (1987) Haematological manifestations of the human immunodeficiency virus (HIV). *British Journal of Haematology*, **66**, 251–256.

20 Schneider D.R. & Picker L.J. (1985) Myelodysplasia in the acquired immunodeficiency syndrome. *American Journal of Clinical Pathology*, **84**, 144–152.

21 Bennett J.M., Catovsky D., Daniel M-T. *et al.* (1982) Proposals for the classification of the myelodysplastic syndromes. *British Journal of Haematology*, **51**, 189–199.

22 Boggs D.R., Wintrobe M.M. & Cartwright G.E. (1962) The acute leukaemias. Analysis of 322 cases and review of the literature. *Medicine (Baltimore)*, **41**, 163–175.

23 Roath S., Israels M.C.G. & Wilkinson J.F. (1964) The acute leukaemias: a study of 580 patients. *Quarterly Journal of Medicine*, **33**, 257.

24 Gross R., Hellriegel K-P. & Heller A. (1973) Zur Definition der Präleukaemia und zur differentiatial Diagnose Fruber Leukaemischer Veranderungen. *Deutsches Medizinisches Wochenschrift*, **98**, 895.

25 Dreyfus B. (1976) Pre-leukaemic states. I. Definition and classification. II. Refractory anaemia with an excess of myeloid blasts in the bone marrow (smouldering acute leukaemia). *Blood Cells*, **2**, 33–55.

26 Joseph A.S., Cinkotai K.I., Hunt L. *et al.* (1982) Natural history of smouldering leukaemia. *British Journal of Cancer*, **46**, 160–166.

27 Saarni M.I. & Linman J.W. (1973) Pre-leukaemia: the haematological syndrome preceding acute leukaemia. *American Journal of Medicine*, **55**, 38–48.

28 Cartwright R.A., Alexander F.E. McKinney P.A. & Ricketts T.J. (1990) *Leukaemias and Lymphomas: an atlas of distribution within areas of England and Wales 1984–1988*. Leukaemia Research Fund, London.

29 Aul C., Gatterman N. & Schneider W. (1992) Age-related incidence and other epidemiological aspects of myelodysplastic syndromes. *British Journal of Haematology*, **82**, 358–367.

30 Williamson P.J., Kruger A.R., Reynolds P.J., Hamblin T.J. & Oscier D.G. (1994) Establishing the incidence of the myelodysplastic syndrome. *British Journal of Haematology*, **87**, 743–745.

31 Levine E.G. & Bloomfield C.D. (1992) Leukaemias and myelodysplastic syndrome secondary to drug, radiation and environmental exposure. *Seminars in Oncology*, **19**, 47–84.

32 Reizenstein P. & Dabrowski L. (1991) Increasing prevalence of the myelodysplastic syndromes: an International Delphi study. *Anticancer Research*, **11**, 1069–1070.

33 Farrow A., Jacobs A. & West R.R. (1988) Myelodysplasia and association with chemicals and other environmental factors (Abstract). *British Journal of Haematology*, **69**, 122.

34 West R.R., Stafford P.A., Farrow A. & Jacobs A. (1995) Occupational and environmental exposures and myelodysplasia: a case control study. *Leukaemia Research*, **19**, 127–139.

35 Prchal J.T., Throckmorton D.W., Carroll A.J. *et al.* (1978) A common progenitor for human, myeloid and lymphoid cells. *Nature*, **274**, 590–591.

36 Pierre P.V. (1974) Pre-leukaemic states. *Seminars in Haematology*, **11**, 73–92.

37 Milner G.R., Testa N.G., Geary C.G. *et al.* (1977) Bone marrow culture studies in refractory cytopenias and 'smouldering' leukaemia. *British Journal of Haematology*, **35**, 251–261.

38 Greenberg P.L. & Mara B. (1979) The pre-leukaemic syndrome. Correlation of *in vitro* parameters of granulopoiesis with clinical features. *American Journal of Medicine*, **66**, 951–959.

39 Lidbeck J. (1980) *In vitro* colony and cluster growth in haemopoietic dysplasia (the pre-leukaemic syndrome). *Scandinavian Journal of Haematology*, **24**, 412–420.

40 Jacobson R.J., Raskind W., Sacher R.A. *et al.* (1982) Refractory anaemia (RA), a myelodysplastic syndrome: clonal development with progressive loss of normal committed progenitors. *Blood*, **60**(Suppl.), 129a.

41 Janssen J.W., Buschle M., Layton M. *et al.* (1989) Clonal analysis of myelodysplastic syndromes; evidence of multipotent stem cell origin. *Blood*, **73**, 245–248.

42 Killmann S.A. (1976) Pre-leukaemia: does it exist? *Blood Cells*, **2**, 81–95.

43 Geary C.G., Catovsky D., Wiltshire E. *et al.* (1975) Chronic myelomonocytic leukaemia. *British Journal of Haematology*, **30**, 289–302.

44 Rowley J.D., Golomn H.M. & Vardiman J.W. (1981) Non-random chromosome abnormalities in acute leukaemia and dysmyelopoietic syndromes in patients with previously treated malignant disease. *Blood*, **58**, 759–767.

45 Tricot G., Boogaerts M.A., De Wolff-Peeters, H. *et al.* (1985) The myelodysplastic syndromes: different evolution patterns based on sequential morphological and cytogenetic investigations. *British Journal of Haematology*, **59**, 659–670.

46 Koeffler H.P. & Golde D.W. (1980) Human preleukaemia. *Annals of Internal Medicine*, **93**, 347–353.

47 Raskind W.H., Tirumali N., Jacobson R. *et al.* (1984) Evidence for a multistep pathogenesis of a myelodysplastic syndrome. *Blood*, **63**, 1318–1323.

48 Beris P. (1989) Primary clonal myelodysplastic syndromes. *Seminars in Haematology*, **26**, 216–233.

49 Bennett J.M., Catovsky D., Daniel M-T. *et al.* (1976) Proposals for the classification of the acute leukaemias. *British Journal of Haematology*, **33**, 451–458.

50 Hamblin T.J. & Oscier D.G. (1987) The myelodysplastic syndrome: a practice guide. *Haematological Oncology*, **5**, 19–34.

51 May S., Smith S.A., Jacos A. *et al.* (1985) The myelodysplastic syndrome: analysis of laboratory characteristics in relation to the FAB classification. *British Journal of Haematology*, **59**, 311–319.

52 Vallespi M.T., Torrabadell M., Irriguible D. *et al.* (1985) Myelodysplastic syndromes: a study of 101 cases according to the FAB classification. *British Journal of Haematology*, **61**, 83–92.

53 Varela B.L., Chuang C. & Bennett J.M. (1982) Clinical significance of the new proposals for the classification of the myelodysplastic syndromes. *Blood*, **60**(Suppl. 1), 140a.

54 Lichtmann M.A. & Brennan J.K. (1995) Myelodysplastic disorders. In: *Williams Hematology* (eds E.B. Beutler, M.A. Lichtman, B.S. Coller & T.J. Kipps), 5th edition, pp. 257–272. McGraw-Hill, New York.

55 Fenaux P., Estienne M.H., Lai J.L. *et al.* (1990) *De novo* myelodysplastic syndromes (MDS) in adults aged 50 or less. Clinical course and comparison with older patients. *Blood*, **76**(No. 10, Suppl. 1), 269.

56 Duguid J.K.M., Mackie M.J. & McVerry B.A. (1983) Skin infiltration associated with chronic myelomonocytic leukaemia. *British Journal of Haematology*, **53**, 257–264.

57 Pagliuca A. & Mufti G.J. (1992) Clinicomorphological features of myelodysplastic syndromes. In: *The Myelodysplastic Syndromes* (eds G.J. Mufti & D.A.G. Galton), pp. 1–13. Churchill Livingstone, Edinburgh.

58 Soppi E., Nousiainen T., Seppa A. & Lahtinen R. (1989) Acute febrile neutrophilic dermatosis (Sweet's syndrome) in association with myelodysplastic syndromes: a report of three cases and a review of the literature. *British Journal of Haematology*, **73**, 43–47.

59 Green A.R., Shuttleworth D., Bowen D.T. & Bentley D.P. (1990) Pathogenesis and clinical variations in patients with myelodysplastic syndromes. *British Journal of Haematology*, **74**, 364–365.

60 Pendry K., Harrison C. & Geary C.G. (1991) Myelodsyplasia

presenting as autoimmune haemolytic anaemia. *British Journal of Haematology*, **79**, 139–140.

61 Enright H., Jacob H.S., Vercellotti *et al.* (1995) Paraneoplastic autoimmune phenomena in patients with myelodysplastic syndromes: response to immunosuppressive therapy. *British Journal of Haematology*, **91**,403–408.

62 Kouides P.A. & Bennett J.M. (1996) Morphology and classification of the myelodysplastic syndromes and their pathological variants. *Seminars in Hematology*, **33**, 95–110.

63 Tuzuner A.V., Cox C., Rowe J.M., Watrous D. & Bennett J.M. (1995) Hypocellular myelodysplastic syndromes: new proposals. *British Journal of Haematology*, **91**, 612–617.

64 Jacobs A. & Clark R.E. (1986) Pathogenesis and clinical variations in myelodysplastic syndromes. *Clinics in Haematology*, **15**, 925–951.

65 Bowen D.T. & Jacobs A. (1989) Primary acquired sideroblastic anaemia in non-anaemic or minimally anaemic patients. *Journal of Clinical Pathology*, **42**, 56–58.

66 Williamson P.J., Oscier D.G., Bell A.J. & Hamblin T.J. (1991) Red cell aplasia in myelodysplastic syndrome. *Journal of Clinical Pathology*, **44**, 431–432.

67 Hast R. (1978) Studies on human preleukaemia. IV. Clinical and prognostic significance of sideroblasts in a regenerative anaemia with hypercellular bone marrow. *Scandinavian Journal of Haematology*, **21**, 396–402.

68 Hast R. & Reizenstein P. (1981) Sideroblastic anaemia and development of leukaemia. *Blut*, **42**, 203–207.

69 Boivin P., Galand C., Hakim J. *et al.* (1975) Acquired erythroenzymopathies in blood disorders: study of 200 cases. *British Journal of Haematology*, **31**, 531–543.

70 Newman D.R. (1973) Studies on the diagnostic significance of hemoglobin F levels. *Mayo Clinic Proceedings*, **48**, 199–205.

71 Boehme W.M. (1978) Acquired haemoglobin H in refractory sideroblastic anaemia. *Archives of Internal Medicine*, **138**, 603–606.

72 Anagnou N.P., Ley J.J., Chesbro B. *et al.* (1983) Acquired α-thalassaemia in pre-leukaemia is due to decreased expression of all four α-globin genes. *Proceedings of the National Academy of Sciences, USA*, **80**, 6051.

73 Salmon C.L. (1976) Blood group changes in pre-leukaemic states. *Blood Cells*, **2**, 211–220.

74 Dreyfus B., Sultan C., Rochant H. *et al.* (1969) Anomalies of blood group antigens and erythrocyte enzymes in two types of refractory anaemia. *British Journal of Haematology*, **16**, 303–312.

75 Xiros, Northoff H., Anger B. *et al.* (1987) Blood group changes in a patient with blast transformation of a myelodysplastic syndrome. *Blut*, **54**, 275–278.

76 Breton-Gorius J. (1979) Abnormalities of granulocytes and megakaryocytes in pre-leukaemic syndromes. In: *Preleukaemia*, (eds F. Schmalzl & K-P. Hellriegel), pp. 24–40. Springer Verlag, Berlin.

77 Davis A.T., Brunning R.D. & Quie P.G. (1984) Polymorphonuclear leucocyte myeloperoxidase deficiency in a patient with myelomonocytic leukaemia. *New England Journal of Medicine*, **285**, 789–790.

78 Heimpel H. (1979) Conventional morphological examination of blood and bone marrow cells in the diagnosis of pre-leukaemic syndromes. In: *Preleukaemia* (eds F. Schmalzl & K-P. Hellriegel), pp. 4–17. Springer Verlag, Berlin.

79 Felman P., Byron P.A., Gentilhomme O. *et al.* (1988) The syndrome of abnormal chromatin clumping in leucocytes: a myelodysplastic disorder with proliferative features. *British Journal of Haematology*, **70**, 49–54.

80 Scott C.S., Cahill A., Bynoe A.G. *et al.* (1983) Esterase cytochemistry in primary myelodysplastic syndromes and megaloblastic anaemias: demonstration of abnormal staining patterns associated with dyserythropoiesis. *British Journal of Haematology*, **55**, 411–418.

81 Schmalzl F. (1979) Cytochemical investigations on the blood and bone marrow cells in pre-leukaemia—demonstration of maturational abnormalities. In: *Preleukaemia* (eds F. Schmalzl & K-P. Hellriegel), pp. 48–55. Springer Verlag, Berlin.

82 Boogaerts M.A., Nelissen V., Roelant C. *et al.* (1983) Blood neutrophil function in primary myelodysplastic syndromes. *British Journal of Haematology*, **55**, 217–227.

83 Goasguen J.E., Bennett J.M. & Cox C. (1991) Prognostic implication and characterisation of the blast cell population in the myelodysplastic syndrome. *Leukaemia Research*, **15**, 1159–1165.

84 Tricot G., De Wolf-Peeters B., Hendrickx B. *et al.* (1984) Bone marrow histology in myelodysplastic syndromes. *British Journal of Haematology*, **57**, 423–430.

85 Weisdorf D.J., Oken M.M., Johnson G.J. *et al.* (1981) Auer rod positive dysmyelopoietic syndrome. *American Journal of Haematology*, **11**, 397–402.

86 Mufti G.J. (1992) A guide to risk assessment in the primary myelodysplastic syndrome. *Hematology/Oncology Clinics of North America*, **6**, 587–606.

87 Hamblin T. (1992) Immunologic abnormalities in myelodysplastic syndromes. *Hematology/Oncology Clinics of North America*, **6**, 571–586.

88 Colombat P., Renoux M., Lamagnere J.P. *et al.* (1984) T-cell function in refractory anaemia with excess blasts. *British Journal of Haematology*, **56**, 171–172.

89 Knox S.J., Greenberg B.R., Anderson R.W. *et al.* (1981) Studies of T-lymphocytes in preleukaemic disorders and acute nonlymphocytic leukaemia: *in vitro* radiosensitivity, mitogenic responsiveness, colony formation and enumeration of lymphocytic subpopulations. *Blood*, **61**, 449–455.

90 Murthy P.B., Kamada N. & Kuromoto A. (1984) Defective ultraviolet induced DNA repair in bone marrow cells and peripheral lymphocytes of patients with RAEB. *Japanese Journal of Clinical Oncology*, **14**, 87–91.

91 Abrahamson G., Boultwood J, Rack K. *et al.* (1990) An investigation of clonality in the myelodysplastic syndromes. *Blood*, **76**(Suppl. 1), 250.

92 Genitsen W.R., Donohue J. & Bauman *et al.* (1992) Clonal analysis of myelodysplastic syndrome: monosomy 7 is expressed in the myeloid lineage but not the lymphoid lineage, as detected by FISH. *Blood*, **80**, 217.

93 Rosenthal D.S. & Moloney W.C. (1984) Refractory dysmyelopoietic anaemia and acute leukaemia. *Blood*, **63**, 314–318.

94 Economopoulos T., Economidou J., Giannopoulos G. *et al.* (1985) Immune abnormalities in myelodysplastic syndromes. *Journal of Clinical Pathology*, **38**, 908–911.

95 Copplestone J.A., Mufti G.J., Oscier D.G. *et al.* (1985) Co-existent myelodysplasia in lymphoproliferative disorders. Proceedings of the British Society for Haematology Warwick. *British Journal of Haematology*, **61**, 557.

96 Monohoran A., Catovsky D., Clein P. *et al.* (1981) Simultaneous or spontaneous occurrence of lympho- and myeloproliferative disorders: a report of four cases. *British Journal of Haematology*, **48**, 111–116.

97 Dacie J.V. & Mollin D.L. (1966) Siderocytes, sideroblasts and sideroblastic anaemia. *Acta Medica Scandinavia*, **445**, 237–242.

98 Rosner F. & Grunwald H. (1974) Multiple myeloma terminating as acute leukaemia. Report of 12 cases and review of the literature. *American Journal of Medicine*, **57**, 922–939.

99 Park D.J. & Koeffler H.P. (1996) Therapy-related myelodysplasia. *Seminars in Hematology*, **33**, 256–273.

100 Copplestone J.A., Mufti G.J., Hamblin T.J. & Oscier D.G. (1986) Immunological abnormalities in myelodysplastic syndromes: II. Co-existent lymphoid or plasma cell neoplasms: a report of 20 cases unrelated to chemotherapy. *British Journal of Haematology*, **63**, 149–159.

101 Sultan Y. & Caen Y.P. (1972) Platelet dysfunction in preleukaemic states and various types of leukaemia. *Annals of the New York Academy of Science*, **201**, 300–306.

102 Maldonado J.E. & Pierre R.V. (1975) The platelets in preleukaemia and myelomonocytic leukaemia: ultrastructural cytochemistry and cytogenetics. *Mayo Clinic Proceedings*, **50**, 573–587.

103 Lintula R., Rasi V., Ikkala E. *et al.* (1981) Platelet function in preleukaemia. *Scandinavian Journal of Haematology*, **26**, 65–71.

104 Russell N.H., Keenen J.P. & Bellingham A.J. (1979) Thrombocytopathy in pre-leukaemia: association with a defect in thromboxane A_2 activity. *British Journal of Haematology*, **41**, 417–429.

105 Gatter K.C., Cordell J.L., Turley H. *et al.* (1988) The immunohistological detection of platelets, megakaryocytes and thrombi in routinely processed specimens. *Histopathology*, **13**, 257–267.

106 Erber W.N., Breton-Gorius J, Villeval J.L., Oscier D.G., Bai Y. & Mason D.Y. (1987) Detection of cells of megakaryocyte lineage in haematological malignancies by immuno-alkaline phosphatase labelling cell smears with a panel of monoclonal antibodies. *British Journal of Haematology*, **65**, 87–94.

107 Bartl R., Frisch B. & Baumgart. (1992) Morphological classification of the myelodysplastic syndromes (MDS): combined utilisation of bone marrow aspirates and trephine biopsies. *Leukaemia Research*, **16**, 15–33.

108 Rosati S., Anastasi J. & Vardiman J. (1996) Recurring diagnostic problems in the pathology of the myelodysplastic syndromes. *Seminars in Hematology*, **33**, 111–126.

109 te Velde J. & Haak H.L. (1977) Aplastic anaemia. Histological investigation of methacrylate embedded bone marrow biopsy specimens: correlation with survival after conventional treatment in 15 adult patients. *British Journal of Haematology*, **35**, 61–69.

110 Kampmeier P., Anastasi J. & Vardiman J.W. (1992) Issues in the pathology of the myelodysplastic syndromes. *Hematology/Oncology Clinics of North America*, **6**, 501–522.

111 Mangi M.H., Salisbury J.R. & Mufti G.J. (1991) Abnormal localisation of immature precursors in the bone marrow of myelodysplastic syndromes: current state of knowledge and future directions. *Leukaemia Research*, **16**, 627.

112 Bain B.J. (1990) *Leukaemia Diagnosis*, p. 48. Gower Medical Publishing, London.

113 Eastman P.M., Schwartz R. & Schrier S.L. (1972) Distinctions between idiopathic ineffective erythropoiesis and di Guglielmo's disease: clinical and biochemical differences. *Blood*, **40**, 487–499.

114 Heimpel H. (1979) Tests for diagnosis of pre-leukaemic states: round table discussion. In: *Preleukaemia* (eds F. Schmalzl & K-P. Hellriegel), pp. 139–146. Springer Verlag, Berlin.

115 Vilter R.W., Will J.J. & Jarrold T. (1967) Refractory anaemia with hyperplastic bone marrow (aregenerative anaemia). *Seminars in Haematology*, **4**, 175–193.

116 Dohy H., Genot J.Y., Imbert M. *et al.* (1980) Myelodysplasia and leukaemia related to chemotherapy and/or radiotherapy—a haematological study of 13 cases. Values of macrocytosis as an early sign of bone marrow injury. *Clinical and Laboratory Haematology*, **2**, 111–119.

117 Beris P.L., Graf J. & Miescher P.A. (1983) Primary acquired sideroblastic and primary acquired refractory anaemia. *Seminars in Haematology*, **20**, 101–113.

118 Craig A., Geary C.G., Love E.M. & Yin J.A.L. (1988) Red cell hypoplasia, thrombocytosis and leucocytosis: myelodysplastic and proliferative syndrome. *Journal of Clinical Pathology*, **41**, 1168–1170.

119 Fitchen J.H. (1985) Pure red cell aplasia: a preleukaemic state? In: *The Preleukaemic Syndrome* (ed. G.C. Bagby), pp. 63–70. CRC Press, Boca Baton, FL.

120 Dumont J. (1974) Clinical studies on 38 cases of chronic red cell aplasia in the adult. In: *Proceedings of the XV Congress International Society of Haematology, Jerusalem*, p. 543.

121 Lacombe C., Casaderall N., Muller O. *et al.* (1984) Erythroid progenitors in adult chronic pure red cell aplasia: relationship of *in vitro* erythroid colonies to therapeutic response. *Blood*, **64**, 71–77.

122 Van de Berghe H., Cassimann J.J., David G. *et al.* (1974) Distinct haematological disorder with deletion of long arm of no. 5 chromosome. *Nature*, **251**, 437–438.

123 Kerkhofs H., Hagemeijer A., Leeksma C.H.W. *et al.* (1982) The 5q- chromosome abnormality in haematological disorders; a collaborative study of 34 cases from the Netherlands. *British Journal of Haematology*, **52**, 365–381.

124 Abe S., Kohno S., Kubonishi I. *et al.* (1979) Chromosomes and causation of human cancer and leukemia XXXIII. 5q- in a case of acute lymphoblastic leukaemia (ALL). *American Journal of Haematology*, **6**, 259–266.

125 Van den Berghe H. (1986) The 5q- syndrome. *Scandinavian Journal of Haematology*, **36**, 78–81.

126 Dewald G.W., Davis M.P., Pierre R.V. *et al.* (1985) Clinical characteristics and prognosis of 50 patients with a myeloproliferative syndrome and deletion of part of the long arm of chromosome 5. *Blood*, **66**, 189–197.

127 Nimer S.D. & Golde D.W. (1987) The 5q- syndrome. *Blood*, **70**, 1705–1712.

128 Boultwood J., Rack K., Buckle V.J. *et al.* (1990) Homozygous deletion of FMS in a patient with the 5q- syndrome. *British Journal of Haematology*, **76**, 310–311.

129 Fenaux P., Morel P. & Luchai J. (1996) Cytogenetics of myelodysplasia. *Seminars in Hematology*, **33**, 127–138.

130 Pederson B. & Jensen I.M. (1991) Clinical and prognostic implications of chromosome 5q- deletions: 96 high resolution studied patients. *Leukemia*, **5**, 556–573.

131 Hast R. (1986) Sideroblasts in myelodysplasia: their nature and clinical significance. *Scandinavian Journal of Haematology*, **36**(Suppl. 45), 53–55.

132 Takeda Y., Sawada H. Sawai H. *et al.* (1995) Acquired hypochromic and macrocytic sideroblastic anaemia responsive to pyridoxine with low value of free erythrocytic protoporphyrin—a possible sub-group of idiopathic acquired sideroblastic anaemia. *British Journal of Haematology*, **90**, 207–209.

133 Jacobs A. (1986) Primary acquired sideroblastic anaemia. *British Journal of Haematology*, **64**, 415–418.

134 Bottomley S.S. & Mullen-Eberhard U. (1988) Pathophysiology of haem synthesis. *Seminars in Hematology*, **25**, 282.

135 Aski Y. (1980) Multiple enzymatic defects in mitochrondria in

hematological cells of patients with primary sideroblastic anaemia. *Journal of Clinical Investigation*, **66**, 43.

136 Bottomley S. (1993) Sideroblastic anaemias. In: *Wintrobe's Clinical Hematology* (eds G.R. Lee *et al.*), 9th edn. pp. 852–871. Lea & Febiger, New York.

137 Linman J.W. & Bagby C.G. (1976) The preleukaemic syndrome: clinical and laboratory features, natural course and management. *Blood Cells*, **2**, 11–31.

138 Carroll A.J., Doon M.C., Robinson N.C. & Gist W.M. (1986) Sideroblastic anaemia associated with thrombocytosis and a chromosome 3 abnormality. *Cancer Genetics and Cytogenetics*, **22**, 183.

139 Foucar K., Langdon R.M. & Armitage J.O. (1985) Myelodysplastic syndromes. A clinical and pathological analysis of 109 cases. *Cancer*, **56**, 553–562.

140 Kushner J.P., Lee G.R., Wintrobe M.M. *et al.* (1971) Idiopathic refractory sideroblastic anaemia. Clinical and laboratory investigation of 17 patients and review of the literature. *Medicine (Baltimore)*, **50**, 139–159.

141 Hussein K.K., Salem Z., Bottomley S.S. *et al.* (1982) Acute leukaemia in idiopathic sideroblastic anemia: response to combination chemotherapy. *Blood*, **59**, 652–656.

142 Lewy R. (1979) Leukemia in patients with acquired idiopathic sideroblastic anemia: an evaluation of prognostic indicators. *American Journal of Hematology*, **6**, 323.

143 Streeten R.R., Present C.A. & Reinhard E. (1977) Prognostic significance of thrombocytosis in idiopathic sideroblastic anemia. *Blood*, **50**, 427–432.

144 Cheng D.S., Kushner J.P. & Wintrobe M.M. (1979) Idiopathic refractory sideroblastic anaemia. Incidence and risk factors for leukaemic transformation. *Cancer*, **44**, 724–731.

145 Cazzola M., Barosi G., Gobbi P.G., Invernizzi R., Riccardi A. & Ascari E. (1988) Natural history of refractory sideroblastic anaemia. *Blood*, **71**, 305–312.

146 Williams M.D., Shinton N.K. & Finney R.D. (1985) Primary acquired refractory sideroblastic anaemia and myeloproliferative disease: a report of 3 cases. *Journal of Clinical and Laboratory Haematology*, **7**, 113–118.

147 Garand R., Gardais J., Bizet M. *et al.* (1992) Heterogeneity of acquired idiopathic sideroblastic anaemia (A.I.S.A.). *Leukaemia Research*, **16**, 463–468.

148 Gattermann N., Aul C. & Schneider W. (1990) Two types of acquired idiopathic sideroblastic anaemia. *British Journal of Haematology*, **74**, 45–52.

149 Sanz G.F., Sanz M.A., Vallespi T. & del Canizo MaC. (1990) Two types of acquired idiopathic sideroblastic anaemia. *British Journal of Haematology*, **75**, 633–634.

150 Hussein K.K., Salem Z., Bottomley S. & Livingstone R.B. (1982) Acute leukaemia in idiopathic sideroblastic anaemia: response to combination chemotherapy. *Blood*, **59**, 652–656.

151 Cazzola M., Barosi G., Berzuini C. *et al.* (1982) Quantitative evaluation of erythropoietic activity in dysmyelopoietic syndromes. *British Journal of Haematology*, **50**, 55–62.

152 May A., De Souza P., Barnes K. *et al.* (1982) Erythroblast iron metabolism in sideroblastic marrows. *British Journal of Haematology*, **52**, 611–621.

153 Greenberg P., Mara B., Bax I. *et al.* (1976) The myeloproliferative disorders: correlation between clinical evolution and alterations of granulopoiesis. *American Journal of Medicine*, **61**, 878–891.

154 Senn J.S., Curtis J.E., Pinkerton P.H. *et al.* (1980) The distribution of marrow granulopoietic progenitors among patients with preleukaemia. *Leukaemia Research*, **4**, 409–413.

155 Cartwright G.E., Edwards C.O. & Skolnick M.H. (1980) Association of HLA-linked hemochromatosis with idiopathic sideroblastic anaemia. *Journal of Clinical Investigation*, **65**, 980–992.

156 Yaouang J., Grosbois B., Jouanolle A.M., Goasquen J. & Leblay R. (1997) Haemochromatosis Cys282Tyr mutation in pyridoxine-responsive sideroblastic anaemia. *Lancet*, **349**, 1475–1476.

157 Dameshek W. (1969) A proposal for considering paroxysmal nocturnal hemoglobinuria (PNH) as a 'candidate' myeloproliferative disorder. *Blood*, **23**, 263.

158 Dacie J.V. & Lewis S.M. (1961) Paroxysmal nocturnal haemoglobin variation in clinical severity and association with bone marrow hypoplasia. *British Journal of Haematology*, **7**, 442.

159 Rotali B. & Luzatto L. (1989) Paroxysmal nocturnal haemoglobinuria. *Seminars in Haematology*, **26**, 201–207.

160 Lewis S.M., Pettit J.E., Tattersall M.H.N. *et al.* (1971) Myelosclerosis and paroxysmal nocturnal haemoglobinuria. *Scandinavian Journal of Haematology*, **8**, 451.

161 Wasi P., Kreutrachue M. & Na-Nakorn K. (1970) Aplastic anaemia–paroxysmal nocturnal haemoglobinuria syndrome-acute leukaemia in the same patient. The first record of such an occurrence. *Journal of the Medical Association of Thailand*, **53**, 656.

162 Orwoll R.L. (1985) Paroxysmal nocturnal haemoglobinuria: a preleukaemic syndrome? In: *The Preleukaemic Syndrome* (ed. G.C. Bagby), pp. 73–86. CRC Press, Boca Raton, FL.

163 Josten K.M., Tooze J.A., Borthwick Clarke C. *et al.* (1991) Acquired aplastic anaemia and paroxysmal nocturnal haemoglobinuria: studies on clonality. *Blood*, **78**, 3162–3167.

164 Zaccania A., Rosti G., Betti S. *et al.* (1982) Normal karyotype in seven patients with paroxysmal nocturnal haemoglobinuria. *British Journal of Haematology*, **57**, 333–334.

165 Van Kamp, Smit J.W., Van den Berg E., Halie R. & Vellenga E. (1994) Myelodysplasia following paroxysmal nocturnal haemoglobinuria: evidence for the emergence of a separate clone. *British Journal of Haematology*, **87**, 399–400.

166 Devine D.V., Gluck W.L., Ross W.F. & Weinberg J.B. (1987) Acute myeloblastic leukaemia in paroxysmal nocturnal haemoglobinuria. *Journal of Clinical Investigation*, **79**, 314–317.

167 Longo L., Bessler M., Beris P., Swirsky D. & Luzzatto L. (1994) Myelodysplasia in a patient with pre-existing paroxysmal nocturnal haemoglobinuria: a clonal disease originating from within a clonal disease. *British Journal of Haematology*, **87**, 401–403.

168 Hillmen P., Lewis S.M., Bessler M., Luzzatto L. & Dacie J.V. (1995) Natural history of paroxysmal nocturnal hemoglobinuria. *New England Journal of Medicine*, **333**, 1253–1258.

169 Dameshek W. (1969) The di Guglielmo syndrome revisited. *Blood*, **34**, 567–572.

170 Kass L. & Schnitzer B. (eds) (1975) *Refractory Anaemia*. C.C. Thomas, Springfield, IL.

171 Kass L. (ed.) (1979) *Preleukaemic Disorders*, C.C. Thomas, Springfield, IL.

172 Bennett J.M., Catovsky D., Daniel M.T. *et al.* (1985) Proposed revised criteria for the classification of acute myeloid leukaemia. *Annals of Internal Medicine*, **103**, 626–629.

173 Hayhoe F.G.J. (1988) Classification of acute leukaemias. *Blood Reviews*, **2**, 186–193.

174 Cuneo A., Van Orshoven A., Michaux J.L. *et al.* (1990) Morphologic, immunologic and cytogenetic studies in erythroleukaemia: evidence for multilineage involvement and identification of two distinct cytogenetic-clinicopathological types. *British Journal of Haematology*, **75**, 346–353.

175 Cohen J.R., Cregor W.P., Greenberg P.L. *et al.* (1979) Subacute myeloid leukaemia. *American Journal of Medicine*, **66**, 959–966.

176 Mufti G.J. & Galton D.A.G. (1986) Myelodysplastic syndromes: natural history and features of prognostic importance. *Clinics in Haematology*, **15**, 953–971.

177 Linman J.W. (1970) Myelomonocytic leukaemia and its pre-leukaemic phase (Editorial). *Journal of Chronic Diseases*, **22**, 713–715.

178 Tefferi A.B., Hoagland H.C., Therneau T.M. & Pierre R.V. (1990) Chronic myelomonocytic leukaemia: natural history and prognostic determinants. *Mayo Clinic Proceedings*, **64**, 1246–1254.

179 Martiat P., Michaux J.L. & Rodhair J. (1991) Philadelphia-negative chronic myeloid leukaemia: comparison with Ph+ CML and chronic myelomonocytic leukaemia. *Blood*, **78**, 205–211.

180 Galton D.A.G. (1992) Haematological differences between chronic granulocytic leukaemia, atypical chronic myeloid leukaemia, and chronic myelomonocytic leukaemia. *Leukaemia and Lymphoma*, **7**, 343–350.

181 Bennett J.M., Catovsky D., Daniel M.T. *et al.* (1994) The chronic myeloid leukaemias: guidelines for distinguishing granulocytic, atypical chronic and chronic myelomonocytic leukaemia. Proposals by the French–American–British Co-operative Leukaemia Group. *British Journal of Haematology*, **87**, 746–754.

182 Meccuci C. & Van den Berghe H. (1992) Cytogenetics in the myelodysplastic syndromes. *Hematology/Oncology Clinics of North America*, **6**, 523–541.

183 Muehleck S.D., McKenna R.W., Arthur D.C. *et al.* (1984) Transformation of chronic myelogeneous leukaemia: clinical morphological and cytogenetic features. *American Journal of Clinical Pathology*, **82**, 1–14.

184 Solal-Celigny P., Desaint B., Himera A. *et al.* (1984) Chronic myelomonocytic leukemia according to the FAB classification: analysis of 35 cases. *Blood*, **63**, 634–638.

185 Hurdle A.D.F., Garso O.M. & Buist D.G.P. (1972) Clinical and cytogenetic studies in chronic myelomonocytic leukaemia. *British Journal of Haematology*, **22**, 773–782.

186 Zittoun R. (1976) Subacute and chronic myelomonocytic leukaemia: a distinct haematological entity (Annotation). *British Journal of Haematology*, **32**, 1–7.

187 Mufti G.J. (1990) Myelodysplastic syndromes. In: *Current Medicine* 2 (ed. D.H. Lawson), pp. 119–136. Churchill Livingstone, Edinburgh.

188 Sexauer J., Kass L. & Schnitzer B. (1974) Subacute myelomonocytic leukemia. Clinical, morphological and ultrastructural studies of 10 cases. *American Journal of Medicine*, **57**, 853–861.

189 Jacobs A. (1989) Annotation: benzene and leukaemia. *British Journal of Haematology*, **72**, 119–121.

190 Young N.S. & Alter P. (1994) Bone marrow failure secondary to genetic injury. In: *Aplastic Anaemia, Acquired and Inherited*, pp. 46–67. W.B. Saunders, London.

191 Abkowitz J.L. & Adamson J.W. (1984) Clonal evolution in the pathogenesis of pancytopenia. In: *Aplastic Anemia—stem cell biology and advances in treatment* (eds N.S. Young, A.S. Levine & R.K. Humphries), pp. 71–82. Alan Liss, New York.

192 Beard M.E.J., Bateman C.J.T., Crowther D.C. *et al.* (1975) Hypoplastic acute myelogenous leukaemia. *British Journal of Haematology*, **31**, 167–176.

193 Howe R.B., Bloomfield C.D. & McKenna R.W. (1982) Hypocellular acute leukemia. *American Journal of Medicine*, **72**, 391–395.

194 Needleman S.W., Burns C.P., Dick F.R. *et al.* (1981) Hypoplastic acute leukaemia. *Cancer*, **48**, 1410–1414.

195 Fohlmeister I., Fischer R., Modder B. *et al.* (1985) Aplastic anaemia and the hypocellular myelodysplastic syndrome: histomorphological, diagnostic, and prognostic features. *Journal of Clinical Pathology*, **38**, 1218–1224.

196 Yoshida Y., Oguma S., Uchino H. *et al.* (1988) Refractory myelodysplastic anaemia with hypocellular bone marrow. *Journal of Clinical Pathology*, **41**, 763–767.

197 Fohlmeister I., Schaefer H.E., Hellriegel K-P. *et al.* (1979) Blood and bone marrow follow-up studies on patients with pre-leukaemic states—observation of different phases of the evolving leukaemic process. In: *Preleukaemia* (eds F. Schmalzl & K-P. Hellriegel), pp. 16–22. Springer Verlag, Berlin.

198 Geary C.G., Dawson D.W., Sitlani P.K. *et al.* (1975) An association between aplastic anaemia and sideroblastic anaemia. *British Journal of Haematology*, **27**, 337–344.

199 Applebaum F.R., Barrall J., Storb R. *et al.* (1990) Clonal cytogenetic abnormalities in patients with otherwise typical aplastic anaemia. *Experimental Haematology*, **15**, 1134–1139.

200 de Planque M.M., Kluin-Nelemans H.C. & van Krieken J.J. (1988) Long term follow up of severe aplastic anaemia patients treated with antithymocyte globulin. *British Journal of Haematology*, **73**, 121–126.

201 de Planque M.M., Kluin-Nelemans H.C. & van Krieken H.J. (1988) Evolution of acquired severe aplastic anaemia to myelodysplasia and subsequent leukaemia in adults. *British Journal of Haematology*, **70**, 55–62.

202 de Planque M.M., van Krieken H.J., Kluin-Nelemans M.C. *et al.* (1989) Bone marrow histopathology of patients with severe aplastic anaemia before treatment and at follow up. *British Journal of Haematology*, **72**, 439–444.

203 Tichelli A., Gratwohl A., Wursh A., Nissen C. & Speck B. (1988) Late haematological complications in severe aplastic anaemia. *British Journal of Haematology*, **69**, 413–418.

204 Narayanan M.N., Geary C.G., Freemont A.J. & Kendra J.R. (1994) Long term follow up of aplastic anaemia. *British Journal of Haematology*, **86**, 837–843.

205 Moormeier J.A., Rubin C.M., Le Beau M.M. *et al.* (1991) Trisomy 6: a recurring cytogenetic abnormality associated with marrow hypoplasia. *Blood*, **77**, 1397–1401.

206 Mikhailova N., Sessarego M., Fugazza G. *et al.* (1996) Cytogenetic abnormalities in patients with severe aplastic anaemia. *Hematologica*, **81**, 418–422.

207 Fohlmeister I., Fischer R. & Schaefer H.E. (1985) Preleukaemic myelodysplastic syndromes (MDS). Pathogenetic considerations based on retrospective clinicomorphological sequential studies. *Anticancer Research*, **5**, 179–188.

208 Marsh J.C.W. & Geary C.G. (1991) Is aplastic anaemia a preleukaemic disorder? Annotation. *British Journal of Haematology*, **77**, 447–452.

209 Van Kamp H., Landegent J.E., Jansen R.P.M., Willemze R. & Fibbe W.E. (1991) Clonal haematopoiesis in patients with acquired aplastic anaemia. *Blood*, **78**, 3209–3214.

210 Young N.S. (1992) The problem of clonality in aplastic anaemia: Dr Dameshek's riddle, restated. *Blood*, **79**, 1385–1392.

211 Shandas G.J., Spier C.M. & List A.F. (1991) Myelodysplastic transformation of polycythaemia vera: case report and review of the literature. *American Journal of Hematology*, **37**, 45–48.

212 Najean Y., Deschamps A., Dresch C. *et al.* (1988) Acute leukaemia and myelodysplasia in polycythaemia vera: a clinical study with long-term follow up. *Cancer*, **61**, 89–95.

213 Sultan C., Sigaux F., Imbert M. *et al.* (1981) Acute myelodysplasia

with myelofibrosis: a report of 8 cases. *British Journal of Haematology*, **49**, 11–16.

214 Lewis S.M. & Szur L. (1963) Malignant mycolsclerosis. *British Medical Journal*, **II**, 472–477.

215 Bearman R.M., Pangalis G.A. & Rappaport H. (1979) Acute ('malignant') mycolsclerosis. *Cancer*, **43**, 279–293.

216 Manohoran A. & Pitney W.R. (1977) Acute mycloblastic leukaemia with marrow fibrosis (malignant mycolsclerosis): acute leukaemia or malignant mycolsclerosis? *Australia and New Zealand Journal of Medicine*, **7**, 638–641.

217 Imbert M., Nguyen D. & Sultan C. (1992) Myelodysplastic syndromes and acute myeloid leukaemia with myelofibrosis. *Leukaemia Research*, **16**, 51–54.

218 Verhoel G.E.C., de Wolf-Peeters C. & Ferrant A. (1990) A case of myelodysplastic syndrome and myelofibrosis. *British Journal of Haematology*, **74**, 373–375.

219 Pagliuca A., Layton D.M., Manohoran A. *et al.* (1989) Myelofibrosis in primary myelodysplastic syndromes: a clinico-morphological study of 10 cases. *British Journal of Haematology*, **71**, 499–504.

220 Levine E.G. & Bloomfield C.D. (1986) Secondary myelodysplastic syndromes and leukaemias. *Clinics in Haematology*, **15**, 1037–1080.

221 Kantarjian H.M. & Keating M.J. (1987) Therapy related leukaemia and myelodysplastic syndrome. *Seminars in Oncology*, **14**, 435–443.

222 Keating M., Cork A., Broach Y. *et al.* (1987) Towards a clinically relevant cytogenetic classification of acute myelogenous leukaemia. *Leukaemia Research*, **11**, 119–133.

223 Foucar K., McKenna R.W., Arthur D.C. *et al.* (1985) Therapy related leukemia—a panmyelosis. *Cancer*, **43**, 1285–1296.

224 Vardiman J.W., Golomb H.M., Rowley J.D. *et al.* (1978) Acute non-lymphocytic leukemia in malignant lymphoma. A morphologic study. *Cancer*, **42**, 229–242.

225 Michels S.D., McKenna R.W., Arthur D.C. *et al.* (1985) Therapy related acute myeloid leukemia and myelodysplastic syndromes: a clinical and morphological study of 65 cases. *Blood*, **65**, 1364–1372.

226 Bennett J.M., Moloney W.C., Greene M.H. *et al.* (1987) Acute myeloid leukaemia and other myelopathic disorders following treatment with alkylating agents. *Haematologic Pathology*, **1**, 99–104.

227 Kantarjian H.M., Keating M.J., Walters R.S. *et al.* (1986) Therapy related leukaemia and myelodysplastic syndrome: Clinical, cytogenetic and prognostic features. *Journal of Clinical Oncology*, **4**, 1748–1757.

228 Renneboog B., Hansen V., Heimann P. *et al.* (1996) Spontaneous remission in a patient with therapy-related myelodysplastic syndrome (t-MDS) with monsomy 7. *British Journal of Haematology*, **92**, 696–698.

229 Cachia P.G., Taylor C., Thompson P.W. *et al.* (1994) Non-dysplastic myelodysplasia? *Leukaemia*, **8**, 677–681.

230 Rieche K. (1984) Carcinogenicity of anti-neoplastic agents in man. *Cancer Treatment Reviews*, **11**, 39–67.

231 Cortes J., O Brien S., Kantarjian H. *et al.* (1994) Abnormalities in the long arm of chromosome 11 (11q) in patients with *de novo* and secondary acute myelogenous leukaemia and myelodysplastic syndromes. *Leukaemia*, **8**, 2174–2178.

232 Pederson-Bjergaard J., Philip P., Larsen S.O. *et al.* (1993) Therapy-related myelodysplasia and acute myeloid leukaemia. Cytogenetic characteristics of 115 consecutive cases and risk in seven cohorts of patients treated intensively for malignant diseases in the Copenhagen series. *Leukaemia*, **7**, 1975–1986.

233 Rubin C.M., Arthur D.C., Woods W.G. *et al.* (1991) Therapy-related myelodysplastic syndrome and acute myeloid leukaemia in children: correlation between chromosomal abnormalities and prior therapy. *Blood*, **78**, 2982–2988.

234 Pederson-Bjergaard J., Daugaard G., Hansen S.W., Philip P., Larsen S.O. & Rorth M. (1991) Increased risk of myelodysplasia and leukaemia after etoposide, cisplatin and bleomycin for germ-cell tumours. *Lancet*, **338**(8763), 359–363.

235 Smith M.A., Rubvinstein L., Cazenave L. *et al.* (1993) Report of the Cancer Therapy Evaluation Program monitoring plan for secondary acute myeloid leukaemia following treatment with epipodophyllotoxins. *Journal of the National Cancer Institute*, **85**, 554–558.

236 Levine E.G. & Bloomfield C.D. (1992) Leukaemias and myelodysplastic syndromes secondary to drug, radiation, and environmental exposure. *Seminars in Oncology*, **19**, 47–48.

237 Devereux S., Selassie T.G., Vaughan Hudson G., Vaughan Hudson B. & Linch D.C. (1990) Leukaemias complicating treatment for Hodgkins disease: the experience of the British National Lymphoma Investigation. *British Medical Journal*, **301**(6760), 1077–1080.

238 Miller J.S., Arthur D.C., Litz C.E. *et al.* (1994) Myelodysplastic syndrome after autologous bone marrow transplantation: an additional late complication of curative cancer chemotherapy. *Blood*, **83**, 3780–3786.

239 Darrington D.L., Vose J.M., Anderson J.R. *et al.* (1994) Incidence and characterization of secondary myelodysplastic syndromes and acute myelogenous leukaemia following high dose chemo-radiotherapy and autologous stem cell transplantation for lymphoid malignancies. *Journal of Clinical Oncology*, **12**, 2527–2534.

240 Lambertenghi-Deliliers G., Orazi A., Luksch R., Annaloro C. & Soligo D. (1991) Myelodysplastic syndrome with increased marrow fibrosis: a distinct clinico-pathological entity. *British Journal of Haematology*, **78**, 47–84.

241 Third MIC Cooperative Study Group (1988) Recommendation for a morphologic, immunologic and cytogenetic (MIC) working classification of the primary and therapy-related myelodysplastic disorders. Report of the Workshop held in Scottsdale, Arizona USA. *Cancer Genetics and Cytogenetics*, **32**, 1–10.

242 Pederson-Bjergaard J. & Preben P. (1987) Cytogenetic characteristics of therapy related acute nonlymphocytic leukaemia, preleukaemia and acute myeloproliferative syndrome: Correlation with clinical data for 61 consecutive cases. *British Journal of Haematology*, **66**, 199.

243 Blank J. & Lange B. (1982) Preleukaemia in children. *Journal of Paediatrics*, **98**, 565–568.

244 Hasle H., Jacobsen B.B. & Pedersen N.T. (1992) Myelodysplastic syndromes in childhood: a population based study of nine cases. *British Journal of Haematology*, **81**, 495.

245 Jackson G.H., Carey P.J., Bown N.P. & Reid M.M. (1993) Myelodysplastic syndromes in children. *British Journal of Haematology*, **84**, 185.

246 Gadner H. & Oscar A.H. (1992) Experience in paediatric myelodysplastic syndromes. *Haematology/Oncology Clinics of North America*, **6**(3), 655–672.

247 Chessells J.M. (1991) Myelodysplasia. *Clinical Haematology*, **4**, 459–482.

248 Haas O.A. & Gadner H. (1996) Pathogenesis, biology and man-

agement of myelodysplastic syndromes in children. *Seminars in Hematology*, **33**, 225–235.

249 Hasle H. (1994) Myelodysplastic syndromes in childhood — classification, epidemiology and treatment. *Leukaemia Lymphoma*, **13**, 11–26.

250 Hardisty R.M., Speed D.E. & Till M. (1964) Granulocytic leukaemia in childhood. *British Journal of Haematology*, **10**, 551–566.

251 Mays J.A., Neerhout R.C., Bagby G.C. & Koler R.D. (1980) Juvenile chronic granulocytic leukaemia. *American Journal of Disease in Children*, **134**, 654–658.

252 Kaneko Y., Maseki N., Sakurai M. *et al.* (1989) Chromosome pattern in juvenile chronic myelogenous leukaemia, myelodysplastic syndrome, and acute leukaemia associated with neurofibromatosis. *Leukaemia*, **3**, 36–41.

253 Brandwein J.M., Horsman D.E., Eaves A.C. *et al.* (1990) Childhood myelodysplasia: suggested classification as myelodysplastic syndromes based on laboratory and clinical findings. *American Journal of Paediatric Hematology/Oncology*, **12**, 63–70.

254 Sieff C.A., Chessells J.M., Harvey B.A.M. *et al.* (1981) Monosomy 7 in childhood: a myeloproliferative disorder. *British Journal of Haematology*, **49**, 235–249.

255 Teasedale J.M., Worth A.J. & Carey M.J. (1970) A missing group C chromosome in the bone marrow cells of three children with myeloproliferative disease. *Cancer*, **25**, 1469–1477.

256 Bader-Meunier B., Rotig A., Mielot F. *et al.* (1994) Refractory anaemia and mitochondral cytopathy in childhood. *British Journal of Haematology*, **87**, 381–385.

257 Creutzig U., Cantu-Rajnoldi A., Ritter J. *et al.* (1987) Myelodysplastic syndromes in childhood. Report of 21 patients from Italy and West Germany. *American Journal of Pediatric Hematology/Oncology*, **9**, 324–330.

258 Passmore S.J., Hann I.M., Stiller C.A. *et al.* (1995) Pediatric myelodysplasia: a study of 68 children and a new prognostic scoring system. *Blood*, **85**, 1742–1750.

259 Eguchi M., Sakakibara H., Suda J. *et al.* (1989) Ultrastructural and ultracytochemical differences between transient myeloproliferative disorder and megakaryoblastic leukaemia in Down's syndrome. *British Journal of Haematology*, **73**, 315–322.

260 Zipursky A., Thorner P., De Herven E., Christensen H. & Doyle J. (1994) Myelodysplasia and acute megakaryoblastic leukaemia in Down's syndrome. *Leukaemia Research*, **18**, 163–171.

261 Greenberg P.L. (1996) Biologic and clinical implications of marrow culture studies in the myelodysplastic syndrome. *Seminars in Hematology*, **33**, 163–175.

262 Linman J.W. & Bagby G.C. (1978) The preleukaemic syndrome (haemopoietic dysplasia). *Cancer*, **42**, 854–864.

263 Todd W.M. & Pierre R.V. (1983) Preleukemia: a long term prospective study of 326 patients. *Blood*, **4**(Suppl. 1), 184a.

264 Tricot G. (1984) *The myelodysplastic syndromes*. MD thesis, University of Leuven, Belgium.

265 Kuriyama K., Tomonaga M., Matsuo T. *et al.* (1989) Diagnostic significance of detecting pseudo-Pelger–Hüet anomalies and micromegakaryocytes in myelodysplastic syndrome. *British Journal of Haematology*, **63**, 665–669.

266 Culligan D.J. & Jacobs A. (1992) Minimal disgnostic criteria for the myelodysplastic syndrome. *Leukaemia Research*, **16**, 4–5.

267 Anttila P., Ihalainen J., Salo A. *et al.* (1995) Idiopathic macrocytic anaemia in the elderly: molecular and cytogenetic findings. *British Journal of Haematology*, **90**, 797–803.

268 Knapp R.H., Dewald G.W. & Pierre R.V. (1985) Cytogenetic studies in 174 consecutive patients with preleukaemic or myelodysplastic syndrome. *British Journal of Haematology*, **63**, 665–669.

269 Heim S. & Mitelman F. (1986) Chromosome abnormalities in myelodysplastic syndromes. *Mayo Clinic Proceedings*, **60**, 507–516.

270 Golub T.R., Barker G.F., Lorett M. & Gilliland D.G. (1994) Fusion of PDGF receptor β to a novel *Ets*-like gene, *tel*, in chronic myelomonocytic leukemia with t(5 : 12) chromosomal translocation. *Cell*, **77**, 307–316.

271 Anderson R.L. & Bagby G.C. (1982) The prognostic value of chromosome studies in patients with preleukaemic syndrome (haemopoietic dysplasia). *Leukaemia Research*, **6**, 175–181.

272 Yunis J.J., Lobell M., Arnesen M.A. *et al.* (1988) Refined chromosome study helps define prognostic subgroups in most patients with primary myelodysplastic syndrome and acute myelogenous leukemia. *British Journal of Haematology*, **68**, 189–194.

273 Rowley J.D., Blaisdell R.K. & Jacobson L.O. (1966) Chromosome studies in pre-leukemia. *Blood*, **27**, 782–799.

274 Clark R., Petas S., Hoy T. *et al.* (1986) Prognostic significance of hypodiploid haemopoietic precursors in myelodysplastic syndromes. *New England Journal of Medicine*, **314**, 1472–1475.

275 Tricot G., Mecucci C. & Van den Berghe H. (1986) Evolution of the myelodysplastic syndromes (Annotation). *British Journal of Haematology*, **63**, 609–614.

276 Brown E.R., Heerema N.A. & Tricot G. (1990) Spontaneous remission in myelodysplastic syndrome. *Cancer Genetics and Cytogenetics*, **46**, 125–130.

277 Benaim E., Hrizdala E.V., Papenhausen P. & Moscinski L.C. (1995) Spontaneous remission in monosomy 7 myelodysplastic syndrome. *British Journal of Haematology*, **89**, 947–948.

278 Kantarjian H.M., Keating M.J., Walters R.S. *et al.* (1986) Therapy related leukaemia and myelodysplastic syndrome. Clinical, cytogenetic and prognostic features. *Journal of Clinical Oncology*, **4**, 1748–1757.

279 Groupe Français de Cytogenetique Hematologique (1984) Chromosome analysis of 63 cases of secondary non-lymphoid blood disorders: a cooperative study. *Cancer Genetics and Cytogenetics*, **12**, 96–104.

280 Whang Peng J., Young R.C., Lee E.C. *et al.* (1988) Cytogenetic studies in patients with secondary leukaemia/dysmyelopoietic syndrome after different treatment modalities. *Blood*, **71**, 403.

281 Johansson B., Mertens F., Heim S., Kristofferson U. & Mitelman F. (1991) Cytogenetics of secondary myelodysplasia (sMDS) and acute nonlymphocytic leukaemia (sANLL). *European Journal of Haematology*, **47**, 17–27.

282 Le Beau M.M., Albain K.S., Larson R.A. *et al.* (1986) Clinical and cytogenetic correlation in 63 patients with therapy-related myelodysplastic syndromes are acute non-lymphocytic leukaemia; further evidence for characteristic abnormalities of chromosomes No 5 and 7. *Journal of Clinical Oncology*, **4**, 325–345.

283 Heim S. (1992) Cytogenetic findings in primary and secondary MDS. *Leukaemia Research*, **16**, 43–46.

284 Tricot G. (1984) *The myelodysplastic syndromes*. MD Thesis, University of Leuven, Belgium.

285 Geary C.G. (1983) The diagnosis of preleukaemia. *British Journal of Haematology*, **55**, 1–6.

286 Pomeroy C., Oken M., Rydell R.E. *et al.* (1991) Infection in the myelodysplastic syndrome. *American Journal of Medicine*, **90**, 338–343.

287 Ariel I., Weiler-Ravell D. & Stalnikowics R. (1981) Preleukaemia

in acute lymphoblastic leukaemia. *Acta Haematologica (Basel)*, **66**, 50–52.

288 Barton J.C., Conrad M.E. & Parmley R.T. (1980) Acute lymphoblastic leukemia in idiopathic refractory sideroblastic anemia: evidence for a common lymphoid and myeloid progenitor cell. *American Journal of Hematology*, **9**, 109–115.

289 Hehlmann R., Zönnchen B., Thiel E. *et al.* (1983) Idiopathic refractory siderachrestic anaemia (IRSA) progressing to acute mixed lymphoblastic myelomonoblastic leukaemia. *Blut*, **46**, 11–21.

290 Hamblin T.J. (1993) Immunological abnormalities in MDS. In: *The Myelodysplastic Syndromes* (eds D.A.G. Galton & G.J. Mufti), pp. 97–114. Churchill Livingstone, Edinburgh.

291 Kohno T., Amenomori T., Atogami S. *et al.* (1996) Progression from myelodysplastic syndrome to acute lymphoblastic leukaemia with Philadelphia chromosome and minor bcr-abl transcript. *British Journal of Haematology*, **93**, 389–391.

292 San Mighel J.F., Hernandes J.M., Gonzalez-Sarmiento R. *et al.* (1991) Acute leukemia after a primary myelodysplastic syndrome: immunophenotypic, genotypic and clinical characteristics. *Blood*, **78**, 764–774.

293 Pereira A.M., De Castro J.T., Santos E.G. *et al.* (1985) T-lymphoblastic transformation of refractory anaemia with excess of blasts. *Clinical and Laboratory Haematology*, **7**, 89–95.

294 Mufti G.J., Stevens J.R., Oscier D.G. *et al.* (1985) Myelodysplastic syndromes: a scoring system with prognostic significance. *British Journal of Haematology*, **59**, 425–433.

295 Worsley A., Oscier D.G. & Stevens J. (1988) Prognostic features of chronic myelomonocytic leukaemia; a modified Bournemouth score gives the best prediction of survival. *British Journal of Haematology*, **68**, 17–21.

296 Sanz G.F., Sanz M.A., Vallespi T. *et al.* (1989) Two regression models and a scoring system for predicting survival and planning treatment in myelodysplastic syndromes: a multivariate analysis of prognostic factors in 370 patients. *Blood*, **74**, 395–408.

297 Aul C., Gattermann N., Heyll A. *et al.* (1992) Primary myelodysplastic syndromes: analysis of prognostic factors in 235 patients and proposals for an improved scoring system. *Leukaemia*, **6**, 52–58.

298 Greenberg P., Cox C., Le Bean M.M. *et al.* (1997) International scoring system for evaluating prognosis in myelodysplastic syndromes. *Blood*, **89**, 2079–2088.

299 Verma D.S., Spitzer G., Dicke K.A. *et al.* (1979) *In vitro* agar culture patterns in preleukaemia and their clinical significance. *Leukemia Research*, **3**, 41–49.

300 Spitzer G., Verma D.S., Dicke K.A. *et al.* (1983) Subgroups of oligoleukaemia as identified by *in vitro* agar culture. *Leukemia Research*, **3**, 29–39.

301 Francis G.E., Miller E.J., Wonke B. *et al.* (1983) Use of bone-marrow culture in prediction of acute leukaemic transformation in pre-leukaemia. *Lancet*, **i**, 1409–1412.

302 Legare R.D. & Gilliland D.G. (1995) Myelodysplastic syndrome. *Current Opinion in Haematology*, **2**, 283–292.

303 Ruutu T., Volin L. & Tenhunen R. (1987) Haemarginate as a treatment of myelodysplastic syndromes. *British Journal of Haematology*, **65**, 425.

304 Hirst W.J.R. & Mufti G. (1993) Management of myelodysplastic syndromes. *British Journal of Haematology*, **84**, 191–196.

305 Hast R., Bevan M. & Reizenstein P.L. (1979) Studies on human pre-leukaemia. VI. Non-specific immunotherapy (BCG) in five patients with aregenerative anaemia and hypercellular bone marrow. In: *Preleukaemia* (eds F. Schmalzl & K-P. Hellriegal), pp. 170–173. Springer Verlag, Berlin.

306 Buzaid A.C., Garewal H.S. & Greenberg B.R. (1986) Management of myelodysplastic syndromes. *American Journal of Hematology*, **80**, 1149–1157.

307 Molldrem J.J., Caples M., Mavroudis D. *et al.* (1997) Antithymocyte globulin for patients with myelodysplastic syndrome. *British Journal of Haematology*, **99**, 699–705.

308 Coutinho L.H., Geary C.G., Chang J.G., Harrison C. & Testa N.G. (1990) Functional studies of bone marrow haemopoietic and stromal cells in the myelodysplastic syndrome. *British Journal of Haematology*, **75**, 16–25.

309 Alasano H., Ohasi H., Ichihara M. *et al.* (1994) Evidence for non-clonal haemopoietic progenitor cell populations in bone marrow from patients with myelodysplastic syndromes. *Blood*, **84**, 588–594.

310 List A.F., Spier C.M., Cline A. *et al.* (1991) Expression of the multidrug resistance phenotype in the myelodysplastic syndromes. *British Journal of Haematology*, **78**, 28–34.

311 Estey E.E. (1993) Prognosis and therapy of myelodysplastic syndromes. In: *Leukaemia: advances, research and treatment* (eds E.J. Freireich & H. Kantarjian), pp. 233–267. Kluwer Academic, Boston.

312 Michels S., Saumur J., Arthur D., Robinson L. & Brunning R. (1989) Refractory anaemia with excess of blasts in transformation: haematologic and clinical study of 52 patients. *Cancer*, **64**, 2340–2346.

313 de Witte T., Muus P., De Pauer B. & Haanen C. (1990) Intensive antileukaemic treatment of patients with myelodysplastic syndromes and secondary acute myeloblastic leukaemia. *Cancer*, **66**, 831–837.

314 Estey E., Thall P., Andreeff M., Beran M. *et al.* (1994) Use of granulocyte colony stimulating factor before, during and after fludarabine plus cytarabine induction therapy of newly diagnosed acute myeloblastic leukaemia or myelodysplastic syndrome. *Journal of Clinical Oncology*, **12**, 671–678.

315 Loeffler H., Schmitz N. & Gassmann W. (1992) Intensive chemotherapy and bone marrow transplantation for myelodysplastic syndromes. *Hematology/Oncology Clinics of North America*, **6**, 619–631.

316 Fenaux P., Morel P., Rose C. *et al.* (1991) Prognostic factors in adult *de novo* myelodysplastic syndrome treated by intensive chemotherapy. *British Journal of Haematology*, **77**, 497–501.

317 Hamblin T.J. & Oscier D.G. (1987) The myelodysplastic syndrome: a practical guide. *Haematological Oncology*, **5**, 19–34.

318 Bagby G.C. (1985) Treatment of patients with the preleukaemic syndrome. In: *The Preleukemic Syndrome (Hemopoietic Dysplasia)* (ed. G.C. Bagby), pp. 219–237. CRC Press, Boca Raton, FL.

319 de Witte T. & Gratwohl A. (1993) Bone marrow transplantation for myelodysplastic syndrome and secondary leukaemia. *British Journal of Surgery*, **84**, 361–364.

320 Anderson J.E., Appelbaum F.R., Fisher L.D. *et al.* (1993) Allogeneic bone marrow transplantation for 93 patients with myelodysplastic syndrome. *Blood*, **82**, 677–681.

321 O'Donnell M.R., Nademanee A.P., Snyder D.S. *et al.* (1987) Bone marrow transplantation for myelodysplastic and myeloproliferative syndromes. *Journal of Clinical Oncology*, **5**, 1822–1826.

322 Baccarani M. & Tura S. (1979) Differentiation of myeloid leukaemic cells: new possibilities for therapy. *British Journal of Haematology*, **42**, 485–487.

323 Tricot G., DeBoc R., Dekker A.W. *et al.* (1984) Low dose cytosine

arabinoside in myelodysplastic syndromes. *British Journal of Haematology*, **58**, 231–240.

324 Cheson B.D., Jasperse D.M., Simon R. & Friedman M.A. (1986) A critical appraisal of low dose cytosine arabinoside in patients with acute non-lymphatic leukaemia and myelodysplastic syndromes. *Journal of Clinical Oncology*, **4**, 1857–1864.

325 Miller K.B., Kim K., Morrison F.S. *et al.* (1988) Evaluation of low-dose ara-C versus supportive care in the treatment of myelodys-plastic syndromes. *Blood*, **72**(Suppl.), 215a.

326 Yoshida Y. (1996) Treatment of the myelodysplastic syndromes: an updated Japanese experience. *Seminars in Hematology*, **33**, 246–255.

327 Oscier D.G., Worsby A., Hamblin T.J. *et al.* (1989) Treatment of chronic myelomonocytic leukaemia with low dose etoposide. *British Journal of Haematology*, **72**, 468–472.

328 Ogata K., Yamada T., Ito T. *et al.* (1992) Low-dose etoposide: a potential therapy for myelodysplastic syndromes. *British Journal of Haematology*, **82**, 354–356.

329 Chitamber C., Libnoch J.A., Matthaeus W.G. *et al.* (1991) Evalua-tion of continuous infusion low-dose 5-azacytidine in the treatment of myelodysplastic syndrome. *American Journal of Haematology*, **37**, 100.

330 Christman J., Mendelsohn N., Heizog D. & Scheiderman N. (1983) Effect of 5-azacytidine on differentiation and DNA methy-lation in human promyelocytic leukaemic cells (HL-60). *Cancer Research*, **43**, 763.

331 Evely R.S. & Burnett A.K. (1996) Differentiation therapy in the myelodysplastic syndromes (MDS). *Royal Society of Medicine, Leukemia Lymphoma*, **IV**(2), 31–47.

332 Zagonel V., Lo Re G. & Marotta G. (1993) 5-Aza-2' deoxycytidine (Decitabine) induces trilineage response in unfavourable myelodysplasia. *Leukemia Research*, **7**, 30–35.

333 Greenberg B., Durie B., Garnett T. & Meyskens F. (1985) Phase I–II study of 113 *cis*-retinoic acid in myelodysplastic syndrome. *Cancer Treatment*, **69**, 1369.

334 Besa E.C., Hyzinski M., Nowell P.C. *et al.* (1985) High dose, prolonged 13-*cis* retinoic acid is required for clinical response in myelodysplastic syndrome (Abstract). *Blood*, **66**(Suppl. 1), 194a.

335 Koeffler H.P., Heitjan D., Mertelsmann R. *et al.* (1988) Ran-domised trial of 13-*cis*-retinoic acid vs placebo in the myelodys-plastic disorders. *Blood*, **71**, 703–708.

336 Kizaki M. & Koeffler H.P. (1992) Differentiation-inducing agents in the treatment of myelodysplastic syndromes. *Seminars in Oncology*, **19**, 95–105.

337 Andreef M., Stone R., Michaeli J. *et al.* (1992) Hexamethylene bisacetamide in myelodysplastic syndrome and acute myelo-geneous leukemia: a phase II clinical trial with a differentiating agent. *Blood*, **80**, 2604–2609.

338 Maiolo A.J., Cortelezzi A., Calori R. & Polli E.E. for the Italian study group (1990) Recombinant gamma-interferon as first line therapy for high risk myelodysplastic syndromes. *Leukemia*, **4**, 480.

339 Hellstrom E., Robert K.H., Gahrton G. *et al.* (1989) Therapeutic effects of low-dose cytosine arabinoside alpha interferon 1-hydroxyvitamin D$_3$ and retinoic acid in acute leukaemia and myelodysplastic syndromes. *European Journal of Haematology*, **40**, 449–459.

340 Paquette R.L. & Koeffler H.P. (1992) Differentiation therapy in myelodysplastic syndromes. *Hematology/Oncology Clinics of North America*, **6**, 687–706.

341 Ganser A. & Hoelzer D. (1992) Treatment of myelodysplastic syn-dromes with haemopoietic growth factors. *Hematology/Oncology Clinics of North America*, **6**, 633–655.

342 Greenberg P.L. (1995) Myelodysplastic syndrome. In: *Hematology, Basic Principles and Practice* (ed. R. Hoffmann), 2nd edn, pp. 1098–1120. Churchill Livingstone, London.

343 Yoshida Y., Hirashima K., Asano S. *et al.* (1991) A phase II trial of recombinant human granulocyte colony-stimulating factor in the myelodysplastic syndrome. *British Journal of Haematology*, **73**, 378–383.

344 Rose E.H., Abels R.I., Nelson R.A., McCullough D.M. & Lessen L. (1995) The use of r-HuEpo in the treatment of anaemia related to myelodysplasia. *British Journal of Haematology*, **89**, 831–837.

345 Ganser A. & Hoelzer D. (1996) Clinical use of hematopoietic growth factors in the myelodysplastic syndrome. *Seminars in Hematology*, **33**, 186–195.

346 Greenberg P.L., Negrin N.S. & Ginzton N. (1992) *In vitro–in vivo* correlations of erythroid responses to G-CSF plus erythropoietin in myelodysplastic syndromes. *Experimental Haematology*, **20**, 733a.

347 Brito-Babapulle F., Catovsky D. & Galton D.A.G. (1987) Clinical and laboratory features of *de novo* acute myeloid leukaemia with trilineage myelodysplasia. *British Journal of Haematology*, **66**, 445–450.

348 Matsuo T., Goasquen J., Cox J.C. & Bennett J.M. (1990) Trilin-eage dysplasia in acute myeloid leukaemia: a study of 332 patients from an ECOG trial (Abstract). *Blood*, **76**(Suppl. 1), 300a.

349 Foucar K., Vanghan W.P., Armitage J.O. *et al.* (1983) Post-leukemic dysmyelopoiesis. *American Journal of Hematology*, **15**, 321–334.

350 Brito-Babapulle F., Catovsky D. & Galton D.A.G. (1988) Myelodysplastic relapse of *de novo* acute myeloid leukaemia with trilineage myelodysplasia: a previously unrecognized correlation. *British Journal of Haematology*, **68**, 411–415.

351 Jowitt S.N., Liu-Yin J.A., Saunders M.J. & Lucas G.S. (1993) Clonal remissions in acute myeloid leukaemia are commonly associated with features of trilineage myelodysplasia during remission. *British Journal of Haematology*, **85**, 698–705.

352 Fialkow P.J., Singer J.W., Adamson J.W. *et al.* (1981) Acute non-lymphocytic leukemia: heterogeneity of stem cell origin. *Blood*, **57**, 1068–1073.

353 Widell S., Auer G., Hast R. & Reizenstein P. (1990) Acute myeloid leukaemia occurring *de novo* and preceded by the myelodysplastic syndrome: two different diseases (Abstract). *Blood*, **76**(Suppl. 1), 335a.

12 Secondary Leukaemias

D.A. Winfield and J.S. Lilleyman

Introduction

For this chapter a leukaemia will be considered to be secondary if it arises following some obvious cytodisruptive insult to the bone marrow or as a recognizable complication of some pre-existing disease. The first type includes leukaemias caused by the use of drugs, chemicals or ionizing radiation, and the second includes leukaemias occurring as part of the natural history of a small group of disorders including chromosome abnormalities, immune deficiencies and nonleukaemic myelodysplasias. Each type will be considered in turn, with emphasis where possible on the nature of the leukaemias encountered and the response to therapy.

Leukaemias induced by cytotoxic drugs

Therapy-related myelodysplasia (t-MDS) and therapy-related acute nonlymphocytic leukaemia (t-ANLL) are now recognized as two of the most serious long-term complications of the use of cytotoxic drugs [1]. The major use of such drugs is in the treatment of malignant disease and potential difficulties may arise in assessing the role of any one individual drug, because they are often given in complex combinations and sometimes in combination with radiotherapy. Nevertheless, from such heterogeneous treatment schedules it has now become apparent that the majority of secondary leukaemias resulting from the use of cytotoxic drugs can be divided into two well-defined groups (Table 12.1), depending on whether the patient has received (i) alkylating agents or (ii) drugs binding to the enzyme DNA–topoisomerase II (Topo II).

Alkylating agents

These drugs are cytotoxic because of their ability to bind to nucleotides in the purine and pyrimidine bases of the DNA molecule and thereby induce their alkylation. In addition, some alkylating agents such as nitrogen mustard may cause covalent cross linkage between the two strands of DNA. The overall result is DNA damage resulting in either cell death or a possible mutagenic effect on cells which are not killed. For the patients developing secondary leukaemia following the use of alkylating agents characteristic features are seen, regardless of the drug used and the condition under treatment. In the majority of instances there is a relatively long interval of the order of 2–8 years [1] between the use of the alkylating agent and the development of MDS/leukaemia.

Almost all alkylating agents in clinical use have been shown to induce leukaemia [2–5] and, although some reports had suggested that busulphan [6] and melphalan [7,8] may be more likely to produce secondary leukaemia, the overall consensus is that alkylating agents are equal in their leukaemogenic potential. The risk appears to increase with the age of the patient [1], and in Hodgkin's disease the risk increases approximately with the square of the age [9]. In several studies there also appears to be an increased risk with the cumulative dose of alkylating agents [1,9].

Between 30 and 60% of patients present with peripheral blood cytopenias [10–12] and bone marrow morphology usually shows the typical features of MDS represented by dyshaemopoiesis and megaloblastosis in the red cell series, degranulation, hypersegmentation and pseudo-Pelger anomaly in neutrophils, and micromegakaryocytes and/or abnormal nuclear lobulation in the megakaryocyte series [13]. In most cases there is trilineage dysplasia and in about 15% of patients the marrow trephine biopsy shows mild to marked fibrosis with increased reticulin [12]. In the patients who develop MDS there is approximately a 30% progression to acute nonlymphocytic leukaemia (ANLL) and this usually occurs within 12 months of diagnosis of the myelodysplastic phase [13].

In the patients who initially present with ANLL, FAB types M_1 and M_2 are most commonly reported, although there are rarer examples of other FAB types and features of trilineage dysplasia are usually present. There may be difficulties in accurate characterization of the leukaemia, because it may be of the acute undifferentiated type (AUL) or multiple cell lines

Table 12.1 Typical features of alkylating agents compared with epipodophyllotoxin/anthracycline secondary leukaemia.

	Alkylating agents	Epipodophyllotoxins/ anthracyclines
Treatment to leukaemia interval	3–8 years	2–3 years
Myelodysplastic phase	Present	Absent
ANLL (FAB) type	Myeloblastic (M$_1$, M$_2$)	Monocytic (M$_4$, M$_5$)
Chromosomal abnormalities	–5, –7, –5q, –7q	11q23 deletion and translocations

may be involved. Cytogenetic analysis is an essential part of investigating secondary MDS and leukaemia, because nonrandom chromosomal abnormalities are present in 75–90% of cases of both secondary MDS and ANLL [14]. Cytogenetics are particularly important in the early stages of MDS with a hypoplastic bone marrow or without an increased percentage of blasts [15].

The most consistent changes involve the loss of entire chromosomes 5 and 7 (–5 and –7) or deletions of these two chromosomes with loss of the whole long arm or various parts of the long arm (5q– and 7q–). Loss of 5q may also be associated with unbalanced translocations of the type t(5;17), in which there is loss of both 5q and 17q, and similarly for chromosome 7 the unbalanced translocation t(1;7), which may result in loss of 7q [16]. In chromosome 5 the deletions are interstitial, the proximal breakpoint varying between bands 5q13 and 5q22 and the distal breakpoint between bands 5q31 and 5q35, with the region between bands 5q22 and 5q31 always missing [1]. Several genes which code for important haemopoietic growth factors have been mapped to a narrow region of the long arm of chromosome 5. Among them are the genes coding for IL-3, IL-4 IL-5, granulocyte macrophage colony-stimulating factor (GM-CSF) and macrophage colony-stimulating factor (M-CSF) [17]. This deletion of the critical bands in 5q may result either in the loss of tumor suppressor genes or in the unopposed expression of an oncogene on the remaining chromosome, with a resultant imbalance in the normal cell cycle.

Other less common, but consistent, findings are trisomy 8 and structural aberrations such as loss of a whole chromosome 18 and rearrangements of the short arm of chromosome 17 [1]. Whereas the presence of characteristic chromosomal abnormalities has been shown to be of major importance in the diagnosis of secondary MDS, their role as a prognostic factor is less apparent. One study has suggested they have no prognostic value [18], but a more recent report has demonstrated that the number of chromosomal aberrations is an independent prognostic factor [15].

Drugs binding to the enzyme DNA–topoisomerase II

DNA–topoisomerase II (Topo II) is an enzyme involved in the unwinding and religation of DNA, and is essential for gene transcription, DNA replication, chromosome segregation and DNA recombination. Cytotoxic drugs binding to Topo II increase chromosome breaks by forming an inhibitor-enzyme–DNA complex that decreases religation, thereby causing cell death [19]. These drugs include.

1 The epipodophyllotoxins, which are semisynthetic derivatives and include etoposide (VP-16) and teniposide (VM-26). Teniposide is reported to be about 10 times more potent than etoposide in causing DNA damage both *in vivo* and *in vitro* [20].

2 The anthracyclins such as doxorubicin and 4-epidoxorubicin.

Since the first paper was published in 1987, suggesting that etoposide had the potential for inducing secondary leukaemia [21], there is now very strong evidence that drugs binding to Topo II are capable of inducing secondary leukaemias which have very different clinical and cytogenetic features compared to those associated with alkylating agents [22–24]. The time interval between the treatment and the development of leukemia is usually short, with a mean value of about 2–3 years, and the ANLL subtype is usually monocytic of FAB groups M$_4$ and M$_5$, although M$_1$ and M$_3$ have also been reported [25,26]. A preceding myelodysplastic phase is absent.

Cytogenetic analysis of this type of secondary leukaemia shows chromosomal deletions or rearrangements, which are most frequently found in 50% of cases on the long arm of chromosome 11 at the 11q23 locus [22,23], and occasionally with translocation affecting 21q22 [27]. This is an important observation, because abnormalities of band 11q23 have also been reported in a number of *de novo* haematological malignancies, including acute lymphoblastic leukaemia (ALL), ANLL, mixed lineage leukaemia and lymphomas [28].

In ALL t(4;11) is found in up to 70% of cases in children under 1 year and in AML t(9;11) and t(11;19) are most common and occur predominantly in infants. 11q23 translocations structurally interrupt the gene variously called *HRX*, *ALL* or *MLL* (myeloid-lymphoid or mixed lineage leukaemia) which spans the breakpoint region. By such translocation two putative DNA binding motifs are disrupted and the *MLL* gene is fused to genes on partner chromosomes such as *LTG4* [29], *LTG9* [30] and *LTG19* [31], resulting in fused mRNA encoding chimeric proteins. Rearrangements of the *MLL* gene have been detected in nine of 10 patients with leukaemia secondary to Topo II-binding drugs and with monocytic morphology and 11q23 translocation [32].

For secondary leukaemia caused by the use of epipodophyllotoxin drugs, the risk of developing leukaemia appears to be dose related [33], and for etoposide the risk occurs with a cumulative dose of more than 2000 mg/m² [34]. Scheduling of drug administration may also be important, with cumulative risk increasing in patients receiving epipodophyllotoxins twice weekly or weekly [33]. There is evidence that other chemotherapy agents given in combination with Topo II-binding drugs may be an important factor in the development of the secondary leukaemia. Thus it is postulated that the administration of methotrexate before epipodophyllotoxin might worsen the resultant DNA damage by reducing purine nucleotide pools available for DNA repair [35]. A synergistic effect of cisplatin and alkylating agents with epidophyllotoxins is also strongly suggested in leukaemia induction [1].

A similar effect of drug interaction has also been reported with the anthracycline group of Topo II binders. Thus 4-epi-doxorubicin has been shown to produce the typical secondary monocytic leukaemias, including 11q23 translocations, but only in treatment arms containing both 4-epi-doxorubicin and either cisplatin [36] or cyclophosphamide [37]. For other anthracyclines the characteristic cytogenetic findings in secondary leukaemia following therapy with doxorubicin-containing combinations also suggest a leukaemogenic effect for this drug [27].

Very occasionally patients receiving both alkylating agents and Topo II-binding drugs may develop secondary leukaemia with chromosome features of 7q– and 11q23 [16].

Therapy-related secondary leukaemia with features of *de novo* acute nonlymphoblastic leukaemia

A small group of patients receiving treatment for solid tumours or haematological malignancies subsequently develop a secondary leukaemia, which is characterized by specific morphological and cytogenetic features. Acute promyelocytic leukaemia (APL) FAB M₃ with t(15;17) is well documented, although the incidence is only 1–2% of reported therapy-related leukaemias [38]. Even more rare are secondary leukaemias with t(8;21) INV(16) and t(8;16) [39]. Common features are a relatively short treatment to leukaemia interval of 2–3 years and the absence of a preceding myelodysplasia, thereby raising the question whether Topo II-binding drugs may also be incriminated in the induction of these leukaemias. There are occasional reports of APL following the use of etoposide alone or in combination chemotherapy for Langerhans' cell histiocytosis [40,41], but the majority of cases of secondary APL have not received epipodophyllotoxins. It is possible that Topo II binding by anthracycline drugs may explain some of these cases, because the majority had received an anthracycline either alone or more often in conjunction with an alkylating agent. However, such a mechanism cannot be the sole explanation, as approximately 25% of APL cases and 10% of the other specific chromosomal abnormalities occur in patients receiving radiotherapy alone [38,39].

Therapy-related acute lymphoblastic leukaemia

There are difficulties in assessing the significance of acute lymphoblastic leukaemia (ALL) developing as a second malignant neoplasm following previous chemotherapy or radiotherapy, because the predominant published work is of single case reports or of small numbers of cases in larger series of secondary ANLL. The incidence is also unclear, although there are suggestions that ALL may comprise about 5% of all cases of secondary leukaemias [10,42]. A review of 17 cases [42] reports previous chemotherapy alone in five cases, previous radiotherapy alone in three cases, combined modality in nine cases. The time interval between treatment and leukaemia is wide and ranges from 1 to 12 years (mean 5.2 years). Despite such heterogeneous findings, there is increasing evidence for a small but distinct subgroup with more characteristic features. These are patients who have received previous etoposide-containing regimens and subsequently develop ALL with cytogenetic characteristics of t(4;11)(q21;q23) [42,43]. The combination of a Topo II binder as a treatment agent with subsequent 11q23 abnormalities therefore closely parallels similar findings in ANLL.

Diseases associated with secondary leukaemia

Malignant conditions are often treated with complex chemotherapy schedules and there may also be associated radiotherapy. The most appropriate way to consider chemotherapy-associated leukaemia is therefore on a disease-by-disease basis rather than drug by drug.

Hodgkin's disease

The first reports of leukaemia developing after treatment for Hodgkin's disease (HD) were in the 1970s [44,45] and since then there have been numerous studies convincingly proving that patients treated with alkylating agents develop acute leukaemia and MDS [46–55].

Despite this extensive literature, there still remain certain questions for which the answers are not clear cut and for which there may be conflicting evidence. Among the most important are whether combined chemotherapy and radiotherapy increases the risk of leukaemia, whether different chemotherapy regimens have different risks of leukaemogenicity and whether factors such as increasing age and splenectomy play a role in the development of secondary leukaemia. Table 12.2 gives details from eight studies analysing the risk of MDS and ANLL developing in patients treated either with chemotherapy or with combined modality treatment. There is general agreement that the risk is increased, although the figures for cumulative risks differ between the series. This is not surprising, because the number of patients studied varies and some are single-centre reports

Reference	Patients (no.)	Cases of MDS/ANLL (no.)	Relative risk of ANLL	Cumulative risk of MDS/AML
Baccarani *et al.*, 1980 [49]	496	7	—	2% at 5–7 years
Pedersen-Bjergaard *et al.*, 1987 [9]	391	20	—	3.9% at 5 years 13.0% at 10 years
Blayney *et al.*, 1987 [46]	192	12	95.7	10 ± 3% at 10 years
Tucker *et al.*, 1988 [47]	648 (adjuvant) 179 (salvage) 80 (CT)	18 5 3	117 — 130	3.3 ± 0.6% at 10 years
Lavey *et al.*, 1990 [55]	78 CT 160 CRT	1 2	36 69	2.0% at 10 years 0.9% at 10 years
Kaldor *et al.*, 1990 [48]	29 552	<1 year: 42 1–4 years: 71 5–8 years: 25	9.6 8.4 6.6	— — —
Andrieu *et al.*, 1990 [50]	441 CRT	10	—	3.5 ± 2.7% at 15 years
Pui *et al.*, 1990 [51]	447 CRT	6	—	1.3% at 10 years

Table 12.2 Recent studies showing the risk of MDS/ANLL in patients receiving chemotherapy for HD.

CRT = chemoradiotherapy; CT = chemotherapy.

and others multicentre. An additional factor which must be considered when analysing these figures is whether cases of myelodysplasia are also included in the overall figures, as this diagnosis may be more difficult to make than typical ANNL [9]. Problems may also arise in interpreting bone marrow biopsies with increased fibrosis, which may develop in MDS or in recurrent Hodgkin's disease [56]. The cumulative incidence of leukaemia progressively rises from the time of stopping chemotherapy, with the highest risk of developing leukaemia occurring between 3 and 10 years. The frequency then appears to decrease or stop after 10 years [46–48].

Alkylating drugs in the chemotherapy schedules seem to be the most important component and there appears to be agreement that the larger the dose of alkylating drug or drugs received the greater the likelihood of secondary leukaemia developing [9,47]. There is a suggestion that the number of individual episodes of chemotherapy is a determinant of leukaemia risk, i.e. 12 cycles of uninterrupted chemotherapy is less leukaemogenic than two separate episodes of 6 cycles each, thus inferring that multiple insults to marrow haemopoiesis of shorter duration are more detrimental than one more prolonged period [57]. There is a suggestion that nonalkylating drug regimens such as ABVD (Adriamycin, bleomycin, vinblastine, dacarbazine) are less leukaemogenic than combinations containing alkylating drugs [58] and, although Kaldor *et al.* [48] found a number of cases of secondary leukaemia in patients receiving ABVD, they had all received other chemotherapy including MOPP (mustine, vincristine, prednisolone, procarbazine). There have been a number of reports of combined modality treatment, with chemotherapy and radiotherapy increasing the risk of sec-

ondary leukaemia compared to chemotherapy alone [44], but on balance the evidence is now favouring the view that there is no synergistic effect between chemotherapy and radiotherapy in increasing leukaemia risk [55,57,59]. One possible explanation for discrepant views may be the extent of irradiation, because limited exposure (e.g. mantle) given in combined modality treatment was found to be less leukaemogenic than larger areas of exposure (subtotal/total nodal irradiation or inverted Y) [50]. Other reports suggest that even total nodal irradiation in combined treatment does not increase the risk of leukaemia [57].

Another controversial area is whether age at time of diagnosis and treatment of HD plays any part in the subsequent development of leukaemia. Kaldor *et al.* [48] suggested that relative risks are higher among younger patients, Tucker *et al.* [47] reported no significant difference in relative risks between those over and under 50 years. Pedersen-Bjergaard *et al.* [9] found that increasing age at diagnosis is a significant and independent risk factor for secondary leukaemia.

An interesting observation which has been made in a number of reports is the increased risk of drug-induced secondary leukaemia in association with previous splenectomy [48,60]. The reason for this finding is unclear, but it is reasonable to speculate a connection with the immunological function of the spleen and its function as a reservoir of recirculating T-lymphocytes.

Myeloma

After HD, the largest number of drug-related secondary

leukaemias has arisen in patients with myeloma [61,62]. Over 150 examples where acute leukaemia (AL) occurred as a terminal event have been reviewed by Rosner & Grunwald [63] and, of these, 146 (97%) had received melphalan, 94 (62%) had had additional or alternative therapy, 55 (36%) had also had radiotherapy, and at least 34 (22%) had received other antineoplastic drugs. Clearer data come from Cuzick *et al.* [64], who reported results of the first two Medical Research Council myeloma trials in which patients received either melphalan or cyclophosphamide. In 648 patients there were 12 cases of secondary myeloid leukaemia, and they were able to demonstrate a significant relationship with the length of melphalan treatment but no relationship was found for cyclophosphamide treatment. The most important determinant in leukaemia risk was the amount of melphalan the patient received both in the 3- and 5-year periods before developing MDS or ANLL. The importance of this observation is that if melphalan is used in the treatment of myeloma, it is preferable to reduce the length of administration to the shortest consistent with optimal control.

The cumulative risk of secondary MDS/ANLL in myeloma is reported as 17.4% at 50 months by Bergsagel *et al.* [61] and 10.0% at 8 years by Cuzick *et al.* [64]; the latter figure agrees more closely with the results in other haematological and non-haematological malignancies (Table 12.3).

MDS is occasionally found in the bone marrow concurrently with the diagnosis of myeloma and may evolve into acute leukaemia [65]. This raises the questions whether an unstable haemopoietic clone is present in some patients with plasma cell neoplasms and whether the risk of subsequently developing AL is independent of the treatment given. This is unlikely, because the pattern of leukaemia is very similar to that found in HD and other conditions treated with cytotoxic drugs, and would not explain the clear relationship found with melphalan treatment [64].

Primary systemic amyloidosis is a plasma cell proliferative disorder that is closely related to multiple myeloma but is not itself a malignant condition. Gertz & Kyle [66] described a series of 153 patients with primary systemic amyloidosis treated with melphalan. They found 10 patients with MDS or ANLL, and chromosome analysis showed eight patients

had the typical secondary leukaemia changes affecting chromosome 7, and three patients had changes affecting chromosome 5.

Macroglobulinaemia

The number of reported cases of macroglobulinaemia subsequently developing ANLL is only 14 [67], but macroglobulinaemia is an uncommon disorder compared to myeloma. The incidence is therefore difficult to assess, but appears to be about 4%, which is similar to secondary leukaemia in other disorders. Exposure to alkylating agents appears to be the predominant factor, because 12 of the reported cases had received treatment with these drugs for varying periods of time before development of the secondary leukaemia.

Non-Hodgkin's lymphoma

The studies listed in Table 12.4 confirm secondary ANLL as being an important long-term complication in patients with non-Hodgkin's lymphoma (NHL) treated with chemotherapy. These series are also large enough to allow calculation of cumulative risks, which vary between 4.6 and 8.0% at 10 years, with the curves for cumulative risk of secondary leukaemia continuing to rise 8–9 years after starting treatment [68]. The most frequently used alkylating agents were cyclophosphamide or chlorambucil [63], and a significantly increased risk of secondary leukaemia was seen in re-treated patients [68] suggesting a dose-related effect. The morphological and cytogenetic findings of secondary leukaemia in NHL [69,72] are exactly the same as those seen in HD and myeloma described above. There was no difference in the risk of inducing leukaemia between patients who had been treated with chemotherapy alone and those treated with combined chemotherapy and radiotherapy [55]. There has not been an effective analysis of whether there is any age-related effect, although in the series reported by Lavey *et al.* [55], all cases occurred in people older than 40 years. The reported cases of Ingram *et al.* [70] all occurred in children and it is of interest that their cumulative risk was similar to the three reports in adults listed in Table 12.4. However, the recent report from St Jude Children's Research Hospital found a lower cumulative risk for children of 1.3% at 10 years.

The type of secondary leukaemia associated with Topo II binders has so far been limited to very few cases, but the increasing use of epipodophyllotoxins in first-line treatment of NHL would suggest that there will be an increased reported incidence of this type of leukaemia. Pedersen-Bjergaard *et al.* [1] have reported a case of M_5 leukaemia with 11q23 abnormality treated with CHOP (cyclophosphamide, vincristine, doxorubicin, prednisolone) therapy containing the anthracycline doxorubicin and there are two reports of Topo II-type leukaemia in children following epipodophyllotoxin treatment [16,23].

Table 12.3 Recent studies showing the risks of MDS/ANLL in patients receiving chemotherapy for myeloma.

Reference	Patients (no.)	Cases of MDS/ANLL (no.)	Cumulative risk of MDS/ANLL
Bergsagel *et al.*, 1979 [61]	364	14	17.4% at 50 months
Cuzick *et al.*, 1987 [64]	648	12	10.0% at 8 years

Reference	Patients (no.)	Cases of MDS/ANLL (no.)	Cumulative risk of MDS/ANLL
Greene et al., 1983 [71]	517 CRT	9	7.9% ± 3.2% at 10 years
Pedersen-Bjergaard et al., 1985 [68]	602	9	8.0 ± 3.3% at 9 years
Ingram et al., 1987 [70]	261 CRT	6	6% at 7 years
Lavey et al., 1990 [55]	322 CT	5	4.6% at 10 years
	292 CRT	4	4.5% at 10 years
Pui et al., 1990 [51]	420	3	1.3% at 10 years

Table 12.4 Recent studies showing the risks of MDS/ANLL in patients receiving chemotherapy for NHL.

CRT = chemoradiotherapy; CT = chemotherapy.

Treatment with high-dose chemotherapy ± radiotherapy and autologous stem cell transplantation

High-dose chemoradiotherapy followed by autologous bone marrow transplantation (ABMT) or peripheral stem cell transplantation (PBSCT) has increasingly been used for treatment in patients with relapsed or poor prognosis HD and NHL. Since both the number of patients has increased, and also the length of their survival posttransplant, the effects of treatment including the incidence of secondary leukaemia is now being assessed. Miller et al. [73] reported nine cases of MDS or ANLL post-ABMT in 206 patients and occurring 5–60 months (median 34 months) post-BMT. Two patients relapsed and received additional treatment. When these were censured from the statistical analysis there was a high cumulative incidence of MDS/ANLL of 14.5% ± 11.6% at 5 years, with similar results for HD and NHL. Karyotypic abnormalities in six cases tested most often involved chromosomes 5 and 7. All patients had received chemotherapy and five had received radiation treatment pretransplant. Darrington et al. [74] have also reported an increased risk of MDS/ANLL following ABMT/PBSCT for lymphoid malignancies. Traweek et al. [75] reported the detection of clonal chromosomal abnormalities in 10 out of 275 patients following transplantation, all of whom had normal chromosomal analysis at the time of stem cell harvest. Abnormalities of chromosomes 5 and 7 occurred in four cases, 11q23 or 21q22 occurred in three cases and a combination of both types of chromosome changes in two cases. Although five of the cases were coexistent with typical morphical features of MDS or ANLL, no such features were found in five. Because the median follow-up time in this latter group is only 8.5 months, it is possible that the cytogenetic abnormalities may have detected an early clonal disease before morphological features become apparent. The problem in interpreting reports of MDS/ANLL post-ABMT is whether pretransplant therapy, rather than the myeloablation associated with the transplant, is the culprit. No definite answer is possible but some involvement of the transplant therapy is suggested by the finding of normal chromosomal analysis at the time of

transplant and also by the report of MDS/ANLL occurring in patients transplanted in first remission and having previously received only limited treatment with CHOP chemotherapy [76].

Acute lymphoblastic leukaemia

There are now large numbers of long-term survivors in patients diagnosed as having acute lymphoblastic leukaemia (ALL), while the development of secondary leukaemia is a relatively rare event. Nonetheless, there are now a number of reports of this complication. Pui et al. [77] showed the cumulative risk of developing ANLL during first bone marrow remission was 1.6% at 3 years, 4.7% at 6 years and, for those patients with T-cell immunophenotype, the cumulative risk was 19.1% at 6 years. Most of these patients had received an epipodophyllotoxin either during induction or continuation therapy. The majority of those patients had the Topo II-related type of secondary leukaemia with typical 11q23 chromosomal features. Similar results with a risk of secondary ANLL at 4 years of 5.9% ± 3.2% and 11q23 abnormalities have been reported in patients with ALL also receiving a protocol with an epipodophyllotoxin given during consolidation and maintenance phases of treatment [35]. The importance of epipodophyllotoxins in leukaemia induction in ALL is indicated by a far lower secondary leukaemia risk in children treated with ALL protocols not containing these drugs [78].

The importance of T-cell immunophenotype is unclear but a relatively high risk of secondary ANLL has also been reported in this group treated with nonepipodophyllotoxin-containing schedules [16]. Whether this risk relates to the T-cell immunophenotype or to the fact that this group may be exposed to more intensive chemotherapy regimens is at present unknown.

Chronic lymphatic leukaemia

There are a very limited number of reported cases of MDS/ANLL in patients with chronic lymphatic leukaemia

(CLL) [79], and it is therefore difficult to determine whether this is an incidental finding.

An analysis of a large number of patients with CLL provided no evidence for an increased risk of secondary leukaemia in CLL, even though these patients had often received alkylating agents such as chlorambucil [80].

Polycythaemia rubra vera

Polycythaemia vera (PV) has been treated for many years with either phlebotomy, radioactive phosphorous or alkylating agents (usually chlorambucil), or any combination of the three. Secondary leukaemia has long been recognized as a complication, but its incidence and the precise role played by the different types of treatment have been hotly debated [81]. Berk *et al.* [82] have done much to dispel these arguments by a carefully constructed study of 431 patients randomized equally to phlebotomy, radioactive phosphorous or chlorambucil and followed up for up to 13 years. One phlebotomy patient, nine phosphorous-treated patients and 16 chlorambucil-treated patients developed a secondary leukaemia — a highly significant result which led to the Polycythaemia Vera Study Group discontinuing the use of chlorambucil.

Additional information is provided by Najean *et al.* [83], who analysed 288 cases of PV with a minimum follow-up of 10 years and found 33 patients with secondary leukaemia. No leukaemia was found in the group treated by phlebotomy alone. The incidence of leukaemia was higher in the group receiving exclusively or mainly chemotherapy than in the group receiving ^{32}P, but the difference was not significant. For patients treated with ^{32}P and followed up for more than 10 years, an overall incidence of ANLL has been reported as 10.3%, with a slowly increasing risk of leukaemia occurring within the first 7 years [84]. Very long-term follow-up of 12–15 years has shown that the risk of leukaemia induction by marrow-suppressive agents was very low after 10 years [85] and no cases were observed more than 16 years after first treatment [84]. For treatment with ^{32}P the question whether leukaemia is dosage dependent is difficult to determine, but it has been suggested that leukaemia induction does not relate to dose administered [84]. It has been suggested that splenic enlargement and marked leucocytosis at presentation are risk factors for the development of secondary leukaemia [86], but Najean *et al.* [83] could not confirm that these were statistically significant predictive factors. Age at presentation was a risk factor for HD but they could not confirm a similar finding for PV. Because the myelofibrotic phase of PV has been reported to precede the appearance of leukaemia [87], the question arises whether increasing marrow fibrosis is part of the disease process. Najean *et al.* [83] concluded that myelofibrosis is part of the natural history of PV and cannot be considered a preleukaemic phase.

In the long-term data from the Polycythaemia Vera Study Group, the highest incidence of myelofibrosis occurred in patients treated with phlebotomy alone. This was possibly a result of failure of this treatment to control myeloid hyperplasia [85].

The clinical and pathological features follow closely the previously reported pattern, and in the review by Najean *et al.* [83] 50% of the patients presented with ANLL and 50% with MDS, half of whom subsequently progressed to ANLL.

Essential thrombocythaemia

Essential thrombocythaemia (ET) is a relatively uncommon disorder but, despite this, Sedlacek *et al.* [88] reported three patients who developed secondary leukaemia in this disease, and in an extensive review of the literature they found 12 other cases of leukaemia in patients with a probable diagnosis of ET. From the total of 15 patients, 14 had been previously treated with alkylating drugs and/or ^{32}P. These findings strengthen the argument for not using such therapeutic agents in asymptomatic patients, especially in the younger age groups.

Nonhaemopoietic neoplasia

The use both of alkylating drugs and of Topo II-binding drugs in a number of nonhaemopoietic malignancies has been shown to be associated with an increased risk of secondary leukaemias. The morphology and the karyotypic abnormalities are the same as those previously described in haematological malignancies.

Breast cancer

Adjuvant chemotherapy is frequently used for the treatment of women with early-stage breast cancer with presumed microscopic disease. Such treatment is now considered to produce a significant increase in disease-free survival and reduction in disease-related mortality in premenopausal women with histologically positive axillary nodes [89]. Against this benefit must be balanced the risk of inducing leukaemia. Melphalan-based adjuvant regimens give cumulative risks of AML of 0.7–1.68% at 10 years [90,91] (Table 12.5). The age at initial diagnosis does not appear to be a risk factor [91]. Because of these results, cyclophosphamide has now replaced melphalan in most adjuvant chemotherapy regimens and, at present, the results on its leukaemogenic potential are conflicting: one study [92] showed no significant leukaemia risk, while others showed an increased risk [8,93].

The study reported by Curtis *et al.* [8] also showed that although there was an increased risk with cyclophosphamide treatment, this was significantly less than compared with melphalan. This is an interesting observation, because in most series of secondary leukaemia in other conditions the consensus view is that various alkylating agents are equal in their

Reference	Patients (no.)	Cases of MDS/ ANLL (no.)	Cumulative risk of MDS/ANLL
Breast cancer			
Fisher *et al.*, 1985 [90]	5 299	34	1.7 ± 0.3% at 10 years
Curtis *et al.*, 1990 [91]	13 734	24	0.7% at 10 years
Andersson *et al.*, 1990 [94]	71	5	25.4 ± 10.3% at 37 months
Lung cancer			
Chak *et al.*, 1984 [97]	158	3	25 ± 13% at 3 years
Pedersen-Bjergaard *et al.*, 1985 [98]	796	6	14.0 ± 6.9% at 4 years
Ratain *et al.*, 1987 [21]	119	4	15 ± 11% at 2 years
Ovarian cancer			
Pedersen-Bjergaard *et al.*, 1980 [101]	553	7	7.6 ± 3.0% at 5 years
Greene *et al.*, 1986 [103]	1 179	21	8.6 ± 2.2% at 10 years

Table 12.5 Recent studies showing the risks of MDS/ANLL in patients receiving chemotherapy for nonhaemopoietic neoplasms.

leukaemogenic potential. In addition, chemotherapy combined with radiotherapy that delivers high doses to the marrow appears to enhance the risk of leukaemia [8].

A surprisingly high cumulative risk of leukaemia of 25.4 ± 10.3% has been reported at 37 months after starting therapy with prednimustine, methotrexate, 5-fluorouracil, mitoxantrone and tamoxifen [94]. Four of the five cases were of alkylating agent type and one suggestive of Topo II type. It is possible that the anthracycline mitoxantrone might be incriminated as the Topo II binder, because the use of the anthracycline 4-epi-doxorubicin in the treatment of breast cancer has been shown to be associated with the development of monocytic or myelomonocytic leukaemias, with balanced translocation at band 11q23 [36].

Lung cancer

Combination chemotherapy, often including alkylating agents, is frequently used in the management of advanced lung cancer, but late complications of therapy [21,95–98] are rarely recognized because of the short survival of most patients. Despite this, Table 12.5 lists three series of secondary leukaemia arising in patients treated for lung cancer and with a cumulative risk higher than in most other haemopoietic and nonhaemopoietic malignancies. Possible explanations are the combined and prolonged use of two alkylating drugs [97,98]. Ratain *et al.* [21] were the first to suggest the leukaemogenic potential of higher doses of etoposide in combination with cisplatin when they described four cases of secondary leukaemia, of which three had monoblastic morphology, a relatively short drug–leukaemia time interval, and two of these had 11q23 abnormalities.

Ovarian cancer

A number of alkylating drugs have been incorporated into the

chemotherapy of ovarian cancer [99–105] and melphalan again appears to be the most leukaemogenic [103,104], although dose–response relationships for leukaemia induction have also been found with cyclophosphamide, chlorambucil, thiotepa and treosulphan [104]. Features of secondary leukaemia have also been described after the use of the nonalkylating regimen of cisplatin and doxorubicin [105], although from this paper it is not possible to determine whether the cases following doxorubicin had the features associated with Topo II-binding drugs. The use of intensive chemotherapy in ovarian cancer needs to be carefully assessed, because the risks of secondary leukaemia might outweigh the survival benefits of the treatment.

Germ cell tumours

The treatment of these tumours with combination chemotherapy comprising etoposide, cisplatin and bleomycin has resulted in a mean cumulative risk of leukaemic complications of 4.7% at 5.7 years after starting chemotherapy. The risk was dose related to etoposide, with leukaemia only occurring in patients receiving a cumulative dose of more than 2000 mg/m^2, and in 60% of the cases there were the typical balanced chromosome translocations affecting bands 11q23 and 21q22 [34].

Other neoplasms

Excluding patients treated with radiotherapy, secondary leukaemia has also been described in drug-treated testicular tumours [106], brain tumours [107,108], Wilms' tumours [109], gastrointestinal cancers [110,111], Ewing's tumour [112], mediastinal teratoma [113], neuroblastoma [114,115] and retinoblastoma [116]. There are also reports of secondary leukaemia with intravesical drug treatment of bladder cancer [117,118].

Nonmalignant disorders

This is perhaps the most disturbing group of all—a small but significant number of patients who have received cytotoxic drug treatment for autoimmune disorders or psoriasis and have probably developed secondary leukaemia as a result [119–127]. Ninety-three patients in this category were reviewed by Rosner & Grunwald [63]: 84 (90%) patients had received single or multiple alkylating drugs, eight had received antipurines and two had received low-dose whole-body irradiation. The type of leukaemia encountered was similar in nearly all cases to that described in haemopoietic and non-haemopoietic malignancies, both in their clinical and pathological features and in their poor response to treatment [124]. Predicting which patients are candidates for such an event in time to stop the offending treatment might be possible by monitoring the number of sister chromatid changes in peripheral blood lymphocytes while on potentially leukaemogenic treatment [128], but whether this or some similar manoeuvre will prove useful in practice remains to be seen. At present, the best advice is to avoid using known leukaemogenic drugs in nonmalignant disorders where possible.

Treatment of secondary leukaemia induced by cytotoxic drugs

Throughout the 1980s the increasing use of intensive chemotherapy has improved remission rates in *de novo* AML to between 60 and 80% and, although this reduces with age, rates of 50–60% have been obtained in patients over 50 years. Results of the Medical Research Council 8th Acute Myeloid Leukaemia Trial showed a median duration of remission of 15 months, with a relapse-free survival at 5 years estimated at 18% [129]. For drug-induced leukaemias, most series report much lower remission rates (Table 12.6). The results of the Medical Research Council 9th Acute Myeloid Leukaemia Trial provide a useful comparative study, because both groups received the same chemotherapy schedules with a remission rate of only 25% in secondary leukaemia, compared to an overall remission rate of 66% in *de novo* cases [130]. The only report of good remission rates is from Priesler *et al.*, who found eight of 11 cases (72%) of secondary leukaemia (three with Hodgkin's disease) had a complete remission following treatment with single-agent high-dose cytarabine [131]. The authors speculated that such treatment might be less toxic to the residual normal haemopoietic stem cells than combined cytarabine+anthracycline chemotherapy, thereby reducing the risk of death in the prolonged marrow hypoplasia phase following chemotherapy in secondary leukaemia. This theory is not supported by the results from the Medical Research Council's 9th Acute Myeloid Leukaemia Trial [130], because death rates in the hypoplastic phase were similar for secondary and *de novo* leukaemias. The poorer results in secondary leukaemia appear simply to be due to a higher level of resistant disease.

Table 12.6 Results of treatment in secondary ANLL.

Reference	Chemotherapy	Patients (no.)	CR rate (%)
Preisler *et al.*, 1983 [131]	HD ara-C	11	72
Pedersen-Bjergaard *et al.*, 1984 [133]	D + ara-C	21	43
Michels *et al.*, 1985 [12]	D + ara-C Dox + ara-C HD ara-C	14	28
Le Beau *et al.*, 1986 [18]	D + ara-C + T	28	18
Larson *et al.*, 1988 [132]	D ara-C	17	47
Hoyle *et al.*, 1989 [130]	D + ara-C + T	20	25

ara-C = cytarabine; CR = complete remission; D = daunorubicin; Dox = doxorubicin; HD ara-C = high dose cytarabine; T = thioguanine.

Larson *et al.* [132] also used a single-agent high-dose cytarabine regimen in a group of 17 patients with secondary leukaemia, comprising 13 with MDS and four with ANLL. Their novel approach in the MDS group was to start chemotherapy when the patients first required platelet transfusion support or frequent red cell transfusions, rather than waiting for a progressive increase in marrow blast cells. The overall remission rate was 47%, but when patients were divided into groups showing good and poor performance status, all seven with good performance status went into remission. Despite using consolidation treatment, the median duration of remission was only 5 months, and similar poor results for remission duration for most patients have been found by others [12,131,133]. At present it is difficult to determine why drug-related cases of leukaemia respond so badly in terms of remission induction and duration. The frequent finding of abnormalities of chromosomes 5 and 7 might suggest that genes localized to these chromosomes may play a part in resistance to chemotherapy drugs. Some support for this theory comes from the finding that patients with abnormalities of chromosomes 5 and 7 in *de novo* AML also have lower response rates. A preliminary analysis of the Medical Research Council's 10th Acute Myeloid Leukaemia Trial has shown a 28% 5-year survival in patients with karyotypic abnormalities of chromosomes 5 and 7 compared to 71% for favourable karyotypes, for example t(8;21), t(15;17) and inv(16), and 41% for all other abnormal karyotypes or normal karyotypes. Although most of the data reporting poor results of treatment relates to secondary leukaemia induced by alkylating agents, a poor clinical outcome has also been found in the epipodophyllotoxin-related myelomonocytic and monocytic leukaemias with 11q23 abnormalities [16,35].

For the relatively small group of patients with secondary leukaemia associated with favourable karyotypes, the results of treatment are far more optimistic. Using standard intensive chemotherapy, patients with t(8;21) had a complete remission (CR) of 76% and actuarial disease-free survival (DFS) of 47%

at 24 months, and for patients with inv(16) the CR was 86% and DFS 56% [39]. Chemotherapy with or without all *trans*-retinoic acid produced a CR of 63% in patients with t(15;17) [38].

Alternative approaches have been described for the treatment of MDS, including low-dose cytarabine [134], *cis*-retinoic acid [135] and GM-CSF [136], but there are few long-term responses and at present their role in treating secondary MDS would appear to be very limited.

In view of the overall poor results with chemotherapy, the role of ABMT has been explored in younger patients with a suitable donor. The recommendations are that marrow transplantation should be performed early, especially for those patients with MDS, and before the disease progresses. This early approach may also reduce transplant-related mortality due to HLA sensitization, iron overload and colonization with fungal organisms [137,138]. The question whether intensive chemotherapy prior to the transplant yields better results is, at present, unanswered [137]. Although ABMT offers the best, and possibly the only, hope for long-term survival in young patients with matched family or unrelated donors, the results in t-MDS are worse than for *de novo* MDS. A single-centre study reports a 5-year actuarial DFS of 25% for secondary leukaemia compared to 41% with *de novo* leukaemia, associated with a higher nonrelapse mortality in the former group [138].

Leukaemias induced by noncytotoxic drugs

There is considerable data suggesting that drugs other than cytotoxic agents can cause leukaemia, although it should be stressed that this evidence is nearly all anecdotal, and formal epidemiological studies have been inconclusive [139]. There are reports of leukaemia developing in patients treated with phenylbutazone [140,141] and chloramphenicol [142,143], with well-documented examples of ANLL following episodes of marrow hypoplasia [144–147]. Because of their potential marrow toxicity both of these drugs are now little used in the UK, but it must be remembered that chloramphenicol is still widely used in many developing countries. A report from China [148] suggested a dose–response relationship between chloramphenicol and subsequent development of ANLL and ALL, with the risk being greater for ANLL and without episodes of marrow aplasia preceding the leukaemia. It could be argued that in some instances the chloramphenicol may be used to treat infections developing in the cytopenic phase of MDS, in which case the antibiotic is not causal in producing the marrow abnormality. However, the failure to demonstrate an increased risk of leukaemia by these authors with other antibiotics is against this idea. Although drug-related marrow aplasia may precede the leukaemia, MDS and ANLL may also occur in severe aplastic anaemia in patients with no history of exposure to drugs or toxins [149].

There are a number of well-documented cases of acute leukaemia occurring in children being treated with growth hormone, with a suggestion that there might be a twofold increased relative risk [150]. The problem with assessing this possible association is that both ALL and ANLL have been reported and no distinct pattern of morphology or karyotypic abnormality has arisen. A second difficulty is that growth hormone is given for short stature, and it has been reported that patients with Fanconi's anaemia, who are known to have an increased risk of secondary leukaemia, may present with short stature with none of the other congenital abnormalities and with normal blood studies initially [151]. There have been reports [152,153] of MDS/ANLL occurring following treatment with granulocyte colony-stimulating factors (G-CSF) in patients with severe aplastic anaemia (SAA) and with congenital neutropenia. Whether this is a true association is difficult to assess, because the numbers of patients are small and progression of SAA to MDS/ANLL can occur as part of the marrow disease and in the absence of G-CSF. Several other drugs have been suggested as possible causes of leukaemia, including chlorpromazine [154], oxymethalone [155], pencillamine [156] and lithium [157,158], but the existence of a true association between drug and disease in these reports is very speculative. Similar speculations have been applied to single cases reports for interferon [159], LSD [160] and amphetamine [161], although a report from the Children's Cancer Study Group suggests that there is an increased risk of childhood ANLL with maternal drug use of marijuana during the *in utero* and postnatal periods [162].

Leukaemia following exposure to chemical myelotoxins

Benzene

In 1982 the International Agency for Research on Cancer (IARC) reviewed the large amount of clinical, epidemiological and experimental data available and concluded that there was sufficient evidence that benzene could cause ANLL. Historically the heaviest benzene exposure used to occur in a small number of industries, including the shoe manufacturing trade, rotogravure printing, dry cleaning, spray painting, the making of imitation leather and rubber processing. In most countries benzene has now been banned as a solvent in inks and glue, but it is still used in large quantities in both the chemical and petrochemical industries [163].

The evidence implicating benzene in leukaemia induction has been based on case-control studies [164,165], American cohort mortality investigations [166] and clinical data from Turkish shoe and leather manufacturing workers. In the latter cases Aksoy *et al.* [167,168] reported a leukaemia incidence of 13.5/100 000 in shoe workers exposed to chronic benzene poisoning in solvents. This leukaemia risk was a statistically significant increase compared to the general population.

With a reduction in benzene usage the leukaemia incidence subsequently fell, implicating benzene as the probable aetiological factor in the earlier report. The problem with most of the published reports is that the relationship between benzene and leukaemia is based upon evaluation of death certificates rather than the medical records or morphological data, and it is therefore difficult to assess the type of leukaemia which occurred and the diagnostic evidence on which the characterization depended. A recent report on a large Chinese cohort study answers this problem, by reviewing patient details and histopathology material and concluding that the majority of benzene-induced leukaemias are ANLL with characteristics similar to treatment-related ANLL, including a preceding myelodysplastic phase in some patients [169].

A further similarity is the presence of nonrandom abnormalities of chromosomes 5 and 7, which have been reported in patients with ANLL, and past occupational exposure to either benzene-containing solvents or petroleum products [170]. A possible explanation for this similarity is that one of the metabolic products of benzene which is considered leukaemogenic is *trans*-muconaldehyde, which has some similarities to the alkylating drugs [171]. Chronic myeloid [169], chronic lymphatic [172] and hairy cell leukaemia [172] have all been reported in individuals exposed to benzene, but because the numbers are small it is not possible to determine whether there is a true association.

The time taken from first benzene exposure of workers to the subsequent development of leukaemia has been enormously variable from 2 to 37 years [173,166], but the duration of exposure has been much shorter and less than 1 year in many cases.

Incidence and degree of exposure

While it is now accepted that there is a relationship between exposure to high concentration of benzene and the risk of developing leukaemia, two important questions which still remain are (i) is there a threshold level of exposure below which there is no risk and (ii) what, if any, is the dose–response relationship? These questions are important in determining legislative requirements for maximum exposure of workers. The current accepted levels in the USA and many other countries, including the UK, is set at 10 µg/g as an 8-hour time-weighted average (TWA) with a ceiling concentration of 25 µg/g. The US Occupational Safety and Health Administration (OSHA) advised reducing the levels to 1 µg/g as an 8-hour TWA, but in 1980 the US Supreme Court invalidated this OSHA standard [174]. In an attempt to clarify the situation, Rinsky *et al.* [174] undertook an extensive quantitative study of leukaemia risk and cumulative exposure to benzene based on historical air-sampling data. They reported a 'strongly positive exposure–response relationship between benzene and leukaemia'. From their data, they constructed a model which

allowed them to calculate that reducing the exposure levels from 10 to 1 µg/g would reduce the leukaemia risk. Despite these results, this area still remains controversial, with conflicting views [175,176].

Other chemicals

Butadiene is one of the chemicals which constitutes the basic substances used in the production of most synthetic rubber polymers. A cohort study of workers in US rubber polymerization plants reported a statistically significant incidence of acute leukaemia (type unspecified) in butadiene workers based on their exposure levels to the chemical [177]. There has been criticism of the interpretation of this study [178] and confirmatory evidence is therefore required. There is no conclusive evidence that any other chemicals are associated with secondary leukaemia, although insecticides, weed killers, wood preservatives, hair dye [179–181] and asbestos [182] have been implicated.

Nonrandom abnormalities of chromosomes 5 and 7 are characteristic findings in MDS and AML secondary to drug-induced leukaemias (see above), but similar abnormalities are also found in *de novo* cases. In these cases it is therefore essential to elicit a full occupational history, to determine whether stronger associations can be found with other possible chemical myelotoxins as well as with benzene [183].

An interesting case–control study from the Children's Cancer Study Group [184] showed an association between ANLL in children and exposure of mothers to pesticides and of fathers to pesticides, solvents and petroleum products. For the mothers it was not possible to determine whether the risk was greatest before, during or after the pregnancy. The significance of these findings in the context of secondary leukaemia is difficult to interpret, especially since abnormalities of chromosomes 5 and 7 were rarely observed in children of exposed parents.

Tobacco

Tobacco smoke contains benzene and radioactive compounds, which are both known leukaemogens in man [185]. Although an early 1976 cohort study of British doctors reported no association between smoking and leukaemia [186], there has been increasing evidence from a number of studies that there may be a relationship. Recent review and meta-analysis papers [187,188] have both concluded that there is a causal relationship between tobacco smoking and ANLL, and have suggested that leukaemia should be added to the list of smoking-related diseases. At present it is unclear how important a contribution is made by tobacco smoking, especially in the context of exposure to other possible occupational leukaemogens, and it is worth noting that in one study [185] the positive association only applied to men and not to women.

Leukaemia following exposure to ionizing radiation

There is no doubt that ionizing radiation can cause leukaemia in man [189], but it is important to qualify such a statement by pointing out that it has only been clearly shown to do so in groups or individuals exposed to relatively high doses, and that little is known of the mechanism of leukaemogenesis.

Radiation exposure can arise in several different ways. It can result from nuclear explosions, from contamination due to nuclear power production or other occupational activities (both industrial and medical), from radiotherapy or diagnostic radiology and from natural sources. Most of the information on radiation-induced leukaemia has been obtained from detailed study of the survivors of the atomic bombs exploded in Hiroshima and Nagasaki in 1945 and from recipients of radiotherapy, particularly for nonmalignant disorders. Information has also been gained from examining patterns of disease in radiation workers, chiefly radiologists, occurring before adequate safety regulations were introduced. Each of these groups will be considered in turn, and brief consideration will also be given to the role (if any) of diagnostic radiology in leukaemogenesis.

Leukaemia following atomic radiation

Three years after the explosion of two atomic bombs at Hiroshima and Nagasaki in 1945, an excess of leukaemia in the surviving inhabitants became apparent and, by 1954, 92 verified cases had been identified from a population at risk of around 200 000 [190]. The total had risen to 209 by 1958 [191] and to 250 by 1965 [192], whereafter by 1972 the leukaemia rate had fallen to that seen in Japan as a whole [189]. By 1979 it was felt that 'the radiation-induced leukaemia experience is essentially over' [193], although an excess of solid tumours was still occurring. It is important to emphasize that only 762 of 82 000 A-bomb survivors studied by Beebe *et al.* in 1978 [194] had died of cancer (0.9%), whereas 19 468 (23%) had died from other causes, which puts a clear perspective on the leukaemogenic effect. Although it is not possible to say exactly how many victims developed leukaemia who would not otherwise have done so, it is less than might be supposed and probably in the region of 100–200.

More precise data available on a smaller, fully documented, aliquot population allow some conclusions to be drawn about the types of radiation-induced leukaemia, the incubation period and the dose effect of received radiation [189].

Clearly excessive rates of leukaemia were seen with (whole-body) doses above 10–50 cGy, but below this the incidence approximated to that of the Japanese national statistics. A similar dose effect was suggested by a relative increase in leukaemia in those exposed within 2000 m of the explosion hypocentre [191]; this was a more crude parameter, which had to be modified according to the degree of shielding the

victims experienced. In the small study population who received more than 10 cGy, there was 54 'excess' leukaemia deaths in Hiroshima and 16 in Nagasaki. This discrepancy has been attributed to the difference between the two bombs; that at Hiroshima produced neutrons and gamma rays, while the bomb at Nagasaki produced almost entirely gamma rays [193]. There were differences, too, in the types of leukaemia seen in the two cities, with 40% of the Hiroshima cases being chronic granulocytic (CGL) in nature compared to only 12% in Nagasaki [192].

The latency period varied with age at exposure, from 9 years in those under 15, to 15 years in those over 30. The types of disease encountered included all varieties, with the singular exception of chronic lymphatic leukaemia. Overall, some 35% were ANLL, 17% were ALL and 48% were CGL [191].

The age distribution among these types broadly resembled that among spontaneous leukaemias, with over half the ALL arising in children under 15 compared to only 25% of the ANLL, and 20% of the CGL [195]. There was also an age effect on the frequency of leukaemia, with the highest rates being seen in those over 50 or under 10 years old and the lowest in those aged 10–20 years.

A reassessment of the acute leukaemia cases [196] has confirmed that the leukaemia developing in the survivors of atomic radiation closely follows the pattern of *de novo* leukaemia, instead of the more typical secondary leukaemia due to cytotoxic drugs. An additional observation is the relatively high incidence of CGL, with the presence of the Philadelphia chromosome [197] and typical evolution of the disease [198]. This again is not a feature of drug-induced leukaemias. Because the long-term consequences of radiation exposure are considered to be the result of interaction between radioactive particles (alpha or beta) or waves (gamma or X-rays) and DNA, this raises the interesting, but unanswered, questions why there should be such differences, and whether atomic radiation and cytotoxic drugs induce leukaemia by different means.

An additional area of controversy is the relationship between radiation dose and leukaemia risk at low exposure levels, especially in the context of military participants in the nuclear tests carried out in the 1950s by the UK and the USA. A statistically significant increase of leukaemia (types not specified) was found in nuclear test participants on military manoeuvres during the US 1957 nuclear test 'Smokey', but accurate information on levels of exposure was not available [199]. Further problems in this area are methods of determining the levels of ingested or inhaled radiation to which these service personnel were exposed.

Leukaemia as a result of radiotherapy

Radiotherapy for nonmalignant conditions

Forty years ago it was first recognized that patients treated with radiotherapy to the spine for ankylosing spondylitis stood an increased risk of developing leukaemia [200]. Ten years later, Court-Brown & Doll [201] amassed a study group of 14 544 patients of whom 52 had died of leukaemia—approximately a 10-fold increase over the expected number. Nearly all cases were myeloid leukaemias, both acute and chronic.

Factors, other than irradiation, involved in the genesis of leukaemia in these patients appeared to be unlikely because of the time relationship (2–15 years after the radiotherapy), and a convincing dose–response curve showed that the incidence of leukaemia rose sharply to over 600 cases/100 000 men/year when the mean dose of radiotherapy to the spinal marrow exceeded 2000 cGy [202]. Review of the case histories and blood and bone marrow morphology of 80% of these cases of leukaemia has shown features of pancytopenia and myelodysplasia closely resembling those of drug-induced leukaemia and in contradistinction to the leukaemia following atomic radiation. Two possible explanations for this are that patients with spondylitis have a predisposition to develop leukaemia [203] or that the patients received orthovoltage treatment that was usually administered over a number of courses.

An excess of leukaemia has also been seen in other non-malignant conditions treated with radiotherapy. Radiation-induced menopause as a treatment for menorrhagia has produced such a result [204], although the risk appears to be very small [205] and the marrow dose of irradiation was much less than in ankylosing spondylitis (mean 134 cGy) [204].

A few cases of leukaemia were thought to follow irradiation of the scalp for tinea capitis in nearly 3000 children during the 1950s, where the cranial marrow was estimated to receive 385 cGy, but the small excess of cases is now considered to be of doubtful significance [189]. However, it is more likely that at least some children given mediastinal irradiation for thymic enlargement in infancy subsequently developed radiation-induced leukaemia [206,207], as a threefold excess of neoplasia was still evident in such children 20 years later [208].

Radiotherapy for malignant disease

Although secondary leukaemia following high-dose radiotherapy for primary cancers has been reported for over 20 years [209], the incidence of this complication appears to be low. One possible explanation is that most reports arise from the era of orthovoltage therapy [210] before the widespread introduction of megavoltage treatment. A second reason may be that for many cancers, only a small percentage of bone marrow is localized within the radiation beam and receives such high concentrated doses of radiation that the marrow stem cells are killed rather than damaged or transformed. One study of leukaemia following radiotherapy for breast cancer [90] did show a cumulative risk of 1.4 ± 0.5% at 10 years, but the numbers studied were relatively small. In a larger series [211] there was no evidence that radiotherapy increased the overall risk of leukaemia, and the series also included a dose–

response analysis which gave no indication that risk varied over discrete categories of radiation dose. Other studies have also found no increased risk [92]. Intensive radiotherapy to the pelvis for cervical cancer has shown only a twofold risk of leukaemia, including CGL as well as ANLL [212]. As previously discussed, there have been conflicting results on the risk of secondary leukaemia following combined treatment with chemotherapy and radiotherapy. The extent of irradiation may be important, because an excess risk of leukaemia has been associated with total nodal irradiation [50], although there are contradictory findings from other studies [57].

Nonrandom chromosome abnormalities are well documented for drug-induced leukaemias, and similar abnormalities of 5q– or –7 have been found for radiotherapy-related ANLL in three of eight cases [214] and five of seven cases [18].

Radioactive isotopes

Phosphorus-32 has been used in the treatment of PV since the early 1940s. Its leukaemogenic potential was more than a suspicion after a few years [86], but the realization was confused by the tendency of the disease itself to progress to leukaemia and by the lack of comparability of patients treated with ^{32}P to those treated by phlebotomy alone [81]. It is now well documented that ^{32}P does result in an excess of secondary ANLL [82,83].

Thorotrast, a colloidal solution of thorium dioxide, emits about 90% of its energy as alpha radiation and has a biological half-life of more than 400 years. It was used between 1930 and 1955 as a radiographic contrast medium, and after injection it is deposited indefinitely in the phagocytes of the reticuloendothelial system. Unfortunately, it was subsequently found to produce local malignancies and a gross excess of leukaemia. By 1976, over 60 cases of various leukaemias and 40 of aplastic anaemia had been reported to be Thorotrast related [215], with a latent period of 2–37 years. This long latent period was confirmed in a Japanese study [216] ranging from 16 to 45 years with a median of 35 years. An additional unusual feature in this report is a high incidence of 42% of erythroleukaemia.

Leukaemia as a result of occupational exposure to radiation

Early workers in medical radiology undoubtedly suffered a highly significant excess of death from leukaemia, myeloma and aplastic anaemia, despite initial concern that such a finding might be spurious [217]. Consequent upon the introduction of adequate safety regulations in the late 1930s (earlier in Great Britain), this excess has disappeared [218], but it does indicate the leukaemogenicity of small doses of X-irradiation over a number of years. Cumulative doses received by these early workers are thought to have been in the region of 1000–2000 cGy [192].

The relationship of secondary leukaemia to other occupations where there may be exposure to radiation is less clear cut, although an apparent excess of leukaemia deaths has been reported in nuclear submarine workers [219].

An even more controversial aspect of occupational radiation is whether there is an increased incidence of childhood leukaemia around nuclear establishments and, if so, whether it relates in any way to radiation. A raised incidence of childhood leukaemias was found in the village of Seascale near the nuclear plant Sellafield [220], and additional reports have suggested a similar excess of leukaemia in children in relation to nuclear establishments at Aldermaston and Burghfield [221] and to the fast breeder reactor and reprocessing operation at Dounreay [222]. Confirmatory evidence for a significant excess mortality from leukaemia in people aged under 25 years living in proximity to a number of nuclear installations was reported by Cook-Mozaffari *et al.* [223]. A more recent report [224] has re-examined the relationship between the risk of childhood leukaemia and proximity of residence to nuclear installations in England and Wales. Leukaemia registration within 25 km of 23 nuclear installations and six control sites was analysed on the basis of observed to expected ratios, and also on a linear risk score test designed to be sensitive to excess incidence in close proximity to a putative source of risk. The conclusion was of no evidence for an increase in leukaemia around nuclear installations, except for a distance-related risk at Sellafield. Despite these conflicting results, there appears to be general acceptance of a definite increased incidence of acute leukaemia in young people under 25 years of age who lived in Seascale during the period 1955–83.

Following the Black Report in 1984, an epidemiological study was commissioned and funded by the UK Department of Health specifically asking whether known causes or factors associated with the nuclear site at Sellafield might have been responsible for the observed excess [225]. The principal findings were an increased leukaemia risk in children relating to total external dose of radiation received by the father before the child's conception. In addition, there was a progressive leukaemia increase with increasing radiation dose for the immediate 6 months prior to conception. The controversial conclusion was that paternal irradiation preconception, via a possible germ-line mutation, was responsible for leukaemia induction (Gardner's hypothesis). Because of the legal consequences of this proposal there has been great interest in further studies from which no support for the hypothesis has been provided from Scotland [226] or Ontario [227]. The conclusion is that Gardner's hypothesis cannot be sustained and that the association between paternal irradiation and leukaemia is a chance finding [228].

If there is no evidence for radiation what other possible mechanisms could explain the 'Seascale cluster'? One hypothesis is that leukaemia induction may be associated with underlying infection, the transmission of which can be facilitated by increases in levels of new social contacts. Nuclear installations are often in isolated areas, requiring a large workforce to come together to build and work at the installation; this therefore introduces an infective cause to a previously isolated community with particular susceptibility [229]. A similar explanation of infection transmission between adults as a result of increased contacts from commuting activity has been postulated to explain the possible excess of childhood leukaemia near to nuclear establishments in West Berkshire [230]. Additional analysis is required before it can be determined whether this hypothesis has any good foundation [231].

Leukaemia as a result of diagnostic radiology

This subject can be briefly dismissed by saying that presently there is no good evidence that diagnostic X-rays cause leukaemia. Twenty years ago it was thought that they might [232,233], and considerable concern also followed the observations of Stewart *et al.* [234] that childhood leukaemia occurred more frequently in children X-rayed *in utero*. Another large study supported the same suggestion [235], and the Oxford group later expanded their original data to show a dose effect where an increasing number of films were shown to correlate with a rising subsequent incidence of childhood malignancy of all types [236]. To keep perspective, however, the risk was never said to be great—less than one case per year per 10 000 children irradiated *in utero*—and by 1975 the same investigators observed the effect to be disappearing [237], a result which they attributed to a general reduction in antenatal X-rays, both in dose and frequency. Whether the effect had ever been significant is debatable. Certainly, the original findings were challenged in a time-matched study [238], and others thought the risks to be overestimated [239]. Interestingly, Jablan & Kato reported that no excess of cases of leukaemia appeared in 1300 children haplessly irradiated *in utero* in Hiroshima and Nagasaki, although they received doses up to several hundred times those given in antenatal radiology [240]. There has been a suggestion that diagnostic radiography might be a risk factor for CGL [241], but the data are inconclusive.

Leukaemia following exposure to nonionizing radiation (electromagnetic fields)

There have been a number of studies on residential exposure to magnetic fields and childhood leukaemia, and at present firm conclusions are difficult to draw. Three studies from Norway, Sweden and Finland have investigated magnetic field exposure generated by high-voltage transmission lines and although there are differences in study design there was a relative leukaemia risk ratio of 2.1 in exposed cases, suggesting that there may be an aetiological role for electromagnetic radiation [242].

Table 12.7 Nonmalignant diseases associated with secondary leukaemia.

Condition	Predominant type of leukaemia	Reference
Group A, association accepted		
Inherited		
Down's syndrome	ANLL/ALL	Robison, 1992 [243]
Ataxia telangiectasia	ALL	Taylor, 1992 [248]
Bloom's syndrome	ALL/ANLL	German, 1993 [250]
Fanconi's anaemia	ANLL	Butturini *et al.*, 1994 [251]
Neurofibromatosis	ANLL/JCML	Stiller *et al.*, 1994 [252]
Acquired		
Marrow transplantation (donor cell leukaemia)	ANLL/ALL	Witherspoon *et al.*, 1989 [254]
Group B, association suspected		
Bruton-type agammaglobulinaemia	ALL	Frizzera *et al.*, 1980 [255]
Wiskott–Aldrich syndrome	AML	Perry *et al.*, 1980 [256]
Congenital agranulocytosis (Kostmann's syndrome)	AML	Rosen & Kang, 1979 [257]
Schwachman's syndrome	ALL	Strevens *et al.*, 1978 [258]
Rubinstein–Taybi syndrome	ALL	Jonas *et al.*, 1978 [259]
Klinefelter's syndrome	ALL	Gürgey *et al.*, 1994 [260]
Poland's syndrome	ALL	Esquembre *et al.*, 1987 [261]
Diamond–Blackfan syndrome	AML	Wasser *et al.*, 1978 [262]
Intestinal lymphangiectasia	ALL	Kay & Lilleyman, 1981 [263]

Diseases predisposing to leukaemia

Several pathological conditions, mostly constitutional and mostly arising in childhood, are known or thought to predispose to the subsequent development of leukaemia. In some the association is strong and well documented, whereas in others it is more tenuous. These disorders are listed in Table 12.7 and divided on the basis of how well an association is established. Some of those in Group A, where there is a strong link, are considered in more detail below.

Down's syndrome

The association between Down's syndrome and leukaemia is well recognized and, although there are widely varying reports on the estimated risk, large studies would suggest that the association occurs 10–15 times more frequently than would be expected by chance [243]. For the cases diagnosed as having ALL there is no evidence that the clinical features are different from those seen in normal children and although there have been suggestions of a higher rate of treatment failures more recent intensive therapy has produced similar results in Down's syndrome and normal children [243]. Patients with Down's syndrome and ANLL are significantly younger at diagnosis, and a large proportion of cases are acute megakaryoblastic leukaemia (FAB M$_7$) with an incidence 600 times greater than expected [244]. There are suggestions that the acute megakaryoblastic leukaemia in Down's syndrome is a unique disease and differs from that found in normal individuals by having a myelodysplastic phase comprising thrombocytopenia and abnormal megakaryocytopoiesis in a high percentage of cases before the leukaemia develops. In addition, there is a higher than expected long-term survival rate [244].

Neonates with Down's syndrome may develop a transient myeloproliferative disorder (TMPD) which, on presentation, is indistinguishable from acute leukaemia and only becomes apparent on follow-up when the condition spontaneously remits without any therapy. Ultrastructural and immunophenotyping studies have shown that the increased blast cells are megakaryoblasts or multipotential progenitor cells and there is increasing evidence that this is a clonal disorder based on cytogenetic abnormalities, inactivation of X-chromosome-linked polymorphic genes [245] and rearrangement of the T-cell receptor B gene [246]. Although spontaneous clinical remission coincides with the disappearance of the clonal characteristics, there is a suggestion that TMPD may be a clonal preleukaemia, because about 20% of cases subsequently develop acute leukaemia [246].

Immunodeficiency syndromes

These may be divided into straightforward immunodeficiencies (e.g. severe combined deficiency, Bruton-type agam-maglobulinaemia and IgA deficiency), more complex syndromes (e.g. ataxia telangiectasia, Bloom's syndrome and Wiskott–Aldrich syndrome) or associated with premature loss or destruction of lymphocytes or immunoglobulins (e.g. intestinal lymphangiectasia). Most of the haematological malignancies which arise in these conditions are lymphomas and leukaemia development is rare and usually of lymphoblastic type. The genesis of the predisposition to malignancy is not fully understood but may, in some instances, be a result of lymphocyte subset imbalances and loss of feedback control mechanism [247].

Ataxia telangiectasia

Ataxia telangiectasia (AT) is a progressive neurological disorder of ataxia, oculomotor dyspraxia and dysarthria combined with immunodeficiency, although the latter is not severe. A majority of patients have a deficiency of cell-mediated immunity with deficiencies of humoral immunity being much more variable [248]. Most patients with AT have spontaneously arising chromosome translocations in their lymphocytes which usually involve breaks at the sites of T-cell receptor genes and some translocation cells can proliferate to produce clones as large as 90% of the circulating T cells. The chromosomal rearrangements seen in these T-cell clones involve one break in a T-cell receptor locus and one break in a non-T-cell receptor locus, for example inv(14)(q11;q32), t(14;14)(q11;q32), t(X;14)(q28;q11) [249]. These clones can be present in the blood for many years but there is the potential for them to develop into leukaemia which, in younger patients (2–12 years), is of the acute lymphoblastic type, whereas in older patients (mean age 33 years) is of the chronic lymphatic type [248]. In both types of leukaemia there is a predominance of T-cell type which is far in excess of the percentage of T-cell leukaemias found in non-AT patients.

Bloom's syndrome

This rare autosomal recessive disorder is characterized by growth retardation, abnormal facies, hypogonadism, variable skin manifestations and reduced levels of immunoglobulin IgM and IgA and, rarely, IgG. The somatic cells of individuals with this syndrome accumulate unusually large numbers of spontaneous chromosome abnormalities of multiple types due to defective DNA replication and repair and there is a marked predisposition for such individuals to develop a large variety of neoplasms at an early age.

From the Bloom's syndrome registry acute leukaemia comprises 21 of the 84 reported malignancies. This occurs predominantly in childhood and comprises ALL in six cases, ANLL in seven and undifferentiated or unspecified in eight, with a poor response to chemotherapy in all types [250].

Fanconi's anaemia

Fanconi's anaemia is an autosomal recessive disease with aplastic anaemia, congenital abnormalities and peripheral blood lymphocytes characterized by an increased frequency of chromatid breaks and hypersensitivity to DNA cross-linking agents. Data from the International Fanconi Anaemia Registry Study shows that the development of myelodysplasia (MDS) and ANLL is a relatively common occurrence, with an acturial risk by 40 years of age of 52% (37–67%) [251]. The median age at detection of MDS and ANLL was 13 years and, although most cases develop after an initial diagnosis of bone marrow failure, in some patients MDS or ANLL may be the first haematological abnormality detected. Evolution of clonal cytogenetic abnormalities may develop often in close temporal proximity to the diagnosis of MDS and ANLL.

Neurofibromatosis

Neurofibromatosis type 1 (NF-1) is an autosomal dominant genetic disorder associated with an excessive incidence of a number of childhood cancers, including leukaemia. The greatest risk is of developing myeloproliferative disorders and ANLL, although a five-fold to 10-fold risk of ALL also occurs [252]. In the myeloproliferative disorders there appears to be a surprisingly high incidence of juvenile chronic myelogenous leukaemia, together with the myeloproliferative syndrome associated with monosomy 7 [253]. For the individuals with myeloid malignancies there is a pattern of inheritance which favours maternal transmission and there is also a marked tendency for males to be affected [253].

In contradistinction for those patients developing ALL, there appears to be a higher proportion of apparently sporadic neurofibromatosis.

Donor cell leukaemia following allogeneic bone marrow transplantation

There have been a number of reports of leukaemia developing in donor cells after allogeneic bone marrow transplantation (ABMT), and because the ratio of observed to expected cases is 40 this indicates a true increase of secondary leukaemia [254]. The donor stem cells have not been exposed to the conditioning regimens of chemoradiotherapy. It is therefore unlikely that this is the causative mechanism. As there is also a definite increase of non-Hodgkin's lymphoma post ABMT [254], the more likely causes are an aberration of the T-cell regulatory mechanism or possible antigenic stimulation arising from differences of HLA and non-HLA between donor and recipient.

References

1 Pedersen-Bjergaard J., Philip P., Larsen S.O. *et al.* (1993) Therapy-related myelodysplasia and acute myeloid leukemia. Cytogenetic

characteristics of 115 consecutive cases and risk in seven cohorts of patients treated intensively for malignant diseases in the Copenhagen series. *Leukaemia*, **7**, 1975–1986.

2 Smith A.G., Prentice A.G., Lucie N.P., Browning J.D., Dagg J.H. & Rowan R.M. (1982) Acute myelogenous leukaemia following cytotoxic therapy. Five cases and a review. *Quarterly Journal of Medicine*, **51**, 227–240.

3 Calabresi P. (1983) Leukemia after cytotoxic chemotherapy — a Pyrrhic victory? *New England Journal of Medicine*, **309**, 1118–1119.

4 Kyle R.A. (1983) Second malignancies and chemotherapeutic agents. *Progress in Clinical and Biological Research (New York)*, **132E**, 45–54.

5 Editorial (1984) Drugs that can cause cancer. *Lancet*, **i**, 261–262.

6 Stott H., Fox W., Girling D.J., Stephens R.J. & Galton D.A.G. (1977) Acute leukaemia after busulphan. *British Medical Journal*, **2**, 1513–1517.

7 Greene M.H., Harris E.L., Gershenson D.M. *et al.* (1986) Melphalan may be a more potent leukemogen than cyclophosphamide. *Annals of Internal Medicine*, **105**, 360–367.

8 Curtis R.E., Boice J.D., Stovall M. *et al.* (1992) Risk of leukemia after chemotherapy and radiation treatment for breast cancer. *New England Journal of Medicine*, **326**, 1745–1751.

9 Pedersen-Bjergaard J., Specht L., Larsen S.O. *et al.* (1987) Risk of therapy-related leukaemia and preleukaemia after Hodgkin's disease: relation to age, cumulative dose of alkylating agents, and time from chemotherapy. *Lancet*, **ii**, 83–88.

10 Grunwald H.W. & Rosner F. (1982) Acute myeloid leukemia following treatment of Hodgkin's disease. A review. *Cancer*, **50**, 676–683.

11 Iurlo A., Mecucci C., Van Orshoven A. *et al.* (1989) Cytogenetic and clinical investigations in 76 cases with therapy-related leukaemia and myelodysplastic syndrome. *Cancer Genetics and Cytogenetics*, **43**, 227–241.

12 Michels S.D., McKenna R.W., Arthur D.C. & Brunning R.D. (1985) Therapy-related acute myeloid leukemia and myelodysplastic syndrome: a clinical and morphologic study of 65 cases. *Blood*, **65**, 1364–1372.

13 Bennett J.M., Catovsky D., Daniel M.T. *et al.* (1982) Proposals for the classification of the myelodysplastic syndromes. *British Journal of Haematology*, **51**, 189–199.

14 Rowley J.D., Golomb H.M. & Vardiman J.W. (1981) Non random chromosome abnormalities in acute leukaemia and dysmyelopoietic syndromes in patients with previously treated malignant disease. *Blood*, **58**, 759–767.

15 Pedersen-Bjergaard J., Philip P., Larsen S.O., Jensen G. & Byrsting K. (1990) Chromosome aberrations and prognostic factors in therapy-related myelodysplasia and acute non lymphocytic leukemia. *Blood*, **76**, 1083–1091.

16 Rubin C.M., Arthur D.C., Woods W.G. *et al.* (1991) Therapy-related myelodysplastic syndrome and acute myeloid leukemia in children: correlation between chromosomal abnormalities and prior therapy. *Blood*, **78**, 2982–2988.

17 Pettenati M.J., Le Beau M.M., Lemons R.S. *et al.* (1987) Assignment of CSF-1 to 5q 33.1: evidence for clustering of genes regulating hematopoiesis and for their involvement in the deletion of the long arm of chromosome 5 in myeloid disorders. *Proceedings of the National Academy of Sciences, USA*, **84**, 2970–2974.

18 Le Beau M.M., Albain K.S., Larson R.A. *et al.* (1986) Clinical and cytogenetic correlations in 63 patients with therapy-related myelodysplastic syndromes and acute non-lymphocytic leukemia. Further evidence for characteristic abnormalities of chromosomes No. 5 and 7. *Journal of Clinical Oncology*, **4**, 325–345.

19 Long B.J. (1992) Mechanisms of action of teniposide (VM-26) and comparison with etoposide (VP16). *Seminars in Oncology*, **19**, S3–S19.

20 Long B.H., Musial S.T. & Brattain M.G. (1985) Single and double strand DNA breakage and repair in human lung adenocarcinoma cells exposed to etoposide and teniposide. *Cancer Research*, **45**, 3106–3112.

21 Ratain M.J., Kaminer L.S., Bitran J.D. *et al.* (1987) Acute non-lymphocytic leukemia following etoposide and cisplatin combination chemotherapy for advanced non-small-cell carcinoma of the lung. *Blood*, **70**, 1412–1417.

22 Ellis M., David M. & Lishner M. (1993) A comparative analysis of alkylating agent and epipodophyllotoxin-related leukemias. *Leukemia and Lymphoma*, **11**, 9–13.

23 Kumar L. (1993) Epipodophyllotoxins and secondary leukaemia. *Lancet*, **342**, 819–820.

24 Ross J.A., Potter J.D. & Robison L.L. (1994) Infant leukemia, topoisomerase II inhibitors and the MLL gene. *Journal of the National Cancer Institute*, **86**, 1678–1680.

25 Nakamura H., Ishizaki T., Itoyama T. *et al.* (1994) Acute myeloid leukaemia with t(9;11)(p22;q23) in a patient treated for adult T cell leukaemia. *British Journal of Haematology*, **86**, 222–224.

26 Hallett J., Aronson I. & Jacobs P. (1995) Therapy-related acute myeloblastic leukaemia (M$_1$) with a 9;11 translocation. *British Journal of Haematology*, **90**, 489–490.

27 Larson R.A., Le Beau M.M., Ratain M.J. & Rowley J.D. (1992) Balanced translocation involving chromosome bands 11q23 and 21q22 in therapy-related leukemia. *Blood*, **79**, 1892–1893.

28 Rowley J.D. (1994) Chromosome translocations: dangerous liaisons. *Leukemia*, **8**, S1–S6.

29 Morrisey J., Tkachuk D.C., Milatovich A., Francke U., Link M. & Cleary M.L. (1993) A serine/proline rich protein is fused to HRX in t(4;11) acute leukaemia. *Blood*, **81**, 1124–1131.

30 Nakamura T., Alder H., Gu Y. *et al.* (1993) Genes on chromosome 4, 9 and 19 involved in 11q23 abnormalities in acute leukemia share sequence homology and/or common motifs. *Proceedings of the National Academy of Sciences, USA*, **90**, 4631–4635.

31 Yamamoto K., Seto M., Komatsu H. *et al.* (1993) Two distinct portions of LTG 19/ENL are involved in t(11;19) leukemia. *Oncogene*, **8**, 2617–2625.

32 Super H.J.G., McCabe N.R., Thirman M.J. *et al.* (1993) Rearrangements of the MLL gene in therapy-related acute myeloid leukaemia in patients previously treated with agents targeting DNA-topoisomerase II. *Blood*, **82**, 3705–3711.

33 Hawkins M.M., Kinnier Wilson L.M., Stovall M.A. *et al.* (1992) Epipodophyllotoxins, alkylating agents, and radiation and risk of secondary leukaemia after childhood cancer. *British Medical Journal*, **304**, 951–958.

34 Pedersen-Bjergaard J., Daugaard G., Hansen S.W., Philip P., Larsen S.O. & Rorth M. (1991) Increased risk of myelodysplasia and leukaemia after etoposide, cisplatin, and bleomycin for germ-cell tumours. *Lancet*, **338**, 359–363.

35 Winick N.J., McKenna R.W., Shuster J.J. *et al.* (1993) Secondary acute myeloid leukemia in children with acute lymphoblastic leukemia treated with etoposide. *Journal of Clinical Oncology*, **11**, 209–217.

36 Pedersen-Bjergaard J., Sigsgaard T.C., Nielsen D. *et al.* (1992) Acute monocytic or myelomonocytic leukaemia with balanced chromosome translocation to band 11q23 after therapy with 4-

epi-doxorubicin and cisplatin or cyclophosphamide for breast cancer. *Journal of Clinical Oncology*, **10**, 1444–1451.

37 Shepherd L., Ottaway J. & Myles J. (1994) Therapy-related leukemia associated with high dose 4-epi-doxorubicin and cyclophosphamide used as adjuvant chemotherapy for breast cancer. *Journal of Clinical Oncology*, **12**, 2514–2515.

38 Detourmignies L., Castaigne S., Stoppa A.M. *et al.* (1992) Therapy-related acute promyelocytic leukemia: a report on 16 cases. *Journal of Clinical Oncology*, **10**, 1430–1435.

39 Quesnel B., Kantarjian H., Pedersen-Bjergaard J. *et al.* (1993) Therapy-related acute myeloid leukemia with t(8;21), inv(16), and t(8;16): a report on 25 cases and review of the literature. *Journal of Clinical Oncology* **11**, 2370–2379.

40 Matsuzaki A., Inamitsu T., Watanabe T. *et al.* (1994) Acute promyelocytic leukaemia in a patient treated with etoposide for Langerhans cell histiocytosis. *British Journal of Haematology*, **86**, 887–889.

41 Egeler R.M. (1995) Acute promyelocytic leukemia with t(15;17) abnormality after chemotherapy containing etoposide for Langerhans cell histiocytosis. *Cancer*, **75**, 134–135.

42 Hunger S.P., Sklar J. & Link M.P. (1992) Acute lymphoblastic leukemia occurring as a second malignant neoplasm in childhood: report of 3 cases and review of the literature. *Journal of Clinical Oncology*, **10**, 156–163.

43 Narayanan M.N., Morgenstern G.R., Chang J.C., Harrison C.J., Ranson M. & Scarffe J.H. (1994) Acute lymphoblastic leukaemia following Hodgkin's disease is associated with a good prognosis. *British Journal of Haematology*, **86**, 867–869.

44 Canellos G.P., de Vita V.T., Arseneau J.C., Whang-Peng J. & Johnson R.E.C. (1975) Second malignancies complicating Hodgkin's disease in remission. *Lancet*, **i**, 947–949.

45 Coleman C.N., Williams C.J., Flint A., Glatstein E.J., Rosenberg S.A. & Kaplan H.S. (1977) Hematologic neoplasia in patients treated for Hodgkin's disease. *New England Journal of Medicine*, **297**, 1249–1252.

46 Blayney D.W., Longe D.L., Young R.C., *et al.* (1987) Decreasing risk of leukemia with prolonged follow-up after chemotherapy and radiotherapy for Hodgkin's disease. *New England Journal of Medicine*, **316**, 710–714.

47 Tucker M.A., Coleman C.N., Cox R.S., Varghese A. & Rosenberg S.A. (1988) Risk of second cancers after treatment for Hodgkin's disease. *New England Journal of Medicine*, **318**, 76–81.

48 Kaldor J.M., Day N.E., Clarke E.A. *et al.* (1990) Leukemia following Hodgkin's disease. *New England Journal of Medicine*, **322**, 7–13.

49 Baccarani M., Bosi A. & Papa G. (1980) Second malignancy in patients treated for Hodgkin's disease. *Cancer*, **46**, 1735–1740.

50 Andrieu J.M., Ifrah N., Payan C., Fermanian J., Coscas Y. & Flandrin G. (1990) Increased risk of secondary acute nonlymphocytic leukemia after extended-field radiation therapy combined with MOPP chemotherapy for Hodgkin's disease. *Journal of Clinical Oncology*, **8**, 1148–1154.

51 Pui C-H., Hancock M.L., Raimondi S.C. *et al.* (1990) Myeloid neoplasia in children treated for solid tumours. *Lancet*, **336**, 417–421.

52 De Vita V.T., Serpick A. & Carbone P.P. (1970) Combination chemotherapy in the treatment of advanced Hodgkin's disease. *Annals of Internal Medicine*, **73**, 881–895.

53 Nicholson W.M., Beard M.E.J., Crowther D. *et al.* (1970) Combination chemotherapy in generalised Hodgkin's disease. *British Medical Journal*, **3**, 7–10.

54 McElwain T.J., Toy J., Smith I.E., Peckham M.J. & Austin D.E. (1977) A combination of chlorambucil, vinblastine, procarbazine and prednisolone for treatment of Hodgkin's disease. *British Journal of Cancer*, **36**, 276–280.

55 Lavey R.S., Eby N.L. & Prosnitz L.R. (1990) Impact on second malignancy risk of the combined use of radiation and chemotherapy for lymphomas. *Cancer*, **66**, 80–88.

56 Gottlieb C.A., Maeda K., Hawley R.C. & Abraham J.P. (1989) Myelodysplasia with bone marrow lymphocytosis and fibrosis mimicking recurrent Hodgkin's disese. *American Journal of Clinical Pathology*, **91**, 6–11.

57 Van Leeuwen F.E., Chorus A.M.J., Belt-Dusebout A.W. *et al.* (1994) Leukaemia risk following Hodgkin's disease: relation to cumulative dose of alkylating agents, treatment with teniposide combinations, number of episodes of chemotherapy and bone marrow damage. *Journal of Clinical Oncology*, **12**, 1063–1073.

58 Valagussa P., Santoro A., Kendra R. *et al.* (1980) Second malignancies in Hodgkin's disease: a complication of certain forms of treatment. *British Medical Journal*, **280**, 216–219.

59 Swerdlow A.J., Douglas A.J., Vaughan Hudson G., Vaughan Hudson B., Bennett M.H. & MacLennan K.A. (1992) Risk of second primary cancers after Hodgkin's disease by type of treatment: analysis of 2846 patients in the British National Lymphoma Investigation. *British Medical Journal*, **304**, 1137–1143.

60 Tura S., Fiacchini M., Zinzani P.L., Brusamolino E. & Gobbi P.G. (1993) Splenectomy and the increasing risk of secondary acute leukemia in Hodgkin's disease. *Journal of Clinical Oncology*, **11**, 925–930.

61 Bergsagel D.E., Bailey A.J., Langley G.R., MacDonald R.N., White D.F. & Miller A.B. (1979) The chemotherapy of plasma cell myeloma and the incidence of acute leukemia. *New England Journal of Medicine*, **301**, 743–748.

62 Buckman R., Cuzick J. & Galton D.A.G. (1982) Long-term survival in myelomatosis. *British Journal of Haematology*, **52**, 589–599.

63 Rosner F. & Grunwald H. (1980) Cytotoxic drugs and leukaemogenesis. *Clinics in Haematology*, **9**, 663–681.

64 Cuzick J., Erskine S., Edelman D. & Galton D.A.G. (1987) A comparison of the incidence of the myelodysplastic syndrome and acute myeloid leukaemia following melphalan and cyclophosphamide treatment for myelomatosis. *British Journal of Cancer*, **55**, 523–529.

65 Mufti G.J., Hamblin T.J., Clein G.P. & Race C. (1983) Coexistent myelodysplasia and plasma cell neoplasia. *British Journal of Haematology*, **54**, 91–96.

66 Gertz M.A. & Kyle R.A. (1990) Acute leukemia and cytogenetic abnormalities complicating melphalan treatment of primary systemic amyloidosis. *Archives of Internal Medicine*, **150**, 629–633.

67 Majumdar G. & Slater N.G.P. (1993) Waldenström's macroglobulinaemia terminating in acute myeloid leukaemia: report of a case and review of the literature. *Leukemia and Lymphoma*, **9**, 513–516.

68 Pedersen-Bjergaard J., Ersboll J., Sorenson H.M. *et al.* (1985) Risk of acute nonlymphocytic leukemia and preleukemia in patients treated with cyclophosphamide for non-Hodgkin's lymphomas. *Annals of Internal Medicine*, **103**, 195–200.

69 Zarrabi M.H., Rosner F. & Bennett J.M. (1979) Non-Hodgkin's lymphoma and acute myeloblastic leukemia. A report of 12 cases and a review of the literature. *Cancer*, **44**, 1070–1080.

70 Ingram L., Mott M.G., Mann J.R., Raafat F., Darbyshire P.J. & Morris Jones P.H. (1987) Second malignancies in children treated for non-Hodgkin's lymphoma and T-cell leukaemia in the UKCCSG regimens. *British Journal of Cancer*, **55**, 463–466.

71 Greene M.H., Young R.C., Merrill J.M. & De Vita V.T. (1983) Evidence of a treatment dose response in acute non lymphocytic

leukaemias which occur after therapy of non-Hodgkin's lymphoma. *Cancer Research*, **43**, 1891–1898.

72 Anderson R.L., Grover C.G. & Richert-Boe K. (1981) Therapy related preleukemic syndrome. *Cancer*, **47**, 1867–1871.

73 Miller J.S., Arthur D.C., Litz C.E., Neglia J.P., Miller W.J. & Weisdorf D.J. (1994) Myelodysplastic syndrome after autologous bone marrow transplantation: an additional late complication of curative cancer therapy. *Blood*, **83**, 3780–3786.

74 Darrington D.C., Vase J.M., Anderson J.R. *et al.* (1994) Incidence and characterization of secondary myelodysplastic syndrome and acute myelogenous leukemia following high dose chemoradiotherapy and autologous stem-cell transplantation for lymphoid malignancies. *Journal of Clinical Oncology*, **12**, 2527–2534.

75 Traweek S.T., Slovak M.L., Nademanee A.P., Brynes R.K., Niland J.C. & Forman S.J. (1994) Clonal karyotypic hematopoietic cell abnormalities occurring after autologous bone marrow transplantation for Hodgkin's disease and non-Hodgkin's lymphoma. *Blood*, **84**, 957–963.

76 Stone R., Neuberg D., Soiffer R. *et al.* (1993) Myelodysplastic syndrome (MDS) as a complication after autologous bone marrow transplantation (ABMT) for non-Hodgkin's lymphoma (NHL). *Blood*, **82**, 196a (abstr.suppl. 1).

77 Pui C-H., Behm F.G., Raimondi S.C. *et al.* (1989) Secondary acute myeloid leukemia in children treated for acute lymphoid leukemia. *New England Journal of Medicine*, **321**, 136–142.

78 Kreissman S.G., Gelber R.D., Cohen H.J., Clavell L.A., Leavitt P. & Sallan S.E. (1992) Incidence of secondary acute myelogenous leukemia after treatment of childhood acute lymphoblastic leukemia. *Cancer*, **70**, 2208–2213.

79 Stern N., Shemesh J. & Ramot B. (1981) Chronic lymphatic leukemia terminating in acute myeloid leukemia. Review of the literature. *Cancer*, **47**, 1849–1851.

80 Robertson L.E., Estey E., Kantarjian H. *et al.* (1994) Therapy related leukemia and myelodysplastic syndrome in chronic lymphatic leukemia. *Leukemia*, **8**, 2047–2051.

81 Landaw S.A. (1976) Acute leukemia in polycythemia vera. *Seminars in Hematology*, **13**, 33–48.

82 Berk P.D., Goldberg J.D., Silverstein M.N. *et al.* (1981) Increased incidence of acute leukemia in polycythemia vera associated with chlorambucil therapy. *New England Journal of Medicine*, **304**, 441–447.

83 Najean Y., Deschamps A., Dresch C., Daniel M.T., Rain J.D. & Arrago J.P. (1988) Acute leukemia and myelodysplasia in polycythemia vera: a clinical study with long-term follow-up. *Cancer*, **61**, 89–95.

84 Brandt L. & Anderson H. (1995) Survival and risk of leukaemia in polycythaemia vera and essential thrombocythaemia treated with oral radiophosphorous: are safer drugs available? *European Journal of Haematology*, **54**, 21–26.

85 Najean Y., Dresch C. & Rain J-D. (1994) The very-long-term course of polycythaemia: a complement to the previously published data of the Polycythaemia Vera Study Group. *British Journal of Haematology*, **86**, 233–235.

86 Tubiana M., Flamant R. & Attie E. (1968) A study of hematological complications occurring in patients with polycythemia vera treated with ^{32}P. *Blood*, **32**, 536–542.

87 Lawrence J.H., Winchell H.S. & Donald W.G. (1969) Leukemia in polycythemia vera: relationship to splenic myeloid metaplasia and therapeutic radiation dose. *Annals of Internal Medicine*, **70**, 763–771.

88 Sedlacek S.M., Curtis J.L., Weintraub J. & Levin J. (1986) Essential thrombocythemia and leukemic transformation. *Medicine*, **65**, 353–364.

89 Concensus Conference (1985) Adjuvant chemotherapy for breast cancer. *Journal of the American Medical Association*, **254**, 3461–3463.

90 Fisher B., Rockette H., Fisher E.R., Wickerham D.L., Redmond C. & Brown A. (1985) Leukemia in breast cancer patients following adjuvant chemotherapy or postoperative radiation: the NSABP experience. *Journal of Clinical Oncology*, **3**, 1640–1658.

91 Curtis R.E., Boice J.D., Moloney W.C., Ries L.G. & Flannery J.T. (1990) Leukemia following chemotherapy for breast cancer. *Cancer Research*, **50**, 2741–2746.

92 Haas J.F., Kittelmann B., Mehnert W.H. *et al.* (1987) Risk of leukaemia in ovarian tumour and breast cancer patients following treatment by cyclophosphamide. *British Journal of Cancer*, **55**, 213–218.

93 Geller R.B., Boone L.B., Karp J.E. *et al.* (1989). Secondary acute myelocytic leukemia after adjuvant therapy for early-stage breast carcinoma. *Cancer*, **64**, 629–634.

94 Andersson M., Philip P. & Pedersen-Bjergaard J. (1990) High risk of therapy-related leukemia and preleukemia after therapy with prednimustine, methotrexate, 5-fluorouracil, mitoxantrone and tamoxifen for advanced breast cancer. *Cancer*, **65**, 2460–2464.

95 Markham M., Pavy M.D. & Abeloff M.D. (1982) Acute leukemia following intensive therapy for small-cell carcinoma of the lung. *Cancer*, **50**, 672–675.

96 Rose V.L., Keppen M.D., Eichner E.R., Pitha J.V. & Murray J.L. (1983) Acute leukemia after successful chemotherapy for oat cell carcinoma. *American Journal of Clinical Pathology*, **79**, 122–124.

97 Chak L.Y., Sikic B.I., Tucker M.A., Horns R.C. & Cox R.S. (1984) Increased incidence of acute nonlymphocytic leukemia following therapy in patients with small cell carcinoma of the lung. *Journal of Clinical Oncology*, **2**, 385–390.

98 Pedersen-Bjergaard J., Osterlind K., Hansen M., Preben P., Pedersen A.G. & Hansen H.H. (1985) Acute nonlymphocytic leukemia, preleukemia and solid tumors following intensive chemotherapy of small cell carcinoma of the lung. *Blood*, **66**, 1393–1397.

99 Reimer R.R., Hoover R., Fraumeni J.F. & Young R.C. (1977) Acute leukemia after alkylating-agent therapy of ovarian cancer. *New England Journal of Medicine*, **297**, 177–181.

100 Kapadia S.B. & Krause J.R. (1978) Ovarian carcinoma terminating in acute non lymphocytic leukemia following alkylating agent therapy. *Cancer*, **41**, 1676–1679.

101 Pedersen-Bjergaard J., Nissen N.I., Sorensen H.M. *et al.* (1980) Acute non-lymphocytic leukemia in patients with ovarian carcinoma following long term treatment with treosulphan (dihydroxybusulphan). *Cancer*, **45**, 19–29.

102 Greene M.H., Boice J.D., Greer B.E., Blessing J.A. & Dembo A.J. (1982) Acute non lymphocytic leukemia after therapy with alkylating agents for ovarian cancer. *New England Journal of Medicine*, **307**, 1416–1421.

103 Greene M.H., Harris E.L., Gershenson D.M. *et al.* (1986) Melphalan may be a more potent leukemogen than cyclophosphamide. *Annals of Internal Medicine*, **105**, 360–367.

104 Kaldor J.M., Day N.E., Pettersson F. *et al.* (1990) Leukemia following chemotherapy for ovarian cancer. *New England Journal of Medicine*, **322**, 1–6.

105 Chambers S.K., Chopyk R.L., Chambers J.T., Schwartz P.E. & Duff T.P. (1989) Development of leukemia after doxorubicin and cisplatin treatment for ovarian cancer. *Cancer*, **64**, 2459–2461.

106 Arlin Z., Schell F. & Gee T. (1982) Long term remission of acute non lymphocytic leukemia in patients with previously treated testicular carcinomas. *Proceedings of the American Association for Cancer Research*, **39**, 339.

107 Vogl S.E. (1978) Acute leukemia complicating treatment of glioblastoma multiforme. *Cancer*, **41**, 333–336.

108 Cohen R.J. (1980) Leukemia after therapy with methyl CCNU. *New England Journal of Medicine*, **302**, 120.

109 Schwartz A.D., Lee H. & Baum E.S. (1975) Leukemia in children with Wilms' tumour. *Journal of Pediatrics*, **87**, 374–376.

110 Wiggans R.G., Jacobson R.J., Fialkow P.J., Woolley P.V., Macdonald J.S. & Schein P.S. (1978) Probable clonal origin of acute myeloblastic leukemia following radiation and chemotherapy of colon cancer. *Blood*, **52**, 659–663.

111 Boice J.D., Greene M.H., Killen J.Y. *et al.* (1983) Leukemia and pre-leukemia after adjuvant treatment of gastrointestinal cancer with semustine (methyl CCNU). *New England Journal of Medicine*, **309**, 1079–1084.

112 Link M.P., Donaldson S.S., Kempson R.L., Wilbur J.R. & Glader B.E. (1984) Acute non lymphocytic leukemia developing during the course of Ewing's sarcoma. *Medical and Pediatric Oncology*, **12**, 194–200.

113 Penchansky L. & Krause J.R. (1982) Acute leukemia following a malignant teratoma in a child with Klinefelter's syndrome. Case report and review of secondary leukemias in children following treatment of primary neoplasms. *Cancer*, **50**, 684–689.

114 Secker-Walker L.M., Stewart E.L. & Todd A. (1985) Acute lymphoblastic leukaemia with t(4;11) follows neuroblastoma: a late effect of treatment? *Medical and Paediatric Oncology*, **13**, 48–50.

115 Weh H.J., Kabisch H., Landbeck G. & Hossfeld D.K. (1986) Translocation (9;11)(p21;q23) in a child with acute monoblastic leukemia following 2 1/2 years after successful chemotherapy for neuroblastoma. *Journal of Clinical Oncology*, **4**, 1518–1520.

116 White L., Ortega J.A. & Ying K.L. (1985) Acute non-lymphocytic leukemia following multi modality therapy for retinoblastoma. *Cancer*, **55**, 496–498.

117 Silberberg J.M. & Zarrabi M.H. (1987) Acute nonlymphocytic leukemia after thiotepa installation into the bladder: report of 2 cases and review of the literature. *Journal of Urology*, **138**, 402–403.

118 Sonneveld P., Kurth K.H., Hagemeyer A. & Abels J. (1990) Secondary hematologic neoplasm after intravesical chemotherapy for superficial bladder carcinoma. *Cancer*, **65**, 23–25.

119 Roberts M.M. & Bell R. (1976) Acute leukaemia after immunosuppressive therapy. *Lancet*, **ii**, 768–770.

120 Chang J. & Geary C.G. (1977) Therapy-linked leukaemia. *Lancet*, **i**, 97.

121 de Bock R.F.K. & Peetermans M.E. (1977) Leukaemia after prolonged use of melphalan for non malignant disease. *Lancet*, **i**, 1208–1209.

122 Kapadia S.B. & Kaplan S.S. (1978) Acute myelogenous leukemia following immunosuppressive therapy for rheumatoid arthritis. *American Journal of Clinical Pathology*, **70**, 301–302.

123 Kahn M.F., Arlet J., Block-Michel H., Caroit M., Chaouat Y. & Renier J.C. (1979) Leucemies aigues apres traitment par agent cytotoxiques en rhumatologie. 19 observations chez 2006 patients. *Nouvelle Presse Medicale*, **8**, 1393–1397.

124 Grunwald H.W. & Rosner F. (1979) Acute leukemia and immunosuppressive therapy for non neoplastic diseases. *Archives of Internal Medicine*, **139**, 461–466.

125 Krause J.R. (1982) Chronic idiopathic thrombocytopenic purpura (ITP): development of acute non lymphocytic leukemia subsequent to treatment with cyclophosphamide. *Medical and Pediatric Oncology*, **10**, 61–65.

126 Horton J.J., Caffrey E.A., Clark K.G.A., MacDonald D.M., Wells R.S. & Daker M.G. (1984) Leukaemia in psoriatic patients treated with razoxane. *British Journal of Dermatology*, **110**, 633–634.

127 Baker G.L., Kahl L.E., Zee B.C., Stolzer B.L., Agarwal A.K. & Medsger T.A. (1987) Malignancy following treatment of rheumatoid arthritis with cyclophosphamide. *American Journal of Medicine*, **83**, 1–9.

128 Palmer R.G., Dore C.J. & Denman A.M. (1984) Chlorambucil induced chromosome damage to human lymphocytes is dose dependent and cumulative. *Lancet*, **i**, 246–249.

129 Rees J.K.H., Gray R.G., Swirsky D. & Hayhoe F.G.J. (1986) Principal results of the Medical Research Council's 8th Acute Myeloid Leukaemia Trial. *Lancet*, **ii**, 1236–1241.

130 Hoyle C.F., De Bastos M., Wheatley K. *et al.* (1989) AML associated with previous cytotoxic therapy, MDS or myeloproliferative disorders. Results from the MRC's 9th AML trial. *British Journal of Haematology*, **72**, 45–53.

131 Priesler H.D., Early A.P., Raza A. *et al.* (1983) Therapy of secondary acute nonlymphocytic leukemia with cytarabine. *New England Journal of Medicine*, **38**, 21–23.

132 Larson R.A., Wernli M., Le Beau M.M. *et al.* (1988) Short remission durations in therapy-related leukemia despite cytogenetic complete responses to high-dose cytarabine. *Blood*, **72**, 1333–1339.

133 Pedersen-Bjergaard J., Philip P., Pedersen N.T. *et al.* (1984) Acute non lymphocytic leukemia, preleukemia and acute myeloproliferative syndrome secondary to treatment of other malignant diseases. II. Bone marrow cytology, cytogenetics, results of HLA typing, response to antileukemic chemotherapy, and survival in a total series of 55 patients. *Cancer*, **54**, 452–462.

134 Baccarani M., Zaccaria A., Bandini G., Cavazzini G., Fanin R. & Tura S. (1983) Low dose arabinosyl cytosine for treatment of myelodysplastic syndromes and subacute myeloid leukemia. *Leukemia Research*, **7**, 539–545.

135 Clark R.E., Jacobs A., Lush C.J. & Smith S.A. (1987) Effect of 13-cis-retinoic acid on survival of patients with myelodysplastic syndrome. *Lancet*, **i**, 763–765.

136 Vadhan-Raj S., Keating M., Le Maistre A. *et al.* (1987) Effects of recombinant human granulocyte-macrophage colony stimulating factor in patients with myelodysplastic syndromes. *New England Journal of Medicine*, **317**, 1545–1552.

137 De Witte T. and Gratwohl A. (1993) Bone marrow transplants for myelodysplastic syndrome and secondary leukaemias. *British Journal of Haematology*, **84**, 361–364.

138 Anderson J.E., Appelbaum F.R. & Storb R. (1995) An update on allogeneic marrow transplantation for myelodysplastic syndrome. *Leukemia and Lymphoma*, **17**, 95–99.

139 Fraumeni J.F. & Miller R.W. Epidemiology of human leukemia. Recent observations. *Journal of the National Cancer Institute*, **38**, 593–605.

140 Bean R.H.D. Phenylbutazone and leukaemia. A possible association. *British Medical Journal*, **2**, 1552–1555.

141 Woodliffe H.J. & Dougan L. (1964) Acute leukaemia associated with phenylbutazone treatment. *British Medical Journal*, **1**, 744–746.

142 Forni A. & Vigliani E.C. (1974) Chemical leukemogenesis in man. *Series Haematologica*, **7**, 211–223.

143 International Agency for Research on Cancer (1982) *Monographs*

on Carcinogenic Risk of Chemicals to Humans, Suppl. 4, IARC, Lyons.

144 Brauer M.J. & Dameschek W. (1967) Hypoplastic anemia and myeloblastic leukemia following chloramphenicol therapy. *New England Journal of Medicine*, **277**, 1003–1005.

145 Cohen T. & Creger W.P. (1967) Acute myeloid leukemia following seven years of aplastic anemia induced by chloramphenicol. *American Journal of Medicine*, **43**, 762–770.

146 Fraumeni J.F. (1967) Bone marrow depression induced by chloramphenicol or phenylbutazone. *Journal of the American Medical Association*, **20**, 828–834.

147 Schmitt-Graff A. (1981) Chloramphenicol-induced aplastic anaemia terminating with acute non lymphocytic leukaemia. *Acta Haematologica*, **66**, 267–268.

148 Shu X.O., Gao Y.T., Linet M.S. *et al.* (1987) Chloramphenicol use and childhood leukaemia in Shanghai. *Lancet*, **ii**, 934–937.

149 De Planque M.M., Kluin-Nelemans H.C., van Krieken H.J.M. *et al.* (1988) Evolution of acquired severe aplastic anaemia to myelodysplasia and subsequent leukaemia in adults. *British Journal of Haematology*, **70**, 55–62.

150 Stahnke N. & Zeisel H.J. (1989) Growth hormone therapy and leukaemia. *European Journal of Paediatrics*, **148**, 591–596.

151 Butturini A., Bernasconi S., Izzi G., Gertner J.M. & Gale R.P. (1994) Short stature Fanconi's anaemia and risk of leukaemia after growth hormone. *Lancet*, **343**, 1576.

152 Izumi T., Muroi K., Takatoku M., Imagawa S., Hatake K. & Miura Y. (1994) Development of acute myeloblastic leukaemia in a case of aplastic anaemia treated with granulocyte colony-stimulating factor. *British Journal of Haematology*, **87**, 666–668.

153 Imashuku S., Hibi S., Kataoka-Morimoto Y. *et al.* (1995) Myelodysplasia and acute myeloid leukaemia in cases of aplastic anaemia and congenital neutropenia following G-CSF administration. *British Journal of Haematology*, **89**, 188–190.

154 Cassileth P.A. (1967) Monocytosis in chlorpromazine-associated agranulocytosis. *American Journal of Medicine*, **43**, 471–476.

155 Delamore I.W. & Geary C.G. (1971) Aplastic anaemia acute myeloblastic leukaemia and oxymethalone. *British Medical Journal*, **2**, 743–745.

156 Gilman P.A. & Holtzman N.A. (1982) Acute lymphoblastic leukemia in a patient receiving penicillamine for Wilson's disease. *Journal of the American Medical Association*, **248**, 467–468.

157 Hammond W.P. & Applebaum F. (1980) Lithium and acute monocytic leukemia. *New England Journal of Medicine*, **302**, 808.

158 Neilson J.L. (1980) More on lithium and leukemia. *New England Journal of Medicine*, **303**, 283–284.

159 Warrell R.P., Krown S.E., Koziner B., Andreeff M. & Kempin S.J. (1983) Acute non lymphocytic leukemia after treatment of nodular lymphoma with human leucocyte interferon. *Annals of Internal Medicine*, **98**, 482–483.

160 Grossbard L., Rosen D., McGilvray E., Capoa A., Miller O. & Bank A. (1968) Acute leukemia with Ph1-like chromosome in an LSD user. *Journal of the American Medical Association*, **205**, 791–792.

161 Berry J.N. (1966) Acute myeloblastic leukemia in a benzedrine addict. *Southern Medical Journal*, **59**, 1169–1170.

162 Robison L.L., Buckley J.D., Daigle A.E. *et al.* (1989) Maternal drug use and risk of childhood non lymphoblastic leukemia among offspring: an epidemiological investigation implicating marijuana. *Cancer*, **63**, 1904–1911.

163 Editorial (1982) Leukemia and benzene. *Annals of Internal Medicine*, **97**, 275–276.

164 Brandt L., Nilsson P.G. & Mitelman F. (1978) Occupational expo-

165 Linos A., Kyle R.A., O'Fallon W.M. & Kurland L.T. (1980) A case-control study of occupational exposure and leukemia. *International Journal of Epidemiology*, **9**, 131–135.

166 Rinsky R.A., Young R.J. & Smith H.B. (1981) Leukemia in benzene workers. *American Journal of Industrial Medicine*, **2**, 217–245.

167 Aksoy M., Erdem S. & Dincol G. (1974) Leukemia in shoe workers chronically exposed to benzene. *Blood*, **44**, 837–851.

168 Aksoy M., Ozeris S., Sabuncu H., Inanici Y. & Yanardag R. (1987) Exposure to benzene in Turkey between 1983 and 1985: a haematological study on 231 workers. *British Journal of Industrial Medicine*, **45**, 785–787.

169 Travis L.B., Chin-Yang L., Zhang Z-N. *et al.* (1994) Hematopoietic malignancies and related disorders among benzene-exposed workers in China. *Leukemia and Lymphoma*, **14**, 91–102.

170 Golomb H.M., Alimena G., Rowley J.D., Vardiman J.W., Testa J.R. & Sovik C. (1982) Correlation of occupation and karyotype in adults with acute non-lymphocytic leukemia. *Blood*, **60**, 404–411.

171 Witz G., Latriano L. & Goldstein B.D. (1989) Metabolism and toxicity of *trans*, *trans*-muconaldehyde an open-ring microsomal metabolite of benzene. *Environmental Health Perspectives*, **82**, 19–22.

172 Aksoy M. (1987) Chronic lymphoid leukaemia and hairy cell leukaemia due to chronic exposure to benzene: a report of three cases. *British Journal of Haematology*, **66**, 209–211.

173 Yin S-N., Li G-L., Tain F-D. *et al.* (1987) Leukaemia in benzene workers: a retrospective cohort study. *British Journal of Industrial Medicine*, **44**, 124–128.

174 Rinksy R.A., Smith A.B., Hornung R. *et al.* (1987) Benzene and leukemia: an epidemiologic risk assessment. *New England Journal of Medicine*, **316**, 1044–1050.

175 Cronkite E.P. (1987) Chemical leukemogenesis: benzene as a model. *Seminars in Hematology*, **24**, 2–11.

176 Swaen G.M.H. & Meijers J.M.M. (1989) Risk assessment of leukaemia and occupational exposure to benzene. *British Journal of Industrial Medicine*, **46**, 826–830.

177 Santos-Burgoa C., Matanoski G.M., Zeger S. & Schwartz L. (1992) Lymphohematopoietic cancer in Styrene-Butadiene polymerization workers. *American Journal Epidemiology*, **136**, 843–854.

178 Acquavella J.F. & Cowles S.R. (1993) Re: lymphohematopoietic cancer in Sytrene-Butadiene polymerization workers. *American Journal of Epidemiology*, **138**, 765–766.

179 Jedlicka V.L., Hermanska Z., Smida I. & Kouba A. (1958) Paramyeloblastic leukaemia appearing simultaneously in two blood cousins after simultaneous contact with gammexane (hexachlorcyclohexane). *Acta Medica Scandinavica*, **161**, 447–451.

180 Timonen T.T.T. & Palva I.P. (1980) Acute leukaemia after exposure to a weed killer, 2-methyl-4-chlorphenoxyacetic acid. *Acta Haematologica*, **63**, 170–171.

181 Mele A., Szklo M., Visani G. *et al.* (1994) Hair dye use and other risk factors for leukemia and pre-leukemia: a case-control study. *American Journal of Epidemiology*, **139**, 609–619.

182 Kishimoto T., Ono T. & Okada K. (1988) Acute myelocytic leukemia after exposure to asbestos. *Cancer*, **62**, 787–790.

183 Fagioli F., Cuneo A., Piva N. *et al.* (1992) Distinct cytogenetic and clinicopathologic features in acute myeloid leukemia after occupational exposure to pesticides and organic solvents. *Cancer*, **70**, 77–85.

184 Buckley J.D., Robison L.L., Swotinsky R. *et al.* (1989) Occupational exposures of parents of children with acute non lymphocytic leukemia: a report from the Children's Cancer Study Group. *Cancer Research*, **49**, 4030–4037.

185 Garfinkel L. & Boffetta P. (1990) Association between smoking and leukemia in two American Cancer Society prospective studies. *Cancer*, **65**, 2356–2360.

186 Doll R. & Peto R. (1976) Mortality in relation to smoking: 20 years observations on male British doctors. *British Medical Journal*, **2**, 1525–1536.

187 Siegel M. (1993) Smoking and leukemia: evaluation of causal hypothesis. *American Journal of Epidemiology*, **138**, 1–9.

188 Brownson R.C., Novotny T.E. & Perry M.C. (1993) Cigarette smoking and adult leukemia. *Archives of Internal Medicine*, **153**, 469–475.

189 United Nations Scientific Committee on the Effects of Atomic Radiation (1977) Sources and effects of ionising radiation. In: *Report to the General Assembly*, pp. 371–377. United Nations, New York.

190 Moloney W.C. (1955) Leukemia in survivors of atomic bombing. *New England Journal of Medicine*, **253**, 88–90.

191 Brill A.A., Tomonaga M. & Heyssel R.M. (1962) Leukemia in man following exposure to ionising radiation. A summary of the findings in Hiroshima and Nagasaki and a comparison with other human experience. *Annals of Internal Medicine*, **56**, 590–609.

192 Gunz F.W. (1983) Ionising radiations and human leukemia. In: *Leukaemia* (eds F.W. Gunz & E.S. Henderson), 4th edn, pp. 359–374. Grune & Stratton, New York.

193 Finch S.C. (1979) The study of atomic bomb survivors in Japan. *American Journal of Medicine*, **66**, 899–901.

194 Beebe G.W., Kato H. & Land E.C. (1978) Studies of the mortality of A-bomb survivors. 6. Mortality and radiation dose. 1950–1974. *Radiation Research*, **75**, 138–201.

195 Mole R.H. (1977) Radiation induced leukemia in man. In: *Radiation-induced Leukemogenesis and Related Viruses*, (ed. J.F. Duplan), pp. 19–36. North Holland Publishing, Amsterdam.

196 Moloney W.C. (1987) Radiogenic leukemia revisited. *Blood*, **70**, 905–908.

197 Kamada N. & Kimio T. (1983) Cytogenetic studies of haematological disorders in atomic bomb survivors. In: *Radiation-induced Chromosome Damage in Man*, (eds T. Ishihara & M.S. Sasaki), pp. 455–474. Alan R. Liss, New York.

198 Moloney W.C. & Lange R.D. (1954) Leukemia in atomic bomb survivors. II. Observations on early phases of leukemia. *Blood*, **9**, 663–685.

199 Caldwell G.G., Kelley D., Zack M., Falk H. & Heath C.W. (1983) Mortality and cancer frequency among military nuclear test (Smokey) participants, 1957 through 1979. *Journal of the American Medical Association*, **250**, 620–624.

200 Van Swaay H. (1955) Aplastic anaemia and myeloid leukaemia after irradiation of the vertebral column. *Lancet*, **ii**, 225–227.

201 Court-Brown W.M. & Doll R. (1965) Mortality from cancer and other causes after radiotherapy for ankylosing spondylitis. *British Medical Journal*, **2**, 1327–1332.

202 Court-Brown W.M. & Doll R. (1965) Leukaemia and aplastic anaemia in patients irradiated for ankylosing spondylitis. In: *Medical Research Council. Special Report*, Series No. 295. HMSO, London.

203 Abbat J.D. & Lea A.J. (1958) Leukaemogens. *Lancet*, **ii**, 880–883.

204 Smith P.G. & Doll R. (1976) Late effects of X-irradiation in patients treated for metropathia haemorrhagica. *British Journal of Radiology*, **49**, 224–232.

205 Alderson M.R. & Jackson S.M. (1971) Long term follow-up of patients with menorrhagia treated by irradiation. *British Journal of Radiology*, **44**, 295–298.

206 Simpson C.L., Hemplemann L.H. & Fuller L.M. (1955) Neoplasia in children treated with X-rays in infancy for thymic enlargement. *Radiology*, **64**, 840–845.

207 Murray R., Heckel P. & Hemplemann L.H. (1959) Leukemia in children exposed to ionising radiation. *New England Journal of Medicine*, **261**, 585–589.

208 Hemplemann L.H., Hall W.J. & Phillips M. (1975) Neoplasms in persons treated with X-rays in infancy: fourth survey in 20 years. *Journal of the National Cancer Institute*, **55**, 519–530.

209 Moloney W.C. (1959) Leukemia and exposure to X-ray: a report of 6 cases. *Blood*, **14**, 1137–1142.

210 Haselow R.E., Nesbit M., Dehner L.P., Khan F.M., McHugh R. & Levitt S.H. (1978) Second neoplasms following megavoltage radiation in a pediatric population. *Cancer*, **42**, 1185–1191.

211 Curtis R.E., Boice J.D., Stovall M. *et al.* (1989) Leukemia risk following radiotherapy for breast cancer. *Journal of Clinical Oncology*, **7**, 21–29.

212 Boice J.D., Blettner M., Kleinerman R.A. *et al.* (1987) Radiation dose and leukemia risk in patients treated for cancer of the cervix. *Journal of the National Cancer Institute*, **79**, 1295–1311.

213 Sullivan K.M., Deeg H.J., Sanders J.E. *et al.* (1984) Late complications after marrow transplantation. *Seminars in Hematology*, **21**, 53–63.

214 Philip P. & Pedersen-Bjergaard J. (1988) Cytogenetic, clinical and cytologic characteristics of radiotherapy related leukaemias. *Cancer Genetics and Cytogenetics*, **31**, 227–236.

215 Johnson S.A.N., Bateman C.J.T., Beard M.E.J. Whitehouse J.M.A. & Waters A.H. (1977) Long term haematological complications of Thorotrast. *Quarterly Journal of Medicine*, **46**, 259–271.

216 Sadamori N., Miyajima J., Okajima S. *et al.* (1987) Japanese patients with leukaemia following the use of Thorotrast including a patient with marked chromosomal rearrangements. *Acta Haematologica*, **77**, 11–14.

217 Lewis E.B. (1963) Leukemia, multiple myeloma, and aplastic anemia in American radiologists. *Science*, **142**, 1492–1494.

218 Matanoski G.M., Seltser R., Sartwell P.E., Diamond E.L. & Elliott E.A. (1975) The current mortality rates of radiologists and other physician specialists. Specific causes of death. *American Journal of Epidemiology*, **101**, 199–201.

219 Najarian T. & Colton T. (1978) Mortality from leukaemia and cancer in shipyard nuclear workers. *Lancet*, **i**, 1018–1020.

220 Report of the Independent Advisory Group. (1984) *Investigation of the Possible Increased Incidence of Cancer in West Cumbria* (Black Report). HMSO, London.

221 Roman E., Beral V., Carpenter L. *et al.* (1987) Childhood leukaemia in the West Berkshire and Basingstoke and North Hampshire District Health Authorities in relation to nuclear establishments in the vicinity. *British Medical Journal*, **294**, 597–602.

222 Heasman M.A., Kemp I.W. & Urquhart J.D. (1986) Childhood leukaemia in Northern Scotland. *Lancet*, **i**, 266.

223 Cook-Mozaffari P.J., Darby S.C., Doll R. *et al.* (1989) Geographical variation in mortality from leukaemia and other cancers in England and Wales in relation to proximity to nuclear installations 1969–78. *British Journal of Cancer*, **59**, 476–485.

224 Bithell J.F., Dutton S.J., Draper G.J. & Neary N.M. (1994) Distrib-

ution of childhood leukaemias and non-Hodgkin's lymphomas near nuclear installations in England and Wales. *British Medical Journal*, **309**, 20–27.

225 Gardner M.J., Snee M.P., Hall A.J., Powell C.A., Downes S. & Terrell J.D. (1990) Results of case-control study of leukaemia and lymphoma among young people near Sellafield nuclear plant in West Cumbria. *British Medical Journal*, **300**, 423–429.

226 Kinlen L.J., Clarke K. & Balkwill A. (1993) Paternal preconceptional radiation exposure in the nuclear industry and leukaemia and non-Hodgkin's lymphoma in young people in Scotland. *British Medical Journal*, **306**, 1153–1158.

227 McLaughlin J.R., King W.D., Anderson T.W., Clarke E.A. & Ashmore J.R. (1993) Partial radiation exposure and leukaemia in offspring: the Ontario case-control study. *British Medical Journal*, **307**, 959–965.

228 Doll R., Evans H.J. & Darby S.C. (1994) Paternal exposure not to blame. *Nature*, **367**, 678–680.

229 Kinlen L. (1988) Evidence for an infective cause of childhood leukaemia: comparison of a Scottish new town with nuclear processing sites in Britain. *Lancet*, **ii**, 1323–1326.

230 Kinlen L.J., Hudson C.M. & Stiller C.A. (1991) Contacts between adults as evidence for an infective origin of childhood leukaemia: an explanation for the excess near nuclear establishments in West Berkshire? *British Journal of Cancer*, **64**, 549–554.

231 Cartwright R.A. (1991) Lifestyle and leukaemia. *British Journal of Cancer*, **64**, 417–418.

232 Gunz F.W. & Atkinson H.R. (1964) Medical radiations and leukaemia: a retrospective survey. *British Medical Journal*, **1**, 389–393.

233 Gibson R.W., Graham S. & Lilienfeld A. (1972) Irradiation in the epidemiology of leukemia among adults. *Journal of the National Cancer Institute*, **48**, 301–311.

234 Stewart A., Webb J. & Giles D. (1956) Malignant disease in childhood and diagnostic radiation *in utero*. Lancet, **ii**, 447–448.

235 McMahon B. (1962) Prenatal X-ray exposure and childhood cancer. *Journal of the National Cancer Institute*, **28**, 1173–1191.

236 Stewart A. & Kneale G.W. (1970) Radiation dose effects in relation to obstetric X-rays and childhood cancer. *Lancet*, **i**, 1186–1188.

237 Bithell J.F. & Stewart A.M. (1975) Pre-natal irradiation and childhood malignancy — a review of British data from the Oxford Survey. *British Journal of Cancer*, **31**, 271–287.

238 Court-Brown W.M., Doll R. & Bradford-Hill A. (1960) Incidence of leukaemia after exposure to diagnostic radiation *in utero*. *British Medical Journal*, **2**, 1539–1545.

239 Lewis T.L.T. (1964) Leukaemia in childhood after ante-natal exposure to X-rays. A survey at Queen Charlotte's Hospital. *British Medical Journal*, **2**, 1551–1552.

240 Jablon S. & Kato H. (1970) Childhood cancer in relation to prenatal exposure to atomic bomb radiation. *Lancet*, **ii**, 1000–1003.

241 Preston-Martin S., Thomas D.C., Yu M.C. & Henderson B.E. (1989) Diagnostic radiography as a risk factor for chronic myeloid and monocytic leukaemia (CML). *British Journal of Cancer*, **59**, 639–644.

242 Ahlbom A., Feychting M., Koskenvuo M. *et al.* (1993) Electromagnetic fields and childhood cancer. *Lancet*, **342**, 1295–1296.

243 Robison L.L. (1992) Down's syndrome and Leukemia. *Leukemia*, **6**(Suppl. 1), 5–7.

244 Zipursky A., Thorner P., De Harven E., Christensen H. & Doyle J. (1994) Myelodysplasia and acute megakaryoblastic leukemia in Down's syndrome. *Leukemia Research*, **18**, 163–171.

245 Kurahashi H., Hara J., Yumura-Yagi K. *et al.* (1991) Monoclonal nature of transient abnormal myelopoiesis in Down's syndrome. *Blood*, **77**, 1161–1163.

246 Kwong Y.L., Cheng G., Tang T.S., Robertson E.P., Lee C.P. & Chan L.C. (1993) Transient myeloproliferative disorder in a Down's neonate with rearranged T-cell receptor B gene and evidence of *in vivo* maturation demonstrated by dual-colour flow cytometric DNA ploidy analysis. *Leukemia*, **7**, 1667–1671.

247 Gershwin M.E. & Steinberg A.D. (1973) Loss of suppressor function as a cause of lymphoid malignancy. *Lancet*, **11**, 1174–1176.

248 Taylor A.M.R. (1992) Ataxia telangiectasia genes and predisposition to leukaemia, lymphoma and breast cancer. *British Journal of Cancer*, **66**, 5–9.

249 Thick J., Mak Y-F., Metcalfe J., Beatty D. & Taylor A.M.R. (1994) A gene on chromosome Xq28 associated with T-cell prolymphocytic leukemia in two patients with ataxia telangiectasia. *Leukemia*, **8**, 564–573.

250 German J. (1993) Bloom syndrome: a Mendelian prototype of somatic mutational disease. *Medicine*, **76**, 393–405.

251 Butturini A., Gale R.P., Verlander P.C., Adler-Brecher B., Gillio A.P. & Auerbach A.D. (1994) Hematologic abnormalities in Fanconi anemia: an International Fanconi Anemia Registry Study. *Blood*, **84**, 1650–1655.

252 Stiller C.A., Chessells J.M. & Fitchett M. (1994) Neurofibromatosis and childhood leukaemia/lymphoma: a population-based UKCCSG study. *British Journal of Cancer*, **70**, 969–972.

253 Shannon K.M., Watterson J., Johnson P. *et al.* (1992) Monosomy 7 myeloproliferative disease in children with neurofibromatosis type 1: epidemiology and molecular analysis. *Blood*, **79**, 1311–1318.

254 Witherspoon R.P., Fisher L.D., Schoch G. *et al.* (1989) Secondary cancers after bone marrow transplantation for leukemia or aplastic anaemia. *New England Journal of Medicine*, **321**, 784–789.

255 Frizzera G., Rosai J., Dehner L.P., Spector B.D. & Kersey J.H. (1980) Lymphoreticular disorders in primary immunodeficiencies. *Cancer*, **46**, 692–699.

256 Perry G.S., Spector B.D., Schuman L.M. *et al.* (1980) The Wiskott–Aldrich syndrome in the United States and Canada (1892–1979). *Journal of Pediatrics*, **97**, 72–78.

257 Rosen R.B. & Kang S.J. (1979) Congenital agranulocytosis terminating in acute myelomonocytic leukaemia. *Journal of Pediatrics*, **94**, 406–408.

258 Strevens M.J., Lilleyman J.S. & Williams R.B. (1978) Schwachman's syndrome and acute lymphoblastic leukaemia. *British Medical Journal*, **2**, 18–19.

259 Jonas D.M., Heilbros D.C. & Albin A.R. (1978) Rubinstein–Taybi syndrome and acute leukaemia. *Journal of Pediatrics*, **92**, 851–852.

260 Gürgey A., Kara A., Tuncer M., Alikasifoglu M. & Tuncibilek E. (1994) Acute lymphoblastic leukaemia associated with Klinefelter syndrome. *Pediatric Hematology and Oncology*, **11**, 227–279.

261 Esquembre C., Ferris J., Verdeguer A., Prieto F., Badia L. & Castel V. (1987) *European Journal of Paediatrics*, **146**, 444.

262 Wasser R.S., Yolken R., Miller D.R. & Diamond L. (1978) Congenital hypoplastic anemia (Diamond–Blackfan syndrome) terminating in acute myelogenous leukemia. *Blood*, **51**, 991–995.

263 Kay A.J. & Lilleyman J.S. (1981) Is intestinal lymphangiectasia a preleukaemic condition? *Clinical and Laboratory Haematology*, **3**, 365–367.

13   Chronic Myeloid Leukaemia

J.M. Goldman

Introduction

Chronic myeloid leukaemia (CML) (also chronic myelogenous leukaemia, chronic granulocytic leukaemia) is a clonal disease that results from an acquired genetic change in a pluripotential haemopoietic stem cell. This altered stem cell proliferates and generates a population of differentiated cells that gradually replaces normal haemopoiesis and leads to a greatly expanded total myeloid mass. The first cases of leukaemia were described in the 1840s [1], but CML was only clearly recognized as distinct from other types of leukaemia with the advent of panoptic stains for blood films at the end of the last century. One important landmark in the study of CML was the discovery of the Philadelphia (Ph) chromosome in 1960 [2] (Table 13.1); the next landmark was the recognition, in 1973, that the Ph chromosome arose as a result of a balanced reciprocal translocation involving chromosomes 9 and 22 [3]. The characterization, in the 1980s, of the *BCR-ABL* chimeric gene was of great importance (Table 13.1). This gene is now believed to play a central role in the pathogenesis of the chronic phase of CML. Until the 1980s, CML was assumed to be incurable and was treated palliatively, first with radiotherapy and, more recently, with alkylating agents, notably busulphan. It has become apparent in the past 10 years that CML can be cured by bone marrow transplantation (BMT), but the proportion of patients eligible for BMT is still relatively small.

Classification

The majority of patients with CML have a relatively homogeneous disease characterized at diagnosis by splenomegaly, leucocytosis and the presence of a Ph chromosome in all leukaemic cells. A minority of patients have a less typical disease that may be classified as atypical CML, as chronic myelomonocytic leukaemia or as chronic neutrophilic leukaemia. Children may have a disease referred to as juvenile chronic myeloid leukaemia. In none of these variants is there a Ph chromosome.

Epidemiology, aetiology and natural history

The incidence of CML appears to be constant worldwide. It occurs in about 1.0–1.5 per 100 000 of the population in all countries where statistics are adequate. CML is rare below the age of 20 years but occurs in all decades, with a median age of onset of 40–50 years. The incidence is slightly higher in males than in females [4,5].

The risk of developing CML is slightly, but significantly, increased by exposure to high doses of irradiation, as occurred in survivors of the atomic bombs exploded in Japan in 1945, and in patients irradiated for ankylosing spondylitis [6–8]. However, in general almost all cases must be regarded as 'sporadic' and no predisposing factors are identifiable. In particular there is no familial predisposition and no association with HLA genotypes has been recognized. No contributory infectious agent has been incriminated.

CML is a biphasic or triphasic disease that is usually diagnosed in the initial 'chronic' or stable phase (Table 13.2). There has been much debate about the duration of disease before the diagnosis is established, a question that is essentially unanswerable. If it is assumed that the disease starts with a 'transformation event' occurring in a single stem cell, it could be 5–10 years before the disease becomes clinically manifest. This estimate depends on the assumption that the leucocyte doubling time in the prediagnosis phase is not fundamentally different from the doubling time after diagnosis (which may not be the case), and the observation that the latent interval between exposure to irradiation from atomic bombs and the earliest identifiable increased incidence of CML was about 7 years. Some evidence suggests that more than one molecular event may be necessary to generate CML [9]. One recent study concluded that a routine blood count might have identified CML on average 6 months before it was actually diagnosed in individual patients.

Patients are usually in the chronic or stable phase when CML is diagnosed (Table 13.2). This chronic phase lasts typically 2–6 years but, on occasions, it may last more than 10 or

Table 13.1 History of the Ph chromosome and the *BCR-ABL* gene.

1960	Discovery of the Ph chromosome
1970	Demonstration that Ph is actually 22q–
1973	Ph is due to a translocation t(9;22)
1973	Discovery of variant Ph translocations
1982	Demonstration that *ABL* is translocated from chromosome 9 to Ph
1984	Description of a [major] breakpoint cluster region (M-bcr) on chromosome 22
1986	Characterization of the *BCR-ABL* fusion gene and *p210*$^{BCR-ABL}$
1989	Characterization of the [minor] m-bcr and *p190*$^{BCR-ABL}$ in ALL
1990	Generation of CML-like disease in mice by transduction of stem cells with *BCR-ABL*
1996	Recognition of μ-bcr and *p230*$^{BCR-ABL}$ in chronic neutrophilic leukaemia

Table 13.2 Classification of disease.

Chronic phase
Ability to reduce spleen size and restore and maintain 'normal' blood count with appropriate therapy

Accelerated phase
Presence of any one of the following:
 Anaemia (<8.0 g/dl)*
 Leucocytosis (>100 × 10^9/l)*
 Thrombocytopenia (<100 × 10^9/l)*
 Thrombocytosis (>1000 × 10^9/l)*
 Splenomegaly*
 >10% blasts in blood or marrow
 >20% blasts plus promyelocytes in blood or marrow
 >20% basophils plus eosinophils in blood
 New cytogenetic changes (in addition to Ph)

Blastic phase
More than 30% blasts plus promyelocytes in blood or marrow

* Classification of the phase of disease must take account of the treatment the patient is receiving. Thus starred features are indications of accelerated phase disease only if a patient is already receiving therapy that would be considered adequate for control of chronic phase disease.

The classification of myelofibrosis is controversial. The presence of myelofibrosis in conjunction with marrow failure may be regarded as an atypical form of accelerated phase disease; when blasts or blasts plus promyelocytes in the blood exceed 30%, the criteria for blastic phase are satisfied.

even 15 years. Very rare spontaneous remissions have been described. In about one-half of cases the chronic phase transforms unpredictably, and abruptly, to a more aggressive phase that used to be referred to as blastic crisis. This phase is now usually described as acute or blastic transformation. In the other half of cases the disease evolves somewhat more gradually through an intermediate phase, described as 'accelerated' disease, which may last for months or occasionally years, before frank transformation. The accelerated and blastic phases may be grouped together under the heading 'advanced phase' disease. Occasional patients have a disease that progresses gradually to a myelofibrotic or osteomyelosclerotic picture, characterized by extensive marrow fibrosis and sometimes gross overgrowth of bony trabeculae; the clinical problems are then due to failure of haemopoiesis rather than to blast cell proliferation. The duration of survival after onset of transformation is usually 2–6 months, so the median survival from diagnosis is 4–5 years.

Many attempts have been made to subclassify or stage CML at diagnosis in a manner that would permit some prediction of the duration of chronic phase in individual patients [10–13]. The most commonly quoted classification, devised by Sokal and colleagues in 1984 [12], is based on a formula that takes account of the patient's age, blast cell count, spleen size and platelet count at diagnosis (Table 13.3), but is still too inaccurate to be clinically useful. At present the best prognostic indicator seems to be the response to initial treatment with interferon alpha (IFNα). Those who achieve haematological control live longer than those who do not, and the longest survival is seen in those patients who convert to Ph-negative (Ph⁻) haemopoiesis.

Table 13.3 Sokal Index for predicting survival.

Exp.[0.0116 (Age – 43.4) +0.0345 (Spleen – 7.51) +0.188 ({Platelets/700}^{2} – 0.563) +0.0887 (Percentage of blasts – 2.10)]	
Good prognosis	<0.8
Moderate prognosis	0.8–1.2
Poor prognosis	>1.2

The Sokal Index is a mathematical expression that gives an approximate guide to the relative risk of death in an individual patient. Those with low indices have relatively good prognoses, while those with high indices have poor prognoses. The correlations are statistically significant, but of limited use, in predicting survival for individual patients. See ref. [12] for further details.

Cytokinetics

The great increase in the peripheral blood leucocyte count in untreated patients is a reflection of the massive increase (by a factor of 10–100) in the total granulocyte mass. The vast quantities of mature and immature myeloid cells, involving especially cells of the granulocytic series, infiltrate the marrow spaces, including peripheral marrow cavities not normally occupied by red marrow in the adult, and underlie the enlargement of the spleen and liver. One might imagine that the number of Ph-positive (Ph⁺) pluripotential stem cells was similarly increased, but this does not appear to be the case. Thus assays of clonogenic progenitor cells, i.e. granulocyte-macrophage colony-forming units (GM-CFU), erythroid burst-forming units (E-BFU) and macrophage colony-forming units (M-CFU), show that their numbers are generally increased but not to the same degree as those of mature granulocytes [14]. Moreover, measurement of more primitive progenitor cell numbers, such as long-term culture-initiating cells, also suggests that the compartmental expansion is not vast. Thus CML must be due to an abnormality at the stem cell level that translates into disordered control of production or destruction of their more mature progeny. In general the response of progenitor cells to those haemopoietic growth factors that have been defined is not fundamentally disturbed. This suggests that growth factors play no primary role in the pathogenesis of CML.

The observation (discussed below) that most patients with CML have only Ph+ metaphases demonstrable in their bone marrow at diagnosis led to the conclusion that all residual normal haemopoiesis had been eradicated by the time a patient was first seen. This is almost certainly erroneous for the following reasons. Firstly, treatment with IFNα restores some degree of Ph- haemopoiesis in 20–40% of patients. Secondly, more than 50% of patients display some degree of Ph- haemopoiesis in the recovery period after administration of cytotoxic drugs at high dosage. Thirdly, Ph- haemopoiesis can be demonstrated in some cases in marrow cells maintained in long-term culture [15]. The best interpretation of these observations is that normal haemopoietic stem cells survive, possibly in normal numbers, but are maintained in G_0 as a result of the proliferation of leukaemia cells. Their continued survival can be demonstrated by appropriate manipulations. The conclusion has important implications for attempts to induce complete remission in CML by autografting (see below).

Cytogenetics

The Ph chromosome is an acquired cytogenetic abnormality that characterizes all leukaemic cells in CML [2,3]. All non-leukaemic cells in the body have normal karyotypes, which is consistent with the concept that the abnormality is acquired in the myeloid lineage. It is formed as a result of a reciprocal translocation of chromosomal material between the long arms of one number 22 chromosome and one number 9 chromosome, an event referred to as t(9;22)(q34;q11). In CML patients the Ph chromosome is present in all myeloid cell lineages, in some B cells and in a very small proportion of T cells.

About 80% of CML patients have a Ph chromosome in association with t(9;22) without other cytogenetic abnormalities at the time of diagnosis [16,17]. About 10% of patients have variant translocations which may be 'simple' involving chromosome 22 and one chromosome other than chromosome 9, or 'complex' involving chromosomes 9, 22 and one or more additional chromosomes. About 8% of patients with haemato-

logically acceptable CML have two morphologically normal number 22 chromosomes; such patients are referred to as cases of Ph- CML. About 40% of Ph- CML patients have a BCR-ABL chimeric gene on the normal-appearing chromosome 22 and are thus referred to as Ph- BCR-ABL-positive cases; the remainder are BCR-ABL-negative and some of these have mutations in the RAS gene.

Some, but not all, patients acquire additional clonal cytogenetic abnormalities during the course of the chronic phase [18]. There is suspicion that some such changes might be caused in part by administration of alkylating agents, but they can undoubtedly occur spontaneously. The observation of nonrandom changes, typically +8, +Ph, iso-17q or +19, usually means that such new clones will expand and that blastic transformation will manifest itself within weeks or months. Eighty per cent of patients in overt blastic transformation have clonal cytogenetic changes in addition to the Ph translocation.

Molecular biology

It was shown in the early 1980s that the ABL protooncogene was located normally on chromosome 9 and was translocated to chromosome 22 in CML patients. In 1984, Groffen and colleagues showed that the precise positions of the genomic breakpoint on chromosome 22 in different CML patients were clustered in a relatively small 5.8 kb region, to which they gave the name 'breakpoint cluster region' (bcr) [19] (or major breakpoint cluster region, M-bcr). Later it became clear that this region formed the central part of a relatively large gene, now known as the BCR gene, whose normal function is unknown. The translocation results in juxtaposition of 5′ sequences from the BCR gene with 3′ ABL sequences derived from chromosome 9. Thus the Ph chromosome carries a chimeric gene, designated BCR-ABL, that is transcribed as an 8.5 kb mRNA and encodes a protein of molecular weight 210 kDa that has greater tyrosine kinase activity than the normal ABL gene product. The p210BCR-ABL must play a pivotal role in the pathogenesis of CML (Table 13.4) (reviewed in refs [20–24]).

The exons within the M-bcr have been numbered b1–b5, although exon b1 is actually the 13th exon (e13) of the BCR gene (Fig. 13.1). In CML the break in the BCR gene occurs nearly always in the intron between exons b2 and b3 or in the intron between exons b3 and b4. The break in the ABL gene is much more variable and may occur at almost any position upstream of exon a2 (also referred to as the first common exon). Once the primary RNA has been spliced, there is, however, remarkable consistency, such that the resulting mRNA almost always contains a b2a2 or a b3a2 junction (Fig. 13.2). About 50% of CML patients have leukaemia cells with a b3a2 junction and 40% have cells with a b2a2 junction; in 10% of cases both junctions are present. It was thought, at one time, that patients with the larger transcript, that included exon b3,

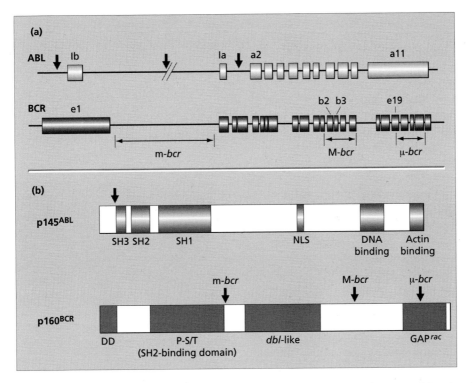

Fig. 13.1 (a) Genomic structure of the *ABL* and *BCR* genes. Exons are shown as blocks and introns are shown as horizontal lines. Note the large first intron between exons Ib and Ia of the *ABL* gene. Vertical arrows show the possible positions of breakpoints. Note also the large intron in the 5′ region of the *BCR* gene, designated m-bcr, in which breaks can occur that lead to the formation of p190BCR-ABL found in Ph-positive ALL. In CML breaks usually occur in a genomic region designated M-bcr, more specifically in the intron between exons b2 and b3 or in the intron between exons b3 and b4. (b) Normal proteins

encoded by *ABL* and *BCR*. The p145ABL (above) and p160BCR (below) are shown schematically. Note the presence in ABL of three SRC-homology domains, designated SH1, SH2 and SH3. SH1 encodes the tyrosine kinase activity. Domains containing a nuclear localization signal (NLS), DNA-binding activity and actin-binding activity are also shown. Note the phospho-serine/threonine rich (P-S/T) SH2 binding domain as well as the dimerization domain (DD), the dbl-like and the GAPrac domains in the BCR protein. (Modified from Melo, 1996 [23].)

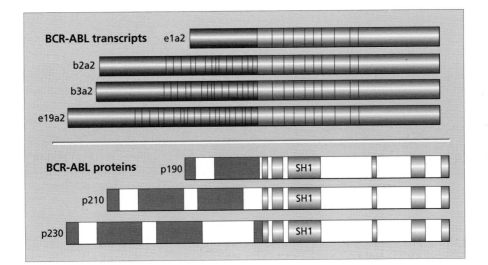

Fig. 13.2 Structure of the BCR-ABL fusion transcripts and proteins. The four types of *BCR-ABL* fusion gene are all expressed in leukaemia cells. The four mRNA transcripts they encode, e1a2, b2a2, b3a2 and e19a2, are shown schematically above; the three corresponding proteins are shown below. Note that the transcript with an e1a2 junction codes for a p190BCR-ABL, and the two types of CML transcripts, b2a2 and b3a2,

encode p210BCR-ABL proteins that are for all practical purposes indistinguishable, although the latter is 25 amino acids larger than the former. The e19a2 transcript encodes the relatively large p230BCR-ABL found in very rare cases of Ph+ chronic neutrophilic leukaemia. (Modified from Melo, 1996 [23].)

might have a generally worse prognosis than those with b2a2 junctions [25,26]. This suggestion has not been confirmed.

The mechanism by which the *BCR-ABL* gene alters stem cell kinetics remains obscure, but there are at least three lines of research that appear promising.

1 Some evidence suggests that the *BCR-ABL* gene, but not the *BCR* gene, can form a complex with the GRB-2/SOS molecular complex that plays a key role in the intracellular second messenger system downstream of *RAS* [27]. Disruption of this pathway with constitutive activation of *RAS* could lead to inappropriate expansion of a progenitor cell compartment.

2 Other evidence suggests that the *ABL* protooncogene, when activated, opposes cellular apoptosis and the *BCR-ABL* gene might act by impeding 'programmed cell death' in target stem cells and might thus 'immortalize' them.

3 CML progenitor cells *in vitro* are less able to adhere to marrow stroma than their normal counterparts, presumably as a result of defective cell–cell adhesion which may be related to the action of *BCR-ABL*; if this defect were expressed *in vivo*, CML cells may be able to escape physiological regulatory mechanisms and thus proliferate semiautonomously.

The molecular basis of disease progression is also poorly defined, but it seems reasonable to infer that one, or more probably a sequence of, additional genetic events occurs in the Ph+ clone. When the critical combination of additional events is achieved, transformation ensues. About 20% of patients with CML in myeloid transformation have point mutations or deletions in the coding sequence of the tumour suppressor gene *p53* [28], a gene implicated in the progression of a variety of solid tumours, notably colonic carcinoma. Deletions in the tumour suppressor gene *p16* are found in about 50% of patients with lymphoid transformations [29]. The retinoblastoma (*RB*) gene is deleted in rare cases of CML in megakaryo-

blastic transformation and changes in *MYC* have been described in one case. Molecular changes underlying the non-random cytogenetic changes described above have not been identified.

Clinical features

Chronic phase

The majority of patients with CML present with disease still in the chronic phase (CP). A small minority, less than 10%, present with advanced-phase disease, although this sometimes only becomes obvious after initial treatment. The commonest symptoms are fatigue or lethargy, but abnormal bleeding, weight loss, splenic discomfort, the feeling of an ill-defined abdominal mass and excessive sweating are all relatively common [30,31] (Table 13.5). Less common are bone pain, headaches and other nonspecific features. Priapism occurs in about 2% of men at diagnosis. Visual disturbances as a result of retinal haemorrhages or hyperviscosity are described. Pleuritic pain because of splenic infarction may be the presenting feature. Very rarely the first symptom is gout associated with hyperuricaemia. In 20–30% of cases the patient is entirely free of symptoms at the time when CML is diagnosed. The diagnosis is then made as an incidental finding, as a result of a 'routine' blood test performed for a variety of unrelated reasons. It is likely that the proportion of patients diagnosed 'incidentally' will increase as automated blood counters become more widely available in medical practice.

The majority of patients are in good general health at the time of diagnosis. They may, however, have nonspecific signs, such as those attributable to weight loss or anaemia. Fever is

Table 13.4 Molecular variants of Ph+ disease.

p190 disease
Usually ALL phenotype
Very rarely CML with monocytosis and dysplasia
p210 disease
Classical CML
About 5% of cases are Ph–
Includes some cases of Ph+ ALL
p230 disease
Chronic neutrophilic leukaemia (Ph+)
Absence of immature cells from peripheral blood

p190BCR-ABL is smaller than p210BCR-ABL and associated almost always with Ph+ acute lymphoblastic leukaemia (see Chapter 3); very rare cases resembling CML have a p190 rather than a p210BCR-ABL protein. Extremely rare cases of Ph+ chronic neutrophilic leukaemia with a p230BCR-ABL protein are described.

Table 13.5 Clinical Symptoms in CML: data from 430 patients referred to the Hammersmith Hospital, London between 1979 and 1995.

Symptom	Patients	
	No.	%
Fatigue	140	34
Bleeding	89	21
Weight loss	84	20
Splenic discomfort	76	18
Abdominal mass	62	14
Sweats	61	14
Bone pain	31	7
Infections	26	6
Priapism	8	2
Others	65	15
Incidental finding	85	20

Table 13.6 Clinical signs in CML: data from 430 patients referred to the Hammersmith Hospital, London between 1979 and 1995.

Signs	Patients	
	No.	%
Spleen palpable	314	76
1–10 cm	153	37
>10 cm	161	39
Spleen not palpable	100	24
Purpura	66	16
Palpable liver	9	2
No signs	85	20

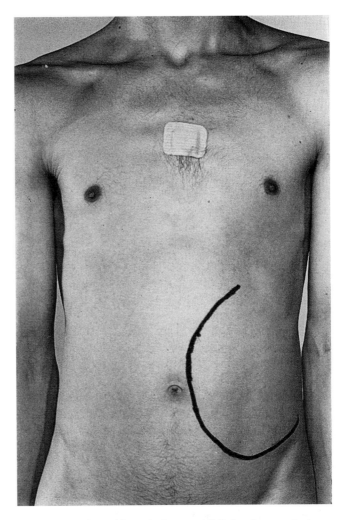

Fig. 13.3 A patient with newly diagnosed CML showing a marked degree of splenomegaly.

very rarely a feature of uncomplicated chronic-phase CML. The spleen is palpable in about 80% of cases (Fig. 13.3) and its size is usually measured in centimetres below the left costal margin (Table 13.6). Occasionally it has enlarged to such an extent that it crosses the midline to the right and it lower pole occupies some of the right iliac fossa. The liver is enlarged in about 20% of cases, usually with a smooth lower border that may be difficult to define. The patient may have various signs of haemorrhage, including purpura and more generalized ecchymoses. Some patients have subcutaneous lumps due, presumably, to extravasation of blood and local deposits of leucocytes. Lymphadenopathy occurs occasionally. About 20% of patients have no abnormal signs at diagnosis.

Advanced phase (comprising accelerated and blastic phases)

Patients may present in advanced phase or more commonly they progress to advanced phase disease after some years in CP. In some cases the symptoms of advanced phase disease may resemble those of untreated CP disease [32–35]. However, they may progress much more rapidly and weight loss, bleeding, excess sweating, splenic pain, sometimes due to splenic infarction, and bone pain may be prominent. The bone pain may be generalized, involving limbs, or may be localized to one or two sites. Fever may be a prominent feature of CML in the advanced phase; it may be low grade and continuous or relatively hectic. Occasionally fever is the only feature, and the diagnosis of advanced phase disease is then a diagnosis of exclusion only after extensive tests for microbial infection have proved negative. The principal abnormal sign characteristic of advanced phase disease is splenomegaly; specifically the spleen may be inappropriately large at a time when the leucocyte count is still reasonably well controlled. Various other signs, principally those as a result of haemorrhage, may be present but are not specific.

A small proportion of patients with CML (perhaps 5%) progress to myelofibrotic transformation. In these cases the main symptoms may be those of anaemia, fever and excessive sweating. The spleen becomes progressively larger and the liver may also enlarge greatly. There may be peripheral lymphadenopathy. The haematological picture is predominantly that of marrow failure.

Haematological and other investigations

Chronic phase

The majority of patients have leucocyte counts between 100 and 300 × 10⁹/l at the time of diagnosis, although a diagnosis of CML can be made in patients with counts as low as 12 × 10⁹/l, and occasional patients present with counts in excess of 500 × 10⁹/l. The predominant leucocyte is a mature neutrophil, which appears morphologically normal, but the lecocyte differential shows a full spectrum, including blasts, promyelocytes, myelocytes and metamyelocytes (see Plate 13.1 between pp.

292 and 293) [36]. There is a chracteristic 'peak' of myelocytes. Basophil numbers are increased and, indeed, the diagnosis of Ph+ CML is uncertain in the absence of this basophilia. Eosinophil numbers are also increased. Monocytes are relatively reduced. The percentage of blast cells is related to the leucocyte count, such that patients with total leucocyte counts less than 100×10^9/l seldom have more than 5% blasts in their blood, while those with higher counts may have up to 10 or 12% blasts. A finding of more than 12% blasts in any patient raises the possibility that the disease is no longer in CP. Platelet numbers are u•ually normal or moderately increased (i.e. $300-600 \times 10^9$/l); some patients are thrombocytopenic at presentation; others may have platelet counts in excess of 1000×10^9/l, a finding that casts doubt on their classification as CP disease. In the absence of iron deficiency or myelofibrosis, the morphology of the red cells is usually normal, but erythroblasts are seen in the blood in some patients.

It has been known for many years that neutrophils from patients with Ph+ CML have low levels or no alkaline phosphatase in their cytoplasm. Thus assay of neutrophil or leucocyte alkaline phosphatase (NAP or LAP) was part of the routine evaluation of all new patients. This low LAP value is not, in fact, a feature that is intrinsic to the leukaemic neutrophil, but rather is related to low ambient levels of granulocyte colony-stimulating factor (G-CSF) [37]. The NAP level is normal or raised in CML patients who achieve neutropenia on treatment or in pregnancy. The test is no longer regarded as particularly helpful in diagnosis, except in the absence of cytogenetic or molecular studies.

It is usual to confirm the diagnosis by examination of the bone marrow by aspiration and trephine biopsy (see Plate 13.2). The aspirate typically reveals multiple small fragments or no clearly defined fragments with intense hypercellularity. Cells of the granulocytic series predominate, with a full spectrum similar to that seen in the peripheral blood. Basophils and eosinophils may stand out. Megakaryocytes are usually increased in number; they may be small and hypolobated. Erythroid cells are relatively decreased. In rare cases large cells resembling Gaucher cells, designated pseudo-Gaucher cells, may be seen. The trephine biopsy parallels the picture seen in the aspirate. The hypercellularity is reflected in complete loss of marrow fat spaces. Special stains usually show that reticulin is normal or modestly increased; in rare cases there is marked collagen deposition or frank fibrosis. Although cytogenetic studies can be carried out on blood specimens if they contain enough dividing cells (i.e. myelocytes or more immature cells), the best preparations are usually obtained from marrow aspirates.

Patients with CML in CP usually have a raised level of vitamin B_{12}; this is because of increased levels of vitamin B_{12}-binding protein (transcobalamin I), which is made by cells of the granulocytic series. Blood urea and electrolyte levels are usually normal. The uric acid is also usually normal or just above the upper limit of normal; very occasionally it is

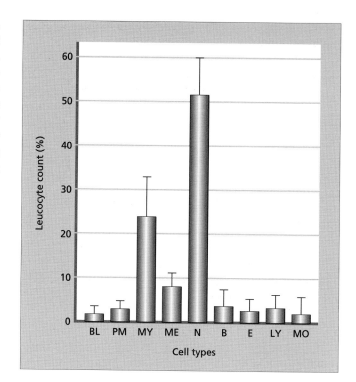

Fig. 13.4 Histogram showing the characteristic differential leucocyte count in untreated high-count CML. Note the 'peaks' of myelocytes and neutrophils. The data were based on examination of peripheral blood films from 50 patients with Ph+ CML. B = basophils; BL = blast cells; E = eosinophils; LY = lymphocytes; ME = metamyelocytes; MO = monocytes; MY = myelocytes; N = neutrophils; PM = promyelocytes. Vertical bars show standard errors.

markedly raised. Tests of liver functions are usually normal but the alkaline phosphatase may be raised. The lactic dehydrogenase is characteristically high.

Advanced phase

The haematological picture in advanced phase disease differs fundamentally from that in CP [33,35,38]. The principal finding in the blood is that the total number of leucocytes is much higher than would be expected in a patient on treatment that should be appropriate for CP disease (Fig. 13.4). Moreover, the percentage of immature granulocytes (mainly blasts or blasts plus promyelocytes) is increased; their precise number may be the basis for separating accelerated phase from blastic transformation (Table 13.2). At this stage the patient is usually anaemic, as a result, partly, of reduced red cell production and, partly, of shortened red cell survival. The platelet numbers are now usually low, but they may still be normal or, occasionally, markedly raised. Erythroblasts may be present in the blood. The marrow aspirate at this stage usually shows a variable degree of replacement with blast cells, with both erythropoiesis and megakaryocytopoiesis reduced.

The blast cells that predominate in transformation are often difficult to characterize by standard morphological methods and do not readily fit the criteria established by the FAB Group for classification of acute leukaemia. However, the predominant blast cell sometimes clearly resembles a lymphoblast; on other occasions it resembles a myeloblast, a monoblast, an erythroblast or a megakaryoblast on the basis of Romanowsky-stained slides. Blast cells of eosinophilic and basophilic lineages are described. However, on more detailed study blasts from patients with CML in transformation prove to be of the myeloid lineage in about 70% of cases, of the lymphoid lineage in 20% of cases and of mixed lineage in the remainder [38]. Immunophenotyping of myeloid blasts shows that they are positive for a series of myeloid markers, including CD13, CD33 and CD34. In some cases the myeloid blasts express markers of the erythroid or megakaryocyte lineages. In contrast, lymphoid blast cells are usually positive for pre-B-cell lymphoid markers, notably CD10, CD19 and CD22. Lymphoid blasts usually stain positively for the nuclear enzyme terminal deoxynucleotidyl transferase (TdT). Very occasional cases of T-lymphoblastic transformation have been described. Blast cells of the lymphoid lineage usually show clonal rearrangements of immunoglobulin heavy-chain and light-chain genes [39]. Some B-lymphoid blasts also show clonal rearrangement of the T-cell receptor.

In patients whose disease has progressed towards myelofibrosis, the peripheral blood appearances are highly informative. The red cells are often hypochromic. Anisocytosis may be obvious and tear-drop forms are conspicuous. There is polychromasia and the reticulocyte count is increased. Nucleated red cells are usually present. Blast cells may be found in the blood, but in much fewer numbers than in frank blastic transformation. Initially platelet numbers may be raised. As transformation progresses anaemia, leucopenia and thrombocytopenia may be seen. Sometimes blast cell numbers increase rapidly as a preterminal event. The marrow is usually inaspirable in myelofibrotic transformation. The findings on trephine biopsy are somewhat unpredictable, partly because the biopsy may or may not reflect the general pattern in the marrow. There is usually a paucity of 'normal' or CP myelopoiesis. The findings range from relatively minor degrees of excess collagen formation to extensive fibrosis; very rarely the most obvious abnormality is new bone formation, a condition referred to as osteomyelosclerosis.

Cytogenetic and molecular studies

It is usual to examine the bone marrow to confirm the presence of a Ph chromosome in newly diagnosed patients. The majority of patients will show a simple t(9;22), as mentioned above, but some will prove to have complex translocations. The clinical courses of patients with simple and complex translocations are indistinguishable. To demonstrate a Ph chromosome it is usually sufficent to use standard cytogenetic techniques with adequately banded chromosomes from

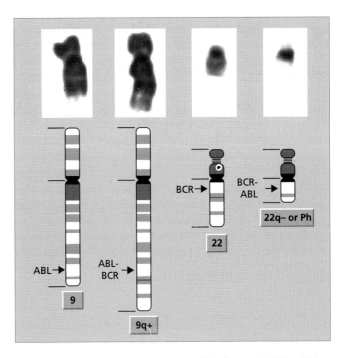
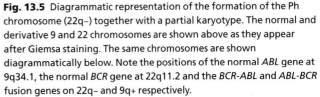

Fig. 13.5 Diagrammatic representation of the formation of the Ph chromosome (22q–) together with a partial karyotype. The normal and derivative 9 and 22 chromosomes are shown above as they appear after Giemsa staining. The same chromosomes are shown diagrammatically below. Note the positions of the normal *ABL* gene at 9q34.1, the normal *BCR* gene at 22q11.2 and the *BCR-ABL* and *ABL-BCR* fusion genes on 22q– and 9q+ respectively.

leukaemia cells in metaphase (Fig. 13.5). In CML, usually 100% of dividing cells from the marrow are found to be Ph+, but occasionally Ph+ positive and Ph– cells coexist in various proportions. This is presumably a reflection of the fact that the Ph+ clone has not yet entirely replaced normal haemopoiesis. It is conventional to assess 30 or more metaphases and to express the findings as the percentage of Ph+ cells. In Ph– cases, or in patients with complex translocations, the use of fluorescence *in situ* hybridization (FISH) with BCR and ABL probes can be informative. In classical CML, FISH studies will demonstrate the presence of a *BCR-ABL* chimeric gene on the Ph chromosome. In patients with complex translocations, *BCR-ABL* is also usually on 22q– but it may found elsewhere in the genome. In Ph– BCR-ABL-positive patients, the *BCR-ABL* gene is usually present on the normal-appearing chromosome 22; very rarely it occurs on the 'normal' chromosome 9.

Various other molecular methods can be used to ascertain directly or indirectly the presence or absence of a *BCR-ABL* gene in material from patents with CML. They include Southern blot analysis, Western blotting and reverse-transcriptase polymerase chain reaction (RT-PCR). Southern blotting is relatively insensitive but is useful as a general screening test. By using a probe for a portion of the *BCR* gene to hybridize to restriction fragments prepared with appropriate enzymes, it can be demonstrated in CML, that there is present, in addition to the normal size fragment, a larger or smaller fragment formed from the *BCR-ABL* fusion gene. This is convincing although indirect evidence for the presence of a *BCR-ABL* gene. The technique is adequate for the study of patient material that consists largely of leukaemia cell DNA, but it is relatively insensitive and is therefore not suitable for the study of minimal residual disease. Western blotting involves the use of an antibody usually directed against ABL sequences to detect the BCR-ABL protein in its characteristic position run on a polyacrylamide gel. The RT-PCR is particularly suitable for the study of minimal residual disease. It relies on the presence of BCR-ABL transcripts in the material to be studied to give a positive signal. Thus mRNA is first isolated from blood leucocytes and then reverse transcribed to cDNA. Using primers carefully selected to span the BCR-ABL junction, the unknown material is then subjected to PCR amplification. If BCR-ABL transcripts were present originally, a specific amplification product will be identified. Its origin can, if necessary, be confirmed by using a radiolabelled probe for BCR or ABL sequences.

Variants of chronic myeloid leukaemia

Ph-negative chronic myeloid leukaemia

About 8% of patients with haematologically acceptable CML have a normal karyotype in the leukaemia cells or a clonal abnormality not involving the long arm of chromosome 22. Such patients are usually referred to as Ph- CML. Those who, on further study, prove to have a cytogenetically undetectable *BCR-ABL* gene usually have clinical features and response to therapy no different from that of Ph+ *BCR-ABL*-positive disease. Patients with Ph-negative, *BCR-ABL*-negative disease usually have an atypical course. They may be asymptomatic at diagnosis or they may present with symptoms similar to those of patient with Ph+ CML. However, the appearance of the blood film distinguishes the disease from classical CML. The numbers of immature and mature granulocytes are increased, but the myelocyte peak typical of Ph+ CML is lacking and the numbers of eosinophils and basophils are normal or reduced. The degree of anaemia may be more severe than is usual in Ph+ CML and thrombocytopenia is common.

Treatment of Ph- *BCR-ABL*-negative CML is usually unsatisfactory. A greatly raised leucocyte count can be controlled to some degree with hydroxyurea or 6-thioguanine, but the duration of benefit may be short. In some patients, however, long-term control of symptoms can be achieved with the use of a single drug. The use of drug combinations appropriate to acute myeloid leukaemia usually induces marrow hypoplasia without achieving complete remission.

Chronic myelomonocytic leukaemia

This is a chronic myeloproliferative disease that has been included in the FAB categorization of myelodysplastic syndromes [40] (see Chapter 11). It affects predominantly the middle aged or elderly and there is a slight male preponderance. Patients often have splenomegaly but the degree of splenic enlargement is less than in CML. The peripheral blood shows an absolute neutrophilia and monocytosis and the serum and urinary lysozyme (muramidase) levels are increased, unlike those in CML. The absence of immature granulocytes in the blood film also distinguishes chronic myelomonocytic leukaemia (CMML) from CML. The neutrophils may be morphologically abnormal with hypogranular, agranular and pseudo-Pelger forms. Platelet numbers are variable. There is no basophilia. The marrow is usually hypercellular with immature monocytes recognizable.

The natural history of CMML is variable. In some patients the leukaemia appears to remain in 'chronic phase' for some years, while in others there is progression to a picture resembling an acute leukaemia within 1 year of diagnosis. Treatment is generally unsatisfactory and should probably be reserved for patients with symptoms. Hydroxyurea may be effective at controlling the leucocyte count, but usually it also causes or aggravates the thrombocytopenia. Regular blood transfusions may be required. Bone marrow transplantation may be successful in younger patients.

Juvenile chronic myeloid leukaemia

Patients with juvenile chronic myeloid leukaemia (jCML) are usually under the age of 5 years and have a disease which bears very little resemblance to Ph+ CML. The clinical picture is characterized by splenomegaly, lymphadenopathy, rashes, septic lesions and haemorrhages. The total leucocyte count is lower than is usually seen in Ph+ CML. Immature granulocytes are present in the peripheral blood, but the differential typical of Ph+ CML is lacking. Thrombocytopenia is the rule. Monocytosis and circulating normoblasts are usually seen. Patients have a persistently high level of fetal haemoglobin. Cytogenetic studies reveal only normal karyotypes in about 80% of cases; other patients have a variety of clonal abnormalities other than the Ph chromosome. Treatment with cytotoxic drugs has not in general been helpful, although symptoms may be controlled for weeks or months. Some patients have been cured by allogeneic bone marrow transplantation, which should certainly be attempted if an HLA-matched sibling donor exists and probably also (in the absence of a matched sibling) if a matched unrelated donor can be identified.

Chronic neutrophilic leukaemia

This disorder is exceedingly rare and is usually diagnosed incidentally [41]. The patient has a raised blood neutrophil count without immature granulocytes and without basophilia or eosinophilia. The neutrophil alkaline phosphatase is usually raised. The marrow is hypercellular but cytogenetic studies are usually normal. The dignosis is based largely on exclusion of other identifiable causes for the leucocytosis. Most patients have no symptoms referable to the neutrophilia and no signs, although some have minor degrees of splenomegaly. Treatment may not be required.

Very rarely patients with a disease resembling chronic neutrophilic leukaemia have been found to have the Ph chromosome. Some such patients have a 'downstream' breakpoint in the BCR gene and a relatively large BCR-ABL protein (p230) [23] (Table 13.4).

Management

Chronic-phase disease

In the nineteenth century there was little effective treatment for CML. Fowler's solution, containing potassium arsenite, was effective in reducing the leucocyte count, but it had little specificity and induced other features of arsenic poisoning. Radiotherapy was introduced at the beginning of the twentieth century and proved to be very effective at controlling symptoms and establishing haematological control. It was given routinely as discrete courses of X-irradiation or gamma-irradiation directed to the spleen. In the 1950s, the oral alkylating busulphan was introduced and a controlled study performed in the UK demonstrated that survival was improved. Busulphan is however a toxic drug, and a more recent study comparing its use with that of hydroxyurea showed that survival is superior with the latter drug [42]. Busulphan has therefore fallen from favour. At the present time evidence is accumulating that suggests that IFNα is better than hydroxyurea. The role of the various grafting procedures also needs to be considered in relation to each patient. Thus the challenge for the clinician today is to determine the best treatment strategy for the newly diagnosed patient (reviewed in refs [43–47]).

General approach

The first important step when a patient is suspected of having CML, is to confirm the diagnosis. This can usually be carried out by careful examination of the peripheral blood, but on occasions cytogenetic and even molecular studies may be necessary before leukaemia can be diagnosed with confidence. The next step is a reasonably frank discussion with the patient and/or appropriate family members. To some patients the diagnosis of CML comes as a considerable surprise in view of the fact that they had only trivial symptoms or felt completely well; in other cases the diagnosis of a serious disorder was already suspected. It is useful to explain some aspects of disease pathogenesis and some patients will seek further information about the Ph chromosome and the *BCR-ABL* gene. A brochure or booklet on CML designed for patients may be useful. The clinician should stress that for all practical purposes CML is not contagious and does not run in families. Some idea of prognosis should be given. A patient can only make an intelligent decision about the need for treatment by transplantation if he/she is aware that CML is a potentially lethal disease and has some idea of the duration of life without a transplant. At this stage the clinician should outline a general strategy of management which may include options for treatment with IFNα, allografting or autografting. Obviously the patient should realize that such a strategy must be flexible. For younger patients who have not yet completed their families, the possible effects of treatment on fertility should be discussed at the earliest opportunity. A man may wish to undertake cryopreservation of semen before any treatment is initiated. In certain circumstances a young woman may regard the completion of a pregnancy as more important than immediate institution of chemotherapy.

Specific measures

It is advisable, but by no means mandatory, to perform leucapheresis with cryopreservation of blood stem cells before any other treatment is undertaken. Such stem cells can be stored indefinitely in liquid nitrogen and can be used as an autograft at a later date if the patient becomes severely pancytopenic in the natural history of the disease or as a result of therapy. Leucapheresis is usually undertaken as an 'emergency' procedure in patients with significant symptoms due to hyperviscosity and in men with priapism. In practice, high-dose hydroxyurea will reduce the leucocyte count almost as rapidly as leucapheresis, and the two approaches can conveniently be combined. It is in fact possible to treat a newly diagnosed patient exclusively by leucapheresis repeated once per week or more often [48]. The spleen size can be reduced and the leucocyte count restored to normal. However, the technique is labour intensive and expensive and is not clearly superior to other methods of treatment.

In patients under the age of 60 years, HLA typing should be undertaken as soon as possible after diagnosis. It is conventional to type all available siblings and both parents if possible. If the patient has children, they too can be typed in the hope of identifying a possible donor who is phenotypically HLA identical or nearly identical with the patient. If no suitable family member is identified, a preliminary search of an unrelated donor panel should be considered.

It is customary today to start treatment as soon a patient's initial evaluation is complete, although a case could be made for delaying treatment in a patient with a low leucocyte count (e.g. <50 × 10^9/l). For the average patient who does not have an HLA-identical sibling and is therefore not a candidate for an early allogeneic transplant, treatment should probably be initiated with IFNα. If a patient cannot tolerate IFNα or is deemed a nonresponder, the use of hydroxyurea is a reasonable alternative. Busulphan should probably be reserved for treatment of patients still in CP whose disease appears refractory to hydroxyurea (Fig. 13.6).

CML is occasionally diagnosed in an asymptomatic woman

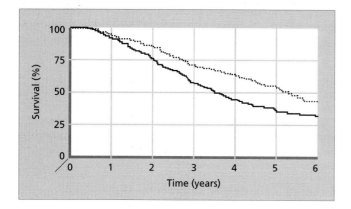

Fig. 13.6 Survival for 557 patients treated with IFNα or cytotoxic drugs for CML in CP. Actuarial survival for 279 patients treated with IFNα (----) compared with survival for 278 patients treated with hydroxyurea or busulphan (——) in the UK Medical Research Council's CML 3 trial. The median survival for patients receiving IFNα vs cytotoxic drugs was 63 vs 43 months, (*P* = 0.0006).

attending an antenatal clinic early in pregnancy. The finding of CML should not be regarded as an automatic reason for terminating the pregnancy and, indeed, once the prognosis is explained, most women will choose to continue the pregnancy to term. If the patient's leucocyte count is below 80 × 10⁹/l and she is not anaemic, treatment may be deferred. If treatment is necessary, leucapheresis once weekly may be adequate to control the leucocyte count. Such data as are available suggest that administration of IFNα early in pregnancy does not harm the fetus [49]. By contrast, hydroxyurea is probably teratogenic and must be avoided at least until the last trimester of pregnancy.

Interferon alpha. Interferon alpha (IFNα) is a member of a large family of glycoproteins of biological origin with antiviral and antiproliferative properties. Studies in the early 1980s using material purified from human cell lines showed that it was active in reducing the leucocyte count and reversing all clinical features of CML in 70–80% of CML patient [50]. Of particular interest was the observation that between 5 and 15% of patients sustained a major reduction in the percentage of Ph+ marrow metaphases with restoration of Ph- (putatively normal) haemopoiesis [51]. This effect is achieved only very rarely with standard cytotoxic drugs. It raised the important question of whether these 'cytogenetic responders' would

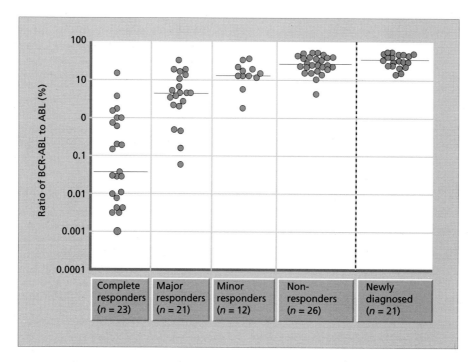

Fig. 13.7 The relationship between BCR-ABL transcript numbers and cytogenetic response to treatment with IFNα in a total of 82 patients treated with IFNα. Values for an additional 21 patients studied at diagnosis are also shown. Note that of the 23 patients who achieved complete cytogenetic responses to IFNα, all still had detectable levels of BCR-ABL transcripts, but the level varied over 4 logs. Note that the numbers of BCR-ABL transcripts are expressed on a log scale as a ratio to the normal ABL transcript as a control for the quality of the cDNA studied. Horizontal lines are mean values for each patient group.

have their life prolonged by treatment with IFNα and prospectively randomized controlled studies were initiated in many European countries and in North America. The results of some of these studies have now been reported and conflict to some extent. The Italian multicentre study compared IFNα with hydroxyurea and concluded that median survival was significantly prolonged in patients randomized to receive IFNα [53]. The British study compared IFNα with cytotoxic drugs (busulphan or hydroxyurea) and concluded that IFNα was significantly better than chemotherapy [54]; when the comparison was performed separately with busulphan and with hydroxyurea, IFNα was significantly superior to busulphan but also superior to hydroxyurea. Further analysis of this study suggested that IFNα conferred survival advantage whether or not a patient achieved a cytogenetic remission (Fig. 13.7). This is potentially an important issue, because the Houston group believed that patients benefit from treatment with IFNα principally as a result of achieving Ph negativity and that consequently this must be the major target of therapy. In contrast to the British and Italian studies, a German multicentre study failed to demonstrate any significant benefit for patients treated with IFNα in comparison with hydroxyurea [55]. Likewise a study performed in North America showed no benefit for IFNα [56].

In summary it appears that treatment with IFNα has two important effects.
1 It identifies, on the basis of speed of haematological response and degree of cytogenetic response, subgroups of patients who will survive longer than others [57].
2 It probably prolongs survival by perhaps 1 or 2 years in the majority of patients [53,54].

Patients who obtain complete cytogenetic response have an extremely low risk of disease transformation and their median survival may exceed 10 years. For the present, it seems reasonable to conclude that IFNα should be offered to all newly diagnosed patients who are not candidates for allogeneic BMT and that treatment should be continued in haematological responders for as long as the drug is tolerated.

IFNα is now available as a preparation purified from a lymphoblastoid cell line (IFNαn1) and in various recombinant DNA forms (IFNα2a and IFNα2b). It must be administered by subcutaneous injection. It may be started at low dosage, for example 3 Mu daily, with gradual increases, or at high dosage, for example 5 Mu/m² daily with dose reduction if necessary. There is some evidence that the greatest chance of cytogenetic response is achieved with the higher dose levels. The drug is not, however, without side effects. Almost all patients experience fevers, shivers, muscle aches and general 'flu-like' features on starting the drug; these last usually 1–2 weeks but may be alleviated by paracetamol. They recur when the dosage is increased. A significant minority of patients cannot tolerate the drug on account of lethargy, malaise, anorexia, weight loss, depression and other affective disorders or alopecia. Autoimmune syndromes, such as thyrotoxicosis, may also

occur. The drug is still very much more expensive than hydroxyurea.

A number of efforts have been made to increase the proportion of patients who achieve Ph negativity by combining IFNα with other drugs. The combination of IFNα with hydroxyurea (see below) has been tested in a number of centres. With this combination it is relatively easy to maintain the leucocyte count in the normal range but the probability of achieving Ph negativity is not increased. In contrast, the combination of IFNα with cytarabine at low dosage has approximately doubled the proportion of the patients who achieve Ph negativity. The toxicity, especially prolonged mucositis, of this combination has been considerable, but a report from the French multicentre group showed that patients treated with IFNα plus cytarabine survived significantly longer than control patients treated with cytarabine alone [58]. Further controlled studies are clearly warranted.

Hydroxyurea. Hydroxyurea is an inhibitor of nucleotide reductase that appears to target specifically the haemopoietic system. It was first used as treatment for CML in the 1960s [42,59], but it only gained widespread popularity in the 1980s. It must be administered by mouth. The usual starting dose is 2.0 g/day but 4.0 or even 6.0 g can be given daily for a short period if rapid reduction of the leucocyte count is required. Maintenance with hydroxyurea must be continued indefinitely if the target is to maintain a normal or slightly subnormal leucocyte count. The usual maintenance dose is between 1.0 and 1.5 g/day.

Hydroxyurea is relatively free of toxicity, which, when it does occur, may be dose related. Most patients tolerate a dose of 1.5–2.0 g daily without problems. Some sustain sore mouths and mucositis with ulceration. Feelings of nausea and diarrhoea may occur. Nonspecific rashes are also seen. Hydroxyurea causes macrocytosis and megaloblastoid changes in the bone marrow. Although overdosage can cause pancytopenia, this reverses very rapidly on stopping the drug. Unlike busulphan, long-lasting marrow aplasia does not occur as a consequence of injudicious treatment.

Busulphan. This is a fat-soluble alkylating agent that is given routinely by mouth. It seems to act as a haemopoietic stem cell poison and has little other clinical utility. It was formerly standard practice to start treatment with 6 or 8 mg daily and to reduce or stop the treatment when the leucocyte count fell to 20×10^9/l. Once the leucocyte count had stabilized in the normal range, treatment could be resumed at a maintenance dose of 1–2 mg daily [60,61]. An alternative approach was to treat the patient only in separate courses. By one or other of these approaches, it was possible to maintain a patient's leucocyte count almost continuously within the normal range.

The administration of busulphan had to be monitored with great care. Occasional patients demonstrated idiosyncratic hypersensitivity to busulphan and could be inadvertently rendered aplastic on standard doses. Continued administration at an inappropriately high dose would render almost any patient permanently aplastic. Busulphan is exquisitely toxic to the gonads. Young women usually stopped menstruating within the first few weeks of treatment and resumption of menstruation was rare. Men were rapidly rendered azoospermic and this change, too, was seldom reversible. After some years of treatment with busulphan, most patients developed cutaneous pigmentation. Occasional patients developed a syndrome characterized by respiratory failure in association with cough, fever and pulmonary infiltrates; this was designated 'busulphan lung' and was usually fatal. There is experimental evidence that busulphan is mutagenic and it is possible, therefore, that its use expedited the onset of blast cell transformation. For these various reasons busulphan is no longer recommended as first-line therapy for CML in CP.

Allogeneic stem cell transplantation using HLA-identical donors. Younger patients with CML in CP who have HLA-identical sibling donors should be offered the opportunity of treatment by haemopoietic stem cell transplantation (HSCT) using blood- or marrow-derived stem cells [62–64]. Most specialist centres exclude from consideration patients over the age of 50 or 60 years, because transplant-related mortality (TRM) in older patients seems to be excessive. The precise timing of the transplantation has, however, been the subject of much debate. There is little argument that the transplantation should be performed before the onset of advanced phase disease, at which point the results are relatively poor (Fig. 13.8) [64]. However, it is now accepted that TRM is lower if the transplantation is performed within 1 year of diagnosis than if it is delayed for some while [65]. The reason for this adverse effect of 'delay to transplant' is unclear, but it could be a result of the generally injurious effect of treatment with cytotoxic drugs, especially with busulphan. It is not yet clear whether treatment with IFNα before transplantation also decreases the chance of survival post-transplantation; a recent report from the International Bone Marrow Transplant Registry in Milwaukee suggests that this is not the case [66]. For the present it can be concluded that for a young patient (e.g. <40 years) with an HLA-identical sibling, for whom transplantation is planned, the procedure should be performed at the earliest convenient opportunity. The main reason is quite simply the risk that, otherwise, transformation will supervene. For a somewhat older patient (age 40–55 years) the choice may also be to proceed to transplantation soon after diagnosis; the alternative is to administer a trial of IFNα and to delay the transplantation if a complete cytogenetic remission is achieved relatively rapidly.

There is no complete agreement about *how* the transplantation should be performed for a patient with CML in CP (see Chapter 22). In general patients are 'conditioned' with cyclophosphamide at high dosage followed by total body irradiation; however, the combinations of total body irradiation and etoposide or busulphan and cyclophosphamide at high

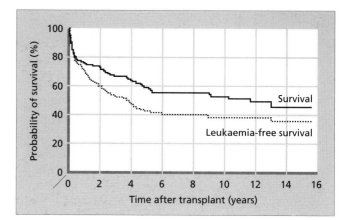

Fig. 13.8 Outcome for allogeneic bone marrow transplantation (BMT) for CML in CP. Actuarial survival and leukaemia-free survival for 229 patients with CML in CP, who were treated with allogeneic BMT with HLA-identical sibling donors at the Hammersmith Hospital (London) between 1981 and 1996. These data include patients treated with marrow depleted *in vitro* of T-lymphocytes, a technique that reduces the risk of GVHD but greatly increases the probability of relapse.

dosage give very similar results [67–69]. The majority of centres use cyclosporin A and methotrexate for the prevention of graft versus host disease (GVHD). Some, however, routinely use some form of T-cell deletion of donor marrow [70,71], either an appropriate monoclonal antibody, soybean lectin agglutination and E-rosette formation or counterflow elutriation. Such methods unquestionably reduce the incidence and severity of GVHD but are uniformly associated with an increased risk of relapse. Relapse can however be treated by donor lymphocyte transfusions (see below). The issue of whether or not to use some form of T-cell depletion has not been resolved.

The clinical results of transplantation for CML in CP using matched sibling donors are relatively consistent in specialist centres worldwide. The major determinants of survival include the age of the patient, his/her CMV serostatus, the age of the donor, the sex of the donor and the precise details of the transplant procedure. In general the probability of survival, of relapse and/or leukaemia-free survival at 5 years are 60–80%, 10–20% and 55–70%, respectively. If a particularly favourable subset of patients was chosen, perhaps those under the age of 40 with male donors and CMV seronegativity, a leukaemia-free survival of 70–80% might be anticipated. The incidence of relapse appears to be maximal at about 2 years post-transplant; a small proportion of patients relapse each year thereafter. It is thus difficult to conclude with complete certainty that any individual patient is truly 'cured', but the probability of relapse has become exceedingly small by 10 years free of leukaemia [72].

Monitoring patients and treatment of relapse. With the availability now of molecular methods to monitor minimal residual disease, complete remission may be defined as the complete absence of evidence of leukaemia at the molecular level [73,74]. For technical reasons even this definition is of course imperfect. The pattern of events in a patient destined to relapse after allogeneic HSCT is relatively consistent [75,76]. The first indication is a rising level of BCR-ABL transcripts in the blood; some months later examination of the marrow reveals partial Ph positivity. After a further interval of months or occasionally years, the patient will manifest a leucocytosis and/or thrombocytosis. Thus relapse proceeds in the sequence molecular → cytogenetic → haematological. The practical implication is that routine cytogenetic studies are probably unnecessary in a patient in molecular remission. Molecular studies should be performed at 2- or 3-month intervals post-transplant. Treatment for relapse should probably be initiated while a patient is still in molecular or cytogenetic relapse.

There are various approaches to the treatment of relapse, including the use of IFNα or hydroxyurea and a second transplant procedure [77,78] but the use of donor lymphocyte transfusions (DLT) currently seems to be the best option [79–82]. They must act by mediating a 'graft-versus-leukaemia' (GVL) effect by a precise immunological mechanism which has not yet been elucidated. Thus if lymphoid cells are collected by leucapheresis from the original transplant donor and transfused to the patient in relapse, complete remission is achieved in about 70% of cases [82]. DLT may however be complicated by marrow aplasia or by initiation or exacerbation of GVHD. For these reasons, it is currently recommended that DLT are started at low cell dosage and the dose is only increased at intervals if no GVL effect is observed [83].

Allogeneic stem cell transplantation using unrelated donors. This qualified success with BMT using matched siblings has led to an increasing use of 'matched' unrelated donors for BMT for patients with CML [84,85]. At present serologically matched unrelated donors can be identified for about 50% of caucasian patients and for lower percentages of patients of other ethnic origins. The results of transplants using such unrelated donors are currently somewhat less good than results when using HLA-identical siblings (Fig. 13.9). In particular patients older than 45 years have a relatively high risk of TRM. Moreover, the incidence of severe viral infections, especially with CMV but also with other usually innocuous viruses, seems higher than after sibling transplants [86,87]. This said, an appreciable proportion of patients lacking HLA-identical sibling donors who received transplants from unrelated donors can expect to have been cured. For very young patients, i.e. those aged less than 20 years, a transplant using an unrelated donor performed within 1 year of diagnosis is a reasonable option. For older patients with suitable volunteer donors, an initial trial of IFNα seems sensible.

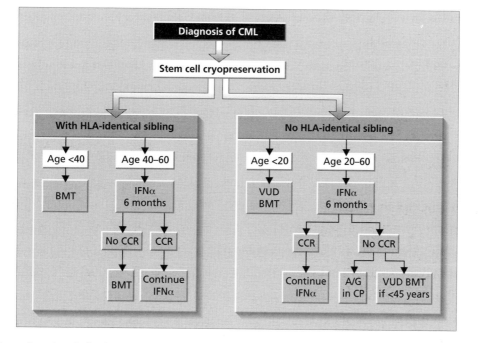

Fig. 13.9 An algorithm or flow chart indicating a possible approach to the management of a newly diagnosed CML patient who has not been entered into a clinical trial. A patient up to the age of 60 years with an HLA-identical sibling should be considered for treatment by allogeneic bone marrow transplantation (BMT) within 1 year of diagnosis. Between the ages of 40 and 60 a trial of IFNα is recommended, so that BMT may be delayed for any patient who achieves a complete cytogenetic response (CCR). All patients who lack an HLA-identical sibling are started on treatment with IFNα unless they are aged less than 20 years, in which case a transplant using an alternative or volunteer unrelated donor (VUD) should be considered as primary treatment. For patients who do not achieve a CCR on IFNα, autografting (A/G) or transplant with a VUD should be considered 6–12 months after diagnosis.

Table 13.7 Methods that may be employed to favour the recovery of predominantly Ph− progenitor cells for use as a subsequent autograft.

In vitro methods
Incubation in liquid culture for 10 days
Incubation with
    Cytotoxic drugs
    Antisense oligodeoxynucleotides
    Ribozymes
    Tyrosine kinase inhibitors

In vivo methods
Initial treatment with interferon alpha
Initial treatment with high-dose chemotherapy

Autografting. Because only a minority of patients are eligible for allogeneic HSCT, much interest has focused recently on the possibility that life may be prolonged and some cures effected by autografting CML patients still in CP. It is possible that the pool of leukaemic stem cells can be substantially reduced by an autograft procedure, and autografting may confer a short-term proliferative advantage on Ph− (presumably normal) stem cells [88]. Thus patients still in CP have been treated in various specialist centres during the past 10 years by high-dose chemotherapy or chemoradiotherapy, followed by transfusion of autologous stem cells that had been collected earlier and cryopreserved in liquid nitrogen [89,90]. These stem cells were collected from the peripheral blood by leucapheresis or by bone marrow harvest. Patients recovered haemopoiesis postautografting in almost every case. In about 50% of cases this haemopoiesis was partially and transiently Ph−. In most cases haemopoiesis had reverted to 100% Ph+ by 6–9 months [91], but very occasionally Ph− haemopoiesis was maintained for a number of years. A recent analysis of survival in patients autografted with 'unmanipulated' stem cells suggested that such patients might survive longer than matched controls [92], but the question can really only be addressed with a properly constructed prospective study. Such studies are now in progress.

The observation that autografting with unmanipulated stem cells might prolong life led, logically, to the concept that additional prolongation might be achieved if the autograft could be performed with stem cells that were predominantly Ph−. There are two contrasting approaches for successful recovery from the patient of Ph− stem cells (Table 13.7), the *in vivo* approach pioneered in Uppsala and Genoa and the *in vitro* approach studied in Vancouver and elsewhere (reviewed in ref. [93]). The former approach involves administration to the patient of IFNα and/or cytotoxic drugs at relatively high dosage. If a patient achieves Ph− haemopoiesis, marrow or blood stem cells are then collected and cryopreserved for future use [94,95]. The latter approach involves collecting blood- or marrow-derived stem cells and incubating them *in vitro* either alone [96] or in conjunction with selected molecules designed to promote the survival of normal stem cells and to inhibit the survival of leukaemia progenitors. A variety of antisense oligodeoxynucleotides have been tested for this purpose [97]. Currently interest focuses on the possibility that incubation of marrow cells with a tyrosine kinase inhibitor manufactured by Novartis might produce a Ph− stem cell product for autografting [98]. In general, the results of autografting with stem cells 'purified' in this manner are too early to evaluate.

Advanced-phase disease

Cytotoxic drugs. Patients in blastic transformation may be treated with combinations of cytotoxic drugs in the hope of prolonging life, but cure can no longer be a realistic objective. Conversely it is not unreasonable to use a relatively innocuous drug such as hydroxyurea at a higher dosage to restrain blast cell numbers and maintain patients at home for as long as possible. If patients have a myeloid transformation, they can be treated with drugs appropriate to the induction of remission in AML, namely daunorubicin, cytosine arabinoside, with or without 6-thioguanine, or etoposide [35]. The blast cell numbers will be reduced substantially in most cases, but their numbers usually increase again within 3–6 weeks. Perhaps 20% of patients are restored to a situation resembling CP disease and this benefit may last for 3–6 months.

Patients in lymphoid transformation may be treated with a little more optimism with drugs applicable to the management of adult acute lymphoblastic leukaemia (e.g. prednisolone, vincristine and daunorucibin, with or without L-asparaginase) [35,99]. More than 50% of patients will be restored to 'second' CP, at which point this status can be maintained with daily 6-mercaptopurine and weekly methotrexate. Patients who achieve second CP are at high risk of developing leukaemic involvement of the central nervous system. They should therefore receive neuroprophylaxis with intrathecal methotrexate weekly for say six consecutive weeks [99], but the administration of cranial irradiation is probably excessive. Some patients treated for lymphoid transformation of CML may sustain long periods of apparent 'remission'.

Allogeneic stem cell transplantation. Allogeneic bone marrow transplantation using HLA-matched sibling donors can be performed in the accelerated phase; the probability of leukaemia-free survival at 5 years is 30–50% [100]. Bone marrow transplantation performed in overt blastic transformation is nearly always unsuccessful. The mortality resulting from GVHD is extremely high and the probability of relapse in those who survive the transplant procedure is very considerable. The probability of survival at 5 years is consequently only 5–10%.

References

1 Bennett J.H. (1845) Case of hypertrophy of the spleen and liver

in which death took place from suppuration of the blood. *Edinburgh Medical and Surgical Journal*, **64**, 413–422.

2 Nowell P.C. & Hungerford D.A. (1960) A minute chromosome in human chronic granulocytic leukemia. *Science*, **132**, 1497.

3 Rowley D. (1973) A new consistent chromosomal abnormality in chronic myelogenous leukemia identified by quinacrine fluorescence and Giemsa staining. *Nature*, **243**, 290–293.

4 Minot J.B., Buckman T.E. & Isaacs R. (1924) Chronic myelogenous leukemia: age incidence, duration and benefit derived from irradiation. *Journal of the American Medical Association*, **82**, 1489–1494.

5 Gunz F.W. (1977) The epidemiology and genetics of the chronic leukaemias. *Clinical Haematology*, **6**, 3–20.

6 Lange R., Moloney W. & Yamawaki T. (1954) Leukemia in atomic bomb survivors. I. General observations. *Blood*, **9**, 574–585.

7 Heysell R., Brill B. & Woodbury L. (1960) Leukemia in Hiroshima atomic bomb survivors. *Blood*, **15**, 313–331.

8 Court Brown W. & Doll R. (1965) Mortality from cancer and other causes after radiotherapy for ankylosing spondylitis. *British Medical Journal*, **2**, 1327–1332.

9 Fialkow P.J. (1981) Evidence for a multistep origin of chronic myeloid leukemia. *Blood*, **58**, 158–163.

10 Tura S., Baccarani M., Corbelli G. *et al.* (1981) Staging of chronic myeloid leukaemia. *British Journal of Haematology*, **47**, 105–119.

11 Cervantes F. & Rozman C. (1982) A multivariate analysis of prognostic factors in chronic myeloid leukemia. *Blood*, **60**, 1298–1304.

12 Sokal J.E., Cox E.B., Baccarani M. *et al.* and the Italian Cooperative CML Study Group (1984) Prognostic discrimination in 'good risk' chronic granulocytic leukaemia. *Blood*, **63**, 789–799.

13 Kantarjian H., Keating M., Smith T. *et al.* (1990) Proposal for a simple synthesis prognostic staging system in chronic myelogenous leukemia. *American Journal of Medicine*, **88**, 1–7.

14 Eaves C.J. & Eaves A.C. (1987) Cell culture studies in CML. *Baillière's Clinical Haematology*, **4**, 931–961.

15 Coulombel L., Kalousek D.K., Eaves C.J. *et al.* (1983) Long term marrow culture reveals chromosomally normal hemopoietic progenitor cells in patients with Philadelphia chromosome positive chronic myelogenous leukemia. *New England Journal of Medicine*, **308**, 1493–1498.

16 Hagemeijer A. (1987) Chromosomal abnormalities in CML. *Baillière's Clinical Haematology*, **2**, 963–981.

17 Bernstein R. (1988) Cytogenetics of chronic myelogenous leukemia. *Seminars in Hematology*, **25**, 20–34.

18 Watmore A.E., Potter A.M., Sokal R.J. *et al.* (1985) Value of cytogenetic studies in prediction of acute phase of CML. *Cancer Genetics and Cytogenetics*, **14**, 293–301.

19 Groffen J., Stephenson J.R., Heisterkamp N. *et al.* (1984) Philadelphia chromosomal breakpoints are clustered within a limited region, bcr, on chromosome 22. *Cell*, **36**, 93–99.

20 Kurzrock R., Gutterman J.U. & Talpaz M. (1988) The molecular genetics of Philadelphia chromosome-positive leukemias. *New England Journal of Medicine*, **319**, 990–998.

21 Gale R.P., Goldman J.M., Grosveld G. & Goldman J.M. (1993) Chronic myelogenous leukemia: biology and therapy. (Meeting Report.) *Leukemia*, **7**, 653–658.

22 Enright H. & McGlave P.B. (1995) Chronic myelogenous leukemia. *Current Opinions in Hematology*, **2**, 293–299.

23 Melo J.V. (1996) The diversity of BCR-ABL fusion proteins and their relationship to leukemic phenotype. *Blood*, **88**, 2375–2384.

24 Melo J.V. (1996) The molecular biology of chronic myeloid leukaemia. *Leukemia*, **10**, 751–756.

25 Mills K.I., MacKenzie E.D. & Birnie G.D. (1988) The site of breakpoint within bcr is a prognostic factor in Philadelphia-positive CML patients. *Blood*, **72**, 1237–1241.

26 Jaubert J., Martiat P., Dowding C. & Goldman J.M. (1990) The position of the M-BCR breakpoint does not predict the duration of chronic phase or survival in chronic myeloid leukaemia. *British Journal of Haematology*, **74**, 30–35.

27 Pendergast A.M., Quilliam L.A., Cripe L.D. *et al.* (1993) BCR-ABL-induced oncogenesis is mediated by direct interaction with the SH2 domain of the GRB-2 adaptor protein. *Cell*, **75**, 175–185.

28 Feinstein E., Cimino G., Gale R.P. *et al.* (1991) p53 in chronic myelogenous leukemia. *Proceedings of the National Academy of Sciences USA*, **88**, 6293–6297.

29 Sill H., Goldman J.M. & Cross N.C.P. (1995) Homozygous deletions of the p16 tumor suppressor gene are associated with lymphoid transformation of chronic myeloid leukemia. *Blood*, **85**, 2013–2016.

30 Spiers A.S.D. (1977) The clinical features of chronic granulocytic leukaemia. *Clinical Haematology*, **6**, 77–95.

31 Savage D.G., Szydlo R.M. & Goldman J.M. (1997) Clinical features of chronic myeloid leukaemia at diagnosis. *British Journal of Haematology*, **96**, 111–116.

32 Karanas A. & Silver R.T. (1968) Characteristics of the terminal phase of chronic granulocytic leukaemia. *Blood*, **32**, 445–459.

33 Kantarjian H.M., Keating M.J., Talpaz M. *et al.* (1987) Chronic myelogenous leukemia in blast crisis: analysis of 242 patients. *American Journal of Medicine*, **83**, 445–454.

34 Kantarjian H.M., Dixon D., Keating M.J. *et al.* (1988) Characteristics of accelerated disease in chronic myelogenous leukemia. *Cancer*, **61**, 1441–1446.

35 Derderian P.M., Kantarjian H.M., Talpaz M. *et al.* (1993) Chronic myelogenous leukemia in the lymphoid blastic phase: characteristics, treatment response and prognosis. *American Journal of Medicine*, **94**, 69–74.

36 Spiers A.S.D., Bain B.J. & Turner J.E. (1977) The peripheral blood in chronic granulocytic leukaemia. Study of 50 untreated Philadelphia-positive cases. *Scandinavian Journal of Haematology*, **18**, 25–38.

37 Chikkappa G., Wang G.J., Santella D. *et al.* (1988) Granulocyte colony-stimulating factor induces synthesis of alkaline phosphatase in neutrophilic granulocytes from chronic myelogenous leukemia patients. *Leukemia Research*, **12**, 491–498.

38 Marks S.M., McCaffrey R., Pippard M.J. *et al.* (1978) Blastic transformation in chronic myelogenous leukemia: experience with 50 patients. *Medical and Pediatric Oncology*, **4**, 159–167.

39 Bakhshi A., Minowada J., Arnold A. *et al.* (1983) Lymphoid blast crisis of chronic myelogenous leukemia represents stages in the development of B-cell precursors. *New England Journal of Medicine*, **309**, 826–831.

40 Bennett J.M., Catovsky D., Daniel T. *et al.* (1982) The French–American–British Cooperative Group: proposals for the classification of the myelodysplastic syndromes. *British Journal of Haematology*, **51**, 189–199.

41 You W. & Weisbrot I.M. (1979) Chronic neutrophilic leukemia: report of 2 cases and a review of the literature. *American Journal of Clinical Pathology*, **72**, 233–242.

42 Hehlmann R., Heimpel H., Hasford J. *et al.* (1993) Randomized comparison of busulfan and hydroxyurea in chronic myelogenous leukemia: prolongation of survival by hydroxyurea. *Blood*, **82**, 398–407.

43 Goldman J.M. (1990) Options for the management of chronic myeloid leukemia—1990. *Leukemia and Lymphoma*, **3**, 159–164.

44 Kantarjian H.M., Deisseroth A., Kurzrock R., Estrov Z. & Talpaz M. (1993) Review: chronic myelogenous leukemia: a concise update. *Blood*, **82**, 691–703.

45 Savage D.G. & Goldman J.M. (1994) Approaches to the management of chronic myeloid leukaemia. *British Journal of Haematology*, **60**, 1–21.

46 Spencer A., O'Brien S.G. & Goldman J.M. (1995) Options for therapy in chronic myeloid leukaemia. *British Journal of Haematology*, **91**, 2–7.

47 Kantarjian H.M., O'Brien S., Anderlini P. & Talpaz M. (1996) Review: treatment of chronic myelogenous leukemia: current status and investigational options. *Blood*, **87**, 3069–3081.

48 Lowenthal R.M., Buskard N.A., Goldman J.M. *et al.* (1975) Intensive leukapheresis as initial therapy of chronic granulocytic leukemia. *Blood*, **46**, 835–844.

49 Delmer A., Rio B., Bauduer F., Ajchenbaum F., Marie J-P. & Zittoun R. (1992) Pregnancy during myelosuppressive treatment for chronic myelogenous leukaemia. *British Journal of Haematology*, **82**, 781–782.

50 Talpaz M., McCredie K.B., Mavligit G.M. & Gutterman J. (1983) Leukocyte interferon-induced myeloid cytoreduction in chronic myelogenous leukemia. *Blood*, **62**, 1052–1056.

51 Talpaz M., Kantarjian H.M., McCredie K.B. *et al.* (1986) Hematologic remission and cytogenetic improvement induced by recombinant human interferon alpha A in chronic myelogenous leukemia. *New England Journal of Medicine*, **314**, 1065–1069.

52 Talpaz M., Kantarjian H.M., McCredie K.B. *et al.* (1986) Hematologic remission and cytogenetic improvement induced by recombinant human interferon A in chronic myelogenous leukemia. *New England Journal of Medicine*, **314**, 1065–1069.

53 Tura S., Baccarani M., Zuffa E. for the Italian Cooperative Study Group on Chronic Myeloid Leukemia (1994) Interferon alfa-2a as compared with conventional chemotherapy for the treatment of chronic myeloid leukemia. *New England Journal of Medicine*, **330**, 820–825.

54 Allan N.C., Richards S.M. & Shepherd P.C.A. (1995) UK Medical Research Council randomised multicentre trial of interferon-αn1 for chronic myeloid leukaemia: improved survival irrespective of cytogenetic response. *Lancet*, **345**, 1392–1397.

55 Hehlmann R., Heimpel H., Hasford J. *et al.* (1994) Randomized comparison of interferon-α with busulfan and hydroxyurea in chronic myelogenous leukemia. *Blood*, **94**, 4064–4077.

56 Ozer H., George S.L., Schiffer C.A. *et al.* (1993) Prolonged subcutaneous administration of recombinant α2b interferon in patients with previously untreated Philadelphia chromosome-positive chronic myeloid leukemia: effect on remission duration and survival: Cancer and Leukemia Group B Study 8583. *Blood*, **82**, 2975–2984.

57 Kantarjian H.M., Smith T.L., O'Brien S., Beran M., Pierce S. & Talpaz M. (1995) Prolonged survival in chronic myelogenous leukemia after cytogenetic response to interferon-α therapy. *Annals of Internal Medicine*, **122**, 254–261.

58 Guilhot F., Chastang C., Michallet M. *et al.* (1997) Interferon alfa combined with cytarabine compared with interferon alone in chronic myelogenous leukemia. *New England Journal of Medicine*, **337**, 223–229.

59 Bolin R.W., Robinson W.A., Sutherland J. *et al.* (1982) Busulfan versus hydroxyurea in the longterm therapy of chronic myelogenous leukemia. *Cancer*, **50**, 1683–1687.

60 Galton D.A.G. (1953) Myleran in chronic myeloid leukaemia. Results of treatment. *Lancet*, **i**, 208–213.

61 Galton D.A.G. (1959) Treatment of the chronic leukaemias. *British Medical Bulletin*, **15**, 79–86.

62 Goldman J.M., Apperley J.F., Jones L.M. *et al.* (1986) Bone marrow transplantation for patients with chronic myeloid leukemia. *New England Journal of Medicine*, **314**, 202–207.

63 Thomas E.D., Clift R.A., Fefer A. *et al.* (1986) Marrow transplantation for the treatment of chronic myelogenous leukemia. *Annals of Internal Medicine*, **104**, 155–163.

64 Gratwohl A., Hermans J., Niederwieser D. *et al.* (1993) Bone marrow transplantation for chronic myeloid leukemia: long-term results. *Bone Marrow Transplant*, **12**, 509–516.

65 Goldman J.M., Szydlo R., Horowitz M.M. *et al.* (1993) Choice of pretransplant treatment and timing of transplants for chronic myelogenous leukemia in chronic phase. *Blood*, **82**, 2235–2238.

66 Szydlo R., Goldman J.M., Klein J.P. *et al.* (1997) Result of allogeneic bone marrow transplants using donors other than HLA-identical siblings. *Journal of Clinical Oncology*, **15**, 1767–1777.

67 Biggs J., Szer J., Crilley P. *et al.* (1992) Treatment of chronic myeloid leukemia with allogeneic bone marrow transplantation after preparation with BuCy2. *Blood*, **80**, 1352–1357.

68 Clift R.A., Buckner C.D., Thomas E.D. *et al.* (1994) Marrow transplantation for chronic myeloid leukemia: a randomized study comparing cyclophosphamide and total body irradiation with busulfan and cyclophosphamide. *Blood*, **84**, 2036–2043.

69 Snyder D., Negrin R., O'Donnell M. *et al.* (1994) Fractionated total-body irradiation and high dose etoposide as a preparatory regimen for bone marrow transplantation for 94 patients with chronic myelogenous leukemia in chronic phase. *Blood*, **84**, 1672–1679.

70 Marmont A.M., Horowitz M.M., Gale R.P. *et al.* (1991) T-cell depletion of HLA-identical transplants in leukemia. *Blood*, **78**, 2120–2130.

71 Goldman J.M., Gale R.P., Horowitz M.M. *et al.* (1988) Bone marrow transplantation for chronic myelogenous leukemia in chronic phase: increased risk of relapse associated with T-cell depletion. *Annals of Internal Medicine*, **108**, 806–814.

72 van Rhee F., Lin F., Cross N.C.P. *et al.* (1994) Detection of residual leukaemia more than 10 years after allogeneic bone marrow transplantation for chronic myelogenous leukaemia. *Bone Marrow Transplant*, **14**, 609–612.

73 Morgan G.J., Hughes T., Janssen J.W.G. *et al.* (1989) Polymerase chain reaction for detection of residual leukaemia. *Lancet*, **i**, 928–929.

74 Hughes T.P., Morgan G.J., Martiat P. & Goldman J.M. (1991) Detection of residual leukemia after bone marrow transplant for chronic myeloid leukemia: role of the polymerase chain reaction. *Blood*, **77**, 874–878.

75 Cross N.C.P., Feng Lin, Chase A., Bungey J., Hughes T.P. & Goldman J.M. (1993) Competitive PCR to estimate the number of BCR-ABL transcripts in chronic myeloid leukemia patients after bone marrow transplantation. *Blood*, **82**, 1929–1936.

76 Lin F., van Rhee F., Goldman J.M. & Cross N.C.P. (1996) Kinetics of increasing BCR-ABL transcript numbers in chronic myeloid leukemia patients who relapse after bone marrow transplantation. *Blood*, **87**, 4473–4478.

77 Arcese W., Gratwohl A., Niederwieser D. *et al.* (1993) Outcome for patients who relapse after allogeneic bone marrow transplantation for chronic myeloid leukemia. *Blood*, **82**, 3211–3219.

78 Cullis J.O., Schwarer A.P., Hughes T.P. *et al.* (1992) Second trans-

plants for patients with chronic myeloid leukaemia in relapse after original transplant with T-depleted donor marrow: feasibility of busulphan alone for re-conditioning. *British Journal of Haematology*, **80**, 33–39.

79 Kolb H.J., Mittermuller J., Clemm C.H. *et al.* (1990) Donor leukocyte transfusions for treatment of recurrent chronic myelogenous leukemia in marrow transplant patients. *Blood*, **76**, 2462–2465.

80 Cullis J.O., Jiang Y.Z., Schwarer A.P., Hughes T.P., Barrett A.J. & Goldman J.M. (1992) Donor leukocyte infusions in the treatment of chronic myeloid leukaemia in relapse following allogeneic bone marrow transplantation (letter). *Blood*, **79**, 1379–1382.

81 van Rhee F., Feng Lin, Cross N.J.P., Bungey J., Chase A. & Goldman J.M. (1994) Relapse of chronic myeloid leukemia after allogeneic bone marrow transplant: the case for giving donor leukocyte transfusions before the onset of hematologic relapse. *Blood*, **83**, 3377–3383.

82 Kolb H.J., Schattenberg A., Goldman J.M. *et al.* (1995) Graft-versus-leukemia effect of donor lymphocyte transfusion in marrow grafted patients. *Blood*, **86**, 2041–2205.

83 Mackinnon S., Papadopoulos E.P., Carabasi M.H. *et al.* (1995) Adoptive immunotherapy evaluating escalating doses of donor leukocytes for relapse of chronic myeloid leukemia following bone marrow transplantation: separation of graft-versus-leukemia responses from graft-versus-host disease. *Blood*, **86**, 1261–1267.

84 Beatty P.G., Anasetti C., Hansen J.A. *et al.* (1993) Marrow transplantation from unrelated donors for treatment of hematologic malignancies: effect of mismatching for one HLA locus. *Blood*, **81**, 249–253.

85 McGlave P., Bartsch G., Anasetti C. *et al.* (1993) Unrelated donor marrow transplantation therapy for chronic myelogenous leukemia: initial experience of the National Marrow Donor Program. *Blood*, **81**, 543–550.

86 Mackinnon S., Hows J.M., Goldman J.M. *et al.* (1989) Bone marrow transplantation for chronic myeloid leukemia: the use of histocompatible unrelated volunteer donors. *Experimental Hematology*, **18**, 421–425.

87 Marks D.I., Cullis J.O., Ward K.N. *et al.* (1993) Allogeneic bone marrow transplantation for chronic myeloid leukemia using sibling and volunteer donors: a comparison of complications in the first two years. *Annals of Internal Medicine*, **119**, 207–214.

88 Daley G.D. & Goldman J.M. (1993) Autologous transplants for CML revisited. *Experimental Hematology*, **21**, 734–737.

89 McGlave P., De Fabritiis P., Deisseroth A. *et al.* (1994) Autologous transplant therapy for chronic myelogenous leukemia prolongs survival: results from eight transplant groups. *Lancet*, **343**, 1486–1491.

90 Reiffers J., Goldman J.M., Meloni G. *et al.* (1994) Autologous stem cell transplantation in chronic myelogenous leukemia. A retrospective analysis of the European Group for Bone Marrow Transplantation. *Bone Marrow Transplant*, **14**, 407–410.

91 Brito-Babapulle F., Bowcock S.J., Marcus R.E. *et al.* (1989) Autografting for patients with chronic myeloid leukaemia in chronic phase: peripheral blood stem cells may have finite capacity for maintaining haemopoiesis. *British Journal of Haematology*, **73**, 76–81.

92 Hoyle C., Gray R., Goldman J.M. *et al.* (1994) Autografting for patients with CML in chronic phase—an update. *British Journal of Haematology*, **86**, 76–81.

93 O'Brien S.G. & Goldman J.M. (1995) Current approaches to hemopoietic stem-cell purging in chronic myeloid leukemia. *Journal of Clinical Oncology*, **13**, 541–546.

94 Simonsson B., Oberg G., Bjoreman M. *et al.* (1992) Intensive treatment in order to minimize the Ph-positive clone in chronic myelogenic leukaemia. *Leukemia and Lymphoma*, **7**(Suppl.), 55–57.

95 Carella A.M., Cunningham I., Lerma E. *et al.* (1997) Mobilization and transplantation of Philadelphia-negative peripheral blood progenitor cells early in chronic myelogenous leukemia. *Journal of Clinical Oncology*, **15**, 1575–1582.

96 Barnett M.J., Eaves C.J., Phillips G.L. *et al.* (1994) Autografting with cultured marrow in chronic myeloid leukemia. Results of a pilot study. *Blood*, **84**, 724–732.

97 de Fabritiis P., Amadori S., Petti M.C. *et al.* (1995) *In vitro* purging with BCR-ABL antisense oligodoxynucleotides does not prevent haematological reconstitution after autologous bone marrow transplantation. *Leukemia*, **9**, 662–664.

98 Druker B.J., Tamura S., Buchdunger E. *et al.* (1996) Effects of a selective inhibitor of the Abl tyrosine kinase on the growth of BCR-ABL positive cells. *Nature Medicine*, **2**, 561–566.

99 Nathwani A. & Goldman J.M. (1993) The management of chronic myeloid leukemia in lymphoid blast crisis. *Haematologica*, **78**, 162–166.

100 Clift R., Buckner C., Thomas E. *et al.* (1994) Marrow transplantation for patients in accelerated phase of chronic myeloid leukemia. *Blood*, **84**, 4368–4373.

14   Myeloma

J.A. Child and G.J. Morgan

Introduction

The incidence of clinically apparent multiple myeloma is of the order of three cases in 100 000 of the population per year. This incidence increases with age and only 2% of all cases occur before the age of 40 years. There must be doubts about the validity of the epidemiological data because of the existence of a large preclinical pool of paraproteinaemias, the size of which is poorly defined. This may directly impinge on incidence and prevalence figures, depending on the extent of clinical investigation performed within a population. However, within these limits, monoclonal gammopathy, which encompasses myeloma and monoclonal gammopathy of uncertain significance (MGUS), seems to account for 10–15% of all haematological malignancies and 1–2% of all malignant disease.

Diagnostic features

The essential clinical features of myeloma can be related to the diffuse or patchy replacement of the bone marrow by neoplastic plasma cells and, in the majority of cases, production of a paraprotein and/or a light-chain moiety. The plasma cells show dysregulated immunoglobulin production which, in the majority of cases, results in a high concentration of paraprotein in the peripheral blood and suppression of immunoglobulin production by normal B cells. In about 80% of cases immunoglobulin light chain is produced in excess of heavy chains. The excess light chain is secreted in the urine and is an important cause of nephrotoxicity and, in some cases, amyloidosis. The infiltrating plasma cells are responsible for disordered bone metabolism which is the presenting feature in most cases. In the later stages of the disease progressive marrow replacement may result in marrow failure.

One measure of the extent of disease is the concentration of paraprotein. The probability of multiple myeloma is high when the monoclonal (M) component exceeds 35 g/l for IgG or 20 g/l for IgA, or kappa or lambda light-chain urinary excretion exceeds 1 g/24 hours. A serum beta-2-microglobulin concentration of greater than 4 mg/l is supplementary evidence of significant disease bulk. In addition, the patient may well have one or more of the typical complications of myeloma — anaemia, hypercalcaemia, bone disease, renal insufficiency or immunosuppression as judged by a reduction of the normal immunoglobulin levels.

In most cases of myeloma the number of plasma cells will exceed 10% of the nucleated cells in a bone marrow aspirate. They show a wide range of cytological abnormalities, including prominent nucleoli, cytoplasmic vacuolation or nuclear inclusions, and have been classified into a number of different types based on their morphological features. This may be helpful diagnostically but is otherwise of limited clinical value. Immunofluorescent detection of cytoplasmic immunoglobulin can identify the immunoglobulin type being produced by the plasma cell and this should correlate with the serum paraproteins and urinary light chains. This can be used diagnostically to confirm the monoclonal nature of the plasma cells.

Increasingly, bone marrow trephine biopsies as well as aspirates are obtained at diagnosis and, although this can provide more information about the degree of infiltration, it is not generally feasible to accurately count the proportion of plasma cells in the biopsy. A differential count would be very time consuming and of doubtful validity, because of the nonrandom distribution of myelomatous plasma cells. The percentage of plasma cells will depend on the cellularity of the other formed elements, i.e. whether the marrow is hyperplastic or hypoplastic. However, within these limits, the trephine can be useful as a tool to monitor the effects of treatment. In addition to the appearance of the abnormal plasma cells, there are diagnostic architectural features. Normal plasma cells accumulate around blood vessels in the bone marrow but in the earliest stage of marrow involvement in myeloma this pattern is lost, the neoplastic plasma cells are found as single cells or small clusters between adipocytes. As the disease progresses, areas of diffuse marrow replacement occur and, ultimately, a 'packed marrow' develops. These stages broadly correspond to the bulk of disease. Two other patterns of infiltration are seen. In a small number of cases early myeloma shows a paratrabecular distribution similar to follicle centre lymphoma and, in some patients with very aggressive disease, tumour nodules, often containing very abnormal plasma cells, may be seen. In assessing the pattern of marrow disease in a trephine biopsy a plasma cell marker, such as VS38c or an anti-light-chain antibody, can be very helpful, as this will often show much heavier infiltration than is apparent by routine staining.

The morphological features of the neoplastic plasma cells seen in trephine biopsies are very variable. In most cases 25% or more of the cells are nucleolated and cells with multiple nuclei or cleaved nuclei may be seen. Cells with abundant foamy or vacuolated cytoplasm may not be readily identified as plasma cells. In some patients with very aggressive disease, especially in relapse, the marrow may be replaced by large lymphoid cells, resembling immunoblasts, with only a small proportion of cells showing features of plasma cell differentiation. The cell-cycle fraction can be determined using Ki67—the proportion of positive plasma cells is low, except in patients with very aggressive disease. In only 10–20% of cases does the proliferating fraction exceed 2% of the plasma cells and even in end-stage disease proliferating fractions of 5% are seldom seem. Relatively few B-lymphocytes are usually present in trephine biopsies infiltrated by myeloma. However, in a few cases one or more large aggregates of small B cells, admixed with occasional proliferating blast cells, may be present; their significance is unknown.

There is a close relationship between MGUS and myeloma, the essential clinical difference being that MGUS is stable and does not require treatment. In MGUS there is no evidence of bone lesions, anaemia, renal failure or immunosuppression, and the paraprotein and marrow plasma cell counts do not meet the criteria for multiple myeloma. In the trephine biopsy, clonal plasma cells may be present, although they are usually sparse and have an interstitial distribution. Because there is often progression from MGUS to myeloma, it is not surprising that intermediate states exist in which the serological and marrow features of myeloma are present but the patient is asymptomatic with minimal or no bone lesions. The terms 'equivocal', 'indolent' or 'smouldering' are variously used in such cases. The diagnostic criteria for MGUS and multiple myeloma are reasonably clearly defined (Tables 14.1 & 14.2). The definition of the intermediate states is artificial and arbitrary but may be of value in the characterization of disease status and patient selection in therapeutic trials (e.g. 'equivocal' myeloma is not eligible for treatment in the Medical Research Council (MRC) trials).

Plasmacytoma and plasma cell tumour variants

A small group of patients present with a solitary bone lesion which on biopsy is found to be a plasmacytoma. These are rare

Table 14.1 Diagnostic criteria for myeloma.

Major criteria

I	Plasmacytoma on tissue biopsy
II	Bone marrow plasmacytosis >30%
III	Monoclonal (M) spike on electrophoresis

>35 g/l (G peaks)
or >20 g/l (A peaks)
or κ or λ light-chain excretion >1.0 g/24 hour

Minor criteria

a	Bone marrow plasmacytosis 10–30%
b	M spike present but less than above
c	Lytic bone lesions
d	The normal immunoglobulin levels decreased:

IgM below 0.5 g/l
or IgA below 1 g/l
or IgG below 6 g/l

Diagnosis of myeloma requires a minimum of one major plus one minor criteria *or* three minor criteria which include both a *and* b

Table 14.2 Diagnostic criteria for MGUS.

I	Monoclonal gammopathy
II	Bone marrow plasma cells <10%
III	Monoclonal (M) component level

IgG ≤35 g/l
IgA ≤20 g/l
κ or λ light chains ≤1.0 g/24 hour

IV	No overt bone lesions
V	No symptoms to suggest myeloma

cases, representing 3–5% of plasma cell neoplasms, and they tend to occur in younger patients. In the majority of cases the lesion is in a vertebral body, which may lead to vertebral collapse fracture and spinal cord compression. The diagnosis of solitary plasmacytoma depends on demonstrating that the lesion consists of a population of clonal plasma cells and that there is no evidence of disseminated disease. This is confirmed by bone marrow aspirate, trephine and skeletal survey. Magnetic resonance image (MRI) scanning may have a role in defining the isolated nature of the lesions. Isolated plasmacytoma may have a paraprotein, but levels are lower than is usual in multiple myeloma; associated immunoparesis is uncommon, as is evidence of myelosuppression. Progression to multiple myeloma is usual, in a period of 3–4 years, indicating that these are variants of the same disease process. Once the lesions have been shown to be isolated, radiotherapy is the treatment of choice and may be curative. If more than one lesion is present the choice of treatment is more difficult. However, radiotherapy may still be the first choice, but it is much less likely to be curative and chemotherapy may eventually be required. A number of patterns of treatment failure may be seen, notably progression to multiple myeloma or the development of further isolated lesions. Occasional patients are identified who relapse repeatedly with bone lesions without evidence of disseminated myeloma and the value of chemotherapy for these cases is unknown. The overall survival duration of cases with solitary plasmacytoma is better than for myeloma.

An area of potential confusion is the relationship of solitary plasmacytoma of bone to plasmacytoma at other sites. The upper respiratory tract is the most common extraskeletal site, but plasmacytomas are also seen in skin, lymph node, thymus and at almost any other site. It is important to remember that most types of B-cell lymphoma can show some evidence of plasma cell differentiation, and in a few cases plasma cells may predominate, for example in marginal zone lymphoma (MALToma). And, unlike plasmacytoma in bone, plasmacytomas at other sites do not progress to myeloma. These tumours should not be confused with nodal or soft tissue spread of myeloma, which occasionally occurs in the context of advanced disease.

In a small number of patients presenting with bone marrow failure with or without lytic bone lesions, bone marrow examination shows replacement of normal marrow by a diffuse large cell lymphoma consisting of rapidly proliferating cells with centroblastic immunoblastic or plasmablastic type morphology. Only a minority of the cells express cIg and a paraprotein is often absent. The tumour cells express CD20 and do not have the typical immunophenotype of myeloma plasma cells. Limited studies suggest that these tumours respond well to CHOP (cyclophosphamide, doxorubicin, vincristine, prednisolone).

Plasma cell leukaemia

An overtly leukaemic phase, with rising plasma cell counts in the peripheral blood and bone marrow failure, represents progressive disease and should not pose a diagnostic problem. However, plasma cell leukaemia may occur as a cause of acute bone marrow failure without a well-documented history of preceding multiple myeloma. The cells in the peripheral blood may be of lymphocyte size without clear evidence of plasma cell morphology, and in some cases monotypic sIg expression may be present which will tend to obscure the detection of cIg. In these instances the key to diagnosis is the identification of other phenotypic features of plasma cell differentiation, such as CD38 and MCA681 positivity with loss of pan B-cell markers.

Bone lesions in myeloma

Lesions of the skeleton represent the most frequent presenting symptom of myeloma. Typically, these are punched-out lytic lesions which are frequently multiple and distributed throughout the skeleton and correspond to focal plasma cell expansions. In addition to this, there is usually generalized osteoporosis, which is often a contributory factor underlying pathological fractures. Collapse fractures of the vertebral column are frequently the net result of erosive bone lesions and diffuse osteoporosis.

The underlying abnormality is excessive bone resorption which is not matched by a comparable amount of bone formation — an imbalance between osteoclastic and osteoblastic activity. The abnormal osteoclastic activity results from increased recruitment of osteoclasts and their stimulation, largely brought about by cytokines, originally termed osteoclast-activating factor (OAF) secreted by the plasma cells. It is now known that one of the major active factors in this is IL-1, although IL-6 may also have an important rôle [1–3]. Osteoblasts are not activated and there is no sclerosis in the bone lesions (which occurs when epithelial malignancies metastasize to bone). Consequently, radioisotopic bone scans which rely on the uptake of activity in new bone formed by osteoblasts do not detect the bone lesions in myeloma.

Understanding the biology of this process, and using this knowledge to help predict patients particularly at risk of bone disease, is an important challenge. This has become particularly relevant in recent years with the advent of bisphosphonate therapy.

Predicting the development of bone disease

There has been recent interest in the assessment of bone resorption in MGUS by the invasive approach of bone histomorphometry and by MRI. In a study of 87 patients with MGUS, bone density was measured, using histomorphometry. Excessive bone resorption was seen at diagnosis in 52% of patients who later went on to develop myeloma, but in only 4% of those with stable MGUS, suggesting that excess resorption is associated with disease progression [4]. A similar study was undertaken in patients with MGUS and stage I myeloma to see whether MRI could be used to predict progression [5]. In both groups an abnormal scan was highly correlated with disease progression. In both studies multivariate analysis showed that MR scanning was an independent variable in the prediction of disease progression.

It would be more useful to use a simple biochemical test to assess bone turnover in the sera. The rate of bone formation is reflected by the measurement of serum alkaline phosphatase, osteocalcin and PICP, a carboxy terminal propeptide which is released into the circulation during the synthesis of type 1 collagen from type 1 procollagen. The rate of bone resorption can be assessed by the measurement of collagen breakdown products, for example ICTP, a serum carboxy terminal cross-linked telopeptide, and studies by several groups of patients with MGUS and myeloma at diagnosis suggest that these may be useful markers [6,7].

Another useful measure of bone resorption is the urinary excretion of collagen breakdown products such as hydroxyproline and pyridinoline cross-links. Unfortunately urinary hydroxyproline also originates from nonosseous collagen and the level is affected by dietary collagen. Measurements of

Table 14.3 Durie–Salmon staging system for myeloma.

Stage I
Low myeloma cell mass ($<0.6 \times 10^{12}$ cells/m²)
Criteria—all of the following:
  Hb >10 g/dl
  Serum calcium (corrected) ⩽3.0 mmol/l
  X-rays: normal bone structure or solitary lesion only
  M-component production rates:
    IgG value <50 g/l
    IgA value <30 g/l
    Urine light-chain excretion <4 g/24 hour

Stage II
Intermediate myeloma cell mass ($0.6–1.2 \times 10^{12}$ cells/m²)
Criteria—fitting neither stage I nor III

Stage III
High myeloma cell mass ($>1.2 \times 10^{12}$ cells/m²)
Criteria—any of the following:
  Hb < 8.5 g/dl
  Serum calcium (corrected) >3.0 mmol/l
  Advanced lytic bone lesions
  M-component production rates:
    IgG value >70 g/l
    IgA value >50 g/l
    Urine light-chain excretion >12 g/24 hour

Subclassified A and B according to renal function; A = serum creatinine <2 mg/100 ml; B = serum creatinine ⩾2 mg/100 ml

Table 14.4 Presenting features: MRC Trials.

Presenting features	%
Performance status	
Asymptomatic	11
Minimal symptoms	39
Restricted activity	50
Lytic bone lesions	
None	25
Isolated	6
Multiple	69
Durie–Salmon Index	
I	3
II	13
III	84
Serum creatinine (μmol/l)	
⩽130	57
>130–⩽200	25
>200	18
Serum β_2m (mg/l)	
⩽4	24
>4–⩽8	42
>8	34

Table 14.5 Relative value of prognostic factors used to stratify patients with myeloma: based on 630 patients entered into the MRC Myeloma V Trial.

Prognostic factor	χ^2	Probability
Serum β_2m	70.8	<0.0001
Cusick Index	46.6	<0.0001
Serum creatinine	38.6	<0.0001
Haemoglobin level	37.5	<0.0001
Durie–Salmon Index	23.0	<0.0001
Age	5.8	<0.017

these variables appear to differentiate patients with myeloma, MGUS and osteoporosis [8] and may be useful for identifying patients at risk of bone disease.

Staging and prognostic factors

The most widely adopted staging system has been devised by Durie & Salmon [9] (Table 14.3). This was based on calculations of tumour cell mass and correlations with clinical and laboratory features considered to carry prognostic significance. Patients with high, intermediate and low tumour cell mass were identified and, in practice, these groups were shown to have significantly different survival patterns [9,10]. The Durie–Salmon index has facilitated comparisons between broadly similar groups of patients, particularly in therapeutic trials, but it has not proved to be an accurate discriminant, as, for example, in determining the need for treatment. Furthermore, either multiple lytic lesions or a high serum paraprotein level, two relatively weak prognostic indicators, will place patients in stage III. Many clinical and investigatory parameters have been shown to have prognostic significance, and their relative frequency and strength has been demonstrated in large-scale trials and studies such as those carried out by the Medical Research Council [11] (Tables 14.4 & 14.5).

The emergence of beta-2-microglobulin (β_2m) as a powerful prognostic indicator has been of particular interest. Beta-2-microglobulin forms the light-chain moiety of the class I major histocompatibility antigens (HLA) on the surface of all nucleated cells [12,13] and cell membrane turnover is probably the principal source of free β_2m in blood and other body fluids [14]. Beta-2-microglobulin is filtered by the renal glomeruli and almost completely (>99%) catabolized to amino acids. The level of β_2m in serum is normally within a fairly narrow range. In the 1970s, increased β_2m levels were reported to occur in various malignancies, including multiple myeloma [15,16]. Subsequent clinical investigations suggested that good and bad prognostic groups could be defined using discriminant levels of β_2m [17], and the studies carried out by Child *et al.* [18] and Bataille *et al.* [19] showed that β_2m was a stronger indicator of prognosis than the current standard parameters, including Durie–Salmon stage (Fig. 14.1). Renal impairment will accentuate the increase in β_2m levels and can be corrected for [20]. In practice, the uncorrected level, reflecting both tumour mass

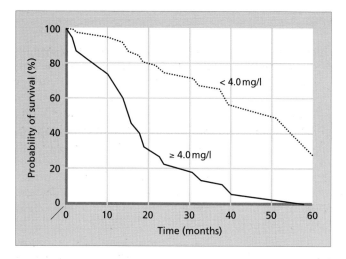

Fig. 14.1 The probability of survival of patients with myelomatosis according to whether the serum β2-microglobulin is ⩾4 mg/l or <4 mg/l at first presentation. *P* ⩽0.0001.

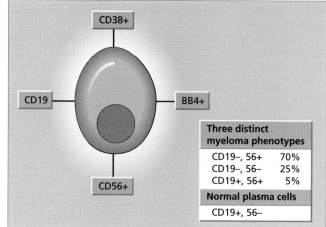

Fig. 14.2 The myeloma cell phenotype.

and renal function, will define risk groups and be predictive of response to treatment. Sequential serum β_2m levels continue to give prognostic information following the institution of treatment and have been shown to reflect disease status [21–23]. This has also been shown to be the case in post-transplantation. However, the principal value of the serum β_2m level appears to be in initial pretreatment stratification. It does not appear to be helpful in clearly distinguishing MGUS from myeloma.

Various terms, equivocal, indolent and smouldering [24], have been used for those states which, although fulfilling the criteria for the diagnosis of myeloma, do not represent progressive disease requiring early treatment. The criteria adopted are clearly arbitrary and artificial, dividing groups of patients in what is probably a continuous spectrum of disease. In therapeutic trials, it is nevertheless clearly important that the criteria for entry and treatment are strictly applied. The proportion of patients with smouldering myeloma, which may continue as such for many years without needing treatment, will influence survival data, and is one reason for the differences in the results of therapeutic studies [11]. A powerful discriminant such as serum β_2m can be used to correct for such bias [21].

The plasma cell labelling index as a measure of cell proliferation is another useful indicator of disease activity, which is of particular value in confirming disease progression and the need to start treatment [25]. The power of β_2m measurement has been shown to be further increased when combined with measurement of the proliferative fraction in the plasma cells, either by pulse labelling or by the use of Ki67 as a marker of cells in the proliferative phase of the cell cycle. Clinical evaluation has suggested that the prognostic value of the β_2m/proliferative fraction is independent of other known prognostic factors.

New prognostic factors

The study of the membrane phenotype of the myeloma cell can provide information about the level of differentiation of the cell and may indicate how it will behave and therefore be prognostically relevant. An additional aim of such an approach is to consider the functional role of membrane markers as adhesion molecules or as signalling molecules and how they affect the behaviour of the tumour cells [26,27].

There is a range of phenotypic characteristics in myeloma, the clinical significance of which is not yet clear. Bone marrow plasma cells can be defined by a high expression of CD38 and Syndecan-1. Normal plasma cells, with a phenotype of CD19+ CD56–, can be distinguished from their myelomatous counterparts which, in the majority of cases, show higher levels of expression of CD56 and a lack of CD19 expression. At presentation approximately 70% of cases have been found to have CD19– CD56+ cells, 25% CD19– CD56– disease and the remainder have CD19+ CD56+ (Fig. 14.2).

The data in the literature are conflicting, and much of this stems from poor methodology. By using methods to adequately define the myeloma cells and then looking at their cell surface, it is now generally accepted that features of pre-B cells such as CD10 are not seen. Furthermore, CD34 is not present on the surface of the myeloma cell, which implies that purging strategies based on positive selection of CD34 stem cells would be appropriate in myeloma.

Cell adhesion molecules

Adhesion molecules expressed on the myeloma cell surface have important interactions with the bone marrow microenvironment and the pattern of their expression may alter the growth and migration pattern of these abnormal plasma cells [28]. Various studies have documented the expression of adhesion molecules on the cell surface. A high expression of CD44, CD29, CD49d(VLA-4) and CD54 have been reported in normal and myelomatous plasma cells, whereas CD56 (NCAM) and CD58 (LFA-3) are expressed on malignant plasma cells rather than on normal plasma cells.

CD56 is an isoform of the neural cell adhesion molecule (NCAM) which, in the haemopoetic system, is expressed on natural killer (NK) cells. In cases where extramedullary disease is a feature, the myeloma cells have been found to lack CD56 expression, which is consistent with the function of CD56 as an adhesion molecule [29]. At relapse the expression of CD56 by myelomatous plasma cells is significantly lower than at presentation.

CD44 appears to be a multifunctional molecule, with involvement in lymphocyte activation and homing, tumour dissemination and the inflammatory reaction. The heterogeneity of function is thought to be a result of the enormous number of isoforms of the molecule, derived from the same gene. In mice, the growth of plasmacytomas has been shown to be dependent on the physical contact of CD44 with the stromal cell feeder layers. In humans, the blockage of this contact leads to inhibited adhesion of cells to the stromal layer and the inhibition of the triggering of IL-6 [30]. CD44 variant isoforms have been detected in myeloma and, in some studies, the presence of larger isoforms is correlated with unfavourable clinical features. Other studies have shown that expression during the different clinical stages shows no significant difference.

It has been suggested that there are two distinct populations of myelomatous plasma cells at different stages of maturation which can be separated on the basis of VLA-5 (CD49e) expression. Clinical response post induction treatment has been related to the percentage of immature myeloma cells (VLA-5–) present, with a significant decrease being noted in the more responsive cases, stable numbers in the nonresponders and a dramatic increase in those cases with progressive disease [31]. The proportion of immature VLA-5– plasma cells at diagnosis was not found, however, to predict the clinical response or prognosis.

Another important set of interactions involves the contact molecules within the germinal centre. CD40 is expressed on normal plasma cells with variable expression on myelomatous plasma cells. In one study all plasma cells from normals expressed CD40 compared to only two-thirds of the myeloma cases, with a high expression in progressive disease [32]. In the presence of IL-4 and IL-10, it has been shown that activation of CD40 can initiate B-cell growth and differentiation. Cross-linking of CD40 has been shown to upregulate the expression of the *BCL2* gene with subsequent rescue from apoptosis. On cross-linking of malignant plasma cells there is proliferation with an autocrine secretion of IL-6. Other adhesion molecules present on the plasma cells, such as VCAM-1, VLA4, CD24 and LFA1, also appear capable of inducing IL-6 production [33].

Cell signalling molecules

A major pathway that is deregulated in malignancy involves the transmission of signals, from the extracellular environment, which regulate cell growth. Such a cell surface marker, which may have prognostic importance in myeloma, is CD20 (which is coexpressed with CD19). In a study of 112 patients, San Miguel *et al.* [34] found an increased incidence of CD19 and CD20 in patients with stage III myeloma. The cases which expressed CD20 had a median survival of 13 months, compared to 25 months for those with CD20– disease ($P = 0.05$). It has been proposed that this difference in behaviour reflects the level of differentiation of plasma cells expressing CD20.

CD117 (C-Kit) is a cell membrane tyrosine kinase receptor and its expression appears to be restricted to myelomatous plasma cells. Antigen expression was found in 18 of 56 untreated myeloma patients, with the range of expression from 75 to 100%. No difference in clinical or haematological variables, however, was observed between positive and negative cases. Both groups showed a similar response to chemotherapy and a similar survival, although follow-up was short [35].

Circulating myelomatous plasma cells

There has been much debate about the presence of circulating cells belonging to the myeloma clone. A consensus view has now begun to emerge. Evidence of clonally related cells within the B-cell compartment can be found using ASO-PCR. These cells are few, of the order of 10% of the total B cells present, and may represent a stage in the evolution of myeloma. It is now generally believed that these cells do not constitute a reservoir of 'stem cells' which continually differentiate and 'feed' the bone marrow myeloma plasma cell population. The most likely proliferative cells against which therapy should be directed are those close to the level of differentiation of a bone marrow plasma cell. Cells with a phenotype identical to these can also be found in the peripheral blood in up to 75% of patients at presentation. The absolute number of these cells varies with disease status in individual patients, with a decrease in patients responding to treatment and a persistent increase in those with refractory disease; stable levels are usual in those who have reached plateau and marked increases are seen at relapse [26]. In a study of 57 patients with newly diagnosed smouldering multiple myeloma, Witzig *et al.* [36] estimated the absolute numbers of circulating plasma cells at presentation and at 6 and 12 months. Disease progression was seen in 16 out of 57 patients during this time and, of these, 63% had abnormal circulating cells, in contrast to only 10% of the patients who had stable disease. The same group subsequently studied 254 newly diagnosed myeloma patients and found the percentage of circulating plasma cells at diagnosis to be an independent prognostic variable. Cases with more than

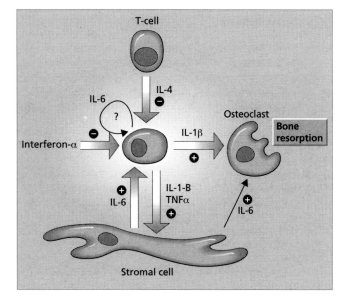

Fig. 14.3 Cytokine networks in myeloma. The interaction of the myeloma cells within their local environment is very important in the pathogenesis of myeloma. IL-6 is central to the growth of the myeloma clone, and there is evidence for both autocrine and paracrine ranks of stimulation. A number of cytokines exert negative influences on the myeloma clone and IFNα has been used therapeutically. Inhibition of other growth-promoting cytokines also has the potential to be useful therapeutically. TNF = tumour necrosis factor.

4% circulating cells had a median survival of 2.4 years, compared to 4.4 years in those cases less than 4% [37].

Cytokine networks as prognostic factors

IL-6 is a multifunctional cytokine originally identified as a B-cell differentiation factor essential for final differentiation of B cells into antibody-producing cells. IL-6 is thought to be central to the growth of the myeloma clone. Prolonging the duration of minimal residual disease states is a major challenge for current therapeutic approaches. Interferon has been used in several recent trials and appears to have a moderate benefit in prolonging the plateau phase. This result suggests that other cytokines might be targets for this approach and IL-6 seems the most obvious to pursue initially (Fig. 14.3).

IL-6 is a multifunctional cytokine originally identified as a B-cell differentiation factor, which induces the final differentiation of B cells into antibody-producing cells. The evidence for IL-6 being a major growth factor in myeloma cells has come from a number of sources. The majority of evidence favours the production of IL-6 by a paracrine mechanism from accessory cells in the bone marrow, rather than by an autocrine loop [1]. Both *in vitro* and *in vivo* studies have shown that by interfering with the IL-6 pathway by the use of anti IL-6 and anti-IL-6 receptor antibodies, the growth of myeloma cells can be inhibited, suggesting a potential therapeutic use [38].

The action of IL-6 is dependent on a 80-kDa membrane-bound specific receptor, IL-6-R, and a transmembrane signal transducer, gp130. A soluble receptor molecule (sIL-6-R) can also mediate the binding of IL-6 to gp130 and hence a signal transduction, without requiring the membrane-bound IL-6 receptor. Soluble IL-6-R and membrane-bound IL-6-R have a similar affinity for IL-6. A number of studies have successfully correlated serum IL-6 and sIL-6 receptor levels with disease activity and survival [39,40].

There is evidence that increased IL-6 is associated with a poor outcome. Bataille *et al.* [2] measured IL-6 levels with a bioassay in 131 patients with plasma cell dyscrasias and showed that levels were related to disease activity. Only 3% of patients with MGUS had elevated levels, 35% of patients with myeloma at presentation and 60% with end-stage disease. Ludwig *et al.* [41] showed disease survival also correlated with IL-6 levels, with 50% of the patients with a level below 7 pg/ml being alive at 53.7 months, compared to a median of only 2.7 months in the patients with higher levels.

sIL-6 receptor levels have also been found to correlate with poor prognosis. Kyrtsonis *et al.* [39] measured levels with an ELISA technique in patients at diagnosis and throughout the course of their disease. Lower levels were seen in patients who responded to treatment compared to those with resistant disease. Using a similar technique, Pulkki *et al.* [40] studied 207 newly diagnosed patients: 47% had elevated levels and the values were significantly higher in patients who died within 3 years. This group also measured IL-6 and β_2m levels, and found that when the patients were stratified into groups, those with increased IL-6 and sIL-6-R levels had a shorter survival than those with normal levels. Interestingly, sIL-6-R levels appeared to be stable throughout the disease and did not correlate with IL-6 levels, which fluctuated with disease activity. This raises concerns about how accurately serum levels reflect activity in the stromal microenvironment.

Another factor that is of relevance to the activity of stimulators of the IL-6 pathway is the concentration of inhibitors of the pathway, in particular sgp130. The gp130 receptor also exists in a soluble nonmembrane-bound form in the plasma, and high levels of this may neutralize the growth-promoting effects of IL-6/sIL-6-R complexes. Pelliniemi *et al.* [42] have published data showing that although sgp130 levels do not correlate with survival, the ratio of sIL-6-R/sgp130 is a prognostic indicator. The interactions of IL-6, its membrane and soluble receptors, with the soluble and membrane-bound signal transducing gp130, is shown in Fig. 14.4.

Among its other functions, IL-6 is a pleotropic cytokine which induces the synthesis of acute-phase reactants in the liver (C-reactive protein, alpha-1-antitrypsin and thymidine kinase). Levels of these have been measured as a surrogate for IL-6 and evaluated for their prognostic role [43,44]. There are a number of problems with these tests, including a poor correlation with disease activity and worries about the accuracy with which they reflect events in the marrow. No clear-cut

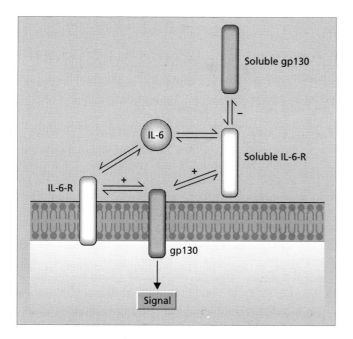

Fig. 14.4 Interactions of IL-6, its membrane and soluble receptors, with the soluble and membrane-bound signal transducing gp130.

answer has emerged and it seems more logical to look at the primary cytokines rather than surrogates.

Genetic abnormalities as prognostic factors

Cytogenetic changes. The search for biologically relevant prognostic variables in many tumour systems, in particular the acute leukaemias and lymphomas, has followed a classic pattern whereby recurrent cytogenetic abnormalities have been identified. These have then been subject to molecular genetic analysis, which has led to the isolation and characterization of genes important in the disease process. This has been difficult in myeloma because of the low proliferation rate of the tumour cells and, consequently, lack of analysable metaphases. Newer techniques utilizing metaphase and interphase cells have shown a diverse group of cytogenetic abnormalities with a mixture of both numerical and structural changes: an abnormal karyotype can be demonstrated in about 50% of myeloma patients. However, by utilizing FISH (fluorescent *in situ* hybridization), abnormalities can be detected in up to 90% of patients [45]. Numerous studies have demonstrated greater cytogenetic abnormalities later in the disease process, suggesting that this could be used prognostically [46].

Numerical chromosomal abnormalities are common, with 61–66% of patients showing hyperdiploidy, 9–20% pseudodiploidy and 10–30% hypodiploidy. Recent data suggests that patients with hyperdiploidy may have a survival advantage [47]. In one study 156 newly diagnosed cases were analysed for DNA content using flow cytometry, 58% showed aneuploidy, with 56% being hyperdiploid and 2% hypodiploid. Those with hyperdiploidy had a median survival of 46 months compared to 21 months in the diploid group [48]. Unfortunately there were only three patients detected with hypodiploidy in this study and hence no comments could be made about the prognostic significance of this.

Structural abnormalities, including deletions and translocations, are also well described, with chromosomes 1, 6, 14, 16 and 19 being most commonly affected [49]. There is a suggestion that patients with partial or complete deletions of chromosome 13q or 11q have an unfavourable karyotype, with a median survival of 11 and 12 months respectively [50].

14q+ and outcome in myeloma. It has been suggested that 14q+ is associated with a poor prognosis, because it is seen mainly in plasma cell leukaemia and stage III disease [45,51,52]. Abnormalities of 14, where a variety of different chromosomal partners are involved in translocation events, are clearly identifiable cytogenetic abnormalities in myeloma. These events are common, with a reported frequency of 10–40%. A number of translocations involving this area have been characterized in myeloma cell lines and genes important in other lymphoid malignancies, such as *BCL1* and *BCL2*, have been identified [53]. The frequency of the dysregulation of such genes in clinical material is unknown. The value of these studies in myeloma has been the realization that the translocations involve the heavy-chain switch region. An elegant cloning strategy, using a Southern blot approach, has meant that cases with an aberrantly rearranged switch region can be identified. Using the switch region as a probe, dysregulated genes have been identified. The noteworthy feature is that a number of genes have been found to be dysregulated rather than a single consistent abnormality.

Tumour suppressor genes and oncogenes as prognostic markers. A number of molecular abnormalities have been described in other lymphoid tumours and have been shown to have important prognostic relevance. There are some data relating to the significance of these in myeloma.

The p53 tumour suppressor gene. The reports of a mutation rate of 2–4% are in accordance with our own studies showing a rate of 3.2% using a polymerase chain reaction – single-stranded conformational polymorphisms (PCR-SSCP) method [49]. Preudhomme *et al.* studied 37 cases and found only one example of a point mutation leading to an amino acid change in the *p53* gene [54]. In cases with end-stage disease and plasma cell leukaemia, the frequency apparently increases appreciably, although this higher frequency may be a reflection of studying myeloma cell lines that have been immortalized *in vitro*. Interestingly when serial samples were examined from patients who had *p53* mutations at the terminal stages of their disease, there was no evidence of these mutations in the earlier samples obtained in plateau phase [55], suggesting a multistep process, with *p53* mutation as a late event in tumour progression. It would seem that *p53* mutations are a rare event in myeloma and are of little use as a prognostic tool, as they appear to be confined to patients with the terminal and leukaemic stages of the disease which are easily identified clinically.

The retinoblastoma tumour suppressor gene. The retinoblastoma (RB) gene codes for a phosphoprotein which is associated with DNA-binding activity and cell proliferation. It appears to have a role in the transcriptional expression of IL-6, and hence inactivation may lead to an increase in IL-6 and growth stimulation. Loss or inactivation of this gene is known to occur by point mutation, gross rearrangement, large area intragenic deletion and complete deletion of the gene. Lack of expression in myeloma may partly be a reflection of the fact that the protein is only detectable in dividing cells [56]. In those cases in which the protein is detected, between 10 and 90% of clonal plasma cells show its expression. DNA rearrangements and deletions appear to be infrequent and studies to define the role of RB in the pathogenesis of myeloma (which would require exhaustive screening of cases for the mutation) have not yet been carried out.

The RAS oncogene. Mutations of the N- and K-*RAS* gene have been seen in up to 47% of cases of myeloma, with the incidence rising to 67% in end-stage disease [57]. Corradini *et al.* looked at the frequency of mutations within the various plasma cell dyscrasia groups. Within the MGUS group 128 cases were analysed, but there was no evidence of mutation. They found 9% of cases of myelomatosis had mutations, but these were seen only in patients with stage III disease. The prevalence of mutation increased markedly in patients with plasma cell leukaemia, where 30% of cases had an identifiable mutation. The frequency of expression also appears to be increased in patients undergoing treatment compared with the findings at diagnosis [58].

The BCL2 gene and resistance to apoptosis. The BCL2 protooncogene has a role in inhibiting apoptopic programmed cell death and hence chemoresistance may be related to increased expression of the BCL2 protein. Studies have shown conflicting results concerning BCL2 expression in chemosensitive and chemoresistant myeloma cell lines. However, overexpression of BCL2 appears to correlate with resistance to interferon [59]. In a group of 40 patients treated with interferon, eight of nine patients who responded had weak or no BCL2 expression. Within the nonresponder group, 16 had strong expression and 14 had weak expression. Clinical studies have shown that protein expression does not appear to be related to a short survival. In a small study of patients who were alive 5 years from diagnosis, there was a tendency towards a higher expression in comparison with a comparative

group who had refractory myeloma and died within a year of diagnosis [60].

Treatment

Conventional chemotherapy

The modern era of treatment of myelomatosis was ushered in with the introduction of the alkylating agents, cyclophosphamide and melphalan, in the early 1960s. Melphalan, which is *p*-di-(2-chloroethyl) amino-L-phenylalanine has, in combination with prednisone/prednisolone, become the standard treatment against which others are tested. After early studies demonstrated cumulative myelotoxicity with continuously administered melphalan [61], intermittent or pulsed treatment became the norm — usually 10 mg daily for 7 days every 4–6 weeks. Although no in-depth studies on the role of corticosteroids or of optimum dose were carried out at the time, prednisone or prednisolone were considered to enhance the response to treatment by several groups [62–65]. However, in the early Medical Research Council (MRC) myelomatosis therapy trials, initiated in 1964, no significant differences in overall survival between patients treated with melphalan or oral cyclophosphamide or melphalan plus prednisolone were observed [66–68].

Although some improvements in supportive care were also being introduced, these developments in chemotherapy were the major reason for the improvement in median survival from, typically, less than 1 year previously, to over 2 years. Using objective response criteria, about half of the patients would respond, with most of these reaching plateau [66–70]. Not surprisingly there were attempts to develop combination regimens. Of particular importance was the report by Alberts and colleagues [71], that the combination of an anthracycline (doxorubicin, Adriamycin) and a nitrosourea (carmustine, BCNU) was active and effective in previously treated patients. Several combination regimens also incorporated the vinca alkaloid, vincristine, with apparent benefit in some studies [72–75], although in a large MRC trial in which vincristine was the single randomized variable, no survival gain was shown [76].

There have been many trials in which melphalan, usually in combination with prednisone/prednisolone (MP), has been tested against combinations, incorporating vincristine, BCNU and an anthracycline. A meta-analysis of trials involving nearly 4000 patients suggested no consistent benefit for combination chemotherapy when compared with melphalan plus prednisone/prednisolone [77], although the data available on anthracycline-containing regimens were limited. In the more recent Myeloma Trialists Collaborative Group overview of worldwide randomized trials, based on individual patient data on nearly 4930 patients and supplementary published data on a further 1703 patients (a total of 27 trials), no significant difference in mortality between the two basic approaches was

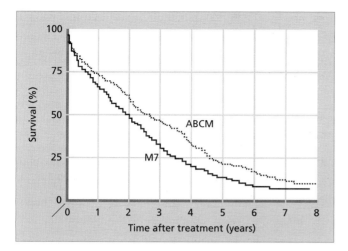

Fig. 14.5 Survival from entry in the MRC Myeloma V Trial. Analysis of 314 patients allocated to ABCM (Adriamycin, BCNU, cyclophosphamide, melphalan) and 316 allocated to M7 (melphalan) ($\chi^2 = 13.2$, $P = 0.0003$).

found [78], either overall or within any subgroup. In both studies there is at least the suggestion that anthracycline-containing regimens may be more effective, although to confirm this would require additional data from trials designed to address this specific issue. In the MRC Myeloma V Trial of ABCM (Adriamycin, BCNU, cyclophosphamide, melphalan), vs melphalan alone, plateau was achieved in 61% of patients given ABCM compared with 49% of those given melphalan alone. Survival of the 314 patients given ABCM was also significantly longer than that of the 316 patients given intermittent melphalan [79] (Fig. 14.5). A cross-trial comparison of VMCP/VBAP (vincristine, melphalan, cyclophosphamide, prednisolone/vincristine, cyclophosphamide, BCNU, prednisolone), as adopted in the Southwest Oncology Group (SWOG) studies, and ABCM suggested that these approaches were likely to be of comparable effectiveness [80].

Infusional chemotherapy

The next step in the evolution of chemotherapeutic approaches stemmed from the investigation of alternative combinations, dose schedules and modes of administration in patients considered resistant to first-line treatment or in relapse. Particularly high response rates were reported with VAD, the combination of vincristine and doxorubicin (Adriamycin), given by 4-day infusion with intermediate dose dexamethasone [81]. Response rates as high as 84% were reported in previously untreated patients [82]. Although the agents incorporated were also included in other 'standard' regimens, the mode of delivery of the doxorubicin and vincristine and the dose of corticosteroid in VAD was appreciably different. Corticosteroids had been given to patients with myeloma for many years and although the relative importance of their contribution had been disputed, the efficacy of higher

doses in refractory disease was reported as long ago as 1967 [83]. Dexamethasone appeared to be the key agent in VAD; it was capable of producing similar responses when given as a single agent to those achieved with VAD—of the order of 27% in patients with primary treatment failure [84], although somewhat less effective in relapsed disease [84], or as initial first-line treatment [85]. Infusional therapy seemed to be particularly appropriate given the low growth fraction of myeloma cells, and the response data on VAD suggested that this regimen could achieve greater cytoreduction and more rapid responses than previously standard chemotherapy [22]. A comparable regimen, VAMP (in which methylprednisolone is substituted for dexamethasone) [86], was further modified by the addition of pulses of intravenous cyclophosphamide in C-VAMP [87,88]. This seemed to further increase response rates, in particular the incidence of complete remission when assessed conventionally.

Melphalan dose escalation

The escalation of the dose of melphalan was pioneered by McElwain & Powles [89]. Doses at the level of 140 mg/m² could achieve a high response rate with considerable reduction in tumour load, with 'complete responses' being reported in about 30% of patients below the age of 60 [90]. Such treatment had its limitations because of toxicity and it became clear that long remissions were not achieved. However, the scene was set for yet more intensive, myeloablative therapy in conjunction with both autologous and allogeneic bone marrow transplantation and, subsequently, peripheral blood stem cell support. Adoption of autologous bone marrow transplantation allowed an increase in the dose of melphalan to 200 mg/m². Preceded by induction chemotherapy with VAMP, this resulted in a complete remission (CR) rate of 50% [91]. In comparable studies this order of response was confirmed [92–95].

The initial follow-up on patients given intensive chemotherapy with supporting autograft, as exemplified by the studies at the Royal Marsden Hospital, was disappointing, as these more complete responses did not lead to prolonged remission or survival. However, on the basis of an assumption that remission might be maintained by the use of interferon alpha (IFNα), patients treated later in the Marsden programme went on to receive IFNα following the recovery of blood counts after the autograft. There is evidence that this approach will result in the prolongation of remission, disease-free survival and overall survival [96,97]. A larger trial has been carried out by the Intergroupe Français du Myelome (IFM), in which patients under the age of 65 with previously untreated myelomatosis were randomized to receive either conventional combination chemotherapy or a regimen including melphalan at 140 mg/m² with total body irradiation (TBI), supported by autologous bone marrow collected after two cycles of initial conventional induction chemotherapy. Patients in both arms received maintenance IFNα. The findings, based on an entry of

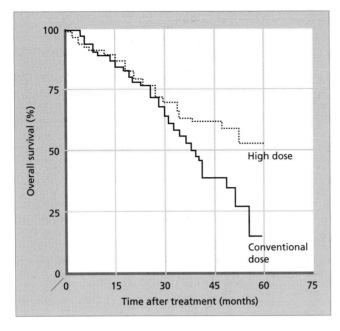

Fig. 14.6 Treatment with IFNα: overall survival according to treatment group. The estimated rate of survival at 5 years was 52% in the high-dose group and 12% in the conventional-dose group (*P* = 0.03). [98].

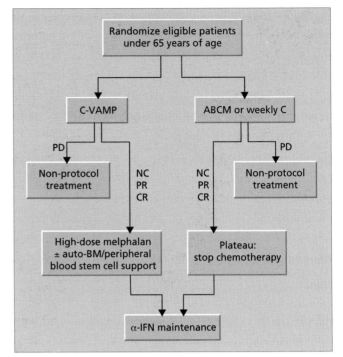

Fig. 14.7 Flow diagram of the MRC Myeloma VII Trial. ABCM = Adriamycin, BCNU, cyclophosphamide, melphalan; BM = bone marrow; C = cyclophosphamide; CR = complete response; C-VAMP = cyclophosphamide, vincristine, Adriamycin, methylprednisolone; IFNα = interferon alpha; NC = no change; PD = progressive disease; PR = partial remission.

200 randomized patients (of which 70 were autografted) and analysis on intention to treat, suggested an advantage for the intensive arm in terms of response rate, duration of response and survival (Fig. 14.6) [98]. In a complementary study, the role of 'up-front' vs delayed autografting (i.e. after disease progression) was investigated. No significant difference in survival between the two arms of the study was found. Several trials designed to confirm the benefit of intensive treatment for myeloma in younger patients (usually taken as less than 65 years of age) are in progress. The current MRC Myeloma VII Trial is illustrated in Fig. 14.7 by a flow diagram.

Exploration of the advantages of yet further intensification of treatment is illustrated by the 'total therapy' of Barlogie *et al.*, which involves multiple courses of intensive chemotherapy supported with autologous stem cells [99]. There is a suggestion that the complete remission rate increases as a result of this approach, but these studies were not randomized and there is no clear-cut evidence of a survival benefit. The IFM Group have pursued such a concept in a randomized trial (IFM 94), and have recently reported the results in an abstract. The study directly randomized 400 patients to either a single autograft, with melphalan 140 mg/m² plus TBI, or a double procedure, initially with melphalan 140 mg/m² alone and subsequently with melphalan and TBI, as in the other procedure. The preliminary analysis of this trial showed no difference in survival between the two procedures, suggesting that this degree of intensification probably confers no advantage (J.L. Harrousseau, personal communication). An interesting

observation, based on the above data, is that the number of complete responses in each arm was the same, suggesting that a double autograft delivered in this way does not increase the response rate, although this had been previously suggested.

Autologous stem cell support

With the introduction of intensive treatment the use of autologous stem cell support became necessary, both to maximize the doses of chemotherapy used and to prevent treatment-related deaths. This raised a number of issues in relation to the source of the cells used, i.e. bone marrow vs peripheral blood. It soon became clear that it was possible to obtain good quality peripheral blood stem cells from patients treated with VAD/VAMP regimens, and that these cells resulted in more rapid engraftment than cells obtained directly from the bone marrow — on average by day 14 after reinfusion of stem cells. Using this approach, transplant-related mortality is less than 1%, although it is unclear whether the use of peripheral blood stem cells has improved survival because of the lack of direct comparisons. Clearly both bone marrow and peripheral blood stem cells can be contaminated with myeloma cells. Using very sensitive PCR oligospecific probes, evidence of contamination by cells belonging to the myeloma clone is present in almost 100% of peripheral blood stem cell harvests. The level of contamination is generally low if the procedure is carried out when the patient is in remission following VAD/VAMP. In the majority of cases (70%), the contamination is less than one tumour cell in 10^{3-4} normal cells. In the remainder of cases, it is present at around this level. It is important to know whether these cells are clonogenic and are capable of leading to disease relapse. This is a difficult question to address, but sensitive immunophenotypic tests have suggested that these cells have a similar phenotype to myelomatous plasma cells from the bone marrow but express lower levels of syndecan-1.

Purging and autologous transplantation

Clonogenic cells reinfused with the stem cells may contribute to relapse, and it is possible, by either selecting for stem cells expressing the CD34 antigen alone or by combining this with a negative selection for myeloma cells, to achieve between 3 and 5 log depletion of these cells. In attempting to understand whether this is worthwhile clinically, a number of theoretical concepts have to be considered. For purging to be successful, there must be no tumour left in the patient despite its presence in the graft. If there is residual tumour in the patient even though none in the graft, or if there is residual tumour in both the patient and the graft, then it cannot be effective. (Table 14.6).

It is already apparent that purging, if it works at all, will only be effective in a minority of cases, and to show that purging is effective in improving patient outcome will require huge studies. Experience with syngeneic transplants (where there is no possibility of any contaminating tumour cells) has suggested that a plateau of survival is not achieved. This suggests that before embarking on extensive studies of purging, it is important to develop better methods of eradicating the myeloma cells left in the patient.

Allogeneic bone marrow transplantation

Against the background of potential cure in other haematological malignancies, particularly the acute leukaemias and chronic granulocytic leukaemia, allogeneic bone marrow

transplantation has been carried out in conjunction with myeloablative conditioning therapy in patients with myeloma, in the hope of achieving similar results. The early reports of small numbers of patients treated in this way indicated that prolonged remissions could be achieved [100–102]. Data on allogeneic bone marrow transplants are systematically collected through the European Group for Bone Marrow Transplantation (EBMT) [103] and the International Bone Marrow Transplant Registry (IBMTR) [104], with some overlap. With the addition of the Seattle group transplants, a reasonable estimate of the total number of patients with myeloma allografted would be 500–600 patients. The 10-year (1983–93) EBMT analysis provided some basic information [103,105]. Patients up to 59 (median 43) years of age were transplanted; 44% of all patients were considered to have entered CR. The stage at original diagnosis, remission status, preconditioning and the extent of previous treatment, together with the serum β_2m level, were important prognostic factors: males and patients with IgG myeloma fared less well. The overall actuarial survival was 32% at 4 years, 25% at 7 years. The Seattle group using Bu–Cy (busulphan, cyclophosphamide) conditioning reported comparable results [106,107]. No clear message about a superior conditioning regimen has emerged, although cyclophosphamide plus TBI is the most frequently adopted. Again there is no data to suggest that T-cell depletion is either advantageous or disadvantageous.

Follow-up of these patients has suggested that, even if they are in complete remission as conventionally assessed, there may be residual clonal myeloma cells detectable by PCR techniques [108]. However, we have observed that some long-term survivors after allogeneic BMT are negative, even using very sensitive polymerase chain reaction (PCR) tests, suggesting that all the disease has been eradicated, possibly by a graft vs myeloma effect. The high incidence of transplant-related mortality and morbidity has tended to inhibit the more widespread adoption of allogeneic BMT in myeloma. The assumption that this mode of treatment is currently the most likely to eradicate the myeloma cells, and the possibility of a significant graft vs myeloma effect, will encourage its further consideration, particularly if immunization, immunomodulation and manipulation of cytokine networks can be used to enhance and maintain the clearance of myeloma cells.

Quality of life assessment

One important aspect of this move towards intensification of treatment is a possible enhancement of quality of life (QOL), resulting from a more effective reduction in tumour load [109]. This has yet to be confirmed systematically. The EORTC QLQ-C30, a general multidimensional cancer-specific questionnaire, appears to be a reliable and valid instrument for assessing QOL [110]. A version of this, incorporating 13 myeloma-specific questions, is the basis of an additional study that is linked to the MRC Myeloma VII Trial.

Table 14.6 Effect of purging depending on the level of residual disease in both the patient and the harvest.

Purging effect	No	No	No	Yes
Residual disease in patient	+	+	–	–
Residual disease in harvest	+	–	–	+

Interferon alpha

In the search for more effective treatment of myeloma, 'biological treatment' was investigated, in particular the activity of human leucocyte alpha interferons (IFNα). Responses in previously untreated patients were reported by Mellstedt *et al.* as early as 1979 [111]. Subsequent studies suggested a dose–response relationship, but also indicated that the higher dose regimens would not be widely applicable because of unacceptable side effects [112]. In the limited number of trials of IFNα as a single agent in induction therapy, response rates were not very different from those seen with either melphalan plus prednisone (MP) or four drug combinations [113–116]. Incorporation of IFNα into various combinations followed, encouraged by *in vitro* studies which suggested that IFNα could enhance the cytotoxic effects of melphalan and corticosteroids [116–123]. Differences in doses and schedules of administration make it difficult to draw any firm conclusions, and the results of the clinical trials carried out have been conflicting. In one large trial, statistically significant prolongation of survival for patients with IgA and Bence Jones myeloma was shown in those who received IFNα, together with an increased response rate for Durie–Salmon stage II patients [121]. In another randomized trial in which patients received either VMCP or VMCP plus IFNα2b in induction, progression-free survival was significantly prolonged in the patients receiving IFNα [120]. However, the value of IFNα as part of induction therapy has yet to be clearly established.

The use of IFNα as maintenance therapy, which was originally stimulated by the findings of Mandelli *et al.* [124], has attracted considerable interest. In a study in 101 patients randomized to observation or IFNα maintenance following a year of conventional chemotherapy, the patients who had shown an objective response to induction therapy and gone on to receive maintenance therapy had longer remissions and a significant prolongation of survival. In a trial carried out by the Myeloma Group of Central Sweden involving 120 patients, there was evidence of prolongation of remission but not of overall survival in patients given IFNα [125]. Data stemming from the series of worldwide trials which followed were conflicting, with some studies finding no benefit from the addition of IFNα [119,126,127], others showing a significantly increased duration of responses and of overall survival [122,128].

There is now an accumulated experience which lends itself to meta-analysis or more detailed overview with compilation of the original data sets. This work is underway. It now seems likely that the benefit from IFNα as maintenance therapy will be significant, but not greatly so, and that this approach should be regarded as simply one important step towards a more sophisticated strategy aimed at decreasing the risk and rate of disease relapse. The use of IFNα following the more intensive treatments [95–97] which achieve states of minimal residual disease may be particularly appropriate, although not easy to substantiate.

Drug resistance and its potential for manipulation in myeloma

As in other lymphoproliferative diseases, the development of drug resistance is an important cause of treatment failure. Although there are probably many underlying factors, one mechanism modulated by the multidrug resistance gene *MDR-1* has been clearly delineated [129,130]. *MDR-1* is associated with increased expression of a membrane glycoprotein (p-170), which decreases intracellular accumulation of cytotoxic agents (notably vinca alkaloids and anthracyclines) via an energy-dependent efflux mechanism.

MDR negativity is usually found at diagnosis in myeloma. There is a progressive increase in MDR expression with response to chemotherapeutic agents, especially vincristine and dexorubicin [3]. Attempts to reverse MDR-related resistance with drugs such as verapamil have tended to be associated with unacceptable toxicities. Cyclosporin-A has been shown to reverse the resistance to VAD in 47% of VAD-refractory patients expressing MDR [131]. Again, toxicity would preclude this as an acceptable routine approach in practice. The cyclosporin analogue PSC-833 appears to be a more effective inhibitor of MDR than cyclosporin-A, and it is less toxic, being neither significantly immunosuppressive nor nephrotoxic. Early studies using this agent [132] have encouraged the initiation of large-scale trials, and the results will be helpful in determining the role of PSC 833 in cases of relapsed myeloma.

Response criteria and definitions

In order to compare the results of the different trials it is important to have standardized response criteria. The definition of response to treatment in myeloma have been numerous and, therefore, potentially more confusing than in other lymphoproliferative diseases. There are several terms which, in effect, describe degrees of partial remission. The paraprotein level, which can be measured in the majority of patients, forms the basis of these definitions, of which 'objective response' may be regarded as the template (Tables 14.7–14.10).

A valuable concept, which emerged as a result of the closer investigation of tumour regression following treatment, was that of plateau. This was characterized, by estimations of tumour load, cell growth and cell death, as a cytokinetically quiescent state associated with a low labelling index and low levels of other markers of proliferation such as serum thymidine kinase (STK) [25,133–136]. In contrast to the kinetically active induction and relapse phase, chemotherapy is likely to be ineffective and unnecessary during plateau. Entry into plateau and its duration, rather than tumour response per se,

Table 14.7 Objective response (OR).

Pretreatment M-protein in:	M-protein must decrease to or be:		24-hour urine excretion of M-protein must decrease to or be:
Serum + urine	≤50% pretreatment level	+	≤50% pretreatment amount
Serum only	≤50% pretreatment level	+	≤150 mg
Urine only	<1.0 g/dl	+	≤10% pretreatment amount

and	No new bone lesions
	No increase in existing lytic lesions
	No new plasmacytomas
	No increase in any existing plasmacytomas
	No recurrence or persistence of hypercalcaemia

Table 14.8 Complete response (CR).

Patients with OR (Table 14.7) who also have complete disappearance of M-protein **and** no evidence of myeloma in the bone marrow (≤3% plasma cells) **and** no evidence of progression of disease by other parameters

Table 14.9 Near complete response (NCR)/partial remission.

Near complete response
Patients with OR (Table 14.7) meeting CR (Table 14.8) criteria except for one of the following:
  lacking repeat bone marrow
  3–6% bone marrow plasma cells remaining
or:
  <3% plasma cells remaining on bone marrow differential count but with marrow aspirate/trephine still showing clear evidence of myeloma (sheets or clusters of malignant plasma cells)

Partial remission
Patients meeting OR criteria but not CR or NCR criteria

Table 14.10 Relapse/progression (PD).

Two of the following criteria:
  increase in serum M-protein (≥50%)
  increase in urine M-protein (≥50%)
  increase in soft tissue plasmacytomas (≥50%, measured)
  Appearance of new lytic lesions or increase in size of existing bone lesions by ≥50%
or:
  ≥50% increase in serum/urine M-protein
plus
  hypercalcaemia
  anaemia
  increase in bone marrow plasma cells by >50%
  generalized bone pain

Table 14.11 Plateau phase: definition adopted in the MRC Myeloma Trials.

Plateau is reached when all of the following three criteria are satisfied:
a. Patient is asymptomatic or has minimal symptoms attributable to active myelomatosis
b. Patient's haemoglobin is stable without requirement for transfusion
c. Patient's serum paraprotein, urinary light-chain output and serum β_2m levels have become stable, as assessed by two samples taken at an interval of 3 months

may be regarded as the main determinant of prognosis. Until the introduction of more effective cytoreductive treatment resulted in an appreciable increase in the number of patients fulfilling the criteria for complete remission (as conventionally assessed), plateau status could be reasonably adopted as an end-point. In the MRC trials, plateau was considered to have been reached when patients were symptomatic or had minimal symptoms attributable to myeloma, did not require blood transfusion and had stable serum paraprotein, urinary light-chain output and serum β_2m levels, as assessed on successive samples at an interval of 3 months (Table 14.11) [11].

With the introduction of high-dose treatment the number of 'complete responses' has increased. Such responses require careful definition. Firstly, it is important to define how the paraprotein is estimated, as there is a difference in sensitivity between standard electrophoresis and immunofixation. Furthermore, it is clear that, of patients obtaining a complete clinical remission, at least 50% will have detectable tumour in bone marrow using a PCR test sensitive to 1 in 10 000 [137]. Even very sensitive tests could be falsely negative because of the patchy nature of the myelomatous marrow involvement and, as the majority of cases eventually relapse, there is bound to be residual disease present.

A consensus IgH PCR has been used by us to monitor disease after both allogeneic and autologous transplantation. This has shown greater numbers of PCR-negative cases after allogeneic BMT than following autograft. This may be a function of either the conditioning used (melphalan vs cyclophosphamide + TBI), which seems unlikely, or it may be a reflection of the contribution of a graft vs myeloma effect in the allogeneic patients. At present the value of such tests to sequentially monitor patients is uncertain. Patients who become PCR positive and remain in remission, as well as those who relapse rapidly following a negative PCR test, have been seen in our own studies. Further investigation of the possible prognostic significance of PCR findings at specific time points post grafting is clearly necessary.

Other problems in patient management

Renal dysfunction and failure

Almost 50% of myeloma patients have some degree of renal impairment at presentation [138]. Although renal failure has generally been regarded to be of adverse prognosis, its incidence is considerably greater than the death rate attributable to it. The great majority of cases are a result of Bence Jones proteinuria or hypercalcaemia, or a combination of the two [139]. Light chains are thought to cause proximal tubular damage through uptake in the endolysosomal system, and to precipitate in the distal tubules with the formation of intra-liminal proteinaceous casts. The chronic secretion of large amounts of Bence Jones proteins does not necessarily result in clinically significant renal impairment [140,141]. However, selective proximal tubular proteinuria is usual and this may persist, even when light-chain output decreases following treatment [142].

Although tubular dysfunction may facilitate the development of renal failure, its precipitation is multifactorial. Difficulties in conserving salt and water, dehydration, hypercalcaemia, proximal tubular acidosis and cast formation may contribute, in various ways, to critical functional changes. Pyogenic infection is one recognizable and relatively common event which can trigger a sequence of changes leading to overt failure. The importance of hydration has been strongly emphasized, based on the experience gained in the MRC myelomatosis trials. It became apparent that although the mechanisms underlying renal dysfunction in myelomatosis were complex, the relatively simple approach of instituting a regimen of high fluid intake (at least 3 l/day) could reverse renal failure in many patients, despite persisting proximal tubular dysfunction and light-chain excretion [143].

In a proportion of patients, only partial recovery of renal function is achieved by vigorous hydration, and some of these patients will require dialysis. Established and nonreversible renal failure requiring continuing frequent dialysis carries a relatively poor prognosis, but some patients can be maintained for prolonged periods of time, usually when the myeloma has responded to treatment and a stable plateau has been achieved. Many patients have been excluded from treatment protocols, particularly the more intensive regimens. In practice, it is often possible to administer chemotherapy with little or no dose modifications, apart from those usually adopted for cytopenias. There is a need for more data in the setting of clinical therapeutic trials. Plasmapheresis as an adjunctive procedure may be helpful as part of the initial treatment approach in acute renal failure, helping to achieve rapid reduction in paraprotein and light-chain levels.

Hypercalcaemia and myeloma-associated bone disease

Hypercalcaemia, reflecting the increased bone resorption in myelomatosis, is an incipient feature of the disease and can become rapidly more severe as a result of coexisting renal dysfunction. This 'vicious circle' is usually compounded by dehydration. The typical clinical features of weakness, nausea, vomiting, thirst, constipation and polyuria progress in the untreated patient, with the development of cardiac arrhythmias, renal failure, increasing encephalopathic features and, ultimately, coma and death.

Vigorous rehydration with saline infusions will rapidly improve the glomerular filtration rate and decrease hypercalcaemia [144]. This is an essential initial aspect of management, although in itself it may prove inadequate because of the degree of bone resorption. Although corticosteroids [145,146], mithramycin [147] and calcitonin [148] have been used to treat and control hypercalcaemia, to date the most effective agents have been the bisphosphonates.

These compounds appear to have a direct effect on osteoclasts, inhibiting function, and an indirect action through the secretion of an inhibitor of osteoclast recruitment by osteoblasts [149]. There is a strong affinity for bone mineral and the skeletal retention is very prolonged. When bisphosphonates are given intravenously in the acute phase they are rapidly effective, and it can be expected that normocalcaemia will be achieved within a few days, particularly if combined with a vigorous rehydration regimen. The duration of effect is variable and depends on the state of the underlying disease; repeated treatment may be necessary. The toxicity of bisphosphonates in this phase is minimal, but it should be noted that renal failure may occasionally be aggravated by rapid infusion [150]. This can be avoided if bisphosphonates given intravenously are diluted in 250–500 ml of saline solution and infused at a rate lower than 200 mg/hour. Given in this way, their use in patients with hypercalcaemia and secondary renal failure usually results in an improvement in renal function.

Bisphosphonates given in this acute phase may also reduce bone pain, and it was this finding which led to the consideration of long-term administration and initiation of therapeutic trials. In the Finnish Myeloma Study [151], patients were randomized to receive oral clodronate (2400 mg/day) or placebo (as well as specific myeloma chemotherapy). In a 2-year period of assessment osteolytic lesions progressed in 24% in the placebo group compared with 12% in the clodronate groups, a significant difference. The trend to fewer vertebral fractures in the clodronate group was not statistically significant. In the largest study to date carried out in conjunction with the MRC Myeloma VI Trial [152], patients were also randomized to receive long-term clodronate (1600 mg/day) or placebo from the time of initial induction chemotherapy.

There was a significant reduction in vertebral fractures in the clodronate group, and those patients also had a lower incidence of pain and better performance status in the long-term assessments. More recently, Berenson *et al.* [153] gave patients with stage III disease, and at least one lytic lesion, either placebo or pamidronate (90 mg) as a 4-weekly infusion for nine cycles, in addition to antimyeloma therapy (first-line or subsequent). The patients given pamidronate had significantly less bone pain, and a reduction in skeletal fractures was recorded in the patients receiving chemotherapy for the first time. Comparable findings have been obtained using parenteral clodronate. The possibility of a survival benefit from long-term bisphosphonate use has been raised, but there are obvious difficulties in separating out the relative contributions of the bisphosphonate and the other treatment given.

While these studies have suggested that treatment with bisphosphonates modifies the bone morbidity associated with myelomatosis, the universal prescription of these agents would represent an appreciable financial burden on health services. The Finnish Group addressed cost–benefit issues and found that length of hospital stay was less in the clodronate-treated patients, although the overall treatment costs were higher in those patients [154]. One approach would be to target patients most at risk of bone changes, but no study to investigate this group has yet been developed. This remains an urgent issue to be addressed.

Supportive care

The immunosuppression associated with myelomatosis, compounded by neutropenia as a result of bone marrow infiltration and/or chemotherapy, results in varying levels of susceptibility to infection [11]. Pyogenic infection is a presenting feature in 10% of myeloma patients, but patients continue to be at risk even when in plateau [155]. Early empirical antibiotic therapy is important and sometimes hospitalization is necessary. Patient education and efficient systems for rapid reassessment should be an integral part of overall management. There is no universally agreed policy for prophylactic measures and the use of immunoglobulins has never been clearly established.

Blood product support may be necessary, as with other lymphoproliferative diseases. Many patients are chronically anaemic and the availability of erythropoietin (rhEPO) has raised the possibility of using this agent to achieve better levels of haemoglobin. The anaemia is often multifactorial, variously reflecting the chronic malignant process with disturbances of cytokine production and function, bone marrow involvement, myelosuppression as a result of myeloma treatment and renal dysfunction. The data, from a series of studies and trials carried out so far, suggest that about 60% of patients with anaemia developing in the course of myeloma will achieve a worthwhile response (increase in haemoglobin level of >2 g/dl), with doses of rhEPO of the order of 500 u/kg/week [156,157]. There is limited evidence about the benefit, although the assumption is that increasing the haemoglobin level will improve the quality of life. Examination of the transfusion requirement would show possible cost-effective benefits [158], and this will obviously be greater if the cost of rhEPO decreases.

The hyperviscosity syndrome (HVS), an occasional complication of IgA or IgG myeloma as a result of polymerization or aggregation of paraprotein, demands prompt intervention. Typical symptoms are mucosal bleeds, purpura, headache, drowsiness and blurring of vision. The finding of vascular congestion with distended veins is an important retinal change which should suggest the diagnosis. Prompt plasmapheresis is required to prevent progressive changes, which may include the aggravation of renal dysfunction.

A wide variety of skeletal and neurological complications may occur during the course of myeloma. A detailed review of their management is outside the scope of this chapter, which is concerned principally with the assessment and treatment of the primary disease process. Spinal cord compression, usually as a result of local extradural or intradural myelomatous

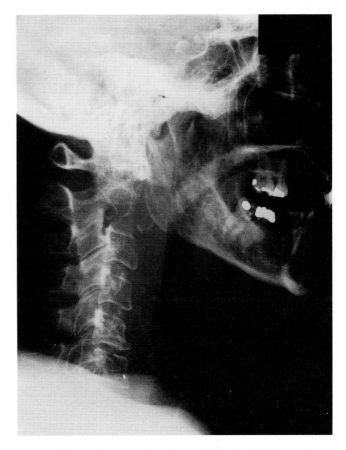

Fig. 14.8 Myelomatosis involving the cervical spine with destruction of C2.

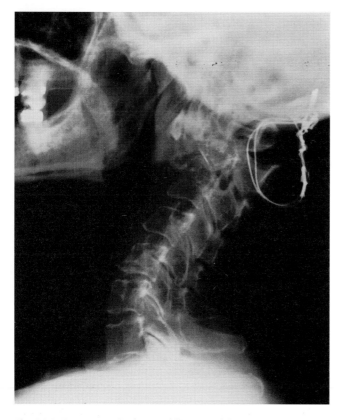

Fig. 14.9 Temporary wire-loop stabilization of the upper cervical spine.

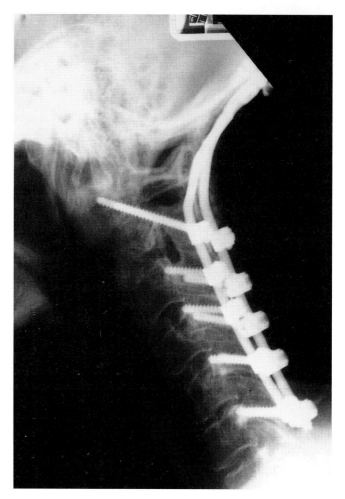

Fig. 14.10 C1–C2 posterior fusion with permanent stabilization.

masses, may be an indication for surgical resection to achieve decompression. Vertebral collapse may also cause spinal cord or nerve root compression and in the neck, particularly, require stabilizing surgical procedures to avoid progressive neurological changes (Figs 14.8–14.10). Local radiotherapy is often instituted as adjunctive treatment, as well as antimyeloma chemotherapy.

True solitary plasmacytoma of bone is best treated with radiotherapy, but multiple lesions without any evidence of progression to true myelomatosis can present management difficulties, particularly if radiotherapy to the several sites involved does not achieve control and there is no satisfactory symptom relief. Although chemotherapy may be instituted, the response is usually suboptimal. There has been little experience of high-dose therapy in such situations. In addition to the valuable contribution of radiotherapy in the treatment of plasmacytomas (of bone and extramedullary), this modality has a particularly important role in the control of bone pain and in effective palliation.

The overall management and care of the myeloma patient is multifaceted, and it often requires a multidisciplinary approach. The importance of ensuring the best possible quality of life during the course of the disease is now well recognized. The objective assessment of this (e.g. using the recently devel-

oped modules) should ideally become an integral aspect of monitoring all forms of treatment in myeloma.

Future developments

Despite the trend to improvement in the survival of patients with myeloma, the long-term outlook remains generally poor. About 20% of patients die within the first year of diagnosis. A greater awareness of the presenting features, earlier diagnosis and the optimization of initial treatment could potentially improve outcome.

The management of relapsed disease also merits closer attention. The median time of survival following relapse is about 18 months, and it is during this period that the patient's quality of life often deteriorates markedly. Improving therapy at this stage should be directed at both improving the quality of life as well as survival. A major therapeutic aim in myeloma should be to prolong the duration of plateau/minimal disease states when the quality of life can be very good. This is particularly so if the progression of bone disease can be inhibited by the use of bisphosphonates. These agents may also have the indirect benefit of prolonging the duration of the plateau phase, presumably by affecting the interaction between the plasma cell and the osteoclasts.

A number of different cytokines signal via gp130, and of those the one central to the pathogenesis of myeloma is IL-6. A number of strategies could be used to inhibit the pathway, with the aim of inhibiting growth of the myeloma clone and prolonging the duration of plateau. Inhibition strategies might include antibody or directed inhibition of gp130, IL-6 or its receptor by super antagonists. A study in end-stage disease has shown a clinical response following inhibition of IL-6.

The data on allogeneic BMT suggest that there is a discernible graft vs myeloma effect. Patients relapsing following allografts have had donor lymphocyte infusions, which have been followed by a return to stable remissions [159]. This combined with some reports of PCR negativity in long-term survivors post allograft would suggest that, if the early mortality associated with the procedure could be overcome, allogeneic BMT would be significantly more effective than autologous transplantation. The potential for idiotypic vaccination of the donor prior to transplant is also being investigated [160]. Such vaccination strategies might be extended into autologous transplantation, although the potential for this after high-dose treatment, in a time frame which would be useful for myeloma patients, is at present questionable because of the immunosuppression which follows these procedures. The procedure demands the generation of T-cell responses to idiotype or other tumour-specific markers in the surface of the myeloma cell. Plasma cells do not express class I on their surface, and it is difficult to conceive how such strategies could be effective when the molecule necessary for presenting the target is absent. This might be an effective approach if a putative myeloma precursor which expressed surface idiotype existed. However, as discussed earlier, it is generally felt that such a precursor would be close to the level of a plasma cell which might not be expected to express such surface molecules. The use of dendritic cells or gene transfer-mediated cytokine immunization remains a possibility. DNA vaccination is being actively explored [161].

The herpes virus KSHV (Kaposi's sarcoma-related herpes virus, alternatively known as HHV-8 — human herpes virus 8), which contains an IL-6 homologue, has recently been found to infect the dendritic cells in the bone marrow of patients with myeloma [162]. In MGUS the virus is less frequent but detectable in about 25% of cases. As the dendritic cells play an important role in the growth and differentiation of mature B cells, KSHV may influence the transformation of MGUS to myeloma and subsequent disease progression. Although KSHV has not yet been shown to be a causative factor in the myeloma disease process, its presence would suggest that antiviral therapy might be an avenue worth exploring.

Acknowledgements

We would like to acknowledge the individual contributions of Dr Andrew Jack, Dr Faith Davies, Mr Andrew Rawstrom and Mrs Gillian Needham in the preparation of this chapter.

References

1 Klein B., Zhang X.G., Jourdan M. *et al.* (1989) Paracrine rather than autocrine regulation of myeloma cell growth and differentiation by interleukin 6. *Blood*, **73**, 517–526.

2 Bataille R., Jourdan M., Zhang X.G. & Klein B. (1989) Serum levels of interleukin 6, a potent myeloma cell growth factor, as a reflection of disease severity in plasma cell dyscrasias. *Journal of Clinical Investigation*, **84**, 2008–2011.

3 Bataille R., Chappard D. & Klein B. (1992) Mechanisms of bone lesions in multiple myeloma. *Haematology and Oncology Clinics of North America*, **6**, 285–295.

4 Bataille R., Chappard D. & Basle M.F. (1996) Quantifiable excess of bone resorption in monoclonal gammopathy is an early symptom of malignancy: a prospective study of 87 bone biopsies. *Blood*, **87**, 4762–4769.

5 Lecouvet F., van de Berg B., Michaux L. *et al.* (1996) Magnetic resonance imaging of the bone marrow to assess the risk of disease progression in patients with monoclonal gammopathy of uncertain significance. *British Journal of Haematology*, **93**(Suppl. 2), 1137.

6 Elomaa I., Virkkunen P., Risteli L. & Risteli J. (1992) Serum concentration of the cross linked carboxyterminal telopeptide of type 1 collagen (ICTP) is a useful prognostic indicator in multiple myeloma. *British Journal of Cancer*, **66**, 337–341.

7 Abildgaard N., Bentzen S.M., Nielson J.L. & Heickenddorff L. (1997) Serum markers of bone metabolism in multiple myeloma: prognostic value of the carboxy-terminal telopeptide of type 1 collagen (ITCP). *British Journal of Haematology*, **96**, 103–110.

8 Pecherstorfer M., Seibel M.J., Woitge H.W. *et al.* (1996) Diagnostic validity of urinary pyridinium crosslinks of collagen in the differentiation of multiple myeloma from monoclonal gammopathy of unknown significance and osteoporosis. *British Journal of Haematology*, **93**(Suppl. 2), 497.

9 Durie B.G. & Salmon S.E. (1975) A clinical staging system for multiple myeloma. *Cancer*, **36**, 842–854.

10 Woodruff R.K., Wadsworth J., Malpas J.S. & Tobias J.S. (1979) Clinical staging in multiple myeloma. *British Journal of Haematology*, **42**, 199–205.

11 MacLennan I., Drayson M. & Dunn J. (1994) Multiple myeloma. *British Journal of Medicine*, **308**, 1033–1036.

12 Cunningham B.A. & Berggard I. (1974) Structure, evolution and significance of β2-microglobulin. *Transplantation Review*, **21**, 3–14.

13 Berggard I., Bjork L., Cigen R. & Lotdbergk L. (1980) β2-microglobulin. *Scandinavian Journal of Clinical and Laboratory Investigation*, **40**(Suppl. 154), 13–45.

14 Creswell P., Springer T., Strominger J.L., Turner M.J., Grey H.M. & Kulo R.T. (1974) Immunological identity of the small subunit of HLA antigens and β2-microglobulin and its turnover on the cell membrane. *Proceedings of the National Academy of Sciences, USA*, **71**, 2123–2127.

15 Evrin P.E. & Wibell L. (1973) Serum β2-microglobulin in various disorders. *Clinica Chimica Acta*, **43**, 183–187.

16 Shuster J., Gold P. & Poulik M.D. (1976) β2-microglobulin levels

in cancerous and other disease states. *Clinica Chimica Acta*, **67**, 307–313.

17 Norfolk D.R., Child J.A., Cooper E.H., Kerruish S. & Milford-Ward A. (1980) Serum β2-microglobulin in myelomatosis: potential value in stratification and monitoring. *British Journal of Cancer*, **39**, 510–515.

18 Child J.A., Crawford S.M., Norfolk D.R., Quigley J., Scarffe J.H. & Struthers L.D.L. (1983) Evaluation of serum β₂-microglobulin as a prognostic indicator in myelomatosis. *British Journal of Cancer*, **47**, 111–114.

19 Bataille R., Durie B.G.B. & Grenier J. (1983) Serum β2-microglobulin and survival duration in multiple myeloma: a simple reliable marker for staging. *British Journal of Haematology*, **55**, 439–447.

20 Cassuto J.P., Krebs B.J., Viot G., Du Jardin P. & Masseyeff R. (1978) β2-microglobulin, a tumour marker of lymphoproliferative disorders. *Lancet*, **ii**, 108.

21 Cuzick J., Cooper E.H. & MacLennan I.C.M. (1985) The prognostic value of serum β2-microglobulin compared with other presentation features in myelomatosis (A report to the Medical Research Council's Working Party on Leukaemia in Adults). *British Journal of Cancer*, **52**, 1–6.

22 Bataille R., Grenier J. & Sany J. (1984) β2-microglobulin in myeloma: optimal use for staging, prognosis and treatment. A prospective study of 160 patients. *Blood*, **63**, 468–476.

23 Garewal H., Durie B.G.M., Kyle R.A., Finley P., Bower B. & Serokman R. (1984) Serum β2-microglobulin in the initial staging and subsequent monitoring of multiple myeloma. *Journal of Clinical Oncology*, **2**, 51–57.

24 Greipp P. & Kyle R.A. (1983) Clinical, morphological and cell kinetic differences among multiple myeloma, monoclonal gammopathy of undetermined significance and smouldering multiple myeloma. *Blood*, **62**, 166–171.

25 Boccadoro M., Gavarotti P., Fossati G. *et al.* (1984) Low plasma cell 3(H) thymidine incorporation in monoclonal gammopathy of undetermined significance (MGUS), smouldering myeloma and remission phase myeloma: a reliable indicator of patients not requiring therapy. *British Journal of Haematology*, **58**, 689–696.

26 Rawstron A., Owen R.G., Davies F.E. *et al.* (1996) Circulating plasma cells in multiple myeloma: characterisation and correlation with disease status. *British Journal of Haematology*, **97**, 46–55.

27 Rawstron A.C., Davies F.E., Owen R.G. *et al.* (1998) B lymphocyte suppression in multiple myeloma is a reversible phenomenon specific to normal B cell progenitors and plasma cell precursors. *British Journal of Haematology*, **100**, 176–183.

28 Pellat-Deceunynck C., Barille S., Puthier D. *et al.* (1995) Adhesion molecules on human myeloma cells: significant changes in expression related to malignancy, tumour spread and immortalisation. *Cancer Research*, **55**, 3647–3653.

29 Van Camp B., Durie B.G.M., Spier C. *et al.* (1990) Plasma cells in multiple myeloma express a natural killer cell associated antigen: CD56. *Blood*, **76**, 377–382.

30 Lokhorst H.M., Lamme T., de Smet M. *et al.* (1994) Primary tumour cells of myeloma patients induce IL-6 secretion in long term bone marrow cultures. *Blood*, **84**, 2269–2277.

31 Kawano M.M., Mahmoud M.S., Huang N. *et al.* (1995) High proportion of VLA-5 immature myeloma cells correlated well with poor response to treatment in multiple myeloma. *British Journal of Haematology*, **92**, 860–864.

32 Pellat-Deceunynck C., Bataille R., Robillard N. *et al.* (1994) Expression of CD28 and CD40 in human myeloma cells: a comparative study with normal plasma cells. *Blood*, **84**, 2597–2603.

33 Urashima M., Chaauhan D., Uchiyma H., Freeman G.J. & Anderson K.C. (1995) CD40 ligand triggered interleukin-6 secretion in multiple myeloma. *Blood*, **85**, 1903–1912.

34 San Miguel J.F., Gonzalez M., Gascon A. *et al.* (1991) Immunophenotypic heterogeneity of multiple myeloma: influence on the biology and the clinical course of the disease. *British Journal of Haematology*, **77**, 185–190.

35 Ocqueteau M., Orfao A., Garcia Sanz R., Almeida J., Gonzalez M. & San Miguel J. (1996) Expression of the CD117 antigen (C-Kit) on normal and myelomatous plasma cells. *British Journal of Haematology*, **95**, 489–493.

36 Witzig T.E., Kyle R.A., O'Fallon W.M. & Greipp P.R. (1994) Detection of peripheral blood plasma cells as a predictor of disease course in patients with smouldering multiple myeloma. *British Journal of Haematology*, **87**, 266–272.

37 Witzig T.E., Gertz M.A., Lust J.A., Kyle R., O'Fallon W.M. & Griepp P.R. (1996) Peripheral blood monoclonal plasma cells as a predictor of survival in patients with multiple myeloma. *Blood*, **88**, 1780–1787.

38 Klein B., Widjenes J., Zhang X.G. *et al.* (1991) Murine anti interleukin 6 monoclonal antibody therapy for a patient with plasma cell leukemia. *Blood*, **78**, 1198–1204.

39 Kyrtsonis M.C., Dedoussis G., Zervas C. *et al.* (1996) Soluble interleukin-6 receptor (sIL-6R), a new prognostic factor in multiple myeloma. *British Journal of Haematology*, **93**, 398–400.

40 Pulkki K., Pelliniemi T.T., Rajamaki A., Tienhaara A., Laakso M. & Lahtinen R. (1996) Soluble interleukin-6 receptor as a prognostic factor in multiple myeloma. *British Journal of Haematology*, **92**, 370–374.

41 Ludwig H., Nachbaur D.M., Fritz E., Krainer M. & Huber H. (1991) Interleukin-6 is a prognostic factor in multiple myeloma (letter). *Blood*, **77**, 2794–2795.

42 Pelliniemi T.T., Hirvonen H., Laakso M. *et al.* (1996) High ratio of serum soluble interleukin 6 receptor (sIL-6R) to soluble glycoprotein 130 (sgp130) at diagnosis predicts poor prognosis in multiple myeloma. *British Journal of Haematology*, **93**(Suppl. 2), 619.

43 Pelliniemi T.T., Irjala K., Mattila K. *et al.* (1995) Immunoreactive interleukin 6 and acute phase proteins as prognostic factors in multiple myeloma. *Blood*, **85**, 765–771.

44 Merlini G., Perfetti V., Gobbi P.G. *et al.* (1992) Acute phase proteins and prognosis in multiple myeloma. *British Journal of Haematology*, **83**, 595–601.

45 Weh H.J., Gutensohn K., Selbaach J. *et al.* (1993) Karyotype in multiple myeloma and plasma cell leukaemia. *European Journal of Cancer*, **29A**, 1269–1273.

46 Smadja V., Louvet C., Isnard F. *et al.* (1995) Cytogenetic study in multiple myeloma at diagnosis: comparison of two techniques. *British Journal of Haematology*, **90**, 619–624.

47 Smadja V., Fruchart C., Dutel J.L. *et al.* (1996) Multiple myeloma: cytogenetic classification. *British Journal of Haematology*, **93**(Suppl. 2), 502.

48 Garcia-Sanz R., Orfao A., Gonzaalez M. *et al.* (1995) Prognostic implications of DNA aneuploidy in 156 untreated multiple myeloma patients. *British Journal of Haematology*, **90**, 106–112.

49 Sawyer J.R., Waldron J.A., Jaganath S. & Barlogie B. (1995) Cytogenetics findings in 200 patients with multiple myeloma. *Cancer, Genetics and Cytogenetics*, **82**, 41–49.

50 Tricot G., Barlogie B., Jaganath S. *et al.* (1995) Poor prognosis in multiple myeloma is associated only with partial or complete deletions of chromosome 13 or abnormalities involving 11q and not with other karyotype abnormalities. *Blood*, **86**, 4250–4256.

51 Lai J.L., Zandecki M., Mary J.Y. *et al.* (1995) Improved cytogenet-

ics in multiple myeloma: a study of 151 patients including 117 patients at diagnosis. *Blood*, **85**, 2490–2497.

52 Philip P., Drivsholm A., Hansen N.E., Jenson M.K. & Kilman S.A. (1980) Chromosomes and survival in multiple myeloma: a banding study of 25 cases. *Cancer, Genetics and Cytogenetics*, **2**, 243–257.

53 Chesi M., Bergsagel P.L., Brents L.A., Smith C.M., Gerhard D.S. & Kuehl W.M. (1996) Dysregulation of Cyclin D1 by translocation into an IgH gamma switch region in two multiple myeloma cell lines. *Blood*, **88**, 674–681.

54 Preudhomme C., Facon T., Zaanddecki M. *et al.* (1992) Rare occurrence of p53 gene mutations in multiple myeloma. *British Journal of Haematology*, **81**, 440–443.

55 Owen R.G., Davis S.A.A., Randerson J. *et al.* (1997) p53 gene mutations in multiple myeloma. *Molecular Pathology*, **50**, 18–20.

56 Corradini P., Inghirami G., Astolfi M. *et al.* (1994) Inactivation of tumour suppressor genes, p53 and Rb1, in plasma cell dyscrasias. *Leukaemia*, **8**, 758–767.

57 Portier M., Moles J.P., Makars G.R. *et al.* (1992) p53 and RAS gene mutations in multiple myeloma. *Oncogene*, **7**, 2539–2543.

58 Corradini P., Ladetto M., Voena C. *et al.* (1993) Mutational activation of N- and K-ras oncogenes in plasma cell dyscrasias. *Blood*, **81**, 2708–2713.

59 Ong F., v. Nieuwkoop J.A., de Groot-Swings G.M.J.S. *et al.* (1995) Bcl-2 protein expression is not related to short survival in multiple myeloma. *Leukaemia*, **9**, 1282–1284.

60 Tsuchiya H., Epstein J., Selvanayagam P. *et al.* (1988) Correlated flow cytometric analysis of H rasp21 and nuclear DNA in multiple myeloma. *Blood*, **72**, 796–800.

61 Alexanian R., Bergsagel D.E., Migliore P.J., Vaughn W.K. & Howe C.D. (1968) Melphalan therapy for plasma cell myeloma. *Blood*, **31**, 1–10.

62 Bergsagel D.E., Griffith K.M., Haut A. & Stuckey J.W. Jr. (1967) The treatment of plasma cell myeloma. *Advances in Cancer Research*, **10**, 311–359.

63 Alexanian R., Haut A., Khan A.U. *et al.* (1969) Treatment for multiple myeloma. Combination chemotherapy with different dose regimens. *Journal of the American Medical Association*, **208**, 1680–1685.

64 Malpas J.S. (1969) Management of multiple myeloma. *British Medical Journal*, **2**, 163–165.

65 Costa G., Engle R.L., Schilling A. *et al.* (1973) Melphalan and prednisone: an effective combination for the treatment of multiple myeloma. *American Journal of Medicine*, **54**, 589–599.

66 Medical Research Council Working Party on Leukaemia in Adults (1971) Myelomatosis: comparison of melphalan and cyclophosphamide therapy. *British Medical Journal*, **1**, 640–641.

67 Medical Research Council Working Party on Leukaemia in Adults (1973) Report on the first myelomatosis trial. Part 1. *British Journal of Haematology*, **24**, 123–139.

68 Medical Research Council Working Party on Leukaemia in Adults (1980) Report on the second myelomatosis trial after five years of follow up. *British Journal of Cancer*, **42**, 813–822.

69 Rivers S.L. & Patno M.E. (1969) Cyclophosphamide versus melphalan in treatment of plasma cell myeloma. *Journal of the American Medical Association*, **207**, 1328–1334.

70 Cooper M.R., McIntyre O.R., Propert K.J. *et al.* (1986) Single, sequential and multiple alkylating agent therapy for multiple myeloma: a CALGB study. *Journal of Clinical Oncology*, **4**, 1331–1339.

71 Alberts D.S., Durie B.G.M. & Salmon S.E. (1975) Doxorubincin/BCNU chemotherapy for multiple myeloma in relapse. *Lancet*, **i**, 926–928.

72 Durie B.G.M., Dixon D.O., Carter S. *et al.* (1986) Improved survival duration with combination chemotherapy induction for multiple myeloma: a Southwest Oncology Group study. *Journal of Clinical Oncology*, **4**, 1227–1237.

73 Peest D., Deicher H., Coldewey R., Schmoll H.J. & Schedel I. (1988) Induction and maintenance therapy in multiple myeloma: a multicentre trial of MP versus VCMP. *European Journal of Cancer and Clinical Oncology*, **24**, 1061–1067.

74 Blade J., San-Miguel J., Alcala A. *et al.* (1990) A randomised multicentre study comparing alternative combination chemotherapy (VCMP/VBAP) and melphalan-prednisolone in multiple myeloma. *Blut*, **60**, 319–322.

75 Hjorth M., Hellquist L., Holmberg E., Magnusson B., Rödjer S. & Westin J. (for the Myeloma Group of Western Sweden) (1990) Initial treatment in multiple myeloma: no advantage of multidrug chemotherapy over melphalan-prednisolone. *British Journal of Haematology*, **74**, 185–191.

76 Medical Research Council Working Party on Leukaemia in Adults (1985) Objective evaluation of the rôle of vincristine in induction and maintenance therapy for myelomatosis. *British Journal of Cancer*, **52**, 153–158.

77 Gregory W.M., Richards M.A. & Malpas J.S. (1992) Combination chemotherapy versus melphalan and prednisolone in the treatment of multiple myeloma: an overview of published trials. *Journal of Clinical Oncology*, **10**, 334–342.

78 The Myeloma Trialists Collaborative Group (1998) Combination chemotherapy versus melphalan plus prednisone as treatment for multiple myeloma: an overview of 6633 patients from 27 randomised trials. (In press.)

79 MacLennan I.C.M., Chapman C., Dunn J. & Kelly K. (1992) Combined chemotherapy with ABCM versus melphalan for treatment of myelomatosis. *Lancet*, **339**, 200–205.

80 Kelly K.A., Durie B.G.M. & MacLennan I.C.M. (1988) Prognostic factors and staging systems for multiple myeloma: comparisons between the Medical Research Council studies in the United Kingdom and the Southwest Oncology Group studies in the United States. *Hematological Oncology*, **6**, 131–140.

81 Barlogie B. & Alexanian R. (1984) Effective treatment of advanced multiple myeloma refractory to alkylating agents. *New England Journal of Medicine*, **310**, 1353–1356.

82 Samson D., Newland A., Kearney J. *et al.* (1989) Infusion of vincristine and doxorubicin with oral dexamethasone as first-line therapy for multiple myeloma. *Lancet*, **ii**, 882–885.

83 Salmon S.E., Shadduck R.K. & Schilling A. (1967) Intermittent high dose prednisone therapy for multiple myeloma. *Cancer Chemotherapy Reports*, **51**, 179–182.

84 Alexanian R., Barlogie B. & Dixon D. (1986) High dose glucocorticoid treatment of resistant myeloma. *Annals of Internal Medicine*, **105**, 8–11.

85 Alexanian R., Dimopoulos M.A., De La Salle K. & Barlogie B. (1992) Primary dexamethasone treatment of multiple myeloma. *Blood*, **80**, 887–890.

86 Forgerson G.V., Selby P., Lakhani S. *et al.* (1988) Infused vincristine and adriamycin with high dose methyl prednisolone (VAMP) in advanced previously treated multiple myeloma patients. *British Journal of Cancer*, **58**, 469–473.

87 Bell J.B.G., Millar B.C., Montes-Borinaga A. *et al.* (1990) Decrease in clonogenic tumour cells in bone marrow aspirates from multiple myeloma patients due to incorporation of cyclophosphamide into treatment with vincristine, adriamycin and methyl prednisolone. *Hematological Oncology*, **8**, 347–353.

88 Raje N., Powles R.L., Milan S. *et al.* (1997) A comparison of

vincristine and doxorubicin infusional chemotherapy with methylprednisolone (VAMP) with the addition of weekly cyclophosphamide (C-VAMP) as induction treatment followed by autografting in previously untreated myeloma. *British Journal of Haematology*, **97**, 153–160.

89 McElwain T.J. & Powles R.L. (1983) High dose intravenous melphalan for plasma cell leukaemia and myeloma. *Lancet*, **ii**, 822–824.

90 Selby P., McElwain T.J., Nandi A.C. *et al.* (1987) Multiple myeloma treated with high-dose intravenous melphalan. *British Journal of Haematology*, **66**, 55–62.

91 Gore M.E., Selby P.J., Viner C. *et al.* (1989) Intensive treatment of multiple myeloma and criteria for complete remission. *Lancet*, **ii**, 879–881.

92 Anderson K.C., Barut B.A., Ritz J. *et al.* (1991) Monoclonal antibody purged autologous bone marrow transplantation therapy for multiple myeloma. *Blood*, **72**, 712–720.

93 Jagannath S., Vesole D.H., Glenn L., Crowley J. & Barlogie B. (1992) Low-risk intensive therapy for multiple myeloma with combined autologous bone marrow and blood stem cell support. *Blood*, **80**, 1666–1672.

94 Attal M., Huguet F., Schlaifer D. *et al.* (1992) Intensive combined therapy for previously untreated aggressive myeloma. *Blood*, **79**, 1130–1136.

95 Reece D.E., Barnett M.J., Connors J.M. *et al.* (1993) Treatment of multiple myeloma with intensive chemotherapy followed by autologous BMT using marrow purged with 4-hydroperoxycyclophosphamide. *Bone Marrow Transplantation*, **11**, 139–146.

96 Cunningham D., Powles R., Malpas J.S. *et al.* (1993) A randomised trial of maintenance therapy with Intron-A following high dose melphalan and ABMT in myeloma. *ASCO Abstracts*, **12**, 364.

97 Powles R., Raje N., Milan S. *et al.* (1997) Outcome assessment of a population based group of 195 unselected myeloma patients under 70 years of age offered intensive treatment. *Bone Marrow Transplantation*, **20**, 435–443.

98 Attal M., Harousseau J., Stoppa A.M. *et al.* for the Intergroupe Français du Myelome (1996) A prospective randomised trial of autologous bone marrow transplantation and chemotherapy in multiple myeloma. *New England Journal of Medicine*, **335**, 91–97.

99 Barlogie B., Jgannath S., Vesole D. *et al.* (1993) Total therapy (TT) for newly diagnosed multiple myeloma (MM). *Blood*, **82**(abstr. Suppl. 1), 193a.

100 Gahrton G., Ringden O., Lönnqvist A., Lindquist R. & Ljungman P. (1986) Bone marrow transplantation in three patients with multiple myeloma. *Acta Medica Scandinavica*, **219**, 523–527.

101 Tura S., Cavo M., Baccarani M., Ricci P. & Gobbi M. (1986) Bone marrow transplantation in multiple myeloma. *Scandinavian Journal of Haematology*, **36**, 176–179.

102 Tura S., Cavo M., Rosti G. *et al.* (1989) Allogeneic bone marrow transplantation for multiple myeloma. *Bone Marrow Transplantation*, **4**, 106–108.

103 Gahrton G., Tura S., Ljungman P. *et al.* (1995) Prognostic factors in allogeneic bone marrow transplantation for multiple myeloma. *Journal of Clinical Oncology*, **13**, 1312–1322.

104 Durie B.G.M., Gale R.P. & Horowitz M.M. (1994) Allogeneic and twin transplants for multiple myeloma: an IBMTR analysis. In: *Multiple Myeloma: from biology to therapy: current concepts. INSERM Mullhouse 24–26 October*, p. 93, abstract.

105 Gahrton G. (1996) Allogeneic bone marrow transplantation in multiple myeloma. *British Journal of Haematology*, **92**, 251–254.

106 Bensinger W.I., Buckner C.D., Clift R.A. *et al.* (1992) A phase I study of busulphan and cyclophosphamide in preparation for allogeneic marrow transplant for patients with multiple myeloma. *Journal of Clinical Oncology*, **10**, 1492–1497.

107 Buckner C.D., Fefer A., Bensinger W.I. *et al.* (1989) Marrow transplantation for malignant plasma cell disorders: summary of the Seattle experience. *European Journal of Haematology*, **43**(Suppl. 51), 186–190.

108 Bird J.M., Russell N.H. & Samson D. (1993) Minimal residual disease after bone marrow transplantation for multiple myeloma; evidence for cure in long-term survivors. *Bone Marrow Transplantation*, **12**, 651–654.

109 Selby P., Zulian G., Forgeson G. *et al.* (1988) The development of high dose melphalan and of autologous bone marrow transplantation in the treatment of multiple myeloma. Royal Marsden and St Bartholomew's Hospital studies. *Hematological Oncology*, **6**, 173–179.

110 Wisloff F. & Svere E. (1996) Measurement of health related QOL in multiple myeloma. *British Journal of Haematology*, **92**, 604–613.

111 Mellstedt H., Åhre A., Björkholm M., Holm G., Johansson B. & Strander H. (1979) Interferon therapy in myelomatosis. *Lancet*, **i**, 245–247.

112 Åhre A., Björkholm M., Osterborg A. *et al.* (1988) High doses of natural α-interferon (α-IFN) in the treatment of multiple myeloma: a pilot study from the Myeloma Group of Central Sweden (MGCS). *European Journal of Haematology*, **41**, 123–130.

113 Åhre A., Björkholm M., Mellstedt H. *et al.* (1984) Human leukocyte interferon and intermittent high dose melphalan/prednisolone administration in the treatment of multiple myeloma: randomized clinical trial. *Cancer Treatment Reports*, **68**, 1331–1338.

114 Ludwig H., Cortelezzi A., Scheithauer W. *et al.* (1986) Recombinant interferon alfa-2b versus polychemotherapy (VMCP) for treatment of multiple myeloma: a prospective randomized trial. *European Journal of Cancer and Clinical Oncology*, **22**, 111–116.

115 Quesade J.R., Alexanian R., Hawkins M. *et al.* (1986) Treatment of multiple myeloma with recombinant α-interferon. *Blood*, **67**, 275–278.

116 Welander C.E., Morgan T.M. & Homesley H.D. (1985) Combined recombinant human interferon alpha-2 and cytotoxic agents studied in the clonogenic assay. *International Journal of Cancer*, **35**, 721–729.

117 Pavlovsky S., Corrado C., Saslavsky J. *et al.* (1989) Randomized trial comparing melphalan-prednisolone with or without recombinant alpha 2 interferon (rα2IFN) in multiple; myeloma. *Proceedings of the American Society of Clinical Oncology*, **8**, 258.

118 Montuoro A., De Rosa L., DeBlasio A., Pacilli L., Petti N. & De Laurenzi A. (1990) Alpha-2a-interferon/melphalan/prednisone versus melphalan/prednisone in previously untreated patients with multiple myeloma. *British Journal of Haematology*, **76**, 365–368.

119 Österborg A. & Mellstedt H. (1991) The mechanisms of action and the role of alpha interferon in the therapy of myeloma. In: *Interferons: mechanisms of action and role in cancer therapy* (eds D. Crowther & U. Veronesi), pp. 25–31. Springer, Berlin.

120 Oken M.M., Kyle R.A., Greipp P.R., Kay N.E., Tsiatis A. & O'Connell M.J. (1992) Possible survival benefit with chemotherapy plus interferon (rIFNα2) in the treatment of multiple myeloma. *ASCO Abstracts*, **11**, 358.

121 Österborg A., Björkholm M., Bjoreman M. *et al.* (1993) Natural interferon-alpha in combination with melphalan/prednisone versus melphalan/prednisone in the treatment of multiple myeloma stages II and III: a randomised study from the Myeloma Group of Central Sweden. *Blood*, **81**, 1428–1434.

122 Ludwig H., Cohen A.M. & Polliak A. (1995) Interferon-alpha for induction and maintenance in multiple myeloma: results of two multicentre randomized trials and summary of other studies. *Annals of Oncology*, **6**, 467–476.

123 Hjorth M. & The Nordic Myeloma Study Group (1996) Interferon-α_{2b} added to melphalan-prednisone for initial and maintenance therapy in multiple myeloma. A randomized, controlled trial. *Annals of Internal Medicine*, **124**, 212–222.

124 Mandelli F., Avvisati G., Amadori S. *et al.* (1990) Maintenance treatment with recombinant interferon alpha2b in patients with multiple myeloma responding to conventional induction chemotherapy. *New England Journal of Medicine*, **322**, 1430–1434.

125 Westin J., Cortelezzi A., Hjorth M., Rödjer S., Turesson I. & Zador G. (1991) Interferon therapy during the plateau phase of multiple myeloma; an update of the Swedish study. *European Journal of Cancer*, **27**(Suppl. 4), 545–548.

126 Peest D., Deicher H., Coldewey R. *et al.* (1990) Melphalan and prednisone (MP) versus vincristrine, BCNU, adriamycin, melphalan and dexamethasone (VBAMDex) induction chemotherapy and interferon maintenance treatment in multiple myeloma: current results of a multicenter trial. The German Myeloma Treatment Group. *Onkologie*, **13**, 458–460.

127 Salmon S.E., Crowley J.J. & Grogan T.M. (1994) Combination chemotherapy, glucocorticoids and interferon alpha in the treatment of multiple myeloma. A Southwest Oncology Group Study. *Journal of Clinical Oncology*, **12**, 2405–2414.

128 Browman G.P., Bergsagel D. & Sicheri D. (1995) Randomized trial of interferon maintenance therapy during plateau phase in multiple myeloma: a randomized study. *British Journal of Haematology*, **89**, 561–568.

129 Arceci R.J. (1993) Clinical significance of P. glycoprotein and multidrug resistance malignancies. *Blood*, **81**, 2215–2222.

130 Sikic B.I. (1993) Modulation of multidrug resistance: at the threshold. *Journal of Clinical Oncology*, **11**, 1629–1635.

131 Sonneveld P., Durie B.G.M., Lokhorst H.M. *et al.* (1992) Modulation of multidrug resistant multiple myeloma by cyclosporin. *Lancet*, **340**, 255–259.

132 Sonneveld P., Marie J.P., Lokhorst H.M., Nooter K. & Schoester M. (1994) Clinical modulation of multidrug resistance in VAD refractory multiple myeloma—studies with cyclosporin and SDZ PSC-833. *Anti-Cancer Drugs*, **5**(Suppl. 1), 72.

133 Durie B.G.M., Russel D.H. & Salmon S.E. (1980) Reappraisal of plateau phase in myeloma. *Lancet*, **ii**, 65–68.

134 Durie B.G.M., Salmon S.E. & Moon T.E. (1980) Pretreatment tumor mass, cell kinetics, and prognosis in multiple myeloma. *Blood*, **55**, 364–372.

135 Hofmann V., Salmon S.E. & Durie B.G.M. (1981) Drug resistance in multiple myeloma associated with high *in-vitro* incorporation of ^{3}[H] thymidine. *Blood*, **57**, 766–782.

136 Brown R.D., Joshua D.E., Ioannides R.A. & Kronenberg H. (1989) Serum thymidine kinase as a marker of disease activity in patients with multiple myeloma. *Australian and New Zealand Journal of Medicine*, **19**, 226–232.

137 Owen R.G., Johnson R.J., Rawstron A.C. *et al.* (1996) Assessment of IgH TCR strategies in multiple myeloma. *Journal of Clinical Pathology*, **49**, 672–675.

138 Kyle R.A. (1975) Multiple myeloma: review of 869 cases. *Mayo Clinic Proceedings*, **50**, 29–40.

139 Alexanian R., Barlogie B. & Dixon B. (1990) Renal failure in multiple myeloma: pathogenesis and prognostic implications. *Archives of Internal Medicine*, **150**, 1693–1695.

140 Woodruff R. & Sweet B. (1977) Multiple myeloma with massive Bence Jones proteinuria and preservation of renal function. *Australian and New Zealand Journal of Medicine*, **7**, 60–62.

141 Kyle R.A. & Greipp P.R. (1982) Idiopathic Bence Jones proteinuria. Long term follow up in seven patients. *New England Journal of Medicine*, **306**, 564–567.

142 Cooper E.H., Forbes M.A., Crockson R.A. & MacLennan I.C.M. (1984) Proximal renal tubular function in myelomatosis: observations in the fourth Medical Research Council trial. *Journal of Clinical Pathology*, **37**, 852–858.

143 MRC Working Party on Leukaemia in Adults (1984) Analysis and management of renal failure in fourth MRC myelomatosis trial. *British Medical Journal*, **288**, 1411–1416.

144 Heyburn P.J., Child J.A. & Peacock M. (1981) The treatment of osteolytic myelomatosis with mithramycin. *Lancet*, **i**, 719–722.

145 Hoogstraten B. (1973) Steroid therapy of multiple myeloma and macroglobulinaemia. *Medical Clinics of North America*, **57**(5), 1321–1330.

146 Delamore L.W. (1982) Hypercalcaemia and myeloma. *British Journal of Haematology*, **51**, 507–509.

147 Stamp T.C.B., Child J.A. & Walker P.G. (1975) The treatment of osteolytic myelomatosis with mithramycin. *Lancet*, **i**, 719–722.

148 Bruatbar N. & Loboshitzky R. (1977) Combined calcitonin and oral phosphate treatment for hypercalcaemia in multiple myeloma. *Archives of Internal Medicine*, **7**, 914–916.

149 Fleisch H. (1997) *Bisphosphonates in Bone Disease. From the laboratory to the patient*, 3rd edn. Parthanon Publishing Group, New York.

150 Adami S. & Zamberlan N. (1996) Adverse effects of bisphosphonates. A comparative review. *Drug Safety*, **14**, 158–170.

151 Lahtinen R., Laakso M., Palva I., Virkkunen P. & Elomaa I. (1992) Randomised placebo-controlled multicentre trial of clodronate in multiple myeloma. *Lancet*, **340**, 1049–1052.

152 McClosky E.V., MacLennan I.C.M., Drayson M.I., Chapman C., Dunn J. & Kanis J.A. (1998) Effect of clodronate on skeletal morbidity in multiple myeloma. *British Journal of Haematology*. (In press.)

153 Berenson J.R., Lightenstein A., Porter L. *et al.* (1996) Efficacy of pamidronate in reducing skeletal events in patients with advanced multiple myeloma. *New England Journal of Medicine*, **334**, 488–493.

154 Laakso M., Lahtinen R., Virkkunen P. & Elomaa I. (1994) Subgroup and cost benefit analysis of the Finnish multicentre trial of clodronate in multiple myeloma. *British Journal of Haematology*, **87**, 725–729.

155 Savage D.G., Lindenbaum J. & Garret T.J. (1982) Biphasic pattern of bacterial infection in multiple myeloma. *Annals of Internal Medicine*, **96**, 47–50.

156 Cazzola M., Messinger D., Battistel V. *et al.* (1995) Recombinant human erythropoietin in the anaemia associated with multiple myeloma or non-Hodgkin's lymphoma: dose finding and identification of predictors of response. *Blood*, **86**, 4446–4453.

157 Birgegård G. (1996) rhEPO treatment for anaemia of multiple myeloma and non-Hodgkin's lymphoma. In: *rh Erythropoietin in Cancer Supportive Treatment* (eds J.F. Smyth, M. Boogaeris & B.R.M. Ehmer), pp. 85–98. Marcel Dekker, New York.

158 Cazzola M., Ponchio L., Beguin Y. *et al.* (1992) Subcutaneous erythropoietin for treatment of refractory anaemia in hematologic disorders: results of a phase I/II clinical trial. *Blood*, **79**, 29–37.

159 Lokhorst H.M., Schattenberg A., Cornelissen J.J., Thomas L.L.M. & Verdonck L.F. (1997) Successful induction of graft versus myeloma by donor leukocyte infusions in relapsed multiple myeloma after allogeneic bone marrow transplantation. In: *Proceedings (syllabus) VI International Workshop on Multiple Myeloma, Boston*, June 1997.

160 Kwak L.W., Jagannath S., Seigel G., Tricot J., Epstein J. & Barlogie B. (1997) Tumor idiotype antigen-specific immunisation of myeloma marrow transplant donors. In: *Proceedings (syllabus) VI International Workshop on Multiple Myeloma, Boston*, June 1997.

161 Stevenson F.K. (1997) DNA vaccines against B cell tumors. In: *Proceedings (syllabus) VI International Workshop on Multiple Myeloma, Boston*, June 1997.

162 Rettig M.B., Ma H.J., Vescio R.A. *et al.* (1997) Kaposi's sarcoma-associated herpesvirus infection of bone marrow dendritic cells from multiple myeloma patients. *Science*, **276**, 1851–1854.

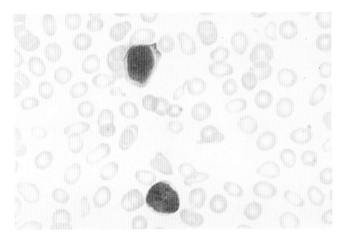

Plate 2.1 Peripheral blood film from a patient with M0 AML supervening in MDS showing two myeloblasts which, on cytological and cytochemical grounds, could not be distinguished from lymphoblasts. Diagnosis was based on immunophenotype. (MGG, ×250.)

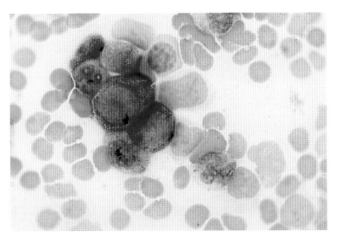

Plate 2.4 Bone marrow film in M1 AML (same case as Plate 2.3) showing a positive reaction for chloroacetate esterase in the majority of blasts. (Chloroacetate esterase reaction, ×250.)

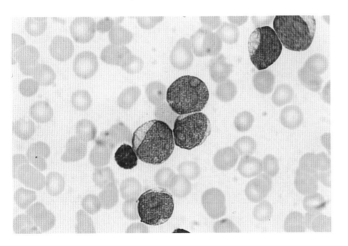

Plate 2.2 Peripheral blood film in M1 AML showing six myeloblasts and a lymphocyte. One blast contains an Auer rod. (MGG, ×250.)

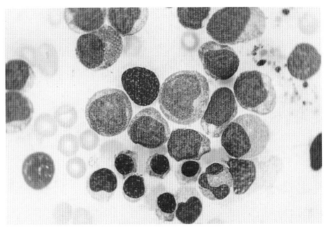

Plate 2.5 Bone marrow film in M2 AML showing a mixture of blasts and maturing cells of granulocyte lineage. The patient had t(8;21) (q22;q22). (MGG, ×250.)

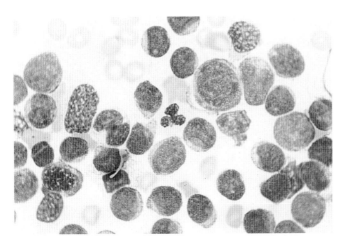

Plate 2.3 Bone marrow film in M1 AML showing blasts which lack granules and Auer rods. The presence of a hypogranular neutrophil and a dysplastic erythroblast suggests that this is M1 AML rather than ALL and this was confirmed by cytochemical reactions. (MGG, ×250.)

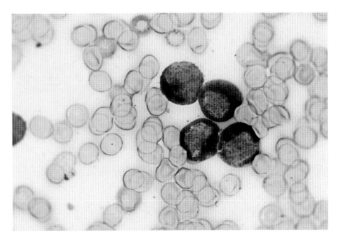

Plate 2.6 Bone marrow film in M2 AML showing Sudan black B-positive cells—one myeloblast and three maturing cells of granulocyte lineage. The patient had t(8;21) (q22;q22). (Sudan black B stain, ×250.)

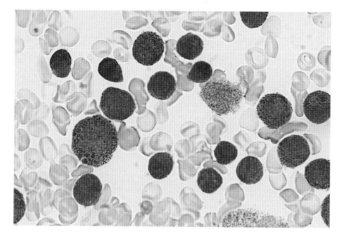

Plate 2.7 Bone marrow film in M3 AML showing hypergranular promyelocytes with large brightly staining granules packing the cytoplasm. A giant granule is apparent in one cell. (MGG, ×250.)

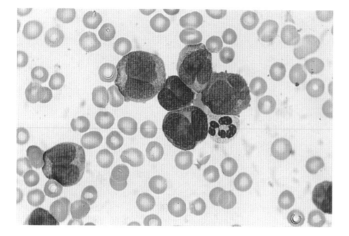

Plate 2.8 Peripheral blood film in M3 variant AML showing variant (hypogranular or microgranular) promyelocytes with characteristic bilobulated nuclei. (MGG, ×250.)

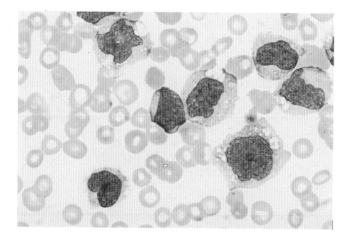

Plate 2.9 Peripheral blood film in M4 AML showing two myeloblasts and four monoblasts. The myeloblasts are relatively small with a high nucleocytoplasmic ratio. The monoblasts are larger with lobulated nuclei and plentiful weakly basophilic vacuolated cytoplasm. (MGG, ×250.)

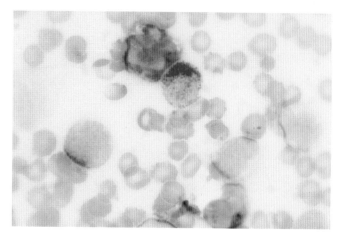

Plate 2.10 Bone marrow film in M4 AML showing one chloroacetate-positive myeloblast (red) and three alpha naphthyl acetate esterase-positive monoblasts (dark brown). (Mixed esterase reaction, ×250.)

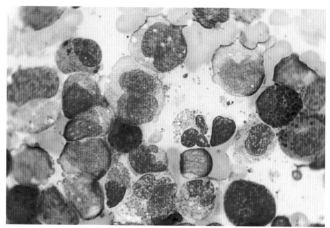

Plate 2.11 Bone marrow film in M4Eo AML (M4 AML with eosinophilia) showing monoblasts, eosinophils and eosinophil precursors with abnormally large basophilic granules. The patient had inv(16) (p13q22). (MGG, ×250.)

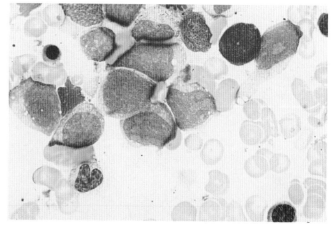

Plate 2.12 Bone marrow film in M5a AML showing that the predominant cell is a monoblast. (MGG, ×250.)

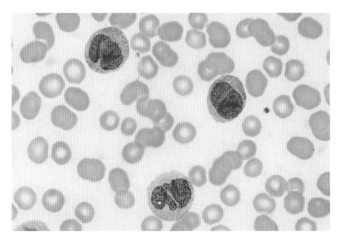

Plate 2.13 Peripheral blood film in M5b AML showing maturing cells of monocyte lineage. (MGG, ×250.)

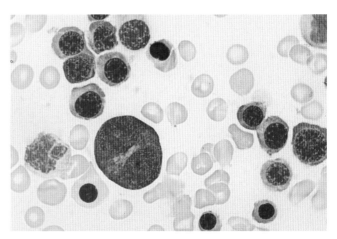

Plate 2.16 Bone marrow film in M6 AML showing a predominance of erythroblasts, one of which is binucleated. More than 30% of nonerythroid cells were myeloblasts. (MGG, ×250.)

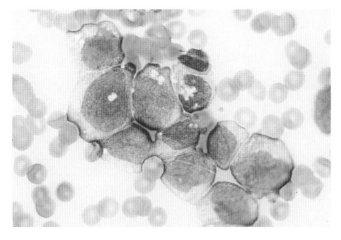

Plate 2.14 Bone marrow film in M5b AML showing a mixture of monoblasts and maturing cells of monocyte lineage. (MGG, ×250.)

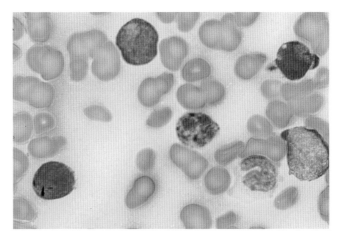

Plate 2.17 Bone marrow film in M6 AML showing primitive cells which are a mixture of proerythroblasts and myeloblasts. One of the myeloblasts contains an Auer rod. (Myeloperoxidase, ×250.)

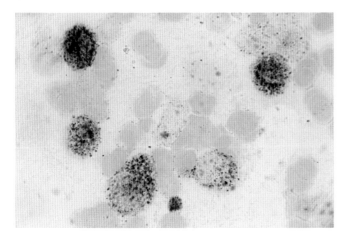

Plate 2.15 Bone marrow film in M5b AML showing a positive reaction with an alpha naphthyl acetate esterase reaction. (Alpha naphthyl acetate esterase reaction, ×250.)

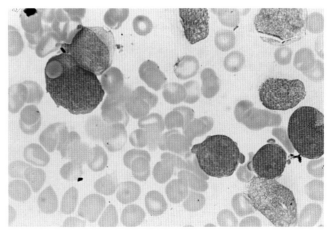

Plate 2.18 Bone marrow film in M7 AML showing megakaryoblasts, some of which have cytoplasmic blebs and one of which has phagocytosed an erythrocyte. (MGG, ×250.)

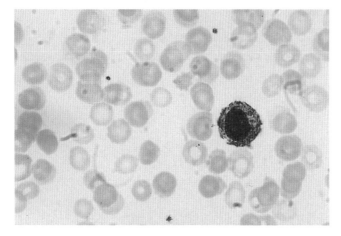

Plate 2.19 Peripheral blood film in acute mast cell leukaemia. The leukaemic cell differs from a normal mature mast cell in having a higher nucleocytoplasmic ratio and fewer granules. (MGG, × 250.)

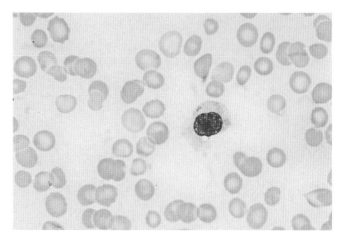

Plate 2.22 Peripheral blood film in MDS showing a neutrophil with the acquired Pelger–Hüet anomaly and a cytoplasmic Döhle body. Döhle bodies are more common in association with reactive neutrophilia but are sometimes present in MDS. (MGG, × 250.)

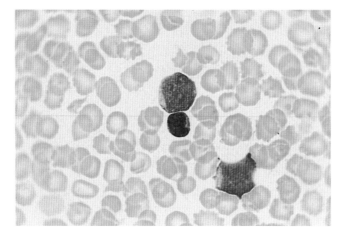

Plate 2.20 Peripheral blood film in transient abnormal myelopoiesis in a neonate with Down's syndrome showing two megakaryoblasts and a lymphocyte. (MGG, × 250.)

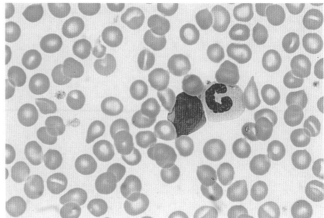

Plate 2.23 Peripheral blood film in MDS showing a myeloblast and a hypogranular neutrophil. There are also poikilocytes including stomatocytes and tear-drop poikilocytes. Platelet numbers are reduced and there is a poorly granulated platelet. (MGG, × 250.)

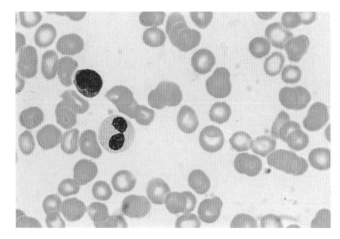

Plate 2.21 Peripheral blood film in MDS showing a neutrophil with the acquired Pelger–Hüet anomaly. There is also macrocytosis. (MGG, × 250.)

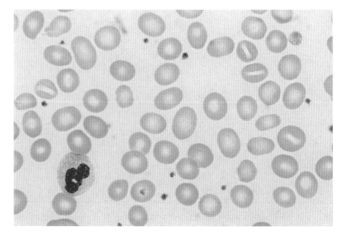

Plate 2.24 Peripheral blood film in MDS (refractory anaemia) showing macrocytosis, ovalocytosis and stomatocytosis. (MGG, × 250.)

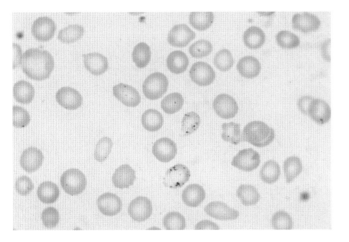

Plate 2.25 Peripheral blood film in MDS (refractory anaemia with ring sideroblasts) showing hypochromic cells and Pappenheimer bodies. (MGG, ×250.)

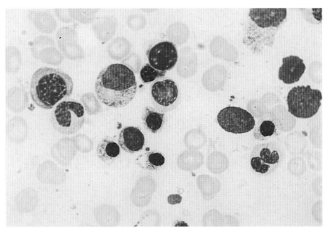

Plate 2.28 Bone marrow film in MDS (refractory anaemia with ring sideroblasts) showing defectively haemoglobinized erythroblasts with Pappenheimer bodies. (MGG, ×250.)

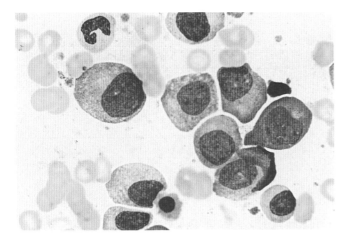

Plate 2.26 Bone marrow film in MDS (refractory anaemia) showing severe erythroid hypoplasia and poorly granulated granulocyte precursors. Erythroid hyperplasia is more typical of MDS but it is important to recognize cases of MDS which simulate pure red cell aplasia. (MGG, ×250.)

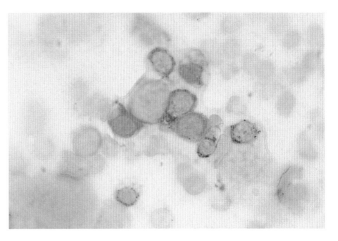

Plate 2.29 Bone marrow film in MDS (refractory anaemia with ring sideroblasts) showing numerous ring sideroblasts. (Perl's stain, ×250.)

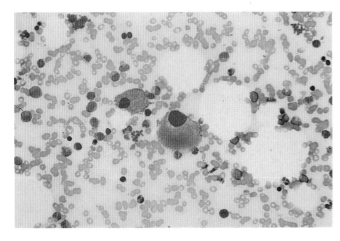

Plate 2.27 Bone marrow film in MDS (refractory anaemia) associated with 5q- showing typical large megakaryocytes with hypolobulated nuclei. This megakaryocyte morphology is typical of the 5q- syndrome. (MGG, ×60.)

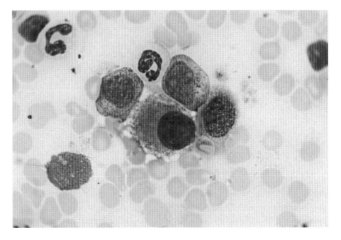

Plate 2.30 Bone marrow film in MDS (refractory anaemia with excess of blasts in transformation) showing a micromegakaryocyte. (MGG, ×250.)

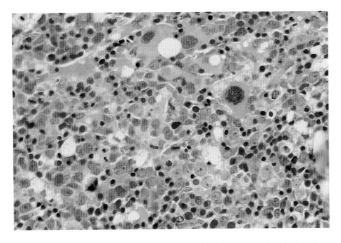

Plate 2.31 Section of bone marrow trephine biopsy in MDS showing ALIP and megakaryocytes with hypolobulated nuclei. (MGG, ×250.)

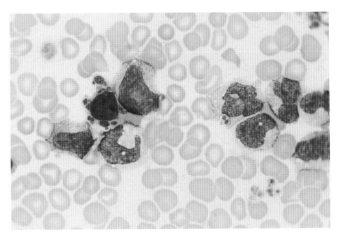

Plate 2.34 Bone marrow film in aCML (same case as Plate 2.33) showing a micromegakaryocyte and dysplastic granulocyte and monocyte precursors. (MGG, ×250.)

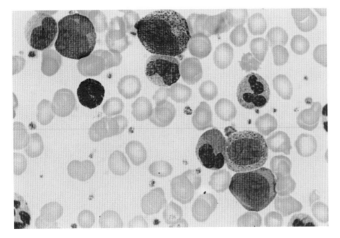

Plate 2.32 Peripheral blood film in chronic granulocytic leukaemia showing a basophil and a spectrum of cells of neutrophil lineage. (MGG, ×250.)

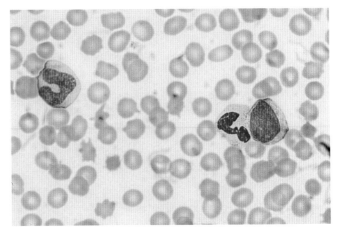

Plate 2.35 Peripheral blood film in CMML showing a neutrophil, a monocyte and an immature cell of uncertain lineage. There is also poikilocytosis as a result of dyserythropoiesis. (MGG, ×250.)

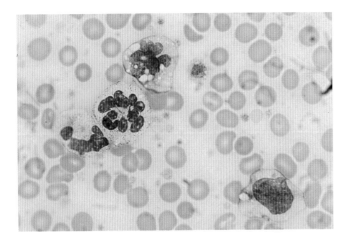

Plate 2.33 Peripheral blood film in aCML showing two neutrophils and two monocytes. One neutrophil is a macropolycyte and one monocyte is immature. There is also a giant platelet. (MGG, ×250.)

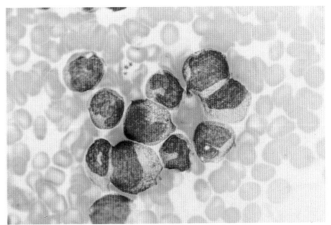

Plate 2.36 Bone marrow film in CMML showing granulocyte and monocyte precursors. (In some cases of CMML monocyte precursors are not so readily detected on an MGG stain, because they may resemble promyelocytes cytologically; esterase cytochemistry is then necesssary to confirm their nature.) (MGG, ×250.)

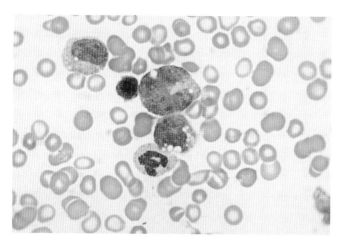

Plate 2.37 Peripheral blood film in juvenile CML showing a neutrophil, a nucleated red cell and large bizarre monocyte precursors. (MGG, ×250.) (Courtesy of Dr O. Oakhill and Dr G.R. Standen, Bristol.)

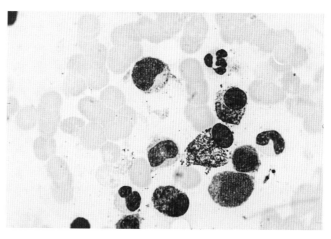

Plate 2.40 Bone marrow film in systemic mastocytosis (same case as Plate 2.39) showing hypogranular neutrophils and highly abnormal mast cells and mast cell precursors. (MGG, ×250.)

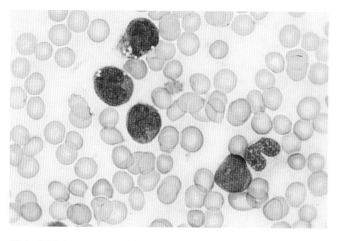

Plate 2.38 Bone marrow film in juvenile CML (same case as Plate 2.37) showing a neutrophil, immature cells of monocyte lineage and a blast cell. (MGG, ×250.)

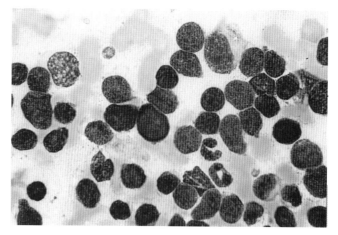

Plate 2.41 Bone marrow film in L1 ALL showing a uniform population of lymphoblasts. (MGG, ×250.)

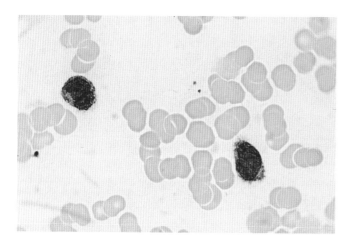

Plate 2.39 Peripheral blood film in systemic mastocytosis showing two very abnormal mast cells. (MGG, ×250.) (Courtesy of Dr D. Thompson.)

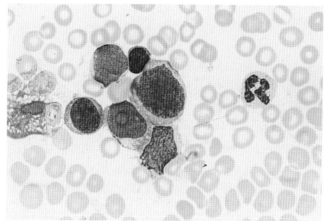

Plate 2.42 Bone marrow film in L2 ALL showing pleomorphic lymphoblasts. (MGG, ×250.)

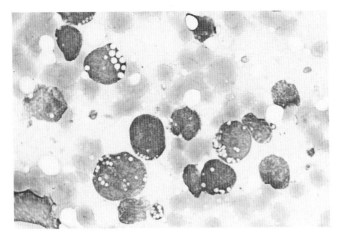

Plate 2.43 Bone marrow film in L3 ALL showing lymphoblasts with moderate cytoplasmic basophilia and heavy vacuolation. (MGG, ×250.)

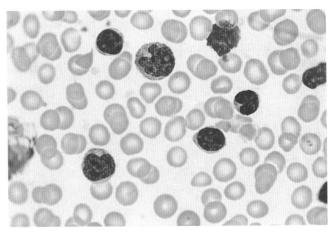

Plate 2.46 Peripheral blood film in CLL, mixed cell type, showing small lymphocytes, pleomorphic prolymphocytes and smear cells. (MGG, ×250.)

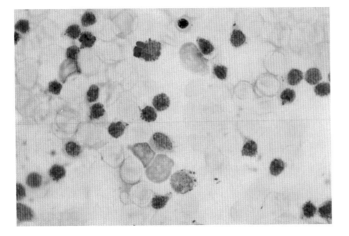

Plate 2.44 Bone marrow film in L1 ALL showing PAS-block positivity. (PAS, ×250.)

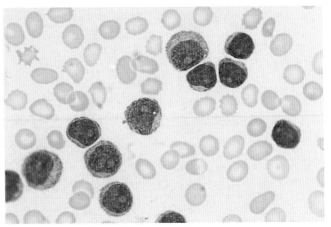

Plate 2.47 Peripheral blood film in B-PLL showing large cells with prominent vesicular nucleoli. (MGG, ×250.)

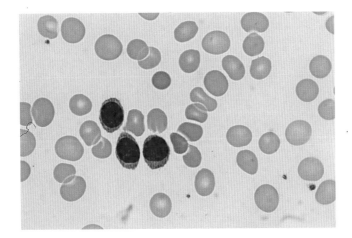

Plate 2.45 Peripheral blood film in CLL showing mature small lymphocytes with chromatin condensed in blocks. The patient had associated autoimmune haemolytic anaemia and spherocytes are present. (MGG, ×250.)

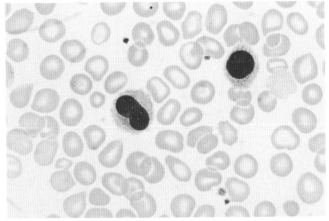

Plate 2.48 Peripheral blood film in HCL showing two hairy cells; one has a peanut-shaped nucleus. (MGG, ×250.)

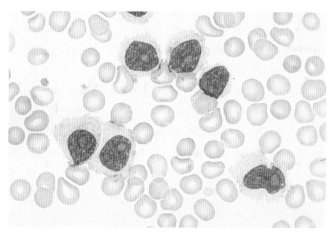

Plate 2.49 Peripheral blood film in the variant form of HCL showing cells with cytoplasm which resembles that of a hairy cell but a nucleus which resembles that of a prolymphocyte. (MGG, ×250.) (Courtesy of Professor D. Catovsky, London.)

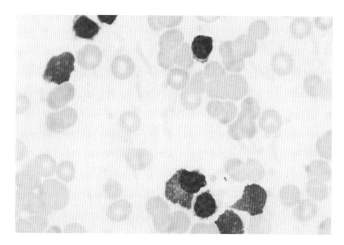

Plate 2.52 Bone marrow film in lymphoplasmacytoid lymphoma showing small lymphocytes, smear cells and a plasma cell. (MGG, ×250.)

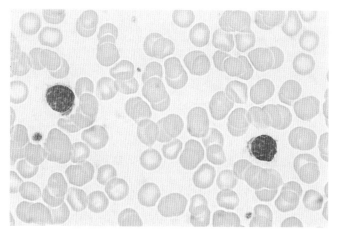

Plate 2.50 Peripheral blood film in SLVL showing two small mature lymphocytes with scanty irregular cytoplasm. (MGG, ×250.)

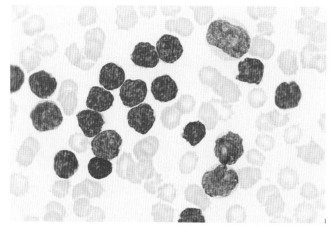

Plate 2.53 Peripheral blood film in mantle cell lymphoma showing somewhat pleomorphic lymphocytes. (MGG, ×250.) (Courtesy of Dr E. Matutes, London.)

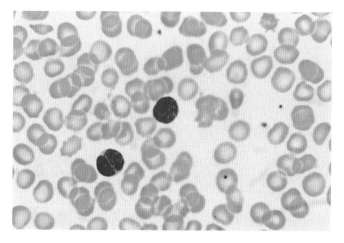

Plate 2.51 Peripheral blood film in follicular lymphoma showing mature small lymphocytes with evenly condensed chromatin and very scanty cytoplasm. One cell has a cleft nucleus. (MGG, ×250.)

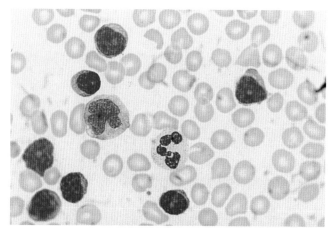

Plate 2.54 Peripheral blood film in T-PLL showing prolymphocytes which are somewhat smaller than those of B-PLL and have smaller nucleoli and denser chromatin. (MGG, ×250.)

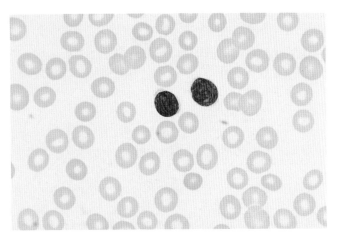

Plate 2.55 Peripheral blood film in Sézary's syndrome showing small Sézary cells with a grooved nucleus. (MGG, ×250.)

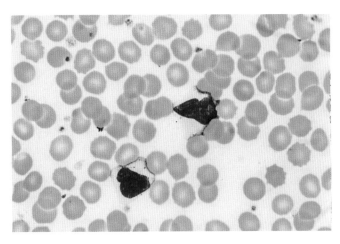

Plate 2.58 Peripheral blood film in large granular lymphocyte leukaemia showing large granular lymphocytes. (MGG, ×250.)

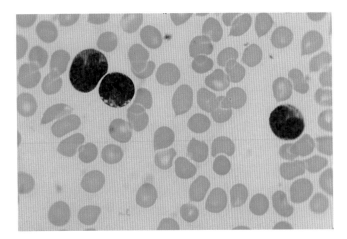

Plate 2.56 Peripheral blood film in Sézary's syndrome showing large Sézary cells with a lobulated and infolded hyperchromatic nucleus. One cell has cytoplasmic vacuoles. (MGG, ×250.)

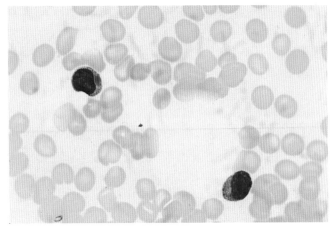

Plate 2.59 Bone marrow film in multiple myeloma showing lymphoplasmacytoid cells, one of which has a cytoplasmic inclusion. A minority of cases of multiple myeloma resemble this case in having neoplastic cells which resemble lymphoplasmacytoid lymphocytes rather than mature plasma cells. When the clinical and pathological features are typical of multiple myeloma the disease is categorized as multiple myeloma rather than as lymphoplasmacytoid lymphoma. (MGG, ×250.)

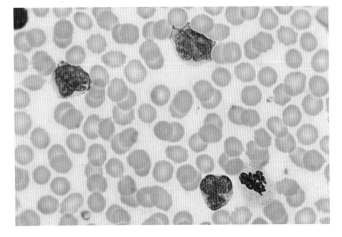

Plate 2.57 Peripheral blood film in ATLL showing pleomorphic lymphoid cells, one of which has a highly lobulated nucleus. (MGG, ×250.)

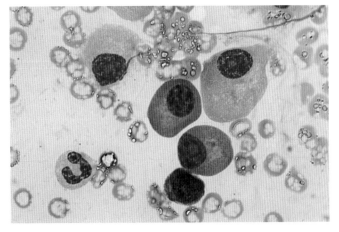

Plate 2.60 Bone marrow film in multiple myeloma showing myeloma cells which have nucleoli but which are otherwise morphologically similar to normal plasma cells. (MGG, ×250.)

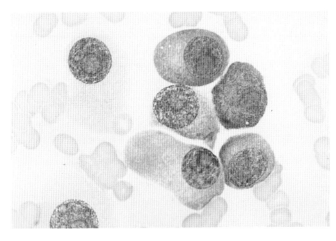

Plate 2.61 Bone marrow film in multiple myeloma showing plasmablasts. (MGG, ×250.)

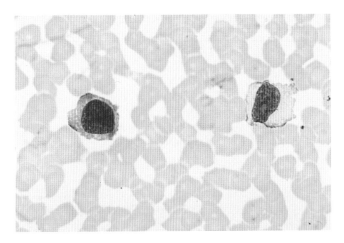

Plate 2.62 Peripheral blood film in plasma cell leukaemia showing two leukaemic cells which have some cytological features in common with normal plasma cells. Cytoplasm of the cells is weakly or moderately basophilic and shows a pink tinge at the periphery. (MGG, ×250.)

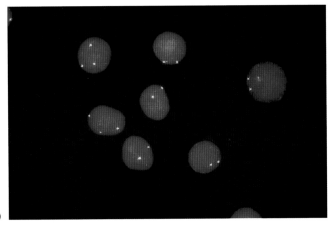

(a)

Plate 3.1 Uses of FISH. (a) Hybridization with a chromosome 8 centromeric probe (Oncor, Ltd, Gaithersburg, USA). Three spots per nucleus indicate trisomy and two spots indicate disomy. (b) Hybridization with a chromosome 12 paint (CAMBIO, Cambridge, UK). The normal chromosome 12 is in the centre of the picture, the smaller signal on the right is an isochromosome for the short arm of chromosome 12, and the larger signal on the left is an isochromosome for the long arm of chromosome 12.

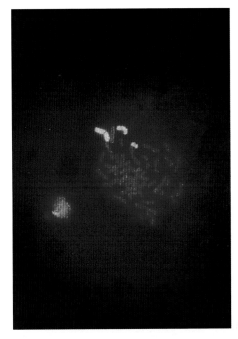

(b)

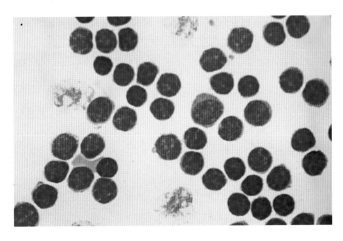

Plate 6.1 CLL cells from a leucapheresis specimen. Note the prolymphocytes and smear cells.

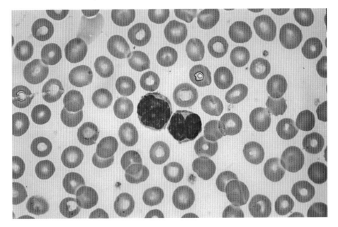

Plate 6.2 Prominent cleaved cells from a patient with CLL.

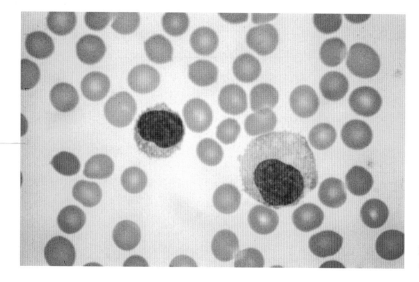

Plate 6.3 Lymphoplasmacytoid cells from a patient with CLL.

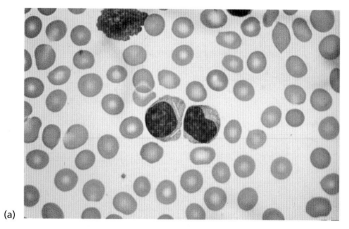

(a)

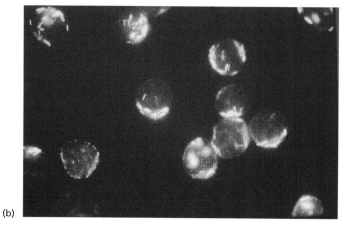

(b)

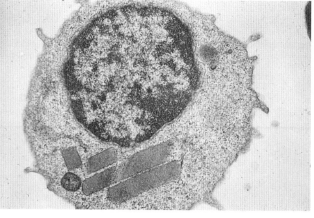

(c)

Plate 6.4 CLL cells showing IgA crystalline inclusions in the cytoplasm by (a) Romanowsky staining, (b) immunofluorescence and (c) electron microscopy.

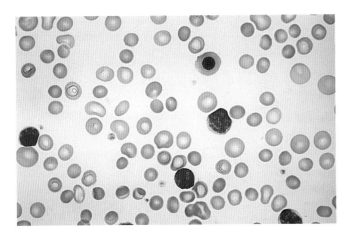

Plate 6.5 Autoimmune haemolytic anaemia complicating CLL. Note spherocytes and nucleated red cells.

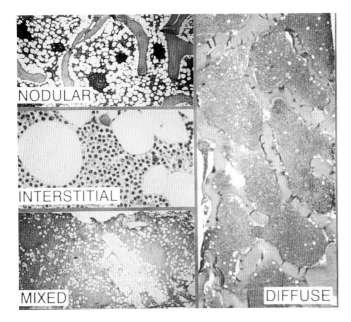

NODULAR

INTERSTITIAL

MIXED

DIFFUSE

Plate 6.6 Four patterns of bone marrow histology in CLL; nodular, interstitial, mixed nodular and interstitial, and diffuse. (Courtesy of Dr E. Montserrat and Dr C. Rozman. Reproduced by permission of *British Journal of Haematology*, Blackwell Science Ltd.)

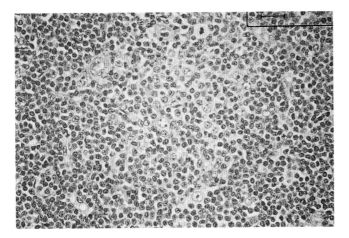

Plate 6.7 Lymph-node histology showing proliferation centre.

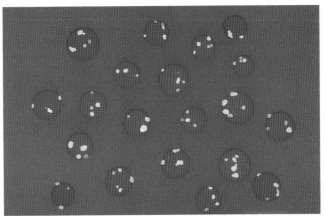

Plate 6.8 Fluorescent *in situ* hybridization in CLL using probes for the centromeric region of chromosome 12 (staining blue) and for Rb on chromosome 13q14 (staining rare). Trisomy 12 and de13q14 are shown in the same cells. This occurs in only 6% of CLLs. (Courtesy of Dr J. Garcia-Marco.)

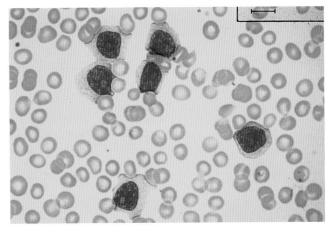

Plate 6.9 Cells from a patient with PLL. Note the more open nuclear chromatin and prominent nucleolus together with more abundant cytoplasm.

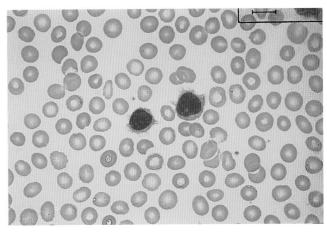

Plate 6.10 Cells from a patient with SLVL. Note the unipolar fine villous cytoplasmic projections. The chromatin is more condensed than in PLL but, as here, a single nucleolus may be seen.

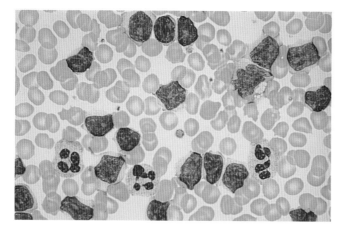

Plate 6.11 Cells from a patient with MCL. The cells are pleomorphic, moderate to large with irregular nuclei and variable nuclear indentation.

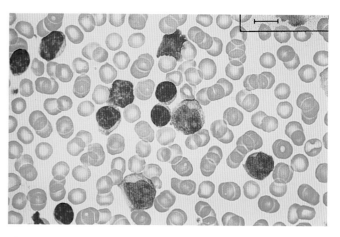

Plate 6.14 Cells from a patient with CLL/PLL.

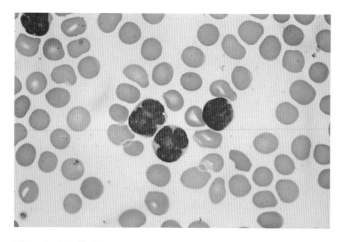

Plate 6.12 Cells from a patient with follicular lymphoma in leukaemic phase. Note the minimal cytoplasm, the smooth nuclear chromatin and the characteristic nuclear clefts.

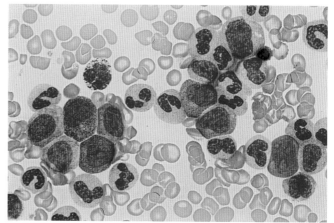

Plate 13.1 Appearances of the peripheral blood of an untreated CML patient. Note the increased numbers of normal-appearing neutrophils, one basophil and the immature granulocytes (myelocytes, promyelocytes and blast cell). There is also one erythroblast. (May-Grunwald Giemsa, × 2500.)

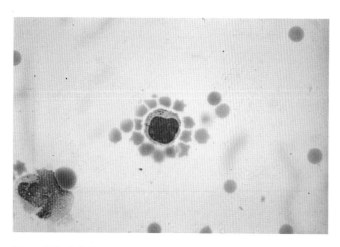

Plate 6.13 Cells from a patient with LGL leukaemia. Note the abundant cytoplasm with multiple azurophil granules, and the rosette formed with sheep red blood cells.

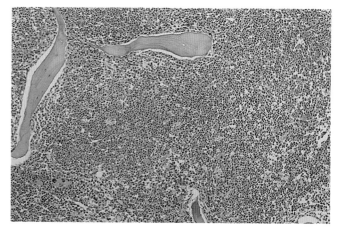

Plate 13.2 Appearances of the bone marrow biopsy of a CML patient. Note the dense cellularity with complete obliteration of normal fat spaces. (May-Grunwald Giemsa, × 25.)

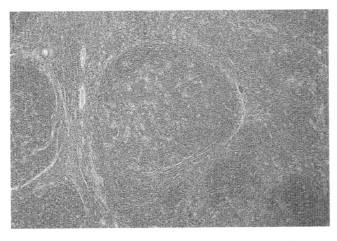

Plate 15.1 Lymphocyte-predominant HD showing a macronodular growth pattern.

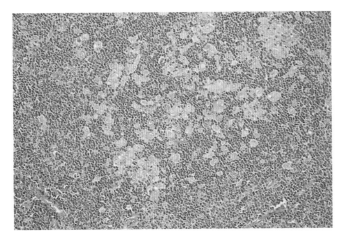

Plate 15.2 Lymphocyte-predominant HD displaying a 'moth-eaten' appearance with admixed small and large lymphoid cells, epithelioid histiocytes and occasional L&H cells.

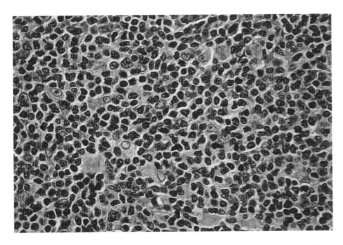

Plate 15.3 Lymphocyte-predominant HD. The cytology of the small B-cell component shows slightly irregular nuclear outlines.

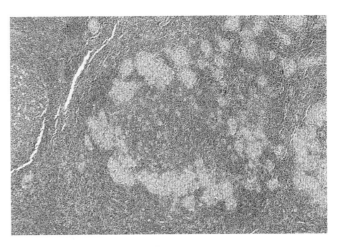

Plate 15.4 Lymphocyte-predominant HD. Sarcoid-like granulomas surround a nodule of LP HD.

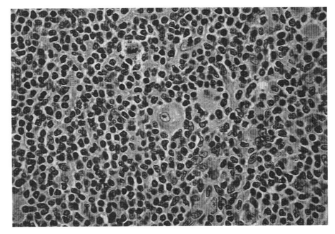

Plate 15.5 Lymphocyte-predominant HD. Typical epithelioid histiocytes showing abundant eosinophilic cytoplasm, and an open nuclear chromatin with a prominent central nucleolus.

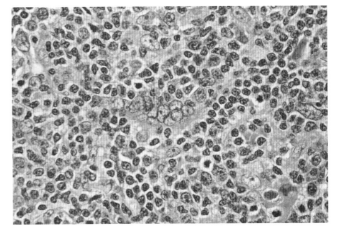

Plate 15.6 Lymphocyte-predominant HD. Multinucleated FDC resembling a Warthin–Finkeldy giant cell.

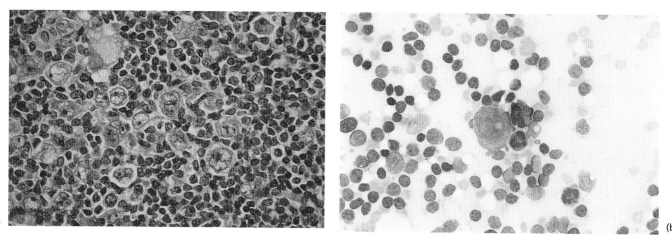

(a)   (b)

Plate 15.7 (a) Lymphocyte-predominant HD. Typical L&H cells showing large, lobulated nuclei and prominent nucleoli. (b) Lymphocyte-predominant HD. Imprint preparation stained with giemsa showing an L&H cell with adherent small lymphocytes.

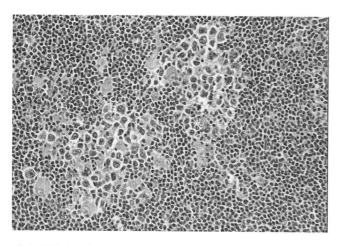

Plate 15.8 Lymphocyte-predominant HD. Numerous L&H cells are present within this nodule; the patient had suffered multiple relapses of LP HD before this biopsy.

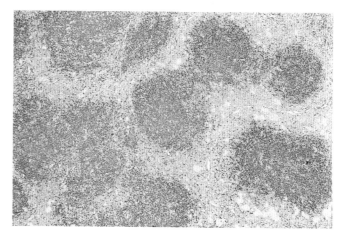

Plate 15.9 Lymphocyte-predominant HD. Immunostained for CD20 showing large B-cell-rich nodules.

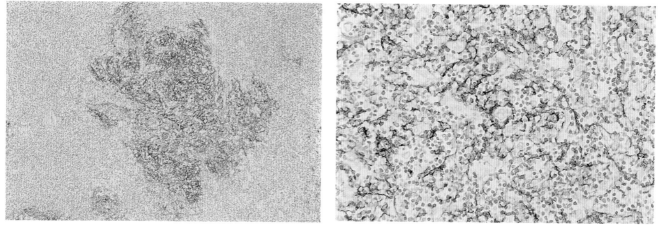

(a)   (b)

Plate 15.10 (a) Lymphocyte-predominant HD. Immunostained for CD21 showing the nodules to contain an abnormal meshwork of FDCs. (b) Lymphocyte-predominant HD. Immunostained for CD21 showing the long processes of FDCs wrapping around an L&H cell.

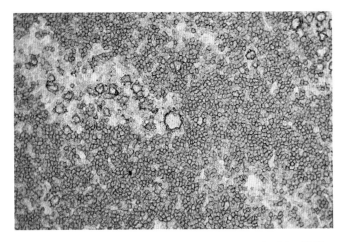

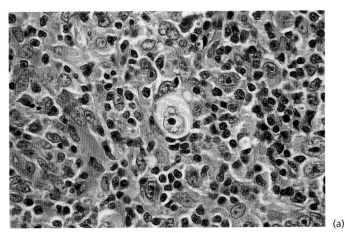
(a)

Plate 15.11 Lymphocyte-predominant HD. Immunostained for CD20 showing a B-cell-rich nodule and an L&H cell strongly stained for CD20; note the corona of unstained lymphocytes immediately adjacent to the L&H cells which represent T cells.

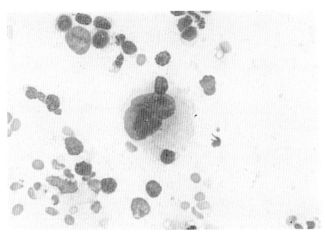
(b)

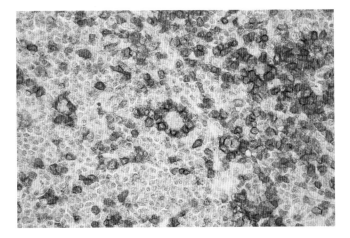

Plate 15.14 Nodular sclerosis. (a) Lacunar cells showing lobulated and twisted nuclei with prominent eosinophillic nucleoli. The cytoplasm has been dissolved during processing to leave a clear space surrounding the nucleus. (b) Imprint preparation stained with giemsa showing a lacunar cell with a large nucleus and prominent nucleolus. The cytoplasm is pale and ill defined.

Plate 15.12 Lymphocyte-predominant HD. Immunostained for CD57 showing the presence of numerous CD57+ T cells which form a corona around the L&H cells.

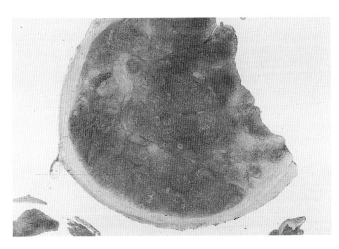

Plate 15.13 Nodular sclerosis. Lymph node showing capsular sclerosis, nodularity and early intranodal collagen band formation.

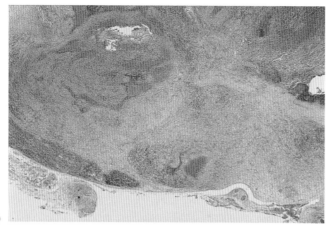

(a)

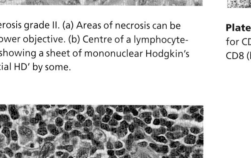

(b)

Plate 15.15 Nodular sclerosis grade II. (a) Areas of necrosis can be seen with the scanning power objective. (b) Centre of a lymphocyte-depleted cellular nodule showing a sheet of mononuclear Hodgkin's cells; this is termed 'syncitial HD' by some.

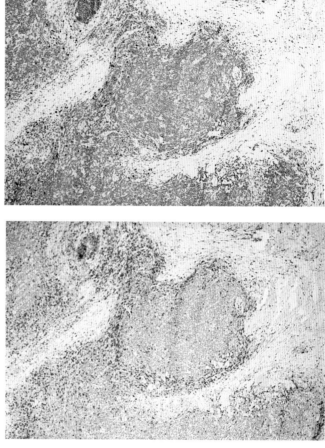

(a)

(b)

Plate 15.17 Nodular sclerosis grade I. Serial frozen sections stained for CD4 (a), showing the majority of the T cells present are CD4+ and CD8 (b) with a peripheral rim of CD8+ cells.

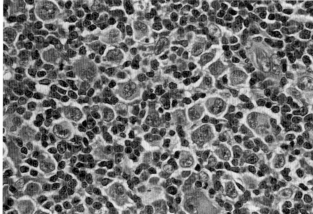

Plate 15.16 Grade II NS showing numerous pleomorphic H-RS and lacunar cells in the absence of lymphocyte depletion.

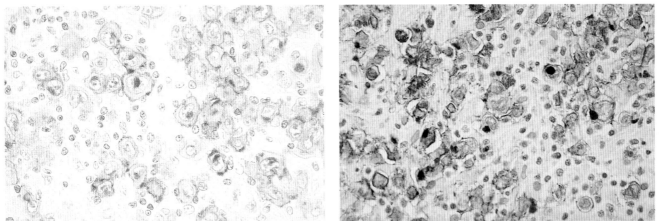

(a)

(b)

Plate 15.18 Nodular sclerosis grade I, immunostained for CD30 (a) and CD15 (b), showing a typical membrane and golgi staining.

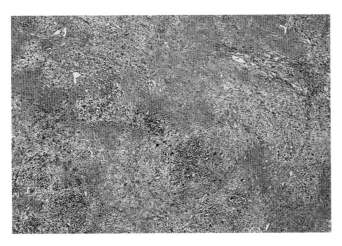

Plate 15.19 Lymphocyte-depleted HD, diffuse fibrosis type. Low power to show hypocellular background with areas of geographic necrosis.

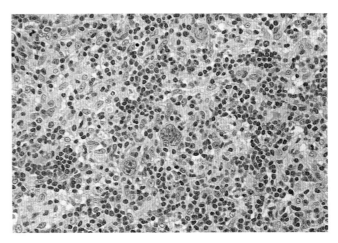

Plate 15.21 Mixed cellularity showing a classical R–S cell and a multinucleate Hodgkin's giant cell. The cellular background contains lymphocytes, histiocytes, eosinophils and plasma cells.

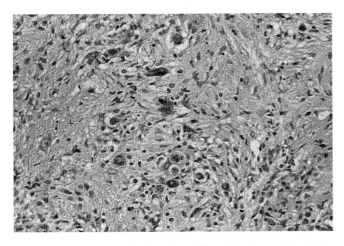

Plate 15.20 Lymphocyte-depleted HD, diffuse fibrosis type. Classic H-RS cells are often difficult to find. In their place is a population of bizarre hyperchromatic giant cells.

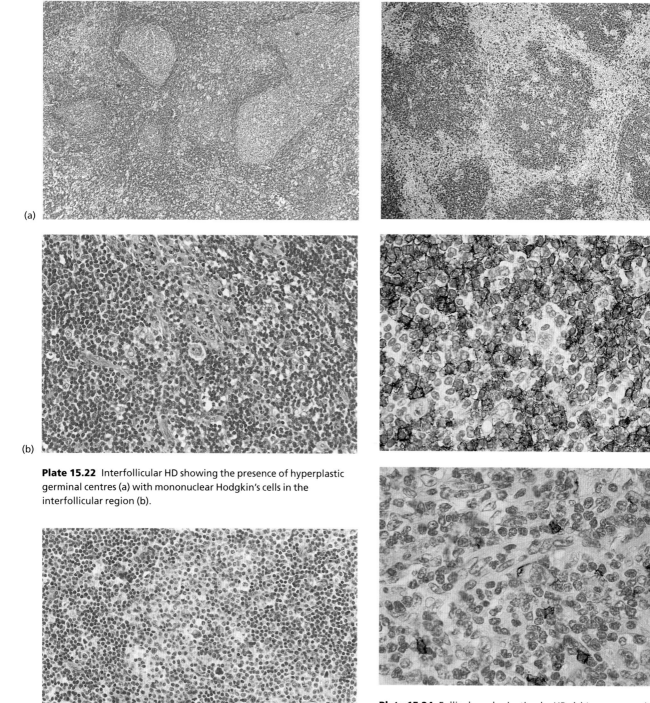

Plate 15.22 Interfollicular HD showing the presence of hyperplastic germinal centres (a) with mononuclear Hodgkin's cells in the interfollicular region (b).

Plate 15.23 H-RS cells within sheets of marginal zone B cells (HD occurring in monocytoid B-cell clusters).

Plate 15.24 Follicular colonization by HD. (a) Low-power view of CD20 immunostain showing numerous B-cell-rich nodules indistinguishable from LP nodular HD. (b) High-power view of CD20 immunostain showing the H-RS cells are negative for B-cell markers. (c) The H-RS cells within the B-cell-rich nodules express CD30.

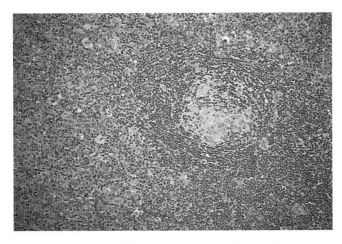

Plate 15.25 Regressive follicular changes resembling hyaline vascular Castleman's disease in response to an interfollicular infiltrate of HD.

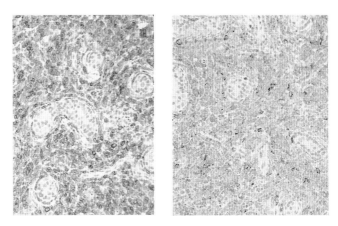

Plate 17.3 Lymph-node biopsy stained for CD20 (right) and CD79a (left). Note that there is only faint positivity for CD20, while CD79a strongly decorates the B-lymphoblasts.

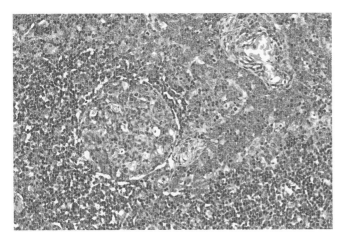

Plate 17.1 Medium-power view of a node infiltrated by B-lymphoblastic lymphoma showing an entrapped reactive follicle centre and blast cells around it and within the sinuses.

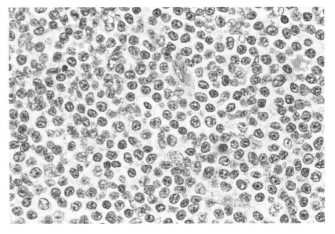

Plate 17.4 Small B-lymphocytic lymphoma. The tumour is composed of a monotonous sheet of small round lymphocytes.

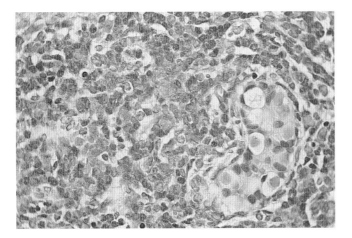

Plate 17.2 Testicular biopsy from a child with B-lymphoblastic lymphoma. Note the residual immature, atrophic seminiferous tubules.

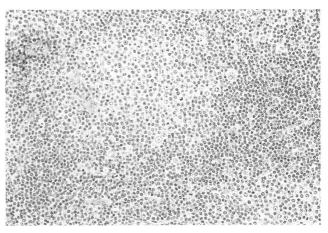

Plate 17.5 Low-power view to show the paler-staining proliferation centres, characteristic of small B-lymphocytic lymphomas.

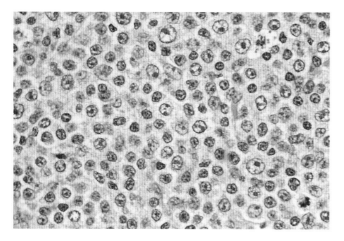

Plate 17.6 High-power detail from the pale proliferation centre seen in Plate 17.5. Note the larger cell size of the prolymphocytes compared to the small lymphocytes in Plate 17.4 and the scattered small immunoblasts.

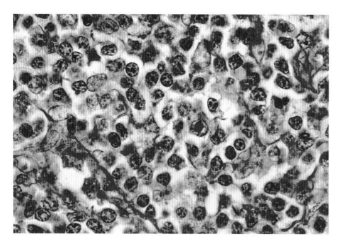

Plate 17.7 Section from a small B-lymphocytic lymphoma with plasmacytoid features. The section is stained by the PAS method, showing up bright pink intranuclear immunoglobulin inclusions (Dutcher bodies).

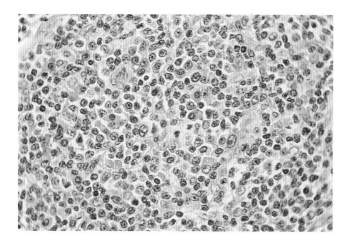

Plate 17.8 Lymph node infiltrated by a lymphoplasmacytoid immunocytoma. Note the varied cytological mix of cells, with many showing frank plasma cell differentiation.

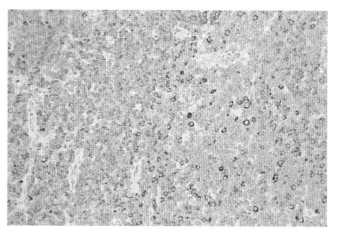

Plate 17.9 Section from the lymphoma seen in Plate 17.8 stained for IgM. Note the strong and widespread cytoplasmic positivity.

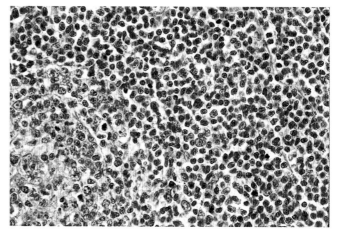

Plate 17.10 Mantle zone growth pattern in a mantle cell lymphoma. Part of the encircled benign reactive germinal centre can be seen (bottom left).

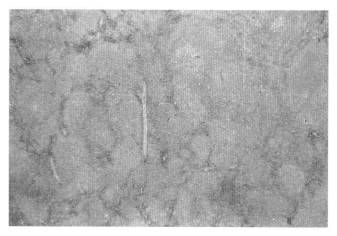

Plate 17.11 Nodular growth pattern in a mantle cell lymphoma low-power magnification.

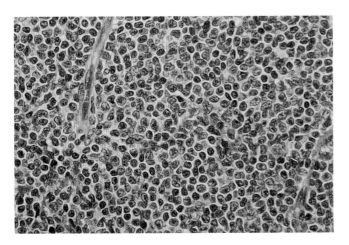

Plate 17.12 Mantle cell lymphoma at high-power magnification. Note the monotony of the neoplastic population of small irregularly shaped lymphoid cells. There are no blast cells present.

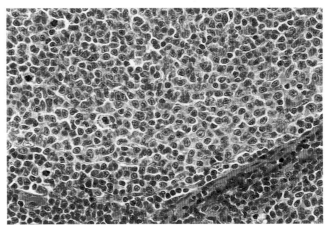

Plate 17.15 Higher magnification view from one of the malignant follicles in Plate 17.14. Note that although there is an admixture of centroblasts and centrocytes, the former are very much in the minority and scattered throughout the field, with no segregation of the two populations.

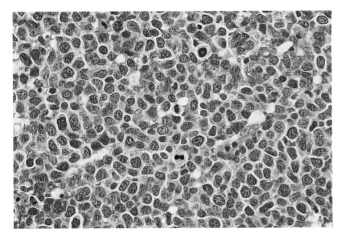

Plate 17.13 Blastoid transformation of a mantle cell lymphoma. Note the increase in cell size compared to Plate 17.12, the increased mitotic activity and the lymphoblast-like nuclear chromatin.

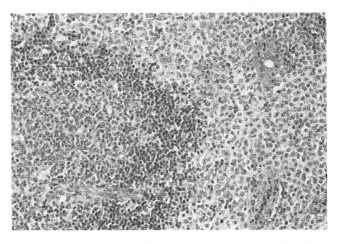

Plate 17.16 Monocytoid B-cell lymphoma in a lymph node. Note the broad zone of pale-staining lymphoma cells external to the mantle of a reactive follicle.

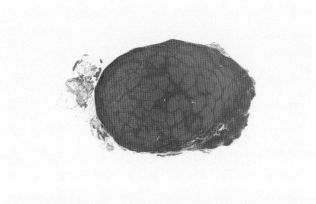

Plate 17.14 Whole-mount preparation from a follicular follicle centre lymphoma showing the complete replacement of the node by a population of even-sized neoplastic follicles.

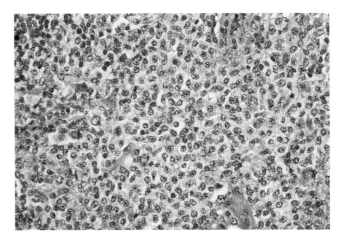

Plate 17.17 High-power view of the monocytoid B-cells seen in Plate 17.16. Note their relatively bland oval to reniform nuclei and abundant pale-staining cytoplasm.

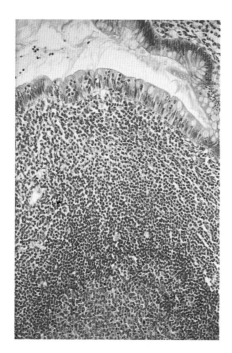

Plate 17.18 Normal Peyer's patch of the small intestine. There is a reactive follicle towards the bottom of the picture with a broad zone of cells above, some of which are infiltrating the dome epithelium.

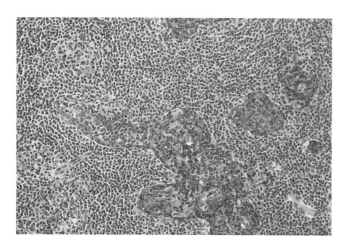

Plate 17.19 Extranodal marginal zone lymphoma of MALT type involving the parotid gland. Small reactive germinal centres are present and the surrounding lymphoma is infiltrating and expanding the parotid ducts to produce epimyoepithelial islands.

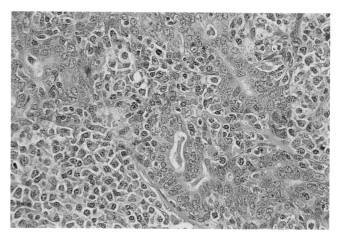

Plate 17.20 Higher magnification view of epimyoepithelial islands (lymphoepithelial lesions) in a MALT-type lymphoma of salivary origin. Neoplastic lymphocytes encircle and infiltrate the epithelium.

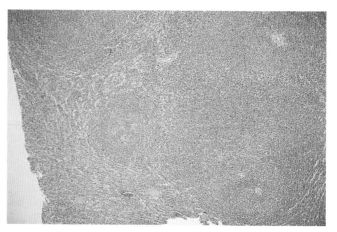

Plate 17.21 Splenic marginal zone lymphoma. Nodular collections of cells with the residua of reactive follicles in their centre are seen studded throughout the section. These nodules have a biphasic pattern imparting a dart-board-like appearance.

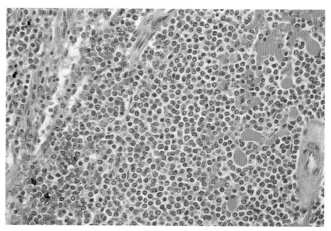

Plate 17.22 Higher-magnification view of the case seen in Plate 17.21 to show the lymphoplasmacytoid appearance of the neoplastic cells at the edge of the nodular collections.

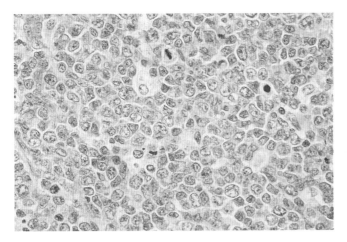

Plate 17.23 Diffuse large B-cell lymphoma composed predominantly of classical centroblasts.

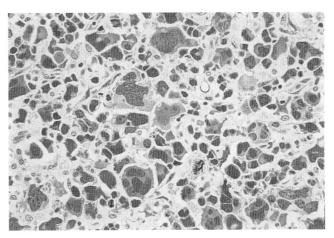

Plate 17.26 Diffuse large B-cell lymphoma composed of bizarre anaplastic giant cells.

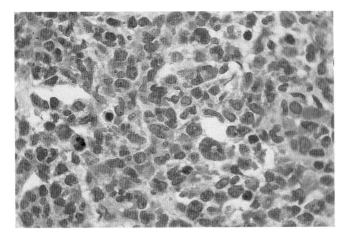

Plate 17.24 Diffuse large B-cell lymphoma composed of multilobated blast cells.

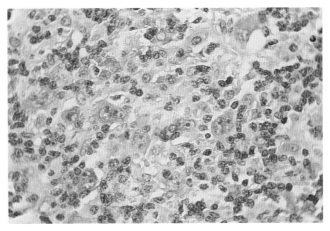

Plate 17.27 Diffuse large B-cell lymphoma with a very high content of reactive T cells; T-cell-rich B-cell lymphoma. The dispersed blast cells are pleomorphic, with some resemblance to Reed–Sternberg cells.

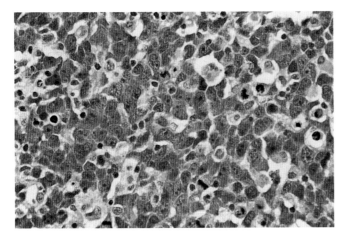

Plate 17.25 Diffuse large B-cell lymphoma composed of immunoblasts.

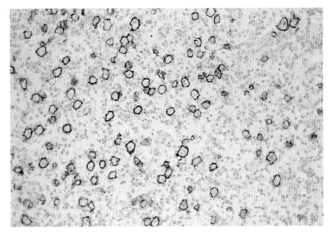

Plate 17.28 T-cell-rich B-cell lymphoma stained with the B-cell marker CD20. Note the dispersed nature of the neoplastic population.

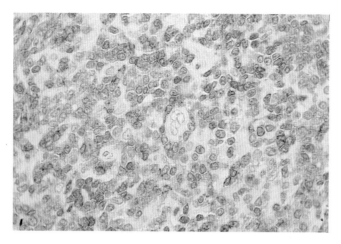

Plate 17.29 T-cell-rich B-cell lymphoma seen in Plate 17.28 stained with the T-cell marker CD3. Reactive T cells greatly outnumber the neoplastic B-blasts.

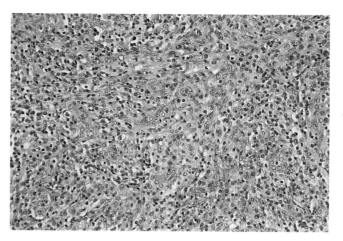

Plate 17.32 Angioimmunoblastic T-cell lymphoma. There is a very dense and abnormally branching vasculature in this field.

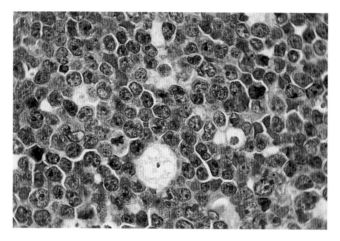

Plate 17.30 High-magnification view of a sporadic Burkitt's lymphoma. The small blasts are tightly packed together, punctuated by scattered 'starry-sky' macrophages.

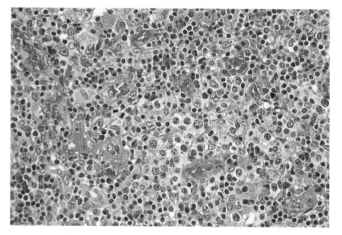

Plate 17.33 High-power view of an angioimmunoblastic T-cell lymphoma. There is a polymorphic mixture of small lymphocytes, plasma cells, eosinophils and larger lymphoid cells, with plentiful water-clear cytoplasm.

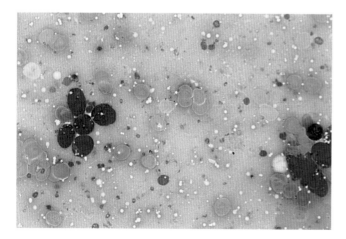

Plate 17.31 Endemic African Burkitt's lymphoma. In this touch preparation the cytoplasmic lipid droplets are well seen.

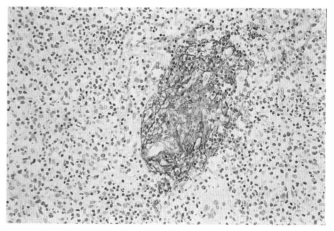

Plate 17.34 Section of an angioimmunoblastic T-cell lymphoma stained for follicular dendritic reticulum cells showing an abnormal mass of these cells in this part of the tumour.

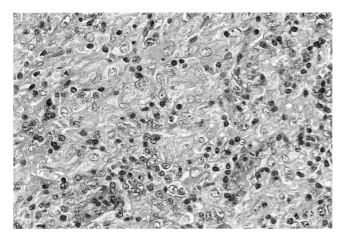

Plate 17.35 Peripheral T-cell lymphoma of Lennert's type with large numbers of reactive epithelioid histiocytes.

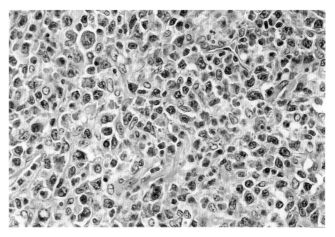

Plate 17.38 Intestinal T-cell lymphoma with a high content of eosinophils. The blast cells are relatively dispersed and exhibit nuclear pleomorphism.

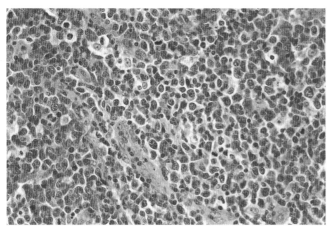

Plate 17.36 Peripheral T-cell lymphoma of pleomorphic medium-size cells. Despite their size, the large cells show considerable traffic through high endothelial venules.

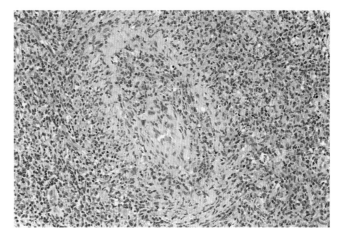

Plate 17.39 Angiocentric lymphoma of possible NK-cell type arising in the nose. There is destructive infiltration of a large venule in the centre of the field by the pleomorphic blast cells.

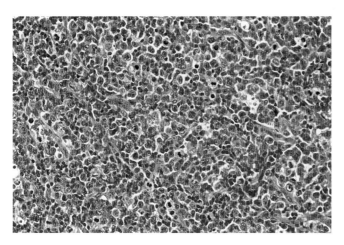

Plate 17.37 Adult T-cell lymphoma/leukaemia in a lymph-node biopsy. The tumour cells are large, bizarre blast forms.

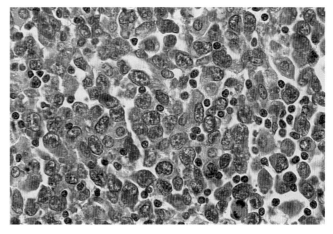

Plate 17.40 Anaplastic large cell lymphoma of T-cell phenotype. The cells are large with reniform nuclei and abundant cytoplasm.

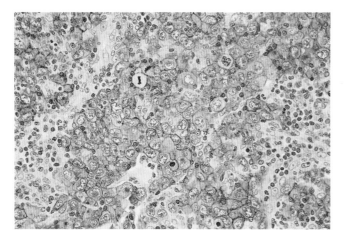

Plate 17.41 Anaplastic large cell lymphoma stained for CD30 antigen and showing widespread strong immunoreactivity.

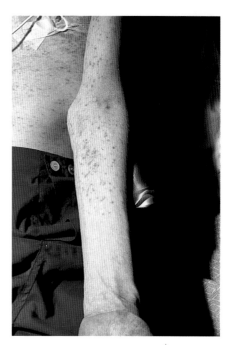

Plate 22.2 Maculopapular form of skin GVHD.

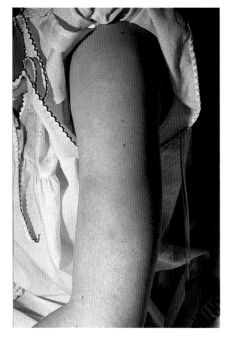

Plate 22.1 Typical early GVHD of the skin.

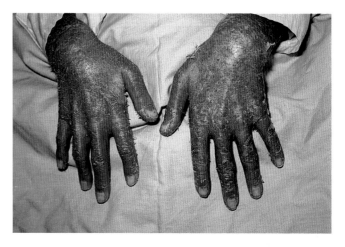

Plate 22.3 Very severe GVHD of the skin with erythroderma and desquamation.

15 Morphology and Classification of Hodgkin's Disease

K.A. MacLennan

Introduction

The first descriptions of the disease currently termed Hodgkin's disease (HD) are attributed to Thomas Hodgkin [1] and the term 'Hodgkin's disease' was generously applied by Sir Samuel Wilks [2]; there are, however, several texts describing a similar disease process which antedate both these workers' manuscripts [3,4]. These early descriptions of HD were all concerned with the macroscopic appearances and distribution of affected lymph nodes, spleen and visceral organs as observed at postmortem examination. Thus there exists some doubt about the exact nature of the disease processes being described. Herbert Fox [5], after histological examination of pathological material from three of Thomas Hodgkin's original cases, believed two were typical of HD and one was an example of lymphosarcoma or leukaemia; other skilled observers have concurred with this view [6,7].

During the latter half of the nineteenth century, many workers undertook histological examination of cases which were felt to be similar to HD [8–11]. From these descriptions, there emerged an awareness that the normal structure of the lymph node was replaced by abnormal tissue, often described as fibrous tissue, and the disease was associated with unusual giant cells. In 1898 Sternberg gave a masterful description of these giant cells [12] which, 4 years later, was followed by the publication of Dorothy Reed's classic paper [13].

Following the meticulous histological descriptions of HD by these early microscopists, terminological confusion was soon to emerge and, by 1933, Walhauser was able to find 52 symptoms for this condition (an unusually large number, even for the field of lymphoreticular pathology) [14]. This ridiculous state of affairs was only resolved by the widespread adoption of the Jackson & Parker classification [15] (see below).

In the early part of the twentieth century, some workers attempted to correlate the histological appearances of HD with the clinical course. Ewing (1919) recognized a rapidly fatal form of the disease, characterized by depletion of lymphocytes and a sheet-like growth of pleomorphic mononuclear and multinuclear cells, which he termed 'Hodgkin's sarcoma' [16].

Rosenthal observed the inverse relationship between the number of lymphocytes and abnormal reticulum cells; he was also able to correlate survival and response to orthovoltage radiotherapy to the histological appearances [17].

Following the work of Rosenthal, Jackson & Parker [15,18–20] proposed their classification of HD. Three histological subtypes were recognized — paragranuloma, granuloma and sarcoma — which showed a good correlation with clinical behaviour and prognosis. Unfortunately, the classification proved to be of limited value, as the majority of cases were classified as Hodgkin's granuloma [17,21], and this subtype showed an extremely variable clinical course [22]. These problems were overcome by the widespread adoption of the Lukes & Butler classification and its modification proposed at the Rye conference [23–26], which has remained essentially unchanged for over 20 years; most pathologists believe they are familiar with the terminology and criteria employed. It is therefore surprising to find high levels of disagreement between pathologists in establishing the diagnosis of HD, and in its classification, which may range from 13% [27,28] to a staggering figure of 47% reported by Symmers [29].

The reasons for the difficulties pathologists experience in the diagnosis of HD are not too difficult to understand. HD is rare, most pathologists will see only a few cases a year, and this, combined with the complexity of the histological picture, which may be closely mimicked by a variety of neoplastic and non-neoplastic lymphoproliferative conditions, will lead to errors in diagnosis. These problems are compounded by our lack of understanding of the basic biology of HD and our ignorance of the precise identity of the Reed–Sternberg cell (R–S cell). Indeed, it now appears that there may be several distinctive biological entities cohabiting under this eponymous term, and the borderline between HD and the non-Hodgkin's lymphomas (NHLs) may not solely be due to our difficulties in pathological diagnosis, but it may represent a real biological interface between the two disease processes [7].

Lymphocyte-predominant Hodgkin's disease

For many years HD with a predominance of lymphocytes has been recognized as having a more indolent natural history [15,17,22–24,30–32] than usual-type HD.

Lukes & Butler [25] described a form of HD which contained a spectrum of cytological appearances, ranging from a predominance of mature lymphocytes to a histiocyte-rich cellular background, which they termed lymphocytic and/or histiocytic (L&H) HD; they recognized nodular and diffuse architectural patterns. These cytological and architectural patterns of L&H HD were amalgamated at the Rye Conference [26] and termed 'lymphocytic predominance' (LP).

Lymphocyte-predominant HD makes up a variable percentage of cases of HD in large series which are dependent on the stringency of the diagnostic criteria applied [33]. In the BNLI series of 4249 cases, LP comprises 5.7%, and in the EORTC–GELA studies of localized HD (H8), which include 722 centrally reviewed cases, LP makes up 4% (M. Henry-Amar & J. Marnay, personal communication). Hodgkin's disease with lymphocyte predominance usually presents with localized, asymptomatic disease and often involves unusual sites such as the suprahyoid neck, the periparotid lymph nodes and the inguinal region. There is a marked male predominance, and patients are usually a decade older than the peak age incidence of usual-type HD [34].

For many years there was a lack of precision in the diagnosis of LP, with many cases of usual-type HD which displayed a lymphocyte-rich cellular background being included in this category. In a seminal paper published in 1979, Poppema and coworkers [35] recognized the cytological similarities between LP nodular HD and a reactive condition affecting germinal centres, termed 'progressive transformation' [36,37]. They postulated that LP nodular HD was a distinct form of HD, which arose in the B-cell regions of the lymph node and was related to progressive transformation of germinal centres. In order to emphasize the differences between LP nodular and other histological subtypes of HD, they proposed the term 'nodular paragranuloma', which has been adopted by some workers.

Morphological features

Lymph nodes affected by LP nodular HD are enlarged and can reach significant sizes (up to 5 cm); their cut surface has a uniform fleshy appearance and, occasionally, residual remnants of lymph node may be observed which are compressed at the periphery of an expansile tumour mass [38].

Microscopically LP nodular HD is characterized by the presence of a macronodular growth pattern, which is expansile rather than infiltrative (see Plate 15.1 between pp. 292 and 293); nodules do not penetrate the lymph-node capsule or extend into perinodal tissue. Diffuse areas are sometimes seen.

Exclusively diffuse LP HD is exceptionally rare in our experience; the majority of cases are, in fact, NHLs of peripheral T cell or T-cell-rich B-cell type [39].

The nodules of LP nodular HD often have a moth-eaten appearance at low power microscopy (see Plate 15.2) and are composed of small round or slightly irregular lymphoid cells with admixed large lymphoid cells, epithelioid histiocytes, dendritic reticulum cells and a Reed–Sternberg cell variant called the L&H or popcorn cell. The lymphocytes within the nodules show a close cytological similarity to mantle zone lymphocytes (see Plate 15.3), which is confirmed by their phenotype. Epithelioid histiocytes may be scattered within the nodules or form loose aggregates; well-formed, sarcoid-like granulomas, if present, are usually seen at the periphery of the nodules and may form encircling rings (see Plate 15.4). The histiocytes bear a close resemblance to those seen in mantle cell lymphoma, and possess an open nuclear chromatin with a single prominent nucleolus and a well-defined eosinophilic cytoplasm (see Plate 15.5). The nuclei of follicular dendritic cells are easily identified and multinucleated forms, resembling Warthin–Finkeldy giant cells, are common (see Plate 15.6).

L&H cells have a characteristic morphology with a large, irregular and often lobulated nucleus, with a prominent nucleolus which is often amphophillic and irregular (see Plate 15.7). Classical R–S cells are rare and are not essential for the diagnosis of LP nodular HD; in fact, if classical R–S cells can be found with ease the diagnosis of LP nodular HD should be changed to one of mixed cellularity, as the clinical behaviour of these cases is different from typical LP [40]. The number of L&H cells is very variable and ranges from scanty to very numerous, making up more than 10% of the cellular composition of the nodules (see Plate 15.8); the latter is often seen in relapses of LP nodular. The number of L&H cells present does not seem to influence the clinical behaviour [34]. L&H cells may be confined to the nodules or may spill out into the internodular region of the node.

Immunocytochemistry

The nodules of LP nodular HD are composed of polytypic small B cells, expressing CD20 and CD79a [41–45] (see Plate 15.9 between pp. 292 and 293), and showing coexpression of IgM and IgD in a similar fashion to mantle zone B cells [45]. Within the nodules is a meshwork of follicular dendritic cells (FDCs), which are revealed by staining for CD21 and CD35, and their processes often wrap around the L&H cells (see Plate 15.10).

The L&H cells uniformly express a B-cell phenotype with strong expression of CD20 and CD79a [46,47] (see Plate 15.11). There is evidence of immunoglobulin synthetic capacity, as shown by the presence of a J-chain within the L&H cells [48], and some workers have shown the presence of kappa light-chain restriction either by immunocytochemistry [49] or by *in situ* hybridization for light-chain messenger RNA [50,51].

The markers of H-RS cells, CD30 and CD15, are not usually detected on L&H cells [52] (there is some evidence for expression of a heavily sialylated form of CD15, which is undetectable without prior neuraminidase digestion [53]), and their presence should prompt consideration of a diagnosis of follicular colonization by usual-type HD (see below). There is frequent expression of epithelial membrane antigen by L&H cells [54], and the presence of EBV is not usually detectable [33,47,55].

Within the nodules are numerous T cells which express CD3; numerous CD57+ T cells are also seen and these may form rosettes around the L&H cells (see Plate 15.12). The number of CD57 has proved useful in the differential diagnosis of LP HD and lymphocyte-rich classic HD (LRCHD). Cases of LP have been shown to have >200 CD57+ cells per high-power field in LRCHD [33].

Non-Hodgkin's lymphoma arising in patients with lymphocyte-predominant nodular Hodgkin's disease

It is now clear from several large studies of patients with LP nodular HD that there is a markedly increased risk of NHL, which ranges from an incidence of 3.8% [56] to nearly 10% [57]. The lymphomas associated with LP nodular HD may occur simultaneously [58–61] or after a period of many years [56,59,62,63]. They are usually of B-cell lineage [56,58,59] and there is some evidence that there may be a clonal relationship between the original LP and the subsequent B-cell NHL [63,64]; other workers have been unable to confirm this [62]. The morphology of these secondary, high-grade B-cell lymphomas is variable, with some showing features typical of diffuse large B-cell lymphoma exhibiting centroblastic or immunoblastic cytology, while others resemble sheets of L&H cells.

Since the first recognition of T-cell lineage NHL following LP nodular HD [56], subsequent reports have confirmed this association [65,66]. Weisenburger and coworkers have reported the concurrent presentation of T-cell NHL and LP nodular HD [67]. These may have a variety of histological patterns, but the majority appear to fall within the peripheral T-cell lymphoma, unspecified group of the revised European–American Classification of lymphoid neoplasms (REAL) [68].

Nodular sclerosis

The presence of fibrosis and the proliferation of fibroblastic cells in HD has been recognized for over a century [10–12,17]. The recognition by Smetana & Cohen [21] of a sclerosing variant of Hodgkin's granuloma [15], and its associated super-

ior survival, were among the first steps in the delineation of nodular sclerosis (NS).

Lukes and coworkers [23–24,69] described the histological features of NS and stressed the importance of nodularity, lacunar cells and birefringent collagen band formation. Rappaport and colleagues emphasized the unique nature of NS by demonstrating the consistency of this histological pattern in sequential biopsies and from different anatomical locations [70,71].

Morphological features

Lymph-node involvement by NS may be partial or complete. There is usually capsular and intranodal fibrosis, which may impart a firm rubbery texture. The cut surface may have a coarsely nodular appearance and areas of necrosis may be macroscopically apparent.

Histologically, capsular thickening is present in the majority of cases (see Plate 15.13 between pp. 292 and 293) and there is a variable degree of intranodal sclerosis, which may range from occasional thin collagen bands to large areas of collagenous sclerosis that obliterate most of the nodal structure.

Nodularity is a constant feature of NS and may be present partially or throughout the lymph node.

NS is associated with a particular H-RS cell variant termed the lacunar cell. The lacunar cell is most obvious in specimens fixed in formalin, in whom paraffin processing dissolves the lipid-rich cytoplasm to leave a clear space; specimens fixed in mercuric-based fixatives do not show this helpful artefact. The nucleus of lacunar cells is typically twisted or lobulated, with a prominent eosinophilic nucleolus (see Plate 15.14).

In recent years there has been considerable confusion over the precise criteria required to diagnose NS, and this has centred around the entity termed cellular phase NS. Lukes [69] required the presence of intranodal collagen band formation in association with lacunar cells to establish a diagnosis of NS and recognized a cellular phase in which only a single band of collagen was found in association with the typical cellular background of NS. Cases lacking collagen band formation were classified as mixed cellularity by Lukes. Other workers have classified cases as cellular-phase NS, when lacunar cells are seen in the absence of collagen band formation [70,72]. The advantage of adhering to the strict criteria proposed by Lukes & Butler [25] is that they do enable pathologists to achieve very high levels of inter- and intra-observer concordance (97%) [73] in the diagnosis of the NS subtype.

The cellular nodules of NS show a wide range of cytological appearances, ranging from a lymphocyte-rich cellular background with scanty lacunar cells to one of lymphocyte depletion and sheets of lacunar and H-RS cells; this later pattern may be associated with areas of necrosis. In many cases there are also admixed histiocytes, eosinophils and plasma cells with the lymphocytes and lacunar cells.

The cytological diversity of the cellular nodules of NS has prompted workers to develop grading systems for NS which might correlate with prognosis (reviewed in ref. [74]). In a series of publications, the BNLI proposed a grading system that recognized low-grade (grade I) and high-grade (grade II) subtypes of NS [34,40,73–76]. The histological criteria for this grading system have been published in detail elsewhere [73] and are only outlined here.

Cases were classified as grade II NS if more than 25% of the cellular nodules showed lymphocyte-depleted cytology. These lymphocyte-depleted nodules are often composed of sheets of mononuclear Hodgkin's and lacunar cells (see Plate 15.15); an appearance which has been termed 'syncytial Hodgkin's disease' by some workers [77,78]. Central necrosis and eosinophilic abscess formation within these LD nodules is sometimes observed. Also, cases in which more than 25% of the cellular nodules contained numerous pleomorphic H-RS cells, in the absence of lymphocyte depletion, were classified as grade II NS (see Plate 15.16). The rarest from of LD cytology was the bland-appearing fibrohistiocytic variety; if more than 80% of the cellular nodules showed this feature, the case was classified as grade II NS [76]. The adverse prognostic significance of fibroblastic proliferation was also reported by Colby *et al.* [79].

All other cases were graded as grade I, including borderline cases. Using this system, significant differences in survival and disease-free survival are seen between the grades of NS (see below). Other workers have confirmed the clinical value of this grading system [80–84]; some have not been able to demonstrate a difference in prognosis between the two grades of NS [85,86].

Immunocytochemistry

The phenotype of NS differs from LP nodular in that the nodules are composed predominantly of T cells [87,88] (CD3+, CD45 Ro+), with a prevalence of CD4+ cells centrally and a rim of CD8+ lymphocytes at the periphery (see Plate 15.17 between pp. 292 and 293). The lacunar cells exhibit strong staining for CD15 in over 80% of cases, and this staining is usually membrane and golgi associated; CD30 is also expressed in the majority of cases [89–93] (see Plate 15.18).

The expression of lymphoid lineage-restricted antigens on H-RS cells remains controversial, with some groups claiming expression of CD3 in a percentage of cases [94,95], while others find expression of B-lineage antigens on a small percentage of H-RS cells [96] which may be seen in up to 60% of cases of HD [97].

Some cases of anaplastic large cell lymphoma (ALCL) may display morphological features which are reminiscent of NS HD, particularly the grade 2 subtype [98]. These similarities may be so close that some workers have introduced the term 'ALCL Hodgkin's like' [68]; other workers feel that the vast majority of these cases are in fact related to classic HD, and

have used the term 'malignant lymphoma with features of Hodgkin's lymphoma' and 'anaplastic large cell lymphoma' [99].

Immunocytochemistry can be helpful in distinguishing between HD and ALCL; while CD30 is usually expressed by both, CD15 staining is uncommon in ALCL and, when present, does not exhibit the membrane and golgi staining characteristic of HD. Leucocyte common antigen (CD45) is expressed in a percentage of ALCL [98], but with us has proved to be of limited value. Recently, antibodies to the p80 NPM-ALK fusion protein, generated by the 2;5 translocation [100] have become available [101,102], which stain just over half the cases of ALCL studied; no case of HD was labelled [102].

Lymphocyte-depleted Hodgkin's disease

Lymphocyte-depleted (LD) HD is the rarest form of HD and its frequency appears to be diminishing. It includes two distinctive morphological entities from the Lukes and Butler classification: diffuse fibrosis and reticular HD. It is now clear from various studies that many of the cases formally classified as LD were, in fact, examples of NHL [103], often of anaplastic large cell type or of other HD subtypes such as the grade II form of NS [40].

In a review of cases from the BNLI, many of which were originally diagnosed as LD were reclassified as NHL, and the incidence of true LD HD was below 2% in this series. Patients with LD tended to be elderly and often presented with advanced symptomatic disease (stage IVb). There was a low attainment of complete remission with combination chemotherapy and survival was poor.

Morphological features

Lymphocyte-depleted Hodgkin's disease has a high frequency of extranodal involvement, in particular the bone marrow is affected in many cases and may be the site of initial diagnostic biopsy. When lymph nodes are affected the architecture is completely effaced. The diffuse fibrosis variant is characterized by hypocellular lymph node, often showing areas of geographic necrosis (see Plate 15.19 between pp. 292 and 293). In the background there is a pink fibrillary appearance of nonbirefringent fibrosis. Lymphocytes are relatively scanty and bizarre mononuclear and multinuclear Hodgkin's cells are seen (see Plate 15.20). Classical R–S cells are often difficult to find.

The reticular subtype of LD HD is characterized by a numerical predominance of H-RS cells. It has been our experience that the majority of cases initially diagnosed as reticular HD represent examples of NHLs.

Mixed cellularity Hodgkin's disease

In the Lukes and Butler classification, mixed cellularity HD was used to classify cases of HD that did not conform to the pathological criteria of LP, NS and LD HD. It thus contained a spectrum of cytological appearances ranging from lymphocyte-rich forms, which contained classical RS cells, to subtypes which showed foci of lymphocyte-depleted cytology not involving the whole lymph node. Many cases of mixed cellularity HD have similarities to nodular sclerosis, such as focal nodularity and the presence of lacunar cells, but lack sufficient criteria to be diagnosed as NS. Other cases show distinctive morphological patterns which often involved alterations in the structure of the germinal centre and the marginal zone B-cell region.

Morphological features

Classical mixed cellularity HD is characterized by a diffuse architecture which effaces the nodal architecture completely. Typically the cytological background contains lymphocytes, macrophages, plasma cells and eosinophils, as well as easy to find mononuclear and classic R–S cells (see Plate 15.21 between pp. 292 and 293). There may be small foci of necrosis, but this is much less common than in either NS or LD HD.

Some cases may show the presence of lacunar cells, or even areas of indistinct nodularity, features which suggest a close association with NS. In the absence of the three essential criteria for the diagnosis of NS (nodularity, intranodal collagen band formation and lacunar cells), these are best classified as mixed cellularity. Some workers prefer to classify these cases with NS features as 'HD unclassified between mixed cellularity and nodular sclerosis' [38], and some even put them into cellular phase of NS.

Several striking morphological patterns have been observed in mixed cellularity HD. One example is interfollicular HD, highlighted by the Stanford Group, which is characterized by florid reactive follicular hyperplasia and an easily overlooked interfollicular infiltrate containing typical mononuclear Hodgkin's cells and R–S cells [104] (see Plate 15.22). A variant of this form of HD is characterized by a marginal zone hyperplasia where the H-RS cells are seen to sit within a sea of marginal zone B cells; this has been termed 'HD occurring in monocytoid B-cell clusters' (see Plate 15.23) [105].

In some cases of mixed cellularity HD the germinal centres are replaced by large expansile masses of mantle zone lymphocytes and, peppered within these, are readily found H-RS cells. Within the mantle cell nodules are an expanded meshwork of FDCs and, in many cases, the Hodgkin's cells express B-cell antigens in addition to CD15 and CD30 (see Plate 15.24). Some workers have termed this 'follicular HD' [106], however, this author prefers the term 'follicular colonization by HD'.

In some cases of HD there are marked regressive changes within germinal centres, which resemble the dendritic cell-only germinal centres that are seen in the hyaline vascular variant of Castleman's disease (see Plate 15.25). These are

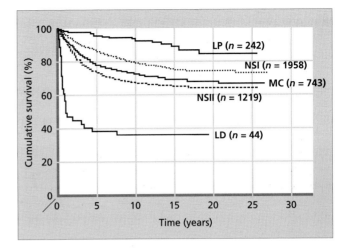

Fig. 15.1 Cause-specific survival for over 4000 patients with HD subdivided by histologic type. (Data from the British National Lymphoma Investigation.) $\chi^2_4 = 160.1$; $P < 0.001$. LD = lymphocyte depleted; LP = lymphocyte predominant; MC = mixed cellularity; NS = nodular sclerosis.

surrounded by H-RS cells which seem to preferentially localize at the junction of the marginal and mantle zones. The reasons for these different patterns of germinal centre reaction in mixed cellularity HD are unknown, but it might be postulated they are related to the pattern of cytokine expression by the H-RS cells. Rare cases with the morphological features of the plasma cell variant of Castleman's disease in association with HD have been described [107].

Clinical significance of morphological pattern in Hodgkin's disease

Many workers believe that histopathology has little part to play in the prognostic assessment of patients with HD and that the role of the pathologist is limited to accurate establishment of the diagnosis of HD and the documentation of involvement of extranodal sites [108–110].

In a series of publications over the past 10 years, the British National Lymphoma Investigation has documented the value of accurate histopathological classification in HD. It has shown that there are marked differences in the clinical presentation, response to therapy, freedom from relapse and overall survival between the different histological subtypes of HD and, in addition, that there is clinical value in the subdivision of NS into two prognostic grades [34,40,73–76,111]. It can be seen from the cause-specific survival curves from over 4000 patients that there are distinct differences in the rate of death from HD in the different histological subtypes (Fig. 15.1).

References

1 Hodgkin T. (1832) On some morbid appearances of the absorbent glands and spleen. *Medical-Chirurgical Transactions*, **17**, 68–114.

2 Wilks Sir S. (1865) Cases of enlargement of the lymphatic glands and spleen (or, Hodgkin's disease), with remarks. *Guy's Hospital Report*, **11**, 56–67.

3 Malpighi (1666) *De Viscerum Structura*. Omnia Opera, Bonn.

4 Craigie D. (1828) *Elements of General and Pathological Anatomy*. Adam Black, Edinburgh.

5 Fox H. (1926) Remarks on microscopic preparations made from some of the original tissue described by Thomas Hodgkin, 1832. *Annals of Medical History* **8**, 370–374.

6 Symmers W. St C. (1978) The lymphoreticular system. In: *Systemic Pathology* (ed W. St C. Symmers), pp. 784–785. Churchill Livingstone, Edinburgh.

7 Lennert K. (1997) Borderlands of pathological entities. In: *The Non-Hodgkin's Lymphomas* (ed I.T. Magrath), 2nd edn, pp. 133–167. Arnold, London.

8 Virchow R. (1864) *Die Krankhaften Geschwuelste*, Vol. 2. Hircwald, Berlin.

9 Murchison C. (1870) Case of lymphadenoma of the lymphatic system, spleen, liver, lungs, heart, diaphragm, dura mater etc. *Transactions of the Pathological Society of London*, **21**, 372–389.

10 Langhans T. (1872) Das maligne lymphosarkom (pseudoleukaemia). *Virchows Archives*, **54**, 509–537.

11 Greenfield W.S. (1878) Specimens illustrative of the pathology of lymphadenoma and leucocythaemia. *Transactions of the Pathology Society London*, **29**, 272–304.

12 Sternberg C. (1898) Uber eine eigenartige unter dem Bilde der Pseudoleukamie verlaufende Tuberculose des lymphatischen Apparates. *Zeitschrift fur Heilk*, **18**, 21–90.

13 Reed D.M. (1902) On the pathological changes in Hodgkin's disease, with especial reference to its relation in tuberculosis. *Johns Hopkins Hospital Report*, **10**, 133–196.

14 Walhauser A. (1933) Hodgkin's disease. *Archives of Pathology*, **16**, 522–562, 672–712.

15 Jackson H. Jr & Parker F. Jr (1947) *Hodgkin's Disease and Allied Disorders*. Oxford University Press, Oxford.

16 Ewing J. (1919) *Neoplastic Diseases*. WB Saunders, Philadelphia.

17 Rosenthal S.R. (1936) Significance of tissue lymphocytes in the prognosis of lymphogranulomatosis. *Archives of Pathology*, **21**, 628–646.

18 Jackson H. Jr & Parker F. Jr (1944) Hodgkin's disease. I. General considerations. *New England Journal of Medicine*, **230**, 1–8.

19 Jackson H. Jr & Parker F. Jr (1944) Hodgkin's disease. II. Pathology. *New England Journal of Medicine*, **231**, 35–44.

20 Jackson H. Jr & Parker F. Jr (1944) Hodgkin's disease. III. Symptoms and course. *New England Journal of Medicine*, **231**, 636–646.

21 Smetana H.F. & Cohen B.M. (1956) Mortality in relation to histologic type in Hodgkin's disease. *Blood*, **11**, 211–244.

22 Jelliffe A.M. & Thompson A.D. (1955) The prognosis in Hodgkin's disease. *British Journal of Cancer*, **9**, 21–36.

23 Lukes R.J. (1963) Relationship of histological features to clinical stages in Hodgkin's disease. *American Journal of Roentgenology*, **90**, 944–955.

24 Lukes R.J., Butler J.J. & Hicks E.B. (1966) Natural history of Hodgkin's disease as related to its pathologic picture. *Cancer* **34**, 317–344.

25 Lukes R.J. & Butler J.J. (1966) The pathology and nomenclature of Hodgkin's disease. *Cancer Research*, **26**, 1063–1081.

26 Lukes R.J., Craver L.F., Hall T.C., Rappaport H. & Rubin P. (1966) Report of the nomenclature committee. *Cancer Research*, **26**, 1311.

27 Chelloul N., Burke J., Motteram R., LeCapon J. & Rappaport H. (1972) HL-A antigens and Hodgkin's disease. Report on the histological analysis. In: *Histocompatability Testing* (eds J. Dausset & J. Colombani), pp. 769–771. Munksgaard, Copenhagen.

28 Miller T.P., Byrne G.E. & Jones S.E. (1982) Mistaken clinical and pathologic diagnoses of Hodgkin's disease. A Southwest Oncology Group study. *Cancer Treatment Reports*, **66**, 645–651.

29 Symmers W. St C. (1968) Survey of the eventual diagnosis in 600 cases referred for a second histologic opinion after an initial biopsy diagnosis of Hodgkin's disease. *Journal of Clinical Pathology*, **21**, 650–653.

30 Harrison C.V. (1952) Benign Hodgkin's disease (Hodgkin's paragranuloma). *Journal Pathology and Bacteriology*, **64**, 513–518.

31 Lumb G. & Newton K.A. (1957) Prognosis in tumours of lymphoid tissue. *Cancer*, **10**, 976–993.

32 Lennert K. & Mohri N. (1974) Histologische Klassifizierung und Vorkommen des M. Hodgkin. *Internist*, **15**, 57–65.

33 von Waielewski R., Werner M., Fischer R. *et al.* (1997) Lymphocyte-predominant Hodgkin's disease: an immunohistochemical analysis of 208 reviewed Hodgkin's disease cases from the German Hodgkin Study Group. *American Journal of Pathology*, **150**, 793–803.

34 MacLennan K.A., Bennett M.H., Bosq J. *et al.* (1990) The histology and immunohistology of Hodgkin's disease: the relationship to prognosis and clinical behavior. In: *Treatment Strategy in Hodgkin's Disease* (eds R. Sommers M. Henry-Amar & P. Carde), pp. 17–25. John Libbey, London.

35 Poppema S., Kaiserling E. & Lennert K. (1979) Nodular paragranuloma and progressively transformed germinal centres: ultrastructural and immunologic findings. *Virchows Archiv. B. Cell Pathology*, **31**, 211–225.

36 Lennert K. & Muller-Hermelink H.K. (1975) Lymphocyten und ihre Funkionsformen — Morphologie, Organisation und immunologische Bedeutung (lecture). *Verhandlungen der Anatomischen Gesellschaft*, **69**, 19–62.

37 Muller-Hermelink H.K. & Lennert K. (1978) The cytologic, histologic and functional basis for a modern classification of lymphomas. In: *Malignant Lymphomas other than Hodgkin's Disease* (K. Lennert in collaboration with H. Stein, N. Mohri, E. Kaiserling & H.K. Muller-Hermelink), pp. 38–41. Springer, New York.

38 Neiman R.S. (1978) Current problems in the histopathologic diagnosis and classification of Hodgkin's disease. *Pathology Annual*, **13**, 289–328.

39 Ramsey A.D., Smith W.J. & Isaacson P.G. (1988) T-cell rich-B-cell lymphoma. *American Journal of Surgical Pathology*, **12**, 433–443.

40 Bennett M.H., MacLennan K.A., Vaughan Hudson B. & Vaughan Hudson G. (1989) The clinical and prognostic relevance of histopathological classification in Hodgkin's disease. *Progress in Surgical Pathology*, **10**, 127–151.

41 Tiemens W., Visser L. & Poppema S. (1986) Nodular lymphocyte predominance type of Hodgkin's disease is a germinal centre lymphoma. *Laboratory Investigation*, **54**, 457–461.

42 Hansmann M.L., Wacker H.H. & Radzun H.J. (1986) Paragranuloma is a variant of Hodgkin's disease with a predominance of B-

cells. *Virchows Archiv. A. Pathological Anatomy and Histopathology*, **409**, 171–181.

43 Coles F.B., Cartun R.W. & Pastuszak W.T. (1988) Hodgkin's disease, lymphocyte predominant type: immunoreactivity with B-cell antibodies. *Modern Pathology*, **1**, 274–278.

44 Pinkus G.S. & Said J.W. (1988) Hodgkin's disease, lymphocytes predominance type, nodular — further evidence for a B-cell derivation. *American Journal of Pathology*, **133**, 211–217.

45 Poppema S. (1991) Lymphocyte-predominance Hodgkin's disease. *International Review of Experimental Pathology*, **33**, 53–79.

46 Kuzu I., Delsol G., Jones M., Gatter K.C. & Mason D.Y. (1993) Expression of the Ig-associated heterodimer (mb-1 and B 29) in Hodgkin's disease. *Histopathology*, **22**, 141–144.

47 Mason D.Y., Banks P.M., Chan J.K.C. *et al.* (1994) Nodular lymphocyte predominance Hodgkin's disease: a distinct clinico-pathological entity. *American Journal of Surgical Pathology*, **18**, 526–530.

48 Stein H., Hansmann M-L., Lennert K., Brandtzaeg P., Gatter K.C. & Mason D.Y. (1986) Reed-Sternberg and Hodgkin's cells in lymphocyte predominance Hodgkin's disease of nodular subtype contain J chain. *American Journal of Clinical Pathology*, **86**, 292–297.

49 Schmidt C., Sargent C. & Isaacson P.G. (1991) L and H cells of nodular lymphocyte predominant Hodgkin's disease show immunoglobulin light chain restriction. *American Journal of Pathology*, **139**, 1281–1289.

50 Hell K., Pringle J.H., Hansmann M-L. *et al.* (1993) Demonstration of light chain mRNA in Hodgkin's disease. *Journal of Pathology*, **17**, 137–143.

51 Stoler M.H., Nichols G.E., Symbula M. & Weiss L.M. (1995) Lymphocyte predominance Hodgkin's disease: Evidence for k light chain restricted monotypic B cell neoplasm. *American Journal of Pathology*, **146**, 812–818.

52 Nicholas D.S., Harris S. & Wright D.H. (1990) Lymphocyte predominance Hodgkin's disease: an immunohistochemical study. *Histopathology*, **16**, 157–165.

53 Hsu S.M., Ho Y.S., Li P.J. *et al.* (1986) L&H variants of Reed–Sternberg cells express sialyated Leu M1 antigen. *American Journal of Pathology*, **122**, 199–203.

54 Jack A.S., Cunningham D., Soukop M., Liddle C.N. & Lee F.D. (1986) Use of Leu M1 and antiepithelial membrane antigen monoclonal antibodies for diagnosing Hodgkin's disease. *Journal of Clinical Pathology*, **39**, 267–270.

55 Bosq J., Audouin J., Henry-Amar M. *et al.* (1995) Relationship between EBV infection, clinical, biological and histologic characteristics and response to therapy in patients with Hodgkin's disease. In: *Proceedings of the Third International Symposium on Hodgkin's Lymphoma*, abstract 9.

56 Bennett M.H., MacLennan K.A., Vaughan Hudson B. & Vaughan Hudson G. (1991) Non Hodgkins lymphoma arising in patients treated for Hodgkins disease in BNLI: a 20 year experience. *Annals of Oncology*, **2**(Suppl. 2), 83–92.

57 Miettinen M., Franssila K.O. & Saxen E. (1983) Hodgkin's disease, lymphocytic predominance nodular increased risk for subsequent non-Hodgkin's lymphoma. *Cancer*, **51**, 2293–2300.

58 Sundeen J.T., Cossman J. & Jaffe E.S. (1988) Lymphocyte predominant Hodgkin's disease with coexistent 'large cell lymphoma': histological progression or composite malignancy? *American Journal of Surgical Pathology*, **12**, 599–606.

59 Hansmann M.L., Stein H., Fellbaum C. *et al.* (1989) Nodular paragranuloma can transform into high-grade malignant lymphoma of B type. *Human Pathology*, **20**, 1169–1175.

60 Whittaker M., Foucar K., Keith T. & McAneny B. (1989) Letter. *American Journal of Surgical Pathology*, **13**, 715–716.

61 Grossman D.M., Hanson C.A. & Schnitzer B. (1991) Simultaneous lymphocyte predominant Hodgkin's disease and large cell lymphoma. *American Journal of Surgical Pathology*, **15**, 668–676.

62 Pan L.X., Diss T.C., Peng H.J., Norton A.J. & Isaacson P.G. (1996) Nodular lymphocyte predominance Hodgkin's disease: a monoclonal or polyclonal B-cell disorder? *Blood*, **87**, 2428–2334.

63 Greiner T.C., Gascoyne R.D., Anderson M.E. *et al.* (1996) Nodular lymphocyte-predominant Hodgkin's disease associated with large cell lymphoma: analysis of Ig gene rearrangements by V-J polymerase chain reaction. *Blood*, **88**, 657–666.

64 Wickert R.S., Weisenburger D.D., Tierens A., Greiner T.C. & Chan W.C. (1995) Clonal relationship between lymphocytic predominance Hodgkin's disease and concurrent or subsequent large cell lymphoma of B lineage. *Blood*, **86**, 2312–2320.

65 Tefferi A., Wiltsie J.C. & Kurtin P.J. (1992) Secondary T cell lymphoma in the setting of nodular lymphocyte predominance Hodgkin's disease. *American Journal of Haematology*, **40**, 232–233.

66 Rysenga E., Linden M.D., Carey J.L. *et al.* (1995) Peripheral T-cell non-Hodgkin's lymphoma following treatment of nodular lymphocyte predominance Hodgkin's disease. *Archives of Pathology and Laboratory Medicine*, **119**, 88–91.

67 Delabie J., Greiner T.C., Chan W.C. & Weisenburger D.D. (1996) Concurrent lymphocyte predominance Hodgkin's disease and T-cell lymphoma. *American Journal Surgical Pathology*, **20**, 355–362.

68 Harris N.L., Jaffe E.S., Stein H. *et al.* (1994) A revised European-American classification of lymphoid neoplasms: a proposal from the International Lymphoma Study Group. *Blood*, **84**, 1361–1392.

69 Lukes R.J. (1971) Criteria for involvement of lymph node, bone marrow, spleen and liver in Hodgkin's disease. *Cancer Research*, **31**, 1755–1767.

70 Strum S.B. & Rappaport H. (1971) Interrelations of the histological types of Hodgkin's disease. *Archives of Pathology*, **91**, 127–134.

71 Strum S.B. & Rappaport H. (1973) Consistency of histological subtypes in Hodgkin's disease in simultaneous and sequential biopsy specimens. *NCI Monographs*, **36**, 253–260.

72 Dorfman R.F. (1990) the enigma of Hodgkin's disease: current concepts based on morphologic, clinical and immunologic observations. In: *Lymphoid Malignances, Immunocytology and Cytogenetics*, (eds M. Hanaoka, M.E. Kadin, A. Mikata & S. Watanabe), pp. 167–176. Field and Wood, New York.

73 MacLennan K.A., Bennett M.H., Vaughan Hudson B. & Vaughan Hudson G. (1992) Diagnosis and grading of nodular sclerosing Hodgkin's disease: a study of 2190 patients. *International Review of Experimental Pathology*, **33**, 27–51.

74 MacLennan K.A., Bennett M.H., Tu A. *et al.* (1985) Prognostic significance of cytologic subdivision in nodular sclerosing Hodgkin's disease: an analysis of 1156 patients. In: *Malignant Lymphomas and Hodgkin's disease: experimental and therapeutic advances* (eds F. Vavallia, G. Bonadonna & M. Rozencweig), pp. 187–200. Martinus Nijhoff, Dordrecht.

75 Bennett M.H., MacLennan K.A., Easterling M.J., Vaughan Hudson B., Vaughan Hudson G. & Jelliffe A.M. (1985) Analysis of histological subtypes of Hodgkin's disease in relation to prognosis

and survival. In: *The Cytobiology of Leukaemia and Lymphomas* (eds D. Quaglino & F.G.J. Hayhoe), Vol. 20, pp. 15–32. Serono publications from Raven Press, New York.

76 MacLennan K.A., Bennett M.H., Tu A., Vaughan Hudson B. & Vaughan Hudson G. (1989) The relationship of histopathology to survival and relapse. A study of 1659 patients. *Cancer,* **64,** 1686–1693.

77 Strickler J.G., Michie S.A., Warnke R.A. & Dorfman R.F. (1986) The 'syncytial variant' of nodular sclerosing Hodgkin's disease. *American Journal of Surgical Pathology,* **10,** 470–477.

78 Ben-Yahuda-Salz D., Ben-Yahuda A., Polliak A., Ron N. & Okon E. (1990) Syncytial variant of nodular sclerosis Hodgkin's disease: a new clinicopathologic entity. *Cancer,* **65,** 1167–1172.

79 Colby T.V., Hoppe R.T. & Warnke R.A. (1981) Hodgkin's disease: a clinicopathologic study of 659 cases. *Cancer,* **49,** 1848–1858.

80 Gartner H.V., Wherman M., Inniger R. & Steinke B. (1987) Nodular sclerosing Hodgkin's disease: prognostic relevance of morphological parameters. In: *First International Symposium on Hodgkin's Lymphoma, Cologne,* abstract 27.

81 Jairam R., Vrints L.W., Breed W.P.M., Wijlhuizen T.J. & Wijnen T.J.M. (1988) Histological subclassification of the nodular sclerotic subtype of Hodgkin's disease. *Netherlands Journal of Medicine,* **33,** 160–167.

82 Wijlhuizen T.J., Vrints L.W., Jairam R. *et al.* (1989) Grades of nodular sclerosis (NSI-NSII) in Hodgkin's disease: are they independent prognostic value? *Cancer,* **63,** 1150–1153.

83 Ferry J.A., Linggood R.M., Convery K.M., Efird J.T., Eliseo R. & Harris N.L. (1993) Hodgkin's disease, nodular sclerosis type implications of histologic subclassification. *Cancer,* **71,** 457–463.

84 Georgii A., Hasenclever D., Fischer R. *et al.* (1995) Histopathological grading of nodular sclerosing Hodgkin's reveals significant differences in survival and relapse rates under protocol-therapy. In: *Proceedings of the Third International Symposium on Hodgkin's Lymphoma, Koln,* abstract 83.

85 Masih A.S., Weisenburger D.D., Vose J.M., Bast M.A. & Armitage J.O. (1992) Histologic grade does not predict prognosis in optimally treated advanced stage nodular sclerosing Hodgkin's disease. *Cancer,* **69,** 228–232.

86 Hess J.L., Bodis S., Pinkus G., Silver B. & Mauch P. (1994) Histopathologic grading of nodular sclerosis Hodgkin's disease: lack of prognostic significance in 254 surgically staged patients. *Cancer,* **74,** 708–714.

87 Borowitz M.J., Croker B.P. & Metzger R.S. (1982) Immunohistochemical analysis of the distribution of lymphocyte subpopulations in Hodgkin's disease. *Cancer Treatment Reports,* **66,** 667–674.

88 Abdulaziz S., Mason D.Y., Stein H., Gatter K.C. & Nash J.R.G. (1984) An immunohistological study of the cellular constituents of Hodgkin's disease using a monoclonal antibody panel. *Histopathology,* **8,** 1–25.

89 Pinkus G.S., Thomas P. & Said J.W. (1985) Leu M1—a marker for Reed–Sternberg cells in Hodgkin's disease. *American Journal of Pathology,* **119,** 244–252.

90 Hall P.A. & D'Ardenne A.J. (1987) Value of CD15 immunostaining in diagnosing Hodgkin's disease: a review of published literature. *Journal of Clinical Pathology,* **40,** 1298–1304.

91 Hall P.A., D'Ardenne A.J., & Stansfield A.J. (1988) Paraffin section immunohistochemistry. II. Hodgkin's disease and large cell anaplastic (Ki1) lymphoma. *Histopathology,* **13,** 161–169.

92 Chittal S.M., Caveriviere R., Schwarting R. *et al.* (1988) Mono-

clonal antibodies in the diagnosis of Hodgkin's disease: the search for a rational panel. *American Journal of Surgical Pathology,* **12,** 9–21.

93 Werner M., Georgii A., Bernhards J., Hubner K., Schwarze E-W. & Fischer R. (1990) Characterization of giant cells in Hodgkin's lymphomas by immunohistochemistry applied to randomly collected diagnostic biopsies from the German Hodgkin trial. *Haematological Oncology,* **8,** 241–250.

94 Cibull M.L., Stein H., Gatter K.C. & Mason D.Y. (1989) The expression of the CD3 antigen in Hodgkin's disease. *Histopathology,* **15,** 597–605.

95 Casey T.T., Olson S.J., Cousar J.B. & Collins R.D. (1989) Immunophenotypes of Reed–Sternberg cells: a study of 19 cases of Hodgkin's disease in plastic-embedded sections. *Blood,* **74,** 2624–2628.

96 Korkolopoulou P., Cordell J., Jones M. *et al.* (1994) The expression of the B-cell marker mb-1 (CD79a) in Hodgkin's disease. *Histopathology,* **24,** 511–515.

97 Isaacson P.G. & Ashton-Key M. (1996) Phenotype of Hodgkin and Reed–Sternberg cells. *Lancet,* **347,** 481.

98 Agnarrson B.A. & Kadin M.E. (1988) Ki1 positive large cell lymphoma: a morphological study of 19 cases. *American Journal of Surgical Pathology,* **12,** 264–274.

99 Stein H. (1997) Hodgkin's disease. *American Journal of Surgical Pathology,* **21,** 119–120.

100 Morris S.W., Kirstein M.N., Valentine M.B. *et al.* (1994) Fusion of a kinase gene, ALK, to a nucleolar protein gene, NPM, in non-Hodgkin's lymphoma. *Science,* **262,** 1281–1284.

101 Shiota M., Nakamura S., Ichinohasama R. *et al.* (1995) Anaplastic large cell lymphomas expressing the novel chimeric protein p80 NPM/ALK: a distinctive clinicopathologic entity. *Blood,* **86,** 1954–1960.

102 Pulford K., Lamant L., Morris S.W. *et al.* (1997) Detection of anaplastic lymphoma kinase (ALK) and nucleolar protein nucleophosphomin (NPM)–ALK proteins in normal and neoplastic cells with the monoclonal antibody ALK1. *Blood,* **89,** 1394–1404.

103 Kant J.A., Hubbard S.M., Longo D.L., Simon R.M., DeVita V.T. & Jaffe E.S. (1986) A critical appraisal of the pathologic and clinical heterogeneity of lymphocyte depleted Hodgkin's disease. *Journal of Clinical Oncology,* **4,** 284–294.

104 Doggett R.S., Colby T.V. & Dorfman R.F. (1983) Interfollicular Hodgkin's disease. *American Journal of Surgical Pathology,* **7,** 145–149.

105 Mohrmann R.L., Nathwani B.N., Brynes R.K. & Sheibani K. (1991) Hodgkin's disease occurring in monocytoid B-cell clusters. *American Journal of Clinical Pathology,* **95,** 802–808.

106 Ashton-Key M., Thorpe P.A., Allen J.P. & Isaacson P.G. (1995) Follicular Hodgkin's disease. *American Journal of Surgical Pathology,* **19,** 1294–1299.

107 Maheswaran P.R., Ramsay A.D., Norton A.J. & Roche W.R. (1991) Hodgkin's disease presenting with the histological features of Castleman's disease. *Histopathology,* **18,** 249–253.

108 Torti F.M., Dorfman R.F., Rosenberg S.A. & Kaplan H.S. (1979) The changing significance of histology in Hodgkin's disease. *Proceedings of the American Association of Cancer Research and ASCO,* **20,** 401 (C-454).

109 Dorfman R.F. & Colby T.V. (1982) The pathologists role in the management of patients with Hodgkin's disease. *Cancer Treatment Report,* **66,** 675–680.

110 Culline S., Henry-Amar H., Diebold J. *et al.* (1989) Relationship of histological subtypes to prognosis in early stage Hodgkin's disease: a review of 312 cases enrolled in a controlled clinical trial. *European Journal of Cancer*, **25**, 551–556.

111 Vaughan Hudson B., Vaughan Hudson G., MacLennan K.A., Bennett M.H. & Jelliffe A.M. (1987) A retrospective evaluation of radiotherapy as a curative agent in localised Hodgkin's disease. *British Journal of Cancer*, **56**, 872.

16 Hodgkin's Disease: Clinical Features and Management

P. Selby and P. Johnson

Introduction

The management of Hodgkin's disease (HD) continues to change and develop. Despite success in curing the majority of patients, the last decade has seen changes in ideas about pathological classification, pathogenesis, appropriate investigation and the choice of management. Emerging late complications in cured patients present new challenges and will influence the choice of primary therapy at all stages of the disease.

The history of the disease is well documented. Thomas Hodgkin from Guy's Hospital described the condition in 1832; Samuel Wilks coined the term 'Hodgkin's disease' in 1865 [1]; Sternberg [2] and Reed [3] identified the pathognomonic giant cells. Modern staging began in the early 1970s with the Ann Arbor Classification [4]. Major steps forward in treatment began with the use of wide-field irradiation by Peters in 1950 [5]; further development of this theme, and the use of the linear accelerator by Kaplan, began at Stanford in the 1960s [6]. The evolution of chemotherapy consisted of single-agent treatment in the 1940s [7], combination chemotherapy to modest effect by Lacher & Durant [8], and then to great effect in the quadruple combination regimen, MOPP (nitrogen mustard, vincristine, procarbazine, prednisone), described first by De Vita et al. in 1970 [9].

Epidemiology

Hodgkin's disease has always been of great interest to epidemiologists, because of its unusual geographical and age distribution. Analysis of risk factors suggests that it should have an infectious aetiology and it is clear now that at least some cases of HD have an intimate link with Epstein–Barr virus (EBV). This topic has been recently reviewed [10].

Broadly, HD occurs with about one-third the frequency of non-Hodgkin lymphomas (NHL), although there is a considerable difference in age distribution. Hodgkin's disease is the commonest cancer in Western Europe in the adolescent age group. The incidence increases as countries become more economically developed and the disease is commoner among affluent populations, in white races and in men. Asians have the lowest incidence. The highest incidence is found among North American whites and Western Europeans. The incidence always exceeds the mortality substantially. Thus, in the USA in the period 1986–90, the age-adjusted incidence was 2.8 cases in every 100 000 people in each year, but the equivalent mortality rate was 0.6, reflecting a high proportion of patients cured [11].

An important feature of HD is the bimodal relationship between incidence and age. In economically advantaged populations, most studies still show a peak incidence in early life between 15 and 25 years, and then a secondary rise after age 55. This pattern has important clinical implications. The frequency of HD in adolescents and young adults is striking and constitutes a major burden of cancer in that group. In patients over 55 years, the proportion of cancer due to HD is, of course, much smaller because of the frequency of epithelial cancers in this age group. The age distribution of HD depends upon the population studied. Correa & O'Connor [12], in their landmark study, showed that in economically disadvantaged groups, the initial peak is in childhood with low rates in young adults [13]. As populations become economically advanced, the transition to the typical bimodal distribution occurs. This was clearly documented by Gutensohn & Cole [14] in the British population as the pattern changed during this century. In younger patients, in countries with developed economies, an association between HD and higher socioeconomic status is seen, particularly for the nodular sclerotic subtype [10].

Epidemiological studies, now supported by serological and molecular studies, suggest an association between EBV infection and HD. Interest in EBV as an aetiological factor in HD stems from the ability of the virus to transform lymphocytes and the presence of multinucleate cells in lymph nodes of patients with infectious mononucleosis. Although the proportion of HD patients with antibodies to EBV is similar to that of controls, there are qualitative differences. HD patients have higher mean IgG titres to EBV capsid and more antibodies against early antigens in the replication cycle of EBV. When populations are followed prospectively, people with high antibody titres against EBV nuclear antigens (EBNA) are more likely to develop HD [10,15]. This field of research took a step forward with the work of Weiss and colleagues [16,17], who showed monoclonal EBV in Hodgkin's tissue localized to the Reed–Sternberg cells.

The localization of EBV in Reed–Sternberg cells by *in situ* hybridization shows that approximately 40–50% of cases are positive in Western populations [18,19] and EBV DNA is both abundant and monoclonal in Reed–Sternberg cells, particularly of the mixed cellularity subtype [20]. The EBV clonality is retained at multiple disease sites and at the time of disease relapse [21]. There has been intensive study of the nature of the EBV latency within HD and, in particular, in Reed–Sternberg cells [19,22,23]. Usually only latent infection is present, but occasionally there are abortive lytic infections [24]. Although the association with a mixed cellularity histological subtype is very strong (about 80% positive), EBV infection is found in the nodular sclerosing subtype in about 20% of patients [18,19,22,24–26]. Nodular lymphocyte-predominant HD, which, as discussed below, has a distinct clinical pattern, is generally EBV negative [27]. Epstein–Barr virus is not the only cause of HD, but it may clearly play a significant part in its molecular pathogenesis.

Hodgkin's disease is also associated with some types of immune deficiency and, more recently, infection with human immunodeficiency virus type 1 (HIV-1). Most of the AIDS-related cases appear to be EBV genome positive and clinically aggressive [28].

The role of genetic factors in the development of HD has been re-emphasized by Mack *et al.* [29], who studied over 300 twin pairs in which one had the disease. The risk of HD occurring in both monozygotic twins greatly exceeds that in dizygotic twins. This important observation is in keeping with the findings that the siblings of patients with HD have a sevenfold higher risk of developing the disease than the general population [30,31], and there is an increased risk in general among relatives of patients with HD. Although there has been much discussion of the association of HD to occupation and exposure to wood dust and chemicals, the data are not clear cut [10,32,33].

Molecular pathology, clonality and cell of origin

The malignant cellular subpopulation of HD consists of mononuclear Hodgkin's cells and multinuclear Reed–Sternberg cells. These together represent less than 1% of the cell population (reviewed in ref. [34]). The cell of origin and clonality of these cells is hotly debated. The debate has been informed considerably by refinements in the pathological subtyping of HD.

In the majority of patients with nodular lymphocyte-predominant HD, the cells express B-lymphocyte markers (CD19, CD20). In nodular sclerosing and mixed cellularity HD, cells may express activation markers such as CD30/Ki-1 (80–90%) and the IL-2 receptor (CD25, 80–90%), transferrin receptor (CD71, 65–90%), CD15 (75–80%) and HLA DR (95%) [34–36]. In these common subtypes of HD, there has been no consistent demonstration of the expression of B- and T-cell-specific markers.

Further information on the cell of origin of HD has emerged since the introduction of polymerase chain reaction (PCR) based genetic analysis of single Hodgkin/Reed–Sternberg cells [37,38]. In the initial report, three patients showed clonal rearrangements of Ig heavy chains, indicating a B-cell monoclonal origin. Other results were less conclusive [39]. Some common subtypes of HD are probably monoclonal B-cell disorders, but uncertainty remains about the proportion or its pathogenetic significance.

Analysis of other molecular genetic abnormalities in HD remains inconclusive. Using the single cell technique, no specific pattern was found by Trumper *et al.* [40]. The claim that Hodgkin/Reed–Sternberg cells frequently contain the *NPM-ALK* fusion gene derived from a chromosomal translocation (2;5) [41] has not been confirmed consistently by other groups [42–45].

Classic cytogenetics (see Chapter 15 and review in ref. [46]) has been relatively uninformative in HD and no consistent pattern has emerged. The distinction between malignant Hodgkin cells and abnormalities in surrounding B cells may be difficult to make. In a typical study, Tilly *et al.* [47] analysed 60 lymph nodes and were able to analyse metaphases in over 80%. There were abnormalities in 55%. Although some, such as the loss of chromosome 13, occurred more frequently than others, no consistent pattern emerged. The use of fluorescence *in situ* hybridization (FISH) will increase the specificity of the analysis of chromosomal abnormalities in HD, and preliminary results [48] show that this method is capable of detecting a much higher proportion of rearrangements.

A radical re-evaluation of the significance of the lymphocyte-predominant pathological subtype has been seen in recent years. The clinical interest lies in the particular pattern of behaviour of this type. The European Task Force on Lymphoma has carried out a multinational project to examine the clinical features and, among 200 patients studied, a clear clinical pattern emerges [49]. The patients have good overall survival, with 95% alive at 10 years, but relapse probability is high, with only 50% of patients remaining disease free at 15 years. Repeated relapse is not uncommon. Extranodal disease is uncommon and few patients have B symptoms. These patients have a relatively high incidence of secondary NHL.

Cell biology

Suitable experimental model systems have been very difficult to establish for the study of HD. Although more than 12 cell lines have been established, this remains a challenging process. The lines resemble the parent tissues in expression of relevant markers such as CD30, CD15 and CD71, but the relationship between the tumour in the patient and the cell line must be established carefully [34,50]. In at least one cell line, the relationship between the parent tumour and the line could be supported by demonstration of identical molecular genetic abnormalities [34]. These lines are capable of forming tumours in severe combined immune deficient mice (SCID mice), but not in T-cell-deficient nude mice [51,52], and these models are proving useful in evaluating novel approaches to therapy.

Clinical presentation

Hodgkin's disease typically presents with lymphadenopathy, most commonly in the neck. However, the involvement of extranodal sites, although infrequent, remains a crucial determinant of treatment. Table 16.1 shows, broadly, the percentage of involved lymph nodes and visceral sites in collected clinical series of HD. The section on 'Imaging investigations' (below) summarizes the distribution of the disease. Lymphadenopathy is typically painless and may wax and wane spontaneously. A few patients experience pain in nodes after drinking alcohol. Systemic symptoms are present in about one-third of patients. Presentation only with systemic symptoms of fever, weight loss, sweats or itching is well recognized but uncommon. Extranodal presentations account for less than 10% of cases. A range of rare syndromes is described (reviewed in refs [53,54]). These include bronchial obstruction, spinal cord compression, gastrointestinal symptoms, thrombocytopenia, leucocytosis, anaemia, jaundice, skin rashes, nephrotic syndrome, neurological deficits and paraneoplastic syndromes.

The diagnosis is normally made by lymph-node biopsy.

Table 16.1 Sites of involvement by HD.

	% involved	% sole site
Right neck nodes	55–60	5
Left neck nodes	60–70	10
Mediastinum	60–65	2
Axillary nodes	20–25	5
Hilar nodes	10–25	<1
Para-aortic nodes	25–35	<1
Iliac nodes	10–15	<1
Inguinal and femoral nodes	5–15	<5
Mesenteric nodes	1	<1
Splenic hilar, coeliac, portal nodes	10–20	<1
Spleen	30	<1
Liver	5–15	<1
Lung	10–20	<1
Bone	5–15	<1
Bone marrow	5–15	<1

Fine-needle aspiration only has a minor role in assessing recurrences.

The extent of HD, described by the Ann Arbor stage (Table 16.2) [4], has been modified by the Cotswold Staging System (Table 16.3) [55].

Table 16.2 The Ann Arbor Staging System of HD.

Stage I
Involvement of a single lymph-node region (I) or of a single extralymphatic organ or site (I_E)

Stage II
Involvement of two or more lymph-node regions on the same side of the diaphragm (II) or localized involvement of an extralymphatic organ or site and of one or more lymph-node regions on the same side of the diaphragm (II_E). An optional recommendation is that the numbers of node regions involved should be indicated by a subscript (e.g. II_3)

Stage III
Involvement of lymph-node regions on both sides of the diaphragm (III) which may also be accompanied by localized involvement of an extralymphatic organ or site (III_E) or by involvement of the spleen (III_S) or both (III_{SE})

Stage IV
Diffuse or disseminated involvement of one or more extralymphatic organs or tissues with or without associated lymph-node enlargement. The reason for classifying the patient as stage IV should be identified further by defining site by symbols

Table 16.3 The Cotswold Staging Classification of HD.

Stage I
Involvement of a single lymph-node region or a lymphoid structure (e.g. spleen, thymus, Waldeyer's ring)

Stage II
Involvement of two or more lymph-node regions on the same side of the diaphragm (i.e. the mediastinum is a single site, hilar lymph nodes are lateralized). The number of anatomical sites should be indicated by a subscript (e.g. II_2)

Stage III
Involvement of lymph-node regions or structures on both sides of the diaphragm:
  III_1 With or without splenic hilar, coeliac or portal nodes
  III_2 With para-aortic, iliac, mesenteric nodes

Stage IV
Involvement of extranodal site(s) beyond that designated E:
  A No symptoms
  B Fever, drenching sweats, weight loss
  X Bulky disease:
      >1/3 the width of the mediastinum
      >10 cm maximal dimension of nodal mass
  E Involvement of a single extranodal site, contiguous or proximal to a known nodal site
  CS Clinical stage
  PS Pathological stage

The approach to the patient with HD will include a careful history, particularly focusing on those symptoms which are used to attribute stage, and physical examination. The patient's emotional state, social and family background will be relevant to future management decisions.

Initial investigations will include a full blood count, erythrocyte sedimentation rate, electrolytes, renal and liver function tests and a serum lactate dehydrogenase. Haematological tests are usually normal but occasionally reveal a Coomb's positive haemolytic anaemia, leucocytosis, lymphopenia or eosinophilia. Abnormalities of liver function tests may reflect hepatic involvement by HD, but are often seen in the absence of infiltration. (For the purposes of staging, a demonstration of focal defects by two imaging modalities or a biopsy are required to confirm liver involvement.)

Current investigations suggest that an understanding of serological changes in cytokines and related molecules may, in the future, give information on the prognosis. Beta-2-microglobulin (β_2m) has been shown to correlate with prognosis in several series [56]. IL-6 has been found to be elevated in 50–75% of patients [57–59], and becomes unmeasurable in most patients after treatment. High concentrations of IL-6 may indicate a poor prognosis. Elevated concentrations of IL-2 receptor (CD25) are seen in many patients and are associated with advanced stage, B symptoms and a poorer outcome [60–63]. Elevated tumour necrosis factor receptors have been described in association with advanced stage and B symptoms [64]. Elevated levels of soluble circulating CD30 are found in between 22 and 87% of patients [65,66], and are also associated with the presence of B symptoms, advanced stage, high tumour burden and poorer survival [64–67].

Imaging investigations

Imaging investigations in HD are designed to describe the pattern of nodal disease and detect extranodal involvement. They have been reviewed recently [68]. Computerized tomography (CT), ultrasonography (US) or magnetic resonance imaging (MRI) indicate lymph-node size. Typically a lymph node can be readily distinguished from surrounding tissues because of its degree of attenuation, which is similar to that of muscle and very distinct from that of fat. Necrosis and calcification are rare in HD in the absence of previous treatment. Hodgkin's disease tends to displace or compress structures nearby rather than invading into them. Even when nodes are enlarged, these imaging techniques cannot discriminate between minor degrees of nodal enlargement resulting from infiltration by HD or, on the other hand, reactive or inflammatory lymphadenopathy.

The accepted normal size of lymph nodes varies from site to site. Mediastinal, hilar, axillary, para-aortic, portocaval and mesenteric lymph nodes are usually less than 10 mm in size. However, lymph nodes further from the diaphragm within the abdomen, such as iliac and inguinal nodes, may be normally

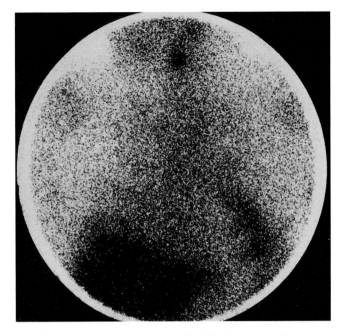

Fig. 16.1 Gallium-67 scan positive on the left side of the neck. Note the normal hepatic excretion.

up to 15 mm. Lymph nodes of 1 cm are probably abnormal in the paracardiac or retrocrural spaces. The acceptable size of lymph nodes decreases with age and interpretation has to take account of this.

Isotopic imaging methods can give information other than the size of the lymph nodes. Gallium is taken up by HD tissues and can be very helpful in distinguishing active from residual fibrotic lymphadenopathy where the uptake is positive (Fig. 16.1) [69], although there is an appreciable false-negative rate. It is most useful in the chest, but images in the abdomen may be obscured by normal uptake into the liver and bowel [68]. Positron emission tomography (PET) holds considerable promise in research applications [70].

Thorax

CT is the cross-sectional imaging investigation of routine choice for patients with HD in the thorax.

The involvement of lymphoid structures in the thorax is common in HD, being found in 65–85% of patients [71,72]. Mediastinal lymphadenopathy is usually located in paratracheal and anterior mediastinal lymph nodes and, much less often, in the posterior mediastinum (Fig. 16.2). Hilar lymphadenopathy is uncommon unless there is associated mediastinal disease, and involvement of lung parenchyma is rare in the absence of mediastinal disease. Enlargement of the thymus is reported in 30–50% of patients with HD [73], and residual enlargement may be seen after treatment. Pulmonary manifestations of HD may be by direct extension from involved lymph nodes or there may be discrete nodular, sometimes

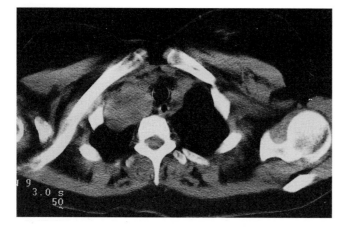

Fig. 16.2 Mediastinal HD with bulky disease to the right of the trachea.

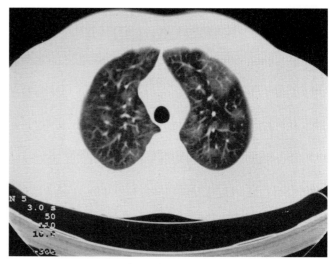

Fig. 16.3 Diffuse pulmonary infiltration with HD.

cavitating, involvement of the lungs (Fig. 16.3). Rarely there may be bronchial obstruction or interstitial infiltration. Between 5 and 10% of patients have pleural effusions.

Abdomen

CT, occasionally supplemented by MRI, will demonstrate the involvement of para-aortic iliac and inguinal lymph nodes if they are enlarged. Lymphangiography was historically thought to be superior to CT in staging para-aortic nodes [74]. Current investigators have not confirmed this [75]. MRI is as good as CT in detecting retroperitoneal and pelvic nodal disease. Neither investigation is reliable for mesenteric lymphadenopathy.

Visceral involvement in the abdomen is most frequently found in the spleen and liver. Within the spleen, involvement is usually diffuse and only occasionally are discrete nodules visible. Splenomegaly does not necessarily indicate involvement by HD and can be found in 30% of patients with the disease who do not have histological involvement [74,76–78]. Similarly, hepatomegaly is not specific for HD and discrete abnormalities in the liver are unusual. Involvement of other intra-abdominal viscera, such as the pancreas, kidneys, bladder, ovaries and the gastrointestinal tract, may be a feature of NHL, but each is only very rarely found in HD and even more rarely as the only site of involvement [68].

Skeleton

Primary involvement of bones by HD does not occur. Secondary involvement in association with extensive disease was seen more frequently prior to the development of effective treatments [79], and most cases arise by direct extension from nodal deposits, particularly in the anterior mediastinum. Sclerosis occurs in bone lesions following treatment. Skeletal radiological survey and isotope scintography are not routinely indicated, unless patients have localized skeletal symptoms or known bone involvement at any site.

Central nervous system

Central nervous system (CNS) involvement by HD is rare at presentation. At relapse, leptomeningeal disease can occur and, occasionally, there are parenchymal brain deposits. However, these occurrences are so uncommon that the diagnosis must be very carefully reconsidered in any patient presenting with CNS masses or infiltration in HD.

Imaging during treatment and follow up

Clinical and plain X-ray assessments of response are made following each cycle of chemotherapy. More detailed assessment is usually made after four cycles by CT scanning, in order to judge whether residual masses after six cycles are continuing to reduce in size. After treatment, all investigations that were previously abnormal should be repeated. Mediastinal masses are a special problem. If a mass continues to regress during treatment, this suggests the presence of active disease. Once it is stable, with no further regression on treatment, then it is labelled a complete remission (uncertain) (CRu). Many patients will be treated with consolidation radiotherapy in this situation, and then followed carefully with CT scans every 3–4 months. An increase in size suggests recurrence but a change in attenuation need not do so. Masses that are static for 1 year are usually regarded as inactive residual tissue.

In patients without a residual mass, routine chest X-rays are normally taken 3-monthly during the first year, 6-monthly until 5 years from the end of treatment and annually thereafter. Many centres use 6-monthly CT scans for the first 3 years and then discontinue cross-sectional imaging investigations unless there is a clinical indication.

Staging laparotomy

With few exceptions the stage of HD is now determined by clinical staging using the clinical, serological and imaging investigations described above. However, staging laparotomy and splenectomy was previously used as a highly accurate method for evaluating the extent of intra-abdominal HD. In patients who were identified as having only supradiaphragmatic involvement clinically, 25–30% showed abdominal involvement after this investigation. If patients were carefully selected, taking account of a wide range of clinical prognostic factors, the probability of detecting abdominal involvement at laparotomy and splenectomy was reduced to under 20%. However, no clinical prognostic factors have yet been identified which can reduce the proportion below this level [80–83]. The diagnostic accuracy of staging laparotomy had to be balanced against the risk of sampling errors, postsplenectomy infection risk, a small but real major complication rate from surgery [84], a possible association with secondary leukaemia [85,86], the cost of the operation and the inevitable delay in instituting therapy.

Determination of clinical prognostic groups allowed the application of chemotherapy for patients with adverse features. This, together with the success of 'salvage' therapy for patients with progressive abdominal disease following extended field radiotherapy to the chest, contributed to the decline of staging laparotomy. A randomized trial demonstrated the equivalent survival of patients staged by laparotomy or clinically when subtotal nodal irradiation was used [87], and such results appear to have been sustained in the long term [88]. The staging laparotomy is therefore no longer used in the great majority of centres worldwide.

Management

Increasingly, the approach to the management of HD considers a broad range of prognostic factors in addition to clinical stage. The aim is to achieve the highest cure rate, which is consistent with the use of the least amount of treatment and the preservation of the best quality of life among cured patients. The choice of treatment modality is now determined not only by the probability of cure, but also by the probability of major long-term toxicities, such as infertility, ischaemic heart disease and second malignancy. Other factors must also be considered in judging the choice of treatment. Patients may have views about the side-effect profile which they are prepared to tolerate, both in the short term and in the long term. Fertility may be a central issue and long-term employment and psychosocial aspects of care must be taken into account. This complex risk/benefit evaluation emphasizes the need for management of patients with HD in multidisciplinary teams.

It is artificial to separate the disease into categories determined only by its anatomical extent. However, treatment can usefully be discussed separately under the headings of localized and advanced disease.

Localized disease

Staging was introduced in order to allow the most appropriate application of radiotherapy, reserving systemic treatment for patients who had little probability of cure by irradiation alone or those in whom the disease recurred. This approach has now changed (reviewed in ref. [83]), with the recognition of the long-term toxicity, particularly second solid cancers, resulting from radiotherapy and the availability of a wider range of effective chemotherapies. Some of these, despite considerable acute toxicity, have much lower probabilities of long-term toxicity than the initial quadruple chemotherapy, MOPP, described by De Vita *et al.* [9].

Localized disease will now be almost always defined by clinical investigation. Factors which influence prognosis have recently been reviewed [83,89,90]. The principal adverse features for localized HD are.

1 The presence of B symptoms and severe pruritus [89–95].

2 Anatomical extent. Even within the Ann Arbor stages, the extent of disease will influence outcome. Unilateral high neck nodes are favourable; bulky mediastinal disease and involvement of more than two sites above the diaphragm are unfavourable, as is the presence of inguinal lymphadenopathy [96–99].

3 Histology: Patients with mixed cellularity of lymphocyte-deplete types have a higher rate of occult spread.

4 Patients of more than 40 or 50 years have a lower probability of survival, even with localized disease.

5 A raised ESR, severe anaemia and lymphocytopenia are unfavourable.

6 Serological abnormalities of IL-6 ferritin, β-2-microglobulin, albumin, lactate dehydrogenase and soluble CD30 may have significant prognostic value, as discussed above.

Radiotherapy

Dose. Complex analyses of the relationship between local control and the dose of radiation have been carried out over many years. Broadly, there is little added value in doses above 35 Gy and daily fraction sizes between 1.5 Gy and 2 Gy are established practice [100–102].

Fields. The use of radiation fields extended beyond apparent sites of disease has been common for many years and is still widely practised [103–105]. The classic extended radiation field is a supradiaphragmatic mantle in which all nodal areas above the diaphragm are irradiated. If this approach is applied to patients with clinical stage I and II disease, then recurrence will occur in up to 45% of patients [83]. Even when staging laparotomy was used to select patients for mantle irradiation, about 30% still had recurrences at some site, usually in non-irradiated areas [82]. This led to the use of prophylactic abdominal irradiation with clinical stage I and II disease.

If patients are selected for a supradiaphragmatic mantle with para-aortic strip using known prognostic factors, then a group is identified with the probability of relapse after irradiation is reduced to about 20% [102]. However, this may no longer be regarded as fully satisfactory, even for this small group. Long-term follow-up of European [93,94,106] and American [106–108] data shows that patients treated with radiotherapy for clinical stage I and II disease have a high late mortality due to radiation, and that this may exceed the mortality from HD. It is not clear, on long-term follow-up, that the extent of the radiation field has a survival impact on patients who have access to effective salvage chemotherapy, and irradiation is a significant contributor to late nondisease-related mortality, which in some cases exceeds 25% [83,109].

The risk–benefit evaluation of the management of localized HD with radiotherapy has now become highly complex. On the one hand, a proportion of these patients, if carefully selected according to prognostic factors, may be freed from the risk of HD with a high probability. On the other hand, they will have an increased risk of cumulative late mortality from other causes.

The value of extended radiotherapy fields compared to less extensive radiotherapy has been evaluated by meta-analysis of randomized trials by Specht & Gray [110]. In this meta-analysis, more extensive radiotherapy reduced the relapse rate. However, because of the success of salvage chemotherapy, the use of more extensive radiation fields was not associated with any improved survival. Since the follow-up in these trials did not exceed 10 years for many patients, the impact of more extensive fields upon late development of secondary solid tumours is not yet evaluable.

Localized Hodgkin's disease below the diaphragm. About 10% of patients will present with nodal disease below the diaphragm [111–116]. Most of these will have palpable femoral or inguinal nodes and a few will have intra-abdominal disease.

The approach to treating these patients is less well defined because of their relative rarity. Patients with isolated stage I disease in femoral, inguinal or superficial iliac regions have been commonly treated with extended irradiation in an inverted Y field, and this would often include splenic irradiation. Such patients develop recurrences in approximately 20% of cases [83]. Patients who have stage II disease below the diaphragm or B symptoms have a high failure rate with radiation therapy and are now treated with chemotherapy.

Mediastinal disease. Involvement of the mediastinum is common and occurs in 60–70% of patients. When this is bulky (defined as greater than one-third of the transthoracic diameter or greater than 10 cm by direct measurement in most

studies), it represents a particular problem [117–119]. When irradiation alone is used there is a high risk of relapse within the thorax. Bulky mediastinal disease is now treated by chemotherapy, with consolidation radiotherapy reserved for treatment of the site of previous bulk or residual masses. The mediastinal contour will frequently remain abnormal after treatment [120–122]. Imaging, particularly using gallium scans, may occasionally be helpful (see above), but often follow-up with chest radiographs and CT scanning are the only ways to determine whether there may be residual active disease. If no change occurs over 1 year of observation, then an assumption of complete remission is usually made.

Radiation to salvage local recurrence of disease. Relapse from radiotherapy is almost always treated by chemotherapy, although isolated local recurrence occurring after involved field radiotherapy or after chemotherapy may sometimes be treated by irradiation alone. Such salvage treatment can result in long-term survival for a small number of carefully selected patients [123–125]. Patients are selected if the relapse appears to be truly localized and nonbulky and there are no systemic symptoms. Patients with a long initial disease-free interval are more likely to be cured by salvage irradiation therapy [125]. This approach should be considered in carefully selected patients who might otherwise receive very complex chemotherapy regimens, including high-dose treatment with autologous haemopoietic support. After the delivery of this treatment it is wise to re-stage patients carefully and consider peripheral blood stem cell harvest and cryopreservation.

Combined modality therapy

The combination of chemotherapy with radiotherapy for patients with localized disease has been in use since the late 1970s. A series of randomized trials has addressed the comparison of irradiation as initial treatment compared to irradiation either preceded or followed by chemotherapy. Even single-agent chemotherapy in an early European Organization for Reseach and Treatment of Cancer (EORTC) trial reduced the probability of relapse following irradiation [80]. However, because of the availability of effective salvage combination chemotherapy, there was no improvement in survival with the combined modality approach. This study pointed the way to subsequent trials comparing extended field radiotherapy to mantle radiotherapy plus MOPP [126]; mantle irradiation to mantle radiotherapy plus MVPP (nitrogen mustard, vinblastine, procarbazine, prednisolone) [127]; extensive radiotherapy to involved field radiotherapy plus vinblastine, bleomycin and methotrexate [128]; extended radiotherapy versus the same radiotherapy plus MOPP [82]; subtotal nodal irradiation compared to involved field radiotherapy plus epirubicin, Bleomycin, vinblastine and prednisolone [129]. All these studies consistently show that chemotherapy can reduce the recurrence rate after radiotherapy. However, none showed any survival advantage from the combined modality approach, presumably due to effective salvage combination chemotherapy after radiotherapy alone.

Specht & Gray [110], in a meta-analysis, combined the data on 12 trials of adjuvant chemotherapy involving 1653 patients. They confirmed that adjuvant chemotherapy had a highly significant impact in reducing the rate of recurrence. However, there was no overall impact on survival, although there was a trend (not statistically significant) towards improved survival in those who received adjuvant chemotherapy (reduction in odds of death $9.3 \pm 9.3\%$). The reduction in deaths in patients who received combined modality treatment was greater when deaths from HD alone were considered (reduction $20 \pm 12\%$).

Three groups have now reported the use of brief Adriamycin-containing chemotherapy followed by radiotherapy, either to involved or extended fields [130,131]. Two have used ABVD (Adriamycin, Bleomycin, vinblastine, dacarbazine), and one a rather similar, short, weekly chemotherapy containing Adriamycin and Bleomycin (VAPEC-B). The reported results are good when this approach is applied to patients with stage I and IIA disease, with disease-free survival and overall survival of over 90%. This simple approach might be expected to have minimal late toxicity in the form of infertility or second malignancies and deserves further evaluation.

Chemotherapy alone vs radiotherapy for localized Hodgkin's disease

The possibility of using chemotherapy alone in localized HD may assume critical importance as the evidence of long-term toxicities from radiotherapy accumulates.

Two questions have been addressed in randomized trials.

1 *Chemotherapy alone vs radiotherapy alone.* Biti *et al.* [132], in a small study of 89 patients with surgically staged localized disease, compared mantle plus para-aortic radiotherapy to six cycles of MOPP combination chemotherapy. The initial control of the disease was similar in the two groups, but with a long follow-up of 8 years median, overall survival was reported to be higher in the radiation-alone group (93%) compared to the chemotherapy-alone group (56%). Longo *et al.* [133], in a group of patients with localized stage IA to IIIA (mainly surgically staged patients), compared subtotal nodal irradiation to MOPP combination chemotherapy and the 10-years disease-free and overall survival rates were significantly higher in the patients treated with MOPP. The difference between these two studies has not been explained and the question remains controversial.

2 *Chemotherapy alone vs chemotherapy plus radiotherapy.* Few randomized trials have addressed this question in localized HD. Pavlovsky *et al.* [134] reported a randomized trial of patients with clinical stage I and II disease, comparing chemotherapy with cyclophosphamide, vinblastine, procarbazine and prednisone against the same regimen with the addition of radiation therapy after the third cycle of combination chemotherapy. A significant advantage in disease-free survival was apparent in those who received radiotherapy, but no overall survival difference was shown. It may be possible to extrapolate from comparisons of chemotherapy to chemotherapy plus radiotherapy carried out in more advanced disease groups. Loeffler *et al.* [135] carried out a meta-analysis, seeking to clarify the role of combined modality treatment compared to chemotherapy alone in intermediate and advanced-stage HD. Although 30 randomized trials were identified in the literature, only 14 were available for the meta-analysis, and varying study designs make interpretation difficult. However, there was a suggestion that when the duration of chemotherapy was limited, radiotherapy may improve long-term disease-free survival. In patients who received more than six cycles of chemotherapy, radiotherapy appeared to add very little. Patients with mediastinal involvement and, in particular, a large mediastinal mass may be those who benefit most from the addition of radiotherapy to chemotherapy.

Advanced disease

Chemotherapy in advanced Hodgkin's disease

Hodgkin's disease which has extended beyond radiotherapy fields can only be treated by chemotherapy. Single-agent activity of drugs has been reviewed [53] and their activities are listed in Table 16.4. Combination chemotherapy is currently the standard approach following the introduction of a cyclical four-drug regimen, MOPP, by De Vita and colleagues [9], which will cure more than half of the patients treated with it [136]. During the past 25 years, work on combination chemotherapy of HD has focused on the introduction of more effective approaches to disease control, on the reduction of

Table 16.4 Single-agent chemotherapy for HD.

	Response (%)	Complete remission (%)
Drugs evaluated before combination chemotherapy		
Chlorambucil	61	16
Cyclophosphamide	54	12
Mustine	63	13
Vinblastine	68	30
Vincristine	58	36
Procarbazine	69	37
Prednisone	60	0
Drugs mainly evaluated after combination chemotherapy		
BCNU	44	5
CCNU	48	12
Adriamycin	30	5
Bleomycin	38	6
Dacarbazine	56	6
Etoposide	27	6

Table 16.5 MOPP regimen and its variants.

MOPP (NCI)
Nitrogen mustard 6 mg/m² days 1, 8 IV
Vincristine 1.4 mg/m² days 1, 8 IV
Procarbazine 100 mg/m² days 1–14 PO
Prednisone 40 mg/m² days 1–14 PO
    q 28 days

MVPP (St Bartholomew's)
Nitrogen mustard 6 mg/m² days 1, 8 IV
Vinblastine 10 mg days 1, 8, 14 IV
Procarbazine 100 mg/m² days 1–14 PO
Prednisolone 40 mg days 1–14 PO
    q 42 days

ChlVPP (Royal Marsden Hospital)
Chlorambucil 6 mg/m² days (not to exceed 10 mg) days 1–14 PO
Vinblastine 6 mg/m² (not to exceed 10 mg) days 1, 8 IV
Procarbazine 100 mg/m² days 1–14 PO
Prednisolone 40 mg days 1–14 PO
    q 28 days

CVPP
Cyclophosphamide 1.0 g/m² IV
Vinblastine 0.1 mg/kg days 1, 8 IV
Procarbazine 100 mg/m² days 1–7 PO
Prednisone 40 mg/m² days 1–7 PO
    q 21 days

CVPP (Minneapolis)
Cyclosphosphamide 300 mg/m² days 1, 8 IV
Vinblastine 10 mg days 1, 8, 15 IV
Procarbazine 100 mg/m² days 1–15 PO
Prednisone 40 mg/m² days 1–15 PO

BCVPP (ECOG)
BCNU 100 mg/m² day 1 IV
Cyclophosphamide 600 mg/m² day 1 IV
Vinblastine 5 mg/m² day 1 IV
Procarbazine 50 mg/day day 1 PO
            100 mg/day days 2–10 PO
Prednisone 60 mg/day days 1–10 PO
    q 28 days

Table 16.6 Doxorubicin-based regimens.

ABVD			
Adriamycin	25 mg/m²		
Bleomycin	10 mg/m²	days 1, 15 IV	Repeat day 29
Vinblastine	6 mg/m²		
Dacarbazine	375 mg/m²		
ABDIC			
Adriamycin	45 mg/m²	day 1 IV	
Bleomycin	5 mg/m²	days 1, 5 IV	
Dacarbazine	200 mg/m²	days 1, 5 V	Repeat day 29
CCNU	50 mg/m²	day 1 PO	
Prednisone	40 mg/m²	day PO 1–5 PO	
B-CAVe			
Bleomycin	5 mg/m²	days 1, 28, 35 IV	
CCNU	100 mg/m²	day 1 PO	
Adriamycin	60 mg/m²	day 1 IV	Repeat day 29
Vinblastine	5 mg/m²	day 1 IV	
HOPE-Bleo			
Adriamycin	40 mg/m²	day 1 IV	
Vincristine	1.4 mg/m²	day 1, 8 IV	
Bleomycin	10 mg/m²	day 1, 8 IV	Repeat day 21
Etoposide	200 mg/m²	days 1–4 PO	
Prednisolone	40 mg/m²	days 1–8 PO	

can be safely tolerated by the patient, in order to achieve the best results.

4 Combinations should be given to complete remission and then two further cycles should be given. No advantage is gained from continuing maintenance chemotherapy in HD beyond this point.

Alkylating-based regimens are no longer regarded as a sufficient therapy when given alone. The introduction of Adriamycin-based regimens, alternating chemotherapy and hybrid regimens have altered the approach to chemotherapy for advanced HD.

Doxorubicin-containing regimens (Table 16.6). The first effective combination chemotherapy containing doxorubicin to achieve wide application was the ABVD regimen, introduced in Milan for the treatment of patients with recurrent disease after therapy with MOPP [137,138]. Once the efficacy of ABVD as a relapse regimen had been established [139–141], it was also tested as initial therapy.

ABVD was compared to MOPP in the pivotal Cancer and Leukaemia Group B study reported by Canellos *et al.* [142], for the treatment of patients who had had no prior chemotherapy. Following six to eight cycles of MOPP, six to eight cycles of ABVD or 12 cycles of alternating MOPP/ABVD, the response rate, failure-free survival and overall survival were all superior in the two anthracycline-containing procedures when compared to MOPP alone. There was no significant difference between alternating and ABVD therapy, except in the

acute and long-term toxicity and, more recently, on the introduction of effective salvage regimens.

The MOPP regimen and its variants. Table 16.5 lists variations that have been introduced on the standard MOPP regimen, containing alternative alkylating agents replacing mustine, or an alternative vinca alkaloid replacing vincristine. These regimens and studies comparing them were reviewed by Selby *et al.* [53] and some general conclusions are possible.

1 None of the alkylating agent-based regimens has been shown to be significantly more effective than any other.

2 Regimens in which mustine is replaced by an oral alkylating agent, particularly chlorambucil, are significantly less acutely toxic than MOPP.

3 Regimens should be delivered in full doses, as intensively as

Table 16.7 Alternating, hybrid and weekly chemotherapy combinations.

Alternating MOPP/ABVD			
Nitrogen mustard	6 mg/m²	days 1, 8 IV	
Vincristine	1.4 mg/m²	days 1, 8 IV	
Procarbazine	100 mg/m²	days 1–14 PO	
Prednisone	40 mg/m²	days 1–14 PO	Cycle repeated
Doxorubicin	25 mg/m²	days 29, 43 IV	q 56 days
Bleomycin	10 mg/m²	days 29, 43 IV	
Vinblastine	6 mg/m²	days 29, 43 IV	
Dacarbazine	375 mg/m²	days 29, 43 IV	
Alternating ChlVPP/PABlOE			
Chlorambucil	6 mg/m²	days 1–14 PO	
Vinblastine	6 mg/m²	days 1, 8 IV	
Procarbazine	100 mg/m²	days 1–14 PO	
Prednisolone	40 mg/m²	days 1–14, 29–38 PO	Cycle repeated
Doxorubicin	40 mg/m²	day 29 IV	q 49 days
Vincristine	1.4 mg/m²	days 29, 36 IV	
Bleomycin	10 mg/m²	days 29, 36 IV	
Etoposide	200 mg/m²	days 29–31 PO	
Hybrid MOPP/ABV			
Nitrogen mustard	6 mg/m²	day 1 IV	
Vincristine	1.4 mg/m²	day 1 IV	
Procarbazine	100 mg/m²	days 1–7 PO	
Prednisone	40 mg/m²	days 1–14 PO	Cycle repeated
Doxorubicin	35 mg/m²	day 8 IV	q 28 days
Bleomycin	10 mg/m²	day 8 IV	
Vinblastine	6 mg/m²	day 8 IV	
Hybrid ChlVPP/EVA			
Chlorambucil	6 mg/m²	days 1–7 PO	
Vincristine	1.4 mg/m²	day 1 IV	
Etoposide	75 mg/m²	days 1–5 PO	
Procarbazine	100 mg/m²	days 1–7 PO	Cycle repeated
Prednisolone	50 mg	days 1–7 PO	q 28 days
Doxorubicin	50 mg/m²	day 8 IV	
Vinblastine	6 mg/m²	day 8 IV	
Stanford V weekly regimen			
Doxorubicin	25 mg/m²	days 1, 15 IV	
Vinblastine	6 mg/m²	days 1, 15 IV	
Nitrogen mustard	6 mg/m²	day 1 IV	Cycle repeated q 28
Vincristine	1.4 mg/m²	days 8, 22 IV	days times 3
Bleomycin	10 mg/m²	days 8, 22 IV	
Etoposide	60 mg/m²	days 15, 16 IV	
Prednisone	40 mg/m²	daily, tapering at week 10	

degree of myelotoxicity, which was greater in the seven-drug procedure.

In the UK, the acute nausea and vomiting associated with ABVD led to the exchange of dacarbazine for etoposide and the introduction of four- or five-drug regimens containing Adriamycin, etoposide, a vinca alkaloid, bleomycin and prednisolone. These have been used to replace ABVD in alternating and hybrid combinations with some success (see below). However, the use of Adriamycin-etoposide containing four- or five-drug regimens alone has not been shown to be equivalent to ABVD in any prospective trial, and recent results suggest that they may be inadequate as initial treatment for advanced HD [143].

Alternating chemotherapy regimens (Table 16.7). The availability of MOPP and related regimens and of ABVD and related regimens, led to the exploration of these given in combination. Theoretical considerations suggest that this might restrict the emergence of drug resistance, and hence of treatment failure [144]. Bonadonna and colleagues in Milan used alternating MOPP/ABVD regimens and showed a significant improvement in outcome, including survival, when compared to MOPP in their initial reports [138] and a persisting favourable trend in longer-term follow up [145]. Similar results are reported from the Cancer and Leukaemia Group B (CALGB) Study, as described above [142], and by the EORTC Study [146], although with a slightly different treatment design. In the UK the British National Lymphoma Investigation (BNLI) used an alternating regimen, consisting of chlorambucil, vincristine, procarbazine and prednisolone (LOPP (Ch1VPP)) with a doxorubicin, etoposide, vinblastine and prednisolone regimen (EVAP). The alternating LOPP/EVAP regimen was superior to LOPP in remission rate, relapse probability and overall survival [147].

A recently completed UK study comparing a doxorubicin, etoposide, Bleomycin, vincristine and prednisolone regimen, known as PABlOE, to the same regimen alternating with Ch1VPP showed significant improvements in complete remission rate and progression-free survival with the alternating regimen [143].

Not all attempts at the development of alternating combination chemotherapy regimens have resulted in improved results when tested in randomized controlled trials. A South Eastern Cancer Study Group trial studied a regimen known as BVCPP-Bleo (cyclophosphamide, BCNU, vinblastine, procarbazine, prednisolone, Bleomycin). The six-drug regimen was compared to the same regimen, alternating with ABVD, with equivalent results [148]. The CALGB Study compared COPP to a regimen known as BAVS (Bleomycin, Adriamycin, vincristine, streptozotocin), and to an alternating treatment containing these two regimens, and again there was no improvement in survival or other outcomes [149]. The US National Cancer Institute compared MOPP to an alternating regimen of MOPP with CABS (CCNU, Adriamycin, Bleomycin, streptozotocin), and similarly showed no improvement in outcome [150]. The comparison of LOPP to an alternating regimen of LOPP/ABOD (Adriamycin, Bleomycin, vincristine, dacarbazine) also showed no improvement [151].

Alternating chemotherapy still has an established role in the management of HD, and the regimen MOPP/ABVD or its derivatives are at least as good as any other published combination chemotherapy treatment schedule. The alternating regimens appear superior to MOPP and related regimens in large trials. It remains unclear whether ABVD will have equivalent efficacy to MOPP/ABVD, although the evidence from the CALGB Study suggests that this may be the case.

Hybrid chemotherapy regimens (Table 16.7). Hybrid regimens integrate the seven or eight drugs from alternating schedules and administer attenuated doses of all the drugs in the course of each cycle [152]. A randomized study comparing a hybrid anthracycline-based regimen with MVPP at the Christie Hospital and St Bartholomew's showed the hybrid to be superior, with 80% 5-year progression-free survival [153].

Two large studies have addressed the relative efficacy of alternating vs hybrid approaches, and both concluded that they were therapeutically equivalent. The longest follow-up (median 9 years) comes from the study in Milan, comparing MOPP alternating with ABVD and half-MOPP/half-ABVD hybrid, with most patients receiving six to eight cycles in total. The complete response rate was high (90%) in both procedures, and actuarial freedom from progression was 68% at

10 years (69% hybrid, 67% alternating). Overall survival was also the same, with an actuarial 10-year survival of 72% in the hybrid and 74% in the alternating procedure [154]. The results of a large Canadian trial addressing the same question are similar, with no difference in response rate, 5-year failure-free survival or overall survival between alternating MOPP/ABVD and hybrid MOPP/ABV [155].

A trial by the German Hodgkin's Disease Study Group, which is now in progress, is examining the efficacy of an alternating regimen, COPP/ABVD, versus a hybrid, BEACOPP (Bleomycin, etoposide, Adriamycin, cytophosphamide, vincristine, prednisolone, procarbazine), the dosage of which is being escalated. An interim analysis has shown the alternating arm to be significantly inferior in terms of progression-free survival [156], but the final results of this study are still awaited. Conversely, a previous BNLI Study suggested that hybrid therapy might be inferior, but the doses used in this schedule were probably suboptimal [157].

Only one study has so far been conducted to compare ABVD with a hybrid schedule. The US Intergroup Study has recently closed, and the results are not yet mature enough for firm conclusions to be made [158]. There was, however, a worrying incidence of secondary leukaemia in the hybrid procedure of this study—a finding not reported from other large trials of hybrid regimens.

Weekly chemotherapy regimens (Table 16.7). Rapid alternating chemotherapy schedules were developed for NHLs as a method of raising dose intensity and the number of different drugs given at an early phase of treatment. Although this approach has not proved to be superior in NHL, there are preliminary results from single-centre pilot studies in HD which appear to hold considerable promise for the future. At Stanford University a 12-week regimen has been used which incorporates mustine, doxorubicin, etoposide, bleomycin, prednisolone and two vincas followed by consolidation radiotherapy, originally given to all sites of involvement, but more recently only to sites of tumour bulk >5 cm. The very high response rate with this regimen is apparently sustained, with 87% 3-year failure-free survival [159]. Although it is difficult to know how much of a role the undoubtedly extensive radiotherapy plays in this success, the initial results seem to be very encouraging.

An alternative weekly therapy, which has been tested in the UK, is VAPEC-B (vinca, Adriamycin, prednisolone, etoposide, cyclophosphamide, Bleomycin) [160]. Although this has been shown to be active against recurrent HD, this regimen, when tested in a randomized trial against a hybrid, has yielded inferior results in terms of progression-free survival [161].

Choice of chemotherapy by prognostic factors

The difficulty of selecting patients for an initial intensive or novel approach to therapy has been emphasized above, in the discussion of prognostic factors. Broadly, the ability to select patients who, at presentation, have features predictive of failure with conventional combination chemotherapy is poor. A large collaborative analysis of prognostic factors in over 5000 patients was only able to identify a small subgroup of less than 5% with a predicted 5-year progression-free survival of less than 50% [162]. Approaches to therapy based upon the risk-adjustment concept are undergoing continuous development [97,163], and may become effective as our understanding of the biology of HD improves.

Radiotherapy in advanced disease

The long-term toxicity of radiotherapy makes it advisable to give the minimum dose necessary. The site of previous bulky disease, in particular in the mediastinum, and residual masses following chemotherapy are now the principal routine clinical indications for radiotherapy, when not considering prospective randomized trials. A recent trial by the German Hodgkins Study Group showed that for patients in complete remission after three cycles of alternating COPP/ABVD, a further cycle of chemotherapy was as effective as involved field radiotherapy for consolidation treatment [164].

Management of recurrent Hodgkin's disease

Recurrence after radiotherapy

Combination chemotherapy is as effective for managing HD recurring after radiotherapy as it is when used in untreated patients. Long-term survival is possible for 50–60% of patients using either MOPP or ABVD regimens, or their derivatives [141,165–167]. The choice of regimen for this treatment is likely to be governed by the same considerations as the choice of regimen for initial chemotherapy. Current conventional preferences must therefore be for either multidrug alternating or hybrid regimens, or for ABVD alone.

Recurrence after chemotherapy

When HD recurs after initially successful chemotherapy, patients' chances of long-term survival are much reduced [168]. A small number may be cured by radiotherapy to localized relapses (see above), but for the majority it is necessary to seek another approach to chemotherapy. Factors prognostic of the outcome following relapse after chemotherapy are less well understood than those for initial treatment [169]. In general, ill patients with rapid recurrence and extensive disease do less well than those with late and localized relapses [170].

Some general principles apply.
1 Patients initially treated with four-drug regimens are usually retreated with the alternative at the time of recurrence. For instance, relapses after MOPP or Ch1VPP may now be treated with ABVD, because this can be regarded as the best treatment option for any patient.

2 Patients previously treated with multidrug regimens pose a difficult problem [171]. They may be retreated with similar drugs but in different schedules, such as weekly regimens, or different drugs altogether, such as BCNU, etoposide, cytosine arabinoside, melphalan (mini-BEAM). There may be a role for the immediate use of high-dose therapy in selected patients in this group, if progenitor cells free of HD can be collected (see below).

3 Patients with short initial remissions or poor prognostic features should be considered for intensive high-dose therapy with autologous haematological support [172]. Patients with chemoresistant disease at second treatment may still be considered for this approach, but the chances of long-term remission or cure are small.

Intensive therapy with haemopoietic support in the treatment of Hodgkin's disease

The management of relapsed HD has been one of the areas of apparent success for the use of intensive high-dose treatment, for which haemopoietic support in the form of autologous bone marrow or peripheral blood progenitor cell rescue is needed (reviewed in refs [173,174]).

The approach has now become widely used for the management of high-risk relapsed patients, and the International Bone Marrow Transplant Registry holds data on 7000 autologous transplants for HD, with about 300 new registrations each year. The worldwide activity is likely to be much greater than this. This treatment approach has thus achieved an established place in the management of HD, although so far only one randomized trial has been conducted to confirm the benefits apparent from case series.

The earliest studies in the 1970s used autologous bone marrow rescue and, because there was relatively little experience in the selection and supportive care of these patients, the treatment carried a significant risk. Some series reported early deaths in 10–20% of patients, with most of them related to the treatment itself. With the improvements in technology, the increasing experience in transplant centres, the introduction of growth factors and peripheral blood progenitor cell harvesting, this treatment approach has become safe within specialist centres that have accumulated the relevant experience [175]. More work is done in outpatient clinics and in older patients [176]. Unfortunately, late complications are now increasingly recognized [177], and the precise place for this approach remains unclear and there is a need for continuing study and, in particular, where possible, for the accumulation of data in randomized prospective trials. More than a dozen phase II trials in relapsed HD have been reported [173,174,178–195]. Published treatment-related mortality ranges from 0 to 23%, and continuous complete remission ranges from 24 to 64%. The different series are not comparable, because they have different case mixes and treatment regimens.

Several studies have been carried out to consider prognostic factors before high-dose therapy. In general, the probability of cure following high-dose therapy is related to prior chemosensitivity, reflected in the number of regimens used previously, and the length of remissions. In one series, patients who had received more than two conventional chemotherapy regimens had a median progression-free survival of 5.1 months compared to 26.9 months for those who had less previous chemotherapy [190]. The response to previous chemotherapy is a powerful determinant, and those with responsive disease, in particular those with treatment leading to a second complete remission with conventional chemotherapy, have a higher probability of cure [179]. Patients with extensive and aggressive disease at recurrence, including systemic symptoms, extranodal sites of disease and short initial remissions, have a poorer prognosis. Reece *et al.* [186] have built these prognostic factors into a model capable of selecting patients with a high probability of long complete remission (no systemic symptoms, long initial remission, no extranodal disease), or a very low probability of prolonged progression-free survival if all of these risk factors are present. O'Brien *et al.* [196], in their analysis of prognostic factors, found little apparent benefit from high-dose chemotherapy in patients who had received three or more chemotherapy regimens and had never achieved complete remission.

In most phase II studies, conventional combination chemotherapy is used at the time of recurrence to reduce the amount of tumour bulk and test the sensitivity of the disease to treatment. The alternative approach of immediate intensive therapy may be feasible in carefully selected patients, such as those with small-volume disease, and the results appear promising [173,174,187]. Radiation to sites of prior disease or residual abnormalities is commonly used after high-dose treatment.

There is a lack of reliable evidence about the use of high-dose therapy. An historical control study was carried out at Stanford University [197], in which 60 patients who underwent high-dose treatment and autografting were compared to 109 matched patients previously treated with conventional therapy. There were some advantages in the high-dose group— event-free survival appeared better (53 vs 27%, P <0.01), although even in this nonrandomized comparison there was no convincing evidence of an overall survival benefit (54 vs 47% at 4 years, P = 0.25). In the only randomized prospective trial, the British National Lymphoma Investigation compared high-dose carmustine, etoposide, cytarabine and melphalan (BEAM) to a similar regimen in smaller doses not requiring haemopoietic rescue. Event-free survival was 53% in the high-dose group compared to 10% in the low-dose group at 3 years and this difference was statistically significant [198]. The trend in overall survival favoured the transplantation group but the difference was not statistically significant then, and is still not now. These results, together with descriptive comparisons of the phase II studies listed above with the results of conventional chemotherapy, are the basis on which the treatment is recommended to patients with recurrent HD after combination chemotherapy. It cannot be said that the results

are conclusive. However, the higher remission rates and the prolonged failure-free survival are indications of the efficacy of treatment. The lack of an impact on overall survival may be due to later cross-over to intensive therapy in patients treated initially with conventional therapy.

In a significant proportion of patients, the primary treatment of HD fails to induce complete remission. Such patients rarely enjoy long survival after conventional second-line therapy. Two studies of high-dose treatment have focused on this difficult group and reported complete remissions with significant progression-free survivals of 42% [199] and 31% [184]. Primary refractory HD of this kind is now usually treated with high-dose therapy and haemopoietic support.

The place of intensive therapy for patients in whom HD recurs after a long complete remission remains unclear. This approach should be considered in patients with recurrences up to 2 years after initial treatment. Patients with relapses after this should probably receive second-line conventional chemotherapy with close monitoring and cryopreservation of cells in remission, rather than routinely receiving intensive treatment, in view of the significant chance of cure with second-line conventional therapy and the risks of myeloablative treatment in both the short and long term [172].

The place of high-dose therapy in first remission for selected patients with HD is also far from established. Studies in NHL have had mixed results, and in HD patient selection is even more difficult [162]. The use of high-dose therapy for those with 'adverse' prognostic factors has been advocated by some groups [180,200]. However, even with the best attempts at selection using prognostic factors, it is difficult to identify the appropriate group of patients for these studies. Two trials are in progress to test the application of high-dose therapy in first remission, and the results of these will be very valuable.

The optimum high-dose regimen for HD has not been determined. In the retrospective studies of the European Bone Marrow Transplant Registry, the results appeared better following melphalan-based regimens when compared to those with high-dose cyclophosphamide [201], but such studies are fraught with difficulties of interpretation. In Europe the melphalan-based BEAM regimen is widely used [195], while in North America CBV is more common [191].

The source of haemopoietic support has changed over the last decade. Autologous bone marrow rescue is now rarely used and most work in HD is done with growth-factor-mobilized peripheral blood progenitors. This avoids the need for general anaesthesia and marrow harvesting, and leads to more rapid marrow reconstitution. The approach has been used in patients with hypocellular bone marrows and in those with bone marrow involvement, although the collection of adequate numbers of progenitors may be problematical in such cases. It is possible that peripheral blood progenitors are less heavily contaminated by malignant cells than bone marrow harvests [202], although this has not been shown conclusively. Most series show that the more rapid marrow reconstitution achieved with peripheral blood progenitors leads to shorter hospital stays and fewer complications. Three randomized studies comparing bone marrow with peripheral blood progenitors have included patients with HD. Two of these [203,204] used peripheral progenitors mobilized with growth factors, and both showed significant reductions in the time to engraftment of neutrophils and platelets, and to discharge from hospital. The third study [205] did not use growth factors for mobilization and showed no significant difference in recovery times. None of the randomized studies has demonstrated any difference in the probability of treatment failure according to the source of progenitors, although a retrospective registry survey did suggest superior results with bone marrow [206]. As with all registry data, the interpretation of these findings is highly uncertain.

Allogeneic bone marrow transplantation has been used in HD in small numbers of patients [207]. Although there is limited applicability, there may be a graft vs lymphoma effect. This approach may be associated with a lower relapse probability [208], but there is no evidence of an overall survival benefit [208–210]. A case-matching exercise carried out by the European Bone Marrow Transplant Registry, comparing 45 matched allogeneic transplants to 45 autologous procedures [211], showed no advantage to allogeneic transplantation, with a higher survival in the autologous transplant group. The procedure-related mortality was 48% in the allogeneic transplantation group compared to 27% in the autologous group.

Antibody-based therapy

Monoclonal antibody-based treatment strategies are beginning to be applied in HD, and preliminary results are now being reported. The markers expressed on HD cells, such as CD30, can be used as potential targets for antibodies directed against them, conjugated in some cases to toxin molecules or radioisotopes. An alternative approach uses bispecific antibodies to link target antigens to surface antigens of cytotoxic T-lymphocytes, such as CD3 or CD28 [212], or antigens of natural killer cells such as CD16 [52]. These approaches are feasible in experimental model systems and show early evidence of efficacy [213].

Special clinical problems

Hodgkin's disease in pregnancy

Patients with HD, particularly those without systemic symptoms, may remain fertile and, occasionally, clinicians will be faced with the problem of the investigation and treatment of a pregnant woman with HD. There is no evidence that pregnancy alters the natural history of HD [53,214–219]. Investigation must be curtailed and ultrasound or magnetic resonance imaging are preferable to plain radiology or computed tomography.

Treatment must be carried out on the assumption that radio-

therapy (including low doses scattered from therapeutic fields) and chemotherapy are significantly teratogenic and carcinogenic in the fetus [220]. This risk, as with all such risks, is worst in the first trimester. It is likely, but unproven, that alkylating agents and procarbazine are more teratogenic than Adriamycin-based regimens.

Following these principles, a pregnancy in the first trimester is at great risk from any therapy given for HD. Most authorities agree that termination of pregnancy, followed by full treatment of HD, is often appropriate in this situation and should be offered to these patients. Some patients will elect to continue in pregnancy, in which case treatment may be deferred if possible into the second trimester. At all stages of pregnancy cervical, mediastinal and axillary HD should be treated with involved radiotherapy fields, thus minimizing exposure to the abdomen [218]. More advanced HD should be treated with combination chemotherapy and the ABVD regimen represents a logical choice, although the long-term risks to the fetus are unknown. Successful pregnancy and treatment for HD can be achieved for many patients.

Patients who are more than 30 weeks pregnant should be given the opportunity to consider early induction and delivery of the fetus before treatment for HD. A careful balance between the risks of prematurity and the risks of chemotherapy or radiotherapy has to be drawn, in consultation with an obstetrician.

Hodgkin's disease in elderly patients

The relatively poor prognosis for older patients with HD has been reviewed recently [221]. Patients over the age of 40 appear to have a higher risk of relapse after radiotherapy alone [222], and the EORTC trial (H5) showed better recurrence-free survival in older patients treated with combined modality therapy than in those treated with only subtotal or total nodal radiation [82]. Relapse after radiotherapy in older patients has a relatively poor outcome when treated with chemotherapy [223]. In general, the management of HD in the elderly should involve combination chemotherapy. Radiotherapy should be reserved for those patients with bulky disease and the extent of the irradiation given should be kept to the minimum possible.

It is not possible to recommend a specific regimen which is appropriate in the elderly. Data increasingly suggests the superiority of regimens containing Adriamycin and related anthracyclines, and it seems likely that this will be a consistent observation for older patients. ABVD is therefore, at this stage, the standard regimen, either on its own or alternating with an alkylating agent-based regimen. The lower toxicity of the chlorambucil-containing regimens, such as ChlVPP, makes these preferable to mustine-containing regimens for elderly patients.

In the future, regimens specifically designed for the elderly should be considered, together with the use of appropriate support measures, to allow the use of full doses at least for the fitter older patients. Although dose reductions will reduce toxicity, they are almost invariably associated with a lower probability of cure [224].

Hodgkin's disease and HIV infection

Hodgkin's disease appears to have an increased incidence in people infected with HIV, with a high odds ratio in some studies [49]. The disease is often aggressive, with mixed cellularity subtype, B symptoms, stage IV disease and bone marrow involvement commonly being found [225–228]. The prognosis is poor with few patients surviving for more than 2 years [227,229]. Epstein–Barr virus involvement in this group is the rule and the prognosis appears to depend on the severity of the HIV infection reflected in CD4 counts [225].

Side effects of therapy

Acute toxicity

Radiotherapy has significant acute and long-term toxicity. For up to 8 weeks following therapy there is a consistent pattern of toxicity, reflecting damage to the proliferating and renewing tissues, such as the bone marrow, gut, oral mucosa, skin and hair. These acute effects resolve over a few weeks. Patients may be tired during therapy and for several weeks following. A dry mouth, parotid swelling and altered taste are frequent in patients receiving irradiation to the base of the skull which includes a substantial proportion of salivary glands. Nausea and emesis occur in a significant minority of patients receiving daily therapy, but these side effects respond well to antiemetics, including 5HT3 antagonists. With modern approaches skin reactions are minimal but dysphagia and mucositis of a minor degree are commonly reported at the dosage used to treat HD. These also resolve spontaneously after 1–2 weeks. Alopecia within the irradiation field is usual but regrowth of hair occurs. Upper abdominal or inverted Y radiotherapy results in fatigue and some myelosuppression. Nausea, emesis and weight loss are commoner than with supradiaphragmatic irradiation.

The acute complications of chemotherapy are well known. Nausea and vomiting are more common with regimens containing dacarbazine and mustine, although the use of 5HT3 antagonists with corticosteroids is usually successful in controlling them. There is nearly always complete alopecia in patients being treated with anthracycline-based regimens. Myelosuppression is a feature of all the regimens used to treat HD, and is the usual dose-limiting factor. Mucositis, particularly mouth ulceration, is often associated with neutropenia.

Late complications

As cure rates exceed 70% and follow-up lengthens for these patients, concern about late nonmalignant complications

increases. This subject has recently been excellently reviewed [230].

The immune deficiency which is characteristic of untreated HD is compounded by aggressive combination chemotherapy and results in prolonged T-cell functional impairment. Immune impairment may be worsened in patients surgically staged with splenectomy. These are therefore vulnerable to a complex mix of infections, including pneumonia, septicaemia, persistent skin infections and meningitis. Common organisms are frequently isolated, including *Streptococcus pneumoniae*, *Staphylococcus aureus*, *Staphylococcus epidermidis* and, less commonly, Gram-negative bacteria. Herpes virus infections and fungal infections, including *Candida*, *Aspergillus* and *Cryptococcosus*, are recognized and obscure clinical problems should always be investigated to exclude infections when patients present with complex syndromes after treatment for HD [231–233].

Thyroid dysfunction

Although thyroid dysfunction has been most commonly attributed to thyroid irradiation, combination chemotherapy can also cause hypothyroidism. In an EORTC study [234], all patients showed elevation of thyroid stimulating hormone, whether treated with irradiation or combination chemotherapy. In a study carried out at Stanford University, the cumulative risk of thyroid disease was 50% at 20 years in patients who mainly received radiotherapy. The proportion of patients with clinical hypothyroidism increases with age and hypothyroidism is associated with female gender, the use of chemotherapy and higher irradiation doses [235–238]. The detection of compensated hypothyroidism is an important part of follow-up, because persistent elevation of thyroid stimulating hormone levels is associated with an increased risk of thyroid cancer, which may be reversed by appropriate replacement therapy.

Cardiovascular damage

Radiation fields which include the heart will induce significant toxicity to the myocardium and coronary vasculature (reviewed in refs [230,239]). The risk of early cardiac toxicity is related to the radiation dose, fraction size and volume treated, and when doses are restricted by careful radiation planning and the dose per fraction is less than 2 Gy, cumulative rates of acute myocardial toxicity are less than 5%. Chronic constrictive pericarditis is now a rare complication. Complete functional studies with long-term follow-up of patients with HD are still uncommon [240–243]. The studies reported above conclude that between 25 and 50% of long survivors, who have had mediastinal irradiation, have a reduction in myocardial function below that expected.

Myocardial infarction is increasingly seen with long follow-up and in the EORTC series [244] the cumulative risk was

4.6% at 15 years. Although comparative data are difficult to obtain, in one study from the Institute Gustave Roussy patients who underwent myocardial irradiation had a 3.9% risk of myocardial infarction at 10 years; this risk is absent from those who had no myocardial irradiation, which is in keeping with the expectation for this age group [245]. The relative risk of cardiac death rises sharply with mediastinal doses of 400 Gy or more, and reached 29.6 in one series [246].

When doxorubicin is used in the primary therapy of HD in regimens such as ABVD, cumulative doses are usually less than 400 mg/m² and should not, therefore, induce cardiomyopathy in patients with otherwise normal hearts. The possibility of additive effects with mediastinal irradiation is a concern however, and whether late congestive cardiac failure will occur in such patients in their sixth, seventh and eighth decades remains to be seen.

Pulmonary toxicity

Mantle radiotherapy, including the paramediastinal and apical lung, results in X-ray changes of acute radiation pneumonitis in these areas 2 or 3 months after treatment. This is usually asymptomatic and resolves, leaving fibrotic change visible on X-rays [247]. The influence of different chemotherapy regimens, given alone or in combined-modality approaches, is of considerable interest, although randomized comparisons are infrequent. Mah *et al.* [248] compared the incidence of radiation-induced lung damage shown on computed tomograms in patients receiving combined-modality treatment comprising thoracic irradiation (35 Gy in 20 fractions) and different chemotherapy regimens. Although the numbers of patients were small, the risk of developing pneumonitis was higher in those treated with ABVD (71%) compared with those treated with MOPP (49%) or MOPP/ABVD (52%).

Infertility

The impact of combination chemotherapy on fertility depends on the regimen used, the dose administered and the age and status of the patient at the time of treatment. In men, testicular damage results in germinal depletion with oligospermia or azoospermia and reduced testicular volume. Less frequently, damage to the epithelium of the seminiferous tubules results in raised follicle stimulating hormone (FSH) and luteinizing hormone (LH). In women, gonadal damage will result in amenorrhoea, symptoms of oestrogen deficiency and raised serum FSH and LH levels. Before puberty, germinal epithelium may be relatively resistant to alkylating agents, but during and after puberty profound damage to germ cells and endocrine cells is induced by such chemotherapy.

In males, alkylating agent-based combination chemotherapy, such as MOPP, or its derivatives, are highly toxic to the testis, and patients who receive six or more cycles are usually azoospermic with testicular atrophy and raised FSH and LH

levels. Regimens such as ABVD without alkylating agents or procarbazine are less likely to produce azoospermia [249,250].

MOPP and related regimens produce amenorrhoea frequently during therapy and this will persist in approximately half of these patients. Younger patients are more likely to recover normal menses and regimens without alkylating agents are much less likely to produce persistent gonadal toxicity in women [250]. Patients who remain fertile after treatment for HD can be reassured that there is no evidence that the outcome of their pregnancies will be abnormal. Aisner *et al.* [251] reviewed pregnancy outcomes in over 200 patients. Among 43 women and 51 men who attempted conception, 35 women and 25 men were successful and there was a total of 84 pregnancies resulting in 68 children. Among the 84 pregnancies there was one premature birth, three spontaneous abortions, 11 elective abortions and two stillbirths. This did not represent an increase in the expected rate of complications and congenital abnormalities were no commoner than in the general population. Similar findings were made among 45 children born to survivors of HD in England: no chromosomal abnormalities were seen in karyotypes prepared from peripheral blood [252]. There appears to be no convincing evidence so far that the risk of HD is increased in offspring [253].

Second malignancies

There is no doubt that patients surviving HD are at increased risk of acute leukaemia, NHL and secondary solid cancers (reviewed in ref. [230]).

Acute nonlymphoblastic leukaemias

Although the relative risk of acute leukaemia is greatly increased after HD, in absolute terms it accounts for a smaller proportion of second malignancies than NHL or solid tumours. Typically it is seen between 2 and 10 years after therapy and is often characterized by pancytopenia, marrow dysplasia and abnormal marrow karyotype. The commonest findings are abnormalities of chromosomes 5q, 7q and 11q. Acute leukaemia is difficult to treat, with the majority of patients dying within a year of diagnosis [254,255]. The cumulative risk of acute myeloid leukaemia varies between series and is higher in patients treated with chemotherapy, particularly with alkylating agent regimens.

The frequency of acute leukaemia appears to depend on the amount of chemotherapy administered [254,256,257]. Acute leukaemia is rare after treatment with radiotherapy alone. In the recent series reported by Biti *et al.* [255] which analysed over 1000 patients from a single institution, the cumulative risk of acute leukaemia was 0.2% in patients treated with radiotherapy alone and 11.1% at 15 years in patients treated with chemotherapy alone. The cumulative risk of acute leukaemia tends to plateau after 10–15 years. Henry-Amar [230] has reviewed in detail factors predicting for the risk of acute leukaemia after chemotherapy, and in particular studies of the relationship between individual drugs and dosage. The risk increases with the use of mustine, cyclophosphamide, procarbazine, nitrosoureas, chlorambucil and vinca alkaloids and with increasing numbers of cycles, total dose and quantity of alkylating agent (references given in ref. [230]). The effect of age is somewhat controversial. Some studies show a higher risk of second acute leukaemia after the diagnosis of HD above 40 years of age but others do not [257]. More extensive disease is associated with an increased risk that is independent of the use of chemotherapy, and splenectomy appears to be a risk factor for acute leukaemia [85,86], although not all studies confirm this association (see recent refs [258,259] for a discussion of this controversy).

Most encouragingly, recent studies have suggested that the incidence of leukaemia in patients cured of HD in the 1980s is lower than that among those treated in the preceding decade, suggesting that newer chemotherapy regimens may be less leukaemogenic [260].

Secondary non-Hodgkin's disease

Krikorian *et al.* [261] first drew attention to the occurrence of NHL after therapy for HD. The increased risk has been confirmed by all other investigators [258,260,262–266]. Typically it occurs between 5 and 15 years after successful treatment for HD, and the cumulative risk at that time ranges between 1 and 5% in the reported studies listed above. They also confirm that the risk is associated with older age, male gender, lymphocyte-predominant histological subtype and combined-modality therapy. In a large North American study, the risk of secondary NHL was also associated with the use of mustine-containing chemotherapy [267].

The factors determining the development of secondary NHL remain unclear. The study reported by Boivin *et al.* [267] suggests a carcinogenic effect from alkylating agents to be one factor. Chronic immune deficiency may well contribute as it does in the development of EBV-positive diffuse large cell lymphomas after immune suppressive therapy. Patients with lymphocyte-predominant histological subtype appear to be biologically predisposed to secondary NHL, although the biological and molecular genetic basis of this evolution remains to be clarified.

Secondary solid tumours

The risk of secondary solid cancers appears to rise in patients with HD towards the end of the first decade of follow-up and continues to increase thereafter. In a large series, 15-year cumulative incidence rates vary between 10 and 15% and are significantly in excess of those expected in the general population, with relative risks between 1.5 and 2.5. Although these relative risks are smaller than those for acute leukaemia or NHL, the absolute numbers of cases are much greater [255,258,260,262,264–266,268]. The excess of solid tumours is usually reported for lung cancer, breast cancer, colorectal cancer, thyroid cancer, tumours of bone and melanoma. The increased risk probably extends to most solid cancers [177,269–272].

The major risk factor for excess second solid tumours appears to be radiation therapy and most sites of increased risk are those that may be included in radiation fields. The majority of patients develop solid cancers within irradiated fields [262].

Chemotherapy is not blameless in relation to second solid cancers. It appears to add to the risk of radiation alone certainly in some studies [255,271]. In the recent studies carried out by Boivin *et al.* [267] and Swerdlow *et al.* [257], chemotherapy was associated with an increased risk of secondary solid cancers in particular sites, including tumours of bone, and these tended to occur earlier than those associated with radiation alone. Several drugs were associated with an increased risk of second tumours, although nitrosoureas were identified as conveying a particularly high risk. They should be used only with caution and after careful selection in patients with HD. Splenectomy appears to be a risk factor for secondary solid cancers [273,274], although not after splenectomy for trauma [275].

The risk of secondary solid tumours after treating HD in childhood and adolescence has now been studied with a long follow-up [177]. This study reported on 1380 patients treated up to 1986, with a median follow-up of over 11 years. Eighty-eight patients developed second cancers (56 solid tumours, 26 leukaemias and four NHLs), so that the cumulative 15-year incidence rates were 3.9, 2.8 and 1.1% respectively. Solid tumours occurred later than leukaemias as expected, and most developed within radiation fields. The most common tumour was breast cancer and the 20-year cumulative incidence of secondary tumours was 12.6% overall. This is in keeping with a large Scandinavian population-based study among 1641 patients treated for HD in childhood or adolescence which revealed a particularly high incidence of breast cancer, with a cumulative risk of 12% at 30 years, and a total cumulative incidence of second malignancies of 18% at the same time point [276].

Psychosocial consequences of Hodgkin's disease and its treatment

A number of groups have studied the psychosocial aspects of HD and its treatment [277–284]. Controlled studies are uncommon, and a particularly valuable French study has used a case-control design to compare psychosocial difficulties among 93 French adult HD survivors with those of 186 case-matched controls [284]. Hodgkin's disease patients were more physically limited, with persistence of dyspnoea and chronic fatigue, compared to the normal population. There was also a significant increase in difficulties with concentration and memory.

In the study carried out by Joly *et al.* (1996) [284] the experience of patients' family life was reported positively. Patients experienced less separations or divorces than controls and a similar level of sexual activity. Social interactions and friendships were also more stable for HD survivors than controls in this study, although others have reported a higher degree of marital disharmony [280–283]. Joly *et al.* [284] found that 64% returned to work after treatment, although job changes were common. Hodgkin's disease survivors appeared to have less ambitious job plans and to set more modest goals, allowing more time for other aspects of life. This was not true in the USA, where patients at Stanford [281] reported an increase in professional ambition after surviving HD, although this study had no control group. Patients with HD who are cured still have difficulties in obtaining insurance and loans.

Causes of death after treatment

In series following large numbers of patients with HD over a long period of time, consistent findings are now reported concerning causes of death [53,93,235,285]. In patients cured of HD, the commonest causes of death are cardiovascular or infective complications. Secondary cancers and treatment-related deaths are less frequent. In the International Database on Hodgkin's Disease, the risk of dying from causes other than HD was analysed and compared to that of the general population matched for gender, age and country [93]. The risk of death from causes other than HD remained twice that of the general population, 2.07 in early-stage patients and 2.13 in advanced-stage patients. This risk increases with time, from 1.79 in the first 5 years to 3.08 between 15 and 20 years. This, of course, is in contrast to the risk of death from HD itself, which decreases with time. The 20-year cumulative risk of dying from HD was less than the risk of dying from some other cause. In the EORTC series of patients treated for early disease, the risk of dying from causes other than HD was three times that of the general population [94], and again increased with time from initial treatment.

Conclusion

Advances in the biology and management of HD are among the most impressive of modern medicine, with a large proportion of patients now being cured. However, treatment choice for the minority of resistant cases, and to minimize late complications, remains difficult. There remain many opportunities for further research and the development of new approaches.

References

1 Wilks Sir S. (1865) Cases of enlargement of the lymphatic glands and spleen (or Hodgkin's disease) with remarks. *Guy's Hospital Report*, **11**, 55–67.
2 Sternberg C. (1898) Uber eine eigenartige unter dem Bilde der Pseudoleukamie verlaufende Tuberculose des lymphatischen Apparates. *Zeitschrer Heilken*, **19**, 21–90.
3 Reed D.M. (1902) On the pathological changes in Hodgkin's disease, with especial reference to its relation to tuberculosis. *Johns Hopkins Hospital Report*, **10**, 133–196.
4 Carbone P.P., Kaplan H.S., Musshoff K. *et al.* (1971) Report of the committee on Hodgkin's disease staging. *Cancer Research*, **31**, 1860–1861.
5 Peters M.V. (1950) A study of survivals in Hodgkin's disease treated radiologically. *American Journal of Roentgenology*, **63**, 299–311.
6 Kaplan H.S. (1962) The radical radiotherapy of regionally localised disease. *Radiology*, **78**, 553–561.
7 Goodman L.S., Wintrobe M.M., Dameshek W. *et al.* (1946) Nitrogen mustard therapy. *Journal of the American Medical Association*, **132**, 126–132.
8 Lacher M.U. & Durant J.R. (1965) Combined vinblastine and chlorambucil therapy of Hodgkin's disease. *Annals of Internal Medicine*, **62**, 468–476.
9 De Vita V.T., Serpick A. & Carbone P.P. (1970) Combination chemotherapy in the treatment of advanced Hodgkin's disease. *Annals of Internal Medicine*, **73**, 881–895.
10 Mueller N.E. (1998) Epidemiology: Hodgkin's disease. In: *Malignant Lymphomas* (eds B. Hancock, P. Selby, K. MacLennan & J.O. Armitage). Chapman and Hall, London. (In Press.)
11 Miller B.A., Ries L.A.G., Hankey B.F. *et al.* (1990) *SEER Cancer Statistics Review: 1973–1990*. National Cancer Institute NIH publ. no. 93–2789. NCI, Bethesda, Washington DC.
12 Correa P. & O'Connor G.T. (1971) Epidemiologic patterns of Hodgkin's disease. *International Journal of Cancer*, **8**, 192–201.
13 Mueller N.E. (1987) The epidemiology of Hodgkin's disease. In: *Hodgkin's Disease* (eds P. Selby & T.J. McElwain), pp. 68–93. Blackwell Scientific Publications, Oxford.
14 Gutensohn N. & Cole P. (1977) Epidemiology of Hodgkin's disease in the young. *International Journal of Cancer*, **19**, 595–604.
15 Rocchi G., Tosato G., Papa G. *et al.* (1975) Antibodies to Epstein–Barr virus associated nuclear antigen and to other viral and non-viral antigens in Hodgkin's disease. *International Journal of Cancer*, **16**, 323–328.
16 Weiss L.M., Strickler J.G., Warnke R.A. *et al.* (1987) Epstein–Barr viral DNA in tissue of Hodgkin's disease. *American Journal of Pathology*, **129**, 86–91.
17 Weiss L.M., Mohaved L.A., Warnke R.A. *et al.* (1989) Detection of Epstein–Barr viral genomes in Reed–Sternberg cells of Hodgkin's disease. *New England Journal of Medicine*, **320**, 502–506.
18 Weiss L.M., Chen Y.Y., Liu X.F. *et al.* (1991) Epstein–Barr virus and Hodgkin's disease: a correlative *in situ* hybridisation and polymerase chain reaction study. *American Journal of Pathology*, **139**, 1259.
19 Herbst H., Steinbrecher E., Niedobitek G. *et al.* (1992) Distribution and phenotype of Epstein–Barr virus harboring cells in Hodgkin's disease. *Blood*, **80**, 484.
20 Gulley M.L., Eagan P.A., Quintanilla-Martinez L. *et al.* (1994) Epstein–Barr virus DNA is abundant and monoclonal in the Reed–Sternberg cells of Hodgkin's disease: association with mixed cellularity subtype and Hispanic American ethnicity. *Blood*, **83**, 1595–1602.
21 Boiocchi M., Dolcetti R., Re V.D. *et al.* (1993) Demonstration of a unique Epstein–Barr virus positive cellular clone in metachronous multiple localizations of Hodgkin's disease. *American Journal of Pathology*, **142**, 33–38.

22 Pallesen G., Hamilton-Dutoit S.J., Rowe M. *et al.* (1991) Expression of Epstein–Barr virus latent gene products in tumour cells of Hodgkin's disease. *Lancet*, **337**, 320–322.

23 Deacon E.M., Pallesen G., Niedobitek G. *et al.* (1993) Epstein–Barr virus and Hodgkin's disease: transcriptional analysis of virus latency in the malignant cells. *Journal of Experimental Medicine*, **177**, 339–349.

24 Pallesen G., Sandvej K., Hamilton-Dutoit S.J. *et al.* (1991) Activation of Epstein–Barr virus replication in Hodgkin's and Reed–Sternberg cells. *Blood*, **78**, 1162–1165.

25 Weiss L.M. & Chang K.L. (1998) Viruses in the etiology and pathogenesis of malignant lymphoma. In: *Malignant Lymphomas* (eds B. Hancock, P. Selby, K. MacLennan & J.O. Armitage). Chapman and Hall, London. (In press.)

26 Brousset P., Schlaifer D., Megetto F. *et al.* (1991) Persistence of the same viral strain in early and late relapses of Epstein–Barr virus associated Hodgkin's disease. *Blood*, **84**, 2447–2451.

27 Stoler M.H., Nichols G.E., Symbula M. *et al.* (1995) Nodular L & H lymphocyte predominance Hodgkin's disease: evidence for a kappa light chain restricted monotypic B cell neoplasm. *American Journal of Pathology*, **146**, 812–818.

28 Knowles D.E., Chamulak G.A., Subar M. *et al.* (1988) Lymphoid neoplasia associated with the Acquired Immunodeficiency Syndrome (AIDS): the New York University Medical Center experience with 105 patients (1981–1986). *Annals of Internal Medicine*, **108**, 744–753.

29 Mack T.M., Cozen W., Shibata D.K. *et al.* (1995) Concordance for Hodgkin's disease in identical twins suggesting genetic susceptibility to the young adult form of the disease. *New England Journal of Medicine*, **332**, 413–418.

30 Grufferman S., Cole P., Smith P.G. *et al.* (1977) Hodgkin's disease in siblings. *New England Journal of Medicine*, **296**, 248–250.

31 Grufferman S., Barton J.W. III & Eby N.L. (1987) Increased sex concordance of sibling pairs with Behcet's disease, Hodgkin's disease, multiple sclerosis and sarcoidosis. *American Journal of Epidemiology*, **126**, 365–369.

32 Grufferman S. & Delzell E. (1984) Epidemiology of Hodgkin's disease. *Epidemiology Reviews*, **6**, 76–106.

33 Hoar S.K., Blair A., Holmes E.F. *et al.* (1986) Agricultural herbicide use and risk of lymphoma and soft tissue sarcoma. *Journal of the American Medical Association*, **256**, 1141–1147.

34 Wolf J. & Diehl V. (1998) The pathogenesis of Hodgkin's lymphoma. In: *Malignant Lymphomas* (eds B. Hancock, P. Selby, K. MacLennan & J.O. Armitage). Chapman and Hall, London. (In press.)

35 Drexler H.G. (1992) Recent results on the biology of Hodgkin and Reed–Sternberg cells. I biopsy material *Leukaemia and Lymphoma*, **8**, 283.

36 Haluska F.G., Brufsky A.M. & Canellos G.P. (1994) The cellular biology of the Reed–Sternberg cell. *Blood*, **84**, 1005.

37 Kuppers R., Rajewsky K., Zhao M. *et al.* (1994) Hodgkin disease: Hodgkin and Reed–Sternberg cells picked from histological sections show clonal immunoglobulin gene rearrangements and appear to be derived from B cells at various stages of development. *Proceedings of the National Academy of Science USA*, **91**, 10962.

38 Hummel M., Ziemann K., Lammert H. *et al.* (1995) Hodgkin's disease with monoclonal and polyclonal populations of Reed–Sternberg cells. *New England Journal of Medicine*, **333**, 901–906.

39 Roth J., Daus H., Trumper L. *et al.* (1995) Detection of immunoglobulin heavy chain gene rearrangement at the single cell level in malignant lymphomas: no rearrangement is found in Hodgkin and Reed–Sternberg cells. *International Journal of Cancer*, **57**, 799.

40 Trumper L., Brady G., Bagg A. *et al.* (1993) Single cell analysis of Hodgkin and Reed–Sternberg cells: molecular heterogeneity of gene expression and p53 mutations. *Blood*, **81**, 3097.

41 Orscheschek K., Merz H., Hell J. *et al.* (1995) Large cell anaplastic lymphoma-specific translocation (t(2;5)(p23;q35)) in Hodgkin's disease: indication of a common pathogenesis? *Lancet*, **345**, 87–90.

42 Elmberger P.G., Lozano M.D., Weisenburger D.D. *et al.* (1995) Transcripts of the *npm-alk*-fusion gene in anaplastic large cell lymphoma, Hodgkin's disease and reactive lymphoid lesions. *Blood*, **86**, 3517.

43 Herbst H., Anagnostoupoulos J., Heinze B. *et al.* (1995) ALK gene products in anaplastic large cell lymphomas and Hodgkin's disease. *Blood*, **86**, 1694.

44 Wellmann A., Otsuki T., Vogelbruch M. *et al.* (1995) Analysis of the t(2;5)(p23;q35) translocation by reverse transcription polymerase chain reaction in CD30+ anaplastic large cell lymphomas in other non-Hodgkin's lymphomas of T cell phenotype and in Hodgkin's disease. *Blood*, **86**, 2232.

45 Johnson P.W.M., Leek J., Swinbank K. *et al* (1997) The use of fluorescent *in situ* hybridisation for detection of the t(2;5)(p23;q35) translocation in anaplastic large cell lymphoma. *Annals of Oncology*, **8**(Suppl. 2), s65–69.

46 Sanger W.G., Dave B.J. & Bishop M.R. (1998) Cytogenetics. In: *Malignant Lymphomas* (eds B. Hancock, P. Selby, K. MacLennan & J.O. Armitage). Chapman and Hall, London. (In press.)

47 Tilly H., Bastard C., Delastre T. *et al.* (1991) Cytogenetic studies in untreated Hodgkin's disease. *Blood*, **77**, 1298.

48 Weber-Matthiesen K., Deerberg J., Poetsch M. *et al.* (1995) Numerical chromosome aberrations are present within the CD30+ Hodgkin and Reed–Stern cells in 100% of analyzed cases of Hodgkin's disease. *Blood*, **86**, 1464.

49 Sextro M., Diehl V., Franklin J. *et al.* (1996) Lymphocyte predominant Hodgkin's disease—a workshop report. European Task Force on Lymphoma. *Annals of Oncology*, **4**, 61–65..

50 Diehl V., von Kalle C., Fonatsch C. *et al.* (1990) The cell of origin of Hodgkin's disease. *Seminars in Oncology*, **17**, 660.

51 Winkler U., Gottstein C., Schon G. *et al.* (1994) Successful treatment of disseminated human Hodgkin's disease in SCID mice with deglycosylated ricin A chain immunotoxins. *Blood*, **83**, 466.

52 Hombach A., Jung W., Pohl C. *et al.* (1993) A CD16/CD30 bispecific monoclonal antibody induces lysis of Hodgkin cells by unstimulated natural killer cells *in vitro* and *in vivo*. *International Journal of Cancer*, **55**, 830.

53 Selby P. & McElwain T. (eds) (1987) *Hodgkin's Disease*. Blackwell Scientific Publications, Oxford.

54 Selby P., Johnson P. & Hancock B. (1998) Hodgkin's disease — clinical features. In: *Malignant Lymphomas* (eds B. Hancock, P. Selby, K. MacLennan & J.O. Armitage). Chapman and Hall, London. (In press.)

55 Lister T.A., Crowther D., Sutcliffe S.B. *et al.* (1989) Report of a committee convened to discuss the evaluation and staging of patients with Hodgkin's disease: Cotswolds meeting. *Journal of Clinical Oncology*, **7**, 1630–1636.

56 Dimopoulos M.A., Cabanillas F., Lee J.J. *et al.* (1993) Prognostic

role of serum beta 2-microglobulin in Hodgkin's disease. *Journal of Clinical Oncology*, **11**, 1108–1111.

57 Gause A., Scholz R., Klein S. *et al.* (1991) Increased levels of circulating interleukin-6 in patients with Hodgkin's disease. *Haematological Oncology*, **9**, 307–313.

58 Gause A., Pohl C., Tschiersch A. *et al.* (1991) Clinical significance of soluble CD30 antigen in the sera of patients with untreated Hodgkin's disease. *Blood*, **77**, 1983–1988.

59 Gorschluter M., Bohlen H., Hasenclever D. *et al.* (1995) Serum cytokine levels correlate with clinical parameters in Hodgkin's disease. *Annals of Oncology*, **6**, 477–482.

60 Hamon M.D., Unal E., Macdonald I. *et al.* (1993) Plasma soluble interleukin 2 receptor levels in patients with malignant lymphoma are correlated with disease activity but not cellular immunosuppression. *Leukaemia and Lymphoma*, **10**, 111–115.

61 Musto P., La S.A., Di R.N. *et al.* (1995) Combined analysis of the soluble antigens (SA) sCD8, sCD25, sCD30 and sCD54 in Hodgkin's disease. *Proceedings of the American Society of Clinical Oncology*, **14**.

62 Gnant M., Mader R.M., Djavanmard M. *et al.* (1995) Soluble interleukin-2 receptor is a powerful prognostic marker in Hodgkin's disease. *Proceedings of the American Society of Clinical Oncology*, **14**.

63 Enblad G., Sundstrom C., Gronowitz S. & Glimelius B. (1995) Serum levels of interleukin-2 receptor (CD25) in patients with Hodgkin's disease, with special reference to age and prognosis. *Annals of Oncology*, **6**, 65–70.

64 Gruss H-J., Dolken G., Brach M.A. *et al.* (1993) The significance of serum levels of soluble 6-kDa receptors for tumor necrosis factor in patients with Hodgkin's disease. *Leukemia*, **7**, 1339–1343.

65 Gause A., Jung W., Schmitz R. *et al.* (1992) Soluble CD8, CD25 and CD30 antigens as prognostic markers in patients with untreated Hodgkin's lymphoma. *Annals of Oncology*, **3**(Suppl. 4), 49–52.

66 Nadali G., Vinante F., Ambrosetti A. *et al.* (1994) Serum levels of soluble CD30 are elevated in the majority of untreated patients with Hodgkin's disease and correlate with clinical features and prognosis. *Journal of Clinical Oncology*, **12**, 793–797.

67 Christiansen I., Enblad G., Kälkner K.M. *et al.* (1995) Soluble ICAM-1 in Hodgkin's disease: a promising independent predictive marker for survival. *Leukaemia and Lymphoma*, **19**, 243–251.

68 Sandrasegran K. & Robinson P.J. (1998) Imaging investigation of lymphoma. In: *Malignant Lymphomas* (eds B. Hancock, P. Selby, K. MacLennan & J.O. Armitage). Chapman and Hall, London. (In press.)

69 Kostakoglu L., Yeh S.D., Portlock C. *et al.* (1992) Validation of gallium-67 citrate SPECT in biopsy confirmed residual Hodgkin's disease in the mediastinum. *Journal of Nuclear Medicine*, **33**, 345–350.

70 Newman J.S., Francis I.R., Kaminski M.S. *et al.* (1994) Imaging of lymphoma with PET with 2-[F-18]-fluoro-2-deoxy-D-glucose: correlation with CT. *Radiology*, **190**, 111–116.

71 Filly R, Blank N. & Castellino R.A. (1976) Radiographic distribution of intrathoracic disease in previously untreated patients with Hodgkin's disease and non-Hodgkins lymphoma. *Radiology*, **120**, 277–281.

72 Castellino R.A., Blank N., Hoppe R.T. *et al.* (1986) Hodgkin's disease: contribution of chest CT in the initial staging evaluation. *Radiology*, **160**, 603–605.

73 Heron C.W., Husband J.E. & Williams M.P. (1988) Hodgkin's disease: CT of the thymus. *Radiology*, **167**, 647–651.

74 Castellino R.A., Hoppe R.T., Blank N. *et al.* (1984) Computed tomography, lymphography and staging laparotomy correlation in initial staging of Hodgkin's disease. *American Journal of Roentgenology*, **143**, 37–41.

75 Stomper P.C., Cholewinski S.P., Park J. *et al.* (1993) Abdominal staging of thoracic Hodgkin's disease: CT-lymphangiography-Ga-67 scanning correlation. *Radiology*, **187**, 381–386.

76 Chabner B.A., Johnson R.E., Young R.C. *et al.* (1976) Sequential nonsurgical and surgical staging of non-Hodgkin's lymphoma. *Annals of Internal Medicine*, **85**, 149–154.

77 Reznek H. & Richards M.A. (1987) The radiology of lymphoma. *Clinical Haematology*, **1**, 77–107.

78 Blackledge G., Bent J.J.K., Crowther D. & Isherwood I. (1980) Computed tomography in the staging of patients with Hodgkin's disease. *Clinical Radiology*, **31**, 143–147.

79 Macdonald J.S., McCready V.R., Cosgrove D.O., Cherryman G.R. & Selby P. (1987) Radiological and other imaging methods. In: *Hodgkin's Disease* (eds P. Selby & T.J. McElwain), pp. 126–159. Blackwell Scientific Publications, Oxford.

80 Tubiana M., Henry-Amar M., van der Werf-Messing B. *et al.* (1985) A multivariate analysis of prognostic factors in early stages Hodgkin's disease. *International Journal of Radiation Oncology, Biology and Physics*, **11**, 23–30.

81 Moormeier J.A., Williams S.F. & Golomb H.M. (1989) The staging of Hodgkin's disease. *Hematology Clinics of North America*, **3**, 237–251.

82 Carde P., Burgers J.M., Henry-Amar M. *et al.* (1988) Clinical stages I and II Hodgkin's disease: a specifically tailored therapy according to prognostic factors. *Journal of Clinical Oncology*, **6**, 239–252.

83 Sutcliffe S.B., Robinson M.H. & Timothy A.R. (1998) Management of localised Hodgkin's disease. In: *Malignant Lymphomas* (eds B. Hancock, P. Selby, K. MacLennan & J.O. Armitage). Chapman and Hall, London. (In press.)

84 Jockovich M., Mendenhall N.P., Sombeck M.D. *et al.* (1994) Long term complications of laparotomy in Hodgkin's disease. *Annals of Surgery*, **219**, 615–624.

85 Van Leeuwen F., Somers R. & Hart A. (1987) Splenectomy in Hodgkin's disease and second leukaemias. *Lancet*, **25**, 210–211.

86 Kaldor J.M., Day N.E., Clarke E.A., Van L.F. & Henry A.M. (1990) Leukemia following Hodgkin's disease. *New England Journal of Medicine*, **322**, 7–13.

87 Carde P., Hagenbeek A., Hayat M. *et al.* (1993) Clinical staging versus laparotomy and combined modality with MOPP versus ABVD in early stage Hodgkin's disease: the H6 twin randomised trials form the European Organisation for Research and Treatment of Cancer Lymphoma Cooperative Group. *Journal of Clinical Oncology*, **11**, 2258–2272.

88 Abrahamsen A.F., Hannisdal E., Nome O. *et al.* (1996) Clinical stage I and II Hodgkin's disease: long-term results of therapy without laparotomy. *Annals of Oncology*, **7**, 145–150.

89 Specht L. (1991) Prognostic factors in Hodgkin's disease. *Cancer Treatment Reviews*, **18**, 21–53.

90 Gospodarowicz M.K., Specht L. & Sutcliffe S.B. (1995) In: *Prognostic Factors in Cancer* (eds P. Hermanek, M.K. Gospodarowicz, D.E. Henson *et al.*), pp. 263–270. UICC, Springer Verlag, Berlin.

91 Cernkovich M., Leopold K. & Hoppe R. (1987) Stage I to IIB

Hodgkin's disease: the combined experience at Stanford University and the Joint Centre for Radiation Therapy. *Journal of Clinical Oncology*, **4**, 1041–1049.

92 Gobbi P.G., Cavalli C., Federico M. *et al.* (1988) Hodgkin's disease prognosis: a directly predictive equation. *Lancet*, **i**, 675–679.

93 Henry-Amar M. & Somers R. (1990) Survival outcome after Hodgkin's disease: a report from the international database on Hodgkin's disease. *Seminars in Oncology*, **17**, 758–768.

94 Henry-Amar M. & Somers R. (1990) Long term survival in early stages of Hodgkin's disease: the EORTC experience. In: *Treatment Strategy in Hodgkin's Disease* (eds R. Somers, M. Henry-Amar, J. Meerwaldt *et al.*), Colloque INSERM, vol. 196, pp. 151–166. John Libbey Eurotext, Paris.

95 Loeffler M., Dixon D.O. & Swindell R. (1990) Prognostic factors of stage III and IV Hodgkin's disease. In: *Treatment Strategy in Hodgkin's Disease* (eds R. Somers, M. Henry-Amar, J. Meerwaldt *et al.*), Colloque INSERM, vol. 196. John Libbey Eurotext, Paris.

96 Hoppe R.T., Cox R.S., Rosenberg S.A. *et al.* (1982) Prognostic factors in pathologic stage III Hodgkin's disease. *Cancer Treatment Reports*, **66**, 743–749.

97 Straus D.J., Gaynor J.J., Myers J. *et al.* (1990) Prognostic factors among 185 adults with newly diagnosed advanced Hodgkin's disease treated with alternating potentially non-cross resistant chemotherapy and intermediate dose radiation therapy. *Journal of Clinical Oncology*, **8**, 1173–1186.

98 Specht L. & Nissen N.I. (1988) Prognostic factors in Hodgkin's disease stage IV. *European Journal of Haematology*, **41**, 80–87.

99 Specht L. (1992) Tumour burden as the main indicator of prognosis in Hodgkin's disease. *European Journal of Cancer*, **28A**, 1982–1985.

100 Hanks G.E., Kinzie J.J., White R.L. *et al.* (1983) Patterns of care outcome studies. Results of the national practice of Hodgkin's disease. *Cancer*, **51**, 569–573.

101 Schewe K.L., Reavis J., Kun L.E. *et al.* (1988) Total dose, fraction size and tumour volume in the local control of Hodgkin's disease. *International Journal of Radiation Oncology, Biology and Physics*, **15**, 25–28.

102 Gospodarowicz M., Sutcliffe S.B., Bergsagel D.E. *et al.* (1992) Radiation therapy in clinical stage I and II Hodgkin's disease: the Princess Margaret Hospital Lymphoma Group. *European Journal of Cancer*, **28A**, 1841–1846.

103 Gilbert R. (1939) Radiotherapy in Hodgkin's disease (malignant granulomatosis): anatomic and clinical foundations; governing principles; results. *American Journal of Roentgenology*, **41**, 198–241.

104 Peters M.V. & Middlemiss K.C.H. (1958) A study of Hodgkin's disease treated by irradiation. *American Journal of Roentgenology*, **79**, 114–121.

105 Rubin P., Keys H., Mayer E. *et al.* (1974) Nodal recurrences following radical radiation therapy in Hodgkin's disease. *American Journal of Roentgenology, Radium and Nuclear Medicine*, **120**, 536–548.

106 Timothy A.R., Van Dyk J. & Sutcliffe S.B. (1987) Radiation therapy for Hodgkin's disease. In: *Hodgkin's Disease* (eds P. Selby & T.J. McElwain), pp. 181–249. Blackwell Scientific Publications, Oxford.

107 Mauch P.M., Canellos G.P., Shulman L.N. *et al.* (1995) Mantle irradiation alone for selected patients with laparotomy—Staged IA–IIA Hodgkin's disease: preliminary results of a prospective trial. *Journal of Clinical Oncology*, **13**, 947–952.

108 Mauch P.M., Kalish L.A., Marcus K.C. *et al.* (1995) Long term survival in Hodgkin's disease: relative impact of mortality, second tumours, infection and cardiovascular disease. *Cancer Journal of Scientific American*, **1**, 33–49.

109 Somers R., Henry-Amar M., Meerwaldt J.K. *et al.* (1990) Treatment strategy in Hodgkin's disease. In: *Proceedings to the Paris International Workshop and Symposium, June 1989 Colloque INSERM*, vol. 196. John Libbey Eurotext, London.

110 Specht L. & Gray R. (1996) Meta-analysis of randomized trials of more extensive radiotherapy and of adjuvant combination chemotherapy in early stage Hodgkin's disease. *Annals of Oncology*, **7** (Suppl. 3); 21.

111 Barrett A., Gregor A., McElwain T.J. *et al.* (1981) Infradiaphragmatic presentation of Hodgkin's disease. *Clinical Radiology*, **32**, 221–224.

112 Mauch P.M., Greenberg H., Lewin A. *et al.* (1983) Prognostic factors in patients with subdiaphragmatic Hodgkin's disease. *Clinical Radiology*, **32**, 221–224.

113 Doreen M., Wrigley P., Jones A. *et al.* (1984) The management of localised infradiaphragmatic Hodgkin's disease: experience of a rare clinical presentation at St Bartholomew's Hospital. *Haematological Oncology*, **2**, 349–357.

114 Lanzillo J., Moylan D., Mohluddin M. *et al.* (1985) Radiotherapy of stage I and II Hodgkin's disease with inguinal presentation. *Radiology*, **154**, 212–215.

115 Specht L. & Nissen N.I. (1988) Hodgkin's disease stages I and II with infradiaphragmatic presentation: a rare and prognostically unfavourable combination. *European Journal of Haematology*, **40**, 396–402.

116 Krikorian J., Portlock C. & Mauch P. (1986) Hodgkin's disease presenting below the diaphragm: a review. *Journal of Clinical Oncology*, **4**, 1551–1562.

117 Mauch P., Goodman R. & Hellman S. (1978) The significance of mediastinal involvement in early stage Hodgkin's disease. *Cancer*, **42**, 1039–1045.

118 Prosnitz L.R., Curtis A.M., Knowlton A.H. *et al.* (1980) Supradiaphragmatic Hodgkin's disease: significance of large mediastinal masses. *International Journal of Radiation Oncology, Biology and Physics*, **6**, 809–813.

119 Lee C.K., Bloomfield C.D., Goldman A.L. *et al.* (1990) Prognostic significance of mediastinal involvement in Hodgkin's disease treated with curative radiotherapy. *Cancer*, **46**, 2403–2409.

120 Jochelson M., Mauch, Balikian J. *et al.* (1985) The significance of the residual mediastinal mass in treated Hodgkin's disease. *Journal of Clinical Oncology*, **3**, 637–640.

121 Radford J.A., Cowan R., Flanagan M. *et al.* (1988) The significance of residual mediastinal abnormality on the chest radiograph following treatment for Hodgkin's disease. *Journal of Clinical Oncology*, **6**, 940–946.

122 Orlandi E., Lazzarino M., Brusamolino E. *et al.* (1990) Residual mediastinal widening following therapy in Hodgkin's disease. *Hematological Oncology*, **8**, 125–131.

123 Leigh B.R., Fox K.A., Mack C.F. *et al.* (1993) Radiation therapy salvage of Hodgkin's disease following chemotherapy failure. *International Journal of Radiation Oncology, Biology and Physics*, **27**, 855–862.

124 Uematsu M., Tarbell N.J., Silver B. *et al.* (1993) Wide field radiation therapy with or without chemotherapy for patients with Hodgkin's disease in relapse after initial combination chemotherapy. *Cancer*, **72**, 207–212.

125 O'Brien P.C. & Parnis F.X. (1995) Salvage radiotherapy following chemotherapy failure in Hodgkin's disease—what is its role? *Acta Oncologica*, **34**, 99–104.

126 Nissen N.I. & Nordentoft A.M. (1982) Radiotherapy versus combined modality treatment of stage I and II Hodgkin's disease. *Cancer Treatment Reports*, **66**, 799–803.

127 Anderson H., Deakin D.P., Wagstaff J. *et al.* (1984) A randomised study of adjuvant chemotherapy after mantle radiotherapy in supradiaphragmatic Hodgkin's disease PS IA–IIB: a report from the Manchester lymphoma group. *British Journal of Cancer*, **49**, 695–702.

128 Horning S.J., Hoppe R.T., Hancock S.L. *et al.* (1988) Vinblastine, bleomycin and methotrexate: an effective adjuvant in favourable Hodgkin's disease. *Journal of Clinical Oncology*, **6**, 1822–1831.

129 Noordijk E.M., Carde P., Mandard A.M. *et al.* (1994). Preliminary results of the EORTC-GPMC controlled clinical trial H7 in early-stage Hodgkin's disease. *Annals of Oncology*, **5**(Suppl. 2), 107–112.

130 Klasa R.J., Connors J.M., Fairey R. *et al.* (1996) Treatment of early stage Hodgkin's disease: improved outcome with brief chemotherapy and radiotherapy without staging laparotomy. *Annals of Oncology*, **7**(Suppl 3), 21.

131 Radford J.A., Cowan R.A., Ryder W.D.J. *et al.* (1996) Four weeks of neo-adjuvant chemotherapy significantly reduces the progression rate in patients treated with limited field radiotherapy for clinical stage IA/IIA Hodgkin's disease. Results of a randomised pilot study. *Annals of Oncology*, **7**(Suppl 3), 10.

132 Biti G.P., Cimino G., Cartoni C. *et al.* (1992) Extended field radiotherapy is superior to MOPP chemotherapy for the treatment of pathologic stage I–IIA Hodgkin's disease: eight year update of an Italian prospective randomised study. *Journal of Clinical Oncology*, **10**, 378–382.

133 Longo D., Glatstein E., Duffey P., *et al.* (1991a) Radiation therapy versus combination chemotherapy in the treatment of early-stage Hodgkin's disease: seven-year results of a prospective randomized trial. *Journal of Clinical Oncology*, **9**, 906–917.

134 Pavlovsky S., Maschio M., Santarelli M.T. *et al.* (1988) Randomised trial of chemotherapy versus chemotherapy plus radiotherapy for stage I–II Hodgkin's disease. *Journal of the National Cancer Institute*, **80**, 1466–1473.

135 Loeffler M., Brosteanu O., Hasenclever D. *et al.* (1996) Combined modality treatment vs chemotherapy alone in Hodgkin's disease: an overview on randomized trials. *Annals of Oncology*, **7**(Suppl 3), 22.

136 Longo D.L., Young R.C., Wesley M. *et al.* (1986) 20 years of MOPP therapy for Hodgkin's disease. *Journal of Clinical Oncology*, **4**, 1295–1306.

137 Santoro A., Bonfante V. & Bonadonna G. (1982) Salvage chemotherapy with ABVD in MOPP resistant Hodgkin's disease. *Annals of Internal Medicine*, **96**, 139–143.

138 Santoro A., Bonadonna G. & Bonfante V. (1982) Alternating drug combinations in the treatment of advanced Hodgkin's disease. *New England Journal of Medicine*, **306**, 770–775.

139 Bonadonna G., Zucali R., Monfardini S. *et al.* (1975) Combination chemotherapy of Hodgkin's disease with adriamycin, bleomycin, vinblastine and imidazole carboxamide versus MOPP. *Cancer*, **36**, 252–259.

140 Bonadonna G. (1994) Modern treatment of malignant lymphomas: a multidisciplinary approach? *Annals of Oncology*, **5**(Suppl 2), S5–S16.

141 Santoro A, Viviani S., Villarreal C.J. *et al.* (1986) Salvage chemotherapy in Hodgkin's disease irradiation failures: superiority of doxorubicin containing regimens over MOPP. *Cancer Treatment Reports*, **70**, 343–348.

142 Canellos G.P., Anderson J.R., Propert K.J. *et al.* (1992) Chemotherapy of advanced Hodgkin's disease with MOPP, ABVD or MOPP alternating with ABVD. *New England Journal of Medicine*, **327**, 1478–1484.

143 Hancock B.W., Cullen M.H. & Vaughan Hudson G. (1997) Alternating ChlVPP/PABlOE is better than PABlOE alone as initial chemotherapy for advanced Hodgkin's disease. *British Journal of Cancer*, **76**(Suppl. 1), 32.

144 Goldie J.H., Coldman A.J. & Gudauskas G.A. (1982) Rationale for the use of alternating non-cross resistant chemotherapy *Cancer Treatment Reports*, **66**, 439–449.

145 Bonadonna G., Valagussa P. & Santoro A. (1986) Alternating non-cross resistant combination chemotherapy or MOPP in stage IV Hodgkin's disease: a report of 8 year results. *Annals of Internal Medicine*, **104**, 739–746.

146 Somers R., Carde P., Henry-Amar M. *et al.* (1994) A randomised study in stage IIIB and IV Hodgkin's disease comparing eight courses of MOPP versus an alternation of MOPP with ABVD: a European Organisation for Research and Treatment of Cancer Lymphoma Cooperative Group and Groupe Pierre et Marie-Curie Controlled clinical trial. *Journal of Clinical Oncology*, **12**, 279–287.

147 Hancock B.W., Vaughan Hudson G., Vaughan Hudson B. *et al.* (1992) LOPP alternating with EVAP is superior to LOPP alone in the initial treatment of advanced Hodgkin's disease: results of a British National Lymphoma Investigation Trial. *Journal of Clinical Oncology*, **10**, 1252–1258.

148 Gams R.A., Omura G.A., Velez-Garcia E. *et al.* (1986) Alternating sequential combination chemotherapy in the management of advanced Hodgkin's disease. A Southeastern Cancer Study Group Trial. *Cancer*, **58**, 1963–1986.

149 Bloomfield C.D., Pajak T.F., Glicksman A.S. *et al.* (1982) Chemotherapy and combined modality therapy for Hodgkin's disease: a progress report on Cancer and Leukemia Group B studies. *Cancer Treat Reports*, **66**, 835–846.

150 Longo D.L., Duffey P.L., DeVita V.T. *et al.* (1991b) Treatment of advanced-stage Hodgkin's disease: alternating noncrossresistant MOPP/CABS is not superior to MOPP. *Journal of Clinical Oncology*, **9**, 1409–1420.

151 Holte H., Mella O., Telhaug R. *et al.* (1995) Randomised study in stage III–IV Hodgkin's disease: ChlVPP is as effective as alternating ChlVPP/ABOD chemotherapy. In: *Abstracts of the Third International Symposium on Hodgkin Lymphoma September 18–23, 1995, Koln, Germany*, p. 113.

152 Klimo P. & Connors J.M. (1985) MOPP/ABV hybrid program: combination chemotherapy based on early introduction of seven effective drugs for advanced Hodgkin's disease. *Journal of Clinical Oncology*, **3**, 1174–1182.

153 Radford J.A., Crowther D., Rohatiner A.Z.S. *et al.* (1995) Results of a randomised trial comparing MVPP chemotherapy with a hybrid regimen: ChlVPP/EVA in the initial treatment of Hodgkin's disease. *Journal of Clinical Oncology*, **13**, 2379–2385.

154 Vivani S., Bonadonna G., Santoro A. *et al.* (1996) Alternating versus hybrid MOPP and ABVD combinations in advanced Hodgkin's disease: ten year results. *Journal of Clinical Oncology*, **14**, 1421–1430.

155 Connors J.M., Klimo P., Adams G. *et al.* (1997) Treatment of advanced Hodgkin's disease with chemotherapy — comparison of MOPP/ABV hybrid regimen with alternating courses of MOPP and ABVD: a report from the National Cancer Institute of Canada Clinical Trials Group. *Journal of Clinical Oncology*, **15**, 1638–1645.

156 Diehl V., Tesch H., Lathan B. *et al.* (1997) BEACOPP, a new intensified hybrid regimen, is at least equally effective compared with copp/abvd in patients with advanced stage Hodgkin's lymphoma. *Proceedings of the American Society for Clinical Oncology*, **16**, 5.

157 Hancock B.W., Vaughan Hudson G., Vaughan Hudson B. *et al.* (1994) Hybrid LOPP/EVA is not better than LOPP alternating with EVAP: a prematurely terminated British National Lymphoma Investigation randomised trial. *Annals of Oncology*, **5**(Suppl. 2), S117–S120.

158 Duggan D., Petroni G., Johnson J. *et al.* (1997) MOPP/ABV versus ABVD for advanced Hodgkin's disease — a preliminary report of CALGB 8952 (with SWOG, ECOG, NCIC). *Proceedings of the American Society for Clinical Oncology*, **16**, 31.

159 Bartlett N.L., Rosenberg S.A., Hoppe R.T. *et al.* (1995) Brief chemotherapy, Stanford V, and adjuvant radiotherapy for bulky or advanced stage Hodgkin's disease: a preliminary report. *Journal of Clinical Oncology*, **13**, 1080–1088.

160 Radford J.A. & Crowther D. (1991) Treatment of relapsed Hodgkin's disease using a weekly chemotherapy of short duration: results of a pilot study in 20 patients. *Annals of Oncology*, **2**, 505–509.

161 Radford J.A., Rohatiner A.Z.S., Dunlop D. *et al.* (1997) Preliminary results of a four-centre randomised trial paring weekly VAPEC-B (V) chemotherapy with the ChlVPP/EVA hybrid (H) regimen in previously untreated Hodgkin's disease (HD). *Proceedings of the American Society for Clinical Oncology*, **16**, 42.

162 Portlock C.S., Rosenberg S.A., Glatstein E. *et al.* (1978) Impact of salvage treatment on initial relapses in patients with Hodgkin's disease stages I–II. *Blood*, **51**, 825–833.

163 Proctor S.J., Taylor P., Donman P. *et al.* (1991) A numerical prognostic index for clinical use in identification of poor risk patients with Hodgkin's disease at diagnosis. *European Journal of Cancer*, **27**, 624–629.

164 Diehl V., Loeffler M., Pfreundschuh M. *et al.* (1995) Further chemotherapy versus low-dose involved-field radiotherapy as consolidation of complete remission after six cycles of alternating chemotherapy in patients with advanced Hodgkin's disease. *Annals of Oncology*, **6**, 901–910.

165 Portlock C.S., Rosenberg S.A., Glatstein E. *et al.* (1978) Impact of salvage treatment on initial relapses in patients with Hodgkin's disease stages I–II. *Blood*, **51**, 825–833.

166 Olver I.N., Wolf M.M., Cruickshank D. *et al.* (1988) Nitrogen mustard, vincristine, procarbazine and prednisolone for relapse after radiation in Hodgkin's disease. An analysis of long term follow up. *Cancer*, **62**, 233–239.

167 Selby P., Patel P., Milan S. *et al.* (1990) ChlVPP combination chemotherapy for Hodgkin's disease: long term results. *British Journal of Cancer*, **62**, 279–285.

168 Longo D.L., Duffey P.L., Young R.C. *et al.* (1992) Conventional-dose salvage combination chemotherapy in patients relapsing with Hodgkin's disease after combination chemotherapy: the low probability for cure. *Journal of Clinical Oncology*, **10**, 210–218.

169 Young R.C., Canellos G.P., Chabner B.A. *et al.* (1978) Patterns of relapse in advanced Hodgkin's disease treated with combination chemotherapy. *Cancer*, **42**, 1001–1007.

170 Brice P., Bastion Y., Divine M. *et al.* (1996) Analysis of prognostic factors after the first relapse of Hodgkin's disease for 187 patients. *Cancer*, **78**, 1293–1299.

171 Bonfante V., Santoro A., Viviani S. *et al.* (1997) Outcome of patients with Hodgkin's disease failing after primary MOPP-ABVD. *Journal of Clinical Oncology*, **15**, 528–534.

172 Desch C.E., Lasala M.R., Smith T.J. & Hillner B.E. (1992) The optimal timing of autologous bone marrow transplantation in Hodgkin's disease patients after a chemotherapy relapse. *Journal of Clinical Oncology*, **10**, 200–209.

173 Bierman P.J., Anderson J.R., Freeman M.B. *et al.* (1996) High dose chemotherapy followed by autologous hematopoietic rescue for Hodgkin's disease patients following first relapse after chemotherapy. *Annals of Oncology*, **7**, 151–156.

174 Bierman P.J., Vose J.M. & Armitage J.O. (1998) High dose therapy for lymphomas. In: *Malignant Lymphomas* (eds B. Hancock, P. Selby, K. MacLennan & J.O. Armitage). Chapman & Hall, London. (In press.)

175 Bennett C.L., Armitage J.L., Armitage G.O. *et al.* (1995) Costs of care and outcomes for high dose therapy and autologous transplantation for lymphoid malignancies: results from the University of Nebraska 1987 through 1991. *Journal of Clinical Oncology*, **13**, 969–973.

176 Miller C.B., Piantadosi S., Vogelsang G.B. *et al.* (1996) Impact of age on outcome of patients with cancer undergoing autologous bone marrow transplant. *Journal of Clinical Oncology*, **14**, 1327–1332.

177 Bhatia S., Ramsay N., Steinbuch M. *et al.* (1996) Malignant neoplasms following bone marrow transplantation. *Blood*, **87**, 3633–3639.

178 Lazarus H.M., Crilley P., Ciobanu N. *et al.* (1992) High dose carmustine, etoposide and cisplatin and autologous bone marrow transplantation for relapsed and refractory lymphoma. *Journal of Clinical Oncology*, **10**, 1682–1689.

179 Harding M., Selby P., Gore M. *et al.* (1992) High-dose chemotherapy and autologous bone marrow transplantation for relapsed and refractory Hodgkins disease. *European Journal of Cancer*, **28A**, 1396–1400.

180 Carella A.M., Carlier P., Congiu A. *et al.* (1991) Autologous bone marrow transplantation as adjuvant treatment for high risk Hodgkin's disease in first complete remission after MOPP/ABVD protocol. *Bone Marrow Transplant*, **8**, 99–103.

181 Phillips G.L., Wolff S.N., Herzig R.H. *et al.* (1989) Treatment of progressive Hodgkin's disease with intensive chemoradiotherapy and autologous bone marrow transplantation. *Blood*, **73**, 2086–2092.

182 Reece D.E., Barnett M.J., Connors J.M. *et al.* (1991) Intensive chemotherapy with cyclophosphamide, carmustine and etoposide followed by autologous bone marrow transplantation for relapsed Hodgkin's disease. *Journal of Clinical Oncology*, **9**, 1871–1879.

183 Crump M., Smith A.M., Brandwein J. *et al.* (1993) High dose etoposide and melphalan and autologous bone marrow transplantation for patients with advanced Hodgkin's disease: importance of disease status at transplant. *Journal of Clinical Oncology*, **1**, 704–711.

184 Gianni A.M., Siena S., Bregni M. *et al.* (1993) High dose sequential chemoradiotherapy with peripheral blood progenitor cell support for relapsed or refractory Hodgkin's disease — a 6 year update. *Annals of Oncology*, **4**, 889–891.

185 Yahalom J., Gulati S.C., Toia M. *et al.* (1993) Accelerated hyperfractionated total lymphoid irradiation, high dose chemotherapy and autologous bone marrow transplantation for refractory and

relapsing patients with Hodgkin's disease. *Journal of Clinical Oncology*, **6**, 1062.

186 Reece D.E., Connors J.M., Spinelli J.J. *et al.* (1994) Intensive therapy with cyclophosphamide, carmustine, etoposide ± cisplatin and autologous bone marrow transplantation for Hodgkin's disease in first relapse after combination chemotherapy. *Blood*, **83**, 1193–1199.

187 Chopra R., McMillan A.K., Linch D.C. *et al.* (1993) The place of high dose BEAM therapy and autologous bone marrow transplantation in poor risk Hodgkin's disease. A single center eight year study of 155 patients. *Blood*, **81**, 1137–1145.

188 Nademanee A., O'Donnell M.R., Snyder D.S. *et al.* (1995) High dose chemotherapy with or without total body irradiation followed by autologous bone marrow and/or peripheral blood stem cell transplantation for patients with relapsed and refractory Hodgkin's disease: results in 85 patients with analysis of prognostic factors. *Blood*, **85**, 1381–1390.

189 Burns L.J., Daniels K.A., McGlave P.B. *et al.* (1995) Autologous stem cell transplantation for refractory and relapsed Hodgkin's disease: factors predictive of prolonged survival. *Bone Marrow Transplantation*, **16**, 13–18.

190 Jagannath S., Armitage J.O., Dicke K.A. *et al.* (1989) Prognostic factors for response and survival after high dose cyclophosphamide, carmustine and etoposide with autologous bone marrow transplantation for relapsed Hodgkin's disease. *Journal of Clinical Oncology*, **7**, 179–185.

191 Armitage J.O., Bierman P.J., Vose J.M. *et al.* (1991) Autologous bone marrow transplantation for patients with relapsed Hodgkin's disease. *American Journal of Medicine*, **91**, 605–611.

192 Bierman P.J., Bagin R.G., Jagannath S. *et al.* (1993) High dose chemotherapy followed by autologous hematopoietic rescue in Hodgkin's disease: long term follow up in 128 patients. *Annals of Oncology*, **4**, 767–773.

193 Spinolo J.A., Jagannath S., Velasquez W.S. *et al.* (1993) Cisplatin-CBV with autologous bone marrow transplantation for relapsed Hodgkin's disease. *Leukaemia and Lymphoma*, **9**, 71–77.

194 Moormeier J.A., Williams S.F., Kaminer L.S. *et al.* (1991) Autologous bone marrow transplantation followed by involved field radiotherapy in patients with relapsed or refractory Hodgkin's disease. *Leukaemia and Lymphoma*, **5**, 243–248.

195 Horning S.J., Chao N.J., Negrin R.S. *et al.* (1997) High dose therapy and autologous haemopoeitic progenitor cell transplantation for recurrent or refractory Hodgkin's disease: analysis of the Stanford University results and prognostic indices. *Blood*, **89**, 801–813.

196 O'Brien M., Milan S., Cunningham D. *et al.* (1996) High dose chemotherapy and autologous bone marrow transplant in relapsed Hodgkin's disease—a pragmatic prognostic index. *British Journal of Cancer*, **73**, 1272–1277.

197 Yuen A.R., Rosenberg S.A., Hoppe R.T. *et al.* (1997) Comparison between conventional salvage therapy and high dose therapy with autografting for recurrent or refractory Hodgkin's disease. *Blood*, **89**, 814–822.

198 Linch D.C., Winfield D., Goldstone A.H. *et al.* (1993) Dose intensification with autologous bone-marrow transplantation in relapsed and resistant Hodgkin's disease: results of a BNLI randomised trial. *Lancet*, **341**, 1051–1054.

199 Reece D.E., Barnett M.J., Shepherd J.D. *et al.* (1995) High dose cyclophosphamide, carmustine (BCNU) and etoposide (VP16-213) with or without cisplatin (CBV ± P) and autologous trans-plantation for patients with Hodgkin's disease who fail to enter a complete remission after combination chemotherapy. *Blood*, **86**, 451–456.

200 Moreau P., Milpied N., Mechinaud-Lacroix F. *et al.* (1993) Early intensive therapy with autotransplantation for high risk Hodgkin's disease. *Leukaemia and Lymphoma*, **12**, 51–58.

201 Fielding A.K., Philip T. & Carella A. (1994) Autologous bone marrow transplantation for lymphomas. *Blood*, **84**, 536A.

202 Shpall E. & Jones R.B. (1994) Relapse of tumor cells from bone marrow. *Blood*, **83**, 623–625.

203 Schmitz N., Linch D.C., Dreger P. *et al.* (1996) Randomised trials of filgrastim mobilised peripheral blood progenitor cell transplantation versus autologous bone marrow transplantation in lymphoma patients. *Lancet*, **347**, 353–357.

204 Hartmann O., Le-Corroller A.G., Blaise D. *et al.* (1997) Peripheral blood stem cell and bone marrow transplantation for solid tumors and lymphomas: hematologic recovery and costs. A randomized, controlled trial. *Annals of Internal Medicine*, **126**, 600–607.

205 Weisdorf D.J., Verfaille C.M., Miller W.J. *et al.* (1997) Autologous bone marrow versus non-mobilized peripheral blood stem cell transplantation for lymphoid malignancies: a prospective, comparative trial. *American Journal of Hematology*, **54**, 202–208.

206 Liberati G., Pearce R., Taghipour G. *et al.* (1994) Comparison of peripheral blood stem cell and autologous bone marrow transplantation for lymphoma patients: a case controlled analysis of the EBMT registry data. *Annals of Oncology*, **5**(Suppl. 2), S151–S153.

207 Gajewski J.L., Phillips G.L., Sobocinski K.A. *et al.* (1996) Bone marrow transplants from HLA identical siblings in advanced Hodgkin's disease. *Journal of Clinical Oncology*, **14**, 572–578.

208 Jones R.J., Ambinder R.F., Piantadosi S. *et al.* (1991) Evidence of a graft versus lymphoma effect associated with allogeneic bone marrow transplantation. *Blood*, **77**, 649–653.

209 Anderson J.E., Litzow A.R., Appelbaum F.R. *et al.* (1993) Allogeneic, syngeneic and autologous bone marrow transplantation for Hodgkin's disease: the 21 year Seattle experience. *Journal of Clinical Oncology*, **11**, 2342.

210 Ratanatharathorn V., Uberti J., Karanes C. *et al.* (1994) Prospective comparative trial of autologous versus allogeneic bone marrow transplantation in patients with non-Hodgkin's lymphoma. *Blood*, **84**, 1050–1055.

211 Milpied N., Fielding A.K. & Pearce R.M. (1996) Allogeneic bone marrow transplant is not better than autologous transplant for patients with relapsed Hodgkin's disease. *Journal of Clinical Oncology*, **14**, 1291–1296.

212 Pohl C., Deneld R., Renner C. *et al.* (1993) CD30 antigen specific targeting and activation of T-cells via murine bispecific antibodies directed against CD3 and CD28: potential use for the treatment of Hodgkin's disease. *International Journal of Cancer*, **54**, 820.

213 Renner C., Jung W., Sahin U. *et al.* (1994) Cure of xenografted human tumors by bispecific monoclonal antibodies and human T-cells. *Science*, **264**, 833.

214 Rothman L.A., Cohen C.J. & Astarloa J. (1973) Placental and fetal involvement by maternal malignancy: a report of rectal carcinoma and review of the literature. *American Journal of Obstetrics and Gynecology*, **116**, 1023–1034.

215 Ward F.T. & Weiss R.B. (1989) Lymphoma and pregnancy. *Seminars in Oncology*, **16**, 397–409.

216 Sadural E. & Smith L.G. Jr (1995) Haematologic malignancies

during pregnancy. *Clinical Obstetrics and Gynaecology*, **38**, 535–546.

217 Lishner M., Zemlickis D., Degendorfer P. *et al.* (1992) Maternal and foetal outcome following Hodgkin's disease in pregnancy. *British Journal of Cancer*, **65**, 114–117.

218 Woo S.Y., Fuller L.M., Cundiff J.H. *et al.* (1992) Radiotherapy during pregnancy for clinical stages IA–IIA Hodgkin's disease. *International Journal of Radiation Oncology and Biological Physics*, **23**, 407–412.

219 Habermann T., Earle J., Johansen K. *et al.* (1993) Synchronous presentation of Hodgkin's disease and pregnancy. *Proceedings American Association of Clinical Oncology*, **12**, A1294.

220 Yahalom J. (1990) Treatment options for Hodgkin's disease during pregnancy. *Leukemia and Lymphoma*, **2**, 151–161.

221 Johnson P.W.M. (1998) Lymphoma in the elderly. In: *Malignant Lymphomas* (eds B. Hancock, P. Selby, K. MacLennan & J.O. Armitage). Chapman and Hall, London. (In press)

222 Sutcliffe S., Gospodarowicz M., Bergsagel D. *et al.* (1985) Prognostic groups for management of localized Hodgkin's disease. *Journal of Clinical Oncology*, **3**, 393–401.

223 Specht L., Horwich A. & Ashley S. (1994) Salvage of relapse of patients with Hodgkin's disease in clinical stages I or II who were staged with laparotomy and initially treated with radiotherapy alone. A report from the international database on Hodgkin's disease. *International Journal of Radiation Oncology, Biology and Physics*, **30**, 805–811.

224 Levis A., Depaoli L., Urgesi A. *et al.* (1994) Probability of cure in elderly Hodgkin's disease patients. *Haematologica*, **79**, 46–54.

225 Levy R., Colonna P., Tourani J.M. *et al.* (1995) Human immunodeficiency virus associated Hodgkin's disease: report of 45 cases from the French registry of HIV-associated tumors. *Leukemia & Lymphoma*, **16**, 451–456.

226 Bellas C., Santon A., Manzanal A. *et al.* (1996) Pathological, immunological, and molecular features of Hodgkin's disease associated with HIV infection: comparison with ordinary Hodgkin's disease. *American Journal of Surgical Pathology*, **20**, 1520–1524.

227 Levine A.M. (1996) HIV-associated Hodgkin's disease: biologic and clinical aspects. *Hematology Oncology Clinics of North America*, **10**, 1135–1148.

228 Errante D., Zagonel V., Vaccher E., Serraino D., Bernardi D. & Sorio R. (1994) Hodgkin's disease in patients with HIV infection and in the general population: comparison of clinicopathological features and survival. *Annals of Oncology*, **2**, 37–40.

229 Tirelli U., Errante D., Dolcetti R. *et al.* (1995) Hodgkin's disease and human immunodeficiency virus infection: clinicopathologic and virologic features of 114 patients from the Italian Cooperative Group on AIDS and Tumors. *Journal of Clinical Oncology*, **13**, 1758–1767.

230 Henry-Amar M. (1998) Long term problems. In: *Malignant Lymphomas* (eds B. Hancock, P. Selby, K. MacLennan & J.O. Armitage). Chapman and Hall, London. (In press.)

231 Bookman M.A. & Longo D.L. (1986) Concomitant illness in patients treated for Hodgkin's disease. *Cancer Treatment Review*, **13**, 77–111.

232 Bjorkholm M., Holm G. & Mellstedt H. (1990) Immunocompetence in patients with Hodgkin's disease. In *Hodgkin's Disease: the consequences of survival* (eds M.J. Lacher & J.R. Redman), pp. 12–150. Lea & Febiger, Philadelphia, PA.

233 Armstrong D. & Minamoto G.Y. (1990) Infectious complications of Hodgkin's disease. In: *Hodgkin's Disease: the consequences of survival* (eds M.J. Lacher & J.R. Redman), pp. 151–167. Lea & Febiger, Philadelphia, PA.

234 Kluin-Nelemans J.C., Henry-Amar M., Carde P. *et al.* (1995) Assessment of thyroid, pulmonary, cardiac and gonadal toxicity in stages I–II Hodgkin's disease. In: *Abstracts of the Third International Symposium on Hodgkin Lymphoma September 18–23, 1995, Koln, Germany*, p. 90, abstract 72.

235 Hancock S.L., Cox R.S. & McDougall I.R. (1991) Thyroid diseases after treatment of Hodgkin's disease. *New England Journal of Medicine*, **325**, 599–605.

236 Peerboom P.F., Hassink E.A.M., Melkert R. *et al.* (1992) Thyroid function 10–18 years after mantle field irradiation for Hodgkin's disease. *European Journal of Cancer*, **28A**, 1716–1718.

237 Desablens B., Alliot C., Dierick A. *et al.* (1995) Hypothyroidism after Hodgkin's disease: pathogenic hypothesis from a study of 51 patients treated by 3 courses of the ABVD-MP regimen and 40 Gy radiotherapy. In: *Abstracts of the Third International Symposium on Hodgkin Lymphoma September 18–23, 1995, Koln, Germany*, p. 117, abstract 99.

238 Redman J.R. & Bajorunas D.R. (1990) Therapy related thyroid and parathyroid dysfunction in patients with Hodgkin's disease. In: *Hodgkin's Disease: the consequences of survival* (eds M.J. Lacher & J.R. Redman), pp. 222–243. Lea and Febiger, Philadelphia, PA.

239 Gerling B., Gottdiener J. & Borer J.S. (1990) Cardiovascular complications of the treatment of Hodgkin's disease. In: *Hodgkin's Disease: the consequences of survival* (eds M.J. Lacher & J.R. Redman), pp. 267–295. Lea and Febiger, Philadelphia, PA.

240 Morgan G.W., Freeman A.P., McLean R.G. *et al.* (1985) Late cardiac, thyroid and pulmonary sequelae of mantle radiotherapy for Hodgkin's disease. *International Journal of Radiation Oncology, Biology and Physics*, **11**, 1925–1931.

241 Pohjola-Sintonen S., Totterman K.J., Salmo M. *et al.* (1987) Late cardiac effects of mediastinal radiotherapy in patients with Hodgkin's disease. *Cancer*, **60**, 31–37.

242 Gustavsson A., Eskilsson J., Landberg T. *et al.* (1990) Late cardiac effects after mantle radiotherapy in patients with Hodgkin's disease. *Annals of Oncology*, **1**, 355–363.

243 Savage D.E., Constine L.S., Schwartz R.G. *et al.* (1990) Radiation effects on left ventricular function and myocardial perfusion in long term survivors of Hodgkin's disease. *International Journal of Radiation Oncology, Biology and Physics*, **19**, 721–727.

244 Cosset J.M., Henry-Amar M. & Meerwaldt J.H. (1991) Long term toxicity of early stages of Hodgkin's disease therapy: the EORTC experience. *Annals of Oncology*, **2**(Suppl. 2), 77–82.

245 Cosset J.M., Henry-Amar M., Pellae-Cosset B. *et al.* (1991) Pericarditis and myocardial infarctions after Hodgkin's disease therapy at the Institut Gustave Roussy. *International Journal of Radiation Oncology, Biology and Physics*, **21**, 447–449.

246 Hancock S.L., Donaldson S.S. & Hope R.T. (1993) Cardiac disease following treatment of Hodgkin's disease in children and adolescents. *Journal of Clinical Oncology*, **11**, 1208–1215.

247 Tarbell N.J., Mauch P. & Hellman S. (1990) Pulmonary complications of Hodgkin's disease treatment: radiation pneumonitis, fibrosis and the effect of cytotoxic drugs. In: *Hodgkin's Disease: the consequences of survival* (eds M.J. Lacher & J.R. Redman), pp. 296–305. Lea and Febiger, Philadelphia, PA.

248 Mah K., Keane T.J., Van Dyk J. *et al.* (1994) Quantitative effects of combined chemotherapy and fractioned radiotherapy on the

incidence of radiation induced lung damage: a prospective clinical study. *International Journal of Radiation Oncology, Biology and Physics*, **28**, 563–574.

249 Bonfante V., Viviani S., Devizzi L. *et al.* (1995) Fertility evaluation in patients with Hodgkin's disease. In: *Abstracts of the Third International Symposium on Hodgkin Lymphoma September 18–23, 1995, Koln, Germany*, p. 88, abstract 70.

250 Hill H., Milan S., Cunningham D. *et al.* (1995) Evaluation of the VEEP regimen in adult Hodgkin's disease with assessment of gonadal and cardiac toxicity. *Journal of Clinical Oncology*, **13**, 387–395.

251 Aisner J., Wiernik P.H. & Pearl P. (1993) Pregnancy outcome in patients treated for Hodgkin's disease. *Journal of Clinical Oncology*, **11**, 507–512.

252 Swerdlow A.J., Jacobs P.A., Marks A. *et al.* (1996) Fertility, reproductive outcomes, and health of offspring, of patients treated for Hodgkin's disease: an investigation including chromosome examinations. *British Journal of Cancer*, **74**, 291–296.

253 Redman J.R., Bajorunas D.R. & Lacher M.J. (1990) Hodgkin's disease: pregnancy and progeny. In: *Hodgkin's Disease: the consequences of survival* (eds M.J. Lacher & J.R. Redman), pp. 244–266. Lea and Febiger, Philadelphia, PA.

254 Henry-Amar M. & Dietrich P.Y. (1993) Acute leukaemia after the treatment of Hodgkin's disease. *Hematology/Oncology Clinics of North America*, **7**, 369–387.

255 Biti G.P., Cellai E., Magrini S. *et al.* (1994) Solid second tumours and leukaemia after treatment for Hodgkin's disease: an analysis of 1121 patients from a single institution. *International Journal of Radiation Oncology, Biology and Physics*, **29**, 25–31.

256 Valagussa P. & Bonadonna G. (1993) Hodgkin's disease and second malignancies (editorial). *Annals of Oncology*, **4**, 94–95.

257 Swerdlow A.J., Barber J.A., Horwich A. *et al.* (1997) Second malignancy in patients with Hodgkin's disease treated at the Royal Marsden Hospital. *British Journal of Cancer*, **75**, 116–123.

258 Swerdlow A.J., Douglas A.J., Vaughan Hudson G. *et al.* (1993) Risk of second primary cancer after Hodgkin's disease in patients in the British National Lymphoma Investigation: relationships to host factors, histology and stage of Hodgkin's disease and splenectomy. *British Journal of Cancer*, **68**, 1006–1011.

259 Mellemkjoer L., Olsen J.H., Linet M.S. *et al.* (1995) Cancer risk following splenectomy. *Cancer*, **75**, 577–583.

260 Van Leeuwen F.E., Klokman W.J., Hagenbeek A. *et al.* (1994) Second cancer risk following Hodgkin's disease: a 20 year follow up study. *Journal of Clinical Oncology*, **12**, 312–325.

261 Krikorian J.G., Burke J.S., Rosenberg S.A. *et al.* (1979) Occurrence of non-Hodgkin's lymphoma after therapy for Hodgkin's disease. *New England Journal of Medicine*, **300**, 452–458.

262 Henry-Amar M. (1988) Quantitative risk of second cancer in patients in first complete remission from early stages of Hodgkin's disease. *National Cancer Institute Monograph*, **6**, 65–72.

263 Bennett M.H., MacLennan K.A., Vaughan Hudson G. *et al.* (1991) Non-Hodgkin's lymphoma arising in patients treated for Hodgkin's disease in the BNLI: a 20 year experience. *Annals of Oncology*, **2**(Suppl. 2), 83–92.

264 Abrahamsen J.F., Andersan A., Hannisdal E. *et al.* (1993) Second malignancies after treatment of Hodgkin's disease: the influence of treatment, follow up time and age. *Journal of Clinical Oncology*, **11**, 255–261.

265 Rodriguez M.A., Fuller L.M., Zimmerman S.O. *et al.* (1993) Hodgkin's disease: study of treatment intensities and incidence of second malignancies. *Annals of Oncology*, **4**, 125–131.

266 Tucker M.A., Coleman N.C., Cox R.S. *et al.* (1988) Risk of secondary malignancies following Hodgkin's disease after 15 years. *New England Journal of Medicine*, **318**, 76–81.

267 Boivin J.F., Hutchinson G.B., Zauber A.G. *et al.* (1995) Incidence of second cancers in patients treated for Hodgkin's disease. *Journal of the National Cancer Institute*, **87**, 732–741.

268 Swerdlow A.J., Douglas A.J., Vaughan Hudson G. *et al.* (1992) Risk of second cancers after Hodgkin's disease by type of treatment: analysis of 2846 patients in the British National Lymphoma Investigation. *British Medical Journal*, **304**, 1137–1143.

269 Hancock S.L., Tucker M.A. & Hoppe R.T. (1993) Breast cancer after treatment for Hodgkin's disease. *Journal of the National Cancer Institute*, **85**, 25–31.

270 Dietrich P.Y., Bellefqih S., Henry-Amar M. *et al.* (1993) Linitis plastica after Hodgkin's disease (letter). *Lancet*, **342**, 57–58.

271 Kaldor J.M., Day N.E., Bell J. *et al.* (1992) Lung cancer following Hodgkin's disease: a case control study. *International Journal of Cancer*, **52**, 677–681.

272 Travis L.B., Curtis R.E., Glimelius B. *et al.* (1995) Bladder and kidney cancer following cyclophosphamide therapy for non-Hodgkin's lymphoma. *Journal of the National Cancer Institute*, **87**, 524–530.

273 Meadows A.T., Obringer A.C., Marrero O. *et al.* (1989) Second malignant neoplasms following childhood Hodgkin's disease: treatment and splenectomy as risk factors. *Medical and Pediatric Oncology*, **17**, 477–484.

274 Dietrich P.Y., Henry-Amar M., Cosset J.M. *et al.* (1994) Second primary cancers in patients continuously disease free from Hodgkin's disease: a protective role for the spleen? *Blood*, **84**, 1209–1215.

275 Robinette C.D. & Fraumeni J.F. Jr (1977) Splenectomy and subsequent mortality in veterans of the 1939–1945 war. *Lancet*, **99**, 127–129.

276 Sankila R., Garwicz S., Olsen J.H. *et al.* (1996) Risks of subsequent malignant neoplasms among 1641 Hodgkin's disease patients diagnosed in childhood and adolescence: a population-based cohort study in the five Nordic countries. *Journal of Clinical Oncology*, **14**, 1442–1446.

277 Devlen J., Maguire P., Phillips P. *et al.* (1987) Psychological problems associated with diagnosis and treatment of lymphomas: prospective study. *British Medical Journal*, **295**, 955–957.

278 Siegal K. & Christ G.H. (1990) Hodgkin's disease survivorship: psychosocial consequences. In: *Hodgkin's Disease: the consequences of survival* (eds M.J. Lacher & J.R. Redman), pp. 383–399. Lea and Febiger, Philadelphia, PA.

279 Yellen S.B., Cella D.F. & Bonomi A. (1993) Quality of life in people with Hodgkin's disease. *Oncology*, **7**, 41–52.

280 Cella D.F. & Tross S. (1986) Psychological adjustment to survival from Hodgkin's disease. *Journal of Consulting and Clinical Psychology*, **54**, 616–622.

281 Fobair P., Hoppe R., Bloom J. *et al.* (1986) Psychosocial problems among survivors of Hodgkin's disease. *Journal of Clinical Oncology*, **4**, 805–814.

282 Kornblith A.B., Anderson J., Cella D.F. *et al.* (1992) Hodgkin's disease survivors at increased risk for problems in psychosocial adaptation *Cancer*, **70**, 2214–2224.

283 Wasserman A.L., Thompson E.I., Wilimas J.A. *et al.* (1987)

The psychological status of survivors of childhood/adolescent Hodgkin's disease. *American Journal of Disease in Children*, **141**, 626–631.

284 Joly F., Henry-Amar M., Arveux P. *et al.* (1996) Late psychosocial sequelae in Hodgkin's disease survivors: a French popula-tion based case control study. *Journal of Clinical Oncology*, **14**, 2444–2453.

285 Vaughan Hudson B., Vaughan Hudson G., Linch D.C. *et al.* (1994) Late mortality in young patients cured of Hodgkin's disease. *Annals of Oncology*, **5**(Suppl. 2), S65–S66.

17 Morphology and Classification of Non-Hodgkin's Lymphomas

A.J. Norton

Introduction

The lymphomas other than Hodgkin's disease (HD) are a heterogeneous group of diseases which are characterized by a wide range of cytomorphologies, immunological marker profiles and genetic anomalies. Careful observance of this triad of features, together with the presence of relatively constant modes of clinical presentation and behaviour, have allowed the terminology of this previously complex and contentious area of tumour pathology to be agreed internationally. This chapter presents a modern classification of these disorders, together with an account of the diagnostic methods available and descriptions of the individual conditions in question.

Classification

Until relatively recently there has been no widely acceptable method of classifying the non-Hodgkin's lymphomas (NHLs) that satisfied all pathologists and clinicians alike. In the early 1970s there was an explosion of new classification schemes each proposed by interested pathologists in the field. The publication of at least five new schemes within a relatively short time span occasioned much dissatisfaction in clinical circles, as there appeared to be no rational means of deciding which of them should be adopted as an international standard to replace the then ageing Rappaport Classification [1–7]. A significant obstacle was that these classifications had appeared with no clinical data to verify their validity. As a result, the National Cancer Institute (NCI) of the USA convened a project to determine which of the proposals was the most suitable for clinical usage. The outcome of this lengthy and complex study was discouraging, because all of the new proposals appeared to be equally good at stratifying lymphomas in the test population into prognostic groups. Thus, as a means of translating between the different classifications, for the purposes of clinical trials, a Working Formulation for clinical usage was devised by the project committee [8]. As such

the Working Formulation, at its instigation, was never intended as a primary classification scheme, but it was only a short time before it was being used for this purpose, principally as a substitute for the Rappaport Classification. By contrast with the other pathologically based classification, the Working Formulation is a curious classification, as morphological diagnostic criteria had to be added to the clinical groupings by subsequent workers in the field [9]. In general, the Working Formulation became popular chiefly in North America, while in Europe there was a mixture of both the Working Formulation and Kiel Classifications in day-to-day usage. This state of affairs persisted with very little attempt at unity or terminological consensus until the early 1990s. By this time, significant progress in the field of lymphoreticular disease had been made. Marker studies had become sophisticated in their ability to discriminate between differing lineages of lymphocytes, and molecular biology and cytogenetics had identified recurring chromosomal anomalies in many individual lymphoma types. Although some of the earlier classifications had been updated as a result of these findings, this had been done in a piecemeal fashion [10–13]. It was against this background that the International Lymphoma Study Group proposed a new method of lymphoma classification based upon a constellation of clinical, morphological, immunophenotypic and molecular features to define individual disease entities. Although they published what they considered to be simply a list of recognizable diseases using present-day technology, the proposal was given the name Revised European American Lymphoma Classification with the provocative acronym REAL (Table 17.1) [14]. Initially this proposal sparked heated debate in the literature, but with time and the completion of a large clinical validation study [15], this scheme has gained ground as a new international standard for classifying lymphoma. It seems likely, however, that the REAL proposal will be overtaken by the new WHO Classification. The WHO Classification will incorporate many of the central ideas of REAL, while addressing many of the earlier criticisms levelled against it, primarily in the areas of leukaemic disease

Table 17.1 The Revised European–American Classification of Lymphoid Neoplasms: lymphoid neoplasms recognized by the International Lymphoma Study Group.

B-cell neoplasms

I Precursor B-cell neoplasm: precursor B-lymphoblastic leukaemia/lymphoma

II Peripheral B-cell neoplasms
  1 B-cell chronic lymphocytic leukaemia/prolymphocytic leukaemia/small lymphocytic lymphoma
  2 Lymphoplasmacytoid lymphoma/immunocytoma
  3 Mantle cell lymphoma
  4 Follicle centre lymphoma, follicular:
    Provisionally cytological grades: I (small cell), II (mixed small and large cell), III (large cell)
    Provisional subtype: diffuse, predominantly small cell type
  5 Marginal zone B-cell lymphoma:
    Extranodal (MALT-type ± monocytoid B cells)
    Provisional subtype: Nodal (± monocytoid B cells)
  6 Provisional entity: splenic marginal zone lymphoma (± villous lymphocytes)
  7 Hairy cell leukaemia
  8 Plasmacytoma/plasma cell myeloma
  9 Diffuse large B-cell lymphoma:
    Subtype: primary mediastinal (thymic) B-cell lymphoma
  10 Burkitt's lymphoma
  11 Provisional entity: high-grade B-cell lymphoma, Burkitt-like

T-cell and putative NK-cell neoplasms

I Precursor T-cell neoplasm : precursor T-lymphoblastic lymphoma/leukaemia

II Peripheral T-cell and NK-cell neoplasms
  1 T-cell chronic lymphocytic leukaemia/prolymphocytic leukaemia
  2 Large granular lymphocytic leukaemia (LGL):
    T-cell type
    NK-cell type
  3 Mycosis fungoides/Sézary's syndrome
  4 Peripheral T-cell lymphomas, unspecified:
    Provisional cytological categories: medium-size cell, mixed medium and large cell, large cell, lymphoepithelioid cell
    Provisional subtype: hepatosplenic γδ T-cell lymphoma
    Provisional subtype: subcutaneous panniculitic T-cell lymphoma
  5 Angioimmunoblastic T-cell lymphoma (AILD)
  6 Angiocentric lymphoma
  7 Intestinal T-cell lymphoma (+/– enteropathy associated)
  8 Adult T-cell lymphoma/leukaemia (ATL/L)
  9 Anaplastic large cell lymphoma (ALCL), CD30+, T- and null-cell types
  10 Provisional entity: anaplastic large-cell lymphoma, Hodgkin's-like

and plasma cell disorders. What seems certain is that lymphomas will no longer be classified according to arbitrary estimates of cell size, private taxonomic lexicons and personal prejudice, but rather by the identification of discrete disease entities which may ultimately deserve a more individualized approach to therapy from the clinicians. For the present, however, the terminology of the REAL scheme will be adopted throughout this account.

Diagnostic methods

Physicochemical stains

Morphology remains central to the diagnosis of lymphoreticular disease. The most commonly used physicochemical stain in use in the UK and USA is haematoxylin and eosin (H&E), while there is a strong tradition of using the Giemsa stain in mainland Europe, especially in centres familiar with the Kiel Classification. Other ancillary stains of value include reticulin stains to outline the sinus architecture and to define the different cellular compartments of organized lymphoid tissue, periodic acid-Schiff (PAS) for demonstrating immunoglobulin inclusions and vascular basement membranes and methyl green pyronin for highlighting cells, such as blasts, lymphoplasmacytoid cells and plasma cells, with large amounts of cytoplasmic RNA.

Enzyme cytochemistry

The use of enzyme cytochemistry is dwindling with the increasing reliance on immunohistochemistry for lymphoma diagnosis. The chloracetate esterase stain is still of very great value for the detection of myeloid cells. Chloroma remains one of the greatest differential diagnostic pitfalls in lymphoma pathology, as the cytoplasmic granulation of myeloblasts is less well seen in tissue sections than in cytological preparations. Other cytochemical stains, such as acid phosphatase, and the greater range of esterase stains have largely been superseded by monoclonal antibodies.

Immunohistochemistry

Without doubt good quality immunohistochemistry is vital for accurate lymphoma diagnosis. Until the late 1980s the only feasible means of demonstrating leucocyte antigens on tissue sections was to perform immunohistochemistry on cryostat sections of fresh snap frozen tissue. Clearly this presented severe limitations to diagnostic histopathologists, as very little tissue, without prior arrangement with the surgeon, ever arrived out of fixative. This problem has been circumvented largely by a number of significant technical advances. Novel reagents tailored to be effective in fixed tissue have steadily appeared in the catalogues of commercial companies, while the use of heating in buffer solutions as a means of retrieving antigens masked by fixation has made many reagents, formerly restricted to the realm of cryostat sections, usable in fixed tissue [16,17]. Lastly, the advent of powerful amplification methods, initially devised for molecular biological applications, have greatly improved detection of weak antigens in fixed and processed tissues [18]. The result is that most histopathology laboratories have forsaken their cryostats in favour of this new generation of antibodies, antigen retrieval techniques and novel amplification methods. Thus, this chapter will largely discuss the tumour phenotypes as determined in routinely processed material, with details of frozen-section work in minor instances only.

B-cell lymphomas

Precursor B-lymphoblastic lymphoma/ B-lymphoblastic leukaemia

Morphology

Lymph nodes. It is quite uncommon to receive lymph-node biopsies from this disease owing to the high frequency of a leukaemic presentation. Characteristically there is diffuse infiltration of the node pulp by a monotonous sheet of small blast cells. These cells overrun the normal architecture, leaving the reticulin framework intact. As well as occupying the node pulp, the blasts distend the node sinuses and also the efferent and afferent lymphatics in some cases. The structures most resistant to the neoplastic infiltrate are the germinal centres, which often remain entrapped within a sea of lymphoma (see Plate 17.1 between pp. 292 and 293). The neoplastic blast cells are usually small and, in poorly fixed samples, may resemble lymphocytes or centrocytes. The nuclear chromatin is dense with a stippled pattern and inconspicuous nucleoli. The cytoplasmic rim is narrow and deeply staining. The mitotic rate is usually very high, but in occasional cases the mitotic rate is deceptively low. The nuclear outline is usually round or oval, but a significant proportion show quite marked nuclear irregularities, corresponding with an FAB ALL L2 morphology on touch preparations of the fresh node.

Bone marrow. The marrow is frequently involved and presents a picture indistinguishable from ALL, with sheets of blast cells occupying the marrow space.

Extranodal disease. Secondary extranodal infiltrates are common in this disease, especially involvement of the CNS and testes. In the testis there is dense interstitial infiltration which pushes the tubules apart (see Plate 17.2). By contrast, with diffuse large B-cell lymphomas there is none of the reduplication of the peritubular basement membranes which is seen in primary and secondary diffuse large B-cell lymphoma of the testis. In soft-tissue deposits the lymphoma infiltrates in an 'Indian-file' pattern, pushing the collagen bundles apart. Primary extranodal precursor B-lymphoblastic lymphoma is quite rare with the single exception of involvement of Waldeyer's ring. Primary involvement of the skin has been reported.

Immunophenotype

Phenotyping these cells in tissue sections can be difficult, depending on the level of maturity of the B-blast cells. CD20 antigen expression is either weak and inhomogeneous or totally absent. A better marker for this disease is the CD79a antigen [19] (see Plate 17.3). There is strong positivity for the CD43 antigen and HLA-DR [20]. In frozen sections the cells express CD10 antigen. By definition there should be nuclear positivity for terminal deoxynucleotidyl transferase (TdT). In a large proportion of cases CD34 antigen is expressed [21]. Many cases, and especially those with a more primitive phenotype, lack CD45 and can stain for the MIC-2 antigen (CD99), which is more commonly associated with primitive neuroectodermal tumours (PNETs).

Differential diagnosis

There can be difficulties in identifying the infiltrate of small blast cells in lymph nodes, especially if much of the normal architecture is still preserved. In adults the differential diagnosis includes mantle cell lymphoma and, in particular, its blastoid variant. The chief problem is choosing the appropriate panel of antibodies for establishing a correct diagnosis. CD20 and CD3 are quite adequate for discriminating between mature T- and B-cell lymphomas, but in lymphoblastic disease both can give false-negative results. The staining for CD99 antigen, as mentioned above, can lead to an erroneous diagnosis of PNET.

Small B-lymphocytic lymphoma

Morphology

Lymph nodes. In tissue sections the majority of examples of this tumour have a very distinctive cytomorphology and architecture. There is complete effacement of the normal lymph-node architecture by a diffuse sheet of small round lymphocytes and these cells often spill into the perinodal fat. The neoplastic lymphocytes show some clumping of their nuclear chromatin, which is similar to that seen in the circulating cells of B-cell chronic lymphocytic leukaemia, (B-CLL) and have a narrow rim of pale eosinophilic cytoplasm (see Plate 17.4 between pp. 292 and 293). Scattered throughout the sheets of tumour cells are many paler staining foci which are best seen at low magnification (see Plate 17.5). These pale areas have very poorly defined boundaries, which seem to disappear as the magnification is increased. The cytology of the cells in these pale zones is different from that in the neighbouring lymphocytes. In these foci the cells have rather more open nuclear chromatin, with small nucleoli and a somewhat broader rim of cytoplasm (see Plate 17.6). These cells have been termed prolymphocytes. The other cell type in the pale zones is a small immunoblast with a prominent eosinophilic nucleolus and a rim of weakly basophilic cytoplasm. These immunoblastic cells have been termed paraimmunoblasts. In total these pale structures are referred to as proliferation centres or pseudofollicles. In a minority of cases the proliferation centres are very poorly formed and only scattered paraimmunoblasts relieve the monotony of the tumour.

Less commonly the lymphoma involves a portion of the lymph node only. In the most subtle form of infiltration the lymphoma replaces the mantle zone or corona of the lymphoid follicles. The mantle zones appear unusually broad and proliferation centres may grow up within them [22]. As the density of the infiltrate increases the neoplastic mantles of neighbouring follicles fuse together, giving a picture of naked germinal centres in a sea of lymphoma.

In a significant proportion of biopsied cases plasma cell differentiation may be evident in the tumour cells. This process is usually focal and tends to be most marked adjacent to the blood vessels. The cytoplasmic volume increases and the nucleus may be eccentrically placed in the cell. Varying degrees of nuclear change, approaching those of true plasma cells, accompany this increase in cytoplasmic volume. In a minority of such cases cytoplasmic immunoglobulin inclusions can be seen, or the inclusions may occupy the nucleus as so-called Dutcher bodies (see Plate 17.7). In addition to cytological alterations in the lymphocytes, a range of characteristic stromal changes occur. The vascular basement membranes may be thickened and mast cell numbers may be increased. Identification of these plasmacytoid small lymphocytic lymphomas is important, as they seem to be more resistant to conventional therapies [23].

Bone marrow. Bone marrow infiltration is common in this disease. The pattern of infiltration is indistinguishable from pure B-CLL, and takes the form of nodules in the centre of the marrow space, or interstitial infiltration, with or without proliferation centre formation.

Extranodal disease. Extranodal deposits of small B-lymphocytic lymphoma are frequently encountered as incidental findings by histopathologists. In some of these cases it is the alerting sign to the presence of a systemic lymphoma. Sites of involvement are quite varied, but include prostatic chippings from transurethral resections of prostate, soft tissue and nodal deposits at breast surgery for carcinoma of breast and skin infiltrates. It is very rare for small B-lymphocytic lymphoma to primarily involve an extranodal site and many cases in the literature are probably extranodal marginal zone lymphomas.

Histological transformation. Transformation of small B-lymphocytic lymphoma to a large cell lymphoma is far less common than in the follicle centre lymphomas. It is estimated by some authorities that approximately 5% of patients will undergo this change. When the tumour assumes a bizarre large cell morphology, this corresponds with what has been termed Richter's syndrome. It is quite common to find residual areas of low-grade disease at the margins of the transformed foci. An unusual mode of transformation is the so-called Hodgkin's disease-like change. In these cases areas strongly resembling a

lymphocyte-depleted form of nodular sclerosis HD are seen [24]. Curiously, the immunophenotype in such instances closely resembles that of Reed–Sternberg cells and Epstein-Barr virus (EBV) is frequently found in the large cells [25].

Immunophenotype

Characteristically the neoplastic cells have a B-cell phenotype with somewhat weaker expression of CD20 antigen than in many other low-grade B-cell lymphomas. The cells are CD5+ and CD43+, usually CD23+, and coexpress surface IgM and IgD [20]. In those cases with plasmacytoid differentiation cytoplasmic immunoglobulin is very strongly expressed (more than one cell per high power field). The proliferation centres lack a well-developed follicular dendritic cell meshwork on appropriate staining, although an occasional follicular dendritic cell may be found [26]. In transformed cases the large cells usually retain their B-cell phenotype but may additionally express a range of activation markers including CD30, and in those cases with Reed–Sternberg-like giant cells the latter may be CD15+.

Relevant molecular genetics

The recurring chromosomal anomalies are identical to those found in B-CLL. However, it is most unusual to have to rely upon these to establish a diagnosis. It is interesting to note that in cases of histological transformation, sequencing of the rearranged immunoglobulin genes sometimes shows that the large cell tumour is clonally related to the low-grade disease, while in a significant proportion the high-grade tumour is a clonally distinct second malignancy [27].

Differential diagnosis

Very early nodal involvement by this disease can easily be overlooked, as can extranodal deposits in a patient with no prior history. In well-established nodal disease cases can be confused with follicle centre lymphomas, especially if the proliferation centres are particularly conspicuous. Similarly, if the proliferation centres are large the author has seen cases erroneously diagnosed as nodular lymphocytic predominance HD, or even high-grade B-cell lymphoma. The latter is a problem compounded by the weak staining for CD20 antigen in the small cells of the tumour and somewhat stronger staining in the paraimmunoblasts and prolymphocytes.

Lymphoplasmacytoid lymphoma

Morphology

Lymph nodes. Nodal disease in this condition is relatively uncommon. When the lymph nodes are infiltrated there is often sparing of the germinal centres, with lymphoma occupying the paracortex and mantle zones of the follicles. Cytologically the tumour is composed of medium-sized lymphocytes with rather open nuclear chromatin and moderate amounts of cytoplasm, together with cells showing frank plasma cell differentiation (see Plate 17.8 between pp. 292 and 293). There may be cytoplasmic Russell bodies and intranuclear Dutcher bodies in a subpopulation of the tumour cells. Proliferation centres are not seen, but occasional scattered transformed cells can be present. Stromal changes include perivascular hyalinization, increased numbers of mast cells and sinus dilatation with darkly staining proteinaceous lymph. In rare cases stromal amyloid deposits are present.

Bone marrow. The bone marrow is the most frequently involved site in this disease. There is interstitial infiltration by lymphocytes and lymphoplasmacytoid cells.

Extranodal disease. After the bone marrow, splenic infiltration is the next most frequent. In splenectomy specimens there is infiltration of red pulp by lymphoma cells and, less often, replacement of the white pulp. Other extranodal sites are only rarely involved and, presently, primary extranodal disease is difficult, if not impossible, to distinguish from extranodal marginal zone lymphomas.

Histological transformation. This is a relatively rare event, but when it occurs the cytology is usually that of a B-cell immunoblastic lymphoma with plasmablastic differentiation.

Immunophenotype

As the cells exhibit marked plasma cell change the tumours show somewhat heterogeneous staining with pan-B-cell markers such as CD20. CD79a is a more reliable marker in such cases, as the antigen persists through to the plasma cell stage of B-cell maturation. There is no expression of CD5 antigen and the CD43 staining is variable. The most frequent heavy-chain type detectable in the cytoplasm of the tumour cells is IgM, with rare cases expressing other heavy-chain types (see Plate 17.9).

Differential diagnosis

The main problem in lymph nodes is distinguishing this from a nonspecific chronic lymphadenitis or the plasma cell variant of Castleman's disease. Careful staining for immunoglobulin heavy and light chains generally facilitates the distinction from a reactive process.

Mantle cell lymphoma

Morphology

Lymph nodes. Mantle cell lymphoma [28] has been known

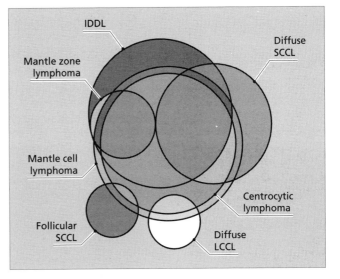

Fig. 17.1 The relation of mantle cell lymphoma to other diagnostic categories in the Working Formulation: diffuse small cleaved cell lymphoma (SCCL), follicular SCCL, diffuse large cleaved cell lymphoma (LCCL), Kiel Classification (centrocytic lymphoma) and two descriptive entities, mantle zone lymphoma and intermediate differentiated lymphocytic lymphama (IDDL).

under a variety of names in the past, reflecting its somewhat varied histological growth pattern. These names include centrocytic lymphoma (Kiel Classification) [29], diffuse small cleaved cell lymphoma (Working Formulation) [8], intermediate differentiated lymphocytic lymphoma [30] and mantle zone lymphoma [31] (Fig. 17.1). The essential starting point in nodal disease is the selective replacement of the normal mantle zones of the follicles by neoplastic cells (see Plate 17.10 between pp. 292 and 293). With time the lymphoma further advances upon the normal follicle, destroying the germinal centre, which results in a nodular growth pattern (see Plate 17.11). Eventually the tumour nodules fuse to produce a sheet-like growth pattern with rare scattered follicular remnants. When large series of cases are examined the growth patterns observed in order of frequency are diffuse, nodular and, lastly, mantle zone [32]. The cytology of the cells is the factor that unifies the disease. The cells are small to medium sized, with darkly staining nuclei containing only occasional small nucleoli (see Plate 17.12). The nuclear contour is usually irregular, cleft or contorted and the degree of monomorphism is high. In badly fixed tissues the cells may have the appearance of small round lymphocytes. The cell cytoplasm is inconspicuous and there are never any inclusions within it. Blast cells are not present in this condition, with the exception of benign blasts remaining from destroyed follicles. The mitotic rate is quite variable and can be focally high. Other features supporting the diagnosis include an increase in reticulin fibres around blood vessels and scattered nonphagocytic epithelioid appearing histiocytes.

Bone marrow. The bone marrow is commonly involved in this disease and this is often accompanied by circulating lymphoma cells. The deposits in bone marrow are often quite extensive and nonparatrabecular. As in other sites, blast cells are not a feature.

Extranodal disease. Extranodal disease is commonly encountered in this disease. Waldeyer's ring and the gastrointestinal tract are the most frequent sites and, in a small proportion of cases, are the sole sites of disease. In Waldeyer's ring the pattern of disease mirrors that in the lymph nodes. Neoplastic cells often infiltrate the squamous epithelium of the palatine tonsils, which should not be interpreted as an extranodal marginal zone lymphoma of mucosa-associated lymphoid tissue (MALT) type; the tonsillar crypt epithelium is quite permissive to all types of lymphoma cells. The large numbers of benign plasma cells in the tonsils can hamper diagnosis and may require light-chain stains to determine their reactive nature. In the gut the lymphoma involves the Peyer's patches and lymphoglandular complexes, again affecting the mantle zones at first. Large deposits of tumour in these sites may produce the syndrome of lymphomatous polyposis of the intestine [33]. By contrast, with MALT-type lymphomas lymphoepithelial lesions are not encountered in this condition, although occasional lymphoma cells may stray into the epithelium overlying large tumour deposits.

Histological transformation. This occurs with a much higher frequency than originally thought, affecting nearly 35% of patients [32]. The cytological changes in a transformed mantle cell lymphoma can be quite subtle. The cells enlarge slightly and the nuclei take on the cytology of lymphoblasts with finely divided, speckled nuclear chromatin [34]. The mitotic rate rises and apoptoses and histiocytes phagocytosing cellular debris become apparent. Small areas of necrosis may be seen. This change has been termed anaplasia in the Kiel Classification and lymphoblastoid or blastoid transformation in the REAL scheme (see Plate 17.13). In a minority of transformed cases, the cells become markedly pleomorphic with the formation of bizarre tumour giant cells.

Immunophenotype

The phenotype is quite close to that of small B-lymphocytic lymphoma. There is expression of pan-B-cell antigens together with CD5 and CD43. Coexpression of IgM and IgD usually occurs, while CD23 antigen is not expressed at high levels. The last marker helps in distinguishing this disease from small B-lymphocytic lymphoma. Latterly antibodies to the overexpressed cyclin-D1 gene product have become available which is only rarely expressed in other low-grade lymphoma types [35]. Other stains of value include BCL2 protein for highlighting the entrapped reactive germinal centres and a follicular dendritic cell marker for highlighting destroyed follicles.

Relevant molecular genetics

The translocation t(11;14) occurs with a very high frequency in this tumour, resulting in overexpression of the cyclin-D1 gene which is present on chromosome 11. The latter can be detected by PCR with a relatively low sensitivity, because of the very wide spread of breakpoints on chromosome 11 [36]. A better method is to stain for the gene product, as indicated above.

Differential diagnosis

Because of the three growth patterns seen in this condition, there is a correspondingly wide differential diagnosis. In the mantle zone growth phase the lymphoma can easily be entirely overlooked, unless care is taken to look at the cytology of the follicle mantle lymphocytes. Examples have also been seen of nodal marginal zone lymphoma (monocytoid B-cell lymphoma) interpreted as mantle cell lymphoma, when the intervening reactive mantle has been overlooked. In the nodular phase of the disease the most frequent misdiagnosis is follicle centre lymphoma or, occasionally, nodular lymphocytic predominance HD. The diffuse phase of the disease must be distinguished from all other diffuse low-grade lymphomas. The absence of any transformed cells differentiates it from diffuse follicle centre lymphoma, while the lack of proliferation centres discriminates this tumour from small B-lymphocytic lymphoma. In the bowel the major differential diagnosis is with extranodal marginal zone lymphoma of the MALT type; the absence of lymphoepithelial lesions and the characteristic phenotype clearly make the distinction.

Follicle centre lymphomas

Morphology

Lymph nodes. Because this is the single most frequent form of low-grade lymphoma, a wide range of variations on the classical histology have been described over the years. In classical examples there is complete replacement of the normal architecture by a population of neoplastic follicles, which often spill over into the neighbouring perinodal fat (see Plate 17.14 between pp. 292 and 293). The follicles, in contrast to those seen in the reactive state, are nearly all of the same size, lack the tingible body macrophages which normally phagocytose apoptotic B-cells and, generally, lack a well-developed corona or mantle of small round B-cells. The mitotic rate is usually much lower than that seen in a reactive germinal centre and there is no spatial segregation of the centroblasts from the centrocytes into the so-called light and dark zones (see Plate 17.15). In the majority of cases the neoplastic follicles are chiefly composed of small- to medium-size centrocytes with a sparse admixture of blast cells. In a minority of cases the blast cells are present in far greater numbers, with a very rare subgroup in which the follicles are almost exclusively composed of blast cells. It is this variation in cellular mix that has produced several grading systems for follicular lymphomas; the most widely used system was devised by Berard for the NCI [37] and applied to the Working Formulation. The follicles are not always sharply defined in this disease, and, as they enlarge, they may merge to confluence in some areas.

Completely diffuse forms of this disease are, in the author's experience, very rare. By definition, there should be no evidence whatsoever of follicle formation and the cytology should resemble either that of predominantly centrocytic follicular lymphoma or a mixed type. If the tumour is diffuse or partly follicular and diffuse with a predominantly blastic cytology, it should be classified as a diffuse large B-cell lymphoma [14].

As mentioned above, histological variants are many and only a few of the more common types will be mentioned here. In nodes taken from the groin or retroperitoneum a marked degree of sclerosis may be evident. This sclerosis is either patchy and intrafollicular or relatively extensive and perifollicular. The latter pattern may closely mimic nodular sclerosis HD on initial inspection at low magnification. Varying degrees of immunoglobulin accumulation may be seen in the neoplastic cells in this disease. In its simplest form the centrocytes develop large brightly eosinophilic Russell bodies. In a rarer variant of the same process the immunoglobulin inclusions are large and water clear, indenting the tumour cell nuclei and thereby imparting a signet ring appearance.

Bone marrow. Classically this disease initially infiltrates the marrow as paratrabecular deposits which are relatively broad based. In more advanced disease the infiltrate spreads out with the rare formation of recognizable follicles.

Extranodal disease. Extranodal spread is not at all uncommon, with deposits containing neoplastic follicles appearing in just about any organ of the body. In very rare instances the tumour presents with a primary extranodal deposit and involvement of the gut may produce polyps.

Histological transformation. Transformation occurs with a high frequency in patients with follicular lymphoma and this process is most apparent in units with a policy of rebiopsying at every relapse. The tumours lose their follicular pattern and take on the cytology of a diffuse large B-cell lymphoma. Very rarely, and usually as a consequence of a further t(8;14), the transformed lymphoma may take on the appearance of a Burkitt's lymphoma [38].

Immunophenotype

The cells express pan-B-cell antigens such as CD20 and CD79a. There is no expression of CD5 or CD43 antigens, but, in contrast to other low-grade B-cell diseases, they express CD10 antigen at a low level which, presently, has to be detected in frozen sections. However, detailed phenotyping is rarely needed for establishing a diagnosis because of the highly characteristic histomorphology. A useful discriminant between follicular lymphoma and reactive follicular hyperplasia is staining for BCL2 protein; this is absent from reactive germinal centres, but is usually strongly expressed in neoplastic follicle centres as a consequence of the t(14;18) [39]. In cases with poorly developed follicularity, stains for follicular dendritic reticulum cells, such as CD21 and CD23, help to reveal the characteristic meshwork of these cells.

Differential diagnosis

Florid reactive follicular hyperplasias can present difficulties and it may be necessary to resort to immunoglobulin light-chain staining and staining for BCL2 protein. The variant of follicular lymphoma with perivascular sclerosis is easily mistaken for nodular sclerosis HD. Mantle cell lymphomas with a nodular growth pattern can easily be misdiagnosed as follicular lymphomas. The diffuse type of follicle centre lymphoma is a diagnosis of exclusion, and entities to be considered include mantle cell lymphoma, lymphoplasmacytoid lymphoma and marginal zone lymphomas.

Marginal zone lymphomas

Morphology

Lymph nodes. Primary nodal marginal zone lymphoma is uncommon and has been included in the REAL scheme as a provisional entity under the name monocytoid B-cell lymphoma [40]. Secondary nodal involvement, in a patient with a primary extranodal marginal zone lymphoma of a mucosal site, is more frequently encountered, however [41,42]. There are some subtle differences between the two processes, and each will be described in turn. In monocytoid B-cell lymphoma there is partial replacement of the lymph-node architecture by a broad band of neoplastic cells which sit external to the follicle mantle zones, often bridging adjacent follicles (see Plate 17.16 between pp. 292 and 293). A significant proportion of the tumour cells actually reside within the lymph-node sinuses, the position normally occupied by reactive monocytoid B cells. The cells are monomorphic and medium sized, with oval or reniform nuclei containing finely divided chromatin and small nucleoli and with a broad rim of pale-staining cytoplasm (see Plate 17.17). It is the latter feature that has earned them the epithet 'monocytoid B cells'. There may be a scanty admixture of neutrophil polymorphs among the tumour cells, but this is not such a constant feature as in reactive monocytoid B-cell collections. Occasional foci of more plasmacytoid-appearing cells may be seen.

In secondary spread of extranodal marginal zone lymphomas the appearances can be identical to a monocytoid B-cell lymphoma and, indeed, some cases of monocytoid B-cell lymphoma in the literature were later found to have an extra-nodal primary [43]. More often, however, the monocytoid features are much less marked or only present in part of the involved node. The distribution of the lymphoma is the same, with the neoplastic cells sitting external to the mantle zones of reactive follicles. A lymphoplasmacytoid of centrocytic cytology may predominate and there can be a heavy admixture of reactive elements, in particular epithelioid histiocytes.

Bone marrow. This site is rarely involved, but on those occasions when disease is present it appears as small interstitial nodules. Rarely the disease occupies the marginal zone of reactive B-cell aggregates.

Extranodal disease. Primary extranodal marginal zone lymphomas are the most common manifestation of this disease. When the disease occurs in a mucosal site the tumours have been termed lymphomas of MALT type [44]. However, a significant minority of cases occur in extranodal sites devoid of a mucosa yet have the same overall architecture. Thus, the term extranodal marginal zone lymphoma has been deemed more appropriate for the group of lymphomas as a whole [14]. In the classical examples occurring at mucosal sites, the lymphoma 'sits' around reactive follicles and their mantle zones in a typical marginal zone distribution [45]. The neoplastic cells which are closest to the overlying epithelial surface infiltrate the epithelium to produce lymphoepithelial lesions. This process can be considered a parody of the lymphocyte migration seen overlying the Peyer's patches of the normal intestine [46] (see Plates 17.18–17.20). Indeed, the presence of lymphoid tissue resembling normal Peyer's patches seems to be a prerequisite for the later development of lymphoma and, in many cases, this has to be acquired at the site in question, either through longstanding chronic inflammation or autoimmunity [45]. Examples of this process are the acquisition of lymphoid tissue in the salivary glands in Sjögren's syndrome and in the stomach in follicular gastritis as a result of *Helicobacter pylori* infection. In all these conditions, B-lymphocytes will infiltrate the overlying epithelium, but, of course, in the early stages of the disease they are purely reactive in nature. For the diagnosis of lymphoma, lymphoepithelial lesions are exaggerated with destruction or distension of the glands. In addition to the perifollicular neoplastic infiltrate and lymphoepithelial lesions, there is often subepithelial plasma cell differentiation of the neoplastic cells and varying degrees of follicular colonization [47]. The latter process is a recapitulation of the normal maturation of marginal zone lymphocytes upon stimulation by antigen [48]. The cytology of the neoplastic cells can vary quite considerably, from small roundish lymphocytes, through centrocyte-like cells to monocytoid B-cells. There are usually dispersed transformed cells and plasma cell differentiation may be quite conspicuous.

In sites devoid of mucosa, extranodal marginal zone lymphomas can occur. Such sites include the orbit and deep sub-

cutis of the skin. The only missing element is the absence of lymphoepithelial lesions in an otherwise typical marginal zone lymphoma. An unusual and notable type of extranodal marginal zone lymphoma of MALT type is the so-called Mediterranean lymphoma, or alpha-chain disease. In this condition the lymphoma involves extensive segments of the small intestine and there is a high degree of plasma cell differentiation of the lymphoma in the lamina propria [49].

Histological transformation

This occurs relatively commonly, and rapid enlargement of the thyroid or salivary gland may be the alerting sign to the presence of an extranodal marginal zone lymphoma with subsequent histological transformation. Cytologically, the transformed tumours fall into the spectrum of diffuse large B-cell lymphoma. It is not unusual to find a low-grade component in an otherwise high-grade lymphoma of a mucosal site, especially if the resection specimen is extensively sampled [50].

Immunophenotype

The immunophenotype of these tumours is not especially distinctive and there are no major differences between the monocytoid B-cell form of the disease and other members of this family of lymphomas. They are usually CD5– and CD43–, with no expression of CD10 in frozen sections. Very rare cases of extranodal marginal zone lymphoma, with a CD5+ positive phenotype, have been described, which have pursued a more aggressive course than usual [51].

Relevant molecular genetics

The tumours do not usually show *BCL2* or *BCL1* gene rearrangements. A common anomaly is the presence of trisomy 3, which can be detected in interphase nuclei either by fluorescence *in situ* hybridization (FISH) or nonfluorescent methods [52].

Differential diagnosis

In lymph nodes monocytoid B-cell lymphoma can be difficult to distinguish from reactive lymphoid proliferations with a high monocytoid B-cell content, such as toxoplasmosis and early HIV infection. Distinction depends upon good quality staining for light chains and the presence of an infiltrative growth pattern by the monocytoid B cells in lymphoma. Another, and relatively common, pitfall is the extensive presence of monocytoid B-cell differentiation external to the neoplastic follicle centres in about one-third of follicular follicle centre lymphomas [53].

In mucosal sites the differential diagnosis includes mantle cell lymphoma, follicular follicle centre lymphomas and florid inflammatory processes, with the production of Peyer's patch-like organized lymphoid tissue [54].

Splenic marginal zone lymphoma

Morphology

Spleen. The marginal zones of the normal spleen are well-developed structures which impart a dartboard-like appearance to the B-cell areas of the white pulp. Lymphomas which appear to selectively occupy this splenic marginal zone have been described by a number of names in the past, and a proportion of these cases have circulating villous B-lymphocytes in the peripheral blood [55–58]. Lymphomas of this type were provisionally included in the REAL Classification as members of the marginal zone group of tumours. However, there is now some doubt about the validity of this decision, which is why they will be discussed separately. In the classic mode of splenic involvement, the B-cell areas of the spleen are expanded by nodular collections of small- to medium-size lymphoid cells. The nodules are chiefly centred upon pre-existing follicles, although some smaller tumour nodules do grow up within the red pulp (see Plates 17.21 & 17.22 between pp. 292 and 293). In many of the nodules the residue of the reactive germinal centre is seen towards the middle of the nodule, this is encircled by a broad band of lymphocytes resembling normal mantle zone cells, and, external to the mantle, a characteristic pale-staining marginal zone. The cells in the marginal zone have relatively plentiful cytoplasm and show varying degrees of lymphoplasmacytoid differentiation. In contrast to marginal zone lymphomas elsewhere, the neoplastic component comprises both the cells in the widened mantle zone as well as those in the marginal zone [59]. Thus, this lymphoma has a curious and unique biphasic growth pattern.

Lymph nodes. The nodal deposits of this disease are most often seen in the splenic hilar lymph nodes at splenectomy. The lymphoma has a nodular growth pattern, centred upon the B-cell follicles, but the curious biphasic histology is not seen, and the tumour has a closer resemblance to a lymphoplasmacytoid lymphoma or mantle cell lymphoma.

Bone marrow. When the marrow is involved it appears as interstitial nodules or diffusely scattered cells. Rarely, the tumour cells are only seen within the marrow sinusoids. The nodular deposits are often centred upon pre-existing benign lymphoid aggregates.

Immunophenotype

The tumour cells express pan-B-cell antigens such as CD20 and CD79a. The more detailed immunophenotype is somewhat inconsistent. Some cases are CD10+, others express CD5, and the majority express neither [59,60]. Whether this is a true heterogeneity or whether there are several lymphomas included in this group is unclear at the present time.

Relevant molecular genetics

Most cases studied lack *BCL2* rearrangements. A small number, however, show rearrangements of the *BCL1* locus with concomitant expression of the cyclin-D1 protein [61].

Differential diagnosis

Most low-grade B-cell lymphomas can produce a nodular growth pattern in the spleen and must be excluded by careful morphology and immunohistochemistry. One of the biggest mimics is follicular lymphoma with a degree of marginal zone differentiation.

Plasmacytoma

Morphology

Lymph nodes. Nodal involvement by plasmacytoma and myeloma is very rare, as is primary nodal plasmacytoma. There is replacement of the paracortex by plasma cells of varying morphology. In many cases there is sparing of the reticulin framework of the node and reactive follicles may remain.

Bone marrow. Plasmacytoma/myeloma diffusely infiltrates the marrow space, ultimately resulting in solid sheets of plasma cells.

Extranodal disease. Extranodal plasmacytoma is relatively common, especially in the upper airways. The tumours vary in cytology from well-differentiated Marschalko plasma cells through to cells closely resembling immunoblasts.

Immunophenotype

As the cells are terminally differentiated B cells, they usually lack CD20 antigen and CD45 antigen on their surface. There is variable staining for CD43 antigen, while CD79a is nearly always present. A number of relatively plasma cell-specific antigens are expressed by these tumours, including that recognized by the antibody VS-38. Difficulties in diagnosis can be caused by the frequent positivity for the epithelial-related antigens EMA and low-molecular-weight cytokeratin [62]. In general, large amounts of cytoplasmic immunoglobulin can be demonstrated.

Differential diagnosis

In most cases the diagnosis is straightforward. Problems in distinguishing a poorly differentiated plasmacytoma from an immunoblastic lymphoma can arise, and the cut-off point between the two conditions is somewhat arbitrary. The most troublesome problem arises as a result of the expression of epithelial markers with the absence of CD45 antigen. This may lead to an erroneous diagnosis of metastatic carcinoma.

Diffuse large B-cell lymphomas

Morphology

Lymph nodes. Diffuse large B-cell lymphomas constitute one of the single largest groups of lymphoma occurring in the Western hemisphere. They have been subclassified with varying degrees of complexity in the Working Formulation [8] and Updated Kiel Classifications [11,12], but it was the view of the International Lymphoma Study Group that such subdivisions were unreproducible and that all such tumours should be placed in a single category of the REAL scheme [14]. While this is a pragmatic decision, it does make the teaching of the different 'faces' of these common tumours somewhat difficult. Apart from these problems, the tumours of this type are composed almost entirely of blast cells, with a variable admixture of small reactive T cells and histiocytes. Cytologically the blasts most frequently resemble those seen in the normal reactive germinal centres—the centroblasts. These cells are large with roundish nuclei, well-defined nuclear membranes, vesicular chromatin and multiple nucleoli which look as though they are adhering to the nuclear membrane itself. The cytoplasmic rim is relatively narrow and, as with all blast cells, is deeply staining as a result of the presence of plentiful cytoplasmic RNA (see Plate 17.23 between pp. 292 and 293). Variations on this basic cell type occur and individual tumours may contain mixtures of these cytological variants or a pure population of either one. The centroblasts may have an irregular rather than a round nuclear shape or they may have a multilobated appearance with nuclei resembling those of neutrophil polymorphs [11] (see Plate 17.24). The second most frequently encountered cytological type of blast cell is the immunoblast. These have round to oval nuclei with distinct nuclear membranes, dispersed chromatin and, usually, one large brightly eosinophilic, centrally placed nucleolus. The cytoplasm is even deeper staining than the centroblasts and, in some cells, a perinuclear hof is apparent, indicating a degree of plasmablastic differentiation (see Plate 17.25). Immunoblasts may be present in variable numbers admixed with centroblasts or, in a relatively rare subgroup, grow as a practically pure culture.

Not all diffuse large B-cell lymphomas conform to the descriptions above and the blast cells may confound subclassification or, in rare instances, may be so bizarre that they resemble an anaplastic large cell lymphoma (see Plate 17.26). However, in the REAL scheme B-cell anaplastic large cell lymphoma is not considered as a separate entity. One perplexing histological variant of nodal diffuse large B-cell lymphoma

deserves further mention. This is the so-called T-cell-rich B-cell lymphoma [63]. In this condition the neoplastic B-blasts are present in very small numbers compared to a very high content of small reactive T cells and variable numbers of histiocytes [64]. The blast cells may have complex nuclear contours and occasional Reed–Sternberg-like giant cells are present, causing confusion with mixed cellularity HD (see Plates 17.27–17.29 between pp. 292 and 293). The exact numbers of infiltrating T cells to qualify for this diagnosis are somewhat arbitrary, but they usually exceed 90% of the cells present. Whether this is a distinct disease entity or not is debatable and some cases will later manifest as more typical diffuse large B-cell lymphomas.

In a small number of cases of diffuse large B-cell lymphoma there is evidence of an underlying low-grade lymphoma in one area of the biopsied lymph node, which is most commonly of the follicular type.

Bone marrow. The tumours usually involve the marrow as interstitial nodules or sheets of cells. In a significant minority the marrow shows a discordant picture with involvement by cytologically low-grade lymphoma, usually of the follicular type.

Extranodal disease. Extranodal involvement is very common in this group of diseases and, as well as being the single most frequent type of nodal lymphoma, they also constitute the single largest group of primary extranodal lymphomas. No site in the body is spared, with Waldeyer's ring and the gastrointestinal tract being the most frequently involved.

One specific type of primary extranodal diffuse large B-cell lymphoma has earned a place in the REAL Classification as mediastinal B-cell lymphoma [14,65–67]. This disease occurs most commonly in young women, as a thymic mass producing superior vena caval obstruction. Histologically, there is often extensive stromal fibrosis, which has earned this tumour the name sclerosing mediastinal B-cell lymphoma in some accounts.

The second peculiar histological variant of primary extranodal diffuse large B-cell lymphoma has the name 'angiotropic large cell lymphoma' [68]. In this rare disease the lymphoma cells are seen exclusively within the vasculature, in the absence of a leukaemic component. The most frequent sites in which this intravascular lymphoma is encountered are the skin and central nervous system.

Immunophenotype

The immunophenotype of these tumours is not especially unique. The tumour cells express one or more pan B-cell antigen such as CD20 and CD79a. There may be expression of monotypic immunoglobulin, but a number of cases fail to make any stainable immunoglobulin, including many of the mediastinal B-cell lymphomas. The results of staining for CD5 and CD10 are variable again, with a minority of cases expressing either of these markers.

Differential diagnosis

Distinction of diffuse large B-cell from large T-cell lymphomas cannot be made with absolute accuracy unless immunophenotyping is performed. A significant histological pitfall is a tissue deposit of acute myeloid leukaemia which, if poorly granulated, can be remarkably similar in appearance to centroblasts. The T-cell-rich variant can readily be confused with a T-cell lymphoma or HD. The differential diagnosis of mediastinal B-cell lymphoma includes thymoma, the epithelial cells of which can be CD20+ in some instances [69].

Burkitt's lymphoma

Morphology

Lymph nodes. Nodal involvement by Burkitt's lymphoma is only rarely encountered, with the majority of cases arising in extranodal locations. There is either complete effacement of the normal architecture by a monomorphic sheet of blast cells or partial involvement of the node. The latter takes the form of selective replacement of follicle mantle zones with the ultimate occupation of the germinal centres by tumour cells. This imparts a follicular appearance to the tumour in some areas. Cytologically the cells are medium-size blast cells with round nuclei with fine nuclear membranes, finely divided nuclear chromatin and between two and five centrally placed small nucleoli (see Plate 17.30 between pp. 292 and 293) [70]. A minority of the cells have a single larger central nucleolus, a feature that is more often seen in the sporadic and AIDS-associated tumours than the endemic type of the disease. The cytoplasmic rim is narrow and darkly staining and contains multiple fine droplets of neutral lipid. The lipid droplets are best seen on touch preparations of nodal tissue or on cytological aspirate specimens (see Plate 17.31). However, with care the droplets can be seen at the very edge of histological sections where the cells tend to have rather more condensed nuclei. The mitotic rate is very high (greater than 10 mitoses per high power field), and there is a correspondingly high rate of apoptosis. The apoptotic tumour cells are contained by plentiful tumour-infiltrating macrophages, which are the cells that impart the 'starry-sky' appearance to these lymphomas.

Bone marrow. Marrow infiltration is in the form of interstitial nodules or sheets of blasts.

Extranodal disease. Extranodal deposits of Burkitt's lymphoma are very common and a significant proportion of cases exclusively involve these sites. The most frequently encountered sites of involvement are the jaws and gonads, in endemic cases, and the ileocaecal region and Waldeyer's ring in sporadic cases.

Immunophenotype

The neoplastic cells have a B-cell phenotype with expression of CD20 and other pan-B-cell antigens. There is positivity for CD10 in frozen sections. In contrast to precursor lymphoblastic lymphomas, the cells lack CD34 antigen and nuclear TdT. Surface IgM can usually be detected. In all endemic and up to 20% of sporadic cases, EBV proteins can be detected in the tumour cells [71]. The repertoire of EBV genes expressed is restricted in Burkitt's lymphoma and *EBNA-1* is the easiest to detect [72]. Burkitt's lymphoma has a proliferative fraction approaching 100% and staining for cell cycle-related proteins, such as Ki-67, decorates nearly every tumour cell.

Differential diagnosis

Burkitt's lymphoma can be distinguished from lymphoblastic lymphomas by the appropriate special stains. The distinction from a centroblastic lymphoma composed of small centroblasts can be difficult at times, and the stains for proliferating fraction are one of the best means of separating these tumours.

T-cell lymphomas and lymphomas of putative NK-cell lineage

Precursor T-lymphoblastic lymphoma/leukaemia

Morphology

Lymph nodes. The pattern of infiltration and cytology is practically indistinguishable from that seen with the precursor B-lymphoblastic lymphomas described above. There are some slight and subtle cytological differences—in the precursor T-lymphoblastic lymphomas the mitotic rate can be unusually low and a small proportion of the cells are nucleolated. The presence of nuclear convolutions, though often present, is an unreliable indicator of a T-cell phenotype.

Bone marrow. The tumour cells infiltrate as sheets within the marrow space.

Extranodal disease. Extranodal deposits are quite often encountered, although rarely biopsied. Thymic involvement occurs in a significant proportion of cases, and, as with the B-cell diseases, the testes may be infiltrated. Primary extranodal disease with the exception of disease in the thymus is extremely rare.

Immunophenotype

The cells have an immature T-cell phenotype. CD3 antigen is usually expressed but can be absent. CD2 in paraffin sections and CD7 in frozen tissue are more reliable markers. As a recapitulation of normal T-cell ontogeny, the cells express CD1a antigen in some instances and variably mark for CD4, CD8 or both CD4 and CD8 antigens. By definition there is expression of nuclear TdT. HLA-DR is not usually expressed at high levels and, similarly, CD34 antigen is only occasionally present. Markers such as CD43 and CD45R0 are usually positive, but they are of poor discriminatory value in precursor lymphoblastic lymphomas.

Differential diagnosis

The major differential diagnosis is with precursor B-lymphoblastic lymphomas. In some instances, especially in children, the morphological distinction from a myeloid leukaemia can be difficult.

Large granular lymphocytic leukaemia

Morphology

Lymph nodes. The lymph nodes are hardly ever sampled in this condition, as it is essentially a haematological diagnosis. In the few cases of the author's experience there has been a subtle expansion of the paracortical T-zones by small round lymphocytes.

Bone marrow. The lymphoma infiltrates as a loosely textured interstitial infiltrate which can be easily overlooked.

Extranodal disease. The spleen is the most likely site of involvement by this disease, other than the nodes and marrow. The spleen is commonly infiltrated and the small round neoplastic cells are seen as relatively widely separated cells in the cords of Bilroth and venous sinuses. Cytoplasmic granulation is not apparent, even in Giemsa-stained tissue preparations, and the characteristic cytology is only seen on touch preparations of fresh tissue.

Immunophenotype

The phenotype in tissue sections varies according to the type of disease present—cytotoxic T cell or NK cell in type [73]. In the cytotoxic T-cell type the tumour cells are CD3+ and CD2+, express CD8 antigen and are usually CD56–. In the NK-cell type the cells are CD2+, lack CD8 and express CD56 antigen. NK cells do produce some cytoplasmic CD3 antigen, which can be detected in tissue sections as a perinuclear zone of staining.

Differential diagnosis

As the spleen is the most likely organ to be encountered, the chief differential diagnostic problem is in actually recognizing the presence of an abnormality, because the red-pulp cellularity is only subtly increased.

T-lymphocytic lymphoma/T-prolymphocytic lymphoma

Morphology

Lymph nodes. The presentation in this group of conditions, as with the large granular lymphocytic proliferations, is principally leukaemic, and the lymph nodes are only rarely removed. In nodal disease the paracortex is expanded by moderately pleomorphic small lymphocytes which eventually grow to confluence, overrunning the normal nodal architecture [74].

Bone marrow. The marrow is infiltrated by sheets of small lymphoid cells.

Extranodal disease. Extranodal deposits are rarely seen in this disease, with the singular exception of cutaneous infiltrates in a significant minority [75].

Immunophenotype

The cells have a mature T-cell phenotype with expression of CD2 and CD3 antigens. Most cases are CD4+.

Differential diagnosis

In spleen and bone marrow the principal differential diagnosis is with diffuse low-grade B-cell lymphomas.

Angioimmunoblastic T-cell lymphoma

Morphology

Lymph nodes. This disease is the archetypal cytologically low-grade T-cell lymphoma. There is complete effacement of the normal nodal architecture by lymphoma. Residual B-cell follicles are not seen, with the exception of occasional small nodular collections of follicular dendritic reticulum cells representing burnt-out germinal centres. There is a complex and abnormally arborizing vascularity composed of high endothelial venules (see Plate 17.32 between pp. 292 and 293). These vessels may be so densely branching as to suggest a vascular neoplasm in some cases. Throughout this background there is an infiltrate which is rich and varied in its cytology. There are small round lymphocytes, dispersed blast cells and lymphocytes with abundant water-clear cytoplasm (see Plate 17.33). Importantly, these clear cells retain their clear cytoplasmic appearance in both haematoxylin and eosin and Giemsa-stained sections. Admixed with these elements are variable proportions of epithelioid histiocytes, plasma cells and eosinophils. Indeed, no two cases have quite the same reactive cytological mix within them. The most constant feature, however, is the presence of proliferating follicular dendritic cells throughout the tumour which require special stains for their demonstration [76] (see Plate 17.34).

Bone marrow. The nodular and diffuse bone marrow infiltrates have an identical appearance to nodal deposits with proliferating vessels and the same rich cytological mix.

Extranodal disease. Extranodal deposits are not uncommon and, as with the bone marrow, the infiltrates in skin and soft tissues carry their blood vessels and reactive elements with them.

Histological transformation. In those rare cases that survive long enough to undergo this process, the cytology alters to that of a pleomorphic diffuse large cell lymphoma with some of the underlying stromal changes still apparent. In rare cases the high-grade lymphoma is of B-cell phenotype and contains the EBV genome in the neoplastic cells [76].

Immunophenotype

The tumour cells have a mature T-cell phenotype, with expression of CD2 and CD3 antigens. The majority of cases are predominantly CD4+ phenotype, but a small proportion are mainly CD8+. The blast cell population is not entirely of neoplastic T-cell type. A significant number of these cells are B-blasts which are polyclonal in nature. On special staining for EBV the B-blasts, and some of the T-cells, contain viral proteins [77,78]. The follicular dendritic cell meshwork alluded to above is readily identified with the appropriate stains, such as for CD21 or CD23.

Differential diagnosis

This disease has long been classified with the reactive lymphadenopathies and has only relatively recently been considered truly neoplastic. Some drugs, notably phenytoin and ACE inhibitors, may produce similar proliferations, albeit with intact residual follicles. The process can be mistaken for HD, especially if the blast cells are large and pleomorphic. Usually the immunophenotype and clinical history help to make the distinction.

Peripheral T-cell lymphoma not otherwise specified

Morphology

Lymph nodes. In the REAL Classification T-cell lymphomas falling into this category are a heterogeneous group of disorders with quite varied cytology. The justification for this decision was the poor reproducibility of the laudable, but complex, Updated Kiel Classification for T-cell lymphoma [10,14,79].

Nevertheless, for teaching purposes it is desirable to retain some of the Kiel distinctions [10]. To that end this section on nodal disease will be divided into tumours with a predominantly small cell cytology and those with a large cell appearance.

1 *Small cell-predominant types.* In the section 'angioimmunoblastic T-cell lymphoma' above, it was stated that its cytology was an archetype for other T-cell lymphomas of small cell type. The cytological mix of peripheral T-cell lymphomas of predominantly small cell type is very similar to tumours of angioimmunoblastic type, with the notable absence of significant numbers of reactive B-blasts, a not so conspicuous high endothelial vascularity and no proliferating follicular dendritic reticulum cells [10]. The pleomorphic small- to medium-size lymphocytes, clear cells and admixture of reactive elements remain a common theme.

In the T-zone pattern of disease, the neoplastic infiltrate is seen expanding the paracortical areas of the node, with conspicuous, well-preserved, relatively widely separated reactive B-cell follicles studded throughout [10].

In the lymphoepithelioid pattern (Lennert's lymphoma), the predominant reactive cellular element is an epithelioid histiocyte. These are present in such large numbers that they obscure the neoplastic infiltrate. Very few residual normal nodal structures remain in this type of lymphoma [10] (see Plate 17.35 between pp. 292 and 293).

In the pleomorphic small cell variant the nodal architecture is either partly or totally replaced by a monomorphic population of small pleomorphic T cells with very few blast cells present [10].

2 *Large cell predominant types.* These tumours are composed of varying mixtures of medium-size and large pleomorphic lymphoid blast cells, together with an admixture of reactive elements and prominent high endothelial venules [10]. The nuclei of the lymphoma cells often show extreme variations in their contour and bizarre giant cells may be seen (see Plate 17.36). Immunoblasts of classic type, but lacking plasmablastic features, may also constitute a part or the entirety of these tumours and, rarely, these have copious water-clear cytoplasm. It is possible to subcategorize these tumours according to the predominant cell type present, but this has been shown to be quite unreproducible [79].

Bone marrow. The lymphomas tend to infiltrate the centre of the marrow space commencing in a perisinusoidal distribution, later producing nodules and sheets.

Extranodal disease. Primary extranodal T-cell lymphomas in a very wide range of sites constitute a high proportion of the large cell cytological variants, while the smaller cell types occur more frequently in lymph nodes or Waldeyer's ring.

Immunophenotype

Most of these tumours have a mature T-cell phenotype. With increasing cell size the chances of one or more pan-T-cell marker failing to 'decorate' the tumour cells increases. Thus, in the large cell types a relatively large panel of reagents is advisable. Most tumours are of CD4+ T-cell type, while a minority are of CD8 type or lack either subset marker [80].

Differential diagnosis

The differential diagnosis is quite wide, depending on the histological growth pattern and cytological mix. The small cell types must be distinguished from infective disorders, in particular viral lymphadenopathies, drug reactions and HD. The large cell types can only be reliably separated from the B-cell lymphomas by immunohistochemistry.

Adult T-cell lymphoma/leukaemia

Morphology

Lymph nodes. In its classic aggressive form, ATL completely effaces the normal nodal architecture with an infiltrate of large, pleomorphic blast forms [10] (see Plate 17.37 between pp. 292 and 293). The nuclear contours of the cells are often extremely complex, earning them descriptive titles such as 'jelly fish cells' and 'fetal cells' [81]. The high endothelial venules are quite conspicuous and, despite the size of the cells, they show marked traffic across the walls of these vessels. The cytology, as with many types of T-cell lymphoma, will vary from case to case and a minority will show a small cell cytology, corresponding with the so-called smouldering phase of the disease.

Bone marrow. The marrow infiltrates are usually heavy and sheet like in this disease.

Extranodal disease. Extranodal infiltration does occur, with the skin being the most frequent site of lymphomatous infiltration, followed by almost all other organ systems. The cutaneous manifestations of the disease may precede the nodal and marrow infiltrates. In such instances the cutaneous disease is almost indistinguishable from mycosis fungoides [82].

Immunophenotype

The tumour cells have a mature T-cell phenotype with expression of CD2 and CD3 antigens. There is usually loss of CD7 antigen on frozen sections. Strong expression of CD25 antigen is almost always found, and CD30 antigen is frequently expressed. The majority of cases will have a CD4+ phenotype [83].

Differential diagnosis

The morphology and immunophenotype do not distinguish this disease from other forms of diffuse large T-cell lymphoma. Only the detection of HTLV-I establishes the diagnosis.

Intestinal T-cell lymphoma

Morphology

Lymph nodes. By definition nodal disease occurs as a secondary process. In many cases the neoplastic blast cells are seen percolating through the lymph node sinuses, only later producing mass lesions.

Bone marrow. Marrow infiltration occurs quite late in the course of the disease and may be quite difficult to detect, with only small collections present adjacent to the marrow sinusoids.

Extranodal disease. The site of predilection for this lymphoma is the jejunum and ileum, but other parts of the bowel may be involved by the same neoplasm. Grossly the tumours appear as annular strictures, fissures or plaques which are frequently multiple [84]. Bowel perforation through one of these deposits is the usual mode of presentation. Cytologically the tumours recapitulate the entire spectrum of high-grade T-cell disease and, rarely, they may be composed of small cells alone. The infiltrate of neoplastic cells can be quite scanty and it requires careful scrutiny of the edges and base of the ulcerated portions of intestine in order to detect them. In addition, the tumour cells are often seen within the epithelium, mimicking the traffic of normal intraepithelial lymphocytes (see Plate 17.38 between pp. 292 and 293). Very often there is an intense reactive intraepithelial lymphocytosis at the ulcer margins and villous atrophy may be present. There is an association between this lymphoma and coeliac disease in a high proportion of cases, and in some instances the coeliac enteropathy only becomes apparent after the lymphoma has manifested itself [84,85].

Immunophenotype

The cells mark as T cells with pan-T-cell markers such as CD3 and CD2. Most cases have a CD4+ phenotype, but contain cytoplasmic proteins associated with activated cytotoxic T cells, such as TIA-1 antigen, granzyme-B and perforin [86]. The large cytological variants often stain for CD30 antigen and other activation markers. Most cases express an integrin molecule associated with intraepithelial lymphocytes (CD103), which is detectable only in frozen sections [87].

Differential diagnosis

The differential diagnosis includes other forms of small bowel ulceration, especially ulcerative ileojejeunitis which can also complicate coeliac disease.

Angiocentric lymphoma

Morphology

Lymph nodes. Lymph nodes are very seldom involved by this principally extranodal condition.

Bone marrow. Marrow infiltration may occur late in this disease, but more often there is a paraneoplastic haemophagocytic syndrome which can be identified on the marrow smears.

Extranodal disease. Angiocentric lymphoma is, almost by definition, an extranodal disease. The most frequent site of involvement is the upper airways in a predominantly midline distribution. The epithet 'angiocentric' refers to the lymphoma's predilection for infiltrating and destroying the walls of veins, venules, small muscular arteries and arterioles [88] (see Plate 17.39 between pp. 292 and 293). This results in widespread necrosis, sometimes with extensive facial deformity. The neoplastic cells are quite variable in their cytology, ranging from small, slightly irregular shaped lymphocytes through to large pleomorphic or bizarre blast forms. There may be heavy admixture of inflammatory elements which can obscure the neoplastic cells, as can the often extensive necrosis. Similar tumours occur in other sites, including the lungs and skin. However, they do not all share the same distinctive phenotypic and virological features listed below.

Immunophenotype

This tumour is the best candidate there is for a true NK-cell tumour. The cells lack surface CD3, but do show some cytoplasmic CD3ε and stain strongly for CD2. There is positivity for one or more NK-cell marker, including CD56. Many cases express activation markers, including CD30, CD25 and HLA-DR. The vast majority of cases contain clonal EBV genome within the tumour cells and viral proteins can be stained for with appropriate antibodies [89].

Relevant molecular genetics

In keeping with a NK-cell derivation clonal immunoglobulin and T-cell receptor gene, rearrangements cannot be detected in these lymphomas [89].

Differential diagnosis

Most problems with establishing a diagnosis rest on the adequacy of the sample from a lymphoma with such a propensity to undergo necrosis. Angioinvasion alone is insufficient for the diagnosis, as many forms of both low- and high-grade lymphoma can destroy vessel walls. Similarly, the presence of a strongly angioinvasive tumour in the skin or lungs does not necessarily indicate the presence of this NK-cell tumour. True T-cell lymphomas can produce this pattern in those sites, and an unusual form of T-cell-rich B-cell lymphoma may closely mimic an angiocentric lymphoma in the lung [90].

Anaplastic large cell lymphoma

Morphology

Lymph nodes. This lymphoma is composed of large cells which have oval or reniform nuclei with finely divided chromatin and one or more small, centrally placed nucleoli. The cytoplasm is voluminous and pale staining, closely resembling the cytoplasm of well-fixed lacunar cells in nodular sclerosis HD (see Plate 17.40 between pp. 292 and 293) [91]. It is this particular cytology that led early investigators into believing that these tumours were of histiocytic derivation. Other variations in the cytology, which are often scattered throughout the main tumour, include multinucleated giant cells with a wreath-like arrangement of their nuclei, thereby resembling a ring doughnut, and bizarre monster giant cells. The growth pattern is highly characteristic of this tumour. In most instances the tumour cells percolate through the lymph-node sinuses as solid cores of cells, only later forming mass lesions. Larger tumour masses may undergo patchy necrosis.

A number of unusual variants of this disease have been described. The most troublesome of these variants is where the neoplastic cells assume a fusiform appearance and cuff blood vessels, producing a picture similar to young granulation tissue [92]. The second histologically taxing variant is where there is a very heavy admixture of peculiar histiocytes with a plasmacytoid appearance obscuring the neoplastic infiltrate. This lymphohistiocytic type is more often seen in the paediatric age group [93].

Bone marrow. Marrow infiltration may be very subtle in this condition. In the early stages the tumour cells infiltrate the marrow space as single cells, which tend to collect around the marrow sinusoids. Only later do the cells produce readily discernible nodules or sheets.

Extranodal disease. This disease shows a predilection for extranodal sites. In primary nodal disease the preferential extranodal site of involvement is the skin. On the other hand, primary cutaneous anaplastic large cell lymphoma is itself not that uncommon. Cutaneous disease may occasionally show a spontaneously remitting picture, and there appears to be a continuum between such types of anaplastic large cell lymphoma and the disorder termed 'lymphomatoid papulosis' [94].

Immunophenotype

The neoplastic cells almost always strongly express lymphocyte activation markers, including CD30 and CD25 antigens,
HLA-DR and transferrin receptors (see Plate 17.41). The staining for CD45 antigen is either weak or completely negative,
while more specific markers of cell lineage may be either negative or very weak. Most cases have a T-cell phenotype, while a
significant number have a null-cell marker profile. Even the T-
cell cases will rarely express a full complement of pan-T-cell
antigens. In the author's experience, CD2 serves as a better
marker than CD3, as the latter is frequently lost. Other antibodies that may decorate these cells include antiepithelial
membrane antigen and antibodies to low-molecular-weight
cytokeratins [95]. In those cases with a t(2;5), there is expression of the p80 NPM-ALK fusion protein in the tumour cells
[96].

Differential diagnosis

The early stages of nodal infiltration mimic metastatic anaplastic carcinoma or malignant melanoma. More troublesome is
metastatic epithelioid embryonal carcinoma, which will lack
CD45 antigen, and stain for both cytokeratin and CD30
antigen [97]. A wide panel of antibodies should be used in
young men for this reason. The peculiar cytological variants
may simply be missed, unless the pathologist is aware of their
existence. Lastly the distinction in primary cutaneous disease
from lymphomatoid papulosis is not always easy and requires
good communication between the dermatologist and pathologist concerned to arrive at a suitable diagnosis [94].

References

1 Dorfman R.F. (1974) Classification of non-Hodgkin's lymphomas.
   Lancet, **i**, 1295–1296.
2 Gérard-Marchant R., Hamlin I., Lennert K. *et al.* (1974)
   Classification of non-Hodgkin's lymphomas. *Lancet*, **ii**, 406–
   408.
3 Bennett M.H., Farrer-Brown G., Henry K. & Jelliffe A.M. (1974)
   Classification of non-Hodgkin's lymphomas. *Lancet*, **ii**, 405–
   406.
4 Lukes R.J. & Collins R.D. (1974) A functional approach to the
   classification of malignant lymphoma. *Recent Results in Cancer
   Research*, **46**, 18–30.
5 Kay H.E.M. (1974) Classification of non-Hodgkin's lymphomas.
   Lancet, **ii**, 586.
6 Higby D.J. (1976) A practical classification of lymphomas. *American Journal of Medicine*, **295**, 1458.
7 Rappaport H. (1966) *Tumors of the Hematopoietic System. Atlas of
   Tumor Pathology, Section III, Fascicle 8*. US Armed Forces Institute of
   Pathology, Washington.
8 Anonymous (1982) National Cancer Institute sponsored study of
   classifications of non-Hodgkin's lymphomas: summary and
   description of a working formulation for clinical usage. The non-

Hodgkin's Lymphoma Pathologic Classification Project. *Cancer*, **49**,
   2112–2135.
9 Nathwani B.N. & Winberg C.D. (1983) Non-Hodgkin's lymphomas: an appraisal of the 'Working Formulation' of non-
   Hodgkin's lymphomas for clinical usage. In: *Malignant Lymphomas:
   a Pathology Annual Monograph* (eds S.C. Sommers & P.P. Rosen), pp.
   1–64. Appleton-Century-Crofts, Connecticut.
10 Suchi T., Lennert K., Tu L-Y. *et al.* (1987) Histopathology and
   immunohistochemistry of peripheral T cell lymphomas: a proposal
   for their classification. *Journal of Clinical Pathology*, **40**, 995–1015.
11 Hui P.K., Feller A.C. & Lennert K. (1988) High-grade non-
   Hodgkin's lymphomas of B-cell type. I. Histopathology. *Histopathology*, **12**, 127–143.
12 Stansfeld A.G., Diebold J., Kapanci Y. *et al.* (1988) Updated Kiel
   classification for lymphomas. *Lancet*, **i**, 292–293, addendum 603.
13 Henry K. (1992) Neoplastic disorders of lymphoreticular tissue. In:
   Systemic Pathology, vol. 7, 3rd edn. *Thymus, Lymph Nodes, Spleen and
   Lymphatics* (eds K. Henry & W. St C. Symmers), pp. 611–690.
   Churchill Livingstone, Edinburgh.
14 Harris N.L., Jaffe E.S., Stein H. *et al.* (1994) A Revised European–
   American classification of lymphoid neoplasms: a proposal from
   the International Lymphoma Study Group. *Blood*, **84**, 1361–1392.
15 Armitage J.O. (1996) Application of the International Lymphoma
   Study Group classification of non-Hodgkin's lymphoma: clinical
   characteristics and outcome of 1400 patients from 8 countries.
   Annals of Oncology, **7**(Suppl. 3), 2.
16 Shi S-R., Key M.E. & Kalra K.L. (1991) Antigen retrieval in formalin-fixed, paraffin-embedded tissues: an enhancement method
   for immunohistochemical staining based on microwave oven
   heating of tissue section. *Journal of Histochemistry Cytochemistry*, **39**,
   741–748.
17 Norton A.J., Jordan S. & Yeomans P. (1994) Brief, high-
   temperature heat denaturation (pressure cooking). A simple and
   effective method of antigen retrieval for routinely processed
   tissues. *Journal of Pathology*, **173**, 371–379.
18 Merz H., Malisius R., Mannweiler S. *et al.* (1995) Immunomax: a
   maximized immunohistochemical method for the retrieval and
   enhancement of hidden antigens. *Laboratory Investigation*, **73**,
   149–156.
19 Mason D., Cordell J., Tse A. *et al.* (1991) The IgM-associated
   protein mb-1 as a marker of normal and neoplastic B-cells. *Journal
   of Immunology*, **147**, 2474–2482.
20 Norton A.J. & Isaacson P.G. (1987) Detailed phenotypic analysis of
   B-cell lymphoma using a panel of antibodies reactive in routinely
   fixed wax embedded tissue. *American Journal of Pathology*, **128**,
   225–240.
21 Hanson C.A., Ross C.W. & Schnitzer B. (1992) Anti-CD34
   immunoperoxidase staining in paraffin sections of acute leukemia:
   comparison with flow cytometric immunophenotyping. *Human
   Pathology*, **23**, 26–32.
22 Ellison D.J., Nathwani B.N., Cho S.Y. & Martin S.E. (1989) Interfollicular lymphocytic lymphoma: the diagnostic significance of
   pseudofollicles. *Human Pathology*, **20**, 1108–1118.
23 Berger F., Felman P., Sonet A. *et al.* (1994) Nonfollicular small B-
   cell lymphomas: a heterogeneous group of patients with distinct
   clinical features and outcome. *Blood*, **10**, 2829–2835.
24 Brecher M. & Banks P.M. (1990) Hodgkin's disease variant of
   Richter's syndrome. Report of eight cases. *American Journal of Clinical Pathology*, **93**, 333–339.
25 Khan G., Norton A.J. & Slavin G. (1993) Epstein–Barr virus in

Reed–Sternberg-like cells in non-Hodgkin's lymphomas. *Journal of Pathology*, **169**, 9–14.

26 Schmid C. & Isaacson P.G. (1994) Proliferation centres in B-cell malignant lymphoma, lymphocytic (B-CLL): an immunophenotypic study. *Histopathology*, **24**, 445–451.

27 Matolcsy A., Inghirami G. & Knowles D.M. (1994) Molecular genetic demonstration of the diverse evolution of Richter's syndrome (chronic lymphocytic leukemia and subsequent large cell lymphoma). *Blood*, **83**, 1363–1372.

28 Banks P.M., Chan J., Cleary M.L. *et al.* (1992) Mantle cell lymphoma. A proposal for unification of morphologic, immunologic, and molecular data. *American Journal of Surgical Pathology*, **16**, 637–640.

29 Lennert K. (1990) Centrocytic lymphoma (mantle cell lymphoma). In: *Histopathology of Non-Hodgkin's Lymphomas (Based on the Updated Kiel Classification)* (eds K. Lennert & A.C. Feller), pp. 93–102. Springer-Verlag, Berlin.

30 Lardelli P., Bookman M.A., Sundeen J., Longo D.L. & Jaffe E.S. (1990) Lymphocytic lymphoma of intermediate differentiation. Morphologic and immunophenotypic spectrum and clinical correlation. *American Journal of Surgical Pathology*, **14**, 752–763.

31 Duggan M.J., Weisenburger D.D., Ye Y.L. *et al.* (1990) Mantle zone lymphoma. A clinicopathologic study of 22 cases. *Cancer*, **66**, 522–529.

32 Norton A.J., Matthews J., Pappa V. *et al.* (1995) Mantle cell lymphoma: natural history defined in a serially biopsied population over a 20-year period. *Annals of Oncology*, **6**, 249–256.

33 Isaacson P.G., MacLennan K.A. & Subbuswamy S.G. (1984) Multiple lymphomatous polyposis of the gastrointestinal tract. *Histopathology*, **8**, 641–656.

34 Zucca E., Stein H., Coiffier B. On behalf of the European Lymphoma Task Force. European Lymphoma Task Force (ELTF) (1994) Report of the workshop on Mantle Cell Lymphoma (MCL). *Annals of Oncology*, **5**, 507–511.

35 Yang W-I., Zukerberg L.R. Motokura T., Arnold A. & Harris N.L. (1994) Cyclin D1 (*Bcl-1*, PRAD1) protein expression in low-grade B-cell lymphomas and reactive hyperplasia. *American Journal of Pathology*, **145**, 86–96.

36 Williams M.E., Swerdlow S.H. & Meeker T.C. (1993) Chromosome t(11;14)(q13;q32) breakpoints in centrocytic lymphoma are highly localized at the bcl-1 major translocation cluster. *Leukemia*, **7**, 1437–1440.

37 Mann R.B. & Berard C.W. (1983) Criteria for the cytologic subclassification of follicular lymphomas: a proposed alternative method. *Hematological Oncology*, **1**, 187–192.

38 Brito-Babapulle V., Crawford A., Khokar T. *et al.* (1991) Translocation t(14;18) and t(8;14) with rearranged bcl-2 and c-myc in a case presenting as B-ALL (L3). *Leukemia*, **5**, 83–87.

39 Pezzella F., Tse A.G.D., Cordell J.L. *et al.* (1990) Expression of the *bcl*-2 oncogene protein is not specific for the 14;18 chromosomal translocation. *American Journal of Pathology*, **137**, 225–232.

40 Sheibani K., Burke J.S., Swartz W.G. *et al.* (1988) Monocytoid B-cell lymphoma: clinicopathologic study of 21 cases of a unique type of low-grade lymphoma. *Cancer*, **62**, 1531–1538.

41 Ngan B.Y., Warnke R.A., Wilson M. *et al.* (1991) Monocytoid B-cell lymphoma. A study of 36 cases. *Human Pathology*, **22**, 409–421.

42 Ortiz-Hidalgo C. & Wright D.H. (1992) The morphological spectrum of monocytoid B-cell lymphoma and its relationship to lymphomas of mucosa-associated lymphoid tissue. *Histopathology*, **21**, 555–561.

43 Nizze H., Cogliatti S.B., Von Schilling C. *et al.* (1991) Monocytoid B-cell lymphoma: morphological variants and relationship to low-grade B-cell lymphoma of the mucosa-associated lymphoid tissue. *Histopathology*, **18**, 403–414.

44 Isaacson P. & Wright D.H. (1984) Extranodal malignant lymphoma arising from mucosa-associated lymphoid tissue. *Cancer*, **53**, 2515–2524.

45 Isaacson P.G. & Spencer J. (1989) Malignant lymphoma of mucosa associated lymphoid tissue. *Histopathology*, **11**, 445–462.

46 Spencer J., Finn T. & Isaacson P.G. (1986) Human Peyer's patches: an immunohistochemical study. *Gut*, **27**, 405–410.

47 Isaacson P.G., Wotherspoon A.C., Diss T. & Pan L. (1991) Follicular colonization in B-cell lymphoma of mocosa-associated lymphoid tissue. *American Journal of Surgical Pathology*, **15**, 819–828.

48 MacLennan I.C.M., Liu Y.J., Oldfield S. *et al.* (1990) The evolution of B-cell clones. *Current Topics in Microbiology and Immunology*, **159**, 37–63.

49 Galian A., Lecestre M.J., Scotto J. *et al.* (1977) Pathological study of alpha-chain disease, with special emphasis on evolution. *Cancer*, **39**, 2081–2101.

50 Chan J.K.C., Ng C.S. & Isaacson P.G. (1990) Relationship between high-grade lymphoma and low-grade B-cell mucosa-associated lymphoid tissue lymphoma (MALToma) of the stomach. *American Journal of Pathology*, **136**, 1153–1164.

51 Ferry J.A., Young W.I., Zukerberg L.R. *et al.* (1996) CD5+ extranodal marginal zone B-cell (MALT) lymphoma. A low grade neoplasm with a propensity for bone marrow involvement and relapse. *American Journal of Clinical Pathology*, **105**, 31–37.

52 Wotherspoon A.C., Finn T.M. & Isaacson P.G. (1995) Trisomy 3 in low-grade B-cell lymphomas of mucosa-associated lymphoid tissue. *Blood*, **85**, 2000–2004.

53 Slovak M.L., Weiss L.M., Nathwani B.N. *et al.* (1993) Cytogenetic studies of composite lymphomas: monocytoid B-cell lymphoma and other B-cell non-Hodgkin's lymphomas. *Human Pathology*, **24**, 1086–1094.

54 Rubin A. & Isaacson P.G. (1990) Florid reactive lymphoid hyperplasia of the terminal ileum in adults: a condition bearing a close resemblance to low-grade malignant lymphoma. *Histopathology*, **17**, 19–26.

55 Spriano P., Barosi G., Invernizzi R. *et al.* (1986) Splenomegalic immunocytoma with circulating hairy cells. Report of eight cases and revision of the literature. *Haematologica*, **71**, 25–33.

56 Narang S., Wolf B.C. & Neiman R.S. (1985) Malignant lymphoma presenting with prominent splenomegaly. A clinicopathologic study with special reference to intermediate cell lymphoma. *Cancer*, **55**, 1948–1957.

57 Melo J.V., Hegde U., Parreira A., Thompson I., Lampert I.A. & Catovsky D. (1987) Splenic lymphoma with circulating villous lymphocytes: differential diagnosis of B cell leukaemias with large spleens. *Journal of Clinical Pathology*, **40**, 642–651.

58 Schmid C., Kirkham N., Diss T. & Isaacson P.G. (1992) Splenic marginal zone lymphoma. *American Journal of Surgical Pathology*, **6**, 455–466.

59 Isaacson P.G., Matutes E., Burke M. & Catovsky D. (1994) The histopathology of splenic lymphoma with villous lymphocytes. *Blood*, **84**, 3828–3834.

60 Matutes E., Morilla R., Owusu-Ankomah K., Houlihan A. & Catovsky D. (1994) The immunophenotype of splenic lymphoma

with villous lymphocytes and its relevance to the differential diagnosis with other B-cell disorders. *Blood*, **83**, 1558–1562.

61 Jadayel D., Matutes E., Dyer M.J. *et al.* (1994) Splenic lymphoma with villous lymphocytes: analysis of BCL-1 rearrangements and expression of the cyclin D1 gene. *Blood*, **83**, 3664–3671.

62 Wotherspoon A.C., Norton A.J. & Isaacson P.G. (1989) Immunoreactive cytokeratins in plasmacytomas. *Histopathology*, **14**, 141–150.

63 Ramsay A.D., Smith W.J. & Isaacson P.G. (1988) T-cell-rich B-cell lymphoma. *American Journal of Surgical Pathology*, **12**, 433–443.

64 Delabie J., Vandenberghe E., Kennes C. *et al.* (1992) Histiocyte-rich B-cell lymphoma. A distinct clinicopathologic entity possibly related to lymphocyte predominant Hodgkin's disease, paragranuloma subtype. *American Journal of Surgical Pathology*, **16**, 37–48.

65 Addis B.J. & Isaacson P.G. (1986) Large cell lymphoma of the mediastinum: a B-cell tumour of probable thymic origin. *Histopathology*, **10**, 379–390.

66 Menestrina F., Chilosi M., Bonetti F. *et al.* (1986) Mediastinal large-cell lymphoma of B-type, with sclerosis: histopathological and immunohistochemical study of eight cases. *Histopathology*, **10**, 589–600.

67 Möller P., Moldenhauer G., Momburg F. *et al.* (1987) Mediastinal lymphoma of clear cell type is a tumor corresponding to terminal steps of B cell differentiation. *Blood*, **69**, 1087–1095.

68 Beal M.F. & Fisher M.C. (1982) Neoplastic angioendotheliosis. *Neurological Science*, **53**, 359–375.

69 Chilosi M., Castelli P., Martiguoni G. *et al.* (1992) Neoplastic epithelial cells in a subset of human thymomas express the B-cell associated CD20 antigen. *American Journal of Surgical Pathology*, **16**, 988–995.

70 Berard C.W., O'Conor G.T., Thomas L.B. & Torloni H. (1969) Histopathological definition of Burkitt's tumour. *Bulletin of the World Health Organization*, **40**, 601–607.

71 Rowe M., Rooney C.M., Rickinson A.B. *et al.* (1985) Distinctions between endemic and sporadic forms of Epstein–Barr virus-positive Burkitt's lymphoma. *International Journal of Cancer*, **35**, 435–441.

72 Rowe D.T., Rowe M., Evans G.I. *et al.* (1986) Restricted expression of EBV latent genes and T-lymphocyte-detected membrane antigen in Burkitt's lymphoma cells. *EMBO Journal*, **5**, 2599–2607.

73 McDaniel H.L., MacPherson B.R., Tindle B.H. & Lunde J.H. (1992) Lymphoproliferative disorder of granular lymphocytes. A heterogeneous disease. *Archives of Pathology and Laboratory Medicine*, **116**, 242–248.

74 Matutes E., Brito-Babapulle V., Swansbury J. *et al.* (1991) Clinical and laboratory features of 78 cases of T-prolymphocytic leukemia. *Blood*, **78**, 3269–3274.

75 Mallett R.B., Matutes E., Catovsky D. *et al.* (1995) Cutaneous infiltration in T-cell prolymphocytic leukaemia. *British Journal of Dermatology*, **132**, 263–266.

76 Leung C.Y., Ho F.C., Srivastava G. *et al.* (1993) Usefulness of follicular dendritic cell pattern in classification of peripheral T-cell lymphomas. *Histopathology*, **23**, 433–437.

77 Abruzzo L.V., Schmidt K., Weiss L.M. *et al.* (1993) B-cell lymphoma after angioimmunoblastic lymphadenopathy: a case with oligoclonal gene rearrangement associated with Epstein–Barr virus. *Blood*, **82**, 241–246.

78 Anagnostopoulos I., Hummel M., Finn T. *et al.* (1992) Heterogeneous Epstein–Barr virus infection patterns in peripheral T-cell lymphoma of angioimmunoblastic lymphadenopathy type. *Blood*, **80**, 1804–1812.

79 Hastrup N., Hamilton-Dutoit S., Ralfkiaer E. & Pallesen G. (1991) Peripheral T-cell lymphomas: an evaluation of reproducibility of the updated Kiel classification. *Histopathology*, **18**, 99–106.

80 Knowles D.M. (1989) Immunophenotypic and antigen receptor gene rearrangement analysis in T cell neoplasia. *American Journal of Pathology*, **134**, 761–785.

81 Suchi T., Tajima K., Nanba K. *et al.* (1979) Some problems on the histo-pathological diagnosis of non-Hodgkin's malignant lymphoma. A proposal of a new type. *Acta Pathologica Japonica*, **29**, 755–756.

82 Detmar M., Pauli G., Anagnostopoulos I. *et al.* (1991) A case of classical mycosis fungoides associated with human T-cell lymphotropic virus type I. *British Journal of Dermatology*, **124**, 198–202.

83 Shoichi D., Nasu K., Arita Y. *et al.* (1989) Immunohistochemical analysis of peripheral T-cell lymphoma in Japanese patients. *American Journal of Clinical Pathology*, **91**, 152–158.

84 Domizio P., Owen R.A., Shepherd N.A. *et al.* (1993) Primary lymphoma of the small intestine: a clinicopathological study of 119 cases. *American Journal of Surgical Pathology*, **17**, 429–432.

85 Swinson C.M., Slavin G., Coles E.C. & Booth C.C. (1983) Coeliac disease and malignancy. *Lancet*, **i**, 111–115.

86 de Bruin P.C., Kummer J.A., van der Valk P. *et al.* (1994) Granzyme B-expressing peripheral T-cell lymphomas: neoplastic equivalents of activated cytotoxic T cells with a preference for mucosa-associated lymphoid tissue location. *Blood*, **84**, 3785–3791.

87 Spencer J., Cerf-Bensussan N., Jarry A. *et al.* (1988) Enteropathy associated T cell lymphoma (malignant histiocytosis of the intestine) is recognized by a monoclonal antibody (HML-1) that defines a membrane molecule on human mucosal lymphocytes. *American Journal of Pathology*, **132**, 1–5.

88 Lipford E.H., Margolick J.B., Longo D.L., Fauci A.S. & Jaffe E.S. (1988) Angiocentric immunoproliferative lesions: a clinicopathologic spectrum of post-thymic T-cell proliferations. *Blood*, **72**, 1674–1681.

89 Kanavaros P., Lescs M-C., Briere J. *et al.* (1993) Nasal T-cell lymphoma: a clinicopathologic entity associated with peculiar phenotype and Epstein–Barr virus. *Blood*, **81**, 2688–2695.

90 Guinee D. Jr, Jaffe E., Kingma D. *et al.* (1994) Pulmonary lymphomatoid granulomatosis. Evidence for a proliferation of Epstein–Barr virus infected B-lymphocytes with a prominent T-cell component and vasculitis. *American Journal of Surgical Pathology*, **18**, 753–764.

91 Chan J.K.C., Ng C.S., Hui P.K. *et al.* (1989) Anaplastic large cell Ki-1 lymphoma. Delineation of two morphological types. *Histopathology*, **15**, 11–34.

92 Chan J.K.C., Buchanan R. & Fletcher C.D. (1990) Sarcomatoid variant of anaplastic large-cell Ki-1 lymphoma. *American Journal of Surgical Pathology*, **14**, 983–988.

93 Pileri S., Falini B., Delsol G. *et al.* (1990) Lymphohistiocytic T-cell lymphoma (anaplastic large cell lymphoma CD30+/Ki-1+ with a high content of reactive histiocytes). *Histopathology*, **16**, 383–391.

94 Willemze R. & Beljaards R.C. (1993) Spectrum of primary cutaneous CD30 (Ki-1)-positive lymphoproliferative disorders. A proposal for classification and guidelines for management and treatment. *Journal of the American Academy of Dermatology*, **28**, 973–980.

95 Gustmann C., Altmannsberger M., Osborn M., Griesser H. & Feller A.C. (1991) Cytokeratin expression and vimentin content in large cell anaplastic lymphomas and other non-Hodgkin's lymphomas. *American Journal of Pathology*, **138**, 1413–1422.

96 Herbst H., Anagnostopoulos J., Heinze B. *et al.* (1995) ALK gene products in anaplastic large cell lymphomas and Hodgkin's disease. *Blood*, **86**, 1694–1700.

97 Pallesen G. & Hamilton-Dutoit S.J. (1988) Ki-1 (CD30) antigen is regularly expressed by tumor cells of embryonal carcinoma. *American Journal of Pathology*, **133**, 446–450.

18   Non-Hodgkin's Lymphoma: Low Grade

S.A.N. Johnson

Introduction

Consistent allocation of an individual patient with lymphoma to a clearly defined diagnostic group has been a longstanding problem which has hindered the interpretation of reports of treatment studies for many years and deprived clinicians of the opportunity to learn how to treat distinct diseases. As the number of active drugs and other forms of treatment for lymphoma increase, it is becoming more important to define particular diseases accurately so that the optimal therapy can be selected for individual patients.

Classification and staging systems

The number of classification systems for lymphomas which have been proposed bears witness to the difficulties involved and those systems derived almost entirely from the morphological appearances of lymph-node biopsy material, such as the Rappaport Classification [1], were replaced in the 1970s by approaches such as the Kiel [2] and Lukes–Collins [3] classifications, which attempted to incorporate newly emerging knowledge of the biology of lymphomas derived from immunological methods. In an attempt to mould together some of the features of the new systems and produce a widely acceptable compromise, the National Cancer Institute (NCI) in the USA sponsored a study of the classification of lymphomas from which emerged a 'Working Formulation' which could be related to diagnoses derived from the other classifications [4] and could also be utilized to determine the long-term prognosis of patients [5]. This achieved wide acceptance and was a useful contribution to the interpretation of clinical publications, despite the fact that it continued to ignore the contribution of immunological data to the final diagnosis [6]. The Working Formulation recognized three broad divisions of clinical aggressiveness categorizing lymphomas as low, intermediate or high grade, on the basis of a histological estimate of malignancy which was not always reflected by the biological behaviour of the diseases described. This classification has also been criticized for grouping together, into a single category, several discrete subtypes of lymphoma [7]. For example, category E, diffuse small cleaved cell lymphoma, encompasses at least three types of lymphoma: (i) rare diffuse counterparts of follicle centre cell-derived lymphomas; (ii) mantle cell lymphomas; (iii) a subset of T-cell lymphomas. The anticipated response to therapy and clinical outcome of these lymphomas is far from uniform. The latest serious attempt to bring some order to the chaos of lymphoma classification emerged from the June 1993 Meeting of the International Study Group in Berlin. This meeting produced a stated intention of using all available diagnostic techniques to identify those diseases which can be recognized and create a lymphoma classification which is simply a list of well-defined, 'real' disease entities [8]. The proposers of this system have expressed the hope that the use of immunophenotyping may improve the poor reproducibility of previous systems which were based on morphological criteria alone [9]. As applied to the low-grade lymphomas, this approach, which is now known as the REAL Classification, is shown in Table 18.1 and is listed together with the equivalent diagnostic categories from the Kiel Classification and the Working Formulation.

Once a firm diagnostic label has been attached to an individual patient with lymphoma, the selection of appropriate therapy is determined by the extent of the disease and an assessment of the prognosis based on the likelihood of response to treatment and the risk of recurrence. Staging of the anatomical distribution of lymphoma using the Ann Arbor System is well established [10] and, despite the fact that this approach was originally intended for patients with Hodgkin's disease (HD), it has been widely applied to the non-Hodgkin's lymphomas (NHLs). While identification of patients with localized disease is important, the majority of patients with NHLs have widespread involvement of lymph nodes and extranodal spread is common. The concept that all patients with a comparable histology and stage would not have the same outcome has led to a search for clinically relevant prognostic factors, and a very large multicentre project has sought

Table 18.1 Equivalent diagnostic categories for low-grade NHL from the Revised European–American Lymphoma (REAL) Classification, the Kiel Classification and the Working Formulation. (Adapted from Harris *et al.*, 1994 [8], with permission.)

Kiel Classification	REAL Classification	Working Formulation
Low-grade NHL B cell B-lymphocytic, CLL B-lymphocytic, prolymphocytic leukaemia Lymphoplasmacytoid immunocytoma	B-cell chronic lymphocytic leukaemia/prolymphocytic leukaemia/small lymphocytic lymphoma	Small lymphocytic, consistent with CLL Small lymphocytic, plasmacytoid
Lymphoplasmacytic immunocytoma	Lymphoplasmacytoid lymphoma	Small lymphocytic, plasmacytoid Diffuse mixed small and large cell
Centrocytic Centroblastic, centrocytoid subtype	Mantle cell lymphoma	Small lymphocytic Diffuse small cleaved cell Follicular, small cleaved cell Diffuse, mixed small and large cell Diffuse, large cleaved cell

Centroblastic–centrocytic, follicular
 	
Centroblastic, follicular
	Follicular centre lymphoma, follicular
	   Grade I
	   Grade II
	   Grade III
		Follicular, predominantly small cleaved cell
		Follicular mixed small and large cell
		Follicular, predominantly large cell

Centroblastic–centrocytic, diffuse	Follicular centre lymphoma, diffuse, small cell (provisional)	Diffuse, small cleaved cell Diffuse, mixed small and large cell
	Extranodal marginal zone B-cell lymphoma (low grade B-cell lymphoma of MALT type)	Small lymphocytic Diffuse small cleaved cell Diffuse mixed small and large cell
Monocytoid, including marginal zone immunocytoma	Nodal marginal zone B-cell lymphoma (provisional)	Small lymphocytic Diffuse, small cleaved cell Diffuse, mixed small and large cell Unclassifiable
Low-grade NHL T cell Small cell cerebriform (mycosis fungoides, Sezary syndrome)	Mycosis fungiodes/Sézary's syndrome	Mycosis fungoides
T-zone Lymphoepithelioid Pleomorphic, small T-cell Pleomorphic, medium-size and large T-cell	Peripheral T-cell lymphomas, unspecified (including provisional subtype; subcutaneous panniculitic T-cell lymphoma)	Diffuse, small cleaved cell Diffuse, mixed small and large cell Diffuse, large cell Large cell immunoblastic

to identify these for patients with high-grade NHL [11]. This index is based on a series of factors—age, performance status, stage, extranodal involvement and serum lactic acid dehydrogenase (LDH) levels, and it is now also beginning to be tested in patients with low-grade NHL [12].

It would seem likely that the era of broad generalizations concerning the 'low-grade lymphomas' has passed. Because of the pattern of continuous relapse with eventual death, which is a feature of many 'low-grade' lymphomas, the survival at 10 years or more from diagnosis in these disorders (particularly follicle centre cell-derived lymphomas) is inferior to that in so-called high-grade NHL [13]. A greater understanding of the molecular biology of the malignant lymphomas is beginning to cast light on the reasons for this anomaly of long-term prognosis and, importantly, it is doing so by identifying distinct forms

of disease which have a defined clinical course and predictable behaviour in response to therapy.

Low-grade non-Hodgkin's lymphoma B-cell types

B-cell chronic lymphocytic leukaemia/prolymphocytic leukaemia/small lymphocytic lymphoma

The characteristic small lymphocyte, which is the cell associated with B-cell chronic lymphocytic leukaemia (B-CLL), also replaces the lymph nodes in that condition, often in association with larger lymphoid cells which produce a pseudofollicular pattern. Most patients whose nodes contain this cellular population will also show evidence of marrow involvement and circulating cells [14], although a small proportion may have disease which remains confined to lymph nodes. Using earlier classifications, this description was applied to at least three other distinct entities — mantle cell lymphoma, centroblastic centrocytic lymphoma and lymphomas of mucosa-associated lymphoid tissue/monocytoid B-cell lymphoma [15]. However, the characteristic immunophenotype of B-CLL cells, which express low amounts of surface membrane immunoglobulin, B-cell associated antigens such as CD19, and CD20 and also express unusual antigens such as CD5 and CD23, enables a clear distinction to be made from the other conditions; this is important in the assessment of outcome and prognosis [16]. If correctly identified, these patients have the features of B-CLL, although the cells presumably do not appear in the circulation because of variation in the pattern of surface adhesion molecules, and their clinical course is described elsewhere in this text (see Chapter 6).

Lymphoplasmacytoid lymphoma/immunocytoma

The cells associated with this disorder are plasmacytoid lymphocytes with abundant basophilic cytoplasm, but lymphocyte-like nuclei which often have an interfollicular growth pattern in the lymph node. Phenotypically the cells have surface and cytoplasmic immunoglobulin, usually of IgM type, and a derived serum paraprotein is also frequently found (Waldenström's macroglobulinemia); they express B-cell associated antigens such as CD19, CD20 and CD22, but they lack CD5 or CD10 [17]. Immunoglobulin heavy and light chains are re-arranged and, in a small number of patients, an associated translocation t(9;14)(p13;q32) has been reported [18]. The age distribution of patients in an elderly population similar to that for B-CLL and disease is generally found in bone marrow, lymph nodes and spleen, with other extranodal sites being less frequently involved. Although the clinical course of the disease is indolent, it may be complicated by hyperviscosity secondary to the IgM paraprotein, requiring plasmapheresis to relieve symptoms [19] or for long-term management [20]. The mainstay of therapy in the past has been low-dose oral alkylating agents such as chlorambucil [21], however, the response to treatment is frequently disappointing and marrow failure may be worsened with treatment. Reports of good responses to therapy with purine analogues bring the hope that fludarabine [22] and, particularly, cladribine may significantly improve the prognosis for patients with this disease, both at presentation [23] and after failure of other forms of treatment [24].

Mantle cell lymphoma

The malignant clone associated with this disease usually consists of small- to medium-size lymphocytes with little cytoplasm and inconspicuous nucleoli, but some irregularity or cleaving of the nuclear outline [15]; an uncommon subset of cases have larger nuclei and a higher mitotic index and can be

identified as a 'lymphoblastoid' variant [25]. Histologically, the pattern of mantle cell lymphoma (MCL) is usually diffuse, with the tumour involving the mantle zones of some reactive follicles. The phenotype of the cells is SIgM+, CD5+, CD10−, CD23−, with CD5 positivity helping to distinguish MCL from follicle centre cell lymphomas [26] and CD23 negativity making a distinction from B-CLL [27]. A chromosomal translocation t(11;14)(q13;q32), which had previously been reported as being associated with a variety of low-grade lymphoid neoplasms, has been identified in the majority of cases of MCL [28]; it seems likely that other diagnostic groups do not demonstrate this anomaly which appears to underlie the biology of MCL. The consequence of t(11;14) is to join the BCL1 gene complex on chromosome 11 to the Ig heavy-chain gene joining region (J_H) on chromosome 14 (Fig. 18.1). This results in the overexpression of a gene, PRAD1 (now known as CCND1), which encodes for cyclin D1, a protein that is not normally expressed in lymphoid cells, and which, if deregulated, may perpetuate the G_1–S transition of the cell cycle [29]. Overexpression of CCND1/PRAD1 is consistently found in MCL, even when the BCL1 rearrangement cannot be demonstrated with techniques utilizing in situ hybridization to cyclin D1 mRNA [30] and immunohistochemical staining [31] both applicable to formalin-fixed paraffin-embedded tissue.

The clinical characteristics of patients with MCL show a male preponderance of between 2:1 and 4:1 and a median age at presentation in the early sixties. Most patients present with generalized disease, so widespread lymphadenopathy, hepatomegaly and splenomegaly are commonly associated with involvement of bone marrow (>75% of patients), blood (>30%) and the gastrointestinal tract as lymphomatous papulosis (>25%) [32]. The incidence of MCL is approximately 5% of all NHLs, with slightly lower figures reported from the USA and higher proportions in Europe [16].

Retrospective analysis of patients has been made simpler by the publication of minimum diagnostic criteria for the purposes of clinical trials [33], which particularly emphasize cytology, histological growth patterns, immunophenotype and molecular markers of the disease, and make it clear that it would be unwise to assume that previous reports of treatment trials apply to a biologically homogeneous population of patients [34].

Regardless of the initial clinical presentation, and apparently equally unrelated to the nature of the treatment given, these patients show a pattern of progression with periods of partial control by treatment but eventual death from disease. The median overall survival is approximately 3 years and conventional prognostic factors (greater age, worse performance status, disseminated disease, high lactate dehydrogenase (LDH) and low albumen) are all associated with a poorer survival rate [35]. The histological growth pattern has been reported to influence survival, with patients whose nodes show the presence of 40 or more large lymphoid cells per 10 high-power fields in the mantle zones having a median

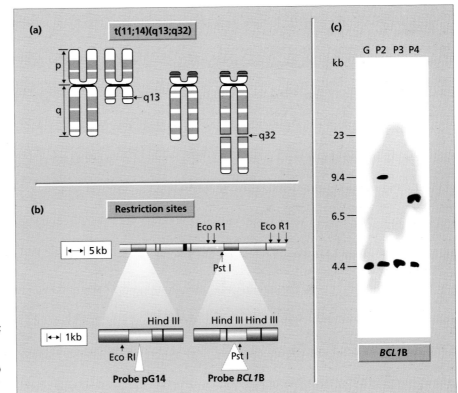

Fig. 18.1 (a) Diagram of t(11;14)(q13;q23). (b) Restriction map of part of the *BCL1* locus at 11q13 showing the location of the *BCL1B* and pG14 probe and restriction endonuclease sites. (c) Southern blot of Pst I-digested DNA hybridized to the *BCL1*B probe. G = placental DNA (germline configuration); P2 and P4 = patient samples showing rearrangement of the major translocation cluster (MTC) of the *BCL1* locus; P3 = patient sample in which rearrangement of the MTC is not detected. (From *Journal of Pathology*, Vandenberghe *et al.*, 1991 [28], © 1991. Reprinted by permission of John Wiley & Sons, Ltd.)

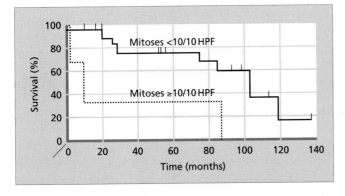

Fig. 18.2 Survival of patients according to the mitotic rate in the mantle zones. (From Duggan *et al.*, 1990 [36].) HPF = high power field.

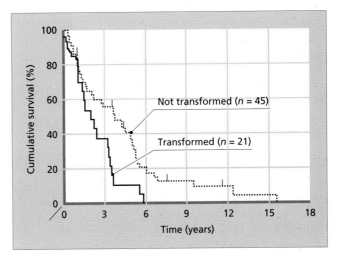

Fig. 18.3 Overall survival of patients with histologically documented blastoid transformation vs those with no evidence of transformation. (From Norton *et al.*, 1995 [39]. Reprinted by permission of Kluwer Academic Publishers.) X: = 5.16; P = 0.02.

survival of 25 months, compared to 103 months (P = 0.04) for those with less (Fig. 18.2) [36]. The series from which this data was drawn included a higher proportion of patients with lower-stage disease than in other comparable studies, which have not achieved any differentiation based on a broad histological division [37]. In a population-based study, those patients with nodal tissue expressing the proliferation marker Ki 67 in more than 10% of the cells pursued a more aggressive course [38]. By contrast, a large sequentially biopsied population of patients from a single centre has emphasized that blastoid change occurs during the clinical course in one-third of

patients and carries a distinct survival disadvantage (Fig. 18.3) [39]. There is also evidence that abnormalities of *p53* expression, involving TP53 mutations which result in an immunohistochemically detectable gene product, may result in a worse prognosis [40].

Guidance on the therapeutic options available for patients

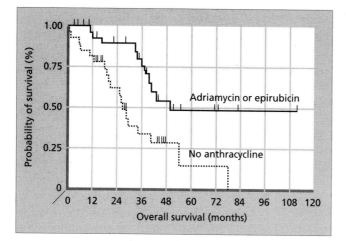

Fig. 18.4 Overall survival of 65 patients with MCL grouped according to the type of chemotherapy given (anthracycline vs no anthracycline). Log rank test: $P = 0.003$. (From Zucca *et al.*, 1995 [42]. Reprinted by permission of Kluwer Academic Publishers.)

with MCL is limited by the shortcomings of the diagnostic criteria applied to entry into older clinical studies. Retrospective analyses include small numbers of patients treated with chlorambucil, COP (cyclophosphamide, vincristine and prednisolone), CHOP (COP + doxorubicin) or more complex combinations, and the results are sufficiently fragmentary to make interpretation difficult. A prospective German study, which accrued 91 patients with centrocytic lymphoma defined by the Kiel Classification, must have contained a high proportion of patients who would now have been diagnosed as having MCL [41]. This trial eventually randomized 63 patients between COP and CHOP, but found no difference in the response rate, relapse-free survival or overall survival between the two groups. Another retrospective analysis again derived data from a population of patients with centrocytic lymphoma, but in this case the patients were morphologically reviewed to confirm the appearances of MCL but not further defined by immunophenotypic or molecular criteria [42]. There was an apparent advantage for patients treated with an anthracycline-containing regimen who had a higher complete response rate (68 vs 25%, $P = 0.0001$) and a longer survival (Fig. 18.4).

The poor results of treatment for this condition make clear recommendations for management difficult to establish. Acknowledging that most treatment modalities are only going to be given with palliative intent, it is appropriate to offer radiotherapy to patients with apparently localized disease and for older patients with disseminated disease to wait until treatment is essential because of disease progression. Initial therapy with single-agent chlorambucil or COP is unlikely to achieve worthwhile responses (complete remission (CR) + good partial remission) in more than half of the patients treated and the median duration of first remission is likely to be under 1 year. The treatment of subsequent recurrences may involve other

cytotoxic agents, and the purine analogues, such as fludarabine [43] or cladribine [44], may contribute to obtaining further responses, although it seems unlikely that these will show as much activity as they have in the management of follicle centre lymphomas. Early results suggest a possible role for interferon alpha IFNα in prolonging the disease-free interval [45]. A retrospective analysis of patients entered in two EORTC phase III studies shows poorer results compared to other lymphomas when treatment with approaches suitable for either low- or intermediate-grade lymphomas is administered, so there is a real need for prospective studies to establish means of obtaining and sustaining better rates of response [46].

Reports of attempts to improve the outcome for patients with MCL by using an initial anthracycline-containing regimen (CAP BOP in various forms, containing cyclophosphamide, doxorubicin or mitozantrone, procarbazine, bleomycin, vincristine and prednisolone or dexamethasone) show limited success, with complete remission obtained in only 29% of patients and no patient graded high/intermediate or high risk by the International Prognostic Index alive and free of disease at 5 years [47]. The same authors report results of high-dose salvage therapy supported by autologous stem cells in nine patients, and, while admitting to small numbers and a short follow-up, found three patients remaining failure free at 7, 12 and 25 months post-transplant [47]. None of these patients underwent procedures involving manipulation of their graft material in an attempt to purge lymphoma cells; although this is technically feasible in a way that is analagous to the high-dose approach to follicular lymphoma (q.v.), there are no specific reports yet of its application to MCL. Once this approach is undertaken it should be possible to monitor elimination of cells from the graft material and also use the same techniques to follow patients for evidence of relapse by seeking to detect the gene t(11;14) rearrangement. Unfortunately, the existing PCR primers do not pick up a very high proportion of cases because the breakpoints on chromosome 11 are spread across a large DNA region, extending up to 63 kbp from the initially identified major translocation cluster [28].

Follicle centre lymphoma (FCL), follicular

This type of lymphoma is composed of a mixture of cells derived from the follicle centre, with both centrocytes and centroblasts identifiable in a pattern which is follicular in at least some areas, although diffuse and commonly somewhat sclerotic in others. The proportion of centroblasts allows a classification of the lymphoma into grade I (predominantly small cell), grade II (mixed small and large cell) and, more rarely, grade III (predominantly large cell) [48]. In addition to the cellular composition, cases may be classified over a spectrum of disease from follicular to diffuse [49], with an uncommon predominantly small cell subtype which is entirely diffuse

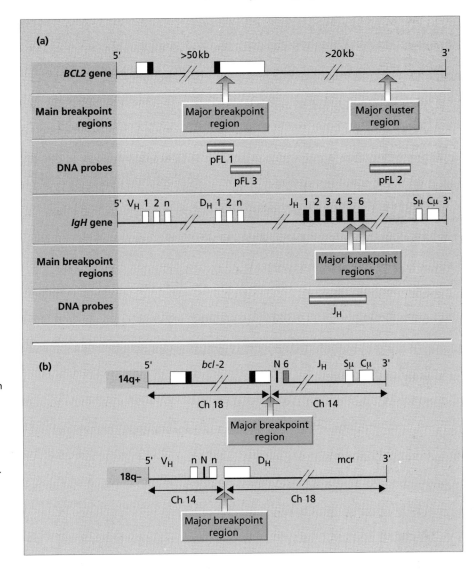

Fig. 18.5 (a) Diagram of the *BCL2* gene (above) and the Ig heavy-chain (*IgH*) gene (below). The main breakpoint regions are shown. The black areas in the *BCL2* gene represent the *BCL2* protein encoding region and the open boxes represent the untranslated segment of the *BCL2* transcriptional unit. (b) Diagram of the derivative 14q+ and 18q− chromosomes resultant from the t(14;18) translocation in lymphoma, at the major breakpoint region. V_H, D_H and J_H represent the Ig heavy-chain gene variable, diversity and joining regions respectively. N = 'N' segment; $S\mu = \mu$ switch region; $C\mu = \mu$ constant region; mcr = minor cluster region; Ch = chromosone. (From Cotter, 1990 [52].)

in pattern. The precise criteria for grading cytology and growth pattern have not been standardized and are likely to vary between institutions. The immunophenotype of these cells shows expression of SIg and B-cell associated antigens (CD19, CD20, CD22), together with variable expression of CD10 which may be useful in distinguishing the cells from marginal zone cell lymphomas. Expression of *BCL2* by lymphoma follicles is useful in distinguishing malignant from reactive follicular patterns, but this protein is also expressed by other types of low-grade lymphoma [50].

A translocation t(14;18)(q32;q21) is present in 70–95% of cases of follicle centre lymphoma and has important effects in defining the biological nature of the disorder [51]. The effect of this translocation is to juxtapose a gene termed *BCL2* on chromosome 18 with the J_H region of the immunoglobin heavy-chain locus on chromosome 14, with the subsequent overexpression of a chimeric *BCL2/IgH* message [52]. Because the chromosomal breakpoint falls outside the translated

portion of the *BCL2* gene, the protein product is identical with the normal BCL2 protein (Fig. 18.5). The physiological role of *BCL2* is to function as a repressor of apoptosis or 'programmed cell death'; transgenic mice bearing a *BCL2*/immunoglobulin minigene, like that produced by the (14;18) translocation, develop polyclonal follicular hyperplasia, in which B cells accumulate because of extended cell survival rather than increased proliferation [53]. The function of BCL2 is not understood in biochemical terms, but it is balanced by a structurally similar partner, BAX (Fig. 18.6) which counters the death-repressing activity of BCL2 by a process of dimerization [54]. It is unclear whether BCL2 blocks a BAX-dependent suicide pathway, whether BAX blocks a BCL2 mediated survival function, or whether the relative levels of BCL2 and BAX simply determine the propensity of an individual cell for programmed cell death.

Although the 14;18 translocation and its effect on BCL2 protein expression provide interesting information on the

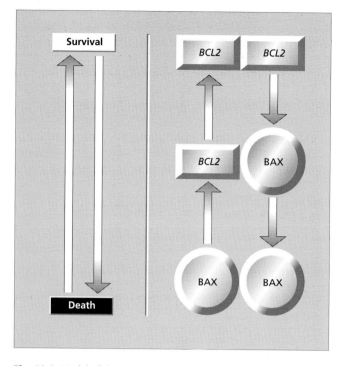

Fig. 18.6 Model of the interrelationship between *BCL2* and BAX and the regulation of programmed cell death. All indicated protein associations may represent dimers or higher oligomers. Free BCL2 is drawn alternatively as a monomer or homodimer. (From Oltrai *et al.*, 1993 [54], ©1993 Cell Press.)

aetiology of follicle centre lymphoma (FCL), these findings have not yet been shown to have prognostic significance. In a retrospective study of 70 cases of FCL, analysis of BCL2 protein expression by immunohistochemistry showed no difference in survival between 55 patients with positive-staining nodes vs nine with negative-staining nodes, and drawn from the same population *BCL2* gene rearrangement detected by Southern blotting or polymerase chain reaction (PCR) had no impact on the survival of 27 positive patients compared with 12 negative patients [55]. Nonetheless, the fact that breakpoints on both the derivative chromosomes fall within two different well-defined areas, known as the major breakpoint region (MBR) and minor cluster region (mcr), has enabled the development of molecular assays for the detection of the DNA rearrangement. These PCR methods utilize primers for areas of the *BCL2* gene and also consensus J_H primers which allow amplification of product to generate the capacity to detect one abnormal cell in 10^5 normal cells. When such sensitive assays are applied to patients who have apparently been disease free for long periods after treatment of their FCL, t(14;18) bearing cells are commonly detectable [56], and this even applies to patients whose disease was apparently localized at presentation [57]. The cells detected by these methods could be quiescent and not represent any threat of clinical recurrence, or alternatively they might not have undergone further genetic events which

would lead to malignant transformation. There is support for the latter hypothesis in the reports of detection of small numbers of PCR-amplifiable t(14;18) rearrangements similar to those associated with lymphoma in benign tonsillar hyperplasia [58] and in the peripheral blood mononuclear cells of healthy donors [59]. This result has also been confirmed by a highly sensitive method involving fluorescence *in situ* hybridization (FISH) to detect both the *BCL2* gene and the *IgH* gene [60]. An attempt to elucidate this further by PCR amplification of a *BCL2/IgH* message in a system involving reverse transcription of RNA appeared to show that, in some patients, treatment was producing downregulation of RNA expression [61], but did not otherwise clarify the sequence of events. Histological transformation of FCL to more aggressive diffuse lymphomas occurs in a high percentage of patients during their clinical course and is generally associated with the development of complex secondary chromosomal abnormalities. In a small proportion of these cases, the transformation appears to be associated with rearrangement of the *MYC* gene at 8q24 [62] or the *BCL3* gene at 17q22 [63], and in a larger proportion of cases mutations of the tumour suppressor gene *p53* are detectable [64].

The FCLs comprise nearly 40% of all NHLs; in most studies they show a slight female preponderance and present at a median age of about 50 years [65]. As a diagnostic group, these diseases are only common in the Western world, with a very low incidence in Asia and the Middle East. No single major environmental factor has been associated with FCL, although epidemiological studies have identified major variations in incidence, with rural areas having an excess of cases [66]. Most patients present with lymphadenopathy, and it is important to appreciate that this may vary without treatment and so a node which spontaneously diminishes in size may still be involved by lymphoma. The majority of patients have disseminated disease at diagnosis which can be documented with appropriate investigations, including detailed examination of Waldeyer's ring, computer tomography (CT) of abdominal nodes and bilateral bone marrow biopsies; routine liver biopsies are not usually undertaken unless clinically indicated. Only 15–20% of patients will have stage I or II disease, which could be possibly managed by local radiotherapy. It is apparent that the Ann Arbor Staging System has a limited capacity to stratify patients into prognostic groups and that other measures are needed. Histological grading of the lymph-node biopsy is able to categorize patients and this has generally resulted in three groups of patients being identified, with progressively shorter median survivals as the proportion of large cells in the node increases. In an early series from the National Cancer Institute (NCI), cytological patterns within the nodes were analysed, those with predominantly small cell disease had a median survival of 78 months, mixed small and large cell disease had a median survival of 55 months and patients with mainly large cells survived for a median of only 29 months [67]. Within the node biopsies there is also a gradation in the areas of diffuse growth, and although this finding was not initially thought to carry adverse prognostic weight [68], it appears that patients whose nodes show a follicular pattern over more than half of the biopsy have a significantly better survival than those with less [69]. Attempts to put the morphological assessment of aggressiveness on a more objective basis have resulted in the use of flow cytometry to measure the proliferative index (the percentage of cells in S + G$_2$ phases of the cell cycle) [70]. The ability of this methodology to identify a high-risk group more reliably than histology alone has been confirmed in studies of S-phase fraction performed on formalin-fixed material [71], but not with fresh tissue [72], although this latter study included only small numbers of patients with FCL.

Clinical features, including age and the presence of constitutional symptoms, have a major impact on survival in most reviews [67,68], and studies based on multivariate analyses have also identified a number of important factors, such as the bulk of disease and extent of extranodal involvement, as well as indirect laboratory estimations which reflect the presence of advanced disease [73]. The importance of obtaining some idea of an individual patient's prognosis at presentation is to give the clinician guidance in selecting appropriate therapy for a disease with an extremely variable natural history. It is important to identify patients whose disease is sufficiently severe to warrant intensive drug treatment and in whom the outcome of such treatment justifies this approach. Although many of the patients with FCLs are elderly and it has been correctly stated that there are no good-prognosis patients over the age of 70 years [74], there remains a need to identify younger patients who also have poor prospects. Among the biochemical markers which reflect prognosis in lymphoma patients, beta-2-microglobulin (β_2m) has a long record of reliability [75], both for monitoring disease activity and identifying patients with a higher risk of treatment failure [76]: however, the serum LDH level appears to have emerged as the most reliable biochemical marker of tumour burden in lymphomas [77]. The International Non-Hodgkin's Lymphoma Prognostic Factors Project has established a predictive model for aggressive NHL [11] which allocates a score on the basis of awarding one point for each of the independent prognostic variables (Table 18.2) established in a series of 2031 patients. This approach has been applied to patients with low-grade lymphomas and, in a study involving over 100 patients with FCL, appeared to achieve good discrimination [12] (Table 18.3), although the proportion of patients identified as being at high risk was rather low. Criticism of this approach to the evaluation of patients with FCL can be made on the grounds that the risk factors were not derived from an appropriate patient population in the original analysis [78], and also by virtue of the association of a high LDH level with rapid histological progression [79], with its inevitable impact on survival. It is not, however, in doubt that clinicians require reliable guidance in the allocation of patients to appropriate therapy. A simple

Table 18.2 International prognostic index. (Adapted from the International Non-Hodgkin's Lymphoma Prognostic Factors Project, 1993 [11].)

Age >60 years
Serum LDH >1 × normal
Performance status >2
Stage III or IV
Extranodal involvement >1 site

Risk group	Score
Low	0 or 1
Low/intermediate	2
High/intermediate	3
High	4 or 5

Table 18.3 International Prognostic Index applied to FCL (*n* = 107). (Adapted from Lopez-Guillermo *et al.*, 1994 [12].)

Risk group	Complete remission (%)	10-year survival (%)
Low	61.5	75
Low/intermediate	41.2	47
High/intermediate	25	55
High	21.4	0

robust scheme based on information readily available at the time of initial evaluation of the patient would be highly desirable, especially if it had been derived from multifactorial analysis of a suitably large population of patients with FCL.

In the 1984 Karnofsky Memorial Lecture, Rosenberg reviewed the extensive experience at Stanford University of the management of low-grade NHLs and emphasized the frustrations involved in treating disorders characterized by relentless recurrence despite sensitivity to therapy [13]. In that address, Rosenberg also reviewed several key issues in the overall management of this group of diseases, drawing attention to the potential curability of localized disease with radiotherapy, the possibility of management of more advanced disease without immediate initial therapy, and the risks associated with histological transformation to more aggressive lymphomas.

There is historical evidence that up to 50% of patients with stage I–II disease may be curable and that involved-field radiotherapy alone may be sufficient to achieve this outcome [80–82]. Because of the acknowledged limitations of clinical staging investigations to exclude occult disease, a number of studies have explored the role of extended radiotherapy/total lymphoid irradiation [80] or adjuvant chemotherapy [83–87], with an apparent improvement in the relapse-free survival rate. Such a result is not surprising, in view of the ease with which circulating cells derived from the malignant lymphoma clone can be detected in patients with ostensibly localized disease, and particularly high rates of durable freedom from relapse have been obtained with treatment schedules involving initial chemotherapy followed by involved-field radiotherapy, followed by further chemotherapy [88]. Molecular methods for monitoring the presence of lymphoma cells involve either the amplification of immunoglobulin (Ig) gene rearrangements [89] or of t(14;18) by PCR. The methods involving detection of Ig gene rearrangement may only pick up about 80% of FCLs, because detection utilizing framework 2 (Fr2) and 3 (Fr3) region primers will not allow PCR amplification of Ig gene configurations if there is partial rearrangement of D (diversity) and J (joining) regions as a consequence of the t(14;18) translocation [90]. Detection of cells bearing t(14;18) is technically straightforward, and using primers which detect both the MBR and mcr results in the capacity to amplify by PCR a *BCL2*/J$_H$ DNA sequence which is unique to the malignant clone [91]. Assessment of patients with localized (stage I and II) FCL by this approach has demonstrated the presence of cells bearing t(14;18) with the same characteristics as those in the diagnostic lymph node in six of eight patients [92]. Although this finding, and the report of three of eight patients with no detectable t(14;18) cells, either at diagnosis or at long-term follow-up [57], implies the existence of a small subgroup of patients whose disease truly lacked a systemic component and was successfully eradicated by primary treatment. The natural corollary is that the large majority of patients have disseminated disease at diagnosis and that, despite this finding, a proportion will have apparently durable remissions with no clinical evidence of disease recurrence. The addition of early adjuvant therapy may well improve the duration of remission [88], but neither the detection of persistent molecular positivity for t(14;18), nor the detection of 'molecular relapse', have been clearly correlated with clinical recurrence [57]. Although this may reflect the slow rate of disease progression, it is in contrast to findings in chronic lymphocytic leukaemia [93]. In the absence of prospective studies to evaluate the molecular monitoring of disease, most clinicians will choose to treat patients with carefully defined clinically localized disease with radiotherapy to involved fields at a dose of 3500 cGy fractionated over 4 weeks and will then expect to give chemotherapy for clinical relapse without having prejudiced their chances of obtaining a response.

It has been known for many years that clinical responses may be achieved by treating patients with advanced stage (III or IV) FCL with corticosteroids [94], radiotherapy or single-agent chemotherapy using cyclophosphamide, chlorambucil or vincristine [95]. The early studies with combination chemotherapy (CVP — cyclophosphamide, vincristine, prednisolone) were conducted in the 1960s [96], and currently practising clinicians should appreciate that this approach was considered to constitute intensive chemotherapy at that time. Before the advent of chemotherapy, the median survival of patients was less than 5 years [97] and, although it is now approaching 10 years, there is little evidence of the plateau on

any survival curve which would indicate that a proportion of patients are being cured. Increasingly intensive treatment produces higher response rates and longer remissions, but the pattern of survival is not much different from those patients managed with a conservative approach.

Because of the lack of curative treatment for advanced FCL, and because many patients at presentation had either an established history of asmptomatic gradually progressive lymphadenopathy or significant intercurrent medical conditions, the group at Stanford began to select some such patients to be followed until therapy was required as indicated by rapid progression, systemic symptoms or marrow compromise. The median time to requiring therapy in this carefully selected and meticulously followed group of patients was 48 months for FCL with small cells and 16.5 months for FCL patients with a significant proportion of large cells [98]. Over the period that these patients were followed, 30% of patients with 'small cell' FCL enjoyed a degree of spontaneous regression of their disease, lasting for a median time of 15 months, and of the histologically more aggressive group regression was noted in 17%, with a median duration of 6 months [99]. The incidence of histological evolution to high-grade lymphomas was the same in initially untreated patients as in those given immediate therapy (approximately 40% with a median time to progression of just under 5 years), implying that histological progression is not induced by therapy. Investigations at the NCI have directly tested the policy of deferred treatment in a trial randomizing selected asymptomatic patients between no initial therapy and ProMACE MOPP chemotherapy plus total lymphoid irradiation [100], and this has not yet demonstrated a survival advantage for those patients given initial therapy. In one retrospective analysis of patients managed with a 'no initial treatment' policy, there was a significantly better survival than in those receiving other approaches to treatment [101].

The historical data relating to the results which can be achieved with chemotherapy must be reviewed. Despite the lack of evidence that conventional-dose cytotoxic chemotherapy, with or without radiotherapy, can prolong the overall survival of patients with widespread FCL, it must be accepted that this is an illness which gives patients symptoms from which they suffer and also visible evidence of enlarged organs which they resent. It has been suggested that disease-free survival is a more realistic standard of success than overall survival, but that the cost in terms of a rise in toxicity must play an important part in assessing the acceptability of any treatment which is not given with curative intent. The treatment trials conducted in the 1970s explored the use of either single-agent alkylator therapy (usually oral chlorambucil), combination chemotherapy (usually CVP) and radiotherapy, frequently given as low-dose total body irradiation [102,103], and failed to demonstrate a convincing advantage for any one choice. The limitations of this approach in terms of poor results obtained with either chemotherapy [104] and compromise of

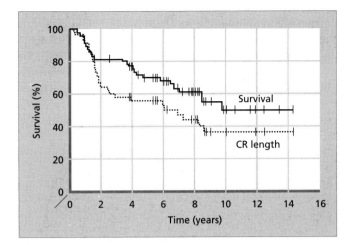

Fig. 18.7 Overall survival of patients with stage III or IV nodular mixed lymphoma, regardless of treatment outcome, and the proportion of patients remaining in their first complete remission (CR), regardless of treatment, are plotted against duration of remission. Of the 64 patients, 26 died, giving a median survival for all patients of 9.6 years. Of the 46 complete responders, 26 had relapses; the median duration of remission is projected to be 6.2 years. (From Longo *et al.*, 1984 [107].)

the haematological tolerance of any subsequent treatment in patients treated with total body irradiation were clearly established. The pattern of relapse for patients with advanced-stage FCL emphasized the inadequacy of initial therapy in eradicating disease, with nodal recurrences tending to be at the site of initial involvement and a high incidence of marrow relapse in those who had infiltration at presentation [105].

In a search for evidence of potentially curative treatment for FCL, attention was given to those lymphomas with a mixture of small and large cells, because these had a shorter time to requiring treatment if not given initial therapy, but longer remission durations once a complete remission had been achieved with combination chemotherapy. In a series of patients treated at the NCI, mainly with nonanthracycline-containing combination chemotherapy, 70% of patients with stage III or IV disease achieved complete remissions lasting for a median of over 6 years [106,107] (Fig. 18.7), and although late relapses occurred, the results were felt to justify optimism about the curative potential of treatment for this subgroup of patients. A contemporaneous Eastern Cooperative Oncology Group (ECOG) study in which patients were randomized between chlorambucil and two more intensive combinations failed to generate comparable results [108]. The next generation of treatment trials in FCL involved the use of anthracycline-based combination chemotherapy, in an attempt to produce results as good in terms of disease-free survival as those that were obtained in patients with high-grade lymphomas. An early nonrandomized study which added doxorubicin to a weekly CVP induction, followed by chlorambucil maintenance, had already established that, although a higher initial response rate could be achieved in FCL (67 vs

25%), there was no improvement in overall survival to match that achieved in the aggressive lymphomas treated with the same schedule [109]. Over a decade from 1972, the South West Oncology Group (SWOG) conducted a series of studies which involved randomization of patients into trials in which a doxorubicin-containing regimen (cyclophosphamide, doxorubicin, vincristine and prednisolone; CHOP) was the initial therapy for some patients; a total of 332 patients had FCL of either small cell or mixed small and large cell grade and the overall complete response rate for all patients with low-grade lymphomas was 64%. A late analysis of this data concentrated on factors affecting survival and indicates a possible plateau for FCL mixed small and large cell patients at about 20%; there was no identifiable plateau for patients with small cell disease and neither maintenance treatment with chemotherapy (chlorambucil) nor immunotherapy (BCG or levamisole) had any significant effect on survival [110]. Other studies with a long follow-up have also documented the fact that although long remissions are obtainable with combination chemotherapy, for example m/M-BACOD, methotrexate, bleomycin, doxorubicin, cyclophosphamide, vincristine and dexamethasone [111], or CHOP + bleomycin [112], late relapses are a feature of FCL with mixed cellular populations and relapses occur steadily among those patients with FCL consisting of small cells [113].

Attempts to isolate the group of patients with FCL consisting mainly of large cells, and define the natural history of this disorder, have shown that higher initial CR rates can be obtained with reasonably intensive anthracycline-containing combinations and that both overall survival and freedom from progression were better than with other treatments [48]. However, this study was not controlled, and nonanthracycline-based treatment may have been assigned to patients with medical contraindications to aggressive therapy. The Stanford group who reported this data subjected their patient population to analysis by the International Prognostic Factors Index, but identified only 10% as having high/intermediate- or high-risk characteristics; it would, therefore, appear that stratification by this means will have limited value in identifying patients for early high-dose treatment approaches. Analysis of patients with lower-risk scores also failed to clearly define a patient group who could have received less intensive therapy, and these investigators have indicated that they feel the achievement of a 10-year overall survival rate of 65% with a freedom-from-progression rate of 55% justifies the use of cyclophosphamide/doxorubicin-based therapy, despite the occurrence of some late relapses.

This pattern of repeated recurrence with response to further treatment has been well documented in a large retrospective analysis undertaken at St Bartholomew's Hospital, London [114]. A summary of their findings (Table 18.4) emphasized that although, at each recurrence, approximately 75% of the patients will respond, these responses become shorter and the expectation of subsequent survival diminishes accordingly.

Table 18.4 Comparison of response rates, response durations and survival times after treatment of consecutive recurrences of FCL. (From Johnson *et al.*, 1995 [114], with permission.)

	Patients treated (no.)	Response rate (%)	Median response duration (months)	Median survival duration (years)	Median survival from response (years)
Presentation	204	88	31	9.2	9.6
Recurrence					
First	110	87	13	4.6	4.9
Second	63	76	13	3.5	3.5
Third	37	68	6	2.0	1.2

Treatment strategies aimed at extending the duration of response to therapy have included the use of IFNα in an attempt to delay disease recurrence or progression, in the same way as can be demonstrated with its use in multiple myeloma. As a single agent, IFNα has modest activity against low-grade lymphoma [115], but it has been shown to be capable of producing responses in up to a third of patients with FCL [112]. Prospective randomized trials of IFNα in either induction therapy, maintenance therapy or both have shown benefit in terms of the time to failure [116–120], but the familiar pattern of continuous relapse is still observed, and there is no evidence that any patients are cured by the additional effect.

The ability of the protein encoded by the *BCL2* gene to protect cells against apoptosis induced by such commonly used cytotoxic agents as dexamethasone, methotrexate, cytosine arabinoside, etoposide, vincristine, hydroperoxy-cyclophosphamide and cisplatin has been clearly demonstrated *in vitro*, and may explain the mechanism by which the activity of these drugs is impaired in the management of FCL [121]. Despite this observation, further responses are readily obtained in patients whose disease recurs; in the series of patients treated at St Bartholomew's Hospital, initial therapy was delayed until the disease became bulky or symptomatic and patients then received either chlorambucil or CVP [122]; 70% responded to initial treatment and, when the disease recurred and progressed, patients were retreated with repeated courses of chlorambucil or CVP until there was evidence of failure to respond. It is not surprising that 68% of patients who responded initially had a further response to treatment, but it is an important observation that 47% of patients who had failed initial therapy responded to further chlorambucil or CVP at the time of recurrence. Continued successful palliation of disease with modest treatment is, therefore, possible for a significant proportion of patients through long periods and over a succession of recurrences, providing there is no evidence of the disease transforming to a more aggressive histological grade. The monitoring of t(14;18) cells in the blood after treatment has not, so far, proved to be either a reliable indicator of clinically significant persistent disease or a useful guide to the timing of further conventional therapy [123].

A large number of cytotoxic drugs have demonstrated activity in the treatment of recurrent FCL. Single-agent activity is well established for mitoxantrone [124], which has now been incorporated into well-tolerated combination therapy [125], but the related compound bisantrene is associated with substantially greater toxicity [126]. An exploration of combinations of drugs incorporating ifosfamide and etoposide, with a variety of other agents, documented a marked reduction in the chances of obtaining a response in those patients who had failed three or more prior treatments, without this being due to any association with histological progression [127]. It seems that this line of reasonably intensive conventional-dose chemotherapy is inappropriate for the palliation of patients with FCL late in the course of their disease.

Activity against FCL has been demonstrated for deoxycoformycin, an adenosine deaminase inhibitor, and its related purine analogues fludarabine and cladribine (2 chloro-deoxyadenosine). The use of deoxycoformycin has been rather limited and although a weekly schedule of 4 mg/m² IV [128] and a schedule of 5 mg/m² IV daily for 3 days every 21 days [129] have received reasonably extensive phase II evaluation, there is no substantial cohort of lightly pretreated patients with FCL in which to assess its activity. Work conducted at the Scripps Institute in La Jolla, California indicated that deoxyadenosine, and its derivative 2 chloro-deoxyadenosine, had substantial toxicity to nondividing human lymphocytes [130]. It was reasoned that this property could be exploited in the treatment of lymphoid malignancies with low rates of proliferation, such as chronic lymphocytic leukaemia and low-grade lymphomas. It was established that fludarabine had clinical activity against NHL by the observation of responses in the phase I studies [131], and this led to further evaluation in a phase II trial [132], which included eight patients with FCL treated on a schedule involving a loading dose of 20 mg/m², followed by a continuous infusion of 30 mg/m² over 48 hours. Schedules involving IV administration by short infusion of 5 consecutive days, repeated every 28 days, were evaluated, and activity was seen at dose levels of 18 mg/m² [133] as well as the currently accepted 25 mg/m² [43,134]. This produced responses in approximately two-thirds of patients with previously treated FCL and even higher proportions of untreated patients [135], although the largest single-agent study of first-line therapy achieved an overall response rate of only 65% and a relatively short median progression-free survival of only 13.6 months [136]. Comparable studies of cladribine have given the drug as a 7-day continuous infusion at a dose rate of 0.1 or 0.15 mg/kg/day and have achieved responses in approximately half the patients treated for recurrent/refractory FCL [44,137,138] and over 80% of those receiving the drug as initial therapy [139]; activity is also noted against CLL when cladribine is given as IV infusions of 0.12 mg/kg on 5 consecutive days [140] and both subcutaneous and oral bioavailability has been documented (Fig. 18.8) [141]. Both fludarabine and cladribine are well tolerated by patients, with virtually no nausea, vomiting or hair loss; however, both produce significant haematological toxicity, which is also associated with a marked and sustained suppression of helper T cells [142], and this may produce a significant incidence of opportunistic infections, especially in patients who are also receiving corticosteroid therapy [143]. A further rare, but serious, consequence of this protracted post-treatment immunosuppression has been the occasional development of transfusion-associated graft vs host disease, which has now been reported with both fludarabine [144] and cladribine [145], and which makes the irradiation of blood products to be transfused to patients obligatory. Despite these limitations, which oblige clinicians using the new purine analogues to exercise care, the activity of these compounds in a wide range of lymphoid malignancies is very considerable and their incorporation into combination therapy is being explored. Results of phase I studies of cladribine and chlorambucil [146], and fludarabine and chlorambucil [147], have defined the maximum tolerated doses of the purine analogues in straightforward combination, and there is some experience with other schedules, such as fludarabine, mitozantrone and dexamethasone [148], fludarabine, cisplatin and cytosine arabinoside [149] and cladribine, cisplatin, bleomycin and prednisolone [140], which suggests that these may offer very high levels of antilymphoma activity. The results achieved with fludarabine, mitozantrone and dexamethasone have been sufficiently encouraging for the investigators to proceed to both an extended phase II evaluation [150] and a phase III comparison with an alternating schedule involving several other combinations of cytotoxics which is being monitored to detect molecular complete responses [151].

Despite the encouraging results which are beginning to be obtained with new chemotherapeutic agents, the mode of cytotoxicity of these drugs probably still involves a pathway in which apoptosis is induced [152], and the potential for curing patients may consequently be limited by the intrinsic protection offered to the malignant cells by overexpression of BCL2.

It has been demonstrated that the mode of action of the immunological cytotoxicity produced by monoclonal antibodies is mediated through Ig receptors on the cell surface inducing cellular protein-tyrosine phosphorylation and that this means of triggering the cascade of events leading to apoptosis is apparently independent of the protective action of high BCL2 levels [153]. This observation is encouraging, because it may mean that immunological approaches will be able to obtain responses at a stage after the failure of conventional treatment. B-cell malignancies arise from cells which have made a genetic commitment to express a unique Ig. In the case of FCL, although the translocation (14;18) appears to be the critical oncogenic event, it occurs after the cell has already rearranged both its functional Ig heavy- and light-chain genes so that its unique idiotypic Ig will be produced. It is possible to generate antibodies which recognize this unique portion of each Ig molecule, and these may arise naturally and be important in regulating the immune response. To exploit this phenomenon therapeutically, it is first necessary to produce sufficient idiotypic Ig to act as an immunogen, and this is achieved by fusing a human lymphoma cell and a mouse myeloma cell to produce a hybrid which secretes the tumour-derived Ig molecule in large quantities [154]. Once the Ig is retrieved, it is purified and used to immunize mice whose spleen cells are fused with a myeloma cell line to make hybridomas from which the appropriately reacting monoclonal antibody can be selected. These custom-made antibodies are highly specific for the lymphoma cells of the individuals to which they are raised [155], and are only suitable for use in the patient for whom they were produced. It has since been shown that it is possible to select antibodies to detect idiotypic structures which are shared by the Ig molecules of different patients and, therefore, a panel of therapeutic antibodies could be manufactured; unfortunately, these reacted with only a

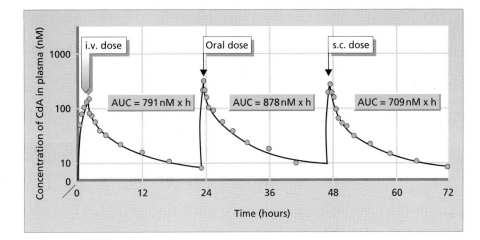

Fig. 18.8 Plasma concentration of 2-chlorodeoxyadenosine (CdA) (cladribine) after IV, SC and oral administration in a patient. The oral dose of CdA was 0.28 mg/kg, the IV infusion and SC doses were 0.14 mg/kg. AUC = area under curve. (From Liliemark *et al.*, 1992 [141].)

minority of all B-cell lymphomas, but at least reduced the necessity for complete individualization of production [156]. The prerequisite for patients to be suitable for therapeutic trials of anti-idiotype antibody are that they should have biopsiable tumour, which secretes an idiotypic Ig into the circulation at only low levels (<50 µg/ml), and which has an Ig receptor on the surface to bind the monoclonal antibody; these requirements exclude a significant proportion of patients with FCL. The Stanford Group, who have conducted much of this work, have performed clinical trials of anti-idiotype antibody alone [157] and in combination with either IFNα [158] or chlorambucil [159], and have been able to obtain responses in approximately half the patients treated. Tolerance of the antibody infusions is reasonable, although chills and fever were frequent; however, the duration of responses was generally short and the efficacy of treatment was limited either by the development of human antimouse antibodies or mutation of the tumour cells to become unreactive with the antibody. Although it is possible to modify the nature of the therapeutic antibody to reduce the risks of an antimouse response [160], the variables involved in determining the outcome of anti-idiotype treatment are extremely complex and make it difficult to predict which patients might benefit from this complicated and expensive form of treatment [161].

Tactics to avoid the necessity of tailoring antibodies to a specific lymphoma include the possibility of exploiting the B-cell antigen CD20 which is expressed on normal B cells and nearly all B-cell lymphomas. This nonmodulating antigen is a promising candidate as a target for antibody-directed therapies, and clinical trials with a chimeric anti-CD20 antibody (IDEC C2B8) [162] have established a dose level for therapeutic trials which have begun recruitment [163,164].

The efficacy of unconjugated antibodies depends on their ability to activate complement and also human effector cells as a means of achieving cytotoxicity. Amplification of the therapeutic efficiency of the antibodies can be achieved by conjugating them to a toxin such as ricin, diphtheria toxin or pseudomonas exotoxin A, or alternatively to a radioisotope [165]. The characteristics of the antibody and the targeted antigen continue to be important, but because of the extreme potency of these compounds idiotype specificity is not required, and the desired properties of the reaction favour internalization of the target antigen after binding, in contrast to the mode of action of unconjugated products. The evaluation of immunotoxin therapy in B-cell NHL has involved phase I studies of anti-CD22 monoclonal antibody bound to a ricin A-chain derivative [166,167] and anti-CD19 bound to a ricin B-chain derivative [168]; dose-limiting capillary-leak syndrome is associated with ricin A-chain administration, and hepatotoxicity with ricin B-chain administration. There are problems associated with the formation of antiricin antibodies and antimurine antibodies which limit the efficacy of repeat dosing, but partial responses of short duration have been achieved in patients highly refractory to chemotherapy. An

anti-CD20 has also been used to deliver iodine-131 to lymphoma cells with encouraging evidence of efficacy [169], including responses in patients with disease which had been resistant to chemotherapy [170].

Immunological means have been used to try to eliminate lymphoma cells *in vitro* from harvested bone marrow prior to its use in autologous bone marrow transplantation. Given the frequency of bone marrow involvement in patients with relapsed FCL, concern about the use of marrow or blood-derived stem cells to support high-dose therapy is understandable. Although autologous bone marrow transplants have been undertaken without any attempt to eliminate occult persistent infiltration by lymphoma [171], other investigators have used immunological purging monitored by PCR detection of the *BCL2* translocation to eliminate contamination by lymphoma. The group at the Dana Faber Cancer Institute [172] in Boston have shown that with a method involving the use of a cocktail of monoclonal antibodies directed against CD10, CD19, CD20 and B5 to label the lymphoma cells, and a goat antimouse antibody conjugated to magnetic beads, it was possible to eliminate lymphoma cells to the point of PCR negativity without damaging haemopoietic stem cells (Fig. 18.9).

The use of high-dose therapy supported by autologous

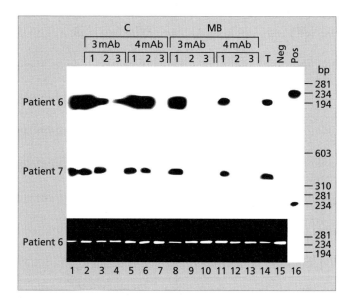

Fig. 18.9 Detection by Southern blot analysis of *BCL2* translocation-specific sequences amplified by PCR. The results of PCR analysis of 1 µg of DNA from samples obtained before and after each of the three treatment cycles, with the three and four monoclonal antibodies (mAb) are shown for two representative patients. The lower panel shows an ethidium bromide-stained agarose gel electrophoresis of 1 µg of DNA from the samples of patient 6 PCR amplified using primers for the B7 gene and show that PCR-amplifiable DNA was obtained in each sample analysed. bp = base pairs; C = complement-mediated lysis; MB = immunomagnetic bead depletion; Neg = negative control; Pos = positive control; T = control sample obtained after three cycles of treatment with four anti-T-cell mAbs. (From Gribben *et al.*, 1992 [172].)

haemopoietic stem cells to ensure marrow reconstitution represents an attempt to cure, rather than palliate, patients with FCL. It is not difficult to define a patient population in whom conventional treatment is completely inadequate. A large cohort entered into the Eastern Cooperative Oncology Group (ECOG) studies yielded a subgroup of 117 patients who were under the age of 60 years and who had an initial response to therapy of less than 1 year; these patients had an age-adjusted mortality in the next year of 30.6% [173] and the short survival of patients after a third or subsequent relapse has also already been noted [114,127]. The poor results to be obtained in treating these patients have readily justified the extensive exploration of intensive chemoradiotherapy, which has been undertaken at the Dana-Faber Cancer Institute in Boston and St Bartholomew's Hospital in London [174]. These investigators have attempted to reduce the level of detectable residual marrow involvement by testing the patients' responsiveness to conventional chemotherapy salvage regimens, while accepting that it would be impossible to eliminate disease detectable by sensitive molecular methods [175]. Harvested autologous bone marrow was then treated by immunological means [176] to try to eliminate residual contamination with lymphoma cells, and patients were subsequently treated with myeloablative cyclophosphamide/total body irradiation before reinfusion of their autologous bone marrow stem cells. It was possible to render approximately half the patients' marrows 'PCR negative' for t(14;18), and the early evidence is that the pattern of recurrence is significantly better if this can be achieved (Fig. 18.10) [176]. Follow-up of this patient population [177], and others treated by similar approaches [178,179,180], is encouraging, but too short to demonstrate confidently that any patients are cured (Fig. 18.11) [174]. The proposition that high-dose therapy with stem cell support will be more effective than conventional chemotherapy for the management of relapsed FCL is being examined in a large collaborative study, the CUP (chemotherapy unpurged purged) trial, co-ordinated through the European Bone Marrow Transplant Working Party. The results of high-dose therapy in open studies are not sufficiently good that it is self-evident that there will be a therapeutic advantage for this approach, especially if it does not result in elimination of the t(14;18) clone [181].

The immediate haematological toxicity of high-dose treatment can be reduced by utilizing growth factor-mobilized peripheral blood stem cells, instead of autologous bone marrow, to effect reconstitution. Although the cost in terms of nonhaematological toxicity to the intestinal mucosa, the long-term effects on fertility and damage to stem cells resulting in a significant incidence of myelodysplasia, remain the same as those for autologous bone marrow transplantation, the improved early tolerance of this technique has allowed treatment of patients up to the age of 60 years. As with the results of autologous bone marrow transplantation, there is little evidence that patients are cured by this procedure [182] and, unfortunately, the problems of contamination of peripheral blood-derived stem cell grafts with cells bearing t(14;18) are not very different from those already encountered in the use of bone marrow [183]. However, one group has reported the phenomenon of patients grafted with PCR-positive harvests who subsequently convert to PCR-negative [184]. As there is uncertainty in the interpretation of PCR detection of persistent lymphoma cells in most cases of FCL, there is, as yet, no rationale for using PCR to direct therapy decisions. Attempts to use molecular means to inhibit BCL2 expression by constructing antisense oligonucleotides that are specific for the sequences

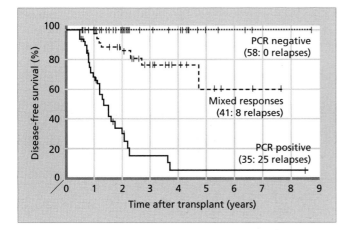

Fig. 18.10 Actuarial probability of disease-free survival after ABMT in 134 patients with B-cell NHL. PCR negative denotes the patients in whom PCR did not detect any residual lymphoma after transplantation; PCR positive denotes patients in whom PCR detected residual lymphoma in all samples; mixed responses denotes the patients in whom PCR detected residual lymphoma in only some of the samples analysed. All BM samples analysed were obtained while patients remained in complete clinical remission (*P* <0.00001). (From Gribben *et al.*, 1993 [176].)

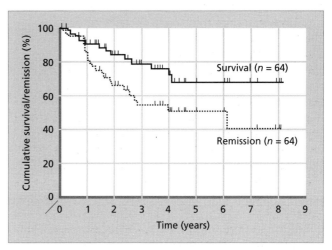

Fig. 18.11 Survival and remission duration of patients receiving CY/TBI/ABMT. (From Rohatiner *et al.*, 1994 [174].)

in the RNAs, have been shown to suppress the proliferation of BCL2-expressing cell lines [185]. It seems likely that much development work will be needed before these substances can be applied *in vivo*, or even used *ex vivo* to selectively inhibit the growth and survival of residual lymphoma cells in graft material. Allogeneic bone marrow represents a guaranteed lymphoma-free source of stem cells, with the theoretical possibility of mediating a therapeutically useful 'graft vs lymphoma' effect (Fig. 18.12) [186]. Current clinical experience is very limited, but suggests that in selected younger patients, long-term disease-free survival can be obtained, even for those with highly refractory disease [187].

Advice on the appropriate management of patients with FCL will clearly vary considerably, according to their clinical features, the assessment of prognosis and, since many patients will need treatment for recurrent disease, on their previous response to therapy. The small minority of patients who present with localized stage I or limited stage II disease should receive irradiation as primary management. Those patients with bulky stage II disease, stage III or stage IV disease at presentation require stratification into risk groups; the features which are likely to aid in this process are shown in Table 18.5, although it has been shown to be possible to use the factors important to the prognosis of patients with high-grade NHL identified in the International Prognostic Index.

Those patients identified as at low risk should probably not receive immediate therapy, but be followed closely for evidence of disease progression, at which time a reassessment of the indications for treatment must be undertaken. Patients at low or intermediate risk, who require therapy because of symptomatic or bulky disease, could be given single-agent alkylator therapy such as oral chlorambucil, either continuously or in pulses with or without corticosteroids. If the response to this is incomplete, the addition of a further cytotoxic such as mitozantrone, or a change to low-intensity combination therapy such as CVP, could be used to obtain better resolution of disease.

Patients with high-risk disease are likely to require more intensive therapy to obtain initial control. An anthracycline-containing combination, such as CHOP, will produce complete responses in a significant proportion of patients, and this could be varied for older patients by substituting either mitozantrone [188] or idarubicin [189] for doxorubicin to improve the tolerance. For those patients at any initial risk level, who obtain a complete response by conventional (nonmolecular) means of assessment, the next issue to be considered is treatment to maintain the response and prevent or delay recurrence. Low-risk patients who have responded well to single-agent therapy probably do not need maintenance treatment; for those patients in whom an initial response was harder to achieve or required more intensive therapy, the principle decision would concern the use of IFNα maintenance, and this should currently be restricted to formal trials. Patients whose predicted survival is limited because they have high-risk features, and

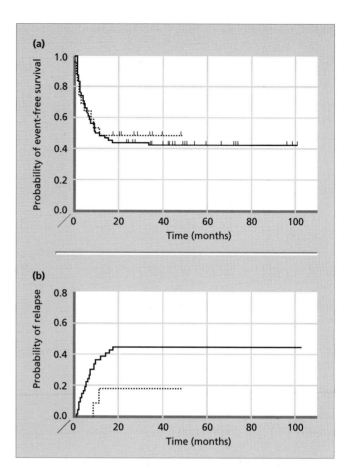

Fig. 18.12 Actuarial probability of (a) event-free survival and (b) relapse in the 61 patients who underwent autologous BMT (——) and the 19 patients who underwent allogeneic BMT (----) for lymphomas in sensitive relapse. The proportions of event-free survival are 41% (28–53%) and 47% (33–60%), respectively ($P = 0.8$). The probabilities of relapse are 46% (33–60%) and 18% (5–55%), respectively ($P = 0.02$). (From Jones *et al.*, 1991 [186].)

who have either not achieved an initial response or whose disease has recurred within a year of treatment, need careful consideration of their management. Those in the younger age group could well be considered for high-dose therapy with autologous stem cell support at this stage, although recruitment to a well-constructed trial testing this approach against conventional treatment should be considered. Patients over the age of 60 years, who would not be suitable candidates either for high-dose therapy or aggressive conventional approach combinations, might well benefit from treatment with a purine analogue such as fludarabine which would have a reasonable chance of offering useful active palliation. To some extent the decisions which are faced in managing patients at the time of first and second relapse are similar to those at presentation. It is important to consider whether patients might have undergone histological transformation which would alter the approach to treatment considerably,

Table 18.5 Prognostic factors in FCL.

Risk	Low	Intermediate	High
Histology of node	Small cell	Small and large cell	Large cell
Age (years)	<40	40–70	>70
Constitutional symptoms	None		B symptoms
Performance status	0, 1	2	3, 4
β_2-Microglobulin	Normal		> Normal
Lactate dehydrogenase	Normal		> Normal

and a low threshold for re-biopsy of recurrent disease is an important aid to selecting therapy. Low-risk patients with limited clinically significant problems can again be followed until progression occurs and again given a trial of single-agent alkylator therapy. Those with inadequate responses at this stage might be changed at a relatively early stage to purine analogue treatment, and evidence of biologically more aggressive behaviour would lead to fairly rapid consideration of anthracycline-based therapy. The threshold for considering high-dose treatment is also lower, and this period in the management of younger patients is likely to involve the careful weighing of risks against possible long-term benefits of treatment given with curative intent. Relapses later in the course of the disease, and those occurring after high-dose treatment, present the clinician with difficult decisions. All therapy given in this situation is likely to be palliative, but there is no reason not to test the responsiveness of the disease to further trials of conventional-dose chemotherapy. Even in the face of extensive extranodal spread, local radiotherapy may have a substantial contribution to make in controlling disfiguring or dangerous areas of lymphoma (e.g. in Waldeyer's ring). For individual patients this might be an appropriate time to explore the possibility of referral to experimental immunotherapeutic studies, and again, for a limited number of patients, high-dose therapy with peripheral stem cell support given at a late stage in the disease may offer the hope of a response of sufficient duration that worthwhile palliation would be obtained. Even a disease which remains responsive to treatment for as long as FCL will eventually cease to show any benefit from active palliation, and a clinician may find that he no longer has even marginally effective therapy to offer a patient who has been under his long-term care. Supportive care at both a psychological and physical level remains an obligation at this period; the expertise of palliative care specialists and the hospice movement may make an important contribution.

Marginal zone B-cell lymphoma

The pathologists of the REAL (Revised European–American

Lymphoma) Classification have proposed that the same cellular origin may be responsible for two related disorders; the low-grade lymphoma of extranodal distribution which has been identified as arising from mucosa-associated lymphoid tissue (MALT) and a disorder with nodal involvement cytologically associated with the presence of monocytoid B-cells [8]. They have postulated that the variation in clinical presentation may be a consequence of different homing patterns of the clonal cells involved, and their proliferation may well depend on the involvement of antigen-driven T cells. Definition of the extranodal lymphoma related to MALT was first made as part of an evaluation of gastrointestinal lymphoma, which contrasted the lesion associated with Mediterranean lymphoma (alpha-chain disease) and that found in patients of non-Middle Eastern origin [190]. The origin of lymphomas of this type, when they arise in the small intestine, is from Peyer's patches, which have a follicle surrounded by a further B-cell zone in which there is also a variable component of macrophages and T cells; the B cells in this marginal zone have morphological and immunophenotypic characteristics of the cells of MALT lymphomas [191]. Extranodal MALT lymphomas may also arise in sites normally devoid of lymphoid tissue, in cases of chronic inflammatory disorders which have resulted in the accumulation of lymphoid infiltrates, and this has been proposed as an explanation for some lymphomas arising in the stomach, lung, salivary gland, thyroid, orbit, skin, breast and kidney [192]. Definition of the nodal equivalent of this disorder has drawn attention to the pattern of parafollicular infiltration by large lymphocytes similar to that seen in toxoplasmosis [193]. In epithelial tissues, there is infiltration producing lymphoepithelial lesions, and plasma cells are often found in distinct subepithelial zones or in interfollicular areas of involved nodes. These features are sufficiently similar to the appearances of lymph nodes involved by spread from primary gastric lymphomas of MALT type, and the two disorders can be firmly linked together [194]. The immunophenotype of these cells shows expression of Ig on the surface, but not always in the cytoplasm, together with the usual B-cell-associated antigens (CD19, CD20, CD22) although not CD5 or CD10 [195]. Immunoglobulin heavy and light chains are rearranged, but neither *BCL1* nor *BCL2* translocations occur [195,196]; trisomy 3 is found in a proportion of patients [197], but the effect of this on the biology of the disease is not established.

Despite the similarities in cytological definition of this form of lymphoma, the natural history of the disease varies considerably according to the initial site of involvement. Low-grade MALT lymphoma of the stomach constitutes a distinct subset of this disease, and attention has focused on the aetiology of this group because of evidence of a rising incidence [198] and a marked variation in geographical distribution [199]. The development of a lymphoid infiltrate in the stomach is almost invariably a consequence of *Helicobacter pylori*-associated chronic gastritis [200], and it seems extremely likely that this provides the aetiological link to the subsequent development of low-grade MALT lymphoma. Further support is provided by laboratory studies, which show that the neoplastic B cells proliferate in response to *H. pylori*, but only of the strain associated with the infection of each individual patient [201]. The mechanism for this phenomenon is dependent on recognition of *H. pylori* antigens by non-neoplastic T cells which provide contact-dependent help to the malignant clone, and it is of great interest that some early lesions of lymphoma will regress and disappear after successful treatment of the *H. pylori* infections, presumably because the antigenic drive is eliminated [202]. In the past, many patients underwent surgical resection following diagnosis, with excellent long-term results which reflect the fact that this disease is often apparently localized at presentation [203]. The future management of these patients may not inevitably involve resection of the primary lesion, and proposals to monitor the response to either treatment of *H. pylori* or cytotoxic chemotherapy, or both by endoscopic surveillance, should take into consideration the fact that clonal lymphoma cells can be readily detected by molecular methods in the regional lymph nodes of a proportion of patients [204,205]. Histologically, some patients with high-grade gastric lymphomas may be viewed as having 'MALT' lymphomas, and it seems likely that the majority of these have arisen from pre-existing low-grade lesions. Although these tumours are also probably related to the effects of previous *H. pylori* infection [204], the cells are no longer responsive to *H. pylori* antigens [201] and the tumour is, therefore, unlikely to respond to eradication of the organism. Anatomical staging of gastrointestinal lymphomas is not ideal using the Ann Arbor Classification [10], so a modification to identify patients as II_{E1} when nodes proximal to the stomach are involved and II_{E2} to acknowledge nodal involvement, which is more distal but still within the abdomen, has been proposed [206]. Patients with high-grade disease are much more likely to have evidence of spread beyond the stomach [207], but in an extensive retrospective study comparing the features of low-grade and high-grade gastric MALT lymphomas, 37% of low-grade patients had evidence of disease beyond the stomach and the incidence of marrow involvement was 14.5% [208]. Stage was the only significant variable affecting survival in this study, and a comparison of patients with disease confined to the abdomen (I, II_{E1}, II_{E2}) showed a 95% 5-year survival, compared to 34% for stages III and IV ($P < 0.001$); disseminated disease does not appear to be curable, but both surgery and radiotherapy are capable of producing long-term disease-free survival for patients with stage I or II disease [209].

Lymphomas arising from extranodal sites other than the stomach, but with the features of marginal zone B-cell lymphoma (MZL) or derivation from MALT, present with particular characteristics attributable to their anatomical location, and in some instances arise in a similar way in cases of reactive lymphoid infiltration. Thus salivary gland MZL lymphoma arising in patients with pre-existing Sjögren's syndrome

[210,211], and similarly thyroid lymphomas arising in glands affected by prior Hashimoto's thyroiditis [212], might be reasonably linked to the pre-existing disorders, while MZL arising in the breast, lung or small intestine do not have such a clear origin [191,194,210,211]. MZL affecting the lacrimal glands and conjunctivae forms a well-defined subgroup of patients in whom the morphological appearance correlates well with the prospects of the disease remaining localized [213]. Rare lymphomas of the skin [214] and thymus [215] may also be derived from B cells of the marginal zone. Management of this group of patients with extranodal marginal zone lymphoma depends on careful anatomical staging; truly localized disease will respond well to initial radiotherapy, but the natural history is of dissemination in about one-third of patients over long periods and with involvement of other extranodal sites [216]; there is also an incidence of transformation to more aggressive histology.

Nodal MZL exists as an entity distinct from the various extranodal forms and may occasionally present with bone marrow involvement and cells in the peripheral blood [217]. Although the clinical course is said to be indolent, a significant proportion of the patients described in papers by pathologists appear to have required combination chemotherapy with anthracycline-containing combinations, and to have had limited responses.

Low-grade non-Hodgkin's lymphoma T-cell types

Mycosis fungoides/Sézary's syndrome (cutaneous T-cell lymphoma)

The tumour cells of this disorder are usually small cells with cerebriform nuclei (occasional similar, but larger cells are seen) which infiltrate the epidermis and, subsequently, the dermis. The cells may also be found in the blood, and the paracortical areas of lymph nodes. In the skin, the infiltrate always features the presence of interdigitating Langerhan's cells. There may be considerable difficulties associated with establishing a firm diagnosis of mycosis fungoides and, in the early stages, the majority of biopsies yield a rather nonspecific picture. Phenotypically, the cells are CD2+ CD3+ CD5+ T cells, usually also expressing CD4 (rarely CD8), and T-cell receptor (TCR) genes are rearranged [218].

Three clinical phases of the disease are recognized—erythematous patches, plaques and tumours. These may present anywhere on the skin, although the covered areas of the trunk and limbs are most commonly involved. Patches are asymmetrical with an irregular outline, pink and sometimes scaly; plaques are similar, but with some degree of induration, and the appearance of tumour nodules which are brownish and may ulcerate is a late stage of the disease. About 15% of patients with mycosis fungoides develop a rapidly progressive form of the disease characterized by generalized erythroderma ('homme rouge') accompanied by intense itching; scaling may be very marked, and alopecia and nail dystrophy may occur. For the full definition of Sézary's syndrome, a triad of erythroderma, lymphadenopathy and more than 10% abnormal peripheral blood mononuclear cells is required. Molecular methods for detecting the TCR rearrangement may be of great help in confirming the diagnosis in morphologically or immunologically indeterminate cases [219], and sensitive reliable PCR approaches based on reverse transcription of RNA are now available [220]. Rearrangements involving other oncogenes, such as *NFKB2/lyt 10*, *tal-1* and *p53*, are reported, but appear to be infrequent [221].

The course of the illness varies considerably from patient to patient; those with low-stage disease have a greater than 80% survival, while patients with high-stage disease have a survival rate of only 20–30% and those with Sézary's syndrome fare particularly badly [222]. For patients with limited local skin involvement, topical treatment with mechlorethamine is effective in controlling the lesions [223], while more extensive disease may respond to total skin electron beam irradiation [224] or 8-methoxypsoralen with ultraviolet A light (PUVA) with or without IFNα [225]; techniques involving extracorporeal photochemotherapy after 8-methoxypsoralen administration to sensitize the lymphoma cells have even been tried for more refractory disease [226]. There is no doubt that IFNα is highly effective therapy for cutaneous T-cell lymphoma (CTL), and as a result of the poor results obtained with conventional chemotherapy [227,228], extensive trials of its activity in early and advanced stage disease have been undertaken [229].

Treatment of CTL with deoxycoformicin and the purine analogues has shown that these agents are highly active and capable of obtaining responses, even in advanced disease. Deoxycoformicin, given on either a weekly low-dose schedule [230,231] or at 5 mg/m² daily for 3 days every 3 weeks [129], can produce durable responses in CTL. However, there is evidence that these patients experience more toxicity than those with other forms of lymphoid malignancy and, therefore, special care must be taken with their management. A similar experience of significant activity, tempered by appreciable toxicity, was noted by investigators using cladribine as a 7-day continuous infusion at doses between 0.05 and 0.15 mg/kg/day [232], while other investigators found less evidence of activity [233]. Fludarabine is also active as a single agent in CTL [234], but appeared to produce unexpected levels of neurological toxicity at conventional doses in patients with mycosis fungoides [235]. Because of the activity of these agents, investigators have utilized IFNα in combination with them, and have shown that it is possible to obtain better response rates with no significant overlap of the toxicities which are anticipated with the use of interferon and either deoxycoformicin [236] or fludarabine [237] alone. The fludarabine study utilized interferon at 5 × 10⁶ U/m² SC on 3 days/week with dose escalation if tolerated, and found this to have acceptable toxicity, while still able to obtain responses

in some patients who had previously received deoxycoformicin/high-dose interferon.

The practical management of patients with this group of disorders can be divided into the management of localized disease and the treatment of either widely disseminated disease involving the skin or disease which has spread to lymph nodes or marrow. Topical therapy of limited skin disease usually starts with the use of moderately potent corticosteroid preparations, such as clobetasol propionate 0.05%, which can be given for repeated local recurrences. More extensive or more refractory disease, for which the cumulative use of topical corticosteroids approaches levels at which systemic toxicity is seen, should be managed with PUVA. Particularly refractory, but well-demarcated, localized skin lesions can be treated with topical mechlorethamine with good palliative results. Control of more extensive disease and the full Sézary syndrome is much more difficult, and the results of conventional alkylating agent-based cytotoxic therapy are not good. Responses may be obtained with superficial radiotherapy with electrons or systemic therapy with IFNα, supplemented by PUVA or purine analogue treatment. The results of treatment in patients whose disease is not controlled by these measures are sufficiently poor that innovative approaches with new drugs, differentiating agents such as retinoids or extracorporeal photochemotherapy are justified [238]. The identification of cytokine dependence of CTL cells on IL-7 and IL-2 may indicate possible means of modifying the proliferation of these cells by interference with the action of these growth factors [239].

A clear understanding of the relationships between CTL and other lymphoproliferative disorders is not yet complete, and an association with HD and lymphomatoid papulosis [240] has been reported which may contain important clues to the aetiology of all three disorders. Lymphomatoid papulosis is histologically distinct from CTL and features large papular lesions which may ulcerate but which generally resolve spontaneously; the behaviour of the lesions is thought to result from secretion by the infiltrating clonal T cells of antiproliferative growth factors of TGFβ type [241].

Peripheral T-cell lymphomas

Histological classification of peripheral T-cell lymphomas (PTCL) is difficult because of their heterogeneity, conceptual difficulties in identifying the malignant clonal population and the marked geographical variation in their incidence. A number of clinical syndromes can be defined, which have sufficiently clear clinical identities to be correlated with morphological subtypes of T-cell lymphoma. However, the assignment of many patients to this group is then a matter of excluding lymphoblastic and anaplastic large cell lymphomas or HD and then seeking positive features in common with other PTCL patients [8]. The cytological range in the lymph node is a mixture of small and large atypical cells, often with

Table 18.6 Clinical variants of PTCL.

	Histology	Phenotype/genotype	Clinical features	Reference
Lennert's lymphoma (Lymphoepitheloid)	Mainly small cell + small clusters of large epithelioid cells	CD4 Ki67 *TCRβ* rearranged variable	Lymphadenopathy + Waldeyer's ring	[244,245]
Angioimmunoblastic lymphoma	Sparse lymphoid cells, many follicular cells	CD4 *TCR* rearranged 75% *IgH* rearranged 10% EBV genomes	Systemic symptoms, fever, weight loss, rash, hypergammaglobulinaemia	[246,247]
Angiocentric lymphoma (?related to lymphomatoid granulomatosis)	Vascular invasion	CD2+ CD− *TCR*—usually genome *IgH*—usually genome EBV genomes	Involvement of lung, nose, palate, skin, haemophagocytic syndrome	[248–250]
Intestinal T-cell lymphoma	Variable cytology with intraepithelial T cells in adjacent mucosa + villous atrophy	CD3+ CD7+ CD8+ *TCRβ* usually rearranged	Usually arises in coeliac disease	[251]
Adult T-cell lymphoma/ leukaemia (ATLL)	Diffuse infiltrate with mixed small/large cells. Hyperlobated cells in blood	CD2+ CD3+ CD5+ CD4+ *TCR* rearranged HTLV 1 genome	Japan/Caribbean/sporadic leukaemia with hepatosplenomegaly and hypercalcaemia	[252]
Hepatosplenic T-cell lymphoma	Medium-size cells infiltrating sinusoids	CD2+ CD3+ CD4− CD8− *TCR* δ or β rearranged	Splenomegaly neutropenia/ thrombocytopenia	[253,254]
Subcutaneous panniculitic T-cell lymphoma	Small and large cells in subcutaneous tissue: necrosis, giant cells	CD2+ CD3+ CD4/8 variable *TCR* rearranged in some	Severe haemophagocytosis	[255]

irregular nuclei, and with variable expression of T-cell antigens (CD3, CD2, CD5, CD7); expression of CD4 is more frequent than CD8, but some tumours are negative for both markers. *TCR* genes are usually, but not invariably, rearranged [242]. The characteristics of some of the more readily identifiable subtypes of PTCL are shown in Table 18.6 and reviewed in other publications [8,243]. A detailed description of ATLL is presented elsewhere in this volume (Chapter 7).

The difficulties encountered in the histological identification of PTCL extend to include problems associated with the criteria by which patients can be graded for the aggressiveness of their disease. It seems likely that many of these disorders undergo histological evolution or progression, with an early stage of clinically relatively unaggressive disease manifested as lymphomatoid papulosis, angioimmunoblastic lymphadenopathy or lymphomatoid granulomatosis, and that during this period clinical responses can be obtained with 'immunosuppressive' therapy consisting of corticosteroids and either azathioprine or cyclophosphamide at low-dose schedules [256,246,249]. Subsequent cytogenetic changes reflect evolution of these clonal processes, and result in an illness that is more readily identifiable as a malignant lymphoma in which the majority of patients have disseminated disease, systemic symptoms are frequent and extranodal involvement is relatively common

[257]. Grading these lymphomas on the basis of the cytology of the lymphoid cells has been undertaken in several series; however, this has not been shown to have an impact on survival (Fig. 18.13) [258]. In most series these patients have been managed with initial radiotherapy if the lesion has been clearly localized, and anthracycline-containing combination chemotherapy for disseminated disease [258–260]. Median survivals in these series were between 2 and 4 years and the results have generally been considered to be poorer than for patients with high-grade NHL, regardless of phenotype. A higher proportion of patients relapse than in series containing exclusively large cell high-grade lymphoma. Although the percentage of second CRs obtained after salvage therapy is not greater for PTCL, there is some suggestion that these patients may live with their disease, without progression, for longer than patients with B-cell lymphomas [261]. In terms of salvage therapy, the anecdotal report of a heavily pretreated patient with Lennert's lymphoma responding to deoxycoformicin [262] will presumably result in assessment of the activity of the other purine analogues in these disorders. The generally bleak view of responsiveness in patients with PTCL may be brightened by observations of clinical activity with *cis*-retinoic acid, which are supported by *in vitro* evidence of the ability to induce differentiation in lymphoma cell lines by a

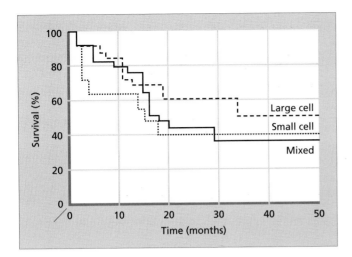

Fig. 18.13 Overall survival of patients with PTCL who received intensive combination chemotherapy regimens grouped by histological subtype. There was no significant difference among the groups. (From Armitage *et al.*, 1989 [258].)

mechanism distinct from that involving the *RARα* gene in acute promyelocytic leukaemia [263]. This data originated from investigators in the Far East, where the geographical incidence of PTCL is greater, but the results of treatment with conventional chemotherapy are no better.

To summarize advice on the treatment of PTCL, those patients in whom there has clearly been evolution to an invasive or disseminated stage should be managed with anthracycline-containing combination chemotherapy as though they were high-grade lymphomas, regardless of the histological assessment of cell size or mix. Consolidation radiotherapy to sites of original major disease involvement may help to prevent recurrence. The outcome with salvage chemotherapy is relatively poor, and innovative chemotherapy with cytotoxic drugs or differentiating agents might be considered early in the management of recurrent disease.

Conclusion

The low-grade NHLs are composed of a number of definable disorders (and, inevitably, also conditions with the manifestations of a malignant, not very aggressive form of lymphoma which resist more accurate definition). The variety arises from the fact that the cells of the immune system from which these disorders originate are varied in appearance, function and preferred site of anatomical location, and further subject to the physiological consequences of reaction to antigenic stimulation or the effects of cytokine secretion by other populations of cells. Given the complexity of this setting, it is more surprising that available forms of therapy may show activity against a number of different forms of malignant proliferation of lymphoid cells than that treatments might be ineffective for indi-

vidual disorders. Of course, radiotherapy and cytotoxic treatment with alkylating drugs are relatively nonspecific means of killing neoplastic cells originating from the lymphoid and many other systems; in fact, these approaches achieve some of their best results when used against lymphomas. Other pharmacological agents also show better activity against lymphoid malignancies than against tumours derived from other organs. Despite these observations, and the range of disorders which may run a very protracted course, the evidence that any available treatment is capable of curing a significant proportion of patients is lacking; the vast majority of patients suffering from these disorders die as a result of their disease, and many of the rest die from the effects of treatment.

The advances in the understanding of the biology of malignant lymphoid cells and their normal equivalents, which have been discussed in this chapter, should form the starting point for the discovery of curative treatment for these diseases. Better comprehension of the limitations of drug treatment, introduction of new active cytotoxic agents, the exploitation of immunological means of targeting lymphoma cells and advances in the handling of the haematological toxicity of high-dose therapy are all important. The possibility of modifying the behaviour of malignant cells by differentiating agents, the manipulation of gene expression or the use of cytokines all constitute exciting areas for future research. Optimism of this sort is an important characteristic for doctors and scientists working in the field of lymphoma treatment, and the energy that it generates will continue to contribute to improving the prospects for patients with these disorders.

It is important that clinicians managing patients with low-grade NHLs do not lose sight of the sad truth that much (if not all) of the treatment they currently give is palliative. This realization should place sensible limits on the toxicity which patients could reasonably be expected to tolerate from any treatment, and the justification that any particular approach is being administered to patients with 'curative intent' should be very carefully examined. It is also central to the relationship between doctors and patients that doctors should not withdraw simply because they have reached the end of their ability to achieve a response from their patients' disease. At this time in the management of patients whose lymphoma is refractory, the trust derived from previous effective treatment must be converted into a belief, by the patients, that their symptoms will be skilfully relieved and that they will not be abandoned to the care of others.

Acknowledgements

Over the years, I have drawn inspiration from Malcolm Phillips, Andrew Lister and Michael Keating, among others; I am especially grateful to Sue McEnroe and Maeve Ewings for checking references, Louise Gwilt and Caroline Ashman for typing the manuscript, and my colleagues, Debbie Richardson, Simon Davies and Simon Rule, for helpful criticism. My daughters, Naomi and Jessica, showed great patience while I was writing this rather than spending my time with them.

References

1 Rappaport H. (1966) Tumors of the hematopoietic system. In: *Atlas of Tumor Pathology*, Section III, Fascicle 8, pp. 97–161. Armed Forces Institute of Pathology, Washington DC.

2 Lennert K. & Mohri N. (1978) Histopathology and diagnosis of non-Hodgkin's Lymphoma. In: *Malignant Lymphomas other than Hodgkin's Disease: histology — cytology — ultrastructure — immunology.* (ed. K. Lennert), pp. 302–313. Springer-Verlag, Berlin.

3 Lukes R.J. & Collins R.D. (1975) New approaches to the classification of the lymphomata. *British Journal of Cancer*, **31**(Suppl. 2), 1–28.

4 The Non-Hodgkin's Lymphoma Pathologic Classification Project, National Cancer Institute sponsored study of classification of Non-Hodgkin's Lymphomas (1982) Summary and description of a Working Formulation for clinical use. *Cancer*, **49**, 2112–2135.

5 Simon R., Durrleman S., Hoppe R.T. *et al.* (1988) The Non-Hodgkin Lymphoma pathologic classification project. Long-term follow-up of 1153 patients with Non-Hodgkin's Lymphomas. *Annals of Internal Medicine*, **109**, 939–945.

6 Sheibani K., Nathwani B.N., Swartz M.S. *et al.* (1988) Variability in interpretation of immunohistologic findings in lymphoproliferative disorders by hematopathologists. A comprehensive statistical analysis of interobserver performance. *Cancer*, **62**, 657–664.

7 Pugh W.C. (1993) Is the working formulation adequate for the classification of the low grade lymphomas? *Leukaemia and Lymphoma*, **10**(Suppl. 1), 1–8.

8 Harris N.L., Jaffe E.S., Stein H. *et al.* (1994) A Revised European-American Classification of lymphoid neoplasms: A proposal from the International Lymphoma Study Group. *Blood*, **84**, 1361–1392.

9 Harris N.L., Jaffe E.S., Stein H. *et al.* (1995) Lymphoma classification proposal: clarification. *Blood*, **85**, 857–860.

10 Carbone P., Kaplan H., Musshoff K., Smithers D.W. & Tubiana M. (1971) Report of the committee on Hodgkin's Disease staging classification. *Cancer Research*, **31**, 1860–1861.

11 The International Non-Hodgkin's Lymphoma Prognostic Factors Project (1993) A predictive model for aggressive non-Hodgkin's Lymphoma. *New England Journal of Medicine*, **329**, 987–994.

12 Lopez-Guillermo A., Montserrat E., Bosch F., Terol M.J., Campo E. & Rozman C. (1994) Applicability of the International Index for aggressive lymphomas to patients with low grade lymphoma. *Journal of Clinical Oncology*, **12**, 1343–1348.

13 Rosenburg S.A. (1985) Karnofsky Memorial Lecture: The Low-Grade Non-Hodgkin's Lymphomas; challenges and opportunites. *Journal of Clinical Oncology*, **3**, 299–310.

14 Ben-Ezra J., Burke J.S., Swartz W.G. *et al.* (1989) Small lymphocytic lymphoma: a clinico-pathologic analysis of 268 cases. *Blood*, **73**, 579–587.

15 Zukerberg L.R., Medeiros L.J.L., Ferry J.A. & Harris N.L. (1993) Diffuse low-grade B-cell lymphomas. Four clinically distinct subtypes defined by a combination of morphologic and immunophenotypic features. *American Journal of Clinical Pathology*, **100**, 373–385.

16 Berger F., Felman P., Sonet A. *et al.* (1994) Non-follicular small B-cell lymphomas: a heterogenous group of patients with distinct clinical features and outcome. *Blood*, **83**, 2829–2835.

17 Harris N.L. & Bhan A.K. (1985) B cell neoplasms of the lymphocytic, lymphoplasmacytoid and plasma cell types: immuno-histological analysis and clinical correlation. *Human Pathology*, **16**, 829–837.

18 Offit K., Parsa N.Z., Filippa D., Jhanwar S.C. & Chaganti R.S.K. (1992) t(9;14)(p13;q32) denotes a subset of low-grade non-Hodgkin's lymphoma with plasmacytoid differentiation. *Blood*, **80**, 2594–2599.

19 Reinhart W.H., Lutolf O., Nydegger U., Mahler F. & Straub P.W. (1992) Plasmapheresis for hyperviscosity syndrome in macroglobulinemia Wäldenstrom and multiple myeloma: influence on blood rheology and the microcirculation. *Journal of Laboratory and Clinical Medicine*, **119**, 69–76.

20 Buskard N.A., Galton D.A.G., Goldman J.M. *et al.* (1977) Plasma exchange in the long term management of Waldenstrom's macroglobulinemia. *Canadian Medical Association Journal*, **117**, 135–137.

21 McCallister B.D., Bayrd E.D., Harrison E.G. Jr & McGuckin W.F. (1967) Primary macroglobulinemia: review with a report on thirty one cases and notes on the value of continuous chlorambucil therapy. *American Journal of Medicine*, **43**, 394–434.

22 Kantarjian H.M., Alexanian R., Koller C.A., Kurzrock R. & Keating M.J (1990) Fludarabine therapy in macroglobulinemic lymphoma. *Blood*, **75**, 1928–1931.

23 Dimopoulos M.A., Kantarjian H.M., Estey E.H. *et al.* (1993) Treatment of Waldenstrom's macroglobulinemia with 2-chlorodeoxyadenosine. *Annals of Internal Medicine*, **118**, 195–198.

24 Dimopoulos M.A., Weber D., Delasalle K.B., Keating M.J. & Alexanian R. (1995) Treatment of Waldenstrom's macroglobulinaemia resistant to standard therapy with 2-chlorodeoxyadenosine: identification of prognostic factors. *Annals of Oncology*, **6**, 49–52.

25 Lardelli P., Bookman M.A., Sundeen J., Longo D.L. & Jaffe E.S. (1990) Lymphocytic lymphoma of intermediate differentiation. Morphologic and immunophenotypic spectrum and clinical correlations. *American Journal of Surgical Pathology*, **14**, 752–763.

26 Harris N.L., Nadler L.M. & Bhan A.K. (1984) Immunohistologic characterization of two malignant lymphomas of germinal center type (centroblastic/centrocytic and centrocytic) with monoclonal antibodies. *American Journal of Pathology*, **117**, 262–272.

27 Banks P.M., Chan J., Cleary M.L. *et al.* (1992) Mantle cell lymphoma. A proposal for unification of morphologic, immunologic and molecular data. *American Journal of Surgical Pathology*, **16**, 637–640.

28 Vandenberghe E., De Wolf-Peeters C., Van den Oord J. *et al.* (1991) Translocation (11;14): a cytogenetic anomaly associated with B-cell lymphomas of non-follicle centre cell lineage. *Journal of Pathology*, **163**, 13–18.

29 Rimokh R., Berger F., Delsol G. *et al.* (1993) Rearrangement and over expression of the *Bcl-1/PRAD-1* gene in intermediate lymphocytic lymphomas and in t(11;q13)-bearing leukaemias. *Blood*, **81**, 3063–3067.

30 Williams M.E., Nichols G.E., Swerdlow S.H. & Stoler M.H. (1995) *In situ* hybridization detection of cyclin D1 mRNA in centrocytic/mantle cell lymphoma. *Annals of Oncology*, **6**, 297–299.

31 De Boer C.J., Schuuring E., Dreef E. *et al.* (1995) Cyclin D1 protein analysis in the diagnosis of mantle cell lymphoma. *Blood*, **86**, 2715–2723.

32 O'Briain D.S., Kennedy M.J., Daly P.A. *et al.* (1989) Multiple lymphomatous papulosis of the gastro-intestinal tract. A clinico-

pathologically distinctive form of non-Hodgkin's lymphoma of B-cell centrocytic type. *American Journal of Surgical Pathology*, **13**, 691–699.

33 Zucca E., Stein H., Coiffier B. on behalf of the European Lymphoma Task Force (1994) European Lymphoma Task Force (ELTF); report on the workshop on Mantle Cell Lymphoma (MCL). *Annals of Oncology*, **5**, 507–511.

34 Segal G.H., Masih A.S., Fox A.C., Jorgensen T., Scott M. & Braylan R.C. (1995) CD5-expressing B-cell non-Hodgkin's lymphomas with *Bcl-1* gene rearrangement have a relatively homogenous immunophenotype and are associated with an overall poor prognosis. *Blood*, **85**, 1570–1579.

35 Coiffier B., Hiddemann W. & Stein H. (1995) Editorial. Mantle cell lymphoma: a therapeutic dilemma. *Annals of Oncology*, **6**, 208–210.

36 Duggan M.J., Weisenburger D.D., Ye Y.L. *et al.* (1990) Mantle zone lymphoma. A clinicopathologic study of 22 cases. *Cancer*, **66**, 522–529.

37 Fisher R.I., Dahlberg S., Nathwani B.N., Banks P.M., Miller T.P., & Grogan T.M. (1995) A clinical analysis of two indolent lymphoma entities; mantle cell lymphoma and marginal zone lymphoma (including the mucosa-associated lymphoid tissue and monocytoid B-cell sub categories): a South West Oncology Group Study. *Blood*, **85**, 1075–1082.

38 Velders G.A., Kluin-Nelemans J.C., De Boer C.J. *et al.* (1996) Mantle cell lymphoma: a population based clinical study. *Journal of Clinical Oncology*, **14**, 1269–1274.

39 Norton A.J., Matthews J., Pappa V. *et al.* (1995) Mantle cell lymphoma: natural history defined in a serially biopsied population over a 20 year period. *Annals of Oncology*, **6**, 249–256.

40 Louie D.C., Offit K., Jastow R. *et al.* (1995) P53 overexpression as a marker of poor prognosis in mantle cell lymphoma with t(11;14)(q13;q32). *Blood*, **86**, 2892–2899.

41 Meusers P., Engelhard M., Bartels H. *et al.* (1989) Multicentre randomized therapeutic trial for advanced centrocytic lymphoma: anthracycline does not improve the prognosis. *Hematological Oncology*, **7**, 365–380.

42 Zucca E., Roggero E., Pinotti G. *et al.* (1995) Patterns of survival in mantle cell lymphoma. *Annals of Oncology*, **6**, 257–262.

43 Whelan J.S., Davis C.L., Rule S. *et al.* (1991) Fludarabine phosphate for the treatment of low grade lymphoid malignancy. *British Journal of Cancer*, **64**, 120–123.

44 Hickish T., Serafinowski P., Cunningham D. *et al.* (1993) 2-Chlorodeoxyadenosine: evaluation of a novel predominantly lymphocyte-selective agent in lymphoid malignancies. *British Journal of Cancer*, **67**, 139–143.

45 Hiddemann W., Unterhalt M., Thiemann M. *et al.* for the German Low Grade Lymphoma Study Group (1994) Characteristics and clinical course of follicle centre lymphomas and mantle cell lymphomas. A study on the clinical relevance of the REAL classification. *Blood*, **84**(Suppl. 1), 449a.

46 Teodorovic I., Pittaluga S., Kluin-Nelemans J.C. *et al.* for the EORTC Lymphoma Co-operative Group (1995) Efficacy of four different regimens in 64 mantle cell lymphoma cases: clinico-pathological comparison with 498 other non-Hodgkin's lymphoma subtypes. *Journal of Clinical Oncology*, **13**, 2819–2826.

47 Stewart D.A., Vose J.M., Weisenburger D.D. *et al.* (1995) The role of high dose therapy and autologous haematopoietic stem cell transplantation for mantle cell lymphoma. *Annals of Oncology*, **6**, 263–266.

48 Bartlett N.L., Rizeq M., Dorfman R.F., Halpern J. & Horning S.J.

49 Hu E., Weiss L.M., Hoppe R.T. & Horning S.J. (1985) Follicular and diffuse mixed small cleaved and large cell lymphoma—a clinicopathologic study. *Journal of Clinical Oncology*, **3**, 1183–1187.

50 Pezzella F., Tse A.G.D., Cordell J.L., Pulford K.A.F., Gatter K.C. & Mason D.Y. (1990) Expression of the *Bcl-2* oncogene protein is not specific for the 14;18 chromosomal translocation. *American Journal of Pathology*, **137**, 225–232.

51 Weiss L.M., Warnke R.A., Sklar J. & Cleary M.L. (1987) Molecular analysis of the t(14;18) chromosomal translocations in malignant lymphomas. *New England Journal of Medicine*, **317**, 1185–1189.

52 Cotter F.E. (1990) The role of the *Bcl-2* gene in lymphoma. *British Journal of Haematology*, **75**, 449–453.

53 McDonnell T.J., Deane N., Platt F.M. *et al.* (1989) *Bcl-2* Immunoglobin transgenic mice demonstrate extended B cell survival and follicular lymphoproliferation. *Cell*, **57**, 79–88.

54 Oltvai Z.N., Milliman C.L. & Korsmeyer S.J. (1993) *Bcl-2* heterodimerizes *in vivo* with a conserved homolog, *Bax*, that accelerates programmed cell death. *Cell*, **74**, 609–619.

55 Pezzella F., Jones M., Ralfkiaer E., Ersboll J., Gatter K.C. & Mason D.Y. (1992) Evaluation of *Bcl-2* protein expression and 14;18 translocation as prognostic markers in follicular lymphoma. *British Journal of Cancer*, **65**, 87–89.

56 Finke J., Slanina J., Lange W. & Dolken G. (1993) Persistence of circulating t(14;18) positive cells in long-term remission after radiation therapy for localised-stage follicular lymphoma. *Journal of Clinical Oncology*, **11**, 1668–1673.

57 Price C.G.A., Meerabux J., Murtagh S. *et al.* (1991) The significance of circulating cells carrying t(14;18) in long remission from follicular lymphoma. *Journal of Clinical Oncology*, **9**, 1527–1532.

58 Limpens J., de Jong D., van Krieken J.H.J.M. *et al.* (1991) *Bcl-2/J*$_H$ rearrangements in benign lymphoid tissues with follicular hyperplasia. *Oncogene*, **6**, 2271–2276.

59 Dölken G., Illerhaus G., Hirt C. & Mertelsman R. (1996) *Bcl-2/J*$_H$ rearrangements in circulating B cells of healthy blood donors and patients with non-malignant disease. *Journal of Clinical Oncology*, **4**, 1333–1344.

60 Poetsch M., Weber-Matthiesen K., Plendl H-J., Grote W. & Schlegelberger B. (1996). Detection of the t(14;18) chromosomal translocation by interphase cytogenetics with yeast-artifical-chromosome probes in follicular lymphoma and non-neoplastic lymphoproliferation. *Journal of Clinical Oncology*, **14**, 963–969.

61 Soubeyran P., Cabanillas F. & Lee M.S. (1993) Analysis of the expression of the hybrid gene *Bcl-2/IgH* in follicular lymphomas. *Blood*, **81**, 122–127.

62 Yano T., Jaffe E.S., Longo D.L. & Raffeld M. (1992) *Myc* rearrangements in histologically progressed follicular lymphomas. *Blood*, **80**, 758–767.

63 Yano T., Sander C.A., Andrade R.E. *et al.* (1993) Molecular analysis of the *Bcl-3* locus at chromosome 17q22 in B-cell neoplasms. *Blood*, **82**, 1813–1819.

64 Sander C.A., Yano T., Clark H.M. *et al.* (1993) p53 mutation is associated with progression in follicular lymphomas. *Blood*, **82**, 1994–2004.

65 Jones S.E., Fuks Z., Bull M. *et al.* (1973) Non-Hodgkin's lymphomas IV. Clinicopathologic correlation in 405 cases. *Cancer*, **31**, 806–823.

66 Cartwright R.A., McKinney P.A. & Barnes N. (1987) Epidemiol-

ogy of the lymphomas in the United Kingdom: recent developments. *Baillière's Clinical Haematology*, **1**, 59–76.

67 Anderson T., DeVita V.T., Simon R.M. *et al.* (1982) Malignant lymphoma II. Prognostic factors and response to treatment of 473 patients at the National Cancer Institute. *Cancer*, **50**, 2708–2721.

68 Rudders R.A., Kaddis M., DeLellis R.A. & Casey H. Jr (1979) Nodular non-Hodgkin's lymphoma (NHL). Factors influencing prognosis and indications for aggressive treatment. *Cancer*, **43**, 1643–1651.

69 Fisher R.I., Jones R.B., DeVita V.T. *et al.* (1981) Natural history of malignant lymphomas with divergent histologies at staging evaluation. *Cancer*, **47**, 2022–2025.

70 Griffin N.R., Howard M.R., Quirke P., O'Brien C.J., Child J.A. & Bird C.C. (1988) Prognostic indicators in centroblastic-centrocytic lymphoma. *Journal of Clinical Pathology*, **41**, 866–870.

71 Macartney J.C., Camplejohn R.S., Morris R., Hollowood K., Clarke D. & Timothy A. (1991) DNA flow cytometry of follicular non-Hodgkin's lymphoma. *Journal of Clinical Pathology*, **44**, 215–218.

72 Lindh J., Jonsson H., Lenner P. & Roos G. (1992) 'Aggressive' low grade lymphocytic lymphomas can be identified by flow cytometric S-phase determinations. *Hematological Oncology*, **10**, 171–179.

73 Richards M.A., Gregory W.M. & Lister T.A. (1987) Prognostic factors in lymphoma. In: *Pointers to Cancer Progress* (ed. B.A. Stoll), pp. 333–357.

74 Leonard R.C.F., Hayward R.L., Prescott R.J., Wang J-X. for the Scotland and Newcastle Lymphoma Group Therapy Working Party (1991) The identification of discrete prognostic groups in low grade non-Hodgkin's lymphoma. *Annals of Oncology*, **2**, 655–662.

75 Child J.A., Spati B., Illingworth S. *et al.* (1980) Serum beta-2 microglobulin and C-reactive protein in the monitoring of lymphomas: findings in a multicentre study and experience in selected patients. *Cancer*, **45**, 318–326.

76 Litam P., Swan F., Cabanillas F. *et al.* (1991) Prognostic value of serum β-2 microglobulin in low grade lymphoma. *Annals of Internal Medicine*, **114**, 855–860.

77 Romaguera J.E., McLaughlin P., North L. *et al.* (1991) Multivariate analysis of prognostic factors in stage IV follicular low-grade lymphoma: a risk model. *Journal of Clinical Oncology*, **9**, 762–769.

78 Bastion Y. & Coiffier B. (1994) Is the International Prognostic Index for aggressive lymphoma patients useful for follicular lymphoma patients? *Journal of Clinical Oncology*, **12**, 1340–1342.

79 Bastion Y., Berger F., Bryon P-A., Felman P., Ffrench M. & Coiffier B. (1991) Follicular lymphomas: assessment of prognostic factors in 127 patients followed for 10 years. *Annals of Oncology*, **2**(Suppl. 2), 123–129.

80 Fuller L.M., Banker F.L., Butler J.J., Gamble J.F. & Sullivan M.P. (1975) The natural history of non-Hodgkin's lymphomata stages I and II. *British Journal of Cancer*, **31**(Suppl. 2), 270–285.

81 Gospodarowicz M.K., Bush R.S., Brown T.C. & Chua T. (1984) Prognostic factors in nodular lymphomas: a multivariate analysis based on the Princess Margaret Hospital experience. *International Journal of Radiation, Oncology, Biology and Physics*, **10**, 489–497.

82 MacManus M. & Hoppe R.T. (1996) Is radiotherapy curative for stage I and II low-grade follicular lymphoma? Results of a long-term follow-up study of patients treated at Stanford University. *Journal of Clinical Oncology*, **14**, 1282–1290.

83 McLaughlin P., Fuller L.M., Velasquez W.S., Sullivan-Halley J.A., Butler J.J. & Cabanillas F. (1986) Stage I–II follicular lymphoma. Treatment results for 76 patients. *Cancer*, **58**, 1596–1602.

84 Gomez G.A., Barcos M., Krishnamsetty R.M., Panahon A.M., Han T. & Henderson E.S. (1986) Treatment of early—stages I and II—nodular poorly differentiated lymphocytic lymphoma. *American Journal of Clinical Oncology*, **9**, 40–44.

85 Monfardini S., Banfi A., Bonadonna G. *et al.* (1980) Improved 5 year survival after combined radiotherapy-chemotherapy for Stage I–II non-Hodgkin's lymphoma. *International Journal of Radiation Oncology, Biology, Physics*, **6**, 125–134.

86 Lawrence T.S., Urba W.J., Steinberg S.M. *et al.* (1988) Retrospective analysis of stage I and II indolent lymphomas at the NCI. *International Journal of Radiation Oncology, Biology, Physics*, **14**, 417–424.

87 Richards M.A., Gregory W.M., Hall P.A. *et al.* (1989) Management of localised non-Hodgkin's lymphoma: the experience at St Bartholomew's Hospital 1972–1985. *Hematological Oncology*, **7**, 1–18.

88 Seymour J.F., McLaughlin P., Fuller L.M. *et al.* (1996) High rate of prolonged remissions following combined modality therapy for patients with localised low-grade lymphoma. *Annals of Oncology*, **7**, 157–163.

89 Corbally N., Grogan L., Dervan P.A. & Carney D.N. (1992) The detection of specific gene rearrangements in non-Hodgkin's lymphoma using the polymerase chain reaction. *British Journal of Cancer*, **66**, 805–809.

90 Diss T.C., Peng H., Wotherspoon A.C., Isaacson P.G. & Pan L. (1993) Detection of monoclonality in low-grade B-cell lymphomas using the polymerase chain reaction is dependent on primer selection and lymphoma type. *Journal of Pathology*, **169**, 291–295.

91 Hickish T.F., Purvies H., Mansi J., Soukop M. & Cunningham D. (1991) Molecular monitoring of low grade non-Hodgkin's lymphoma by gene amplification. *British Journal of Cancer*, **64**, 1161–1163.

92 Lambrechts A.C., Hupkes P.E., Dorssers L.C.J. & Van't Veer M.B. (1993) Translocation (14;18) positive cells are present in the circulation of the majority of patients with localized (stage I and II) follicular non-Hodgkin's lymphoma. *Blood*, **82**, 2510–2516.

93 Richardson D.S., Johnson S.A., Hopkins J.A., Howe D. & Phillips M.J. (1994) Absence of minimal residual disease detectable by FACS, Southern blot or PCR in patients with chronic lymphocytic leukaemia treated with fludarabine. *Acta Oncologica*, **33**, 627–630.

94 Ezdinli E.Z., Stutzman L., Aungst C.W. & Firat D. (1969) Corticosteroid therapy for lymphomas and chronic lymphocytic leukaemia. *Cancer*, **23**, 900–909.

95 Jones S.E., Rosenberg S.A., Kaplan H.S., Kadin M.E. & Dorfman R.F. (1972) Non-Hodgkin's lymphoma II—single agent chemotherapy. *Cancer*, **30**, 31–38.

96 Bagley C.M. Jr, DeVita V.T., Berard C.W. & Canellos G.P. (1972) Advanced lymphosarcoma: intensive clinical combination chemotherapy with cyclophosphamide, vincristine and prednisolone. *Annals of Internal Medicine*, **76**, 227–234.

97 Gall E.A. & Mallory T.B. (1942) Malignant lymphoma: a clinicopathological survey of 618 cases. *American Journal of Pathology*, **18**, 381–429.

98 Portlock C.S. & Rosenberg S.A. (1979) No initial therapy for Stage III and IV non-Hodgkin's lymphomas of favourable histologic types. *Annals of Internal Medicine*, **90**, 10–13.

99 Horning S.J. & Rosenberg S.A. (1984) The natural history of initially untreated low-grade non-Hodgkin's lymphoma. *New England Journal of Medicine*, **311**, 1471–1475.

100 Young R.C., Longo D.L., Glatstein E., Ihde D.C., Jaffe E.S. &

DeVita V.T. (1988) The treatment of indolent lymphomas: watchful waiting v aggressive combined modality treatment. *Seminars in Hematology*, **25**, 11–16.

101 O'Brien M.E.R., Easterbrook P., Powell J. *et al.* (1991) The natural history of low grade non-Hodgkin's lymphoma and the impact of a no initial treatment policy on survival. *Quarterly Journal of Medicine*, **80**, 651–660.

102 Hoppe R.T., Kushlan P., Kaplan H.S., Rosenberg S.A. & Brown B.W. (1981) The treatment of advanced stage favourable histology non-Hodgkin's lymphoma: a preliminary report of a randomized trial comparing single agent chemotherapy, combination chemotherapy and whole body irradiation. *Blood*, **58**, 592–598.

103 Brereton H.D., Young R.C., Longo D.L. *et al.* (1979) A comparison between combination chemotherapy and total body irradiation plus combination chemotherapy in non-Hodgkin's lymphoma. *Cancer*, **43**, 2227–2231.

104 Lister T.A., Cullen M.H., Beard M.E.J. *et al.* (1978) Comparison of combined and single-agent chemotherapy in non-Hodgkin's lymphoma of favourable histological type. *British Medical Journal*, **1**, 533–537.

105 Hoppe R.T. (1983) Patterns of failure after treatment for the non-Hodgkin's lymphomas. *Cancer Treatment Symposia*, **2**, 133–136.

106 Anderson T., Bender R.A., Fisher R.I. *et al.* (1977) Combination chemotherapy in non-Hodgkin's lymphoma: results of long term follow up. *Cancer Treatment Reports*, **61**, 1057–1066.

107 Longo D.L., Young R.C., Hubbard S.M. *et al.* (1984) Prolonged initial remission in patients with nodular mixed lymphoma. *Annals of Internal Medicine*, **100**, 651–656.

108 Glick J.H., Barnes J.M., Ezdinli E.Z., Berard C.W., Orlow E.L. & Bennet J.M. (1981) Nodular mixed lymphoma; results of a randomised trial failing to confirm prolonged disease-free survival with COPP chemotherapy. *Blood*, **58**, 920–925.

109 Parlier Y., Gorin N.C., Najman A., Stachowiak J. & Duhamel G. (1982) Combination chemotherapy with cyclophosphamide, vincristine, prednisolone and the contribution of adriamycin in the treatment of adult non-Hodgkin's lymphoma. A report of 131 cases. *Cancer*, **50**, 401–409.

110 Dana B.W., Dahlberg S., Nathwani B.N. *et al.* (1993) Long-term follow-up of patients with low-grade malignant lymphomas treated with doxorubicin-based chemotherapy or chemoimmunotherapy. *Journal of Clinical Oncology*, **11**, 644–651.

111 Licht J.D., Bosserman L.D., Andersen J.W. *et al.* (1990) Treatment of low-grade and intermediate grade lymphoma with intensive combination chemotherapy results in long-term disease-free survival. *Cancer*, **66**, 632–639.

112 McLaughlin P., Cabanillas F., Hagemeister F.B. *et al.* (1993) CHOP-Bleo plus Interferon for Stage IV low-grade lymphoma. *Annals of Oncology*, **4**, 205–211.

113 Morel P., Dupriez B., Plantier-Colcher I. *et al.* (1993) Long-term outcome of follicular low-grade lymphoma. A report of 91 patients. *Annals of Hematology*, **66**, 303–308.

114 Johnson P.M.W., Rohatiner A.Z.S., Whelan J.S. *et al.* (1995) Patterns of survival in patients with recurrent follicular lymphoma: a 20 year study from a single centre. *Journal of Clinical Oncology*, **13**, 140–147.

115 Foon K.A., Sherwin S.A., Abrams P.G. *et al.* (1984) Treatment of advanced non-Hodgkin's lymphoma with recombinant leukocyte A Interferon. *New England Journal of Medicine*, **311**, 1148–1152.

116 Smalley R.V., Andersen J.W., Hawkins M.J. *et al.* (1992) Interferon alfa combined with cytotoxic chemotherapy for patients with non-Hodgkin's lymphoma. *New England Journal of Medicine*, **327**, 1336–1341.

117 Price C.G.A., Rohatiner A.Z.S., Steward W. *et al.* (1991) Interferon-alpha 2 B in the treatment of follicular lymphoma; preliminary results of a trial in progress. *Annals of Oncology*, **2**(Suppl. 2), 141–145.

118 Hagenbeek A., Carde P., Somers R. *et al.* (1992) Maintenance of remission with human recombinant alpha-2 interferon (Roferon-A) in patients with Stages III and IV low grade malignant non-Hodgkin's lymphoma. Results from a prospective randomised phase III clinical trial in 331 patients. *Blood*, **80**(Suppl. 1), 74a.

119 Peterson B.A., Petroni G., Oken M.M. & Ozer H. (1993) Cyclophosphamide versus cyclophosphamide plus interferon alpha-2b in follicular low-grade lymphomas: a preliminary report of an intergroup trial (CALGB 8691 and EST 7486). *Proceedings of the American Society of Clinical Oncology*, **12**, 1240 (abstract).

120 Solal-Celigny P., Lepage E., Brousse N. *et al.* for GELA. (1993) Recombinant interferon alfa-2b combined with a regimen containing doxorubicin in patients with advanced follicular lymphoma. *New England Journal of Medicine*, **329**, 1608–1614.

121 Miyashita T. & Reed J.C. (1993) *Bcl*-2 oncoprotein blocks chemotherapy-induced apoptosis in a human leukaemia cell line. *Blood*, **81**, 151–157.

122 Gallagher C.J. & Lister T.A. (1987) Follicular non-Hodgkin's lymphoma. *Baillière's Clinical Haematology*, **1**, 141–155.

123 Lambrechts A.C., Hupkes P.E., Dorssers L.C.J. & Van't Veer M.B. (1994) Clinical significance of t(14;18)-positive cells in the circulation of patients with stage III or IV follicular non-Hodgkin's lymphoma during first remission. *Journal of Clinical Oncology*, **12**, 1541–1546.

124 Gams R.A., Bryan S., Dukart G. *et al.* (1985) Mitoxantrone in malignant lymphomas. *Investigational New Drugs*, **3**, 219–222.

125 Bernard T., Johnson S.A., Prentice A.G., Jones L., Phillips M.J. & Newland A.C. (1994) Mitoxantrone, chlorambucil and prednisolone in the treatment of non-Hodgkin's lymphoma. *Leukemia and Lymphoma*, **15**, 481–485.

126 McLaughlin P., Cabanillas F., Hagemeister F.B. & Velasquez W. (1987) Activity of bisantrene in refractory lymphoma. *Cancer Treatment Reports*, **71**, 631–633.

127 Spinolo J.A., Cabanillas F., Dixon D.O. *et al.* (1992) Therapy of relapsed or refractory low grade follicular lymphomas: factors associated with complete remission, survival and time to treatment failure. *Annals of Oncology*, **3**, 227–232.

128 Duggan D.B., Anderson J.R., Dillman R., Case D. & Gottlieb K.J. (1990) 2 Deoxycoformycin (Pentostatin) for refractory non-Hodgkin's Lymphoma. A CALGB phase II study. *Medical and Pediatric Oncology*, **18**, 203–206.

129 Cummings F.J., Kim K., Neiman R.S. *et al.* (1991) Phase II trial of pentostatin in refractory lymphomas and cutaneous T cell disease. *Journal of Clinical Oncology*, **9**, 565–571.

130 Seto S., Carrera C.J., Kubota M., Wasdon D.B. & Carson D.A. (1985) Mechanism of deoxyadenosine and 2-chlorodeoxyadenosine toxicity to non-dividing human lymphomas. *Journal of Clinical Investigation*, **75**, 377–383.

131 Grever M.R., Kraut E.H., Neidhart J.A. & Malspeis L. (1984) 2-Fluora-ara-AMP; a phase I clinical investigation. 4th NCI-EORTC symposium on new drugs in cancer therapy Brussels 1984. *Investigational New Drugs*, **2**, 116.

132 Leiby J.M., Snider K.M., Kraut E.H. *et al.* (1987) Phase II trial of 9-β-D-arabinofuranosyl-2-fluoroadenine 5 — monophosphate in

non-Hodgkin's lymphoma: prospective comparison of response with deoxycytidine kinase activity. *Cancer Research*, **47**, 2719–2722.

133 Hochster H.S., Kim K., Green M.D. *et al.* (1992) Activity of fludarabine in previously treated non-Hodgkin's low grade lymphoma: results of an ECOG study. *Journal of Clinical Oncology*, **10**, 28–32.

134 Redman R.J., Cabanillas F., Velasquez W.S. *et al.* (1992) Phase II trial of fludarabine phosphate in lymphoma: an effective new agent in low grade lymphoma. *Journal of Clinical Oncology*, **10**, 790–794.

135 Zinzani P.L., Lauria F., Rondelli D. *et al.* (1993) Fludarabine: an active agent in the treatment of previously-treated and untreated low-grade non-Hodgkin's lymphoma. *Annals of Oncology*, **4**, 575–578.

136 Solal-Celigny P., Brice P., Brousse N. *et al.* (1996) Phase II trial of fludarabine monophosphate as first-line treatment in patients with advanced follicular lymphoma: a multicenter study by the Groupe d'Etude des lymphomes de l'Adulte. *Journal of Clinical Oncology*, **14**, 514–519.

137 Kay A.C., Saven A., Carrera C.J. *et al.* (1992) 2 Chlorodeoxyadenosine treatment of low-grade lymphomas. *Journal of Clinical Oncology*, **10**, 371–377.

138 Hoffman M., Tallman M.S., Hakimian D. *et al.* (1994) 2 Chlorodeoxyadenosine is an active salvage therapy in advanced indolent non-Hodgkin's lymphoma. *Journal of Clinical Oncology*, **12**, 788–792.

139 Betticher D.C., Zucca E., Von Rohr A. *et al.* (1996) 2 Chlorodeoxyadenosine (2-CdA) therapy in previously untreated patients with follicular stage III–IV non-Hodgkin's lymphoma. *Annals of Oncology*, **7**, 793–799.

140 Beutler E., Piro L.D., Savan A. *et al.* (1991) 2 Chlorodeoxyadenosine (2-CdA): a potent chemotherapeutic and immunosuppressive nucleoside. *Leukemia and Lymphoma*, **5**, 1–8.

141 Liliemark J., Albertioni F., Hassan M. & Juliusson G. (1992) On the bioavailability of oral and subcutaneous 2-chloro-2-deoxyadensine in humans: alternative routes of administration. *Journal of Clinical Oncology*, **10**, 1514–1518.

142 Keating M.J. (1993) Immunosuppression with purine analogues — the flip side of the gold coin. *Annals of Oncology*, **4**, 347–348.

143 O'Brien S., Kantarjian H., Beran M. *et al.* (1993) Results of fludarabine and prednisolone therapy in 264 patients with chronic lymphocytic leukaemia with multivariate analysis-derived prognostic model for response to treatment. *Blood*, **82**, 1695–1700.

144 Maung Z.T., Wood A.C., Jackson G.H., Turner G.E., Appleton A.L. & Hamilton P.J. (1994) Transfusion associated Graft-versus-Host disease in Fludarabine treated B-chronic lymphocytic leukaemia. *British Journal of Haematology*, **88**, 649–652.

145 Zulian G.B., Roux E., Tiercy J-M. *et al.* (1995) Transfusion-associated graft-versus-host disease in a patient treated with Cladribine (2-chlorodeoxyadenosine): demonstration of exogenous DNA in various tissue extracts by PCR analysis. *British Journal of Haematology*, **89**, 83–89.

146 Tefferi A., Witzig E.T., Reid J.M., Li C-Y. & Ames M.M. (1994) Phase I study of combined 2-chlorodeoxyadenosine and chlorambucil in chronic lymphoid leukaemia and low-grade lymphoma. *Journal of Clinical Oncology*, **12**, 569–576.

147 Elias L., Stock-Novack D., Head D.R. *et al.* (1993) A phase I trial of combination fludarabine monophosphate and chlorambucil in chronic lymphocytic leukaemia: a Southwest Oncology Group Study. *Leukaemia*, **7**, 361–365.

148 McLaughlin P., Hagemeister F.B., Swan F. Jr. *et al.* (1994) Phase I study of the combination of fludarabine, mitoxantrone and dexomethasone in low grade lymphoma. *Journal of Clinical Oncology*, **12**, 575–579.

149 Robertson L.E., Kantarjian H., O'Brien S. *et al.* (1993) Cisplatin, fludarabine and ara C (CFA): a regimen for advanced fludarabine — refractory chronic lymphocytic leukaemia (CLL). *Proceedings of the American Society of Clinical Oncology*, **12**, A1014.

150 McLaughlin P., Hagemeister F.B., Romagnera J.E. *et al.* (1996) Fludarabine, mitoxantrone and dexamethasone: an effective new regimen for indolent lymphomat. *Journal of Clinical Oncology*, **14**, 1262–1268.

151 McLaughlin P., Cabanillas F., Younes A. *et al.* (1996) Stage IV low-grade lymphoma: randomized trial of two innovative regimens, with monitoring of *BCL*-2 by PCR. *Annals of Oncology*, **7**(Suppl. 3), A109, 34.

152 Robertson L.E., Chubb S., Meyn R.E. *et al.* (1993) Induction of apoptotic cell death in chronic lymphocytic leukaemia by 2-chloro-2-deoxyadenosine and 9β-D-arabinosyl-2-fluoroadenine. *Blood*, **81**, 143–150.

153 Vuist W.M.J., Levy R. & Maloney D.G. (1994) Lymphoma regression induced by monoclonal anti-idiotypic antibodies correlates with their ability to induce Ig signal transduction and is not prevented by tumor expression of high levels of Bcl-2 protein. *Blood*, **83**, 899–906.

154 Carroll W.L., Thielemans K., Dilley J. & Levy R. (1986) Mouse × human heterohybridomas as fusion partners with human B cell tumors. *Journal of Immunological Methods*, **89**, 61–72.

155 Thielemans K., Maloney D.G., Meeker T. *et al.* (1984) Strategies for production of monoclonal anti-idiotype antibodies against human B-cell lymphomas. *Journal of Immunology*, **133**, 495–501.

156 Levy R. & Miller R.A. (1990) Therapy of lymphoma directed at idiotypes. *Journal of the National Cancer Institute Monographs*, **10**, 61–68.

157 Meeker T.C., Lowder J., Maloney D.G. *et al.* (1985) A clinical trial of anti-idiotype therapy for B-cell malignancy. *Blood*, **65**, 1349–1363.

158 Brown S.L., Miller R.A., Horning S.J. *et al.* (1989) Treatment of B-cell lymphomas with anti-idiotype antibodies alone and in combination with alpha Interferon. *Blood*, **73**, 651–661.

159 Maloney D.G., Brown S., Czerwinski D.K. *et al.* (1992) Monoclonal anti-idiotype antibody therapy for B-cell lymphoma: the addition of a short course of chemotherapy does not interfere with the anti-tumor effect nor prevent the emergence of idiotype-negative variant cells. *Blood*, **80**, 1502–1510.

160 Hamblin T.J., Cattan A.R., Glennie M.J. *et al.* (1987) Initial experience in treating human lymphoma with a chimeric univalent derivative of monoclonal anti-idiotype antibody. *Blood*, **69**, 790–797.

161 Lowder J.N., Meeker T.C., Campbell M. *et al.* (1987) Studies on B lymphoid tumors treated with monoclonal anti-idiotype antibodies: correlation with clinical response. *Blood*, **69**, 199–210.

162 Maloney D.G., Liles T.M., Czerwinski D.K. *et al.* (1994) Phase I clinical trial using escalating single-dose infusion of chimeric anti-CD20 monoclonal antibody (IDEC-C2B8) in patients with recurrent B-cell lymphoma. *Blood*, **84**, 2457–2466.

163 Grillo-Lopez A.J., Varns C., Waldichuk C. *et al.* (1996) IDEC-C2B8: clinical development of a chimeric anti-CD20 antibody for the treatment of patients with relapsed low-grade or follicular NHL. *Annals of Oncology*, **7**(Suppl. 1), A190, 56.

164 Czuczman M., Grillo-Lopez A.J., McLaughlin P. *et al.* (1996) The

anti-CD20 antibody IDEC-C2B8 clears lymphoma cells bearing the t(14;18) translocation from the peripheral blood and bone marrow of a proportion of patients with low-grade or follicular non-Hodgkin's lymphoma. *Annals of Oncology*, **7**(Suppl. 5), A532P, 111.

165 Grossbard M.L., Press O.W., Appelbaum F.R., Bernstein I.D. & Nadler L.M. (1992) Monoclonal antibody-based therapies of leukaemia and lymphoma. *Blood*, **80**, 863–878.

166 Vitetta E.S., Stone M., Amlot P. *et al.* (1991) Phase I immunotoxin trial in patients with B-cell lymphoma. *Cancer Research*, **51**, 4052–4058.

167 Amlot P.L., Stone M.J., Cunningham D. *et al.* (1993) A Phase I study of an anti CD22-deglycosylated ricin A chain immunotoxin in the treatment of B-cell lymphomas resistant to conventional therapy. *Blood*, **82**, 2624–2633.

168 Grossbard M.L., Freedman A.S., Ritz J. *et al.* (1992) Serotherapy of B-cell neoplasms with anti-B4-blocked ricin: a phase I trial of daily bolus infusion. *Blood*, **79**, 576–585.

169 Kaminski M.S., Zasadny K.R., Francis I.R. *et al.* (1993) Radioimmunotherapy of B-cell lymphoma with [^{131}I] anti-B1 (anti CD20) antibody. *New England Journal of Medicine*, **329**, 459–465.

170 Kaminski M.S., Zasadny K.R., Francis I.R., *et al.* (1996) Iodine-131-antiB1 radioimmunotherapy for B-cell lymphoma. *Journal of Clinical Oncology*, **14**, 1974–1981.

171 Armitage J.O. (1989) Bone marrow transplantation in the treatment of patients with lymphoma. *Blood*, **73**, 1749–1758.

172 Gribben J.G., Saporito L., Barber M. *et al.* (1992) Bone marrows of non-Hodgkin's lymphoma patients with a *Bcl*-2-translocation can be purged of polymerase chain reaction-detectable lymphoma cells using monoclonal antibodies and immunomagnetic bead depletion. *Blood*, **80**, 1083–1089.

173 Weisdorf D.J., Andersen J.W., Glick J.H. & Oken M.M. (1992) Survival after relapse of low-grade non-Hodgkin's lymphoma: implications for marrow transplantations. *Journal of Clinical Oncology*, **10**, 942–947.

174 Rohatiner A.Z.S., Johnson P.W.M., Price C.G.A. *et al.* (1994) Myeloblative therapy with autologous bone marrow transplantation as consolidation therapy for recurrent follicular lymphoma. *Journal of Clinical Oncology*, **12**, 1117–1184.

175 Gribben J.G., Freedman A.S., Woo S.D. *et al.* (1991) All advanced stage non-Hodgkin's lymphomas with a polymerase chains reaction amplificable breakpoint of *Bcl*-2 have residual cells containing the *Bcl*-2 rearrangment at evaluation and after treatment. *Blood*, **78**, 3275–3280.

176 Gribben J.G., Neuberg D., Freedman A.S. *et al.* (1993) Detection by polymerase chain reaction of residual cells with the *Bcl*-2 translocation is associated with increased risk of relapse after autologous bone marrow transplantation for B-cell lymphoma. *Blood*, **81**, 3449–3457.

177 Zwicky C.S., Maddocks A.B., Andersen N. & Gribben J.G. (1996) Eradication of polymerase chain reaction detectable immunoglobin gene rearrangement in non-Hodgkin's lymphoma is associated with decreased relapse after autologous bone marrow transplantation. *Blood*, **88**, 3314–3322.

178 Fouillard L., Gorin N.C., Laporte J.P. *et al.* (1991) Feasibility of autologous bone marrow transplantation for early consolidation of follicular non-Hodgkin's lymphoma. *European Journal of Haematology*, **46**, 279–284.

179 Colombat P., Binet C.H. & Linassier C. (1992) High dose chemotherapy with autologus marrow transplanation in follicular lymphoma. *Leukemia and Lymphoma*, **7**, 3–6.

180 Freedman A.S., Ritz J., Neuberg D. *et al.* (1991) Autologous bone marrow transplantation in 69 patients with a history of low-grade B-cell non-Hodgkin's lymphoma. *Blood*, **77**, 2524–2529.

181 Johnson P.M.W., Price C.G.A., Smith T. *et al.* (1994) Detection of cells bearing the t(14;18) translocation following myeloablative treatment and autologous bone marrow transplantation for follicular lymphoma. *Journal of Clinical Oncology*, **12**, 798–805.

182 Bastion Y., Brice P., Haioun C. *et al.* (1996) Intensive therapy with peripheral blood progenitor cell transplantation in 60 patients with poor-prognosis follicular lymphoma. *Blood*, **86**, 3257–3262.

183 Hardingham J.E., Kotasek D., Sage R.E. *et al.* (1995) Significance of molecular marker-positive cells after autologous peripheral-blood stem-cell transplantation for non-Hodgkin's lymphoma. *Journal of Clinical Oncology*, **13**, 1073–1079.

184 Haas R., Moos M., Karcher A. *et al.* (1994) Sequential high-dose therapy with peripheral blood progenitor cell support in low-grade non-Hodgkin's lymphoma. *Journal of Clinical Oncology*, **12**, 1685–1692.

185 Reed J.C., Stein C., Subasinghe C. *et al.* (1990) Antisense-mediated inhibition of *Bcl*-2 proto-oncogene expression and leukaemic cell growth and survival: comparison of phosphodiester and phosphorothioate oligodeoxynucleotides. *Cancer Research*, **50**, 6565–6570.

186 Jones R.J., Ambinder R.F., Piantadosi S. & Santos G.W. (1991) Evidence of a graft versus lymphoma effect associated with allogeneic bone-marrow transplantation. *Blood*, **77**, 649–653.

187 Van Besien K.W., Khouri I.F., Giralt S.A. *et al.* (1995) Allogeneic bone marrow transplantation for refractory and recurrent low-grade lymphoma: the case for aggressive management. *Journal of Clinical Oncology*, **13**, 1096–1102.

188 Bezwoda W.R. & Rastogi R.B. (1994) A randomized comparative study of cyclophosphamide, vincristine, doxorubicin and prednisolone and cyclophosphamide, vincristine, mitoxantrone and prednisolone regimens in the treatment of intermediate and high-grade lymphoma with 8 years follow up. *Seminars in Hematology*, **31**(Suppl. 3), 3.

189 Zinzani P.L., Tura S., Cajozzo A. *et al.* (1993) Anthracycline containing regimens in intermediate grade lymphoma. *Leukemia and Lymphoma*, **10**(Suppl.), 39–41.

190 Isaacson P. & Wright D.H. (1983) Malignant lymphoma of mucosa-associated lymphoid tissue. A distinctive type of B-cell lymphoma. *Cancer*, **52**, 1410–1416.

191 Isaacson P.G. & Spencer J. (1987) Malignant lymphoma of mucosa-associated lymphoid tissue. *Histopathology*, **11**, 445–462.

192 Pelstring R.J., Essell J.H., Kurtin P.J., Cohen A.R. & Banks P.M. (1991) Diversity of organ site involvement among malignant lymphomas of mucosa-associated tissues. *American Journal of Clinical Pathology*, **96**, 738–745.

193 Cousar J.B., McGinn D.L., Glick A.D., List A.F. & Collins R.D. (1987) Report of an unusual lymphoma arising from parafollicular B-lymphocytes (PBLs) or so-called 'monocytoid' lymphocytes. *American Journal of Clinical Pathology*, **87**, 121–128.

194 Nizze H., Cogliatti S.B., Von Schilling C., Feller A.C. & Lennert K. (1991) Monocytoid B-cell lymphoma: morphological variants and relationship to low-grade B-cell lymphoma of the mucosa-associated lymphoid tissue. *Histopathology*, **18**, 403–414.

195 Sanchez L., Algara P., Villuendas R. *et al.* (1993) B-cell clonal detection in gastric low-grade lymphoma and regional lymph nodes: an immunohistologic and molecular study. *American Journal of Gastroenterology*, **88**, 413–419.

196 Wotherspoon A.C., Pan L.X., Diss T.C. & Isaacson P.G. (1990) A

genotypic study of low grade B-cell lymphomas, including lymphomas of mucosa associated lymphoid tissue (MALT). *Journal of Pathology*, **162**, 135–140.

197 Wotherspoon A.C., Finn T.M. & Isaacson P.G. (1995) Trisomy 3 in low-grade B-cell lymphomas of mucosa-associated lymphoid tissue. *Blood*, **85**, 2000–2004.

198 Severson R.K. & Davis S. (1990) Increasing incidence of primary gastric lymphoma. *Cancer*, **66**, 1283–1287.

199 Doglioni C., Wotherspoon A.C., Moschini A., De Boni M. & Isaacson P.G. (1992) High incidence of primary gastric lymphoma in North Eastern Italy. *Lancet*, **339**, 834–835.

200 Genta R.M., Hamner H.W. & Graham D.Y. (1993) Gastric lymphoid follicles in *Helicobacter pylori* infection: frequency, distribution, and response to triple therapy. *Human Pathology*, **24**, 577–583.

201 Hussell T., Isaacson P.G., Crabtree J.E. & Spencer J. (1993) The response of cells from low-grade B-cell gastric lymphomas of mucosa-associated lymphoid tissue to *Helicobacter pylori*. *Lancet*, **342**, 571–574.

202 Wotherspoon A.C., Doglioni C., Diss T.C. *et al.* (1993) Regression of primary low-grade B-cell gastric lymphoma of mucosa-associated lymphoid tissue type after eradication of *Helicobacter pylori*. *Lancet*, **342**, 575–577.

203 Shepherd F.A., Evans W.K., Kutas G. *et al.* (1988) Chemotherapy following surgery for stages I E and II E non-Hodgkin's lymphoma of the gastrointestinal tract. *Journal of Clinical Oncology*, **6**, 253–260.

204 Parsonnet J., Hansen S., Rodriguez L. *et al.* (1994) *Helicobacter pylori* infection and gastric lymphoma. *New England Journal of Medicine*, **330**, 1267–1271.

205 Zucca E. & Roggero E. (1996) Biology and treatment of MALT lymphoma: the state of the art in 1996. *Annals of Oncology*, **7**, 787–792.

206 Mussholff K. (1977) Klinische Stadieneinteilung der nicht-Hodgkin's Lymphoma. *Strahlentherapie*, **153**, 218–221.

207 Cogliatti S.B., Schmid U., Schumacher U. *et al.* (1991) Primary B-cell gastric lymphoma: a clinicopathological study of 145 patients. *Gastroenterology*, **101**, 1159–1170.

208 Montalban C., Castrillo J.M., Abraira V. *et al.* (1995) Gastric B-cell mucosa-associated lymphoid tissue (MALT) lymphoma. Clinicopathological study and evaluation of the prognostic factors in 143 patients. *Annals of Oncology*, **6**, 355–362.

209 D'Amore F., Brincker H., Gronbaek K. *et al.* for the Danish Lymphoma Study Group (1994) Non-Hodgkin's lymphoma of the gastro-intestinal tract: a population-based analysis of incidence, geographic distribution, clinicopathologic presentation features and prognosis. *Journal of Clinical Oncology*, **12**, 1673–1684.

210 Ngan B-Y., Warnke R.A., Wilson M., Takagi K., Cleary M.L. & Dorfman R.F. (1991) Monocytoid B-cell lymphoma: a study of 36 cases. *Human Pathology*, **22**, 409–421.

211 Sheibani K, Burke J.S., Swartz W.G., Nademanee A. & Winberg C.D. (1988) Monocytoid B-cell lymphoma: clinicopathologic study of 21 cases of a unique type of low-grade lymphoma. *Cancer*, **62**, 1531–1538.

212 Hyjek E. & Isaacson P. (1988) Primary B-cell lymphoma of the thyroid and its relationship of Hashimoto's thyroiditis. *Human Pathology*, **19**, 1315–1326.

213 Medeiros L.J., Harmon D.C., Linggood R.M. & Harris N.L. (1989) Immunohistologic features predict clinical behaviour of orbital and conjunctival lymphoid infiltrates. *Blood*, **74**, 2121–2129.

214 Santucci M. Pimpinelli N. & Arganini L. (1991) Primary cutaneous B-cell lymphoma: a unique type of low-grade lymphoma. *Cancer*, **67**, 2311–2326.

215 Isaacson P.G., Chan J.K.C., Tang C. & Addis B.J. (1990) Low grade B-cell lymphoma of mucosa-associated lymphoid tissue arising in the thymus. *American Journal of Surgical Pathology*, **14**, 342–351.

216 Mattia A., Ferry J. & Harris N. (1993) Breast lymphoma: a B-cell spectrum including the low-grade B-cell lymphoma of mucosa associated lymphoid tissue. *American Journal of Surgical Pathology*, **17**, 574–587.

217 Carbone A., Gloghini A., Pinto A., Attadia V., Zagonel V. & Volpe R. (1989) Monocytoid B-cell lymphoma with bone-marrow and peripheral blood involvement at presentation. *American Journal of Clinical Pathology*, **92**, 228.

218 Weiss L.M., Hu E., Wood G.S. *et al.* (1985) Clonal rearrangements of T-cell receptor genes in mycosis fungoides and dermatopathic lymphadenopathy. *New England Journal of Medicine*, **313**, 539–544.

219 Xerri L., Horschowski N., Boudaouara T., Grob J.J., Lejeune C. & Hassoun J. (1991) Cutaneous lymphomas of phenotypically undetermined lineage: contribution of genotypic analyses. *Journal of the American Academy of Dermatology*, **25**, 33–40.

220 Lynas C., Howe D., Copplestone J.A., Johnson S.A.N. & Phillips M.J. (1995) A rapid and reliable PCR method for detecting clonal T-cell populations. *Journal of Clinical Pathology Molecular Pathology*, **48**, M101–M104.

221 Neri A., Fracchiolla N.S., Roscetti E. *et al.* (1995) Molecular analysis of cutaneous B and T-cell lymphomas. *Blood*, **86**, 3160–3172.

222 Bunn P.A. Jr, Hoffman S.J., Norris D., Golitz L.E. & Aeling J.L. (1994) Systemic therapy of cutaneous T-cell lymphomas (mycosis fungoides and the Sézary syndrome). *Annals of Internal Medicine*, **121**, 592–602.

223 Vonderheid E., Tan E., Kantor A., Shrager L., Micaily B. & Van Scott E.J. (1989) Long-term efficacy, curative potential and carcinogenicity of topical mechlorethamine chemotherapy in cutaneous T-cell lymphoma. *Journal of the American Academy of Dermatology*, **20**, 416–428.

224 Hoppe R., Cox R., Fuks Z., Price N.M., Bagshawe M.A. & Farber E.M. (1979) Electron beam therapy for mycosis fungoides: the Stanford experience. *Cancer Treatment Reports*, **63**, 691–700.

225 Roenig H, Kuzel T. & Skoutelis A. (1990) Photo chemistry alone or combined in interferon alpha 2A in the treatment of cutaneous T-cell lymphoma. *Journal of Investigative Dermatology*, **95**(Suppl.), 1985–2055.

226 Heald P., Rook A., Perez M. *et al.* (1992) Treatment of erythrodermic cutaneous T-cell lymphoma with extra-corporeal photochemotherapy. *Journal of the American Academy of Dermatology*, **27**, 427–433.

227 Kaye F.J., Bunn P.A., Steinberg S.M. *et al.* (1989) A randomized trial comparing combination electron beam radiation and chemotherapy with topical therapy in the intital treatment of mycosis fungoides. *New England Journal of Medicine*, **321**, 1784–1790.

228 Winkler C.F., Sausville E.A., Ihde D.C. *et al.* (1986) Combined modality treatment of cutaneous T-cell lymphoma: results of a 6 year follow-up. *Journal of Clinical Oncology*, **4**, 1094–1100.

229 Papa G., Tura S., Mandelli F. *et al.* (1991) Is interferon alpha in cutaneous lymphoma a treatment of choice? *British Journal of Haematology*, **79**(Suppl. 1), 48–51.

230 Grever M.R., Bisaccia E., Scarborough D.A., Metz E.N. & Neidhart J.A. (1983) An investigation of 2-deoxycoformycin in the treatment of cutaneous T-cell lymphoma. *Blood*, **61**, 279–282.

231 Ho A.D., Thaler J., Willemze R. *et al.* (1990) Pentostatin (2-deoxy-coformicin) for the treatment of lymphoid neoplasms. *Cancer Treatment Reviews*, **17**, 213–215.

232 Saven A., Carrera C.J., Carson D.A., Beutler E. & Piro L.D. (1992) 2-Chlorodeoxyadenosine: an active agent in the treatment of cutaneous T-cell lymphoma. *Blood*, **80**, 587–592.

233 O'Brien S., Kurzrock R., Duvic M. *et al.* (1994) 2-Chlorodeoxyadenosine therapy in patients with T-cell lympho-proliferative disorders. *Blood*, **84**, 733–738.

234 Von Hoff D.D., Dahlberg S., Hartstock R.J. & Eyre H.J. (1990) Activity of fludarabine monophosphate in patients with advanced mycosis fungoides: a South West Oncology Group study. *Journal of the National Cancer Institute*, **82**, 1353–1355.

235 Cohen R.B., Abdallah J.M., Gray J.R. & Foss F. (1993) Reversible neurological toxicity in patients treated with standard dose fludarabine phosphate for mycosis fungoides and chronic lymphocytic leukaemia. *Annals of Internal Medicine*, **118**, 114–116.

236 Foss F.M., Ihde D.C., Breneman D.L. *et al.* (1992) Phase II study of pentostatin and intermittent high dose recombinant interferon alfa 2A in advanced mycosis fungoides/Sézary syndrome. *Journal of Clinical Oncology*, **10**, 1907–1913.

237 Foss F.M., Ihde D.C., Linnoila I.R., *et al.* (1994) Phase II trial of fludarabine phosphate and interferon alfa-2A in advanced mycosis fungoides/Sézary syndrome. *Journal of Clinical Oncology*, **12**, 2051–2059.

238 Diamandidou E., Cohen P.R. & Kurzrock R. (1996) Mycosis fungoides and Sézary syndrome. *Blood*, **88**, 2385–2409.

239 Foss F.M., Koc Y., Stetler-Stevenson M.A. *et al.* (1994) Costimulation of cutaneous T-cell lymphoma cells by interleukin 7 and interleukin 2: potential autocrine or paracrine effectors in the Sézary syndrome. *Journal of Clinical Oncology*, **12**, 326–335.

240 Davis T.H., Morton C.C., Miller-Cassman R., Balk S.P. & Kadin M.E. (1992) Hodgkin's disease, lymphomatoid papulosis and cutaneous T-cell lymphoma derived from a common T-cell clone. *New England Journal of Medicine*, **326**, 1115–1122.

241 Newcom S.R., Kadin M.E. & Ansari A.A. (1988) Production of transformation growth factor-beta activity by Ki-1 positive lymphoma cells and analysis of its role in the regulation of Ki-1 positive lymphoma growth. *American Journal of Pathology*, **131**, 569–577.

242 Takagi N., Nakamura S., Ueda R., Osada H. *et al.* (1992) A phenotypic and genotypic study of three node-based, low-grade peripheral T-cell lymphomas: angioimmunoblastic lymphoma, T-zone lymphoma and lymphoepithelioid lymphoma. *Cancer*, **69**, 2571–2582.

243 Suchi T., Lennert K., Tu L-Y. *et al.* (1987) Histopathology and immunohistochemistry of peripheral T-cell lymphomas: a proposal for their classification. *Journal of Clinical Pathology*, **40**, 995–1015.

244 Feller A.C., Griesser G.H., Mak T.W. & Lennert K. (1986) Lympho-epithelioid lymphoma (Lennert's lymphoma) is a monoclonal proliferation of helper/inducer T-cells. *Blood*, **68**, 663–667.

245 Patsouris E., Noel H. & Lennert K. (1988) Histological and immuno-histological findings in lymphoepithelioid cell lymphoma (Lennert's lymphoma). *American Journal of Surgical Pathology*, **12**, 341–350.

246 Cullen M.H., Stansfeld A.G., Oliver R.T.D., Lister T.A. & Malpas J.S. (1979) Angioimmunoblastic lymphadenopathy: report of ten cases and review of the literature. *Quarterly Journal of Medicine*, **189**, 151–177.

247 Weiss L.M., Jaffe E.S., Liu X-F., Chen Y-Y., Shibata D. & Medeiros L.J. (1992) Detection and localisation of Epstein–Barr viral genomes in angioimmunoblastic lymphadenopathy and angioimmunoblastic lymphadenopathy-like lymphoma. *Blood*, **79**, 1789–1795.

248 Lipford E.H. Jr, Margolick J.B., Longo D.L., Fauci A.S. & Jaffe E.S. (1988) Angiocentric immunoproliferative lesions: a clinicopathologic spectrum of post-thymic T-cell proliferations. *Blood*, **72**, 1674–1681.

249 Fauci A.S., Haynes B.F., Costa J., Katz P. & Wolff S.M. (1982) Lymphomatoid granulomatosis: prospective clinical and therapeutic experience over 10 years. *New England Journal of Medicine*, **306**, 68–74.

250 Chan J.K.C., Ng C.S., Lau W.H. & Lo S.T.H. (1987) Most nasal/nasopharyngeal lymphomas are peripheral T-cell neoplasms. *American Journal of Surgical Pathology*, **11**, 418–429.

251 Isaacson P.G., Spencer J., Connolly C.E. *et al.* (1985) Malignant histiocytosis of the intestine: a T-cell lymphoma. *Lancet*, **ii**, 688–691.

252 Kikuchi M., Mitsui T., Takeshita M., Okamura H., Natoh H. & Eimoto T. (1986) Virus associated adult T-cell leukaemia (ATL) in Japan: clinical, histological and immunological studies. *Hematological Oncology*, **4**, 67–81.

253 Farcet J-P., Gaulard P., Marolleau J-P. *et al.* (1990) Hepatosplenic T-cell lymphoma: sinusal/sinusoidal localization of malignant cells expressing the T-cell receptor γ. *Blood*, **75**, 2213–2219.

254 Kruskall M.S., Weitzman S.A., Stossel T.P., Harris N. & Robinson S.H. (1982) Lymphoma with autoimmune neutropenia and hepatic sinusoidal infiltration: a syndrome. *Annals of Internal Medicine*, **97**, 202–205.

255 Gonzalez C.L., Medeiros L.J., Braziel R.M. & Jaffe E.S. (1991) T-cell lymphoma involving subcutaneous tissue: a clinicopathologic entity commonly associated with hemophagocytic syndrome. *American Journal of Surgical Pathology*, **15**, 17–27.

256 Karp D.L. & Horn T.D. (1994) Continuing medical education: lymphomatoid papulosis. *Journal of the American Academy of Dermatology*, **30**, 379–395.

257 Schlegelberger B., Zwingers T., Hohenadel K. *et al.* (1996) Significance of cytogenetic findings for the clinical outcome in patients with T-cell lymphoma of angioimmunoblastic lymphadenopathy type. *Journal of Clinical Oncology*, **14**, 593–599.

258 Armitage J.O., Greer J.P., Levine A.M. *et al.* (1989) Peripheral T-cell lymphoma. *Cancer*, **63**, 158–163.

259 Chott A., Augustin I., Wrba F., Hanak H., Ohlinger W. & Radaszkiewicz T. (1990) Peripheral T-cell lymphomas: a clinicopathologic study of 75 cases. *Human Pathology*, **21**, 1117–1125.

260 Remotti D., Pescarmona E., Burgio V.L. *et al.* (1992) Prognostic value of the histologic classification of peripheral T-cell lymphoma: a clinicopathologic study of 71 HTLV-1 negative cases. *Leukemia and Lymphoma*, **8**, 371–380.

261 Coiffer B., Brousse N., Peuchmaur M. *et al.* for the GELA (1990) Peripheral T-cell lymphomas have a worse prognosis than B-cell lymphomas: a prospective study of 361 immunophenotyped patients with the LNH-84 regime. *Annals of Oncology*, **1**, 45–50.

262 Lowenthal R.M., Wiley J.S., Rooney K.F., Challis D.R. & Woods G.M. (1990) Lennert's lymphoma: response to 2-deoxycoformicin. *British Journal of Haematology*, **76**, 555–556.

263 Cheng A-L., Su I-J., Chen C-C. *et al.* (1994) Use of retinoic acids in the treatment of peripheral T-cell lymphoma: a pilot study. *Journal of Clinical Oncology*, **12**, 1185–1192.

19 Non-Hodgkin's Lymphoma: Histologically Aggressive

D.C. Linch

Introduction

The term 'histologically aggressive non-Hodgkin's lymphoma' (NHL) is used here to encompass NHL with 'nonindolent' histology or 'non-low-grade' lymphomas. The histologically aggressive lymphomas include the intermediate-grade and high-grade NHLs, as classified in the Working Formulation, with the exception of the diffuse small cleaved lymphomas, most of which are mantle cell lymphomas or marginal cell lymphomas (Revised European–American Lymphoma (REAL) Classification) and are discussed in the preceding chapter. The proportion of histologically indolent and histologically aggressive lymphomas shows marked geographic variation [1]. In the UK, the incidence of NHL is 8.2/100 000 per annum, and approximately half are histologically aggressive [2]. In the USA the incidence of NHL is higher, at 13.7/100 000 in 1989, and the proportion of histologically aggressive lymphomas is greater. Histologically indolent lymphomas are relatively rare in Japan, even in HTLV-I nonendemic areas. The incidence of NHL in the USA appears to be rising, although the trend is less convincing in Europe [3].

Aetiology

The cause of the large majority of histologically aggressive NHLs is unknown. Only rarely can ionizing irradiation or chemical carcinogens be clearly implicated, although it has been hypothesized that exposure to solvents and herbicides may be relevant in some localities [4]. Several viruses are also involved in the pathogenesis of histologically aggressive NHL. The Epstein–Barr virus (EBV) was originally implicated in endemic Burkitt's lymphoma [5], but it also plays an important role in B-cell lymphomas arising in immunosuppressed individuals, and in some post-thymic T-cell lymphomas [6]. EBV is most readily detected in tumour cells by *in situ* hybridization using probes specific for EBV small RNAs (EBERs). In Burkitt's lymphoma the typical pattern of latent gene expression is *EBNA1+, EBNA2–, LMP1–*, whereas in B-cell lymphomas arising in immunodeficient patients, it is typically *EBNA1+, EBNA2+, LMP1+*, and in HD *EBNA1+, EBNA2–, LMP +* [5]. The consistent finding is the expression of *EBNA1*, suggesting that this is of importance in the pathogenesis of the malignancy. *EBNA1* transgenic mice have been generated with the transgene expression directed to the B-cell compartment using the mouse heavy-chain intron enhancer, and indeed these mice do develop monoclonal follicular centre cell-derived lymphomas [7]. The mechanism of EBV-induced lymphomagenesis is still not fully clear however. EBV induces polyclonal B-cell activation and can immortalize some B cells *in vitro*. *In vivo* it may cause a block in differentiation, with continued proliferation and cell survival. Expression of LMP-1 upregulates a range of cell surface molecules, including the adhesion molecules ICAM-1, LFA-1 and LFA-3. The LMP-1 molecule is able to act like a constitutively activated surface receptor, in similar way to CD40 (a member of the TNF receptor family), and is able to activate NFκB [8].

Lymphomas, nearly always of the histologically aggressive variety, have become more common in immunosuppressed patients since the advent of AIDS and the increase in organ transplantation. Lymphoma has been reported to occur in 4–10% of patients with AIDS and the pathogenesis is almost certainly multifactorial. Apart from the increased risk of infections with oncogenic viruses such as EBV, chronic antigen exposure and cytokine stimulation arising from repeated infections results in polyclonal B-cell activation and, therefore, a greater chance of mutations that develop randomly during mitosis. Approximately 20% of centroblastic lymphomas, 35% of Burkitt-like lymphomas, 75% of immunoblastic lymphomas and virtually all small noncleaved cell lymphomas and cases of HD arising in the immunosuppressed are EBV+. Lymphomas arise in less than 1% of allogeneic bone marrow transplant recipients, although the risk is higher in those cases where rigorous T-cell depletion has been carried out and heavy postgraft immunosuppression given. In heart/lung transplants the incidence is as high as 4–7% [9]. Most post-transplant lymphomas are EBV related. In the early stages they may be polyclonal or oligoclonal and only later become monoclonal, but the clonal nature of the proliferation does not appear to predict closely for the response to withdrawal of immunosuppression, which may result in spontaneous remission.

HTLV-I is an RNA-containing 'c-type retrovirus' involved in the development of adult T-cell leukaemia/lymphoma, which has been predominantly described in individuals from Japan and the Caribbean basin. The virus conforms to the usual retroviral structure of 'LTR-gag-pol-env-LTR', and between the env and 3'LTR is a region referred to as pX. This contains four overlapping open-reading frames, one of which codes for a protein known as Tax. This appears to transactivate the transcription of a set of cellular genes involved in T-cell growth. This includes the IL-2 receptor and, in the early stages, possibly also IL-2, giving the potential for autocrine growth [10]. This would be polyclonal but could facilitate malignant progression (multistep pathogenesis) in a small number of infected individuals.

Classification of histologically aggressive non-Hodgkin's lymphoma

Two classification systems have been most widely used in recent years — in Europe the Kiel Classification (Table 19.1)

Table 19.1 Kiel Classification (updated).

B-cell lymphomas	T-cell lymphomas
Low grade	
Lymphocytic—chronic lymphocytic and prolymphocytic leukaemia	Lymphocytic—chronic lymphocytic and prolymphocytic leukaemia
Hairy cell leukaemia	Small, cerebriform cell, mycosis fungoides, Sézary's syndrome
Lymphoplasmactic (cytoid) (lymphoplasmacyte immunocytoma)	Lymphoepithelioid (Lennert's lymphoma)
Plasmacytic	Angioimmunoblastic
Centroblastic centrocytic Follicular ± diffuse Diffuse	T zone
Centrocytic	Pleomorphic, small cell (HTLV±)
High grade	
Centroblastic	Pleomorphic, medium and large cell (HTLV-I±)
Immunoblastic	Immunoblastic (HTLV-I±)
Large cell anaplastic (Ki-1±)	Large cell anaplastic (Ki-1±)
Burkitt's lymphoma	
Lymphoblastic	Lymphoblastic
Rare types	

Table 19.2 Working Formulation.

Grade	Types of malignant lymphoma (ML)	Subcategories
Low	a ML Small lymphocytic	Consistent with CLL / Plasmacytoid
	b ML Follicular predominantly small cleaved cell	Diffuse areas / Sclerosis
	c ML Follicular mixed small cleaved and large cell	Diffuse areas / Sclerosis
Intermediate	d ML Follicular predominantly large cell	Diffuse areas / Sclerosis
	e ML Diffuse small cleaved cell	Sclerosis
	f ML Diffuse mixed small and large cell	Sclerosis / Epithelioid cell component
	g ML Diffuse large cleaved cell, noncleaved cell	Sclerosis
High	h ML Large cell immunoblastic	Plasmacytoid / Clear cell / Polymorphous / Epithelioid cell component
	i ML Lymphoblastic	Convoluted cell / Nonconvoluted cell
	j ML Small noncleaved cell Burkitt's	Sclerosis / Follicular areas
Miscellaneous	Composite / Mycosis fungoides / Histiocytic / Extramedullary plasmacytoma / Unclassifiable / Other	

Table 19.3 The REAL Classification of NHL.

A *B-cell neoplasms*
  i Precursor B-cell neoplasms
     B-lymphoblastic leukaemia/lymphoma
  ii Peripheral B-cell neoplasms
     1 B-cell chronic lymphocytic leukaemia
        B-cell prolymphocytic leukaemia
        Small lymphocytic lymphoma
     2 Lymphoplasmacytoid lymphoma/immunocytoma
     3 Mantle cell lymphoma
     4 Germinal centre lymphoma
     5 Marginal zone B-cell lymphoma
        Extranodal (MALT type ± monocytoid B cells)
        Nodal ± monocytoid B cells
        Splenic ± villous lymphocytes
     6 Hairy cell leukaemia
     7 Plasmacytoma/myeloma
     8 Diffuse large B-cell lymphoma
        Subtype: primary mediastinal (thymic) B-cell lymphoma
     9 Burkitt's lymphoma
    10 *High grade B-cell lymphoma, Burkitt-like*

B *T-cell and putative NK-cell neoplasms*
  i Precursor T-cell neoplasms
     T-lymphoblastic lymphoma/leukaemia
  ii Peripheral T-cell and NK-cell neoplasms
     1 T-cell chronic lymphocytic leukaemia
        T-cell prolymphocytic leukaemia
     2 Large granular lymphocyte leukaemia (LGL)
        T-cell type
        NK-cell type
     3 Mycosis fungoides/Sézary's syndrome.
     4 Adult T-cell lymphoma/leukaemia (ATLL)
     5 Angioimmunoblastic T-cell lymphoma (AILD)
     6 Angiocentric lymphoma
     7 Intestinal T-cell lymphoma (± enteropathy associated)
     8 Peripheral T-cell lymphomas not otherwise specified.
        (small, mixed/medium, large)
        Lymphoepithelioid cell lymphoma (Lennert's)
     9 Anaplastic large cell lymphoma (ALCL)
        CD30+, T- and null-cell types
    10 *Anaplastic large-cell lymphoma, Hodgkin-like*

Categories/subtypes in italics are provisional.

Table 19.4 Classification of cutaneous lymphomas.

B-cell lymphomas
  Histologically indolent
    B-cell chronic lymphocytic leukaemia (B-CLL)
    Marginal zone B-cell lymphoma (MALT-like)
    Follicle centre lymphomas
  Histologically aggressive
    Follicle centre lymphomas (large cell)

T-cell lymphomas
  Histologically indolent
    Mycosis fungoides/Sézary's syndrome
    T-cell chronic lymphocytic leukaemia/prolymphocytic leukaemia
      (T-CLL/PLL)
  Histologically aggressive
    CD30+ anaplastic lymphomas
    Adult T-cell leukaemia/lymphoma (ATLL)
    Other

and in the USA the Working Formulation (Table 19.2) [11,12]. Neither system is ideal. In the Working Formulation distinction between low-, intermediate- and high-grade lymphoma is supposed to be clinically based and yet the categories are not in accord with current practice. Immunoblastic lymphomas, for instance, have the same prognosis as other large cell lymphomas, and are treated in the same way in nearly all centres. The entity of follicular large cell lymphoma is a difficult diagnostic category, as these lymphomas usually show areas of diffuse large cell lymphoma and are often classified as such by many histopathologists. No account is taken in the Working Formulation of immunophenotype and various distinct

biological entities are not recognized, including angioimmunoblastic lymphoma, which may appear as either diffuse mixed small and large cell lymphoma or as diffuse large cell immunoblastic lymphoma in the Working Formulation, and anaplastic CD30+ large cell lymphomas, which have a frequent specific chromosomal translocation. These entities are recognized in the Kiel Classification, but other specific histologically aggressive lymphomas, such as the enteropathy-associated T-cell lymphomas (EATCLs) of the gut, are not. The Kiel classification has also been criticised for its complexity and lack of reproducibility in certain categories. The distinction between centroblastic, B-immunoblastic and B-large cell anaplastic lymphomas, can for instance be quite subjective. In response to such criticisms the International Lymphoma Study Group proposed a Revised European and American Lymphoma (REAL) Classification (Table 19.3) [13]. This classification is reproducible and recognizes most distinctly biological entities, which will become increasingly important as and when specific therapies for distinct entities are developed. It is, however, very complex and includes the lymphoid leukaemias, over 20 major categories of lymphoma and other additional subtypes and provisional types. The REAL Classification does not ascribe 'grade' to the different entities, and this can be problematical for the clinician. Defining eligibility for trial entry using the REAL Classification can be quite cumbersome.

The large majority of histologically aggressive lymphomas are of B-cell type. Lymphoblastic lymphomas are usually of T-cell type, but account for less than 5% of adult lymphomas. Adult T-cell leukaemia/lymphoma is rare, except in HTLV-I endemic areas. In a recent immunophenotypic analysis of cases of stages II–IV histologically aggressive lymphomas carried out by the British National Lymphoma Investigation (BNLI), only 43 out of 337 (12%) were thought to be of T-cell origin (K. MacLennan *et al.*, unpublished data). This concurs with other series, where the reported proportion of T-cell lymphomas varies between 10 and 20%.

The REAL Classification did not deal specifically with primary cutaneous lymphomas and there is some debate about whether a specific cutaneous classification is required. A possible classification is shown in Table 19.4. The cutaneous follicular cell lymphomas are both phenotypically and genotypically distinct from the nodal follicular centre cell lymphomas, with t(14;18) being rare, and some authorities consider these to be B-cell marginal zone lymphomas rather than follicular centre cell derived.

Chromosomal abnormalities

Cytogenetic abnormalities can usually be found in the histologically aggressive NHL, although it can be difficult to obtain good quality karyotypes. The abnormalities are often numerical or structurally complex, but a number of common translocations have now been defined (Table 19.5). The rearrangements frequently involve the TcR genes (α and δ genes on chromosome 14q11; β gene on chromosome 7q35; γ gene on 7q15) and the immunoglobin genes (heavy chain on chromosome 14q32; Kappa chain on chromosome 2p12; lambda chain on chromosome 22q11), which rearrange normally as part of the process to T- and B-cell generation. In some cases the aberrant recombination may be a result of structural similarities between the regions close to the breakpoints and the heptamer nonamer recombinase-recognition sequences bordering the normally rearranged genes [14]. The rearrangements typically mediate the expression of either fusion proteins encompassing tyrosine kinases or transcription factors or the dysregulated expression of structurally normal transcription factors.

The t(14;18) translocation, typically found in histologically indolent follicular lymphomas (see Chapter 18), is also found in approximately 20% of disseminated large cell lymphomas. In addition, a significant proportion of large cell lymphomas express relatively high levels of BCL2 protein without a t(14;18). The presence of BCL2 protein predicts for a higher relapse rate and a lower overall survival [15,16].

The BCL6 gene on chromosome 3q27 is rearranged in about 30% of all large cell lymphomas and there are many possible translocation partners, although the Ig heavy-chain, and, to a lesser extent, light-chain loci account for over 50% of cases [17,18]. Point mutations within the BCL6 regulatory regions have also been found [19]. Such mutations appear to be extremely frequent in AIDS lymphomas [20]. The BCL6 gene is a transcription factor of the zinc finger family and the BCL6 protein is usually expressed in the nuclei of normal germinal centre cells, although its precise function is not known. The presence of translocations upregulating BCL6 are associated with an increased tendency to extranodal disease. One study suggested this was also associated with an improved prognosis [17], but this was not confirmed in another study [18]. BCL6

Table 19.5 Selected translocations present in histologically aggressive NHL.

Translocations	Genes involved		Type of lymphoma
t(8;14)(q24;q32)	C-MYC	IgH	Burkitt's lymphoma
t(8;2)(p11/2;q24)	C-MYC	Igκ	
t(8;22)(q24;q11)	C-MYC	Igλ	
t(14;18)(q32;q21)	BCL2	IgH	Some large cell lymphomas, but more common in follicular lymphomas
t(3;14)(q27;q32)	BCL6	IgH	Large cell
t(3;v)(q27;v)	BCL6	v	
t(2;5)(p23;q35)	ALK	Nucleophosmin	CD30+ anaplastic large cell lymphoma (ALCL)

rearrangements were also found in 14% of follicular lymphomas and were associated with a good prognosis [21].

A high proportion of the anaplastic CD30+ large cell lymphomas have a t(2;5)(p23;q35) translocation [22]. This translocation is also found in some cases of lymphomatoid papulosis and pleomorphic large cell lymphomas of the skin. The translocation is not found in HD, which is another CD30+ tumour, nor in the Hodgkin's-like anaplastic large cell lymphomas. The genes involved in this translocation are a receptor tyrosine kinase (anaplastic lymphoma kinase (ALK) on chromosome 2 and nucleophosmin on chromosome 5 [23]. This results in high-level expression of a fusion protein (NPM/ALK) with kinase activity; this kinase is usually silent in lymphoid cells.

The usual cytogenetic abnormality in Burkitt's lymphoma is a translocation involving chromosome 8 and 14, which is found in over 80% of cases t(8;14)(q24;q32). Although both the endemic and sporadic forms of Burkitt's lymphoma have the same gross translocations, there are subtle differences at the molecular level. Variant translocations involve chromosome 8 with either chromosome 2 or 22 [24]. In all cases there is upregulation of C-MYC, which is a nuclear transcription factor involved in cell proliferation, and the regulation of apoptosis, brought about by the vicinity of immunoglobulin gene enhancer sequences to the C-MYC gene.

T-cell lymphomas are rarer than B-cell lymphomas and have been less studied at the molecular level. T-cell lymphoblastic lymphomas may have similar abnormalities to those found in T-cell acute lymphoblastic leukaemia (T-ALL) such as abnormalities of the TAL 1 gene on chromosome 11. The anaplastic CD30+ lymphomas referred to above are usually of T-cell origin.

The presence of a common translocation where the break-

Table 19.6 The Ann Arbor Staging System.

Stage I	Disease in one lymph-node area only
Stage II	Disease in two or more lymph-node areas on the same side of the diaphragm
Stage III	Disease in lymph-node areas on both sides of the diaphragm (the spleen is considered to be nodal)
Stage IV	Extensive disease in liver, bone marrow or other extranodal sites
Substage E	Localized extranodal disease
Symptom status A	Absence of fevers, sweats or weight loss
Symptom status B	Unexplained fevers >38°C
	Drenching night sweats
	Weight loss of >10% in preceding 6 months

Table 19.7 The St Jude Staging System for childhood NHL.

Stage 1	A single tumour (extranodal or single anatomical nodal area) with the exclusion of the mediastinum or abdomen
Stage 2	A single extranodal tumour with regional node involvement Two or more nodal areas on the same side of the diaphragm Two single extranodal tumours ± regional node involvement on the same side of the diaphragm A primary gastrointestinal tumour ± mesenteric nodes (not extensive)
Stage 3	Two or more extranodal tumours on opposite sides of the diaphragm Two or more nodal areas on opposite sides of the diaphragm Primary intrathoracic tumours Extensive primary intra-abdominal disease Paraspinal or epidural tumours
Stage 4	Any of the above with CNS and or bone marrow involvement

point falls within a well-defined and limited region(s), allows specific PCR analysis either to assist diagnosis or for the detection of minimal residual disease (MRD). The clinical significance and value of such MRD studies in histologically aggressive lymphomas is yet to be determined.

Staging

Anatomical staging is central to defining prognosis and determining appropriate treatment. The Ann Arbor Staging System is used in adults (Table 19.6) [25] and the St Jude Staging System is usually used in children (Table 19.7) [26]. Inspection of Waldeyer's ring is important, and a bone marrow biopsy should be performed in all patients. Although a laparotomy may sometimes be required to relieve a gut obstruction, or stop a haemorrhage or to make a diagnosis of disease restricted to the abdomen, a staging laparotomy per se is not indicated. Computerized tomography is the standard approach for staging intrathoracic and intra-abdominal disease, although in specific circumstances, such as bone or nervous system involvement, magnetic resonance imaging may be useful. Positron emission tomography, using [18]fluoradesoxyglucose, appears to be valuable for the evaluation of residual masses, and may therefore find a role in initial staging to determine which tumours are 'hot' [27].

Risk of central nervous system disease

Post-mortem studies have shown that central nervous system (CNS) involvement is frequently found in patients, with histologically aggressive lymphomas who die of disseminated disease. From a therapeutic standpoint, however, what matters is the likelihood of developing isolated CNS relapse, or of this being the initial site of more widespread relapse. The risk of spread to the CNS is closely related to the histological type, with the biggest risk being in lymphoblastic lymphoma and Burkitt's (and Burkitt-like) lymphoma (Table 19.8) [28], and in HTLV-I lymphomas [29]. Patients with bone marrow

Table 19.8 Risks of CNS relapse in different histological entities. (Based on data from Finsen Institute, 1985 [28].)

Lymphoma type (Working Formulation)	Incidence
Small lymphocytic	<5%
Follicular-SC	<5%
Follicular-M	<5%
Follicular-L	<5%
Diffuse-SC	<5%
Diffuse-M	<5%
Diffuse-L	5%
Immunoblastic	<5%
Lymphoblastic	24%
SNC	19%

infiltration, testicular lymphomas and lymphoma of the central facial sinuses also have a raised incidence of developing CNS disease, although this relates, in part, to the histological type. CNS disease is also relatively common in immunosuppressed patients, including those infected with HIV [30]. Rarely, histologically aggressive NHL presents as isolated parenchymal CNS disease. This entity is discussed later.

Prognostic factors

Various prognostic factors have been used to identify patients with different long-term prognoses, In 1993 the International Non-Hodgkin's Lymphomas Prognostic Factors Project reported 'a predictive model for aggressive non-Hodgkin's lymphoma', based on an analysis of presenting features and outcome in 2031 patients [31]. Four risk groups were identified on the basis of age, stage, serum LDH levels, performance status and number of extranodal sites. The Eastern Cooperative Oncology Group (ECOG) scale of performance status is shown in Table 19.9. In the low-risk groups (35% of patients), the complete remission (CR) rate was 87% and the overall survival at 5 years was 73%. In the high-risk group the CR rate was 44% and the overall survival at 5 years was only 26%. Age is a major determinant of outcome, but it is of limited value to use this parameter in a predictive model, as it results in the identification of 'poor-risk patients' who might be candidates for more intensive therapy, but are too old to receive it.

For this reason an age-adjusted index was also developed. The index for patients 60 years of age or younger is shown in Table 19.10. The International Index predicted for both CR rate and relapse from CR, which is relevant to considerations of consolidation therapy given in remission. The value of the Prognostic Index was confirmed in the analysis of the GELA LNH 87 trial [32], although it should be noted that the prediction of relapse probably refers to very early relapse rather than that occurring months after completing therapy.

Management

The histologically aggressive lymphomas were once all treated in a similar way. With increasing understanding of the different biological entities and prognostic factors, risk-adjusted approaches to therapy have been adopted (Fig. 19.1).

Table 19.9 ECOG performance status.

0   Able to carry out normal activity without restriction

1   Restricted in physically strenous activity but ambulatory and able to carry out light work

2   Ambulatory and capable of self-care, but unable to carry out any work; up and about more than 50% of waking hours

3   Capable of only limited self-care; confined to bed or chair for more than 50% of waking hours

4   Completely disabled; cannot carry out any self-care; totally confined to bed or chair

Treatment of stage IA lymphomas with a low risk of central nervous system disease

There is a consensus that patients with bulky stage IA lymphomas or patients with stage IB disease should receive combination chemotherapy. Localized lymphoblastic lymphoma, Burkitt's or Burkitt-like lymphomas should also receive disease-specific chemotherapy regimens. Pathologically staged I/IE histologically aggressive lymphomas of other types, without bulky disease or B symptoms, can be cured in over 90% of cases by local radiotherapy [33], but few centres would consider a staging laparotomy to be justified in this condition. There is uncertainty about the appropriate treatment of clinical stage I lymphomas. In a large series of 243 stage I/IE patients without bulk disease or B symptoms reported by the BNLI, 84% obtained a CR, with most of the non complete responses being a result of the rapid appearance of disease outside of the radiation field [34]. The relapse rate was considerable, with less than half the patients achieving and maintaining a CR, but effective salvage with chemotherapy was possible in many patients, especially the non-elderly. In patients under 60 years of age at diagnosis the cause-specific actuarial survival at 10 years was 80%, which is a challenging yardstick by which to judge other therapeutic approaches. Some centres claim better results with combination chemotherapy [35,36], but data from randomized trials are lacking. A Southwest Oncology Group trial of three courses of CHOP alone, followed by involved field radiotherapy vs eight courses of CHOP, in patients with stage I and nonbulky stage II disease, showed a survival advantage for the combined modality arm [37], although the survival difference was a result of excess deaths in the CHOP-alone arm rather than worse disease control. Furthermore, the benefit of three cycles of CHOP plus radiotherapy was only in the 'good prognosis subgroup', and it is not certain that the results are better in terms of survival than would have been achieved with initial radiotherapy alone. Interestingly, a Yugoslavian group has reported on a series of 41 patients in whom the localized disease was totally removed at diagnostic surgery and a watch and wait policy was subsequently adopted [38]. With a median follow-up of 43.5 months, only eight patients had relapsed,

Table 19.10 Age-adjusted index for patients less than 60 years of age.

Index	Risk factors* (no.)	Proportion of patients (%)	CR rate (%)	RFS at 5 years (%)	OS at 5 years (%)
Low	0	22	92	86	83
Low–intermediate	1	32	78	66	69
High–intermediate	2	32	57	53	46
High	3	14	46	58	32

* Risk factors are: stage III/IV; performance status 2–4; raised LDH.
CR = complete remission; OS = overall survival; RFS = relapse-free survival.

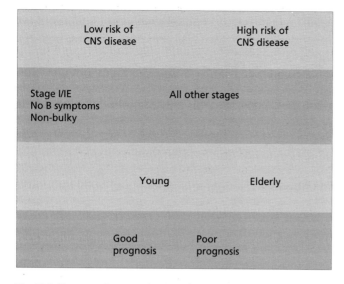

Fig. 19.1 Therapeutic categorization of the histologically aggressive lymphomas in adults.

Table 19.11 Results of the SWOG/ECOG Trial in histologically aggressive NHL. (Data from Fisher *et al.*, 1993 [46].)

	CR rate (%)	OS (at 3 years) (%)
CHOP (*n* = 225)	44	54
MACOP-B (*n* = 218)	51	50
mBACOD (*n* = 223)	48	52
ProMACE CytaBOM (*n* = 233)	56	50

CR = complete remission; OS = overall survival.

and at least half had attained a second CR with subsequent chemotherapy.

Stage II–IV disease with low risk to the central nervous system

Initial therapy

In bulky stage IIA or IIB, and all stage III and IV patients, combination chemotherapy is required. Most centres also give combination chemotherapy to nonbulky stage IIA disease. The standard regimen CHOP, which is the combination of cyclophosphamide, hydroxydaunorubicin, oncovin and prednisolone, was introduced over 20 years ago [39]. In patients with stage II–IV disease, about 50–60% of patients will attain a CR, with about 60% of these patients remaining disease free. This means that only about one-third of patients will be cured. The role of radiotherapy to consolidate a response to chemotherapy is not clear. In a recent ECOG Trial, 345 patients with bulky or extranodal Stage I and II disease were randomized to receive either eight cycles of CHOP or eight cycles of CHOP followed by radiotherapy in remission to sites of previous disease. The long-term disease-free survival was significantly better in the radiotherapy arm [40], but there is less evidence for giving consolidation radiotherapy in more advanced stages.

Attempts to improve on the results obtained with CHOP have focused on increasing the number of cytotoxic agents used, in line with the Goldie–Coldman hypothesis [41], and increasing the dose intensity of the therapy administered. Initial studies suggested that such approaches could be successful [42–44]. However, retrospective analyses failed to take adequate account of the fact that those patients who received suboptimal therapy may often have been those whose general condition was poorest (one of the most potent poor prognostic indicators), and the excellent results obtained with several second- and third-generation regimens from single centres, in nonrandomized trials, may have represented patient selection (often determined before referral to specialist centres) as much as treatment efficacy.

The ECOG Trial comparing CHOP and m-BACOD showed no difference in CR rate or in survival [45], and the analysis of the South-West Oncology Group/Eastern Co-operative Oncology Group (SWOG/ECOG) Trial comparing CHOP with m-BACOD, MACOP-B and ProMACECytabom shows no significant advantage, to date, for any regimen over CHOP (Table 19.11) [46]. A similar lack of superiority of third-generation regimens over CHOP has been found in some other randomized trials, but not all trials have been negative. In a comparison of CHOP vs PACEBOM, an 11-week multiagent weekly regimen, conducted by the BNLI in stage II–IV patients, there was a small non-significant improvement in CR rate with PACEBOM (57 vs 63%) and a similar small difference overall in survival. However, a subset analysis of stage IV patients revealed a significant advantage to PACEBOM in terms of both response and survival [47]. A similar advantage was apparent for a poor prognostic group defined by other factors, but the International Prognostic Index was not used on the entire series due to the lack of complete lactate dehydrogenase (LDH) measurements at diagnosis. The Australian and New Zealand Lymphoma Group carried out a randomized comparison of CHOP and MACOP-B. An initial analysis showed equivalent results, with less toxicity in the CHOP arm [48], but an update of this study shows that the MACOP-B-treated patients have a better actuarial 5-year progression-free survival (44 vs 29%, *P* = 0.03) [49]. It is difficult to consolidate these different results, but if there is an advantage for any of the third-generation regimens over CHOP, it is likely to be small. Clearly better front-line regimens are required, and one approach has been to intensify therapy yet further. A number of groups are testing intensified CHOP with the aid of haemopoietic growth factors. Several national and international groups are exploring three cycles of CHOP or CHOP-like therapy, followed by high-dose therapy with haemopoietic stem cell support in poor prognosis patients, and the results of these trials are awaited with interest. The GELA LNH 93-3 compared their standard ACVB arm in poor prognosis patients, with a short intensified treatment of three cycles of intensified therapy followed by high-dose BEAM (BCNU, etoposide, ara-C, melphalan) therapy with peripheral blood stem cell support [50]. The complete remission rate was no higher in the high-dose arm and the actuarial overall survival, albeit with a short follow-up, was worse. This very disappointing result contrasts with data from Milan and Turin, where 75 patients with 'high-risk' diffuse B-cell lymphomas were randomized to receive MACOP-B or high-dose sequential chemotherapy, culminating in an autologous transplant [51,52]. The complete remission was significantly higher in the high-dose arm (94 vs 61%, $P = 0.001$), and the time to treatment failure (73 vs 40%, $P = 0.008$) and overall survival were also better in the high-dose arm. A large randomized trial of this approach is clearly warranted.

The GELA group have also examined the value of high-dose therapy with autologous stem cell transplantation as consolidation in a randomized trial involving 464 patients achieving CR on the ACVB protocol. It was reported that such high-dose consolidation conferred no significant advantage overall, although there was a trend to an improved disease-free survival with transplantation in the high-intermediate- and high-risk groups [32]. A subsequent abstract, with longer follow-up, has confirmed that there is a significant disease-free survival advantage for the high-dose therapy recipients with poor prognostic factors at presentation and a trend towards improved overall survival [53]. This result clearly requires further confirmation. A notable feature of this trial is that, of the 174 autologous bone marrow transplantation (ABMT) procedures, there were only two procedure-related deaths, attesting to the safety of high-dose therapy for patients in complete remission.

Special comment is required about a number of disease subgroups that have been recently defined. The CD30+ anaplastic large cell lymphomas (ALCL) were initially considered to be a very aggressive form of lymphoma, but it now appears that the prognosis of adult primary ALCL is at least as good as other forms of histologically aggressive NHL [54–56]. In those patients with nodal disease and skin involvement, it has been suggested that the disease in more indolent, but it relapses more frequently. In a Japanese study the p80 NPM/ALK protein, arising from the t(2;5)(p23;q35), was expressed in 29% of cases, was found mainly in children and was associated with a better clinical outcome compared to the p80 NPM/ALK negative cases [56]. Limited information on the most appropriate form of chemotherapy can be deduced from the literature. The Italian study [55] used either F-MACHOP or MACOP-B with similar results, and concluded that 'ALCLs benefit from application of third-generation protocols for high-grade non-Hodgkin's lymphomas'. This statement must, however, be viewed with caution in the absence of data from randomized trials. A particular problem arises with ALCLs with bulky mediastinal disease, as residual masses are often present at the end of therapy. It is thus tempting to consolidate therapy in such patients with radiotherapy, or even high-dose

therapy with stem cell support, especially as bone marrow involvement is relatively uncommon. It should be noted that, in the successful Italian series, a conservative approach was usually taken in the management of residual masses [55]. It has also been suggested that other subgroups of lymphomas, such as T-cell-rich B-cell lymphomas and mediastinal sclerosing B-cell lymphomas [57], might benefit from individualized therapeutic approaches, but once again there is insufficient data to support such claims. Within the major category of the large cell lymphomas, the immunophenotype appears to have little independent prognostic significance, and again does not influence the choice of therapy [58].

Salvage therapy

Once a patient has failed initial chemotherapy the outlook is poor and long-term overall survival is less than 10%. Some of the best results were reported with the IMVP16 regimen; 14 out of 41 (34%) patients with resistant or relapsed disease obtained a CR, although over half of these had relapsed within 18 months [59]. In a BNLI Study using the same drugs (albeit with some minor dose modifications) for salvage therapy, only one out of 47 patients has remained disease free [60]. Cisplatin, in combination with other drugs, is a valuable second-line agent. Fifty-eight patients with resistant or relapsed diffuse large cell/immunoblastic lymphomas were treated with the DHAP regimen, and 17 (29%) achieved a CR; however, by 2 years approximately half of these patients had relapsed [61]. Using the ESHAP regimen, 32 out of 85 patients (38%) with relapsed or resistant intermediate-grade lymphomas achieved a complete remission, although again the majority of patients had relapsed by 2 years [62]. The mini-BEAM regimen, containing BCNU, etoposide, ara-C and melphalan, was originally designed as an HD salvage regimen [63], but it is also efficacious in NHLs.

Many centres have explored high-dose therapy with autologous stem cell support as salvage therapy, and it is clear that this strategy is only effective in those patients with disease that shows some chemosensitivity to conventional-dose therapy, i.e. partial response without progression on first-line therapy or responding relapse [64]. In a series from UCLH, the actuarial overall survival at 5 years following BEAM plus ABMT in patients with chemosensitive disease was 49%, compared to 13% in those with chemoresistant disease [65]. In this series the best results were in those patients who had achieved a partial remission (PR) on first-line therapy, although this raises the issue of whether some of the patients with nonbiopsied residual mediastinal or abdominal masses at the time of transplant might have already been cured of their disease, with the residual masses representing fibrosis rather than disease.

An Italian group randomized a series of patients obtaining a (PR) but not a CR with two-thirds of F-MACHOP or MACOP-B therapy to either an autograft or conventional-dose salvage and there was a significant disease-free advantage in favour of ABMT [66]. A Dutch multicentre group carried out a randomized trial in patients achieving a PR but not a CR after three courses of CHOP. Sixty-nine patients were randomized to receive either a further five courses of CHOP or an autograft after the fourth course of CHOP [67]. In contrast, to the Italian study there was no significant difference in the attainment of complete remission, the event-free survival or overall survival. It should be noted, however, that the outcome in the slow responders treated with CHOP alone was the same as that in the fast responders who were in CR after three courses of CHOP, indicating that the speed of CR may not be a good indicator on which to base further therapy.

For patients with responding relapse the pivotal study has been the Parma Trial [68]. Two hundred and fifteen patients with relapsed histologically aggressive lymphomas were given two courses of DHAP. One hundred and twenty-five patients (58%) had a response to therapy and 109 of these were randomized to receive either four additional courses of DHAP (+ radiotherapy) or high-dose chemotherapy and autologous bone marrow transplantation (+ radiotherapy). Of these 109 patients, 45 were in CR at the time of randomization. The actuarial event-free survival at 5 years was 46% in the transplant arm (intention to treat) and 12% in the conventional chemotherapy arm ($P = 0.001$). The actuarial overall survivals were 53 and 32% respectively ($P = 0.038$). Eighteen patients randomized to receive conventional therapy later underwent ABMT, but at the time of reporting only four remained alive, with only two disease free from the time of transplantation. There is little doubt that for patients with relapsed disease that is still chemosensitive, high-dose therapy with autologous stem cell rescue is the treatment of choice. It must, however, be pointed out that this improved salvage has a relatively small impact overall in the disease, because of the age restrictions of high-dose therapy and the high degree of selection for this type of treatment.

Patients who have no response to first-line therapy tend to fare very poorly, although occasional patients can still be rescued. Verdonk and colleagues [69] treated 31 patients who had failed to respond to CHOP (17 primary refractory and 14 resistant first relapse) with Pro-MACE-MOPP. Twenty-eight patients responded, with five achieving a CR. Seventeen of the 28 responders then proceeded to total body irradiation and ABMT; this included only one patient already in CR. Following high-dose therapy, 14 patients were in CR. The actuarial disease-free survival at 3 years in the transplanted patients was 50%, and 25% in the whole cohort of CHOP failures. This has not been a general experience however, and novel approaches to this category of patient are required.

Allogeneic transplantation, when available, has the potential advantage that the graft will definitely not be contaminated by lymphoma and there is the possibility of a graft vs leukaemia effect. The disadvantages are the greater toxicity, which restricts the age range of such procedures, and the limited number of patients who have a matched sibling donor. Evaluation of allogeneic transplants for lymphoma is made difficult by the fact that few centres have carried out a large number of procedures and the recipients have often been highly selected. A case-control comparison of 101 allograft–autograft pairs in the European Group for Bone Marrow Transplantation (EBMT) database showed a similar overall survival with both types of transplant. The procedure-related mortality was higher in the allograft arm (25 vs 10%), but the relapse rate was lower (20 vs 35%) [70]. The possible graft vs lymphoma effect was most apparent in patients with lymphoblastic lymphomas. Two other studies have suggested that there is a lower relapse rate in allogeneic transplant recipients [71,72], again suggestive but not conclusive of a graft vs lymphoma effect.

Extranodal lymphomas

Extranodal lymphomas do not, in general, behave very differently from nodal lymphomas, and the treatment is usually similar. Lymphomas affecting the gut, skin and brain are often distinct entities, however, which merit special consideration.

Gut lymphomas

There is considerable uncertainty about the optimal management of histologically aggressive gastrointestinal lymphomas. At one time, gastrointestinal lymphomas were mainly diagnosed following a laparotomy, at which time a complete resection was usually carried out. Today, increasing numbers of gastric lymphomas, in particular, are diagnosed following endoscopic biopsy, and this raises the question whether a resection should then be performed if the disease appears to be localized to the stomach (stage IE). Surgery allows debulking to be carried out, and may reduce the risks of therapy-induced bleeding or perforation, but gastrectomy has an appreciable intrinsic mortality and a significant long-term morbidity. A retrospective analysis by Taal and colleagues of 119 patients with localized gastric lymphoma, treated with either radiotherapy alone (no surgery) or surgery followed by adjuvant radiotherapy, revealed no difference in outcome [73], suggesting that surgery is not required as initial therapy and might be better reserved for patients not achieving a CR or who later relapse. A similar conclusion that surgery was not necessary in localized disease was also made by the German Multicenter Study Group on GI-NHL [74]. The actuarial 5-year survival in the Taal series was 70% in stage I disease, but only 37% in stage II disease. The unsatisfactory results in stage II disease suggest that chemotherapy might be preferable to radiotherapy and some centres would also advocate the use of chemotherapy, either alone or in combination with radiotherapy, in stage I disease. For more advanced disease arising from the stomach, treatment is the same as in other forms of histologically aggressive NHL, and the outcome is similar [75]. When a high-grade mucosa-associated lymphoid tissue (MALT) lymphoma of the stomach is diagnosed, it is advisable to also give patients a course of triple anti-*Helicobacter*, although this will not induce remission in the way that frequently occurs in the low-grade gastric MALT lymphomas. It should be noted that MALT lymphomas have a relatively good prognosis, regardless of their histological grade, with an overall survival at 10 years in excess of 70% in gastric disease and over 50% in intestinal disease [76].

In immunoproliferative small intestinal disease, a trial of broad-spectrum antibiotics is worth trying but, contrary to early optimism, chemotherapy is usually required. Enteropathy-associated T-cell lymphomas have a very ominous reputation, but this may relate to the poor performance status of many patients at diagnosis. The large series from the National Cancer Institute in Milan suggests that, when matched for prognostic index, intestinal lymphomas do no worse than gastric lymphomas [75].

Cutaneous-lymphomas

Mycosis fungoides is treated initially with local therapies, such as electron beam radiotherapy or PUVA with or without retinoids. Topical chemotherapy, such as nitrogen mustard or BCNU, is occasionally used. Nearly half of the patients with very localized disease may be cured by electron beam therapy, but once the disease occupies more than 10% of the skin or there is a circulating clone of T cells, the disease is rarely curable [77]. Early aggressive treatment of those patients with the more disseminated disease does not appear to improve the ultimate outlook [78]. For systemic disease chemotherapy is used, including alkylating agents, anthracycline-containing combination chemotherapy, deoxycoformycin and 2-chlorodeoxyadenosine [79]. There have also been reports of responses to interferon alpha [79]. Extracorporeal photophoresis may also be helpful, but no treatment is satisfactory for advanced disease. The median survival for mycosis fungoides is over 10 years from the appearance of the first lesions (not diagnosis), but is considerably less than this from the development of Sézary's syndrome. The precise prognosis of Sézary's syndrome is difficult to ascertain precisely because of the widely different definitions of this disease entity used in the published series.

Some other localized primary skin lymphomas of T-cell origin can be cured by local excision and radiotherapy. In the series reported by Beljaards and colleagues, large cell lymphomas expressing CD30 were usually responsive to local therapies, but the CD30– tumours were not [80]. Aggressive multiagent chemotherapy would seem to be justified in the latter case, at least in the younger patients.

Primary B-cell lymphomas of the skin can be successfully treated by surgery, if solitary, or radiotherapy, if localized. Only low doses of radiotherapy are required, for example 15 cGy. If the disease is more widespread and, possibly, if the leg is involved in older patients, combination chemotherapy should be considered.

Primary central nervous system lymphoma

Rarely lymphoma may be confined exclusively to the cranial spinal axis at presentation, and this entity diffusely infiltrates and spreads along the white-matter neuronal tracts and rarely spreads outside of the CNS, even in the terminal stages. Primary central nervous system lymphoma (PCNSL) is more frequent in immunosuppressed patients. Traditional therapy has been with whole-brain irradiation, but the results are not good, with the median survival only being about 1 year and with very few long-term survivors [81]. Most relapses are a result of failure within the radiation field. In view of these results, combined modality therapy has frequently been used. A number of studies have demonstrated the efficacy of chemotherapy, sometimes with hyperosmolar disruption of the blood–brain barrier [82], which, when combined with irradiation, resulted in median survivals between 2 and 5 years [83,84]. The US Radiation Therapy Oncology Group (RTOG) found that preradiation CHOP therapy gave very disappointing results [85], but this is hardly surprising as, once the blood–brain barrier is re-established, these drugs would not be expected to gain access to the tumour. Drugs that are likely to be effective at penetrating the blood–brain barrier include the anthracycline idarubicin, high-dose methotrexate, high-dose rapid infusion Ara-C, the nitrosoureas and dexamethasone, and CNS-directed chemotherapy regimens must be designed with this aspect of pharmacokinetics in mind.

Lymphomas with a high risk of central nervous system disease

Patients with T-cell lymphoblastic lymphomas, small non-cleaved cell lymphomas, immunodeficiency and HTLV-I-associated disease all have a high risk of developing CNS disease. The latter two entities are dealt with separately in a subsequent section, and only lymphoblastic, Burkitt's and Burkitt's-like lymphomas are discussed here.

In lymphoblastic lymphomas it is essential that CNS-directed prophylactic therapy is given and, for this reason, many centres use acute lymphoblastic leukaemia regimens, although similar results have been obtained with CHOP-like regimens supplemented by intrathecal methotrexate, and cranial irradiation followed by a maintenance phase [86]. The CR rates in lymphoblastic lymphomas are very high (75–95%), but the long-term disease-free and overall survival is less satisfactory, the latter being reported at between 35 and 55% [86–88]. Attempts have been made to analyse the prognostic factors at presentation, but each study is too small alone to allow reliable interpretation, and there is lack of conformity between the studies in terms of entry criteria and the apparent factors of significance.

Several studies have reported encouraging results with the use of total body irradiation (TBI) and ABMT in first remission [89,90], but randomized trials are required to determine the true value of this treatment modality. Such a study has now been completed in Europe. Similar encouraging results were reported with allogeneic transplatation [89,91], and a case–control study from the EBMT Group Registry, comparing autologous ABMT with allogeneic transplant, suggested that an allogeneic graft vs lymphoma effect may be operative in lymphoblastic lymphoma [70]. Allogeneic transplantation certainly merits further consideration in younger adults.

There is limited data available about treatment outcomes in small noncleaved cell lymphomas in adults. Many centres use lymphoblastic leukaemia-type regimens, often including cyclophosphamide. In other studies, sequential lymphoma regimens have been used with cranial prophylaxis. With most such intensive therapies, approximately 60% of patients are reported to be long-term survivors [92–94]. Patients with stage IV disease fare considerably worse than those with stages I–III disease, and bulky intra-abdominal disease and a raised LDH are probably also poor prognostic features. In poor-risk patients it may be reasonable to consider high-dose therapy and bone marrow transplantation during the first CR. An analysis by the EBMT Group of patients autografted in first CR showed that the actuarial disease-free survival was only 46% [95]. This is not obviously better than with standard chemotherapy. Furthermore, considerably better results have recently been reported from the NCI using CODOX-M or the very intensive CODOX-M/IVAC regimen [96]. For patients purported to have 'good-prognosis' disease, three cycles of CODOX-M, are given over 10–12 weeks. For patients with more advanced disease, two complete cycles of CODOX-M, alternating with IVAC (etoposide, ifosfamide, cytarabine) are given with growth factor support. Of the 20 adult HIV-negative patients treated with this regimen, 15 were in the high-risk group, and yet with a median follow-up of 30 months all obtained CR and have remained disease free. This result clearly needs confirmation in other studies. As alluded to above, Burkitt's lymphoma is relatively common in HIV-positive individuals and in some geographical areas a significant proportion of patients with small noncleaved cell lymphomas are HIV positive; this will of, course, affect the long-term outcome and influence treatment choices.

There may be other categories of patients with histologically aggressive NHL who merit CNS prophylaxis, including patients with testicular disease, involvement of the facial sinuses and infiltration of the bone marrow. At the very least these patients should have a staging lumber puncture (and intrathecal methotrexate) at initial diagnosis.

Treamtent of HTLV-I-associated lymphomas

HTLV-I infection is endemic to parts of Japan, Africa, the Carribean basin and the south-eastern USA, transmission being vertical and by sexual intercourse and the receipt of contaminated blood products. A proportion of immigrants in Europe originating from these areas have also been infected. A small proportion of infected individuals (up to 4%) [97] develop a T-cell malignancy referred to as adult T-cell leukaemia/lymphoma (ATLL). This disease has a very variable clinical phenotype and is divided into acute, chronic and smoldering ATLL and a 'lymphoma-type' [98]. The acute form of ATLL and the lymphoma-type are much the most common, the difference between them being the extent of lymphadenopathy and of blood and bone marrow involvement. Organomegaly, skin infiltration and hypercalcaemia are frequent findings. Central nervous system disease occurs in about 10%.

The results with standard chemotherapy are poor. The rate of complete remission is generally below 30%, relapse is the rule, and the median survival is about 6 months [99]. The use of purine analogues has not been successful [100]. Some response has been observed with the interferons [101,102], and two reports have suggested that the combination of the antiretroviral agent zidovudine and INFα is moderately effective. In the report by Gill and colleagues [103], 19 patients received this therapy, seven having previously failed on multi-agent cytotoxic regimens. Eleven patients had a major response, with five achieving a CR and six surviving for more than 1 year. In the report by Hermine and colleagues [104], three out of six patients were alive at or beyond 1 year. As HTLV-I associated lymphomas express high levels of IL-2 receptors, antibodies to this receptor, either alone or as radio-conjugates, have been tried with some minor success [105].

Treatment of lymphoma in immunodeficient patients

In those patients in whom the immunosuppression is iatrogenic, the level of immunosuppression should be reduced as much as possible. This is obviously not possible in individuals with HIV infection. In these patients the treatment is, in principle, the same as in other types of histologically aggressive lymphomas, but it must be borne in mind that there is a high degree of regimen-related toxicity, especially in those individuals with a very low CD4 count. In such cases it may be appropriate to consider palliative therapy only [106], although Hagemeister and colleagues have emphasized that the infective complications of therapy can usually be overcome, and the response to chemotherapy is not dissimilar to that in HIV-negative individuals [107].

Treatment of the elderly

Approximately half the patients with histologically aggressive NHL are over the age of 60 years and these older patients pose a particular therapeutic problem. They have a worse prognosis than younger patients, partly because they tolerate therapy less well and require more dose modifications, and partly because the disease appears to behave in a more aggressive manner. Because of the reduced tolerability of standard therapy, a number of groups are testing the use of prophylactic haemopoietic growth factors, to determine whether improved dose delivery will translate into improved tumour response and survival. Others have developed specific protocols for the elderly, some of which are curtailed to only 8 weeks [108].

Salvage therapy can be very problematical in the elderly, but age per se should not be a bar to further treatment. With careful patient selection, patients up to the age of 70 years can safely be given high-dose therapy with an autologous stem cell transplant. In many patients, of course, such a strategy is inappropriate and only palliation is indicated.

Childhood lymphomas

Indolent lymphomas almost never occur in childhood. Small noncleaved cell lymphomas, T-cell lymphoblastic lymphomas and diffuse large cell lymphomas account for over 90% of cases. The results of treatment in all these entities has improved dramatically in the last two decades [109].

In the small noncleaved cell lymphomas, intensive multi-agent chemotherapy regimens, such as the LMB 84 regimen or the CODOX-M/IVAC regimen, given over a few months have proved highly effective, with cure rates in excess of 75% in advanced disease, providing there was no CNS involvement at diagnosis [96,110]. The CNS prophylaxis used in these protocols is high-dose systemic methotrexate with intrathecal cytotoxics and cranial irradiation is not necessary. Even when there is CNS and bone marrow involvement, good results have been achieved using aggressive treatment, including high-dose ara-C and craniospinal irradiation. In those patients who only achieve a PR to initial therapy, a significant proportion may still be rescued by very intensive therapy with haemopoietic stem cell rescue. Relapses, if they occur, usually happen within 9 months. If the tumours still show chemosensitivity, a transplant procedure is worthwhile.

T-lymphoblastic lymphomas require different therapy from the small noncleaved cell lymphomas. A number of intensive ALL regimens give equivalent results, with long-term survivals of 60–80% reported [109].

There is not widespread agreement on the treatment of large cell lymphomas in childhood, but those of B-cell origin are usually treated as for small noncleaved cell lymphomas, and those of T-cell origin are treated as for T-lymphoblastic lymphomas. Between 60 and 80% of patients achieve long-term survival [109].

Novel therapies

A number of treatment modalities, other than conventional cytotoxic drugs, are being evaluated, including the use of monoclonal antibodies. Initial studies used antibody alone, either unmodified rodent antibodies or humanized antibodies, to reduce the production of antirodent antibodies. The antibodies were either directed against broad lineage-specific antigens [111–114], or were anti-idiotype antibodies raised against specific B-cell tumours [115]. The results have generally been disappointing, in part as a result of escape by antigen or idiotype-negative cells, and in part because of problems of biodistribution, and the limitations of the host effector mechanisms (complement lysis and antibody dependent cellular cytotoxicity) [116]. Other studies have used antibodies conjugated to either toxins or radioisotopes with modest response and some toxicity, particularly myelosuppression with the ^{131}I-labelled antibodies and fever and rigors with the ricin-conjugated antibodies [117,118]. Encouraging results have been reported from Seattle using ^{131}I-labelled antibodies and autologous marrow infusions to overcome the toxicity of severe myelosuppression [119]. Such strategies might be advantageously combined with high-dose chemotherapy, as the ^{131}I-labelled antibodies, by virtue of a bystander effect, might be particularly effective in the treatment of the larger masses which are less amenable to chemotherapy. The CD30 antigen is an attractive additional target for similar strategies in ALCL, because of its limited expression on normal lymphoid cells. Studies are in progress [120].

Cytokine therapy, with the exception of IFNα in the indolent lymphomas, has not yet proved effective, but the range of potentially useful factors, and their combinations, have not been exhausted.

Some lymphomas may also be amenable to infusion (vaccination) of irradiated tumour cells overexpressing cytokines [121] or appropriate immune-recognition molecules, such as members of the B7 family [122], in the hope of augmenting the host antitumour response. A further vaccination strategy is to inject lymphoma-specific immunoglobulin genes into muscle, where it is hoped that a potent immune response will be generated to the exogenous protein that will subsequently eliminate the tumour cells [123].

There is the theoretical possibility that tumour cells with a known genetic defect (e.g. specific translocation or mutant p53) could be directly targeted *in vivo*, with the intention of correcting the genetic defect. Although conceptually attractive, there are formidible technical issues to resolve. It will be necessary to target any systemically administered agent to the tumour cells, and one possibility is to use retroviruses genetically engineered, to bind alternative receptors to the usual amphotropic retroviral receptor, which are expressed in a tumour or tissue-specific way [124]. Alternative approaches include the use of tissue-specific promotors in the retroviral or plasmid vectors. Unfortunately, retroviruses are rapidly destroyed *in vivo*, although the recent discovery that inactivation of murine retroviruses by human complement is due to cross-species glycosylation differences means that this problem can be overcome by the use of human, rather than murine, packaging lines [125]. Administration of antisense oligonucleotides provides a potential alternative to gene correction, although again there are many technical problems to overcome [126]. Studies in patients with overexpression of *BCL2* have commenced, and a number of other genes could be similarly targeted. However, it will probably be another decade before any judgement can be made on the likely utility of these approaches.

References

1 Magrath I.T. (1990) The non-Hodgkin's lymphomas: an introduction. In: *The Non-Hodgkin's lymphomas.* (ed. I.T. Magrath), pp. 1–14. Edward Arnold, London.

2 *Leukaemia and Lymphoma: the epidemiology of haematological malignancies in the UK* (1990) Leukaemia Research Fund, London.

3 Morgan G.J., Jack A., Claydon A.D. *et al.* (1996) Trends in the incidence of lymphoma in Europe. *Annals of Oncology,* 7(Suppl. 3), abstract 27.

4 Weisenburger D.D. (1990) Environmental epidemiology of non-Hodgkin's lymphoma in eastern Nebraska. *American Journal of Internal Medicine,* 18, 303–305.

5 Joske D. & Knecht H. (1993) Epstein Barr virus in lymphomas: a review. *Blood Reviews,* 7, 215–222.

6 d'Amore F., Johansen P.M., Mortensen L.S. *et al.* (1996) Epstein–Barr virus in T cell lymphomas: frequency distribution and prognostic significance. *Annals of Oncology,* 7(Suppl. 3), abstract 30.

7 Wilson J.B., Bell J.L. & Levine A.J. (1996) Expression of Epstein–Barr virus nuclear antigen-1 induces B-cell neoplasia in transgenic mice. *EMBO Journal,* 15, 3117–3126.

8 Kieff E. (1995) Epstein–Barr virus. Increasing evidence of a link to carcinoma. *New England Journal of Medicine,* 333, 724–726.

9 Swerdlow S.H. (1992) Post-transplant lymphoproliferative disorders: a morphologic, phenotypic and genotypic spectrum of disease. *Histopathology,* 20, 373–385.

10 Divine M. & Farcet J-P. (1993) Adult T-cell leukemia/lymphoma: a model of retrovirus-induced I lymphomagenesis. In: *Non-Hodgkin's Lymphomas* (eds P. Solal-celigny, N. Brousse, F. Reyes, C. Gisselbrecht & B. Coiffier), pp. 31–40. Manson, Paris.

11 Stansfeld A., Diebold J., Kapanci Y. *et al.* (1988) Updated Kiel classification for lymphomas. *Lancet,* i, 292–293.

12 Non Hodgkin's Lymphoma Pathologic Classification Project (1982) National Cancer Institute sponsored study of classifications of non-Hodgkin's lymphomas: summary and description of a Working Formulation for clinical usage. *Cancer,* 49, 2112–2135.

13 Harris N.L., Jaffe E.S., Stein H. *et al.* (1994) A Revised European–American Classification of lymphoid neoplasms: a proposal from the International Lymphoma Study Group. *Blood,* 84, 1361–1392.

14 Ramsden D.A., McBlane J.F., van Gent D.C. & Gellert M. (1996) Distinct DNA sequences and structure requirements for the two steps of V(D)J recombination signal cleavage. *EMBO Journal,* 15, 3197–3206.

15 Hermine O., Haioun C., Lepage E. *et al.* (1996) Prognostic significance of *bcl*-2 protein expression in aggressive non-Hodgkin's lymphoma. *Blood,* 87, 265–272.

16 Hill M.E., MacLennan K.A., Cunningham D.C. *et al.* (1996) Prognostic significance of *BCL*-2 expression and *bcl*-2 major breakpoint region rearrangement in diffuse large-cell non-Hodgkin's lymphoma. *Blood,* 88, 1046–1081.

17 Offit K., LoCoco F., Louie D.C. *et al.* (1994) Rearrangement of the *bcl*-6 gene as a prognostic marker in diffuse large cell lymphoma *New England Journal of Medicine,* 331, 74–80.

18 Bastard C., Deweindt C. & Kerckaert J.P. (1994) LAZ3 rearrangements in non-Hodgkin's lymphoma: correlation with histology, immunophenotype, karyotype and clinical outcome in 217 patients. *Blood,* 83, 2423–2427.

19 Migliazza A., Martinotti S., Chen W. *et al.* (1995) Frequent somatic hypermutation of the 5′ non coding region of the *bcl*

20 Gaidano G., Pastore C., Migliazza A. *et al.* (1996) Mutations of *bcl*-6 regulating regions in AIDS-related lymphoma. *Annals of Oncology,* 1996. 7(Suppl. 3), abstract 49.

21 Louie D.C., Hochauser D., Schluger A. *et al.* (1996) Bcl6 and bcl2 rearrangement and p53 overexpression as prognostic factors in follicular lymphoma. *Annals of Oncology,* 7(Suppl. 3), abstract 51.

22 Lamant L., Megetto F. & Saati T. (1996) High incidence of the t(2;5)(p23;q35) translocation in anaplastic large cell lymphoma and its lack of detection in Hodgkin's disease. Comparison of cytogenetic analysis, reverse transcriptase-polymerase chain reaction and p80 immunostaining. *Blood,* 87, 284–291.

23 Morris S.W., Kirstein M.N. & Valentine M.B. (1994) Fusion of a kinase gene, ALK, to a nucleolar protein gene, NPM, in non-Hodgkin's lymphoma. *Science,* 263, 1281–1284.

24 Magrath I. (1990) The pathogenesis of Burkitt's lymphoma. *Advances in Cancer Research,* 55, 133–270.

25 Carbone P.P., Kaplan H.S., Musshof K., Smithers D.W. & Tubiana M. (1971) Report of the committee on Hodgkin's disease staging classification. *Cancer Research,* 31, 1860–1861.

26 Murphy S.B. (1980) Classification, staging and end results of treatment of childhood non-Hodgkin's lymphomas: dissimilarities from lymphomas in adults. *Seminars in Oncology,* 7, 332–340.

27 Bangerter M., Kocher F., Binder T. *et al.* (1995) Total body positron emission tomography (PET) for staging and follow-up of lymphoma. *Proceedings of the American Society of Clinical Oncology,* 14, abstract 1206.

28 Nissen N.I. & Ersboll J. (1985) Treatment of non-Hodgkin's lymphoma in adults. In: *Leukaemia and Lymphomas* (ed. P.H. Wiernik), pp. 97–126. Churchill Livingstone, Edinburgh.

29 Takatsuki T. (1995) Adult T-cell leukaemia. *Internal Medicine,* 34, 947–952.

30 Ziegler J.L., Beckstead J.A., Volberding P.A. *et al.* (1984) Non Hodgkin's lymphoma in 90 homosexual men. Relation to generalised lymphadenopathy and the aquired immunodeficiency syndrome. *New England Journal of Medicine,* 311, 565–570.

31 Anon (1993) A predictive model for aggressive non-Hodgkin's lymphoma. *New England Journal of Medicine,* 329, 987–994.

32 Haioun C., Lepage E., Gisselbrecht C. *et al.* (1994) Comparison of autologous bone marrow transplantation with sequential chemotherapy for intermediate-grade and high-grade non-Hodgkin's lymphoma in first complete remission. A study of 464 patients. *Journal of Clinical Oncology,* 12, 2543–2551.

33 Miller T.D. & Jones S.E. (1980) Is there a role for radiotherapy in localised diffuse lymphomas? *Cancer Chemotherapy and Pharmacology,* 4, 67–70.

34 Vaughan Hudson B., Vaughan Hudson G., MacLennan K.A., Anderson L. & Linch D.C. (1994) Clinical stage I non-Hodgkin's lymphoma: long term follow up of patients treated by the British National Lymphoma Investigation with radiotherapy alone as initial therapy. *British Journal of Cancer,* 69, 1088–1093.

35 Jones S.E., Miller T.P. & Connors J.M. (1989) Long-term follow-up and analysis for prognostic factors for patients with limited stage diffuse large cell lymphoma treated with initial chemotherapy with or without radiotherapy. *Journal of Clinical Oncology,* 7, 1186–1191.

36 Longo D.L., Glatstein E., Duffey P.L. *et al.* (1989) Treatment of localised aggressive lymphoma with combination chemotherapy followed by involved-field radiation therapy. *Journal of Clinical Oncology,* 7, 1295–1302.

gene in B-cell lymphoma. *Proceedings of the National Academy of Sciences USA,* 92, 12520–12524.

37 Miller T.P., Dahlberg S. & Cassady J.R. (1996) Superiority of a brief course of CHOP plus radiotherapy (RT) over CHOP alone in localised unfavourable non-Hodgkin's lymphoma is seen in lowest risk subgroups: a Southwest Oncology Group Study. *Annals of Oncology*, **7**(Suppl. 3), abstract 76.

38 Jelic S., Frim O., Jovanovic V., Gilgorijevic G., Opric M. & Gavrilovic D. (1996) Watch and wait policy for patients with non-Hodgkin's lymphoma clinical stage I or IE with no lymphoma left following diagnostic surgery. *Annals of Oncology*, **7**(Suppl. 3), abstract 188.

39 McKelvey E.M., Gottlieb J.A., Wilson H.E. *et al.* (1976) Hydroxyl-daunomycin (adriamycin) combination chemotherapy in malignant lymphoma. *Cancer*, **38**, 1484–1493.

40 Glick J.H., Kim K., Earle J. & O'Connell M.J. (1995) An ECOG randomised Phase III trial of CHOP vs CHOP + radiotherapy for intermediate grade early stage non-Hodgkin's lymphoma. *Proceedings of the American Society of Clinical Oncology*, **14**, 391.

41 Goldie H. & Coldman R.A. (1979) A mathematical model for relating the drug sensitivity of tumours to their spontaneous mutation rate. *Cancer Treatment Reports*, **63**, 1727–1733.

42 Shipp M.A., Harrington D.P., Klatt M.M. *et al.* (1986) Identification of major prognostic subgroups of patients with large cell lymphoma treated by m-BACOD or M-BACOD. *Annals of Internal Medicine*, **104**, 757–765.

43 Longo D.L., Devita V.T., Duffey P.I. *et al.* (1991) Superiority of ProMACE-CytaBOM over ProMACE-MOPP in the treatment of advanced diffuse aggressive lymphoma: results of a prospective randomised trial. *Journal of Clinical Oncology*, **9**, 25–38.

44 Klimo P. & Connors J.M. (1985) MACOB-B chemotherapy for the treatment of diffuse large-cell lymphoma. *Annals of Internal Medicine*, **102**, 596–602.

45 Gordon L.I., Harrington D., Andersen J. *et al.* (1992) Comparison of a second generation combination chemotherapeutic regimen (m-BACOD) with a standard regimen (CHOP) for advanced diffuse non Hodgkin's lymphoma. *New England Journal of Medicine*, **327**, 1342–1349.

46 Fisher R.I., Gaynor E.R., Dahlberg S. *et al.* (1993) Comparison of a standard regimen (CHOP) with three intensive chemotherapy regimens for advanced non-Hodgkin's lymphoma. *New England Journal of Medicine*, **328**, 1002–1006.

47 Linch D.C., Vaughan Hudson B., Hancock B.W. *et al.* (1996) A randomised comparison of third generation regimen (PACEBOM) with a standard regimen (CHOP) in patients with histologically aggressive non Hodgkin's Lymphoma: a British National Lymphoma Investigation Report. *British Journal of Cancer*, **74**, 318–322.

48 Cooper I.A., Wolf M.M., Robertson T.I. *et al.* (1994) Randomized comparison of MACOP-B with CHOP in patients with intermediate-grade non-Hodgkin's lymphoma. *Journal of Clinical Oncology*, **12**, 769–778.

49 Wolf M., Cooper I., Robertson T., Fox R., Matthews J. & Stone J. (1996) A randomised comparison of MACOP-B with CHOP for intermediate grade non Hodgkin's lymphoma: long-term follow-up. *Annals of Oncology*, **7**(Suppl. 3), abstract 77.

50 Gisselbrecht C., LePage E., Morel P. *et al.* (1996) Short and intensified treatment with autologous stem cell transplantation (ASCT) versus ACVB regimen in poor prognosis aggressive lymphoma. Prognostic factors of induction failure. *Annals of Oncology*, **7**(Suppl. 3), abstract 56.

51 Gianni A.M., Bregni M., Siena S. *et al.* (1994) 5-year update on the Milan Cancer Institute randomised trial of high-dose sequen-tial vs MACOP-B therapy for diffuse large cell lymphomas. *Proceedings of the American Society of Clinical Oncology*, **13**, abstract 1263.

52 Gianni A.M., Bregni M., Siena S. *et al.* (1996) Is high dose better than standard dose chemotherapy as initial treatment of poor risk large-cell lymphomas? A critical analysis from available randomised trials. *Annals of Oncology*, **7**(Suppl. 3), abstract 37.

53 Haioun C., Lepage E., Gisselbrecht C. *et al.* (1985) Autologous bone marrow transplantation versus sequential chemotherapy for aggressive non-Hodgkin's lymphoma in first remission. *Blood*, **86**(Suppl. 1), 1816.

54 Shulman L.N., Frisard B., Antin J.H. *et al.* (1993) Primary Ki-1 anaplastic large cell lymphoma in adults: clinical characteristics and therapeutic outcome. *Journal of Clinical Oncology*, **11**, 937–942.

55 Pileri S., Bocchia M., Baroni C.D. *et al.* (1994) Anaplastic large cell lymphoma (CD30+/Ki1+): results of a prospective clinico-pathological study in 69 cases. *British Journal of Haematology*, **86**, 513–523.

56 Shiota M., Nakamura S., Ichinohasama R. *et al.* (1995) Anaplastic large cell lymphomas expressing the novel chimeric protein p80$^{NPM/ALK}$: a distinct clinicopathologic entity. *Blood*, **86**, 1954–1960.

57 Todeschini G., Ambrosetti A., Meneghini V. *et al.* (1990) Mediastinal large B-cell lymphoma with sclerosis: a clinical study of 21 patients. *Journal of Clinical Oncology*, **8**, 804–808.

58 Armitage J.O., Vose J.M., Linder J. *et al.* (1989) Clinical significance of immunophenotype in diffuse aggressive non-Hodgkin's lymphoma. *Journal of Clinical Oncology*, **12**, 1783–1790.

59 Cabanillas F., Hagemeister F.B., Bodey G.P. & Freireich E.J. (1982) IMVP-16: an effective regimen for patients with lymphoma who have relapsed after initial combination chemotherapy. *Blood*, **60**, 693–697.

60 De Lord C., Newland A.C., Linch D.C., Vaughan Hudson B. & Vaughan Hudson G. (1992) Failure of IMPV-16 as second line treatment for relapsed or refractory high grade non-Hodgkin's lymphoma. *Haematological Oncology*, **10**, 81–86.

61 Velasquez W.S., Cabanillas F., Salvador P. *et al.* (1988) Effective salvage therapy for lymphoma with cisplatin in combination with high dose Ara-C and dexamethasone (DHAP) *Blood*, **71**, 117–122.

62 Velasquez W.S., McLaughlin P., Tucker S. *et al.* (1994) ESHAP—an effective chemotherapy regimen in refractory and relapsing lymphoma: a 4-year follow-up study. *Journal of Clinical Oncology*, **12**, 1169–1176.

63 Chopra R., Linch D.C., McMillan A.K. *et al.* (1982) Mini-BEAM followed by BEAM and ABMT for very poor risk Hodgkin's disease. *British Journal of Haematology*, **81**, 197–202.

64 Philip T., Amitage J.O., Spitzer G. *et al.* (1987) High dose therapy and autologous bone marrow transplantation after failure of conventional chemotherapy in adults with intermediate grade or high grade non-Hodgkin's lymphoma. *New England Journal of Medicine*, **316**, 1493–1497.

65 Mills W., Chopra R., McMillan A., Pearce R., Linch D.C. & Goldstone A.H. (1995) BEAM chemotherapy and autologous bone marrow transplantation for patients with relapsed or refractory non-Hodgkin's lymphoma. *Journal of Clinical Oncology*, **13**, 588–595.

66 Martelli M., Vignetti M., Zinzani P.L. *et al.* (1996) High-dose chemotherapy followed by autologous bone marrow transplantation versus dexamethasone, cisplatin and cytarabine in aggressive non-Hodgkin's lymphoma with partial response to front-line

chemotherapy: a prospective randomised Italian multicenter study. *Journal of Clinical Oncology*, **14**, 534–542.

67 Verdonk L.F., van Patten W.L.J., Hagenbeek A. *et al.* (1995) Comparison of CHOP chemotherapy with autologous bone marrow transplantation for slowly responding patients with aggressive non-Hodgkin's lymphoma. *New England Journal of Medicine*, **332**, 1045–1051.

68 Philip T., Guglielmi C., Hagenbeek A. *et al.* (1995) Autologous bone marrow transplantation as compared with salvage chemotherapy in relapses of chemotherapy-sensitive non-Hodgkin's lymphoma. *New England Journal of Medicine*, **333**, 1540–1545.

69 Verdonk L.F., Dekker A.W., de Gast G.C. *et al.* (1992) Salvage therapy with Pro-MACE-MOPP followed by intensive chemoradiotherapy and autologous bone marrow transplantaion for patients with non-Hodgkin's lymphoma who failed to respond to first-line CHOP. *Journal of Clinical Oncology*, **10**, 1949–1954.

70 Chopra R., Goldstone A.H., Pearce R. *et al.* (1992) Autologous versus allogeneic bone marrow transplantation for non-Hodgkin's lymphoma: a case controlled analysis of the European Bone Marrow Transplant Registry data. *Journal of Clinical Oncology*, **10**, 1690–1695.

71 Jones R.J., Ambinder R.F., Piantadosi S. & Santos G.W. (1991) Evidence of graft-versus-lymphoma effect associated with allogeneic transplantation. *Blood*, **77**, 649–653.

72 Ratanatharathorn V., Uberti J., Karanes C. *et al.* (1994) Prospective comparative trial of autologous versus allogeneic bone marrow transplantation in patients with non-Hodgkin's lymphoma. *Blood*, **84**, 1050–1055.

73 Taal B.G., Den Hartog Jager F.C.A., Butgers J.M.V. *et al.* (1989) Primary non-Hodgkin's lymphoma of the stomach: changing aspects and therapeutic choices. *European Journal of Cancer and Clinical Oncology*, **25**, 439–450.

74 Koch P., Grothaus-Pinke B., Hiddemann W. *et al.* (1996) Primary lymphoma of the stomach: 3-year results of a prospective multicenter study. *Annals of Oncology*, **7**(Suppl. 3), 81.

75 Tondini G., Giardini R., Buzzetti F. *et al.* (1993) Combined modality treatment for primary gastrointestinal non Hodgkin's lymphoma. The Milan Cancer Institute experience. *Annals of Oncology*, **4**, 831–837.

76 Morton J.E., Leyland M.J., Vaughan Hudson G. *et al.* (1993) Primary gastrointestinal non-Hodgkin's lymphoma: a review or 175 British National Lymphoma Investigation cases. *British Journal of Cancer*, **67**, 776–782.

77 Jones G.W., Hoppe R.T. & Glatstein E. (1995) Electron beam therapy for cutaneous T-cell lymphoma. *Haematology/Oncology Clinics of North America*, **9**, 1057–1076.

78 Kaye F., Bunn P., Steinberg H. *et al.* (1989) A randomised trial comparing combination electron beam radiation and chemotherapy with topical therapy in the initial treatment of mycosis fungoides. *New England Journal of Medicine*, **321**, 1784–1790.

79 Holloway K., Flowers F. & Ramos-Caro F. (1992) Therapeutic alternatives in cutaneous T-cell lymphoma. *Journal of the American Academy of Dermatology*, **27**, 367–378.

80 Beljaards R.C., Meijer C.J.L.M., Scheffer E. *et al.* (1989) Prognostic significance of CD30 expression of primary cutaneous large cell lymphomas of T-cell origin. A clinicopathologic and immunohistochemical study of 20 patients. *American Journal of Pathology*, **135**, 1169–1178.

81 Loeffler J.S., Ervin T.J., Mauch P. *et al.* (1985) Primary lymphomas of the central nervous system: patterns of failure and factors that influence survival. *Journal of Clinical Oncology*, **3**, 490–497.

82 Neuwelt E.A., Goldman D.L., Dahlberg S.A. *et al.* (1991) Primary CNS-lymphoma treated with osmotic blood–brain barrier disruption: prolonged survival and preservation of cognitive function. *Journal of Clinical Oncology*, **9**, 1580–1586.

83 Fine H.A. (1995) Treatment of primary central nervous system lymphoma: still more questions than answers. *Blood*, **86**, 2873–2875.

84 Blay J-L., Bouhour D., Carrie C. *et al.* (1995) A regimen of high dose chemotherapy and radiotherapy in primary cerebral non-Hodgkin's lymphoma of patients with no known cause of immunosuppression. *Blood*, **86**, 2922–2928.

85 Schultz C., Scott C.T.W., Fisher B. *et al.* (1994) Pre-irradiation chemotherapy with cyclophosphamide, adriamycin, vincristine and decadron for primary central nervous system lymphoma: initial report of Radiation Therapy Oncology Group protocol 88-06. *Proceedings of the American Society of Clinical Oncology*, **485**, abstract 174.

86 Coleman C.N., Picozzi V.J., Cox R.S. *et al.* (1986) Treatment of lymphoblastic lymphoma in adults. *Journal of Clinical Oncology*, **4**, 1629–1637.

87 Slater D.E., Mertelsmann R., Koriner B. *et al.* (1986) Lymphoblastic lymphoma in adults. *Journal of Clinical Oncology*, **4**, 57–67.

88 Bernasconi C., Brusamoline E., Lazzarino M. *et al.* (1990) Lymphoblastic lymphoma in adult patients; clinicopathological features and response to intensive multi agent chemotherapy analogous to that used in acute lymphoblastic leukaemia. *Annals of Oncology*, **1**, 141–146.

89 Milipied N., Ifrah N., Kuentz M. *et al.* (1989) Bone marrow transplantation for adult poor prognosis lymphoblastic lymphoma in first complete remission. *British Journal of Haematology*, **73**, 82–87.

90 Santini G., Coser P., Chiesi T. *et al.* (1991) Autologous bone marrow transplantation for advanced stage lymphoblastic lymphoma in first complete remission. *Annals of Oncology*, **2**(Suppl. 2), 181–185.

91 Santini G., Congiu A., D'Amico T.D. *et al.* (1989) Lymphoblastic lymphoma and acute lymphoblastic leukaemia in adults: relationship and therapeutic perspective. *Bone Marrow Transplantation*, **4**(Suppl. 1), 106–107.

92 Lopez T.M., Hagemeister F.B., McLaughlin P. *et al.* (1990) Small non-cleaved cell Burkitt's lymphoma in adults: superior results for Stage I–III disease. *Journal of Clinical Oncology*, **8**, 615–622.

93 McMaster M.L., Greer J.P., Greco A. *et al.* (1991) Effective treatment of small non-cleaved cell lymphoma with high-intensity, brief duration chemotherapy. *Journal of Clinical Oncology*, **9**, 941–946.

94 Longo D.L., Duffey P.L., Jaffe E.S. *et al.* (1994) Diffuse small non-cleaved cell Burkitt's lymphoma in adults: a high-grade lymphoma responsive to ProMACE-based combination chemotherapy. *Journal of Clinical Oncology*, **12**, 2153–2159.

95 Sweetenham J.W., Proctor S.J., Blaise D. *et al.* (1994) High dose therapy and autologous bone marrow transplantation in first complete remission for adult patients with high-grade non-Hodgkin's lymphoma: the EBMT experience. *Annals of Oncology*, **5**, S155–S159.

96 Magrath I.T., Adde M., Shad A. *et al.* (1996) Adults and children with small non-cleaved cell lymphoma have a similar excellent outcome when treated with the same chemotherapy regimen. *Journal of Clinical Oncology*, **13**, 222–246.

97 Schultz T. & Weber J. (1990) Epidemiology of HTLV-I. In: *AIDS*

and the New Viruses (eds A. Dalgliesh & R. Weiss), pp. 135–162. Academic, London.

98 Shimoyama M. (1991) Diagnostic criteria and classification of clinical subtypes of adult T-cell leukaemia-lymphoma: a report from the Lymphoma Study Group (1984–87). *British Journal of Haematology*, **79**, 428–437.

99 Bunn P.A. Jr, Schecter G.P., Jaffe E. *et al.* (1983) Clinical course of retrovirus-associated adult T-cell lymphoma in the United States. *New England Journal of Medicine*, **309**, 257–264.

100 Brogden R.N. & Sorkin E.M. (1993) Pentostatin. A review of its pharmacodynamic and pharmakinetic properties and therapeutic potential in lymphoproliferative disorders. *Drugs*, **46**, 652–677.

101 Tamura K., Makino S., Araki Y., Imamura T. & Seita M. (1987) Recombinant interferon beta and gamma in the treatment of adult T-cell leukaemia. *Cancer*, **59**, 1059–1062.

102 Ichimaru M., Kamihiri S., Moriuchi Y. *et al.* (1988) Clinical study on the effect of natural α-interferon (HLBI) in the treatment of adult T-cell leukaemia. *Japanese Journal of Cancer and Chemotherapy*, **15**, 2975–2981 [in Japanese].

103 Gill P.S., Harrington W., Kaplan M.H. *et al.* (1995) Treatment of adult T-cell leukaemia-lymphoma with a combination of interferon alfa and zidovudine. *New England Journal of Medicine*, **332**, 1744–1748.

104 Hermine O., Bouscary D., Gessain A. *et al.* (1995) Brief report: treatment of adult T-cell leukaemia-lymphoma with zidovudine and interferon alfa. *New England Journal of Medicine*, **332**, 1749–1751.

105 Waldmann T.A., White J.D., Carrasquillo J.A. *et al.* (1995) Radioimmunotherapy of interleukin-2RA-expressing adult T-cell leukaemia with yttrium-90-labeled anti-Tac. *Blood*, **86**, 4063–4075.

106 Sparan J.A. (1995) Treatment of AIDS-related lymphomas. *Current Opinions in Oncology*, **7**, 442–449.

107 Hagemeister F.B., Khetan R., Allen P. *et al.* (1994) Stage, serum LDH, and performance status predict disease progression and survival in HIV-associated lymphomas. *Annals of Oncology*, **5**(Suppl. 2), 41–46.

108 O'Reilly S.E., Connors J.M., Howdle S. *et al.* (1993) In search of an optimal regimen for elderly patients with advanced stage diffuse large-cell lymphoma: results of a phase II study of P/DOCE chemotherapy. *Journal of Clinical Oncology*, **11**, 2250–2257.

109 Blay J.L., Louis D., Buffet E. *et al.* (1991) Management of paediatric non-Hodgkin's lymphoma. *Blood Reviews*, **5**, 90–97.

110 Patte C., Philip T., Rodary C. *et al.* (1991) High survival rate in advanced stage B cell lymphomas and leukaemias without CNS involvement with a short intensive polychemotherapy: results from the French Paediatric Oncology Society of a randomised trial of 216 children. *Journal of Clinical Oncology*, **9**, 123–132.

111 Dillman R.O., Shawler D.L., Dillman J.B. *et al.* (1984) Therapy of chronic lymphocytic leukaemia and cutaneous T-cell lymphoma with T101 monoclonal antibody. *Journal of Clinical Oncology*, **2**, 881–891.

112 Bertram J.H., Gill P.S., Levin A.M., *et al.* (1986) Monoclonal antibody T101 in T-cell malignancies: a clinical, pharmacological and immunological correlation. *Blood*, **68**, 752–761.

113 Hale G., Clark M.R., Marcus R.E. *et al.* (1988) Remission induction in non-Hodgkin's lymphoma with reshaped human monoclonal antibody CAMPATH-1H. *Lancet*, **ii**, 1394–1399.

114 Hekman A., Honselaar A., Vuist W.M.J. *et al.* (1991) Initial experience with treatment of human B-cell lymphoma with anti-CD19 monoclonal antibody. *Cancer Immunology, Immunotherapy*, **32**, 364–372.

115 Brown S.L., Miller R.A., Borning S.J. *et al.* (1989) Treatment of B-cell lymphomas with anti-idiotype antibodies alone and in combination with alpha interferon. *Blood*, **73**, 651–661.

116 Lim S.H. & Marcus R.E. (1992) Monoclonal antibody therapy in non-Hodgkin's lymphoma. *Blood Reviews*, **6**, 157–162.

117 Grossbard M.L., Freedman A.S., Ritz J. *et al.* (1992) Serotherapy of B-cell neoplasms with anti-B4 blocked ricin: a phase I trial of daily bolus infusion. *Blood*, **79**, 576–585.

118 Czuczman M.S., Straus D.J., Divgi C.D. *et al.* (1993) Phase I dose-escalation trial of iodine 131-labeled monoclonal antibody OKB7 in patients with non-Hodgkin's lymphoma. *Journal of Clinical Oncology*, **11**, 2021–2029.

119 Press O.W., Eary J.F., Appelbaun F.R. *et al.* (1993) Radiolabelled-antibody therapy of B-cell lymphoma with autologous bone marrow support. *New England Journal of Medicine*, **329**, 1219–1224.

120 Terenzi A., Bolognesi A., Pasqualucci L. *et al.* (1996) Anti-CD30 immunotoxins containing the type-1 ribosome-inactivating proteins momordin and PAP-S (pokeweed antiviral protein from seeds) display powerful antitumour activity against anti-CD30 tumour cells *in vitro* and in SCID mice. *British Journal of Haematology*, **92**, 872–879.

121 Bubenik J. (1996) Cytokine gene modified vaccines in the therapy of cancer. *Pharmacological Therapeutics*, **69**, 1–14.

122 Schultze J., Nadler L.M., & Gribben J.G. (1996) B7-mediated co-stimulation and immune response. *Blood Reviews*, **10**, 111–127.

123 Hawkins R.E., Winter G., Hamblin T.J. *et al.* (1993) A genetic approach to anti-idiotype immunisation. *Journal of Immunotherapy*, **14**, 273–278.

124 Takeuchi Y., Porter C., Strahan K. *et al.* (1996) Sensitization of cells and retroviruses to human serum by (α1–3) galactosyl transferase. *Nature*, **379**, 85–99.

125 Kasahara N., Dozy A.M. & Kan Y.W. (1994) Tissue-specific targeting of retroviral vectors through ligand–receptor interactions. *Science*, **266**, 1373–1376.

126 Cotter F., Johnson P., Hall P. *et al.* (1994) Antisense oligonucleotides suppress B-cell lymphoma growth in SCID-hu mouse model. *Oncogene*, **9**, 3049–3055.

20 The Lymphomas: Current Clinical Trials

S.J. Proctor and P.R.A. Taylor

Introduction

Improving treatment in any form of malignant disease is inevitably a slow and painstaking process. However, within haematological oncology, a few areas exist where there is intrinsic chemosensitivity and in which chemocurability is possible, and often attainable. Within the diverse group of diseases designated the lymphomas, including all forms of non-Hodgkin's lymphoma (NHL) and Hodgkin's disease (HD) everyone concerned can look back over the past 20 years with some degree of satisfaction when considering the results of treatment with radiotherapy for localized disease and the various forms of combination chemotherapy for more advanced forms of disease. The details of such approaches have been reviewed in Chapters 16, 18 and 19.

Hodgkin's disease

The general conclusions about what has been achieved so far vary, according to the disease group. By 1980 substantial progress had already been made in HD, with the vast majority of patients with localized forms of the disease being cured by local radiotherapeutic treatment. The MOPP schedule (mustine, vincristine, prednisolone, procarbazine), introduced by DeVita, had demonstrated that, if given in appropriate doses according to schedule, 65% of patients might be cured at 10 years [1], although the more accepted figure is 50% [2]. Subsequent activity during the 1980s was aimed at further intensification of conventional treatment, usually in the form of various phase II studies, although the occasional randomized trial suggested improved event-free survival for hybrid schedules when compared to more conventional approaches [3] — ABVD (Adriamycin*, bleomycin, vinblastine, DTIC) was found to be as effective as alternating MOPP/ABVD in this study. However, it must be noted that substantially larger amounts of drug were utilized in some of the hybrid schedules,

in comparison to the normal schedules with which they were compared. In the late 1980s attention began to focus more on the role of chemotherapy intensification with bone marrow rescue, and debate has centred on whether such intensifications should be conducted as part of planned primary treatment or as part of salvage regimens. In relapsed chemosensitive disease intensification appeared to be of value when tested in a randomized trial [4]. Preliminary results suggested that such intensification treatments might provide some added therapeutic value, but uncertainties existed, and still exist, about which patient populations should be included in early intensifications.

Low-grade non-Hodgkin's lymphoma

As indicated in Chapter 18 on low-grade lymphomas, if overall survival is looked at in the 1970s and 1980s, following all forms of treatment, there has, essentially, been no shift in the survival curves. As each new agent enters the field, hopes arise that the increased response rate might translate not only into prolonged event-free survival, but also into overall survival in the longer term. Once again, towards the end of the 1980s, attention began to focus on the role of intensification therapy in relapsed patients and current treatment is described in Chapter 19.

High-grade non-Hodgkin's lymphoma

It is now well accepted that within the group of disorders that are known as the intermediate- and high-grade NHLs, there is remarkable heterogeneity, once more highlighted by the recent updating of pathological and immunological perceptions of the Revised European–American Lymphoma (REAL) Classification Group [5]. In essence, in large cell lymphomas there is universal agreement that the introduction of CHOP (cyclophosphamide, Adriamycin, vincristine, prednisolone)

---

* Adriamycin = doxorubicin for all chemotherapy schedules in this chapter.

chemotherapy was a milestone in lymphoma treatment and that a large minority of patients can be cured by the use of this combination therapy. During the late 1970s, and throughout the 1980s, the 'third-generation' chemotherapeutic regimens were tried both as phase II and in randomized phase III studies, as described in Chapter 19, and so far there has been disappointment that the introduction of additional drugs at conventional doses has not made any radical difference in therapeutic outcome [6]: CHOP remains the 'gold standard'. Once again the concept of intensification, using bone marrow or peripheral stem cell rescue, has been put through various phase II and phase III studies. In the two major published studies to date, from the French/Belgian Group and the Dutch Group, there appears to be no advantage over aggressive chemotherapy vs early intensification with marrow or stem cell support, if intermediate- and high-grade NHLs are included together [7,8]. There are proposals for the more consistent identification of risk groups using prognostic indices [9–11], in order to identify better those with poor-risk disease so that early intensification treatments can be given appropriately and responses assessed more accurately.

In summary, this is the current state of progress in clinical trials as we enter the mid 1990s. It is against this 'backcloth' that this chapter attempts to summarize the current studies available for investigating new therapeutic approaches in NHL and HD within the UK.

Organization of clinical trials in the UK

The logical approach to lymphoma trials within the UK started with the development of the British National Lymphoma Investigation (BNLI) Group. Over the years, the BNLI Group has accrued large numbers of patients in pilot studies and randomized trials, and they have published results at regular intervals. More than any other organization in lymphoma work, the Group has brought to lymphoma treatment a degree of uniformity and clarity, and deserves huge credit for this major contribution. The Group has often been criticized for reporting lower response rates than those claimed by single-centre institutions elsewhere, but it has become evident that the BLNI data represents the reality of practice as perceived within most hospitals in the UK. During the late 1970s and early 1980s, additional regional and supraregional organizations were formed, particularly in areas that were not submitting cases to BNLI studies. Thus the Scotland and Newcastle Lymphoma Group, the Central Lymphoma Group, the Bart's–Manchester Combined Group, the South West Group and the Wessex Group have all been involved in phase II and phase III studies over the past decade and a half.

Recently, the Cancer Research Campaign (CRC), looking at the overall situation, invited participants from the main groups to attempt a more coordinated approach by forming an 'umbrella' organization known as the UK Lymphoma Group. The UK Lymphoma Group is a loose affiliation of individuals involved in the other lymphoma groups, who meet to try and draw common threads together within the UK, and thus facilitate involvement in clinical trials and introduce specific studies where they seem to be necessary and appropriate.

Because of historical groupings in relation to lymphoma activity within the UK, it has not hitherto proved possible to form a coordinated national approach. While individual groups might have differences of opinion on how specific questions ought to be addressed, all agree that because progress is difficult to engender and assess, it is critically important that patients treated for lymphoma in the UK should, wherever possible, be incorporated into either a national or regional protocol. It is the intention of this chapter to highlight the currently available and active protocols within the UK and, at the time of writing (1996), to define briefly the rationale for each specific protocol. All treatment schedules discussed below have been placed in summary format in a short publication with the title *Current Lymphoma Protocols in the UK*, Volume 1, and can be obtained free of charge from the author.*

Hodgkin's disease

Early-stage Hodgkin's disease

Within the UK, there is currently little coordinated activity of studies in early-stage HD. Where studies are being conducted, the questions asked relate to the value of the utilization of chemotherapy as an adjunct to the use of radiotherapy in terms of event-free interval and overall outcome.

1 The combined Bart's–Manchester Group have investigated the use of minimal initial therapy for low-risk clinical stage I and II HD. This was a randomized trial comparing radiotherapy alone against the new adjuvant chemotherapy VAPEC-B (vincristine, Adriamycin, prednisolone, etoposide, cyclophosphamide, bleomycin) and radiotherapy. Initial results were promising, so this study now forms the basis for the current UK Lymphoma Group Study (LY07), which aims to compare the short neoadjuvant chemotherapy (VAPEC-B) plus involved-field radiotherapy vs mantle radiotherapy in early-stage HD (IA and IIA), the principle exclusion criteria being bulky disease. It is hoped that the study will demonstrate, firstly, whether a short course of chemotherapy before involved-field radiotherapy reduces the recurrence rate compared with

---

* Proctor S.J. & Sweetenham J. (1995) *Current Lymphoma Protocols in the UK*, Vol. 1. Booklet produced on behalf of the UK Lymphoma Group providing precise details of all the studies described in this chapter, in particular indicating the contact numbers so that full protocols can be obtained. To obtain a copy contact: Professor S.J. Proctor, Department of Haematology, Royal Victoria Infirmary, Newcastle upon Tyne NE1 4LP, UK; tel. +44 191 232 5131 ext. 25042, fax +44 191 201 0154.

mantle field radiotherapy alone and, secondly, whether this approach is associated with a better long-term survival. The potential benefit of reduced late effects in the test arm (combined modality) on cardiac and pulmonary function, and the incidence of second malignancy, will also be assessed. This study opened in autumn 1996.

2 The only other major active protocol available in the UK is a phase III study of radiotherapy vs ABVD plus radiotherapy vs ABVD alone in the treatment of early-stage HD. This is a Canadian Study Group protocol run by the NCIC (National Cancer Institute of Canada) Clinical Trials Group, with involvement of the Wessex Lymphoma Group which has opened it up for UK participation. Patients are divided initially into low- and high-risk groups. Low-risk patients are randomized to radiotherapy alone or ABVD × 2, with reassessment at 1 and 3 months. Good responders are administered a further ABVD × 2, with ABVD × 4 for partial responders. High-risk patients (essentially those with bulk disease) are randomized to ABVD × 2 and radiotherapy with reassessment at 1 and 3 months or ABVD × 2 with reassessment; again a further ABVD × 2 is given to good responders and ABVD × 4 to partial responders. This study remains open and it is anticipated that input will be required for several years, as a substantial number of patients will be required for any difference to be proven.

Advanced Hodgkin's disease

There is more trial activity in advanced HD than in the early form of disease within the UK at the present time. The majority of studies relate to comparisons of differing forms of hybrid schedules in clinical subgroups of HD, according to the Ann Arbor Classification. The exception to this approach is the Scotland and Newcastle Lymphoma Group's utilization of the 'SNLG' Prognostic Index [12]. This study is different, because it compares conventional hybrid therapy with early intensification therapy as part of a planned primary approach.

Initial treatment studies

1 The BNLI and the Central Lymphoma Group have combined to produce a study* to assess the validity of a randomized comparison of cyclical anthracyline-based chemotherapy (PA(BI)OE — prednisolone, Adriamycin, bleomycin, vincristine, etoposide) with alternating chemotherapy (CLVPP(LOPP) (chlorambucil, vinblastine, prednisolone, procarbazine)/PA(BI)OE) in advanced HD. There is a second randomization between radiotherapy or observation alone in patients in complete remission (CR) or with minimal residual masses on computed tomography (CT). This trial is an extension of the previous BNLI Group study, which found that the hybrid schedule was of more overall value than CLVPP alone [13]. The purpose of this study is to evaluate whether it is nec-

essary to have CLVPP in the combination at all. It is the intention to assess whether there is an improvement in the frequency of second malignancy, in fertility, pulmonary and cardiac toxicity, and also to assess in a randomized study the role of radiotherapy following chemotherapy-induced CR.

2 The Bart's–Manchester Group are involved in a randomized trial* comparing a frontal hybrid schedule with VAPEC-B chemotherapy (a combination used by this group in non-Hodgkin's lymphoma (NHL)) in advanced HD. The essential end points are the standard ones: assessment of remission rates and progression-free survival, with the impact of both regimens on testicular and ovarian function and incidence of second tumours.

3 The Southampton and Wessex Group are involved in assessing PACE-BOM (prednisolone, Adriamycin, etoposide, bleomycin, vincristine, methotrexate), a new combination chemotherapy regimen for advanced HD. This is not a randomized trial and the aim is to assess the efficacy of this approach in patients with advanced disease, and to measure treatment-related toxicity, especially in relation to fertility.

4 Over the last 10 years, the Scotland and Newcastle Lymphoma Group (SNLG) developed a prognostic index, separate from, but including, Ann Arbor Staging, which they found had a better predictive value than Ann Arbor Staging alone in their patients [12,14]. The accuracy of the approach has been confirmed independently [15], and is utilized for selecting patients for a trial (HD3) to assess the value of early intensification. Patients receive 3 months of a hybrid schedule PVACE-BOP (prednisolone, vinblastine, Adriamycin, chlorambucil, etoposide, bleomycin, vincristine, procarbazine) [16], similar to Stanford V [17], and after appropriate response and radiotherapy to bulk disease, a randomization then takes place to either two further courses of hybrid chemotherapy or an early intensification with melphalan/etoposide preconditioning. The subablative approach to intensification is less toxic than regimens utilized for salvage approaches and can be used without cryopreserving the rescue product [18,19]. The SNLG Index for assessing the risk status in Hodgkin's disease (HD) patients is shown in Table 20.1. A recent observation has been made of retained female fertility after the autotransplant procedure [20].

Studies in relapsed/progressive Hodgkin's disease

There are few studies reported in a coordinated way for relapsed and progressive HD. The Royal Marsden Lymphoma Group have a randomized trial, which is currently active, for difficult relapsed or refractory HD stages II–IV comparing platinum-based chemotherapy (ECP — etoposide, cisplatin, prednisolone) plus or minus granulocyte colony-stimulating factor (G-CSF) in relapsed HD and NHL.

It is probably necessary to develop far more coordinated approaches for the production of specific protocols for this very

---

* These studies have recently closed and new protocols have not been activated.

Table 20.1 The SNLG HD Index.

To calculate the index, patient's age (Age), clinical stage (CS), absolute lymphocyte count (LC), haemoglobin (Hb) and bulk disease are required:

The index (I) + 1.5858 − 0.0363 Age + 0.0005 (Age²)*
+ 0.0683 CS − 0.086 LC − 0.0587 Hb
+ additional factor if bulk disease is present†

Age is entered as an absolute figure in the equation

Clinical stage is entered according to the key (Ann Arbor Classification):

IA, IIA, IIA = 1
IB, IIB = 2
IIIB = 3
IV = 4

Absolute lymphocyte count is entered as a score:

<1.0 × 10⁹/l = 1
1.0–1.5 × 10⁹/l = 2
1.5–2.0 × 10⁹/l = 3
>2.0 × 10⁹/l = 4

Haemoglobin (Hb) in g/dl is entered as an absolute figure in equation

Bulk disease (>10 cm) – index score add 0.3†

Patients with index 0.5 have risk of death from progressive HD of 60–70% in 4 years. Such patients are being entered on a trial protocol in first remission

This index is not for use in patients <15 years of age

---

* In the original publication of the index [12], a typographical error was made in the factor relating to age.
† The index published in ref. [14], and reproduced above, corrects the error and adds the additional factor for bulk disease.

difficult group of early progressive HD patients. It may well be that, in time, many of these patients will be found to have subvariants of lymphoproliferative disorders and will not be truly classified as HD cases.

Low-grade non-Hodgkin's lymphoma

As discussed in Chapter 18, results over the past 10–20 years essentially show that new treatment modalities have not radically changed event-free or overall survival patterns. It is perhaps true that insufficient attention has been given to trying to identify appropriate risk groups within the categories designated 'low-grade NHL'. Recently, various prognostic indices have been introduced [21,22], and the application of the index which was produced for high-grade disease may provide a basis for the stratification of patients for trial purposes [9]. The currently active trials and studies in low-grade lymphoma within the UK are summarized below.

Initial treatment studies

1 The BNLI and EORTC (European Organization for Treat-

ment of Cancer) are presently running a combined protocol comparing the newer agent fludarabine, which has been shown to have activity in low-grade NHL as a single agent [23], to the well-known combination of cyclophosphamide, vincristine and prednisolone (CVP) in advanced low-grade NHL. Most categories of 'low-grade' are included, but diffuse centrocytic (mantle cell) disease and follicular large cell disease are specifically excluded.

2 The Southampton Group have an open study of fludarabine therapy as a single agent in newly diagnosed patients with low-grade B-cell lymphoma, which also includes those with Waldenström's macroglobulinaemia and low-grade peripheral T-cell lymphoma. This is a phase II study aimed to assess the safety of the drug, the duration of response, time to disease progression and overall survival.

3 The Scotland and Newcastle Lymphoma Group are conducting a study in low-grade B-cell lymphoma which contains two randomizations. The first phase utilizes an all-oral induction therapy, with short-course higher-dose chlorambucil linked with oral idarubicin and dexamethasone (CID) vs higher-dose chlorambucil and dexamethasone alone. This randomized study follows an initial study on 72 patients who demonstrated good efficacy and acceptable toxicity to the CID combination. The second randomization in this study is to no further therapy after 6 courses vs interferon (IFN) 3 Mu three times a week or IFN at low dose of 1 Mu three times a week for a period of 36 months as 'maintenance' treatment. The aim of the study is to:

(a) assess the value of adding idarubicin in the CID combination, and

(b) to assess whether IFN has any impact on relapse rate.

4 The Royal Marsden Group have a randomized trial of alpha-calcidol as maintenance therapy in low-grade (Working Formulation) NHL. This is for patients who have achieved a first or subsequent remission, and they are then randomized to no further treatment or alpha-calcidol given orally. No additional medication may be given to the control arm and patients receive the alpha-calcidol until disease progression. In addition, this study will try to determine the role of polymerase chain reaction (PCR) by monitoring *BCL2* rearrangements in peripheral blood and bone marrow in this disease.

Studies in relapsed patients

1 The St Bartholomew's Group continue with their study of high-dose therapy with marrow rescue and marrow 'clean-up' in selected patients following relapse. The results of this study are mentioned in Chapter 18.

2 Similarly, the Central Lymphoma Group have a pilot study to evaluate the potential for mobilizing peripheral blood stem cells (PBSCs) in patients who have been pretreated for follicular lymphoma. It aims to evaluate the success of CD34 selection in bringing about a purge of circulatory B cells in this condition and to assess the time to engraftment with these selected cells. A limited number of patients are being sought to give pilot information (and certain patients with 'poor-risk disease' at presentation are also eligible), and if this study looks promising a randomized study will commence.

3 In the European Cooperative Trial known as the 'European CUP Trial' (which is an European Group for Bone Marrow Transplantation (EBMT) Working Party Study) there is a randomized study comparing the efficacy of chemotherapy with purged or unpurged autologous transplantation in adults with poor-risk relapsed follicular NHL. Patients are given three cycles of chemotherapy and then reassessed; if they have achieved CR/PR, they are then randomized to receive either three further cycles of chemotherapy, or high-dose chemotherapy with either unpurged or purged stem cell rescue.

Thus the general pattern of trials in relapsed low-grade NHL is now divided into those assessing new agents, such as fludarabine, and those assessing therapy intensification. Whilst intensifications may be applicable to a selected few patients with low-grade NHL in the younger age groups, toxicities in relation to second tumours, and the age range of patients with follicular lymphoma, seem destined to limit the usefulness of the technique [24]. It is disappointing that so few trials are pursuing the relevance of the use of cytokines such as IFN as maintenance, in spite of some interesting preliminary data for this particular agent [25,26].

High-grade non-Hodgkin's lymphoma

Within the high-grade NHL protocols, there is a tendency to include both intermediate- and high-grade histologies (Working Formulation) in many of the protocols for primary treatment. However, the lymphoblastic lymphomas of Burkitt or non-Burkitt type tend to have separate protocols in the majority of cases. The first group laid out below relates to the primary studies for high grade and lymphoblastic disease followed by the few studies available for subsequent salvage therapy. In essence, as discussed previously in this volume, it is now accepted that CHOP chemotherapy remains the 'gold standard' and that any assessment of successes of new approaches must relate to risk assessment for which, at the moment, the international prognostic index is utilized [9].

Initial treatment studies

1 The UK Lymphoma Group has a trial (LYO5) available for patients with localized stage I and II disease comparing radiotherapy alone vs CHOP × 3 plus radiotherapy vs CHOP × 6 plus radiotherapy. This is for intermediate- or high-grade lymphoma (Working Formulation), excluding lymphoblastic disease of all types. The study aims to assess time to progression, site of relapse and survival.

2 Another UK Lymphoma Group study (LYO2) is being conducted in a randomized form to evaluate early high-dose therapy and autologous stem cell transplantation as part of

planned initial therapy for poor- and intermediate-risk patients (as defined by the International Prognostic Index) with intermediate-/high-grade NHL. In this study all patients receive three courses of CHOP chemotherapy. Responders proceed to bone marrow harvest and are then randomized to either high-dose therapy plus autologous bone marrow transplantation (ABMT) or continued conventional therapy.

3 A similar approach is being taken in an EBMT/UK Lymphoma Group study in patients with lymphoblastic lymphoma (non-Burkitt type). This is a prospective randomized trial of high-dose therapy and autologous transplantation vs continuing conventional chemotherapy. Randomization takes place after a response to induction chemotherapy. For patients who are given standard chemotherapy, ABMT in second remission is allowed.

4 The BNLI Group have a trial of CHOP vs CIOP (cyclophosphamide, idarubicin, vincristine, prednisolone) in good-risk stage II–IV patients with histologically aggressive NHL. The aims of the study are:

(a) to assess the efficacy in a randomized trial of idarubicin compared to doxorubicin in combination with cyclophosphamide, oncovin and prednisolone;

(b) to compare the long-term toxicity of the anthracyclines;

(c) to prospectively evaluate the prognostic factors used to differentiate good- and poor-risk disease.

5 The SNLG are conducting a randomized study to assess the role of autologous bone marrow transplantation in patients with advanced high-grade lymphoma, based on their risk grouping according to both the International Index and the SNLG Lymphoma Index [21,22]. For 'good-risk' patients therapy induction is standard treatment with CHOP or VAPEC-B, radiotherapy to bulk is allowed and then randomization is between no further treatment vs a modest intensification with melphalan 3 mg/kg using marrow or PBSC rescue. The intermediate- and poor-risk-group patients receive the same induction and radiotherapy to bulk, but in these groups the randomization is between a modest intensification with melphalan 3 mg/kg alone vs an ablative autotransplant using either melphalan/total body irradiation (TBI) or BEAM (BCNU, etoposide, ara-C, melphalan) (i.e. all intermediate- and poor-risk patients receive some intensification).

High-grade non-Hodgkin's lymphoma in the elderly

1 In the elderly age group, studies for treatment of high-grade lymphoma are not easy to conduct, even though large numbers of patients exist in this category. The BNLI are conducting a study of short-course therapy in elderly patients. The chemotherapy is either PAdriaCEBO (prednisolone, Adriamycin, cyclophosphamide, etoposide, bleomycin, vincristine) or PMitCEBO (prednisolone, mitoxantrone, cyclophosphamide, etoposide, bleomycin, vincristine). The aims of the study are to create a database on unselected elderly patients with high-grade NHL and to establish the CR rate, overall survival and disease-specific survival obtained from an 8-week, seven-drug regimen. The study includes a randomization between mitoxantrone and Adriamycin, because it is also hoped to establish whether there is any difference in toxicity and improved quality of life between the two arms.

2 A similar study in the elderly run by the Central Lymphoma Group is a trial of modified therapy for patients in the age group of 65 years and over with intermediate- or high-grade lymphoma. Patients are randomized between receiving six courses of 'modified' CHOP or MCOP. The aims of this study are to assess the toxicity and acceptability of the two 'gentle' therapies and to compare toxicities between the two anthracyclines (Adriamycin and mitoxantrone).

Burkitt's lymphoblastic lymphoma

Burkitt's lymphoblastic lymphoma in its advanced form was, until recently, a disease with an extremely poor prognosis. However, some interesting results are emerging from intensive treatment protocols for L3 leukaemia and lymphoma, particularly in children [27]. It is hoped to extend these promising results in children to the treatment of adults, and the UK Lymphoma Group is currently developing their own brief, high-dose therapy schedule which is a modification of the National Cancer Institute Protocol 89-C-41 [28]. This new protocol (LYO6) is available for use.

In LYO6, patients are divided into a 'low-risk' category (low stage, normal LDH, no bulk) and receive three courses of CODOX-M (a regimen containing high-dose methotrexate and cyclophosphamide, vincristine, doxorubicin, cytarabine). All other patients are categorized as 'poor risk' and will receive CODOX-M alternating with IVAC, a non-cross-resistant protocol (etoposide, ifosfamide, ara-C), for a total of four courses. The aims of this UK study are to assess the treatment toxicity and efficacy and to see if the successful results obtained at the National Cancer Institute (NCI), from their 89-C-41, can be repeated elsewhere.

Studies in relapsed high-grade non-Hodgkin's lymphoma

Once patients with high-grade NHL relapse following primary treatment, it is generally accepted that the outlook is very poor and perhaps this is one reason why relatively few ideas for studies in the relapsed state are currently active in the UK.

1 A phase II study of idarubicin as a single agent for patients with relapsed intermediate- and high-grade lymphoma is being conducted by the Southampton Group, utilizing idarubicin alone at 21-day intervals at a dose of 15 mg/m², with dose escalation to a maximum of 20 mg/m². Response rates, toxicity and survival rates are being assessed.

2 The Royal Marsden Group are running a randomized trial of platinum-based chemotherapy with ECP with or without G-CSF for use in relapsed high-grade NHL and also in HD. This study aims to determine the maximum tolerated number of days of oral etoposide, with and without G-CSF, and the effect of this on response rate, and also to evaluate the efficacy and toxicity of ECP as a combination treatment in relapsed lymphoma patients.

3 The South West and Yorkshire Groups are running a pilot collaborative study utilizing dexamethasone, ara-C and cisplatinum with fludarabine phosphate (FLUDAP) in patients with relapsed refractory intermediate- and high-grade lymphoma. This is a 3-day course of treatment repeated every 3 weeks, and the drugs are all given as infusions of various lengths. The study aims to assess the toxicity and efficacy to this approach and entry to the study is restricted.

Extranodal non-Hodgkin's lymphoma

Extranodal NHL accounts for some 30% of presentations, with the commonest site being the gastrointestinal tract. A very useful review of the types of extranodal disease and approaches to treatment has recently been produced by Sutcliffe & Gospodarowicz [29]. While all workers in the lymphoma field have recognized, for some time, that the gastrointestinal lymphomas are a major problem, the difficulties associated with case accrual, staging and evaluation of treatment have been substantial. Thus, at the present time, only three major trials are in place for extranodal lymphomas in the UK.

Gastrointestinal lymphoma

Maltoma

The UK Lymphoma Group has recently activated a trial for low-grade gastric lymphoma (maltoma) (LYO3). In this study, the patients are randomized either to observation or chlorambucil following anti-*Helicobacter* therapy. This is to determine whether a 'wait and watch' policy is superior to oral chlorambucil when given to patients in remission following adequate anti-*Helicobacter* treatment.

Intermediate/high-grade lymphoma

The UK Lymphoma Group is also carrying out a study into the role of adjuvant therapy in intermediate- and high-grade gastrointestinal lymphoma. This study (LYO4) is for patients with gastrointestinal lymphoma who have had complete surgical resection of their tumour. Patients are again divided into risk groups. Those with low-stage disease (T_{1-2}, N_0, M_0) are randomized between CHOP × 3 and no further treatment. Those at high risk (T_{3-4}, N_{1-2}, M_0) are randomized between three and six cycles of CHOP. Patients with Burkitt's/lymphoblastic histology are excluded from this study. At the time of writing, this study is failing to recruit and may not proceed.

Cerebral lymphoma

Primary cerebral lymphoma is a rare tumour. There is a Medical Research Council trial (MRC BR6) which aims to assess if there is any difference in outcome (disease-free and overall survival) utilizing adjuvant chemotherapy in these patients. Following operative treatment and whole-brain radiotherapy, patients are randomized to receive six courses of CHOP or no further treatment.

Skin lymphomas

Within the UK there are also groups of individuals, attached to the main lymphoma groups, who have an interest in skin lymphomas. A number of protocols are in development, but none are available at the time of writing.

Conclusion

In many of the areas of lymphoma management, a classical trial structure can be extremely difficult to establish, and adherence to trial treatments can be very variable from centre to centre. The selection of patients within centres for any study can have a favourable effect on treatment results [30], and perhaps more effort should be made to audit what happens to those eligible patients who are excluded from the study in any participating centre. An alternative population-based practical method has been proposed, and provides an excellent vehicle for study where trials do not exist [31].

Progress in lymphoma treatment has slowed over the past decade and this has, in part, been because of insufficient numbers of patients being entered into appropriate studies and also partly because of the inconsistent design of some investigations. It is extremely important that, where a new treatment looks promising, it should be tested in a logical and formal way, so that any advantage can be proven beyond reasonable doubt. For rare tumours, national (or international) studies are required and in these instances the collaboration of regional groups is essential; an example of this is the 'Burkitt's' lymphomas and some of the extranodal lymphomas.

Alternative strategies include the assessment of outcome of particular diseases in population-based studies. When combined with detailed audit on presentation details and treatment, these can provide valuable information on the true incidence and patterns of survival, particularly in older patients and those with rare tumours who would not normally be entered into formal studies or placed on formal protocols [31]. In these patients this information would be unavailable from any other source, and in the absence of major studies could provide useful treatment guidelines. A similar approach might also prove useful in assessing the impact of newer, novel treatments, where formal trials are proving difficult to implement, for example assessing the impact of high-dose chemotherapy and bone marrow rescue, since recruitment for formal randomized trials can sometimes be difficult.

After a period of stagnation, a potentially exciting era of treatment for lymphoma is being entered, with newer strategies, including the use of cytokines, intensive treatments with growth factors and stem cell transplantation, which will all provide hope for the future. It is vital that these new opportunities are not wasted; national and international collaboration has never been easier or of more importance, and consultants within the UK can make major contributions in this field if such opportunities are grasped enthusiastically.

References

1 DeVita V.T., Simon R.M., Hubbard S.M. *et al.* (1980) Curability of advanced Hodgkin's disease with chemotherapy: long term follow-up of MOPP treated patients at the NCI. *Annals of Internal Medicine*, **92**, 587–595.
2 Coltman C.A. Jr. (1980) Chemotherapy of advanced Hodgkin's disease. *Seminars in Oncology*, **7**(2), 155–173.
3 Canellos G.P., Anderson J.R., Propert K.J. *et al.* (1992) Chemotherapy of advanced Hodgkin's disease with MOPP, ABVD, OR MOPP alternating with ABVD. *New England Journal of Medicine*, **372**, 1478–1484.
4 Linch D.C., Winfield D.A., Goldstone A.H. *et al.* (1993) Dose intensification with autologous bone marrow transplantation in relapsed and resistant Hodgkin's disease: results of a BNLI randomised trial. *Lancet*, **341**, 1050–1054.
5 Harris N.L., Jaffe E.S., Stein H. *et al.* (1994) A revised European–American classification of lymphoid neoplasms: a proposal from the International Lymphoma Study Group. *Blood*, **84**, 1361–1392.
6 Fisher R.I., Gaynor E.R., Dahlberg S. *et al.* (1993) Comparison of a standard regimen (CHOP) with three intensive chemotherapy regimens for advanced non-Hodgkin's lymphoma. *New England Journal of Medicine*, **328**, 1002–1006.
7 Verdonck L.F., Van Putten W.L.J., Hagenbeek A. *et al.* (1995) Comparison of CHOP chemotherapy with autologous bone marrow transplantation for slowly responding patients with aggressive non-Hodgkin's lymphoma. *New England Journal of Medicine*, **332**, 1045–1051.
8 Haioun C., Lepage E., Gisselbrecht C. *et al.* (1994) Comparison of autologous bone marrow transplantation with sequential chemotherapy for intermediate-grade and high-grade non-Hodgkin's lymphoma in first complete remission: a study of 464 patients. *Journal of Clinical Oncology*, **12**, 2543–2551.
9 Shipp M.A. on behalf of the International Non-Hodgkin's Lymphoma Prognostic Factors Project (1993) A predictive model for aggressive non-Hodgkin's lymphoma. *New England Journal of Medicine*, **329**, 987–994.
10 Vose J.M., Anderson J.R., Kessinger A. *et al.* (1993) High-dose chemotherapy and autologous haematopoietic stem-cell transplantation for aggressive non-Hodgkin's lymphoma. *Journal of Clinical Oncology*, **11**, 1846–1851.
11 Leonard R.C.F., Prescott R.J., Mao J.-H., White J.M. with members of the SNLG Therapy Working Party and Pathology Working Party: Allan N.C. *et al.* (1993) Successful application of a previously derived prognostic index in the analysis of a randomised trial of 281 patients with high grade non-Hodgkin's lymphoma (HIGNHL). *Annals of Oncology*, **4**, 853–856.
12 Proctor S.J., Taylor P.R.A., Donnan P. *et al.* with members of the Scotland and Newcastle Lymphoma Group (SNLG) Therapy Working Party (1991) A numerical prognostic index

for clinical use in identification of poor-risk patients with Hodgkin's disease at diagnosis. *European Journal of Cancer*, **27**, 624–629.

13 Haycock B.W., Vaughan Hudson G., Vaughan Hudson B. *et al.* (1992) LOPP alternating with EVAP is superior to LOPP alone in the initial treatment of advanced Hodgkin's disease: results of a British National Lymphoma Investigation Trial. *Journal of Clinical Oncology*, **10**, 1252–1258.

14 Proctor S.J. & Taylor P.R.A. (1993) Classical staging of Hodgkin's disease is inappropriate for selecting patients for clinical trials of intensive therapy: the case for the objective use of prognostic factor information in addition to classical staging. *Leukemia*, **7**, 1911–1920.

15 Bezwoda W.R., McPhail A.P., Dansey R. *et al.* (1995) Hodgkin's disease and its treatment in sub-Saharan Africa. In: *Cambridge Medical Reviews: haematological oncology*, pp. 21–40. Cambridge University Press, Cambridge.

16 Proctor S.J., Taylor P.R.A., Mackie M.J., Donnan R.B., Lennard A. & Prescott R.J. (1992) A numerical prognostic index for clinical use in identification of poor-risk patients with Hodgkin's disease at diagnosis. *Leukaemia and Lymphoma*, **7**, 17–20.

17 Horning S.J., Rosenberg S.A. & Hoppe R.T. (1996) Brief chemotherapy (Stanford V) and adjuvant radiotherapy for bulky or advanced Hodgkin's disease: an update. *Annals of Oncology*, **7**, 105–108.

18 Seymour L.K., Dansey R.D. & Bezwoda W.R. (1994) Single high-dose etoposide and melphalan with non-cryopreserved autologous marrow rescue as primary therapy for relapsed, refractory and poor-prognosis Hodgkin's disease. *British Journal of Cancer*, **70**, 526–530.

19 Taylor P.R.A., Jackson G.H., Lennard A.L., Lucraft H., Proctor S.J. on behalf of the Newcastle and Northern Region Lymphoma Group (1993) Autologous transplantation in poor risk Hodgkin's disease using high dose melphalan/etoposide conditioning with non-cryopreserved marrow rescue. *British Journal of Cancer*, **67**, 383–387.

20 Jackson G.H., Wood A.M., Taylor P.R.A. *et al.* (1997) Early high dose chemotherapy intensification with autologous bone marrow transplantation in lymphoma associated with retention of fertility and normal pregnancies in females. *Leukaemia and Lymphoma*, **28**, 127–132.

21 Leonard R.C.F., Hayward R.L., Prescott R.J. *et al.* (1991) The identification of discrete prognostic groups in low grade non-Hodgkin's lymphoma. *Annals of Oncology*, **2**, 655–662.

22 Cameron D.A.Y., Leonard R.C.F., Jian-Hua Mao *et al.* (1993) Identification of prognostic groups in follicular lymphoma. *Leukemia and Lymphoma*, **10**, 89–99.

23 Keating M.J., O'Brien S., Robertson L.E. *et al.* (1994) The expanding role of fludarabine in hematologic malignancies. *Leukemia and Lymphoma*, **14**, 11–16.

24 Johnson P.W.M., Rohatiner A.Z.S., Whelan J.S. *et al.* (1995) Patterns of survival in patients with recurrent follicular lymphoma: a 20 year study from a single centre. *Journal of Clinical Oncology*, **13**, 140–147.

25 Solal-Celigny P., Lepage E., Brousse N. *et al.* (1993) Recombinant interferon alfa-2b combined with a regimen containing doxorubicin in patients with advanced follicular lymphoma. *New England Journal of Medicine*, **329**, 1608–1613.

26 Smalley R.V., Andersen J.W., Hawkins M.J. *et al.* (1995) Interferon alfa combined with cytotoxic chemotherapy for patients with non-Hodgkin's lymphoma. *New England Journal of Medicine*, **327**, 1336–1349.

27 Patte C., Michon J., Frappaz D. *et al.* (1994) Therapy of Burkitt and other B-cell acute lymphoblastic leukaemia and lymphoma: experience with the LMB protocols of the SFOP (French Paediatric Oncology Society) in children and adults. *Ballière's Clinical Haematology*, **7**, 339–348.

28 McGrath I.T., Adde M., Eliad A. *et al.* (1996) Adults and children with small non-cleaved cell lymphoma have a similar excellent outcome when treated with the same chemotherapy regimen. *Journal of Clinical Oncology*, **14**, 925–934.

29 Sutcliffe S.B. & Gospodarowicz M.K. (1992) Clinical features and management of localized extranodal lymphomas. *Hematological Oncology*, **2**, 189–222.

30 The Toronto Leukaemia Study Group (1986) Results of chemotherapy for unselected patients with acute myeloblastic leukaemia: effect of exclusions on interpretation of results. *Lancet*, **i**, 786–788.

31 Charlton B.G., Taylor P.R.A. & Proctor S.J. (1997) The PACE (population-adjusted clinical epidemiology) strategy: a new approach to multi-centred clinical research. *Quarterly Journal of Medicine*, **90**, 147–151.

21 Allogeneic Bone Marrow Transplantation: Donor Selection

J. Hows and B. Bradley

Introduction

Over the last decade, the prevalence of allogeneic bone marrow transplantation (BMT) in Europe has increased from 880 in 1983 to 3639 in 1994 [1]. This is a result of the widening indications for the procedure and the increasing availability of unrelated volunteer donors [2]. Allogeneic BMT remains a costly high-risk procedure, to be carried out by experienced teams in centres with appropriate facilities and staffing equating to a 'level four' unit, which has been recently defined elsewhere [3]. This chapter addresses current theoretical, immunogenetic and clinical aspects of allogeneic marrow donor selection. The selection of HLA genotypically identical siblings, other relatives and unrelated volunteers as bone marrow donors is discussed, and recent data on banked cord blood and adult peripheral blood as alternative sources of haemopoietic stem cells are reviewed. Microbiological, psychosocial, medicolegal and ethical aspects of donor selection are not discussed in detail, as they have been recently and expertly reviewed elsewhere [4,5].

Patient selection—the first logical step in donor selection

At the outset, before a treatment plan is formulated, the haematologist must discuss with the patient and their family whether allogeneic transplantation is the clear treatment of choice, assuming a suitable donor can be found. Careful patient selection is the first step towards appropriate donor selection and a successful transplant. At present, it is difficult to know the precise place of allogeneic BMT compared with nonallograft treatment, not only because insufficient trials have been carried out, but also because the results of both allograft and nonallograft therapy are slowly improving as new therapeutic regimens are developed. Currently, there are relatively few disorders in which allogeneic BMT is the undisputed treatment of choice but many in which it has been used with a degree of success. For this reason, when a patient is considered a potential candidate for allogeneic BMT but doubt exists whether allografting is superior to nonallograft therapy, entry into national or international prospective randomized studies is important and advisable. The decision to enter patients into an appropriate study will often be made by the patient's primary haematologist. Where ongoing studies do not exist and a BMT is carried out, the transplant centre should submit the results to one of the two international BMT registries maintained by the European Group for Blood and Bone Marrow Transplantation (EBMT) and the International Bone Marrow Transplant Registry (IBMTR).

Deciding when not to proceed with a search for an allogeneic donor

It is often difficult for haematologists to take an objective decision not to initiate a donor search, as patients and their families may see BMT as the only chance of survival. It would be inappropriate to raise false hope of a 'cure' by searching for an HLA-identical sibling donor for a 60-year-old diabetic with ischaemic heart disease, chronic renal failure and chronic myeloid leukaemia, or for a child with persistent acute lymphoblastic leukaemia and septicaemia 1 month after failure of a first unrelated volunteer donor transplant.

Alternative donors are defined as family donors other than HLA genotypically identical siblings and all unrelated volunteer donors. Making the decision whether or not to embark on a search for an alternative donor for patients who lack an HLA-identical sibling can be even more problematical, as the only completely clear-cut indication for alternative donor transplantation is in infants with severe combined immunodeficiency [6]. Clinical guidelines dealing with selecting patients for unrelated donor BMT have been produced and published [7]. These guidelines are disease orientated and are shown in a modified form in Table 21.1. The recommendations in Table 21.1 may also be used as guidelines for selecting patients for partially HLA-matched family donor BMT. Developments in allogeneic BMT occur frequently, and current

Table 21.1 Patient criteria for unrelated donor search: assuming patient age of less than 55 years, patient informed consent and agreement by accredited transplant centre to treat patient. (Adapted from Schmitz *et al.*, 1996 [7].)

Category 1: BMT by accredited unit in research programme with ethics committee approval	Category 2: BMT by accredited unit for indication generally accepted on basis of published data from other centres
ALL in CR high risk	ALL in CR high risk
AML in CR high risk	AML in CR high risk
CML in chronic phase	CML in chronic phase
MDS (RA) poor risk	MDS (RA) poor risk
Lymphoma	Lymphoma
Myeloma	Myeloma
AML relapse	
CML accelerated phase	
RAEB	
RAEB-t	
SAA ($<0.2 \times 10^9$/l neutrophils) 3–6 months postimmunosuppression no response	SAA 3–6 months postimmunosuppression no response
Fanconi's anaemia, other congenital bone marrow failure	Fanconi's anaemia, other congenital bone marrow failure,
Inborn errors	Inborn errors
SCID, Wiscott–Aldrich syndrome	SCID, Wiscott–Aldrich syndrome
Chediack–Higashi syndrome	Chediack–Higashi syndrome
Hurler's disease	Hurler's disease
Gaucher's disease	Gaucher's disease
Osteopetrosis	Osteopetrosis
SAA ($>0.2 \times 10^9$/l neutrophils) >6 months postimmunosuppression no response	
Sickle cell disease, thalassaemia major	

ALL = acute lymphoblastic leukaemia; AML = acute myeloid leukaemia; CML = chronic myeloid leukaemia; CR = complete remission; MDS = myelodysplasia syndrome; RA = refractory anaemia; RAEB = refractory anaemia with excess of blasts; RAEB-t = refractory anaemia with excess of blasts in transformation; SAA = severe aplastic anaemia; SCID = severe combined immunodeficiency.

experimental treatment regimens will quickly be brought into the realms of established clinical trials. Increasingly there will be a choice of donor source for allogeneic stem cells as the use of peripheral blood progenitor cells [8,9] and cord blood cells [10,11] becomes established.

Cellular aspects of alloreactivity

Direct and indirect pathways of alloreactivity

Conceptually there are two pathways of alloreactivity — the direct and indirect pathways [12,13]. The distinction lies in the way donor and recipient cells interact to generate alloreactivity. Initially naive CD4+ T-helper-cell clones interact with dendritic cells carrying antigenic 'nonself' peptide. The T-cell clones with receptors for these antigens are activated, secrete cytokines and trigger a cascade of cellular responses that lead to graft rejection or graft vs host disease (GVHD). Antigenic peptide on dendritic cells are endogenously produced molecules synthesized by the genome (or latent viruses), that have been degraded and assembled in the endoplasmic reticulum into molecular complexes with newly formed HLA molecules. These complexes are expressed on the cell membrane, and form an extracellular array of HLA–peptide complexes that together constitute the histocompatibility phenotype of the individual. This array is surveyed by T cells that selectively bind to the complexes according to the avidity of their T-cell receptors (TCR). Antigenic peptide may, in addition, be acquired from extracellular histocompatibility proteins, microorganisms and oncogene products. These proteins are endocytosed, degraded and assembled with newly formed HLA molecules, before expression as HLA–peptide complexes at the cell surface. Direct activation occurs when donor T cells are stimulated by host dendritic cells. Indirect activation occurs when donor T cells are activated by donor dendritic cells that have acquired nonself peptide. These two pathways are not mutually exclusive, but may differ in timing of onset and duration. The direct pathway may be operational immediately after transplantation and may not persist after host dendritic cells have been replaced by donor cells. The indirect pathway will take longer to evolve, presumably because the frequency of specifically reactive donor T cells is low in the early posttransplant period. However, this pathway will continue to operate for as long as the graft persists, and may be responsible for acute and chronic GVHD, graft versus leukaemia activity, immunity against microbial pathogens and specific donor/recipient tolerance.

Proinflammatory and anti-inflammatory cytokine responses

According to one concept, naive CD4+ T-helper cells, termed TH_0 in the mouse, interact with dendritic cells bearing antigenic HLA–peptide complexes [14]. TH_0 cells then differentiate along one of two alternative pathways, termed TH_1 and TH_2. The predominance of one pathway dictates whether the evolving response is aggressive or anergic. TH_1 clones secrete 'proinflammatory cytokines' (interleukin-2 (IL-2), tumour necrosis factor alpha (TNFα), interferon gamma (IFNγ)), characteristically found in association with aggressive allograft rejection, life-threatening GVHD and the clinically recognizable 'cytokine storm' that can follow BMT from donors other than HLA genotypically identical siblings. TH_2 clones secrete 'anti-inflammatory' cytokines (IL-10, IL-4) that damp down cellular alloimmunity but favour humoral alloimmunity and are found in situations where tolerance and stable chimerism persist. Typically, anti-inflammatory (TH_2) cytokines predominate in mice that have been rendered tolerant by neonatal injection of foreign spleen cells (classical tolerance). In man, TH_2 cytokines predominate in children born with severe combined immunodeficiency disease (SCID) who have been successfully cured following the transplantation of unmatched embryonic liver cells at birth [15].

NK-cell function

Mature NK cells are polyclonal cytotoxic lymphocytes that lack the phenotypic markers of both T cells (TCR, CD3) and B cells (membrane immunoglobulin, CD19). Morphologically they are large granular lymphocytes. They bear Fc RIII (CD16) and CD56 markers *in vitro*. They kill cells infected with microorganisms (viruses, bacteria, fungi) and certain sensitive tumour cell-lines that lack expression of HLA (K562). The mechanism of killing is via the perforin/granzyme pathway. Their *raison d'être* is poorly understood, but they are thought to have a unique role in the immune system to detect and eliminate cells with absent or aberrant expression of HLA-Class I molecules. In healthy individuals, NK-cell clones are inhibited via specific receptors, known as 'killer inhibitor receptors' (KIR), that bind to ligands on HLA-Class I molecules (HLA-A, B and C). Failure of inhibition and killing by NK clones occurs if expression of a specific HLA molecule on the cell under surveillance is altered or absent. NK cells play an important role in defence against a wide range of microorganisms, because they are able to synthesize IFNγ and activate macrophages [16]. Donor-derived NK cells peak around 28 days after BMT, even where donor T cells have been depleted from the graft. These cells may play an important part in recovery of immune competence after BMT. For many years it has been suggested that NK cells have an antitumour cell function. When expanded *in vitro* with IL-2 to create populations of so-called 'lymphokine-activated killer' (LAK) cells, there is evidence that autologous NK cells have antitumour activity [17]. There are limited *in vitro* data to support an NK-cell-mediated graft versus leukaemia effect after BMT [18], although an *in vivo* antileukaemic role remains unproven. The contribution of NK cells to rejection or GVHD in situations where HLA-Class I is mismatched is also poorly understood, but deserves further investigation. At present NK-cell activity is not taken into consideration in clinical donor selection.

Molecular aspects of alloreactivity

HLA–peptide complex assembly

Newly synthesized proteins are processed within cytoplasmic proteasomes and transported, in association with TAP1/TAP2 heterodimeric proteins, into the endoplasmic reticulum. They then become associated with maturing HLA-Class I β2-microglobulin molecules, with which they are transported to the cytoplasmic membrane. Exogenous proteins are processed entirely in endocytic compartments and are bound to HLA-Class II heterodimers before transport to the cytoplasmic membrane. Thus, HLA molecules form stable complexes with peptides that are either produced endogenously or exogenously in relation to the cell's genome. The allogeneic peptide component of these complexes are the degraded products of non-HLA genes (the minority) and other HLA genes (the majority). Class I-associated peptides tend to be nine amino acids in length (nonamers) and Class II-associated peptides are 12–25 amino acids in length. Together, these HLA–peptide complexes constitute the histocompatibility phenotype of the individual. Following BMT, many components of the host peptide pool are seen as 'nonself' by mature donor T cells, despite close HLA matching between donor and recipient [19].

Polymorphism of histocompatibility genes

The histocompatibility phenotype of an individual includes an array of HLA–peptide complexes which are the products of HLA and non-HLA genes. Apart from monozygotic twins, no two individuals carry exactly the same phenotype. The HLA region spans 4000 kilobases on the short arm of chromosome 6 [20]. It contains more than 50 loci; alloreactivity *in vitro* can be elicited by 11 of these. These loci are divided into HLA-Class I (HLA-A, B, C) and HLA-Class II (HLA-DRA1, DRB1, DRB3, DRB4, DRB5, DQA1, DQB1, DPB1). The number of alleles discovered at each of these loci increases monthly as different populations are typed by sensitive genotyping techniques. Each offspring inherits two codominantly expressed alleles at each locus, one from the mother and one from the father. Within families, the HLA region tends to be inherited *en bloc* and each paternal or maternal set of alleles is termed a 'haplotype'. Occasionally recombination occurs during meiosis (one in 60 meiotic divisions), causing rearrangement of alleles in juxtaposition and the creation of new 'recombined' haplo-

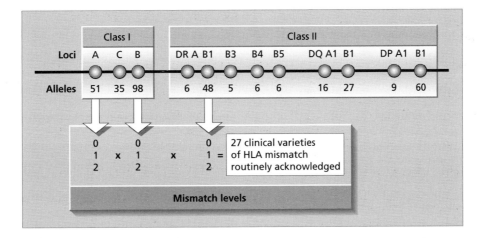

Fig. 21.1 Diagram of an HLA haplotype showing the loci that code for histocompatibility antigens and the total number of alleles identified at each, plus one for the unidentified 'null' gene. Given that each individual inherits one allele from each parent, the theoretical number of HLA phenotypes is given by: $(51 \times 35 \times 98 \times 6 \times 48 \times 5 \times 6 \times 6 \times 16 \times 27 \times 9 \times 60)^2 = 4.5 \times 10^{30}$. In routine tissue typing for most clinical transplantation purposes, mismatches at only three loci (HLA-A, B, DR) are considered. Knowledge of the influence of mismatches at different HLA loci is therefore confined to the 27 varieties of mismatch at these loci.

types in the offspring. Rarely mutations occur at an HLA locus to create a new allele. Thus three evolutionary mechanisms conspire to create a vast range of HLA polymorphisms, simple codominant inheritance, recombination and mutation. The impetus behind this diversity is the need for a flexible immune system, to counteract the vast range of pathogens that require elimination if an individual is to survive [21]. In this way pathogen-driven diversity is creating a vast range of histocompatibility phenotypes (Fig. 21.1).

In families the parental HLA haplotypes, represented by *ab* and *cd*, are inherited as four possible combinations, *ac, ad, bc* and *bd*, giving a 25% probability of any two offspring being HLA identical. More distant relatives have a correspondingly lower probability, and unrelated pairs of individuals have the lowest probability of being HLA identical. However, ethnic groups have different size HLA gene pools and, in addition, founder effects and promotion of first-cousin marriages can restrict HLA polymorphism, increasing the chances of finding an HLA phenotypically matched related donor.

The phenomenon of linkage disequilibrium, whereby sets of linked HLA genes tend to occur more often than expected within a population, ensures that some histocompatibility phenotypes recur more frequently than expected. Each ethnically distinct population is characterized by a set of 'common haplotypes' that ensure an uneven distribution of histocompatibility types (Table 21.2). For these reasons, searching for an HLA-matched donor within a defined ethnic

group becomes a realistic exercise [22]. The products of non-HLA genes that code for the peptide pool are either monomorphic or polymorphic. The immunogenicity of non-HLA gene products depends on the individual's HLA genotype. Experimental evidence indicates that different HLA alleles selectively bind different non-HLA peptide segments from the same 'parent' protein, according to the avidity of their anchor sites. This accounts for the lack of immunogenicity between certain non-HLA mismatches. The male-linked histocompatibility antigen, H-Y, is an example, as it appears to be immunogenic when presented in the context of HLA-A2 but nonimmunogenic when presented in the context of many other HLA-Class I alleles [23]. This suggests that in a large family where the patient expresses HLA-A2, and both a brother and sister are HLA identical, the same-sex donor should be selected to avoid host versus graft and graft versus host reactions resulting from alloreactivity associated with the H-Y antigen. Polymorphic non-HLA gene products so far implicated in acute GVHD are: HA-1 [24], PECAM-1 (CD31) [25] and a gene product coded on the long arm of chromosome 22 between the platelet-derived growth factor beta (PDGFβ) and the beta chain of the IL-2 receptor (IL-2Rβ) genes. The chromosome 22 peptide has only been identified in a limited number of HLA-B7 individuals [26]. The HA-1 antigen has an antigen frequency of approximately 20% in HLA-A2 individuals. PECAM-1 (CD31) polymorphisms are attributed to a single base change in codon 125 giving two alleles, CD31.L and CD31.V. Homozygotes for CD31.L have a frequency of 0.30, homozygotes for CD31.V 0.28 and heterozygotes 0.42.

The T-cell repertoire

This refers to the entire range of epitopes recognized by an individual's T cells. Each clone carries a distinct T-cell receptor (TCR), controlled by a number of different TCR-region genetic sequences [27]. The T-cell repertoire is tailored by the thymus during fetal ontogeny, so that clones directed towards the self-HLA-peptide pool are cut out, thereby giving it a negative

Population (no. typed)	A	Cw	B	DR	DQ	HF (%)*
North American Negroid (312)	36	4	53	11	1	1.1
Cornish (101)	1	7	8	3	2	8.4
Dane (122)	3	7	7	15	1	3.6
French (244)	1	7	8	3	2	2.5
German (203)	1	7	8	3	2	4.8
Greek (176)	2	4	35	11	7	2.0
Italian (483)	2	4	35	11	7	2.3
Spanish (192)	29	—†	44	7	2	3.0
USA (226)	1	7	8	3	2	4.5
Canadian (142)	1	7	8	3	2	5.2
Brazilian (286)	24	4	35	11	7	1.4
Japanese (893)	24	—	52	15	1	8.3
Korean (235)	33	—	44	13	1	4.5
Thais (235)	2	11	46	9	3	4.5
Vietnamese (140)	29	—	7	10	1	4.6
Inuit (144)	24	—	48	4	7	9.4

Table 21.2 The most common HLA haplotypes in various ethnic groups.

* Haplotype frequency.
† Null or unidentified allele.

imprint of the individual's own histocompatibility phenotype. The antigen-binding specificity of each TCR is determined by the total genetic contribution of both TCR and (or) V, D and J segment genes, as well as N-region genes. The V-region repertoire is considered synonymous with the T-cell repertoire, even though it is only one measure of diversity within T-cell populations. The V-region repertoire mirrors the self-HLA–peptide pool. The influence of histocompatibility phenotype on V-region repertoire is unequivocally demonstrated in pairwise comparisons between HLA-identical siblings, who have more homology in their V-segment distribution than HLA-mismatched siblings. The similarity between monozygotic twins is greater than HLA genotypically identical sibling pairs, reflecting the contribution of non-HLA peptides to the TCR repertoire [28,29]. The CD4+ T-cell subpopulation possesses higher frequencies of certain Vβ alleles, Vβ.2, 5, 19, 20, whereas CD8+ T cells use other alleles, Vβ.7, 14. The former are 'instructed' by the thymus to interact with HLA-Class II–peptide and the latter with HLA-Class I–peptide complexes. After BMT, the importance of the host T-cell repertoire dwindles over a period of months as host lymphocytes die off and donor T cells become established [30]. The donor repertoire contains clones recognizing mismatched HLA–peptide complexes of host origin; these trigger the synthesis of proinflammatory cytokines, leading to acute GVHD and other complications [31]. Studies of immunological reconstitution after adult BMT indicate that the donor's mature T-cell repertoire is adopted by the host [32]. In the event of T-cell depletion, however, immune reconstitution will depend on the naive donor T-cell repertoire derived from freshly differentiated T cells programmed through the host's thymus. There are data which indicate that immune reconstitution is slower after unrelated-donor compared with HLA-identical sibling trans-

plants [33]. Thymic function declines with age, but in paediatric recipients its continuing function might explain, in part, why children tolerate HLA-mismatched BMT better than adults [34].

Donor T-cell sensitization to alloantigens

Another major influence on the T-cell repertoire is prior sensitization of the donor to histocompatibility antigens through pregnancy or blood transfusions. Selected, high-avidity T-cell clones, directed to certain epitopes, become disproportionately represented compared with the naive T-cell repertoire. In clinical practice, the risk of acute GVHD after HLA-identical sibling BMT is higher with parous female donors compared with non-sensitized male donors, probably as a result of pregnancy-induced sensitization [35]. In clinical donor selection, where more than one potential donor is matched for HLA and has negative cytomegalovirus (CMV) serology (see below), prior sensitization of the donor should be considered as a selection criterion. When this opportunity arises, a nonsensitized donor should be selected.

T-cell sensitization to viral antigens

It is of interest that accumulative exposure of the donor to herpes viruses prior to donation is associated with increasingly severe acute GVHD [36]. It is likely that clones of virus-specific mature donor T cells are responsible for recognition of virally infected cells in the recipient, and these trigger a T-cell-mediated graft versus host reaction. There is a high probability that all haemopoietic stem cell donors, apart from cord blood donors, will have been exposed to one or more herpes virus. This means that, in most cases, transfer of virally primed donor

T cells cannot be avoided. Where there is a choice of donors because a number are histocompatibile, the donor's exposure to cytomegalovirus (CMV) should be considered as a selection criterion. This is not only because of the GVHD association with latent donor CMV virus, but also because of the small risk that recipient CMV infection in the post-transplant period may occur as a result of transferred donor virus.

Cytokine polymorphisms

TNFα is a proinflammatory cytokine released by activated macrophages and, together with IFNγ and IL-1, it causes endothelial cell activation, leading to increased expression of cell adhesion molecules (ICAM-1, VCAM-1, E-selectin), and upregulation of HLA expression, leading to activation of allogeneic T cells [37]. The genes responsible for TNFα map between HLA-B and DR and certain haplotypes are associated with different levels of TNFα production. HLA-DR2, DQ1 individuals give consistently lower TNFα levels than HLA-DR3 and DR4 individuals [38]. These differences are associated with a single base substitution (A/G) at position −308 in the TNFα promoter gene. The two alleles created by this substitution are associated with a sevenfold difference in the level of TNFα transcription [39]. In HLA-identical sibling BMT, recipient TNFα levels measured before and during pretransplant conditioning therapy are higher in recipients who subsequently develop clinically severe transplant-related complications, including GVHD, than in those who do not [40,41]. This difference is associated with allelic differences at the −308 site in the TNFα promoter. It is not yet known how the donor TNFα polymorphism affects the incidence of transplant-related complications. In unrelated donor BMT, where minor degrees of HLA mismatch are very frequent, the influence of TNFα promoter gene polymorphisms is likely to be greater, although there are no clinical reports, as yet, to confirm this hypothesis.

IL-10 is an anti-inflammatory cytokine that counteracts the effects of TNFα. The spontaneous release of IL-10 from the mononuclear cells of patients, who were sampled prior to commencing pretransplant conditioning, shows a striking association with survival and transplant-related complications after BMT. Those with low levels of secretion are at greater risk of dying from transplant-related complications than those with high levels [42]. To date, three allelic polymorphisms have been found at positions −1082, −879 and −592 in relation to the transcription start site of the IL-10 gene. Each of these sites is associated with high or low levels of production in Con A-stimulated peripheral blood lymphocytes *in vitro* [43]. At present, there are no data relating IL-10 promoter polymorphisms to donor selection or clinical outcome after BMT. Other pro- and anti-inflammatory cytokine promoters are known to be polymorphic, including TGFβ and IL-4.

Theoretical considerations influencing donor selection

Selection of the 'ideal' allogeneic bone marrow donor would lead to the following desirable post-transplant events: (i) optimal engraftment and immune reconstitution; (ii) minimal acute and chronic GVHD; (iii) minimal probability of relapse.

Important characteristics of the graft which predict transplant outcome are highly interactive. An attempt has been made to summarize major interactions between graft variables and transplant outcome in Table 21.3. The universal ideal donation does not exist in reality. Most patients, and many physicians, would consider a syngeneic twin as the ideal donor. This might be so for a patient receiving a transplant for severe aplastic anaemia, where prompt engraftment, good immune reconstitution and complete lack of GVHD are the ideal. It is debatable whether the same dogma applies to all patients with leukaemia, where the probability of relapse is significantly higher after syngeneic transplantation than after T-cell-replete HLA genotypically identical sibling BMT in the presence or absence of acute and chronic GVHD. This emphasizes the need for clinical or subclinical donor T-cell alloreactivity, to provide extra antileukaemic activity in addition to that provided by the pretransplant conditioning protocol [44].

In practice, patients rarely have the choice between a syngeneic twin and an HLA genotypically identical sibling, and at least two-thirds of patients only have the choice of an unrelated volunteer who may or may not be well matched for HLA. Thus the main objective in clinical donor selection is to use the donor who best matches the patient for HLA. Where mismatch exists, it should be defined as carefully as possible with the available techniques, this being the first step towards 'intelligent mismatching'. In the future, intelligent mismatching will only be possible when there is a better understanding

Table 21.3 Graft variables which affect haemopoietic cell transplant outcome.

	Engraftment	Immune reconstitution	GVHD	Relapse
Donor sensitization	?	?	Increased	?
HLA/non-HLA mismatch	Reduced	Reduced	Increased	Reduced
High cell dose	Increased	?	?	?
Donor T-cell depletion	Reduced	Reduced	Reduced	Increased

of which HLA (and non-HLA) mismatches lead to alloreactivity and which may be associated with immunological tolerance.

Application of typing and matching techniques

The outcome of BMT is associated with better results when all HLA loci are matched, which is only certain when the donor is a well-typed HLA genotypically identical sibling. Avoidance of mismatches for non-HLA loci may be feasible in situations where the patient or the donor are known to be sensitized to single epitopes (e.g. female patients sensitized to H-Y), but otherwise it is not routinely possible. A more pragmatic goal is to identify the levels of tolerable mismatch that can be controlled by current immunosuppressive drug regimens. Current ignorance of which mismatches are tolerable should not prevent the defininition of donor and recipient genotypes as precisely as current techniques will allow. Only by studying such data in a wide range of transplants will optimal donor selection be developed. Many cytokine genes are associated with polymorphisms at promoter gene level, leading to different rates of mRNA transcription and varying levels of cytokine production. At least one of these, the TNFα promoter gene, is known to have a major effect on BMT outcome [45]. Knowledge of polymorphisms of both donor and recipient promoter genes for TNFα, and possibly IL-10, will be of prognostic value for predicting transplant-related complications. For reasons of economy and speed, not all tests can be carried out before transplantation, so sufficient viable cells and DNA must be stored prior to the transplant for further retrospective studies. At present, a pragmatic approach to defining acceptable mismatches is required. The following sections describe the principles underlying typing and matching donors during the selection procedure.

HLA typing by serology

During the 1960s, a 'simple' genetic system responsible for kidney transplant rejection and BMT success was discovered. It had a few alleles, similar to the ABO blood group system. Leukoagglutinins found in the sera of some parous women were used as the reagents to select compatible siblings for most of the early bone marrow transplants reported in the literature [46,47]. As the complexity of this human leukocyte antigen (HLA) system emerged, a more practical microlymphocytotoxicity test was developed that required a battery of highly selected sera from parous women. Lymphocytes to be typed were added to the typing sera, followed by a fresh rabbit serum as a source of complement. Rabbit serum is not inhibited by human decay accelerating factor (DAF), and allows cell lysis to proceed to completion. After incubation a viability stain, ethidium bromide, was added to measure the degree of cell death. Lymphocytotoxicity was assessed microscopically by a skilled technician. Patterns of positive wells were interpreted

against known HLA specificities and a phenotype deduced. A standardized version of this method, known as the 'NIH method', was, until recently, widely used for routine HLA typing and matching for transplantation.

The major drawback of microlymphocytotoxicity typing is the complexity of the typing sera used. These are derived from pregnant women who often respond to all paternal HLA-Class I and II mismatches on fetal tissues. Another complication is that, whereas all peripheral blood lymphocytes (PBL) express HLA-Class I antigens, HLA-Class II antigens are only expressed on B cells constituting 10% of PBL. Hence an enrichment step for B cells is required for HLA-Class II typing. Class II typing of some patients fails, because B cells have been depleted by the disease [48]. The technological limitations of serological typing are exaggerated with certain HLA molecules that are weakly expressed on the cell membrane, such as HLA-C and DP. Interestingly, sera from patients who rejected organ transplants are considered unsuitable for typing, even though they contain high titres of antibodies directed to relevant HLA mismatches. The reason is that such sera are 'too complex', because they react with multiple epitopes, many of which are shared between different HLA alleles. For typing, focused allele-specific sera are required; the ideal is a specific monoclonal antibody and there are several commercially available. HLA alleles of different loci in high linkage disequilibrium, such as HLA-DR and DQ, are often very difficult to serotype accurately, because the polyclonal sera used contain antibodies to linked products of adjacent loci. Furthermore, ethnic groups are characterized by different sets of linked alleles, causing serological reagents from one ethnic group to be less accurate when tested on another. As most HLA typing sera are Caucasian, difficulties arise when serotyping non-Caucasian individuals and those of mixed ethnic background.

Lymphocytotoxic antibody crossmatching

A cytotoxic crossmatch is performed routinely before unrelated cadaveric renal transplantation to avoid hyperacute rejection. Patient serum is crossmatched against lymphocytes from the potential donor in a lymphocytotoxicity assay similar to that used for serotyping by the NIH method. Humoral sensitization against mismatched HLA antigens is acquired through prior transplantation, transfusion or pregnancy. Virtually all lymphocytotoxic antibodies are directed to HLA gene products, hence in HLA-identical sibling BMT a cytotoxic crossmatch is unhelpful. However, a cytotoxic crossmatch is invaluable in detecting prior sensitization to HLA mismatches when partially matched related and unrelated donors are considered. Multifactorial analysis of variables affecting engraftment failure has shown a strong association between this complication and a positive cytotoxic crossmatch [49]. Non-HLA histocompatibility antigens rarely elicit humoral antibody production, but commonly give rise to T-cell sensitization that can be detected in a cell-mediated lympholysis assay (CML)

[23]. This technique has not been used for routine donor selection.

HLA typing by DNA technology

The recent introduction of DNA typing methods for HLA has exposed the technical limitations of serological typing [50]. DNA and amino acid sequences of all known HLA-A, B, C, DR, DQ and DP alleles are documented and it is clear that as typing sera are limited rarer alleles will be missed or mistyped by serology. In a limited comparison of serological and DNA typing, it emerged that rarer alleles are often misassigned to poorly defined serological types such as HLA-DR6, leading to false assumptions of matching. Over the past 5 years, DNA typing methods have become routine for HLA-Class II typing of marrow donors and recipients [51]. Initially this was carried out by analysis of restriction fragment length polymorphisms (RFLP). Genomic DNA is digested using endonucleases that cut the DNA in the introns (restriction sites) to give fragments of variable length. The precise location of these sites is specific to each HLA allele or set of alleles. For RFLP typing, the DNA digest is treated with alkali to render it single stranded, and then electrophoresed on a gel to separate the fragments according to size. The gel is then blotted onto a membrane that is incubated with a radioactive phosphorus-labelled single-stranded locus-specific probe. The probe binds to the gene fragments and is visualized autoradiographically as a banding pattern. The number of bands, and their distance from the origin, gives a unique pattern for each HLA-DR allele. In principle, RFLP analysis seldom detects alleles that cannot be detected serologically with very high quality reagents, but it has advantages over *routine* serology. The clinical relevance of RFLP analysis was shown in kidney transplant studies, where grafts that were HLA-DR matched by RFLP and serology had a significantly higher survival rate than those matched by serology alone [52]. The main disadvantage of RFLP typing is that it is slow, taking 14 days to complete, and has largely been superseded by polymerase chain reaction (PCR) based techniques.

PCR methods are in routine use for HLA-Class II and are increasingly used for HLA-Class I typing. The different techniques so far developed have been recently reviewed [51] and are summarized in Table 21.4. Locus-specific primers or sets of allele-specific primers are incubated with single-stranded genomic DNA along with Taq polymerase. In situations where rapid results are required on relatively small batches of samples, an appropriately selected set of sequence-specific primers are used in the PCR. Consequently allelic products are amplified several million fold, but only those allelic products present in the genome will be expanded. Genotyping is then a simple matter of electrophoresing the products to see which reactions have yielded an amplified product. This technique is known as PCR sequence-specific primer (PCR-SSP) typing. An alternative technique, more suitable for large batches of samples where only intermediate resolution typing is required, involves the use of locus-specific PCR primers. The product is converted into single-stranded DNA and tested against an appropriately selected set of labelled allele-specific oligonucleotide probes. Positive hybridization with an allele-specific probe indicates the presence of that allele in the genome. This approach is known as PCR sequence-specific oligonucleotide (PCR-SSO) typing. Both PCR-SSP and PCR-SSO have been developed with nonradioactive readouts utilizing colorimetric or chemiluminescent labels. Reagents required for PCR-SSP and PCR-SSO typing have been assembled into kits by expert research laboratories in association with organizations such as Eurotransplant and the British Society for Histocompatibility and Immunogenetics. This policy has allowed a large number of smaller laboratories to take advantage of standardized, cost-effective current technology for typing donors and recipients for BMT.

A more elaborate approach to HLA typing is nucleotide sequencing of the specific hypervariable region of each allele of interest in exons 2 and 3 of the HLA genes. Sequence-based

Table 21.4 Polymerase chain reaction-based HLA typing methods. (Adapted and updated from Bidwell, 1994 [51].)

Method	Multiple PCR	Multiple probes	Post-PCR manipulations	Applications described
PCR-SSO dot blot	−	+	H, AR/CD	HLA-A, B, DRB, DQA, DQB, DPB
PCR-SSO reverse dot blot (automated variations)	−	+	H, CD	HLA-DRB, DQA, DQB, DPB
PCR-RFLP	−	+	RE, AGE	HLA-DRB, DQA, DQB, DPA, DPB
PCR-SSP	+	−	AGE	HLA-A, B, C, DRB, DQA, DQB
PCR-SBT	−	−	DD, DP	HLA-A, B, C, DRB
PCR-SSCP	−	−	NDP	HLA-DRB, DQB
PCR-heteroduplex analysis	−	−	NDP, CM	HLA-DRB, DQA, DQB, DPB

AGE = agarose gel electrophoresis; AR = autoradiography; CD = colometric or chemiluminesence detection; CM = crossmatch; DD = dideoxynucleotide chain termination sequencing; DP = denaturing polyacrylamide gel electrophoresis; H = hybridization; NDP = nondenaturing polyacrylamide gel electrophoresis; RE = restriction endonuclease digestion.

typing (SBT) is a PCR technique, in which the product is either analysed using Dynabeads in solid phase or by utilizing cDNA copies of the polymorphic exons of HLA synthesized by reverse transcriptase from total cellular RNA. Although SBT is now fully automated, it is not currently a cost-effective method for HLA of typing donor–recipient pairs in routine laboratories.

HLA matching by DNA technology

Serological typing, PCR-SSP and PCR-SSO typing all rely on the assignment of a genotype to assess donor–recipient compatibility. The absence of reagents for rarer alleles means that in cases where they are present, practically always as heterozygotes, they will be misclassified or given a 'blank' assignment. This leads to matching errors and poor clinical outcome. One way to detect rare alleles is to use a form of DNA matching. The relevant exons of HLA-Class I and II genes are PCR amplified using locus-specific primers, and the single-stranded products are snap cooled on ice before electrophoresing on polyacrylamide minigels. Rapid cooling causes the single-stranded PCR product to anneal to itself via stretches of complementary nucleotides, to form uniquely shaped molecules that migrate to specific sites on the gel. These are known as sequence-specific conformational polymorphisms (SSCP). In addition to SSCP, single-stranded products reanneal to partially complementary antisense products of adjacent genes in both *cis* and *trans* to form heteroduplexes, or with complementary strands to form homoduplexes. These products (SSCP, heteroduplexes and homoduplexes) migrate to specific sites in the gel by virtue of their shape and charge, giving a reproducible and unique banding pattern for each HLA phenotype at each locus (Fig. 21.2). Banding patterns are revealed by ethidium bromide or silver staining and can be compared visually or by densitometry and stored electronically. Image analysis techniques can then be applied to reveal differences resulting from undetected mismatches. This method is simple, exquisitely sensitive, fast and inexpensive. It is known as DNA conformational analysis (DNA-CA). Alternative forms of this approach have been developed for Class II [53] and Class I [54] genes, and applied to the detection of clinically relevant mismatches [55].

Analysis of cytokine profiles

This is performed in specialist laboratories. Serum levels of TNFα and IL-10 are assayed by an enzyme-linked immunoabsorbent assay [42]. The quantitation of cytokine messenger RNA can be carried out using competitive reverse transcriptase PCR (RT-PCR) assays. Genotyping for the TNFα promoter mutation at position −308 is by DNA-RFLP analysis using the endonuclease NcoI, or by PCR techniques. PCR techniques have also been used to investigate IL-10 promoter polymorphisms.

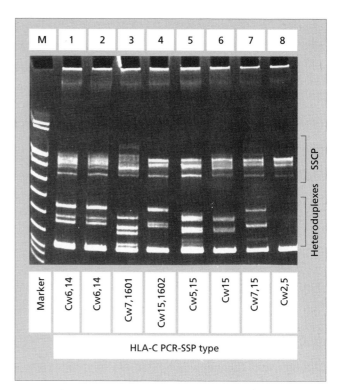

Fig. 21.2 A PCR-SSCP analysis of the HLA-C locus in eight normal individuals. The HLA-C PCR-SSP types of these individuals are shown at the bottom of the figure. The PCR-SSCP analysis shows a unique banding pattern made up of both SSCP and hetereoduplex bands for each individual.

Non-HLA histocompatibility antigen and gene typing

This is performed in specialist laboratories, where the only important associations with graft failure and graft versus host disease identified have been with H-Y [23] and HA-1 [24], respectively, in HLA-identical sibling BMT. HA-1 typing is carried out by a lymphocytolysis assay. Cloned T-killer-cell lines recognizing the HLA–peptide complex (HLA-A2; HA-1) are used as reagents to test for the presence of the epitope on radioactive chromium-labelled PHA lymphoblasts from the individual to be typed. Typing is currently confined to HLA-A2-positive individuals. The peptide identified on the long arm of chromosome 22 has been typed in a similar lymphocytolysis assay using cloned T-killer-cell lines (MD2), and here the restricting type is the HLA-B7 allele, but the peptide has yet to be characterized [26]. PECAM 1 (CD31) typing is by a PCR-SSP applied to genomic DNA using pairs of primers designed to recognize the CD31.L and CD31.V alleles [25]. Typing for non-HLA antigens is not currently carried out in clinical donor selection.

Functional assays for donor selection

All *in vitro* functional tests of alloreactivity are based on the 'one-way' mixed lymphocyte reaction (MLR). Peripheral blood mononuclear cells from one individual, designated the responder, are placed in tissue culture with similar cells from another individual, designated the stimulator. Stimulator cells are irradiated (2000–3000 cGy) or treated with mitomycin C. This allows these cells to express HLA–peptide complexes and to stimulate the responder lymphocyte population, but prevents them proliferating. In a standard MLR, the readout is the amount of lymphocyte proliferation at 3–5 days measured by the incorporation of radioactive thymidine into the DNA of proliferating responder cells. The MLR is a polyclonal reaction involving activation mainly of T-cell clones with many different functions. MLR studies involving partially HLA-matched sibling pairs, where recombination has occurred between the HLA-B and DR loci, indicate that mismatched HLA-Class II region gene products (especially HLA-DR) are the strongest stimulus for proliferation. However, CD8+ killer T cells capable of killing HLA-Class I mismatches on the stimulator cell also proliferate and differentiate in MLR. Studies with unrelated partially matched individuals show that all HLA-Class I and II gene products contribute to proliferation by the responding T-cell population. Although the MLR is a good indicator of mismatch, it is of limited prognostic value in the selection of unrelated donors for reasons that are not fully understood [56].

In the cell-mediated lympholysis (CML) assay, cells are cultured in a one-way MLR, but the readout is a measure of the cultured responder cell's ability to lyse target cells of the stimulator phenotype. Target cells are lymphoblasts generated by culturing nonirradiated mononuclear cells from the stimulator individual with phytohaemaglutinin (PHA). When PHA blast transformation is optimal, they are labelled with radioactive chromium and added to the MLR-primed responder cells. The level of chromium released into the supernatant is a semi-quantitative measure of the cytotoxic cells specific for the original stimulator generated. CML assays reflect mismatches for HLA-Class I gene products and the 'allopeptides' carried by these molecules.

Cytotoxic T-cell precursor frequency assay

The cytotoxic T-cell precursor (CTL-p) frequency assay is a quantitative form of the CML. It may, in certain clinical settings, provide information of prognostic value with regard to the outcome of BMT. The CTL-p assay is performed using limiting dilutions analysis to measure the frequency of T cells capable of lysing target lymphoblasts. Assays are set up in 96-well culture plates with a standard number of irradiated stimulator cells, excess IL-2 and serial dilutions of responder cells. After 7 days, radioactive chromium-labelled PHA lymphoblasts of stimulator type are added to each well and the chromium release in the supernatant measured. A high level of chromium release signifies the presence of at least one clone of killer cells in a well, which corresponds to a single cell in the

original population of cells. By counting the proportion of negative wells at each dilution, and by applying Poisson statistics, the frequency of cytolytic T-cell precursors is estimated [57]. Unlike MLR and CML tests, CTL-p frequencies correlate with the outcome of unrelated donor BMT when conducted in some, but not all, centres [58–60]. It is possible that this correlation is highly dependent on the transplant centre's immunosuppressive protocol for GVHD prophylaxis. So far, all centres finding the CTL-p frequency assay predictive of unrelated donor BMT outcome have used T-cell depletion protocols [58,59]. In contrast, the Seattle group, who rely on the cyclosporin and methotrexate protocol for prevention of GVHD after unrelated donor BMT, have failed to correlate CTL-p frequency with transplant outcome [60]. The CTL-p frequency analysis is not sensitive enough to be used as a predictive test of outcome after HLA-identical sibling BMT [58]. The CTL-p assay is expensive and labour intensive and, until it is standardized between laboratories, its value in unrelated marrow donor selection is controversial.

Helper T-cell precursor frequency analysis

The helper T-cell precursor (HTL-p) frequency is measured by limiting dilution analysis and is calculated in exactly the same way as CTL-p, except that the readout is a measure of whether or not IL-2 is released into the supernatant, which indicates the proliferation of one or more responder T-helper cells present in individual wells. Replicate cultures at several different responder cell dilutions and fixed numbers of irradiated stimulator cells are set up in 96-well plates and cultured for 64 hours, followed by the addition of cells from the IL-2-dependent CTLL-2 cell-line. After a further 16 hours' incubation, proliferation of the indicator cell line is measured by the uptake of radioactive thymidine. Wells that produce IL-2 are assumed to contain one or more clones of helper T cells, each of which corresponds to a precursor cell in the original population. Preliminary reports suggest that HTL-p frequency assays predict GVHD after HLA-identical sibling BMT [61]. Unfortunately, HTL-p is difficult to standardize between different BMT centres which use diverse immunosuppressive transplant protocols. HTL-p frequency analysis remains an interesting research tool, and is not currently used in routine donor selection.

Finding an 'acceptable' donor

Immunogenetic aspects

The probability of finding an HLA genetically identical sibling will depend on family size. Any two siblings have a 25% chance of being HLA identical, but the average number of siblings in families in Europe and North America means that only 30% of patients have an HLA-identical sibling donor. Countries with a smaller average sibling number per family have

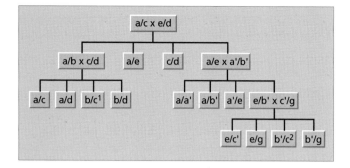

Fig. 21.3 HLA phenotypically matched donor BMT using a distant relative discovered by an extended family search. Here the phenotypically matched pair are second uncle/aunt (b/c^1) and second niece/nephew (b'/c^2), respectively. Haplotype c is inherited in the blood line, whereas b and b' are similar but unrelated common haplotypes that recur in distant relatives of the same family. Hence the probability of success of an extended family search depends on the size of the family and whether or not the patient carries a common HLA haplotype.

correspondingly lower chances and those with larger families a greater chance. In Ireland, 60–70% of potential recipients have an HLA-identical sibling (S. McCann, personal communication). A patient's extended family (blood-related aunts, uncles, nieces, nephews and first cousins) may yield an HLA phenotypically matched donor. This is more likely if the patient carries one or more 'common' HLA haplotype. The higher the frequency of the haplotype in the population, the higher the probability it will be introduced into the extended family from two separate branches (Fig. 21.3). Mathematical formulae have been developed that predict the probability of success in finding an extended family donor if there is prior knowledge of the HLA haplotype frequency *in the associated ethnic group* [62]. Recently a computer-based simulation program has been developed to predict the probability of finding a phenotypically matched donor in the patient's extended family [63]. This program requires input of the nuclear family HLA types and the number of first cousins, uncles, aunts, nephews and nieces available on both the maternal and paternal sides of the family. Extended family donor searches are only justified when the patient possesses one, or preferably two, HLA-A, B, DR haplotypes that are common within their ethnic group. They are also more likely to succeed in societies where first-cousin marriages are customary. Extended family donor searches should be limited to the situations described as, if applied inappropriately, serious delay may occur in the identification of an acceptable unrelated donor.

Over the past 10 years there has been massive recruitment to unrelated donor panels worldwide, resulting in over three million HLA-typed volunteers being registered on computer files by December 1995. As already stated, the capacity of the

HLA system to generate diverse phenotypes far exceeds the world population. Whereas HLA could yield more than 10^{30} different phenotypes, the world population is unlikely to rise above 10^9 by the year 2050. If we assume that 25% of the population carry common HLA phenotypes, this leaves 0.75×10^9 individuals to carry relatively rare or unique HLA types. Calculations based on the known frequency of HLA phenotypes within homogeneous populations give some indication of the relationship between panel size and the theoretical probability of finding closely HLA-matched donors [64,65]. These estimates show that the relationship between probability and panel size is nonlinear. However, a panel of 150 000 Caucasians should yield one or more acceptable donor for 50% of Caucasoid patients for whom a search is initiated. This probability is increased if the stringency of the match requirements is relaxed to allow one or two HLA mismatches. These calculations are based on the known HLA phenotype distribution in a random sample of 2000 UK organ donors, and they take no consideration of the efficiency of the donor search procedure or the clinical urgency of the transplant. Such theoretical estimates will vary between ethnic groups according to the frequency of HLA alleles and the population size.

Laboratory aspects

The minimal typing necessary to screen siblings for HLA genotypic identity is a full HLA-A, B, DR, DQ type on the patients and all available full siblings. However, confirmation of HLA genotypic identity should be based on more definitive typing, to exclude an undetected mismatch occurring through recombination or initial mistyping. The commonest recombination event in HLA-A, B, DR, DQ identical siblings occurs between DQ and DP, leading to DP mismatching in 7% of otherwise HLA identical siblings [66]. Interestingly, no definite effect on transplant outcome has been attributed to DP mismatching, and this observation should not deter clinicians from using such donors for transplantation in preference to other family members or well-matched unrelated donors. If parents are available, it is very helpful to type them to assist with HLA haplotype assignment. This may be essential when the patient has an unusual HLA phenotype, is homozygous at one locus, or is technically difficult to type because of an abnormal blood picture. Haplotype assignment is essential in families with rare or previously unidentified HLA alleles. Such families are often non-Caucasian, have a mixed ethnic background or possess rare HLA alleles, which may initially be recorded as 'blanks' leading to a false assumption of homozygosity. If no HLA-identical sibling is found, after discussion with an expert immunogenetics laboratory, an extended family donor search may be indicated based on the immunogenetic criteria defined above. Unless these criteria exist, an extended family donor search may be dangerous because it will delay a search for a well-matched unrelated donor during which time the patient will undergo disease progression and become unsuitable for BMT, or even die from their disease.

If no family donor can be found, a search for an unrelated donor may be indicated depending on the clinical status of the patient. Initially, full family HLA typing, including haplotypes, is required. A detailed knowledge of the ethnic background of the patient will help to guide the search. A search begins with a request from the physician in charge of the patient to the national volunteer registry. In countries which do not have a donor registry, the initial search should be of a large panel known to contain individuals of the same ethnic origin as the patient. The National Marrow Donor Program (NMDP) is actively recruiting large numbers of black, Hispanic, Asian and oriental donors. Failure to find a donor will result in the search being extended internationally. Searching is greatly facilitated through *Bone Marrow Donors Worldwide* (BMDW), which is a continuously updated computerized register of donor HLA types from all major volunteer registries. The registry where the donor is located can then be approached to obtain samples for further high-resolution DNA typing, usually by PCR-SSP typing at the laboratory serving the BMT centre. Final typing and matching should always be carried out in the immunogenetics laboratory serving the patient's BMT centre. HLA-DNA typing of HLA-A, B, C, DR and DQ to the highest possible resolution should be applied to the ultimate donor, as well as DNA crossmatching in centres where the technique is available. Although current information from Petersdorf and others suggests that HLA-DP mismatch does not influence transplant outcome [66,67], there are preliminary data to suggest that HLA-C mismatching may be associated with poor outcome of unrelated donor transplantation [68]. It is possible that alloreactivity may be associated with C-locus mismatch, which, until the advent of high-resolution DNA typing, was difficult to define. If HLA mismatch detectable by intermediate-resolution DNA techniques or by serology is present, a negative cytotoxic crossmatch between recipient serum and donor PBL should be demonstrated. Functional tests such as the CTL-p and HTL-p frequency assays are optional, as their predictive value for transplant outcome is uncertain and the acquisition of the large number of viable cells required to perform the tests may introduce unacceptable delay into the selection procedure. However, if appropriate cells can be obtained from the recipient and definitive donor immediately pretransplant, the results of CTL-p and HTL-p frequency analysis may provide valuable retrospective information. It is now apparent that HLA typing can be usefully supplemented with recipient and, possibly, donor TNFα promoter gene typing, which, in the near future, may be used as a guide to protocol selection for low and high producers. Non-HLA typing is still of academic interest, mainly because of the complexity and limitations of current typing techniques (see above). In the future, routine typing for non-HLA may be of value if all clinically relevant non-HLA histocompatibility genes are cloned and simple DNA-based typing tests developed.

Logistic and clinical aspects of HLA-identical sibling donor selection

Donor age limits, the contraindication for selecting donors with physical or psychological disorders and procedures for informed consent vary, according to whether or not the donor is related to the recipient [5,4].

It is essential to take a careful family history from all new patients under the approximate age of 55 to establish whether or not siblings are available. Once the haematologist has decided that allogeneic BMT is the treatment of choice for a newly diagnosed patient, either at diagnosis or as a consolidation treatment, it may be clinically urgent to establish whether the patient has an HLA-identical sibling. The patient and family members chosen by the patient should be counselled in advance about the probability of finding an HLA-identical sibling, the probable results of HLA-identical sibling transplantation should be discussed, as well as a realistic alternative treatment plan, should a sibling not be available. The need to HLA type newly diagnosed patients and their families becomes urgent when an immediate BMT is deemed to have a greater chance of success than a delayed BMT. A good example of this is when a patient below the age of 45–50 years presents with severe acquired aplastic anaemia (SAA). In this situation, a delay may prejudice the outcome, because cure by *early* BMT is 70–90% with an HLA-matched sibling donor [69,70]. If sibling BMT is delayed, the probability of survival decreases through graft rejection secondary to sensitization to minor histocompatibility antigens acquired through multiple blood transfusions [71]. There is an equally urgent need to know that a patient with newly diagnosed SAA does not have an HLA-identical sibling, so that effective alternative treatment with optimal immunosuppression can be commenced as soon as possible before the onset of sensitization leading to resistance to platelet transfusions or to systemic infection. Although clinically less urgent, it is good management practice to perform early HLA typing on young patients with diseases controllable by conservative therapy but only curable by BMT. The classic example is the young patient with newly diagnosed chronic myeloid leukaemia (CML) in the chronic phase, where there is clear evidence that results of BMT performed in the first year after diagnosis are superior to the results of later BMT [72]. It is reasonable to manage the few young patients with myelodysplasia [73], multiple myeloma [74] and stage II and III chronic lymphatic leukaemia [75] in the same way. In myelodysplastic syndrome there are preliminary data that *early* HLA-identical sibling BMT results in improved post-transplant survival [73].

Another commonly encountered situation within clinical trials is when patients with acute leukaemia are selected for HLA-identical sibling BMT based on whether or not an HLA-identical sibling is available [76]. In this situation, it is usually most cost effective to delay HLA typing the patient and their family until complete remission is attained. Using conventional serological methods, the patient's HLA-Class I results may not be clear cut if typing is done at diagnosis, because of aberrant expression of HLA on the surface of leukaemic blasts. With the routine use of DNA typing for HLA-Class I, this caveat will no longer apply.

Logistic and clinical aspects of selection of partially HLA-matched family donors

In clinical practice the level of acceptable HLA mismatch varies according to donor source, patient diagnosis, disease status and age. At one extreme, infants with SCID may be successfully transplanted from a one-haplotype-mismatch parent or sibling [6]. However, this level of mismatch is unacceptable for family donor BMT for adult leukaemia, because of a high probability of fatal graft failure or GVHD [49,77]. In a single-centre retrospective study from Seattle, it was shown that survival after one-antigen-mismatched transplants for young adults with acute leukaemia in remission or chronic myeloid leukaemia in chronic phase was not significantly different from HLA-identical sibling transplants for patients with the same clinical characteristics [77]. Unfortunately, the favourable outcome of one-antigen-mismatched family donor transplants for good-risk leukaemia has not been confirmed in a large multicentre analysis by the International Bone Marrow Transplant Registry [78]. In practice, such donors only extend the family donor pool by 5% over that provided by HLA-identical siblings. To summarize, the only related donor who is likely to be superior to a well-matched unrelated donor is an HLA 'phenotypically matched family donor'. The unusual situations, in which an extended family donor search for such a donor is worthwhile have been defined above.

Logistic and clinical aspects of selection of 'matched' unrelated donors

In the clinical situation, actual donor yield as a proportion of the number of searches undertaken was studied in 700 consecutive searches in the UK between 1989 and 1991 [79]. Clinical search failure was predicted by progressive disease, ethnic mismatching between donor and recipient and uncommon recipient HLA phenotype. Half the searches initiated were discontinued, either because the patient's condition deteriorated or logistic problems were encountered in the search procedure; only 10% of searches resulted in BMT.

Recent advances in HLA typing and matching technology [51] and improvements in the donor search procedures have taken place since the late 1980s. By 1993–94 there was a 30–40% probability of an unrelated donor transplant at 2 years after a search request directed initially to the UK-unrelated volunteer donor registries, and this is rising every year (Fig. 21.4) [80]. More and more patients will benefit from the rapid growth of donors and access through the BMDW. Unfortunately, little improvement in the success of searches

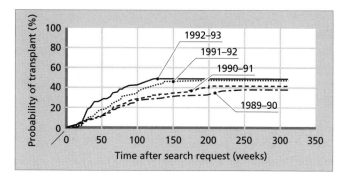

Fig. 21.4 The probability of being able to have an unrelated donor transplant following a search request to UK registries.

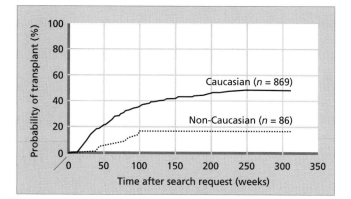

Fig. 21.5 The probability of Caucasian and non-Caucasian patients being able to have an unrelated donor transplant.

initiated for non-Caucasian patients has been demonstrated, and the probability of success in this situation is less than 10% at 2 years (Fig. 21.5) [80]. All searches are first performed nationally, and if no donor is found the search may be extended internationally on behalf of the clinician through their national unrelated donor registry or 'HUB'. Guidelines for international searches have recently been published by the World Marrow Donor Association [4]. Unrelated donor searches add costs to the transplant [81], therefore the clinician should identify a source of funding before proceeding. Unfortunately, the median time to complete an unrelated donor search is still 3–6 months, which, in some cases, leads to clinical deterioration or disease progression before the transplant can be carried out.

Allogeneic peripheral blood progenitor cell donors

Relative efficacy of autologous peripheral blood progenitor cell and marrow transplantation

The results of autologous peripheral blood progenitor cell (PBPC) transplantation for haematological malignancies, especially lymphoma and myeloma, show clear-cut benefits compared with marrow autografts. The reduction of time to platelet transfusion independence has been particularly impressive, and prompt neutrophil recovery has allowed earlier discharge from hospital compared to marrow autografting procedures.

To date, late graft failure and the occurrence of leukaemia attributed to the administration of recombinant haemopoietic growth factors has not been documented. An EBMT survey of transplant procedures in Europe showed that the recent increase in the number of autografts performed has been associated with the use of PBPC [1], demonstrating that many investigators see both medical and logistic advantages of this source of haemopoietic stem cells over autologous bone marrow.

Related allogeneic peripheral blood progenitor cell donors

The development of protocols using recombinant growth factors to enhance the quantity and quality of progenitor cells mobilized has lead to the interesting possibility of mobilizing PBPC from healthy allogeneic donors. Most experience of the available recombinant growth factors has been gained with granulocyte colony-stimulating factor (G-CSF). Phase I trials with normal donors indicated a dose of 4–12 μg/kg/day of G-CSF over 5–7 days [82]. In 1994, 215 allogeneic PBPC transplants were reported to the EBMTG Registry. Retrospective pilot data from single centres [82], and the collected EBMT experience [9], have been reported. This report consists of a mixed group of 59 patients who received allogeneic PBPC grafts, of whom 39 had poor-risk disease at the time of transplant. This was predominantly an adult group of patients, with a median age of 39 (range 2–54) years. Conditioning protocols were the standard allogeneic transplant protocol used by the reporting centres, as conditioning was similar to that in patients undergoing HLA-identical sibling BMT. All donors were HLA-identical siblings and were given G-CSF between 4.5 and 24 μg/kg/day for 4–7 days to mobilize PBPC. Donations contained a median of 9.65×10^8 nucleated cells (range 2.3–22.4) and 6.47×10^6 CD34+ cells (range 1.44–68.8). Engraftment occurred in 56 of the 59 patients who survived beyond day 16 post-transplant. Both neutrophil and platelet recovery were prompt, with median times to engraftment of 17 days and 16 days for peripheral blood neutrophil (>20 × 10^9/l) respectively. As a result of these pilot data, the EBMT Group is undertaking a prospective randomized study to compare both the effects of donation and transplant outcome in HLA-identical sibling transplantation performed either using PBPC or marrow.

Unrelated peripheral blood progenitor cell donors

There is controversy concerning the ethical considerations of PBPC mobilization in unrelated volunteer donors. Different registries have different policies, which are currently under review. The main issues are whether there are sufficient data on the long-term safety of G-CSF and whether central venous catheters may be inserted if the volunteer donor has poor venous access. In general, the use of a continuous-flow cell separator for the collection of leucocytes from volunteer donors is not an issue, as many volunteer donors are already apheresis platelet donors.

Umbilical cord blood donations

The ultimate value of human umbilical cord blood (UCB) for clinical transplantation will depend on whether single donations can reliably engraft adults, who constitute around 80% of all allograft recipients. Certain inherent advantages of cord blood (CB) over adult marrow donations are potentially attractive. Cord blood collected from healthy full-term cord and placenta is likely to be virus free. This is associated with a naive immunophenotype of CB lymphocytes, [83] and a low level of mature cytotoxic T cells [84]. The immunophenotype and functional naivety of CB may allow HLA partially mismatched transplants without inducing life-threatening GVHD. In addition, CB may be conveniently banked after collection [85] and, in the future, banks may be networked worldwide. Cord blood banking could dramatically reduce the search-to-transplant interval for patients who lack a family donor and at present rely on volunteer marrow donors. Although, in recent years, there has been some improvement in the search success in the UK, there has been little improvement in searches for patients from ethnic minority groups (Fig. 5) [80]. It may be that non-Caucasian patients will benefit most from CB banks.

Related umbilical cord blood donations

The first successful CB transplant documented with sustained engraftment was performed in Paris, as a result of close collaboration between French and American scientists and clinicians [86]. The patient, who was transplanted for Fanconi's anaemia, received HLA-identical sibling CB. Initial peripheral blood recovery was satisfactory and engraftment sustained. There was no clinically significant acute or chronic GVHD, and immune reconstitution was good, The patient was well and disease free 8 years after the transplant. In 1995 pilot data were reported on 44 paediatric CB transplants from sibling donors, 34 from HLA-identical and 10 from partially HLA-mismatched siblings. Importantly, despite a low median nucleated cell dose of 5.2×10^7/kg (range: $1–33 \times 10^7$) of recipient body weight, engraftment was satisfactory. Graft versus host disease was unremarkable in this paediatric group.

Unrelated cord blood donations

Over 200 unrelated CB transplants have now been performed

worldwide from donations stored in CB banks. To date, 6682 CB donations have been made available to the transplant community through BMDW. Unfortunately, valid clinical data on the results of these transplants are sparse. A recent report from the USA describes a single-centre, predominantly paediatric, CB-transplant experience of 25 patients utilizing donations collected and stored in the New York Cord Blood Bank [11]. The median nucleated cell dose was low at 3×10^7/kg (range: $0.7–11 \times 10^7$) of recipient body weight, however engraftment was satisfactory. All but one of the donations was overtly HLA mismatched but, despite this, GVHD was not a major problem. However, eight of the 25 patients died of late infections, which suggests that immune reconstitution after mismatched CB transplants may be unsatisfactory. Until a controlled study comparing CB with marrow in matched groups of patients is performed, it will not be possible to fully evaluate engraftment, GVHD, relapse or post-transplant immune reconstitution after CB transplants.

Impact of current research on donor selection

Role of intelligent mismatching

It is unlikely that the unrelated donor pool can be enlarged enough to significantly increase the proportion of fully HLA-matched unrelated donors worldwide. Thus a policy for intelligent mismatching is required if alternative donor BMT is to be safely extended to a higher proportion of potential recipients. Such a policy would require cost-effective routine methods of identifying occult HLA mismatches between superficially HLA-matched donor recipient pairs [67]. Methods to detect HLA epitopes, which are associated with low T-cell alloreactivity, are required. Ultimately, a series of routine methods for defining the individual patient's potential to produce proinflammatory (TH_1 type) and anti-inflammatory cytokines (TH_2 type) in response to the donor's alloantigens may improve the safety of BMT in the absence of an HLA-identical sibling.

HLA molecular epitope analysis

Mismatches defined by serological typing correlate poorly with functional tests of T-cell reactivity [87]. Parham and others have suggested that the amino acid sequences within the HLA molecule which define antigenic epitopes reactive with cytotoxic antibodies, may be partially or completely different from the epitopes which stimulate T cells [87]. Short sequences of amino acids have been shown to define molecular epitopes and, when mismatched in the transplant situation, these can trigger alloreactive responses. By contrast, other epitopes have been identified which are associated with nonreactivity after mismatched transplants [88]. The first step towards intelligent mismatching using epitope analysis is precise HLA typing, as described above. Secondly, pilot studies to correlate

quantitative measure of T-cell alloreactivity and BMT outcome have to be undertaken. The ultimate aims are to establish which HLA epitopes are important and to develop *in vitro* tests of T-cell function that will predict whether or not donor/recipient alloreactivity is likely to develop after stem cell transplantation.

References

1 Gratwohl A., Herman J. & Baldowero H. (1996) Haematopoietic precursor cell transplant in Europe: activity in 1994. Report of the European Group for Blood and Marrow Transplantation (EBMT). *Transplantation*, **17**, 137–149.
2 Downie T.R., Hows J.M., Gore S.M., Bradley B.A. & Howard M.R. (1995) A survey of the use of unrelated volunteer donor bone marrow transplantation at 46 centres worldwide 1989–1993. *Bone Marrow Transplantation*, **15**, 499–503.
3 Whittaker J.A., Summerfield G.P., Clough J.V. *et al.* (1995) Guidelines on the provision of facilities for the care of adult patients with haematological malignancies (including leukaemia and lymphoma and severe bone marrow failure). *Clinical and Laboratory Haematology*, **17**, 310.
4 Goldman J.M. (1994) For the WMDA Executive Committee (1994) A special report: bone marrow transplants using volunteer donors — recommendations and requirements for a standardized practice throughout the world — 1994 update. *Blood*, **84**, 2833–2839.
5 Buckner C.D., Peterson F.B. & Bolonski B.A. (1995) Bone marrow donors. In: *Bone Marrow Transplant* (eds S. Foreman, K. Blume & E. Donnall Thomas). pp. 259–271. Blackwell Science, Cambridge, Massachusetts.
6 Fischer A., Landais P., Friedrich W. *et al.* (1990) European experience of bone marrow transplantation for severe combined immunodeficiency. *Lancet*, **336**, 850–854.
7 Schmitz N., Gratwohl A. & Goldman J.M. (1996) For Accreditation Sub-committee of the European Group for Blood and Marrow Transplantation (EBMT). *Bone Marrow Transplantation*, **17**, 471–477.
8 Aversa F., Tabilo A., Terenzi A. *et al.* (1994) Successful engraftment of T-cell depleted haploidentical 'three loci' incompatible transplants in leukaemia patients by addition of recombinant human granulocyte colour-stimulating factor-mobilized peripheral blood progenitor cells to bone marrow inoculation. *Blood*, **84**, 3948–3955.
9 Schmitz N., Bacigalupo A., Labopin M. *et al.* (1996) Transplantation of allogeneic peripheral blood progenitor cells — the EBMT experience. *Bone Marrow Transplantation*, **17**(Suppl. 2), 40–45.
10 Wagner J.E., Kernan N.A., Steinbuch M. *et al.* (1995) Allogeneic sibling umbilical cord blood transplantation in forty-four children with malignant and non-malignant disease. *Lancet*, **346**, 214–220.
11 Kurtsberg J., Laughlin M., Graham M. *et al.* (1996) Placental blood as a source of hematopoietic stem cells for transplantation into unrelated recipients. *New England Journal of Medicine*, **335**, 157–165.
12 Shoskes D.A. & Wood K.J. (1994) Indirect presentation of MHC antigens in transplantation. *Immunology Today*, **15**, 32.
13 Sayegh M.H., Watschinger B. & Carpenter C.B. (1994) Mechanisms of T cell recognition of alloantigen. The role of peptides. *Transplantation*, **57**, 1295–1302.
14 Mosmann T.R. & Sad S. (1996) The expanding universe of T-cell subsets: Th1, Th2 and more. *Immunology Today*, **17**, 138–146.

15 Bacchetta R., Bigler M., Touraine J.L. *et al.* (1994) High levels of IL-10 production *in vivo* are associated with tolerance in SCID patients transplanted with HLA mismatched hematopoietic stem cells. *Journal of Experimental Medicine*, **179**, 493.

16 Lanvier L.L. & Phillips J.H. (1996) Inhibitory MHC Class I receptors on NK cells and T cells. *Immunology Today*, **17**, 86–91.

17 Miller J.S., Klingsorn S., Lund J. *et al.* (1994) Large scale *ex vivo* expansion and activation of human natural killer cells for autologous therapy. *Bone Marrow Transplantation*, **14**, 555–562.

18 Xun C.Q., Thompson J.S., Jennings C.D. & Brown S.A. (1995) The effect of human IL-2 activated natural killer and T cells on graft-versus-host disease and graft-versus-leukaemia in SCID mice bearing human leukaemic cells. *Transplantation*, **60**, 821–827.

19 Sherman L.A. & Chattopadheay S. (1993) The molecular basis of allorecognition. *Annual Review of Medicine*, **11**, 385–402.

20 Campbell R.D. & Trowsdale J. (1993) Map of the human MHC. *Immunology Today*, **14**, 349–352.

21 Kaufman R. (1995) HLA prediction model for extended family matches. *Bone Marrow Transplantation*, **15**, 279–282.

22 Loffell M.S., Steinberg A., Bias W.B., Macham C. & Zachary A.A. (1994) The distribution of HLA antigens and phenotypes among donors and patients in the UNOS Registry. *Transplantation*, **58**, 1119–1130.

23 Goulmy E., Termijtelen A., Bradley B.A. & van Rood J.J. (1977) Y-antigen killing by T cells of women is restricted by HLA. *Nature*, **266**, 544–545.

24 Goulmy E., Schipper R., Pool J. *et al.* (1996) Mismatches of minor histocompatibility antigens between HLA-identical donors and recipients and the development of graft versus host disease after bone marrow transplantation. *New England Journal of Medicine*, **334**, 281–286.

25 Behar E., Nelson J., Chao M.D. *et al.* (1996) Polymorphism of adhesion molecule CD31 and its role in acute graft versus host disease. *New England Journal of Medicine*, **334**, 286–291.

26 James C., Jenkin M., Gubarev I. *et al.* (1994) Proposed localization of genes encoding minor histocompatibility antigens. *Journal of Cellular Biochemistry*, Suppl. 18B, 70 (abstract G205).

27 Paul A., Moss A. & Bell J.I. (1995) The human T cell receptor repertoire. In: *T Cell Receptors* (eds J.I. Bell, M.J. Owen & E. Simpson), pp. 11–132. Oxford University Press, Oxford.

28 Elliott J.I. (1993) The identity of the cells that positively select thymocytes. *Immunological Reviews*, **135**, 215–225.

29 Elliott J.I. (1993) Thymic selection reinterpreted. *Immunological Reviews*, **135**, 227–241.

30 Roosneck E., Roux E., Helgm C., Damount F.G., Chapuis B. & Jeannet M. (1996) Analysis of T cell repopulation after allogeneic bone marrow transplantation: significant difference between recipients of T cell depleted and unmanipulated grafts. *Bone Marrow Transplantation*, **17**(Suppl. 1), abstract 481, 109.

31 Antin J.H. & Ferrara J.L.M. (1992) Cytokine dysregulation and accute graft versus host disease. *Blood*, **80**, 2964–2968.

32 Walter E.A., Greenberg P.D., Gilbert M.J. *et al.* (1995) Reconstitution of cellular immunity against cytomegalovirus in recipients of allogeneic bone marrow by transfer of T-cell clones from the donor. *New England Journal of Medicine*, **333**, 1038–1044.

33 Marks D.I., Cullis J.O., Ward K.N. *et al.* (1993) Allogeneic bone marrow transplantation for chronic myeloid leukemia using sibling and volunteer unrelated donors: a comparison of complications in the first 2 years. *Annab of Internal Medicine*, **119**, 207–212.

34 Casper J., Camitta B., Truitt R. & Baxterlowe N.A. (1995) Unre-lated bone marrow transplants for children with leukemia or mylodysplasia. *Blood*, **85**, 2354–2363.

35 Gale R.P., Bortin M.M. & van Beckum B.W. (1987) Acute graft versus host disease following bone marrow transplantation in humans: assessment of risk factors. *British Journal of Haematology*, **67**, 397–406.

36 Bostrom L., Ringden O., Sarberg B. *et al.* (1988) Pretransplant herpes virus serology and graft versus host disease. *Transplantation*, **46**, 548–557.

37 Vassalli P. (1992) The pathophysiology of tumour necrosis factors. *Annual Review of Medicine*, **10**, 411–452.

38 Jacob C.O., Fronek Z., Lewis G.D., Koo M., Hansen J.A. & McDevitt H.O. (1990) Heritable major histocompatibility complex II associated differences in production of tumour necrosis factor α: relevance to genetic predisposition to systemic lupus erythematosis. *Proceeding of the National Academy of Sciences, USA*, **87**, 1233.

39 Wilson A.G., DiGiovine F.S., Blackemore A.I.F. & Duff G.W. (1992) Single base polymorphism in the human tumour necrosis factor alpha (TNFα) gene detectable by NcoI restriction of PCR product. *Human Molecular Genetics*, **1**, 353.

40 Holler E., Kolb H.J., Müller A. *et al.* (1990) Increased serum levels of tumour necrosis factor α precedes major complications of bone marrow transplantation. *Blood*, **75**, 1011–1016.

41 Remberger M., Ringden O. & Markling L. (1995) TNFα levels are increased during Bone Marrow Transplant conditioning in patients who develop acute GVHD. *Bone Marrow Transplantation*, **15**, 99–104.

42 Holler E., Roncarolo M.G., Hintermeier-Knabe R. *et al.* (1995) Low incidence of transplant related complication in patients with high spontaneous cellular IL-10 production prior to conditioning—evidence for a protective role of IL-10 in allogeneic BMT. *Bone Marrow Transplantation*, **15**(Suppl. 2), 59 (abstract 256).

43 Williams D.M., Turner D.M., Dyer P.A., Sinnott P.J. & Hutchinson I.V. (1996) Polymorphism in the interleukin-10 (IL-10) promoter. *European Journal of Immunogenetics*, **23**, 80 (abstract 4.2).

44 Horowitz M.M., Gale R.P., Sandel P.M. *et al.* (1990) Graft versus host leukemia after bone marrow transplantation. *Blood*, **75**, 555–562.

45 Mayer F.R., Messer G., Knabe H. *et al.* (1996) High response of TNF α secretions *in vivo* in patients undergoing BMT may be associated with the − 308 bp TNF-α − gene enhancer polymorphism. *Bone Marrow Transplantation*, **17**(Suppl. 1), 101 (abstract 448).

46 Bach F.H., Albertini R.J., Joo P., Anderson J.L. & Bortin M.M. (1968) Bone marrow transplantation in a patient with the Wiskott–Aldrich syndrome. *Lancet*, **ii**, 1364–1366.

47 Gatti R.A., Meuwissen H.J., Allen H.D., Hong R. & Good R.A. (1968) Immunological reconstitution of sex linked, lymphopenic immunological deficiency. *Lancet*, **ii**, 1366–1369.

48 Gordon-Smith E.C., Fairhead S.M., Chipping P.M. *et al.* (1982) Bone marrow transplantation for severe aplastic anaemia using histocompatible unrelated volunteer donors. *British Medical Journal*, **285**, 835.

49 Anasetti S., Amos D., Beatty P.G. *et al.* (1989) Effect of HLA compatibility on engraftment of bone marrow transplants in patients with leukemia or lymphoma. *New England Journal of Medicine*, **320**, 197–204.

50 Clay T.M., Bidwell J.L., Howard M.R. & Bradley B.A. (1991) PCR fingerprinting for selection of HLA matched unrelated marrow donors. *Lancet*, **337**, 1049–1052.

51 Bidwell J. (1994) Advances in DNA-based HLA typing methods. *Immunology Today*, **15**, 303–307.

52 Opelz G., Mytilincos J., Scherer S. *et al.* (1993) Analysis of HLA-DR matching in DNA typed cadaver kidney transplants. *Transplantation*, **55**, 782–785.

53 Clay T.M., Culpan D., Pursall M.C., Bradley B.A. & Bidwell J.L. (1995) HLA-DQB1 and DQA1 matching by ambient temperature PCR-SSCP. *European Journal of Immunogenetics*, **22**, 467–478.

54 Pursall M.C., Clay T.M. & Bidwell J.L. (1995) Combined PCR-heteroduplex and PCR-SSCP analysis for matching of HLA-A, B and C allotypes in marrow transplantation. *European Journal of Immunogenetics*, **26**, 41–53.

55 Bradley B.A. (1996) Prognostic genotyping and matching for BMT. *Bone Marrow Transplantation*, **17**(Suppl. 1), A232.

56 Hows J., Bradley B., Gore S., Downie T., Howard M. & Gluckman E.(1993) Prospective evaluation of unrelated donor bone marrow transplantation. *Bone Marrow Transplantation*, **12**, 371–380.

57 Kaminski E., Hows J.M., Goldman J.M. *et al.* (1991) Optimising a limiting dilution culture system for quantitating frequencies of alloreactive cytotoxic T lymphocyte precursors. *Cell Immunology*, **137**, 88–95.

58 Kaminski E., Hows J.M., Man S. *et al.* (1989) Prediction of graft-versus-host-disease by frequency analysis of cytotoxic T cell after unrelated donor marrow transplantation. *Transplantation*, **48**, 608–613.

59 Spencer A., Szydlo R.M., Brookes P.A. *et al.* (1995) Bone marrow transplantation for chronic myeloid leukemia with volunteer unrelated donors using *ex-vivo* or *In-vivo* T-cell depletion: major prognostic impact of Class I identity between donor and recipient. *Blood*, **86**, 3590–3597.

60 Pei J., Masewicz S., Anasetti C. *et al.* (1993) Analysis of correlation between alloimmune cytotoxic responses generated from unrelated donors and seventy acute graft versus host disease. *Human Immunology*, **37**(Suppl. 1), 37a.

61 Schwarer A.P., Jiang Zheng Y., Brookes P.A. *et al.* (1993) Frequency of anti-recipient alloreactive helper T cell precursors in donor blood and graft versus host disease after HLA identical sibling bone marrow transplantation. *Lancet*, **341**, 203–209.

62 Kaufman J., Volk H. & Walling H-J. (1995) A 'minimal essential MHC' and an 'unrecognised MHC': two extremes in selection for polymorphism. *Immunological Reviews*, **143**, 63–88.

63 Schipper R.F., D'Amaro J. & Oudshoorn M. (1996) The probability of finding a suitable related donor for bone marrow transplantation in extended families. *Blood*, **87**, 800–804.

64 Bradley B.A., Gilks W.R., Gore S.M. *et al.* (1987) How many HLA typed volunteer donors for bone marrow transplantation (BMT) are needed to provide an effective service? *Bone Marrow Transplantation*, **2**(Suppl. 1), 79.

65 Beatty P.G., Dahlberg S., Michelson E.M. *et al.* (1988) Probability of finding HLA-matched unrelated donors. *Transplantation*, **45**, 714.

66 Petersdorf E.W., Perkins H., Sekiguchin S. *et al.* (1992) Marrow transplantation. In: *HLA 1991, Proceedings of the Eleventh International Histocompatibility Workshop and Conference* (eds K. Tsuji, M. Aizawa & T. Sasazuki), Vol. 1, pp. 812–820. Oxford Scientific Publications, Oxford.

67 Speiser D.E., Tiercy J.M., Rufer N. *et al.* (1996) High resolution HLA matching associated with decreased mortality after unrelated bone marrow donor transplantation *Blood*, **87**, 4455–4463.

68 Scott I., Bunce M., Brookes P. *et al.* (1995) The role of cellular and molecular Class I HLA typing in selection of unrelated bone marrow donors. *Experimental Hematology*, **23**, 744 (abstract 11).

69 Bacigalupo A., Hows J., Gluckman E. *et al.* (1988) Bone marrow transplantation (BMT) versus immunosuppression for the treatment of severe aplastic anaemia (SAA): a report of the EBMT SAA Working Party. *British Journal of Haematology*, **70**, 531–535.

70 Storb R., Etzioni R., Anasetti C. *et al.* (1994) Cyclophosphamide combined with antilymphocyte globulin in preparation for allogeneic marrow transplants in patients with aplastic anemia: *Blood*, **84**, 941–950.

71 Champlin R.E., Horowitz M.M., van Beckum D.W. *et al.* (1989) Graft failure following bone marrow transplantation for severe aplastic anemia: risk factors and treatment results. *Blood*, **73**, 606.

72 Thomas E.D., Clift R.A., Fefer A. *et al.*(1986) Marrow transplantation for the treatment of chronic myelogenous leukemia. *Annals of Internal Medicine*, **104**, 155–163.

73 Anderson J.E., Appelbaum F.R., Fisher C.D. *et al.* (1993) Allogeneic bone marrow transplantation for 93 patients with myelodysplastic syndrome. *Blood*, **82**, 677–681.

74 Gahrton G., Tura S., Ljungman P. *et al.* (1991) Allogeneic bone marrow transplantation in multiple myeloma. European Group for Bone Marrow Transplantation. *New England Journal of Medicine*, **325**, 1267–1273.

75 Rabinowe S.N., Soiffer R.J., Gribben J.G. *et al.* (1993) Autologous and allogeneic bone marrow transplantation for poor prognosis patients with B cell chronic lymphatic leukemia. *Blood*, **82**, 1366–1376.

76 Zittoun R.A., Mandelli R., Willemze R. *et al.* (1995) Autologous or allogeneic bone marrow transplantation compared with intensive chemotherapy in acute myelogenous leukemia. *New England Journal of Medicine*, **332**, 217–223.

77 Beatty P.G., Clift R.A. & Michelson E.M. (1985) Marrow transplantation from related donors other than HLA identical siblings. *New England Journal of Medicine*, **313**, 765–771.

78 Szydlo R., Goldman J., Klein J. *et al.* (1997) Results of allogeneic bone marrow transplantation for leukemia using donors other than HLA-identical siblings. *Journal of Clinical Oncology*, **15**, 1767–1777.

79 Howard M.R., Gore S.M., Hows J.M., Downie T.R. & Bradley B.A. (1994) A prospective study of factors determining the outcome of unrelated marrow donor searches: report from the International Marrow Unrelated Search and Transplant Study Working Group on behalf of collaborating centres. *Bone Marrow Transplantation*, **13**, 389–397.

80 Hows J., Downie T., Nunn A. *et al.* (1996) The fate of 1026 patients undergoing unrelated marrow donor searches through UK registries. *Bone Marrow Transplantation*, (Suppl. 1), A451.

81 Ottinger H., Grosse-Wilde A. & Grosse-Wilde H. (1994) Immunogenetic marrow donor search for 1012 patients: a retrospective analysis of strategies outcome and costs. *Bone Marrow Transplantation*, **14**(Suppl. 4), 34–39.

82 Bensinger W.I., Weaver C.H., Appelbaum F.R. *et al.* (1995) Transplantation of allogeneic peripheral blood stem cells mobilized by recombinant human granulocyte colony-stimulating factor. *Blood*, **85**, 1655–1658.

83 Rabian-Hertzog C., Lesage C. & Gluckman E. (1992) Characterisation of lymphocytes populations in cord blood. *Bone Marrow Transplantation*, **9**(Suppl. 1), 64–68.

84 Risdon G., Gaddy J., Stehman F.B. & Broxmeyer H.E. (1994) Proliferative and cytotoxic responses of human umbilical cord blood lymphocytes following allogeneic stimulation. *Cellular Immunology*, **154**, 14–20.

85 Rubinstein P., Rosenfield R.E., Adamson J.N. *et al.* (1993) A review

— stored placental blood for unrelated bone marrow reconstitution. *Blood*, **81**, 1679–1690.

86 Gluckman E., Broxmeyer H.E., Auerbach A.D. *et al.* (1989) Hematopoietic reconstitution in a patient with Fanconi's anemia by means of umbilical cord blood from an HLA-identical sibling. *New England Journal of Medicine*, **321**, 1174–1178.

87 Parham P. (1992) Typing for Class I HLA polymorphism: past, present and future. *European Journal of Immunogenetics*, **19**, 347–359.

88 Laundy G.J. & Bradley B.A. (1995) The predictive value of epitope analysis in highly sensitized patients awaiting renal transplantation. *Transplantation*, **59**, 1207–1213.

22 Allogeneic Bone Marrow Transplantation: Clinical Management

I.M. Franklin

Introduction

The most intensive and physically demanding therapy, in terms of the potential complications and their duration, that can be applied to a patient with leukaemia is the transplantation of haemopoietic bone marrow progenitors from a healthy donor. The intensity of the chemo/radiotherapy required to eradicate residual disease and to permit engraftment, the risk of immune-mediated events, such as graft-vs-host disease (GVHD), the associated prolonged immune suppression, and the potential for damaging late effects of the procedure, conspire to make allogeneic bone marrow transplantation (BMT) a daunting prospect for even the fittest of potential patients. In this chapter, the background, rationale, indications, technique and complications of allogeneic BMT will be considered. Recent advances have the potential for confusion in the nomenclature of BMT. Throughout this chapter the term bone marrow transplantation will be used to denote a transplantation of haemopoietic cells, whether they be of bone marrow, peripheral blood or umbilical cord origin. Where peripheral blood- or umbilical cord-derived cells are referred to specifically, this will be made explicit. Other terms warrant explanation. Various categories of a donor for allogeneic BMT are possible. Allogeneic refers to the donor being genetically different from the recipient. Thus all related and unrelated donors are allogeneic, whatever the degree of HLA identity. In the rare case of a monozygotic (identical) twin transplant this is termed syngeneic. When the person's own marrow cells are used this is an autologous transplant, or autograft. Although the number of allogeneic BMTs reported to the International Bone Marrow Transplant Registry (IBMTR) is increasing steadily (a total of 8000 in 1994), since 1990 the numbers have been surpassed by autologous transplants, of which over 12 000 were reported in 1994 (Fig. 22.1). Autologous transplantation for leukaemias and other disorders is discussed in Chapter 23.

The past 5 years have been a period of great innovation and excitement in allogeneic BMT. Although the most common

donor in an allogeneic BMT is a related sibling, increasingly, over the past 5 years, donors may be unrelated volunteers. The great increase in the number of unrelated donors used for such transplants has been a direct result of the increased size and efficiency of the donor registries (see Chapter 21). Nevertheless, unrelated donors comprise less than 20% of allogeneic bone marrow transplants (Fig. 22.2). The use of peripheral blood-derived progenitor or stem cells (PBSC), collected after stimulation of the donor with, usually, granulocyte colony-stimulating factor (G-CSF), is becoming more frequent [1] and may be producing a significantly more rapid engraftment post-transplant. It seems likely that this technique will soon become the harvest method of choice. In addition, the management of relapse following allogeneic BMT, particularly for chronic myeloid leukaemia, has been greatly improved by the recognition that infusions of donor lymphocytes may reinduce complete responses without the need for a second transplant [2]. Finally, our understanding of the mechanisms and management of GVHD have also improved greatly, in particular our ability to identify and separate the positive component of the GVH reaction, the graft-versus-leukaemia effect [3]. Although the innovations mentioned above have, as yet, not changed the outlook for large numbers of patients undergoing allogeneic marrow transplantation, they are likely to do so over the next decade.

In addition to leukaemia and associated neoplastic disorders, some nonmalignant conditions will be considered in this chapter, because information that has been gained from the transplantation of severe aplastic anaemia and severe combined immunodeficiency, for example, is of relevance to, and has influenced, transplantation practice for leukaemia.

Historical background

The initial studies in BMT were supported by the US government in response to concerns about nuclear warfare and nuclear accidents in the 1950s [4]. While the applications of

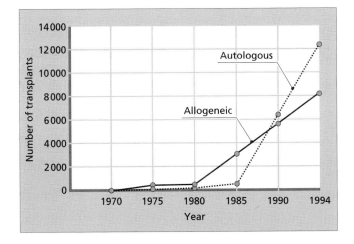

Fig. 22.1 Annual number of transplants worldwide: 1970–94. (Data from the International Bone Marrow Transplant Registry (IBMTR) and the Autologous Blood and Marrow Transplant Registry (ABMTR) of North America.)

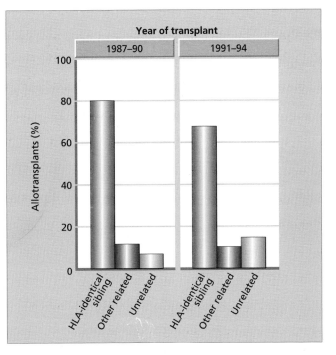

Fig. 22.2 Donor type for allotransplants. (Data from the IBMTR and the ABMTR of North America.)

BMT in such circumstances are now known to be limited [5], many thousands of allogeneic BMTs are now undertaken for acute leukaemia and other disorders each year.

Until the early 1970s, acute leukaemia in adults or children was an essentially incurable disorder. As early as the 1950s, attempts had been made to carry out transplants of healthy bone marrow from donors into leukaemia sufferers in order to try to cure them [6]. These initial attempts were unsuccessful, mainly because the essential knowledge about the HLA system did not develop sufficiently until the 1960s.

The potential problems in transplantation had been recognized in experiments of BMT between outbred strains of mice. Following BMT, mice initially suffer from disease caused by the radiotherapy toxicity ('primary disease'), but the survivors of this primary disease then develop a 'secondary disease' that is immunologically mediated. This secondary or 'runt' disease is caused by an attack by immune-competent bone marrow cells on the immunodeficient host and is analogous to GVHD seen in human transplantation [7].

In 1968 Thomas began his series of transplants in Seattle, USA [8], following extensive preliminary work on dogs. The first human transplants were carried out in patients with end-stage leukaemia who had a survival estimated at a few weeks only. Despite the poor risk status in these patients and the relatively rudimentary, by today's standards, antibiotics and blood products support available, 10% of the first series of over 100 patients survived long term. This justified extension of BMT to better-risk patients, and in particular those in first complete remission of acute myeloid leukaemia (AML). Publication by the Seattle group of these initial encouraging data [9] in 1975 lead to the acceptance of BMT as a mainstream element in leukaemia management and removed it from the wholly experimental sphere. Thomas' contribution over the

40-year period was rewarded by the Nobel Prize for Medicine in 1990.

The transplantation regimen originally described by Thomas in the two-part paper of 1975 [9], consisted of cyclophosphamide to a total dose of 120 mg/kg over 2 days followed by total body irradiation (TBI) of 1000 cGy. After this treatment, known as conditioning, the patient then received an infusion of unmanipulated bone marrow followed by a GVHD prevention regimen of intravenous methotrexate in the 2 weeks posttransplant. The first substantial development on this protocol occurred with the introduction of cyclosporin A (cyclosporin) prophylaxis for GVHD [8]. This appeared to make BMT safer, mainly by reducing the period of neutropenia and thrombocytopenia, and better tolerated, mainly by reducing mucositis, but increased survival only marginally [10]. These apparent benefits of cyclosporin were offset, to some degree, by nephrotoxicity [11]. The major trial comparing cyclosporin directly with methotrexate showed that cyclosporin did appear superior, although the study closed when only a relatively small number of patients had entered [12]. The combination of cyclosporin together with methotrexate has subsequently been shown to be more effective than either agent used singly [13,14]. This combination may now be considered to be the standard therapy for allogeneic BMT between siblings. The issue of GVHD and its prevention and treatment is dealt with later in this chapter. The introduction of cyclosporin made a particular contribution to the transplantation of severe aplastic anaemia (SAA). Before 1980, rejection of donated bone marrow in SAA transplants was a common risk [15], but cyclosporin acts not only to prevent GVHD but also promotes engraftment and reduces the risk of rejection in good-risk minimally transfused SAA patients to the order of 10% [16].

The cells responsible for causing the GVH reaction are immune-competent T-lymphocytes [17], and initial attempts to transplant bone marrow depleted of these cells were made from 1981 onwards [18–20]. These studies of bone marrow T-depletion showed that not only could GVHD be prevented by the removal of T-lymphocytes, but also that transplantation across at least some HLA barriers could be successful, particularly if the sibling was unable to reject the graft because of inherited immunodeficiency [20]. The short-term results of T-cell-depleted BMT were particularly impressive in chronic myeloid leukaemia (CML) [21]. However, it became clear over the next few years that T-cell-depleted BMT for CML lead to a significantly increased risk of relapse [22]. This evidence that an absence of GVHD seemed to be associated with the loss of graft-vs-leukaemia (GVL) effect was the final definitive proof that such a GVL effect existed [22,23]. Subsequent BMT studies suggest that when GVHD prophylaxis is most effective, then the relapse rates are higher and this also appears to be the case for combinations of cyclosporin with methotrexate [24,25]. However, such relapse rates are never as high as in T-cell-depleted transplants.

In the past few years attempts have been made to induce the GVL effect in patients who have a molecular or cytogenetic relapse following allogeneic BMT for CML [2]. Initial attempts at infusing donor lymphocytes tended to be successful in reinducing remission, but are often complicated by inducing aplasia or GVHD. More recently, Mackinnon *et al.* [26] have shown that by giving a specific dose of donor T-lymphocytes, it may be possible to induce an effective GVL effect without inducing GVHD or aplasia. A similar strategy may also have benefit in multiple myeloma [27].

A further development that has occurred since 1994 is the use of haemopoietic progenitors from donors collected from peripheral blood after stimulation with G-CSF [28–29]. Such peripheral blood progenitor cell (PBPC) transplants appear, in preliminary studies, to be associated with more rapid engraftment, particularly of platelets, without an obvious increase of acute GVHD. However, it will require several years of follow-up and many more patients before it can be confirmed that such transplants are equivalent, in terms of long-term survival, to transplantation using conventional bone marrow. A recent report from the Seattle group has shown that chronic GVHD is increased using this technique [30].

Experience gained over the past 25 years has lead to increased confidence in tackling more complex transplant cases, in particular those in which there is no family donor available [31,32]. It is now possible to search for an unrelated donor in a coordinated manner using a network of national donor panels [33]. The ease of obtaining unrelated donors has been the major factor in the increased transplant activity using such donors. An improvement in the results has also been a major factor [34], although many problems remain, such as GVHD, post-transplant neoplasms secondary to the profound immunosuppression [35] and poor immune recovery.

Recently the possibility of using family donors mismatched at three HLA A, B or DR loci (haplo-identical donors) has been explored [36] using an increased intensity of conditioning to overcome rejection, combined with profound T-cell depletion to prevent GVHD. Aversa *et al.* [36] have shown good engraftment associated with minimal GVHD in poor-risk patients, although long-term survival was disappointing, and with this degree of immune suppression there must be concern that survivors will be at risk of Epstein–Barr virus (EBV) related lymphoproliferative disease [37].

These recent developments in allogeneic BMT suggest that the technique will remain a major component of antileukaemic therapy during the next decade and, certainly, utilization of allogeneic as well as autologous BMT continues to increase [38–40]. The precise role of many of the experimental treatments, however, remains to be determined, and in each case the transplant physician must be aware of the respective merits of alternative therapies, including autologous transplants [41–43] and intensive chemotherapy without marrow support [43,44], before recommending family or unrelated donor allogeneic BMT.

Technique for allogeneic bone marrow transplantation

The indications for allogeneic BMT change progressively over time and, in addition, the alternative therapies available are also changing. When considering whether a patient may be suitable for allogeneic BMT, it will be important to obtain the advice of a physician expert in allogeneic BMT to determine the appropriate treatment options for any individual patient. The European Group for Blood and Marrow Transplantation (EBMT) has formulated proposals for the appropriate indications for all types of BMT [45]. These are divided into 'routine', 'clinical research protocol based', 'pilot studies' and 'not recommended.' The number and variety of complications associated with allogeneic BMT is very great and so it is important that these are communicated appropriately to the patient and their family. This can only be done by a physician experienced in allogeneic BMT. In order to make clear the procedures that patients and their physician must go through in preparing for and undergoing an allogeneic BMT, the procedure for what may be considered a 'standard' BMT is described here. The principles of management have been summarized recently in a number of publications. The technical aspects have been addressed by the Eastern Cooperative Oncology Group (ECOG) in guideline format [46], as has the supportive care appropriate for marrow transplantation [47]. The facilities considered necessary in the UK for undertaking BMT procedures have also been considered [48].

Pretransplant period

The issue of whether allogeneic BMT is suitable for a patient with acute leukaemia or other haematological disorder will often arise soon after diagnosis. On many occasions this will be raised by the patient or their family. The range of indications and, especially, the upper age limit for allogeneic BMT has been extended significantly in the past decade. In addition, the range of, often experimental, alternative therapies for patients who may not have a family donor may make the decision more difficult.

It is therefore important at an early stage that the physician caring for the patient discusses the case with a local transplant physician in order to decide whether allogeneic BMT may be an important option for future care. The search for a donor should then be made initially among any available siblings, but in certain circumstances this may include the extended family. The initial discussions with the transplant centre will have determined whether the search should thereafter be extended to donor registries seeking an unrelated donor (see Chapter 21). Once a donor has been identified the timing of any transplant procedure should be agreed in general and, at an early stage, the donor should be examined to ensure that they are fit to donate. This is particularly important now that upper age limits in excess of 55 years are acceptable for allogeneic BMT recipients and therefore their sibling donors will be of a similar age group. Until recently, donation of bone marrow required a general anaesthetic and the aspiration of bone marrow material from the posterior iliac crests and other bones as appropriate. However, in the past few years it has been found possible to administer haemopoietic growth factors, usually G-CSF, to normal donors in order to mobilize haemopoietic progenitors into the peripheral blood for subsequent collection. The precise technique is described in Chapter 23. It is now necessary, therefore, to discuss with the donor the options for bone marrow or PBSC donation; ideally, at a similar time, these issues are discussed with the recipient. It will usually be most appropriate to obtain the consent of both donor and recipient to donation and receipt of either bone marrow or peripheral blood, so that the subsequent decision can be made on clinical grounds.

At the time of HLA typing, suitable donors should be screened for previous virus exposure, in particular to cytomegalovirus (CMV) and toxoplasma, but also to other herpes group viruses such as herpes simplex and herpes zoster. At some point the donor will require to be screened for hepatitis viruses A, B and C and also for HIV and HTLVs, but it may be most appropriate to delay such tests until tissue-type identity has been determined.

Prospective recipients should, by now, have been referred to the transplant centre where they should be seen by a suitably experienced physician, who is able to discuss the risks and benefits of allogeneic BMT and also the alternative treatments available for their condition. Increasingly, such interviews take place within a structured interview format, although the precise level of information given depends upon the country in which the transplant is being carried out. Counselling about infertility must be provided and sperm sample testing and banking offered to males. For females it is currently not possible to cryopreserve ova, although fertilized eggs (embryos) may be cryopreserved. Women with a stable longstanding partner should be referred for such embryo storage and, depending on the ethical constraints upon the service locally, other women referred also. Clearly such procedures may take some time, and may be impossible when patients have acute leukaemia or SAA, as the optimum timing of the transplant does not permit such techniques.

The whole counselling and advice-giving procedure may have to take as little as a few days in the case of SAA or may, on occasion, be extended to months in patients with first chronic phase CML or with early myelodysplasia.

Once the patient and donor have given their consent, the allogeneic BMT should be scheduled in a unit experienced in the technique. Venous access will be secured with at least a double-lumen Hickman-type catheter [49,50]. At this point, consideration should be given to taking a back-up bone marrow harvest. This decision will be affected by the primary diagnosis and the mode of transplant proposed. Back-up autologous harvests are more likely to be used for patients undergoing T-cell-depleted transplants, in which the risk of graft rejection is higher, and also in patients who are undergoing unrelated donor transplants.

It is recommended that a written timetable be produced for the critical events in the early stage of the transplant (Table 22.1). Such a timetable should clarify the decisions taken concerning anti-infection protocols (viral, bacterial and fungal), the anti-GVHD protocol to be used, the conditioning regimen, blood product support required, donor care and any other specific requirements. These pretransplant aspects are considered further in more detail later in this chapter.

Post-transplant period

It is convenient to divide the post-transplant period into three stages. Most of the major complications of allogeneic BMT occur at specific times and these have been documented by the IBMTR [51].

Phase I—the period of bone marrow failure

Up to the first 30 days post transplant, the patient must achieve bone marrow engraftment and, before doing so, will be at risk of haemorrhage and infection. Regimen-related toxicity tends to be foremost in this period, in particular gut toxicity and Gram-positive infections related to the indwelling venous

Table 22.1 Representative timetable for a patient undergoing a sibling allograft using PBSCs for acute lymphoblastic leukaemia (ALL).

Patient name:	Jane Doe		Donor name:	Andy N. Other (brother of Jane Doe)
Date of birth:	22.06.72		Date of birth:	11.11.68
Blood group:	O Rh D positive		Blood group:	O Rh D positive
CMV status:	Positive		CMV status:	Negative
Height:	158 cm		Start G-CSF (650 µg/day):	12.04.99
Weight:	62 kg		PBSC collections:	16.04.99; 17.04.99; ?18.04.99
Surface area:	1.62 m²			
UPN no:	GRI 888			

Diagnosis	Acute lymphoblastic leukaemia (UK ALL XII)
1 Conditioning	Etoposide 60 mg/kg + TBI 1320 cGy
	Give etoposide undiluted by syringe driver over 4 hours through Hickman line, use ECG monitor through this time
2 Antimicrobials	Ciprofloxacin 500 mg b.d. + acyclovir 400 mg b.d. + fluconazole 100 mg o.d.
3 PCP prophylaxis	Co-trimoxazole ii tabs b.d. days –6 to –1; when WBC >1.0 × 10⁹/l commence co-trimoxazole i tab. 3 × weekly for 6 months
4 Blood products	Irradiated CMV negative, group O positive
5 Marrow/PBSC	PBSC. Collected on: 16.04.99; 17.04.99; ?18.04.99
6 Haemopoietic growth factors	None as routine
7 Anti-GVHD therapy	Cyclosporin + methotrexate
8 Antiemetics	Tropisetron + dexamethasone
9 CMV prophylaxis	CMV-negative blood products + IV immunoglobulins 400 mg/kg day +7, then 200 mg/kg days +21, +35, +49, +63, +77, +91
	Ganciclovir 500 mg daily IV day –7 to day –1, then 500 mg Monday, Wednesday and Friday when neutrophils >1.0 × 10⁹/l until day + 100 post BMT

Timetable

(NB: If donor cells have not arrived on the ward by *4 p.m.* on day of transplant, please contact Marrow Processing Laboratory on ext. 4024.)

Day	Date	Event/procedure
–8		Admit. Measuring for TBI
–7		Insertion of Hickman line (today or tomorrow)
–6		Confirm all investigations complete and functioning Hickman line
		Start ganciclovir
–5		Rest day
–4		Etoposide 60 mg/kg = 3720 mg as single dose over 4 hours with cardiac monitor throughout; give etoposide undiluted via syringe pump or similar into central vein
–3		Rest day
–2		TBI
–1		TBI
		Commence cyclosporin IV 3 mg/kg daily as two divided doses
0		TBI. Last day. Return from radiotherapy and enter isolation
		PBSC transplant with cells collected as above
+1		Methotrexate 15 mg/m² = 24.3 mg IV. (Check renal and hepatic function.) Then, starting 12 hours after methotrexate, folinic acid 15 mg/m² =24.3 mg 6 hourly for three doses
+3		Methotrexate 10 mg/m² = 16.2 mg IV. (Check renal and hepatic function.) Then, starting 12 hours after methotrexate, folinic acid 10 mg/m² = 16.2 mg 6 hourly for six doses
+6		Methotrexate 10 mg/m² = 16.2 mg IV. (Check renal and hepatic function.) Then, starting 24 hours after methotrexate, folinic acid 10 mg/m² = 16.2 mg 6 hourly for eight doses
+7		IV immunoglobulin 400 mg/kg = 24.8 g
+11		Methotrexate 10 mg/m² = 16.2 mg IV. (Check renal and hepatic function.) Then, starting 24 hours after methotrexate, folinic acid 10 mg/m² = 16.2 mg 6 hourly for eight doses

This table is intended as an example providing the sort of information that should be included within a transplant timetable. It should be distributed to those departments in the hospital that have a need for the information, e.g. radiotherapy, pharmacy, stem cell processing laboratory, ward. It does not replace the requirement for these areas to be fully consulted about the procedure nor for appropriate clinical consultations.

catheter are especially common. Gram-negative infections, although potentially life threatening, are relatively rare in this period.

The period to engraft depends on the method of GVHD prophylaxis and also on the quality and HLA identity of the stem cell material used for transplants. Patients receiving haemopoietic stem cell growth factor-mobilized PBSCs tend to engraft more quickly than patients receiving bone marrow, and anti-GVHD prophylaxis regimens containing methotrexate are more likely to delay engraftment. Most patients will have engrafted neutrophils in excess of $0.5 \times 10^9/l$ by day 14 if given adequate numbers of PBSCs and by day 21 with bone marrow.

Phase II—the early engraftment phase

With recovery of the peripheral blood counts there is a risk of GVHD. Management of acute GVHD is particularly important. At this stage all patients, but especially those who require high doses of corticosteroids to treat GVHD, will be at risk of fungal infections and also of life-threatening viral and protozoal (*Pneumocystis*) infections. The management of graft failure may become critically important at this stage.

Phase III—post 100 days

By tradition the first 100 days is the period in which acute GVHD may occur and any GVHD occurring after this time is termed chronic. Other late complications include virus infections, particularly with CMV (Fig. 22.3), and herpes zoster. In patients with high-risk disease recurrence may be a concern here and in addition there will be a continuing requirement for monitoring complications, including recovery from alopecia, hormone replacement in young women and, later, post-transplant, cataracts, infertility and the risk of second malignancies.

The allogeneic donor

The selection of the donor has been covered in some detail in Chapter 21. In allogeneic BMT, the safety of the donor must remain the paramount feature of management. Donors must be reassured that there will be no attempt to encourage them to donate if they are not completely fit. If the transplantation is likely to be some months ahead, it may be prudent to take bone marrow for cryopreservation in advance if there is any likelihood that the donor may become transiently unfit, in particular as a result of pregnancy. Donors from overseas may require to return home and marrow material should be cryopreserved before they do so. Any medical problems detected in the donor should be referred to an independent physician, who will make the decision whether it is suitable for them to proceed. A fairly common example includes hypertension and ischaemic heart disease. At this stage, it should be decided

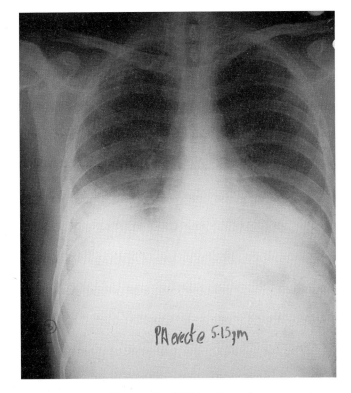

Fig. 22.3 Pneumonitis caused by CMV; the diagnosis was proven by bronchoalveolar lavage and the patient survived after therapy with ganciclovir and foscarnet.

whether the patient is fit for either or both bone marrow and PBSC donation. Many thousands of bone marrow donations have taken place worldwide and there is an extremely good safety record [52]. However, significant morbidity can occur and a minor degree of morbidity, particularly lower back pain, is not infrequent [53]. The technique is important [54,55], and marrow harvesting of allogeneic donors, especially if unrelated, should not be delegated to inexperienced junior staff. Following donation, the donor should be checked to exclude evidence of iron deficiency and outpatient follow-up should be arranged to ensure there are no lasting complications of donation.

The short-term and longer-term consequences of growth factor-mobilized PBSC donation are less clear. The technique of PBSC donation is covered in detail Chapter 23. It seems likely that this form of donation will prove to be at least as safe as donating bone marrow, but at present there is too little experience to be completely certain of this. The use of G-CSF or other growth factors in normal donors should be followed with more formal and prolonged follow-up, to provide the appropriate reassurance that the use of such factors is as safe as anticipated.

Bone marrow donation

Once the donor has been counselled appropriately, and their fitness to donate established, the decision whether the donor will give bone marrow or peripheral blood must be made. For patients who are planning to give bone marrow it will be appropriate, in most cases, 7–14 days before the procedure, for a unit of blood to be withdrawn for autologous transfusion at the time of bone marrow donation. It is important that a safe clinical system is in operation for identifying this unit of blood. Autologous transfusion will reduce the risk of virus transmission to the donor and remove risks of alloimmunization. The alternative procedure is to process the marrow donation at the time of collection and return the red cells to the donor. For the harvest itself, the donor will usually be admitted to hospital on the previous day. In some centres it is routine to admit the donor to hospital, or keep them under some other form of observation, as soon as the patient commences irrevocable bone marrow ablative therapy (radiotherapy or high-dose busulphan). The transplant procedure itself involves anaesthetizing the donor, then turning them into the prone position to enable access to the posterior iliac crests. General anaesthesia is usual, but regional anaesthesia has been used successfully, and outpatient harvesting is entirely feasible [56]. Bone marrow is collected by multiple puncture of the posterior iliac crests and 2–5 ml of bone marrow blood is removed from each puncture. Removing small volumes of bone marrow will produce a higher relative yield of bone marrow progenitors over contaminating blood [54], but can also lengthen the time required to obtain the necessary amount of marrow. It is therefore more practical to take 5–10 ml at each puncture. In order to avoid disfiguring marks, it is usually possible to aspirate sufficient bone marrow using only one to three skin punctures on each side. After approximately 300 ml have been withdrawn and placed into either heparinized or citrated medium in a sterile container, a small aliquot should be removed for nucleated cell counting. This will give an estimate of the cellularity of the donation and enable a calculation to be made of the necessary volume likely to be required. The usual minimum number of cells required is 2×10^8 nucleated cells/kg recipient body weight for a fully HLA-matched sibling donor. When an unrelated donor is used, an absolute minimum of 3×10^8 nucleated cells/kg would be more usual, but more if a degree of mismatch was present. The volume required can easily be calculated from the formula:

$$\text{Total volume required (litres)} = \frac{\text{Recipient weight in kilograms} \times (2 \times 10^8)}{\text{Nucleated cell counts } (\times 10^9/\text{l})}$$

At the conclusion of the procedure, the washings from the aspirations are added to the blood bag and a final sample taken for counting. It is at this point that any postdonation manipulation of the marrow, such as T-cell depletion or red cell depletion, may be undertaken. The use of filters to remove large particles of marrow has been advised, but there appears little evidence to support this, and all bone marrow may be in-fused safely through a central venous catheter by conventional blood giving sets. Pulmonary complications in the recipient have been described but are uncommon [57]. Postoperative management of the donor involves attention to analgesia, the reinfusion of autologous blood and subsequent iron therapy if necessary. Only very occasionally should it be necessary for patients to receive red cells other than the autologous unit, and this should not be done without discussion with the transplant physician responsible for the harvest procedure. Donors may often feel neglected, and their own concerns and anxieties perceived as minor in relation to the predicament of the recipient. Therefore it is important to recognize the needs of the donor.

Peripheral blood stem cells donation

The first use of PBSC in allogeneic BMT was in 1993 [58]. Most protocols for collecting PBSC from normal donors uses 5 days pretreatment with G-CSF at 10 μg/kg, collecting stem cells on the fifth day and subsequent days as necessary [28–30]. The target dose required is of the order of 4×10^6/kg CD34+ cells, based on data collected from the UK experience of PBSC allografting. Patients who received more than 4×10^6/kg had prompt engraftment, whereas with fewer cells recovery was more variable [59]. For an unrelated donor there are no data available, although intuitively one may wish to obtain at least 6×10^6/kg, although there is little data available about the ideal cell number in this situation. At the time of writing, most donor registries will not permit the collection of PBSC from volunteer donors using G-CSF for 'primary' transplants, although some will permit the use of PBSC for regrafts. It seems inevitable that the use of PBSC for unrelated BMT will become the usual technique over the next decade.

Umbilical cord cells

Transplantation using umbilical cord cells is beginning to develop momentum, although long-term follow-up data is very limited for paediatric cases and absent for adults. Cord cells will usually be provided from a cord blood bank [60], although most transplants performed so far have been directed donations from normal siblings born after the index child. The number of cells required to engraft an adult is not yet known, but it does appear [61] that there are sufficient cells in a good umbilical cord cell collection to encourage pilot studies in adults. Engraftment appears to be slower than for PBSC, more like a marrow donation [62], and although hopes that cord blood cells would be so naive as to be incapable of GVHD have not proved correct, it remains possible that cord blood might be transplanted across greater HLA disparity than adult marrow or PBSC may be [63]. It is too soon to know whether cord blood transplants will replace adult matched unrelated donor (MUD) donations for adult transplants, or whether they are a passing fashion. The next 5 years will tell.

Conditioning regimens

The original protocol developed in Seattle using cyclophosphamide 120 mg/kg over 2 days, followed by total body irradiation (TBI) of between 1000 and 1440 cGy, remains the standard against which other regimens are judged [64,65]. In many cases the evidence for the improved efficacy of other regimens is lacking, but there will be a significant proportion of patients who may be unable to receive total body radiotherapy by virtue of having prior radiation therapy or other relevant illness. Therefore it is important to be aware of alternative conditioning regimens for transplantation and to be able to select the appropriate treatment for a specific patient. Some examples are summarized in Table 22.2.

Total body irradiation

In transplants for leukaemia, regimens including TBI will usually be used, and the Seattle protocol referred to above is the most common variant [65]. There is evidence that if TBI is given in fractions, efficacy is maintained and toxicity reduced and hyperfractionation may be further beneficial [66,67]. Giving TBI in fractions over a few days enables better recovery of normal tissue between fractions and reduces toxicity such as pneumonitis. It was previously thought that cataracts may also

be reduced in frequency, but it is now felt that this complication may simply be delayed by fractionation of TBI. Any BMT programme will require the assistance of an experienced radiation therapist, who will be responsible for supervising the planning of the radiotherapy and the delivery. There is little evidence to suggest that there is any difference in outcome between different radiotherapy sources, for example linear accelerator or cobalt. If fractionated TBI can be given in more than six fractions, the rate of delivery of the radiation appears to be unimportant. However, if single-fraction radiotherapy is given then the dose rate is highly important and maintaining this at more than 5 cGy per minute will reduce significantly the incidence of interstitial pneumonitis [68]. Alternatively, the dose rate may be maintained and the total dose reduced to 750–800 cGy. Maintaining low-dose rates prolongs the procedure and skilled medical and nursing attention are essential, particularly for younger patients.

Chemotherapy

Cyclophosphamide. The inclusion of cyclophosphamide in conditioning regimens for allogeneic BMT is based on the premise that it would provide 'space' for the incoming marrow to regenerate. Cyclophosphamide is a poor stem cell poison and therefore unlikely to have a major role in the eradication of

Table 22.2 Chemotherapy and radiotherapy regimens for allogeneic BMT.

Regimen	Description (total doses)	Indication	Reference
CY/TBI	sTBI 10 Gy; CY 120 mg/kg	Leukaemia	[9]
	sTBI 9.5–11.5 Gy; CY 120 mg/kg	AML	[75]
	fTBI 12–15.75 Gy; CY 120 mg/kg	AML	[257]
Ara-C/TBI	sTBI 8.5 Gy; Ara-C 36 g/m²	ALL	[83]
Etop/TBI	fTBI 13.2 Gy; etoposide 25–70 mg/kg	Leukaemia	[76]
	fTBI 13.2 Gy; etoposide 60 mg/kg	ALL	ECOG/MRC Trial
Mel/TBI	TBI 9.5–11.5; melphalan 110 mg/m²	Acute leukaemia	[75]
CY/Etop/TBI	TBI; cyclophosphamide, high-dose etoposide in various doses	Acute leukaemia	[77]
		AML	[79]
		CML	[80]
BuCY	Busulphan 16 mg/kg; CY 120 mg/kg	CML	[70]
	Busulphan 14 mg/kg; CY 200 mg/kg	Thalassaemia	[72]
BuCY/Thiotepa	Thiotepa 250 mg/m² × 3; busulfan 12 mg/kg; cyclophosphamide 120 mg/kg	Allogenic BMT, myeloma	[81,86]
CY	CY 200 mg/kg	Aplastic anaemia	[15]

There is no convincing evidence that any regimen can provide improved long-term DFS over conventional fractionated TBI given with cyclophosphamide 120 mg/kg, although some regimens have been shown to be similar. For practical purposes, 16 mg/kg of busulphan should be the maximum dose outwith a clinical trial. Personal experience with CY/Etop/TBI has shown it to be effective in eradicating leukaemia in poor-risk transplant patients, but produces very severe mucositis.

Ara-C = cytosine arabinoside; CY = cyclophosphamide; Etop = etoposide; fTBI = fractionated total body irradiation; sTBI = single fraction total body irradiation.

leukaemia. However, as mentioned above, there is little evidence to support other regimens replacing cyclophosphamide with other chemotherapy agents as being significantly better. Cyclophosphamide is a good immunosuppressive drug and may therefore be important in preventing rejection. A major complication of cyclophosphamide is haemorrhagic cystitis, which is caused by irritation of the bladder lining by byproducts of cyclophosphamide metabolism. The detoxifying agent mesna may be given during and following the cyclophosphamide infusion and will largely prevent such haemorrhagic cystitis, although patients should be advised that cystitis may still occur and on rare occasions may be serious. It may be exacerbated by concomitant CMV infection or by GVHD [69].

Busulphan. This is given orally and is therefore a convenient drug to use in conditioning patients for BMT. It has been particularly used in the transplantation of CML [70], in which it has been shown to be equivalent to TBI [71], and also for thalassaemia [72]. For thalassaemia a total dose of 14 mg/kg, with 200 mg/kg cyclophosphamide, can safely be given without radiotherapy with good engraftment. Because the toxicity between radiotherapy and busulphan tends to be cumulative, it is usual to use only one or the other. Lower doses, however, of busulphan, for example 5 mg/kg, may be added to TBI without a significant increase in the risk of toxicity. There is a tendency for regimens containing high-dose busulphan (16 mg/kg total dose) to produce more hepatic toxicity, particularly veno-occlusive disease (VOD) of the liver, than lung toxicity [73], although Bearman has suggested recently that there is little evidence to support the idea of busulphan increasing the risk of hepatic VOD [74].

Because busulphan in very high doses can produce epileptic seizures, it is important that patients receive prophylactic medication with an antiepileptic drug such as phenytoin.

Melphalan. This is a good stem cell poison and it also has a relatively limited range of side effects, mainly affecting the bone marrow, gut and, transiently, renal function. These acute effects on renal function have tended to limit its use, and its combination with TBI, although effective in eradicating leukaemia, has been associated with an increased incidence of acute toxicity [75].

Etoposide. This has been used in a number of regimens in high dose, usually combined with TBI [76–80]. Doses as high as 60 mg/kg have been given, and with such doses it must be given undiluted by syringe driver. Dilution of such a large dose would result in such a high volume that this would be impractical. However, etoposide is not licensed in the UK for delivery in this way, and physicians need to be aware of this. It is acutely cardiotoxic and patients require cardiac monitoring while receiving such high doses. There is some evidence to suggest that it may be more effective, particularly in acute lymphoblastic leukaemia (ALL), and for this reason it has been included in the

on-going joint trial in acute lymphoblastic leukaemia run by the Eastern Cooperative Oncology Group (ECOG) and the UK Medical Research Council (MRC ALL 12 Trial).

Other regimens

A large number of other regimens has been used for conditioning prior to BMT. Usually, these have been introduced in order to target a specific disease or, for example, advanced stage disease [81]. Very few trials have addressed the specific issue of efficacy of conditioning regimen, the best known being the Seattle comparison between BuCy and cyclophosphamide TBI [71]. Early experiments with chemotherapy regimens [82] produced greater regimen-related toxicity than those incorporating TBI. Cytosine arabinoside in high dose is an effective therapy in AML and might appear a useful adjunct to conditioning regimens. Its toxicity profile is such that it is possible to add it to conventional conditioning regimens or in place of other agents such as cyclophosphamide. It is important that new conditioning regimens are evaluated carefully in large transplant centres, preferably in controlled trials, because some may be of inferior efficacy or have a worse toxicity than conventional cyclophosphamide + TBI [83,84].

Toxic effects of conditioning regimens— regimen-related toxicity

This section reviews aspects of chemo/radiotherapy conditioning that are commonly encountered. Toxicity related to some specific regimens has been considered [85,86]. In 1990, exciting data were presented, suggesting that the use of pentoxiphylline could dramatically reduce regimen-related toxicity (RRT) and even GVHD after allogeneic bone marrow transplantation [87]. However, subsequent studies have failed to reproduce these data and, at present, there is a general view that pentoxiphylline has little value for this purpose [88–91].

Gut toxicity

Most patients suffer nausea, vomiting and diarrhoea during and after chemo/radiotherapy. It was apparent, after the earliest studies [92], that the optimal use of 5-HT3 receptor antagonists, such as ondansetron, would revolutionize the management of chemotherapy-induced emesis. Together with dexamethasone [93], these agents have reduced substantially the degree of sickness, although most patients will experience some nausea and loss of appetite. Other agents, such as high-dose metoclopramide, lorazepam, prochlorperazine and methotrimeprazine, may be useful for breakthrough or prolonged nausea. Not all of these agents are licensed as antiemetics, and methotrimeprazine use is stated to be contraindicated in bone marrow depression. Diarrhoea and loss of appetite become worse during the first and second weeks after total body irradiation, tending to improve with the recovery of peripheral blood counts. Gut toxicity is more severe if melphalan is added to TBI [75], and in more intensive regimens designed for poor-risk disease categories. Severe mucositis is another distressing complication of intensive chemo/radiotherapy schedules, and may be helped somewhat with prostaglandin E2 [94]. The use of topical granulocyte macrophage colony stimulating factor (GM-CSF) to prevent or treat oral mucositis has been advocated [95], but randomized controlled trials are lacking.

Skin toxicity

All conditioning regimens for allogeneic BMT cause reversible alopecia. Occasionally patients may have lasting alopecia, especially if they have received prior cranial radiotherapy. Many patients suffer transient nail dystrophy, which persists until the nails grow out some months later. Desquamation of the skin is seen frequently and it can be quite severe, particularly over the hands and feet. On occasions, this can cause confusion with GVHD, and a skin biopsy is essential to clarify the cause. Dry skin is usual for a few months after BMT, and is best managed with emollients. After TBI, patients should be warned about hypersensitivity of the skin to sunlight, and advised to avoid such exposure for at least the first year. Skin malignancies are the most common second neoplasm to afflict survivors of BMT, and these are discussed below in the section on second malignancies.

Gonad toxicity

Total body irradiation produces irreversible sterility for males and females in almost all cases, as does high-dose busulphan [96]. Patients need to be counselled about this and give informed consent before BMT. Females will suffer irradiation-induced menopause and require gynaecological advice after the first 100 days [97]. Hormone replacement therapy will be required in premenopausal women, and this should be considered in all women after BMT. Some women who are very young at the time of BMT may recover some fertility later, but this occurs at too low a level to provide reassurance, and all women should be advised that infertility is effectively permanent. Occasional pregnancies have been reported, however [98–100]. Sexual dysfunction is common after BMT, and this appears to be worse than that experienced by patients with AML, who become long-term survivors after chemotherapy only (unpublished data from the UK MRC 10th AML Trial). In children the stunting of growth and sterility will be a problem that will require the attention of a paediatric endocrinologist and intensive counselling support at a later date [101].

Other endocrine organs are also affected by the conditioning regimens [102]. Hypothyroidism is common, and requires regular screening post BMT [103].

Bone marrow toxicity

This is obviously universal and is the intention of the conditioning treatment. The regimens have been chosen to be intensive enough that recovery without bone marrow rescue is not possible, although a small proportion of patients will develop autologous recovery postallogeneic BMT, despite treatments which include TBI. In an era in which the use of haemopoietic stem cells to support less intensive chemotherapy schedules is becoming more common, a working definition of a transplant would be the use of haemopoietic stem cells with chemo/radiotherapy that would not be survivable without the stem cell support. The duration of profound bone marrow failure varies greatly, from about a week in some cases receiving PBSC allografts, to many weeks in the more difficult unrelated donor transplant. Bone marrow chimerism, where populations of donor and recipient cells coexist, is also not infrequent [104]. These states are not necessarily associated with subsequent relapse of the primary disease. Chimeric states associated with the detection of a specific tumour marker, especially if the marker did become undetectable at some stage post BMT, is more sinister and usually associated with relapse. Examples are detection of BCR/ABL by polymerase chain reaction (PCR) in CML [105], and of specific immunoglobulin gene rearrangements in childhood ALL.

Hepatotoxicity

Transient rises of serum liver enzyme levels are not uncommon at the time of conditioning for BMT. During the post-transplant period, there are numerous causes of liver dysfunction, and determining the precise reason can be difficult. Since by definition patients are thrombocytopenic, liver biopsy is difficult, and even if attempted by the transvenous route, samples may be inadequate. The major causes of liver function abnormalities relate to drug reactions (especially cyclosporin), hepatic VOD and GVHD.

Risk factors for developing VOD include patients who have been heavily pretreated and who receive regimens containing high doses of busulphan or more than 1200 cGy TBI and who have pre-existing evidence of liver disease [106,107]. Recent trials have not confirmed the special risk associated with busulphan rather than TBI, nor that any specific GVHD prophylaxis regimen is more likely to induce VOD [74]. Mortality rates in allogeneic BMT are about 2–5% from VOD of the liver, but the variation in figures given in the medical literature suggests that there are major differences in the criteria used to diagnosis it. The most severe forms manifest themselves within 10 days of BMT with fluid retention, abdominal distension due to ascites and the rapid descent of the patient into hepatic coma. On occasions, jaundice may be a relatively minor feature because of the rapid progression of the liver failure. More commonly, the condition is milder and associated with transient and less severe changes in liver function and enlargement of the liver with or without ascites. No treatment has been shown to affect the course of the condition once it has occurred, but there is some evidence that the use of heparin in the pretransplant period around the time of chemo/radiotherapy, until the platelet count has dropped below 30 × 10⁹/l, is helpful in preventing VOD [108,109], although Bearman concluded that its role remains uncertain [74]. Another agent that appeared to have promise in preventing VOD and other regimen-related toxicity is pentoxifylline, but again there is little convincing evidence for its efficacy [74]. Established hepatic VOD may respond to fibrinolytic therapy [110,111] and, since the initial case, recombinant tPA has been used in some 18 patients. While there is some evidence of effect, severe haemorrhage can occur [110], and a randomized trial is required to confirm its effect.

An important factor in the pretransplant assessment of patients is to avoid transplanting patients with active hepatitis. Patients who have had an episode of overt hepatitis in the period before BMT should have a liver biopsy and the transplant delayed until their liver histology shows at least some signs of recovery or has fully recovered. Both radiotherapy and busulphan-containing regimens carry a risk of VOD of the liver and therefore modifying transplantation regimens to accommodate prior hepatic dysfunction is unlikely to be an appropriate management strategy. It is possible to proceed, if essential, using TBI with liver shielding to reduce the dose to the liver. Such a strategy is clearly appropriate only if the target disease is not thought to reside in the liver. However, patients who are positive for hepatitis B antigen may be transplanted successfully [112].

Many patients who survive BMT continue to have deranged liver function tests. This syndrome has been little investigated, but it appears probable that it is caused by a combination of hepatitis viruses, especially HCV [113], which can present as an acute infection [114]. Hepatic iron overload as a result of transfusions also plays an important part. Whatever the HCV status, liver function tests improve after venesection in iron-loaded subjects [115].

Renal toxicity

Minor changes in renal function around the time of chemo/radiotherapy are common. These mainly relate to the excretion of large amounts of uric acid and, before transplantation, patients must be well hydrated with attention paid to their fluid balance, and pretreated with allopurinol. Regimens containing high-dose melphalan are particularly likely to cause renal impairment [75] and patients with any pre-existing renal disease should have their chemotherapy doses reduced. Pretransplant investigation should include measurement of the glomerular filtration rate, and further investigations should be undertaken if this is abnormal.

The most common cause of renal impairment is toxicity from cyclosporin [11], although acute renal failure may result from septicaemic episodes. Broad-spectrum antibiotics, par-

ticularly aminoglycosides, and amphotericin B, all conspire to make renal impairment one of the most common toxic complications of bone marrow transplantation.

Complications of specific chemo/radiotherapy agents

Cyclophosphamide

High doses of cyclophosphamide, such as those used in allogeneic BMT (120 mg/kg for acute leukaemia; 200 mg/kg for aplastic anaemia) and for mobilization of peripheral blood stem cells (6 g/m²), are associated with specific complications, especially cystitis, skin pigmentation and antidiuretic hormone effects.

Cystitis may largely be prevented by the use of mesna, which will inactivate the cyclophosphamide metabolites which cause inflammation to the urothelium [69]. It is important to calculate the appropriate dose of mesna (two-thirds of the total cyclophosphamide dose in four divided doses) and to give this precisely at times prescribed between 0 and 12 hours after the cyclophosphamide dosage. This prevents cystitis in about 90% of patients, although a few patients develop minor degrees of haematuria which may continue throughout the transplant period.

Late cystitis (2–3 weeks post-BMT) should be investigated, since GVHD of the bladder has been described and can be confused with cyclophosphamide-induced cystitis. Urine should be investigated for evidence of cytomegalovirus. On occasions, haemorrhagic cystitis can be life threatening, requiring catheterization, bladder washouts and repeated blood and platelet transfusions. The use of alum washouts may have a place, but occasionally haemorrhage has been so torrential that it has been necessary to resort to cystectomy. Intravesical carboprost has also been used successfully [116]. Other viruses, especially adenovirus, may cause or contribute to haemorrhagic cystitis [117,118].

Skin pigmentation occurs occasionally, but it is usually transient and confined to the flanks. On occasions, patients have a more florid rash which appears to be maculopapular, but this is usually easy to distinguish from GVHD.

Cyclophosphamide has an antidiuretic effect and therefore it is important that fluid balance is measured on an hourly basis during the preceding 6 hours before cyclophosphamide is given and also in the 12 hours after its administration. Urine output should be maintained at greater than 100 ml per minute, by frusemide injections if necessary. Most patients can tolerate this regimen without bladder catheterization, particularly now that nausea and vomiting is better controlled using H3 receptor antagonists.

Total body irradiation

Acute problems related to TBI affect the skin, which may develop a sunburned appearance which usually fades over 2 or 3 days. This is particularly common with single-fraction radiotherapy and is quite commonly associated with transient fever. Sometimes the fever is greater than 39°C and may require antibiotic cover to ensure that an infection has not been overlooked. The salivary glands and the pancreas are often inflamed following TBI and transient elevations in serum amylase are not uncommon. However, in the great majority of cases facial tenderness and abdominal discomfort disappears over the following day or two, and it is simply necessary to reassure the patient that the cause of their facial swelling is the radiotherapy.

Significant late complications may occur. Lens cataracts occur in up to 60% of patients following single-fraction TBI and perhaps 20% of patients who receive fractionated TBI [119]. It now seems more likely that fractionation of TBI serves to delay rather than prevent the onset of cataract. Surgical implantation of a new lens is usually successful, but occasionally it may be a more complicated procedure if it is associated with dry eyes.

Reduced tear production may be a feature of chronic GVHD but it can also be a long-term effect of the radiotherapy on exocrine glands. Dry skin in the absence of chronic GVHD is also common and advice about the use of emollient and rehydrating cream and oils is often required. Occasionally, patients will suffer accelerated tooth decay following radiotherapy, although with the doses used in allogeneic BMT this will affect only about 10% of patients.

Interstitial pneumonitis

This remains a major complication following allogeneic BMT [120] and, although it is usually possible to diagnose cytomegalovirus (CMV) or other viral infections to be the cause of 70% of the cases, a proportion of patients have pneumonitis of undetermined cause. The onset may be very varied, including an extremely rapid presentation over 24–48 hours. However, other patients will have an indolent phase with a preceding illness of perhaps a few weeks associated with a dry cough and some tightness in the chest which progresses inexorably to diminishing lung function, deterioration in oxygenation and death. The early diagnosis of interstitial pneumonitis is most important and centres around two main procedures. Bronchoscopy with bronchoalveolar lavage [121] will identify pathogens positively, although negative results in patients who continue to progress to respiratory failure are not uncommon. This procedure is especially useful for aspergillus and pneumocystis detection. In those patients with a more indolent course, an open lung biopsy should be considered at an early stage, because this is the most reliable method of diagnosis. CMV infections are more common in patients with GVHD and may even precipitate GVHD by increasing the expression of HLA antigens [122]. The incidence of clinical CMV infections has reduced substantially since the introduction of ganciclovir prophylaxis [123,124], although the optimum regimen remains to be defined fully.

The three main causes of interstitial pneumonitis are non-specific fibrosis, possibly related to TBI, viral infections, particularly CMV and, rarely, GVHD associated with infiltration of the lung by lymphocytes. As each of these may require different management, correct diagnosis is of great importance. Radiation-induced pneumonitis is treated with corticosteroids, as is GVHD. Late effects are not uncommon [125]. Although a few years ago it seemed that human herpes virus 6 (HHV-6) might be a major pathogen, more recent studies suggest that although infections may be frequent, serious morbidity is unusual [126]. The management of virus infection is considered below.

Prevention of infection

The detailed management of specific infections in leukaemias is discussed in Chapter 25 and the broad principles of management specific to allogeneic BMT will be discussed here.

Patients undergoing allogeneic BMT are at profound risk of infection from bacteria, fungi, viruses and protozoa for most of the first year after transplant, and in relation to some organisms such as pneumococci and meningococci, this susceptibility may be lifelong. The prevention and management of infections following transplantation therefore requires prophylaxis against all these pathogens and the prompt treatment of any infections that occur. On occasions, these infections will be apparent and easy to diagnose, but equally often infective organisms will not be isolated and empirical treatment will be necessary.

On admission to the transplant unit the patient is examined and swabs and viral cultures taken to exclude the presence of active infections prior to transplantation. A careful search for resistant Gram-negative bacteria and methicillin-resistant *Staphylococcus aureus* (MRSA) is especially important. In the pretransplant period the exposure profile of patients to viruses such as CMV and other herpes viruses will have already been ascertained.

Traditionally, combinations of oral nonabsorbable antibiotics and agents, with acronyms such as NEOCON and FRACON [127], have been used in the prophylaxis of bacterial and fungal infections. These incorporate neomycin or colistin and framycetin, together with the antifungals amphotericin and nystatin, to attempt to 'sterilize' the gut of Gram-negative pathogens and pathogenic fungi. To prevent fungal overgrowth, it is usual to commence the antifungals first. Such regimens can be effective, but they consist of many tablets and compliance may be poor.

The use of co-trimoxazole orally to prevent Gram-negative infections was described some years ago [128] and, although it is effective and simple, it does have the disadvantage of increasing the time to engraftment because of its antifolate effect. The antibiotic ciprofloxacin has been used to prevent bacterial infections and has been extremely effective [129,130].

The most common bacterial infections are related to colonization of central venous catheters with, usually, coagulase-negative staphylococci or diphtheroids. Meticulous line care from insertion to removal is the only effective prophylactic measure. Infusions of vancomycin at the time of insertion may help. Those patients receiving high-dose corticosteroids for the treatment or prevention of acute GVHD are at special risk [131] and may be best treated expectantly with broad-spectrum therapeutic antibiotics.

The use of oral imidazole drugs such as ketoconazole, fluconazole and itraconazole to prevent fungal infections [132,133] has been a significant advance. Ketoconazole and itraconazole in prophylactic dosage have the disadvantage that they can interfere with the metabolism of cyclosporin if this is being used for the prophylaxis or treatment of GVHD. Fluconazole, which appears to have less interaction with cyclosporin A, has become widely used, leading to a simplification of antibacterial and antifungal prophylaxis to ciprofloxacin or a related compound plus fluconazole or a related compound. Of these agents, only itraconazole has activity against aspergillus, but this agent may have less activity against some more unusual candida species, and so the final decision will depend upon the spectrum of fungal infections seen locally. Aerosols of amphotericin B may also be considered as part of the antifungal regimen [134], although at present there is little evidence that the use of intravenous amphotericin B at less than therapeutic doses has any prophylactic benefit.

The prevention of virus infections is of particular importance. Those patients who have had previous exposure to herpes simplex virus should receive acyclovir [135]. Dosage regimens vary, but 400 mg twice daily is well tolerated, although it is possibly less effective than 200 mg five times daily. Attempts to prevent CMV infection should be active and commence at the diagnosis of leukaemia if possible [136]. Patients who are negative for previous CMV exposure should be protected from future exposure by the use of CMV-negative blood products [137,138] or by giving blood products that have been filtered using a high-efficiency white cell filter [139]. Patients who have had evidence of previous CMV exposure or whose donor has had previous exposure, should be considered for an active prophylactic regimen. High-dose acyclovir has been shown to have some benefits [136,140], while prophylaxis and treatment with ganciclovir and/or CMV-specific immunoglobulin have also been studied [141–143]. The regimen described by Atkinson *et al.* [124] involves treatment for 1 week pretransplant, followed by thrice weekly treatment. The author has found this to be tolerable to 100 days after BMT, and CMV incidence dramatically reduced, although Przepiorka *et al.* did not find thrice weekly ganciclovir sufficient [144]. Two subsequent studies have confirmed the benefit of ganciclovir [145,146].

Prevention of *Pneumocystis carinii* pneumonia is important, because the disease has been all but eradicated using co-trimoxazole. This should be given for 1–2 weeks before transplantation and then again from engraftment (neutrophils greater than 1×10^9/l) at doses of 960 mg twice a day on 2–3 days each week [147]. An alternative for patients with slow engraftment, or whose blood counts fall on therapy, is inhaled pentamidine [148,149]. It is less effective than optimal therapy with co-trimoxazole, however. Co-trimoxazole prophylaxis for *P. carinii* pneumonia appears to be effective against toxoplasma also, although Fansidar may be more specific and effective [150,151]. Varicella zoster is a major problem in the post-BMT period [152], and although prophylaxis with acyclovir is effective, zoster reactivation may occur when stopping the prophylaxis. The wide range of rare but potential pathogens in allogeneic BMT recipients is probably endless, and so levels of surveillance and suspicion must remain high at all times. Adenoviruses are often identified as pathogens [153], and as mentioned earlier, HHV-6 may reactivate in the post-transplant phase [126].

Patients who receive TBI as conditioning are rendered functionally asplenic and should receive appropriate life-long support thereafter [154].

Intravenous infusions of polyvalent immunoglobulins have also been used to prevent infection after allogeneic bone marrow transplantation [155] and, additionally, have been shown to affect the incidence of GVHD [156]. These studies have generally used very high doses of product that would be prohibitively expensive to use routinely. Therefore the potential benefits [157] must be weighed against the additional costs. The use of immunoglobulin therapy after allogeneic bone marrow transplantation has been reviewed recently [158], and the consensus view of the ECOG group [46] is that allogeneic BMT recipients should receive this therapy post-transplant.

Treatment of infection

Following allogeneic BMT, most patients will develop a fever requiring antibiotic or antifungal therapy. It is important to use an empirical protocol based on the local spectrum of organisms encountered [159]. If an organism is isolated, it is important that this is treated, but not at the expense of sacrificing a broad spectrum of antibiotic cover because more than one organism may be present. The frequency of central-line-associated infection is so great that most centres use intravenous vancomycin or teicoplanin very early in the regimen [160], and some groups have used vancomycin prophylactically [161]. If control of infection is not gained within 48–72 hours and the patient remains unwell, then intravenous amphotericin should be started [162]. The use of 5-flucytosine is toxic to the bone marrow but may, on occasions, be important for particularly invasive or CNS-related fungal infections. Newer strategies for treating invasive fungal infections using liposomal amphotericin [163] are effective and appear to have less side effects [164,165]. However, each is substantially more expensive than amphotericin.

Broad-spectrum antibiotics should be continued at least

until the neutrophils have recovered to greater than $0.5 \times 10^9/l$ and antifungal therapy is usually required even after sustained engraftment, depending on the severity of the initial fungal infection. The time at which prophylactic antibiotics and antifungals can be stopped is very variable and depends upon other factors related to the transplant. For instance, patients who have good engraftment, but have continuing active acute GVHD requiring treatment with corticosteroids, should remain on prophylactic antibiotics and antifungals for a significantly longer period of time than patients who engraft without GVHD.

Immunization post bone marrow transplantation

Subsequent prevention of infection should be considered, in particular in considering the immunization of patients [166]. At 12 months post transplant, it is safe to give pneumococcal 23 valent vaccine and meningococcal vaccine. The HIB protein conjugate and diphtheria and tetanus toxoid are also safe. At 24 months, the patient can be given measles, mumps and rubella vaccine unless receiving treatment for chronic GVHD [167]. The killed Salk polio vaccine is also safe at this stage. Live polio has generally been avoided post transplant. It is therefore important that BMT recipients are not sent home to an environment in which children have recently received live polio vaccine.

One issue that is not well addressed is the response to vaccination. Patients with active chronic GVHD are unlikely to respond well to vaccination, and should be monitored to assess their response. If these patients fail to mount an adequate response, the options available are limited to repeat vaccination, however, and monitoring the response only provides the awareness that an individual patient remains essentially nonimmune to a specific antigen.

Blood product support

Blood product support of patients with bone marrow failure is discussed in detail in Chapter 24. Specific transfusion measures need consideration for allogeneic BMT patients in the pretransplant period, including support during the induction of remission of acute leukaemia, the management of any donor–recipient incompatibility, avoidance of transfusion-related GVHD and plans for blood product support during and after transplantation.

Pretransplant measures

It is important to avoid alloimmunization of the recipient, particularly against closely related family HLA types, but also against white cells and platelets if febrile nonhaemolytic transfusion reactions and platelet refractoriness are to be avoided. Blood products are screened for HIV and hepatitis viruses, but CMV-negative patients who may be candidates for BMT should be transfused with filtered CMV-negative products [137], or filtered (leucocyte-depleted) products if these are unavailable [138,168].

ABO incompatibility between donor and recipient

The main transfusion problem for BMT recipients is the transfusion with the bone marrow graft of incompatible red blood cells. This usually occurs when an O recipient receives A- or B-group red cells, although A into B or B into A may also cause problems. If ABO incompatibility is detected during the donor assessment, then the anti-A or anti-B titres in the recipient need to be determined. Depending on whether the antibody titre is very high and whether or not there is a lytic component, the necessary measures to prevent a haemolytic reaction can be undertaken.

Various measures can be used. The first to be used involved plasmapheresis of the recipient [169]. This is time consuming, quite arduous for the patient and often must take place at a time when chemotherapy and radiotherapy are being administered and the patient is feeling unwell. However, this may be necessary if the antibody titres are very high, for example greater than $1:256$, and there is significant haemolysin present. Plasmapheresis should attempt to reduce the antibody titre to $1:8$ or less by the time of bone marrow infusion.

A much more satisfactory alternative is to deplete the donor bone marrow of red cells [170]. It is of great importance to monitor the recovery of bone marrow nucleated cells at each stage of any manipulation and no part of the donation should be discarded until the final, adequate, satisfactory product is obtained and infused.

In the post-transplant phase a transfusion policy needs to be followed. Blood products of the recipient's blood group should be used while monitoring antibody titres. It is also important to monitor mixed-field red cell patterns and reticulocyte counts, so that engraftment can be identified and the change then made to donor blood group transfusions. Red blood cell chimerism can be monitored using flow cytometry. In general in the post-transplant phase, haemolytic reactions are less of a problem than those seen in solid organ transplants involving passenger lymphocytes. In cases where the donor is group O and may have anti-A or anti-B antibodies that could react with an A or B recipient, the antibody titre must be determined and any potential for haemolysis through passive immunization considered. If this is a possibility, then the donor bone marrow should be centrifuged and as much plasma as possible expressed and replaced with AB plasma, albumin or saline.

Transfusion policy for the bone marrow transplant recipient

The plan for blood product support needs to consider three issues.

1 *The CMV antibody status of the recipient and the donor.* Cases where both the recipient and the donor are negative for CMV should receive CMV-negative blood products [137] or products filtered through a high-efficiency white cell filter [138]. If both the donor and the recipient are CMV positive, there is little evidence to support giving CMV-negative products. If either is negative, then negative products should be given, although there is less strong evidence for their importance. In addition, donor–recipient pairs in which either is CMV positive should be considered for specific anti-CMV prophylaxis.

2 *Irradiation of blood products.* All blood products must be irradiated [171,172] to at least 2500 cGy and under no circumstances must unirradiated products be given because of the risk of transfusing immune-competent alloreactive T-lymphocytes with the potential for the development of fatal GVHD [173,174]. Such a transfusion policy should probably be lifelong, although the safety of unirradiated products in patients who relapse after allogeneic BMT and need further cytoreductive therapy has not been formally assessed.

3 *The blood groups acceptable for transfusion* need to be considered in case there is a shortage of specific groups.

Transfusion regimen

Red cell transfusions. Plasma-reduced red cells should be given to maintain the haemoglobin above 10 g/dl.

White blood cells. Neutropenia and lymphopenia are managed by protocols for the prevention and treatment of infection, as discussed above. Occasional patients who are suffering from localized infection may respond to white blood cell transfusions from single donors or, rarely, from buffy coats from multiple donors [175]. The necessity for such manoeuvres will be most unusual now with improvements in antibiotics and antifungal therapy. G-CSF-mobilized granulocytes are more likely to be useful, especially if they can be obtained from the transplant donor [176]. The issue of promoting white cell engraftment using cytokines and PBSCs is considered below.

Platelets. Platelet count should be maintained above $15 \times 10^9/l$, although on occasions patients with higher counts may bleed, and they should receive additional support. Guidelines are available [177]. Patients with a history of platelet refractoriness should be considered for platelet crossmatching and the selection of specific single donors from within the family before the transplant period. Refractoriness to platelets should be assessed by measuring platelet recovery at 1 hour postinfusion. On occasions, patients may appear refractory, but they may have received an inadequate dose of platelets. There is a trend, in many centres, to move away from the use of multiple random donor platelet support towards apheresis platelets, in order to reduce the exposure to such large numbers of donors when pooled random products are used. If specific HLA-matched platelets are needed, donors from a transfusion centre donor panel may be utilized.

Post-transplant immune cytopenias

These phenomena are uncommon but may affect red cells [178], platelets [179] or all cell lineages [180]. It is important to identify the cause of any late cytopenia to ensure that appropriate management is instituted. The most common cause is drug-induced toxicity, but virus and other infections are also common, and much more so than immune destruction.

Graft-vs-host disease

This condition was first described in mice when it was known as 'secondary disease' or 'runt disease' [7]. It is caused by alloreactive T cells in the transplant reacting against foreign antigens in the recipient [17]. The removal of T cells from the bone marrow graft will prevent GVHD [18,19], and new T-cell clones will develop from progenitors which acquire tolerance of host antigens in the thymus. The preliminary studies of T-cell depletion, especially in CML, showed that removal of these T cells lead to increased relapse and increased graft failure [16,21]. These data provided evidence both that there was a graft-vs-leukaemia (GVL) effect, and also that T cells play a role in both the GVL effect and engraftment. GVHD is conventionally divided into acute and chronic; these often merge, but the two conditions at the ends of the spectrum each have a quite distinct pathophysiology [181].

Acute graft-vs-host disease

This has been well described by the Seattle BMT Group [182], who have developed a scoring system for its degree of severity (Table 22.3). Acute GVHD mainly affects the skin, liver and gut, with an onset 3–30 days post BMT, but it can be delayed for up to 100 days post-transplant. GVHD appearing more than 100 days after transplant is termed by convention chronic GVHD [9]. Those patients who have grades of GVHD greater than II have a worse survival [183,184]. The incidence of acute GVHD varies between 5 and 70%, depending on the preventative regimens used, the donor's age, the recipient's age, the sexes of donor and recipient, and the degree of HLA matching between them [185].

Skin graft-vs-host disease

This usually starts with minor erythema, particularly of the palms of the hands and soles of the feet. The skin over the chest, back and face is also commonly involved. The rash may extend to generalized erythema and, in the most severe forms, bullae and skin desquamation occur. The pathology of the later and more severe grades is well established [182], but earlier stages may be quite difficult to diagnose [186]. Very occasional patients will have severe GVHD in demarcated rather than generalized areas (see Plates 22.1–22.3 between pp. 292 and 293).

Table 22.3 Grading of severity of GVHD by clinical and laboratory criteria. (Adapted from Glucksberg *et al.*,1974 [182].)

Grade	Skin	Liver function	Intestine
<I	Mild erythema <10% of body surface area	Normal	<500 ml diarrhoea/24 hours
I	Maculopapular rash <25% body surface area	Bilirubin 25–40 µmol/l. Alkaline phosphatase 2 × normal Alanine transaminase 3 × normal	>500 ml/24 hours
II	Maculopapular rash 25–50% body surface area	Bilirubin 41–74 µmol/l	>1000 ml/24 hours
III	Generalized erythroderma	Bilirubin 75–300 µmol/l	>1500 ml/24 hours
IV	Generalized erythroderma with desquamation and bullae	Bilirubin >300 µmol/l	Severe abdominal pain, ileus, bloody diarrhoea

This is the most practical guide to the assessment of the severity of GVHD and has stood the test of time. It is not a substitute for clinical judgement, however. Patients do not necessarily, or even usually, develop organ involvement in a synchronous manner. For instance, it is common for a patient to have grade III GVHD of one system with minimal or no involvement elsewhere.

Skin GVHD should be confirmed with a diagnostic skin biopsy to distinguish it from drug-related and nonspecific eruptions. However, more severe forms are quite characteristic and are often associated with tenderness of the palms of the hands and the soles of the feet, and, if confined to these areas, biopsy may be inappropriate. Minor degrees of skin GVHD may not be directly related to alloreactive T-lymphocytes, because similar skin changes may be seen in patients following autologous bone marrow rescue procedures.

Liver graft-vs-host disease

Acute liver GVHD tends to be a biliary tract disease with the picture of obstructive jaundice [182]. Bilirubin and alkaline phosphatase levels increase, with hepatitis being a less common feature. Differential diagnosis of these abnormalities is often complicated by the possibility of cyclosporin toxicity, VOD of the liver, and virus infections, particularly CMV. Liver biopsy is extremely important in the diagnosis of liver abnormalities post-BMT [187], and in those patients with abnormal coagulation and/or low platelet counts the transjugular approach may be helpful. More recently, laparoscopic biopsy has been shown to be safe in experienced hands and provides larger biopsies. Severe progressive liver GVHD that is resistant to corticosteroids has a poor prognosis.

Gut graft-vs-host disease

This most commonly presents as diarrhoea which may be anything from mild to torrential, with up to 10–15 litres of watery and bloody diarrhoea passed daily. In the early stages of severe GVHD of the gut, stools may take on a characteristic mincemeat appearance, although this is not a particularly reliable sign. Another presentation is with upper gastrointestinal symptoms such as nausea, abdominal discomfort and cramps.

Biopsy of the rectum or upper gastrointestinal tract, as appropriate, is important to confirm the diagnosis and, in difficult cases, upper gastrointestinal endoscopy and contrast radiology series may be required. Virus infections of the gut must be excluded, as must bacterial pathogens.

Chronic graft-vs-host disease

Recipients of allogeneic BMT develop chronic GVHD in 25–50% of cases [184]. This is an autoimmune disorder associated with scleroderma-like changes and tends to be progressive [188]. It often emerges from acute GVHD that has not been completely controlled by treatment but can develop *de novo*. By convention, GVHD occurring after 100 days is termed chronic GVHD. Acute GVHD and increased age of recipient or donor are important prognostic indicators, as is any mismatching between recipient and donor and, in aplastic anaemia recipients, the use of donor buffy coat cells [184]. A common manifestation is a sicca syndrome with dry eyes and mouth and this may also affect the vulva in females. Skin changes involve thickening of the skin with dryness and loss of hair. Tethering of the skin overlying bony prominences is particularly common, and a reduction in skin elasticity can lead to joint contractures. Hyperpigmentation and hypopigmentation, which can cause confusion with fungal disorders of the skin, are common, and skin biopsy is appropriate in such cases. Chronic GVHD of the gut leads to a malabsorption syndrome with wasting of the patient; immune incompetence in particular to bacterial and fungal infections is extremely common. Limited skin or liver involvement has a favourable outcome, but patients with extensive chronic GVHD have a less than 20% long-term survival free of disability [189]. Persistent thrombocytopenia carries an especially poor prognosis, in part because poor bone marrow function causes difficulties in delivering optimal therapy. The one benefit of chronic

GVHD is that there is a significantly reduced risk of leukaemia relapse.

Prevention of graft-vs-host disease

The available methods for GVHD prevention are legion, and their very multiplicity explains the dilemma. No one method can clearly be considered the best in all situations. In general, the more effective the technique is at preventing GVHD, the greater the risk of recurrent leukaemia post-BMT [21,22,25], or, to a lesser degree, the greater the risk of rejection [16] or secondary lymphoproliferative disorders [37]. Some newer techniques reflect knowledge about the role of cytokines in the production of the GVHD reaction [190]. The efficacy of preventive regimens may also be influenced by reporting of the severity of GVHD, which has been shown to have a variation between centres [191].

The ability to predict those donor–recipient pairs who are most likely to get clinically significant grades of GVHD (grades III–IV) would be helpful. It is certainly known that giving no GVHD prophylaxis leads to early and severe disease in adults [192]. Similarly, using donors mismatched at more than one Class I or II HLA locus will lead to an unacceptable incidence of GVHD, despite early optimism [193], unless very intensive T-cell depletion is used with a large progenitor cell dose [36]. Other risk factors have been identified [194], and various techniques have been developed to predict severity [195–197], but none has been universally adopted or proven to be unequivocally effective. It seems most likely that developments in the molecular histocompatibility typing of donors and recipients, whether related or not, will prove to be the most useful predictor of complications.

Four regimens have been used commonly for the prevention of GVHD in allogeneic BMT [185]: methotrexate, cyclosporin, a combination of methotrexate and cyclosporin A and *ex vivo* T-cell depletion of bone marrow. In addition, some regimens have included agents such as prednisolone [198] and antilymphocyte (ALG) or thymocyte (ATG) globulin as part of the conditioning. The use of ALG/ATG tends to be limited to patients undergoing MUD transplants and it is mainly an adjunct to engraftment which prevents donor rejection of the incoming graft [199]. *In vivo* T-cell depletion (the effect that using ATG/ALG has) may also be affected by using a monoclonal antibody, Campath [200,201], although numerous other techniques are available [18,202], some of which only deplete certain T-cell subsets [198].

Methotrexate prophylaxis was originally used in Seattle [9] and includes intravenous methotrexate at 10–15 mg/m² per dose in the 11 days post-transplant ('short' methotrexate). Acute GVHD will still develop in 70% of patients conditioned in this way, and, of these, approximately 20% will have severe life-threatening GVHD. Cyclosporin was introduced in 1980 [10] and is associated with a slightly lower incidence of acute GVHD which tends to be less severe. There is a slight improvement in the short-term outcome, but this may not be significant [12]. The combination of cyclosporin and methotrexate was first used in 1985 [13] and appears, now, to be the most used treatment. It is probably the most effective way of preventing acute GVHD without T cells depleting the bone marrow graft, but it does lead to a small but significant increase in relapse risk when compared with methotrexate alone [25]. Higher doses of cyclosporin also lead to an increased relapse risk [24]. Indeed, the interaction between GVHD and GVL is such that almost all techniques that reduce significantly the risk of acute GVHD will also lead to an increase in relapse risk [23,203]. However, a large number of patients may be needed to detect this effect, and the freedom from acute GVHD, in particular, remains a very strong prognostic factor in favour of long-term survival.

T-cell depletion of bone marrow using either soyabean agglutinin and red cell rosetting or monoclonal antibodies with or without immunotoxins [18] is a very effective way of preventing acute GVHD. The efficacy is proportional to the degree of T-cell depletion, and the T cells are reduced to less than 0.1% of the original number, then the incidence of acute GVHD will be less than 5%. However, the penalty to pay is a 10% rejection rate, and in CML an unacceptable increased relapse rate of 50% [21,22]. New techniques using positive selection of CD34+ haemopoietic progenitors can also deplete the marrow, or PBSC, collection of 2 to 3 logs of T cells. The concerns about the relapse rate after completely T-cell-depleted transplants has lead some groups to explore the concept of delayed reinfusion of T cells some time after the graft [204], or the addition of a known low dose of T lymphocytes [205].

At the present time adult patients undergoing allogeneic BMT for malignant disease are, in the absence of an approved research protocol, best managed with a combination of cyclosporin A and methotrexate if their donor is an HLA-matched relative. T-cell depletion should be considered for patients receiving transplants from unrelated donors, although the evidence for this remains tentative. There are numerous protocols for these transplants [206–208]. Research protocols looking at the use of CD34 selection for T-cell depletion should be supported in appropriate patients. Measures may then be necessary to prevent graft rejection by suppressing or reducing the number of T cells in the recipient or, by using PBSC, increasing the number of haemopoietic stem cells transplanted. The emergence of post-transplant immune modulation, using donor lymphocyte infusion for example, also provides an opportunity to attempt to reduce the risk of relapse after a T-cell-depleted transplant (see below). The increasing knowledge abut the immune responses involved in the development of graft-vs-host reactions has prompted a number of new approaches in this area [209–211]. Careful evaluation of new techniques is required to ensure that they do not have a worse outcome than current practice [212].

Complications of anti-graft-vs-host disease therapy

Methotrexate

The toxicities seen in patients receiving cyclosporin and methotrexate have recently been reviewed [213]. Methotrexate produces an increased risk of severe oral mucositis which should be managed with local measures and opiate analgesia as required. There is also delayed engraftment, over nonmethotrexate-containing treatments, of between 5 and 7 days to reach neutrophil counts of $0.5 \times 10^9/l$ [11]. Methotrexate is also hepatotoxic, although evidence for an increased risk of hepatic VOD [214] now seems to be disputed [74]. Its use is associated with less relapse post BMT [215].

Cyclosporin

This is a notoriously toxic drug [213], particularly to the kidney [11]. It produces initially reversible renal impairment and, commonly, this is associated with hypertension. Fits are common, particularly in younger patients. Regular monitoring of cyclosporin levels in the blood should be carried out in the immediate post-transplant phase, as much to ensure levels are adequate as to avoid toxicity, and monitoring should continue intermittently while the patient is on cyclosporin. Chronic irreversible nephrotoxicity can also occur in patients on long-term cyclosporin. Other common and more chronic side effects of cyclosporin A are hirsuties, tremor and rhinitis. It is usual to continue cyclosporin for 6 months post-transplant and then to reduce the dose gradually over the following 3 months so that cyclosporin is withdrawn 9 months post transplant [10]. Patients who have no GVHD can probably have the drug withdrawn more quickly. If possible, it should be given by the oral route throughout, because this is likely to reduce the incidence of side effects, but patients who are unable to eat because of mucositis, or who have gut malabsorption because of radiation-induced gut dysfunction or GVHD, may require intravenous therapy. Cyclosporin combined with prednisolone on an alternate-day basis is effective therapy for chronic GVHD [216], but long-term toxicity may still occur and careful monitoring remains essential.

T-cell depletion

There is very little immediate toxicity related to this, because the procedure is usually carried out *in vitro* and any antibodies used are usually washed from the cells prior to reinfusion. However, because many of the monoclonal antibodies, for example OKT3 [217] and Campath [200], are of mouse and rat origin, respectively, there is a possibility of allergic reactions at the time of reinfusion of marrow. Campath may also be given intravenously to deplete T cells both pre- and post-BMT [201],

and humanized versions are now available. The most important adverse effects of T-cell depletion relate to the indirect effects [218] of graft failure [219] and relapse [220].

Treatment of graft-vs-host disease

Acute graft-vs-host disease

Grades of acute GVHD of I or less can be treated expectantly by observation. Patients with grade II disease should receive steroid therapy, and clinical judgement will determine whether this should be low-dose 1 mg/kg oral prednisolone or high-dose $1 g/m^2$ daily (or even twice daily) methyl prednisolone [185]. For patients with severe GVHD of grades III or IV, high-dose methylprednisolone is the treatment of choice, and this should be continued for 3 days and then a reduction attempted. The original protocol suggested suddenly stopping high doses of steroids, but this tends to lead to recrudescence of acute GVHD, therefore stepwise reduction of dosage is usually necessary. The rate at which steroids may be withdrawn will depend upon the degree and rapidity of response, but reducing it by 50% every 3–4 days is usual. Patients on high doses of corticosteroids following transplantation have an increased risk of bacterial infection and, particularly, of fungal infection. This may be compounded if diabetes mellitus is induced. Catabolic effects are usual at high dose, and enteral, or parenteral if gut GVHD is present, feeding should be instituted if already discontinued. The risk of gastrointestinal haemorrhage should be reduced by using an H2 receptor antagonist, for example cimetidine or ranitidine. Patients on $1 g/m^2$ methlyprednisolone or equivalent doses should receive broad-spectrum intravenous antibiotics to prevent bacterial infection and should also receive intensive surveillance for fungal infection. High-dose corticosteroids can also occasionally precipitate viral infections, particularly CMV pneumonitis, as a result of the intensive immunosuppression.

As the dose of steroids is reduced, it is often possible to give alternate doses on different days between high and low dose to minimize the side effects. Occasional patients may require prolonged corticosteroid therapy extending into many months or, occasionally, years if chronic GVHD follows.

In vivo T-cell depletion. The most usual way to do this is to use ALG or ATG for a 4- or 5-day course [221]. This is very effective in depleting the peripheral blood of T-lymphocytes and will usually result in a satisfactory initial response of the acute GVHD. However, a significant proportion of patients will relapse following this treatment, but some will gain a durable response and it will be possible to reduce the corticosteroid doses to an acceptable and less toxic level following the course of ALG or ATG. Longer courses of ATG (10 days) appear to be more effective but they bring associated problems of immune suppression. No randomized trials exist to guide therapy. Other antibodies such as Campath IG [200], IL-2 receptor antibody [222,223], XomaZyme H65 (anti CD5) [224], anti CD8 and OKT3 (CD3) [217] are also available, but few data are available on these products. Most treatments will produce transient responses, but few patients with severe steroid-resistant GVHD will become long-term survivors. The use of *in vivo* T-cell depletion is highly immunosuppressive and similar precautions to those taken when patients are receiving high-dose steroids are required. Since ALG or ATG are often used in steroid-resistant cases of acute GVHD, vigilance is particularly important. Progression to chronic GVHD does not appear to be prevented by these measures.

Cyclosporin. Initial studies failed to show any benefit for cyclosporin in treating GVHD. However, it does appear to have some effect [225] if the dose is increased for those patients already receiving cyclosporin for GVHD prophylaxis. Chronic GVHD may respond to alternate-day dosing of cyclosporin and steroids [216], particularly if the patient did not receive cyclosporin as part of the prophylactic regimen.

Azathiaprine. This is only moderately effective in acute to chronic GVHD [189]. Myelosuppression is the usual problem with this compound, and it is often in the early stages after transplantation that the patient requires additional anti-GVHD effect. However, in those patients with a good bone marrow graft and established GVHD that is moderately resistant to steroids, azathiaprine can be dramatically effective in controlling the GVHD. Doses up to 2.5 mg/kg should be attempted, but a reduction of neutrophil counts often occur at this dosage, and it is often necessary to decrease the dose to between 1 and 2 mg/kg. Recurrence, especially of chronic liver GVHD, appears common after stopping azathiaprine.

Chronic graft-vs-host disease

Patients who develop chronic GVHD from acute GVHD will usually have been receiving continuing corticosteroid therapy. In addition, they may or may not have been given azathiaprine. The cornerstone of the treatment of chronic GVHD is to commence treatment early, because once scleroderma-like skin changes or sicca syndrome are established they are difficult to reverse. Patients with good bone marrow engraftment will often respond to prednisolone and azathiaprine [189], and those patients with low platelet counts (less than 100×10^9/l) appear to respond better with cyclosporin and corticosteroids given on alternate days [216] at a dose of cyclosporin 6 mg/kg twice daily and prednisolone 1 mg/kg daily. Even with active treatment, patients with low platelet counts will have a 35% mortality, whereas those patients with a robust bone marrow graft (platelet count greater than 100×10^9/l) have a relatively low mortality (6%), with only 8% failing to respond. The actuarial survival of chronic GVHD patients who respond to treatment is 80%. The overall survival for those with low platelets is 43% and they have a very high risk of life-threatening septicaemia over a 3-year period of 40% [226]. The use of thalidomide is helpful, because it is relatively nonmyelotoxic and it has been particularly useful in skin chronic GVHD [227,228]. For intractable cases, immunosuppressive treatment such as total lymphoid irradiation have been tried with anecdotal success, but data are limited. Tretinoin [229], ultraviolet light (PUVA) [230] or extracorporeal T-cell depletion using phototherapy [231] may help resistant skin disease. The overall management of chronic GVHD was reviewed in 1994 [232]. The factors that predict for developing chronic GVHD are various, but most patients will have had pre-existing acute disease [233,234].

Bone marrow engraftment

The median time postallogeneic BMT to achieve a count of 1×10^9/l neutrophils and 50×10^9/l platelets varies greatly and depends on the regimen used to prevent GVHD. Most patients will engraft between 10 and 30 days post-transplant, with an average time of 14–24 days. Treatments containing methotrexate or involving T-cell depletion of the marrow graft will extend the period of time to engraftment, while cyclosporin tends to reduce this period [19,235]. The recent introduction of haemopoietic growth factor mobilized PBSC for allografts appears to reduce the time to engraftment, particularly for platelet recovery [1,59]. The existence of early acute GVHD may also extend the time for full engraftment, as will virus infections, particularly herpes simplex. The use of co-trimoxazole to prevent infection in the post-transplant period will extend the time to engraftment. Mismatching between donor and recipient will also slow engraftment [104]. The recovery of normal or near normal peripheral blood counts is only the first stage in the restitution of full lympho-haemopoiesis. Immune recovery may be much slower, especially in the presence of significant GVHD [236]. In the post-BMT period, examination of the chimeric (donor; recipient proportions) status can either reassure the physician that engraftment is proceeding satisfactorily or confirm rejection [237,238]. Although mixed chimerism by no means always predicts for subsequent relapse, it appears to do so if T-cell chimerism is present in cases of CML [239].

Graft failure

Graft failure may be a primary, complete failure to engraft in which no donor cells are ever identified, or it may be secondary, in which the graft has been observed, may or may not become stable, and then is lost. Patients who require intensive management because of acute GVHD or severe fungal or viral infection, may often be receiving drugs that compromise engraftment, and this may be associated with a deterioration in blood counts. Predictors of graft failure are T-cell-depleted BMT [19,235], degrees of mismatch between donor and recipient [104] and BMT for aplastic anaemia [16]. It may be possible to reverse secondary graft failure with intensive immunosuppression with corticosteroids [240], or ATG [157].

When graft failure has become irreversible, various options for rescuing the patient are available, although none is very satisfactory. These may include autologous marrow infusions or a second transplant. Second BMT for graft failure in leukaemia gives disappointing results, with only a 9% survival at 2 years in one study of 80 patients [241]. The main problem relates to treatment-related complications, including secondary graft failure, GVHD, interstitial pneumonitis and hepatic VOD. Because the mechanism of graft failure is rejection, some form of further immunosuppressive therapy is required, usually cyclophosphamide at a high dose. This is being given to a patient who will have endured some weeks of profound bone marrow failure and probably, a period of further intensive immunosuppression with corticosteroids and ATG/ALG. The survivability of such a second transplant therefore depends on the clinical condition of the patient at the time. The poor results in leukaemia contrast with the outlook of second transplants for aplastic anaemia in the same study [241] in which 63 patients were studied, with 53% alive at 2 years. These data would suggest that in leukaemia it is difficult to justify second allogeneic transplants for graft failure, with autologous rescue being preferable, whereas in aplastic anaemia this is clearly an appropriate course of action in which, by definition, autografting is not available.

Promoting engraftment

The use of haemopoietic growth factors in allogeneic BMT for leukaemia was initially limited, because of the concern that stimulation of myeloid leukaemia clones may occur. Although it is known that stimulation of leukaemic blasts *in vitro* by these agents does happen, there is no evidence that the use of G- or GM-CSF after allogeneic BMT has any adverse effect on outcome [242]. A reduction in the period of neutropenia is seen, but in allogeneic BMT this is not an important index of successful outcome. The use of haemopoietic growth factors after BMT is encouraged in the ECOG guidelines [46]. Cytokines which have a broader spectrum of effect, such as IL-3 which has the capacity to stimulate both myeloid and megakaryocyte cytopoiesis, might appear to be more useful, because poor platelet engraftment is common after bone marrow allografts [243,244]. However, IL-3 has yet to find its place in the routine therapy of neutropenia and thrombocytopenia after conventional-dose therapy or for PBSC mobilization, and it appears unlikely that this agent will transform engraftment after allogeneic BMT. The recently cloned and isolated megakaryocyte colony stimulator shows more promise [245]. In mice, this agent accelerates the recovery of platelets after PBSC transplantation [246]. Preliminary phase I/II studies in humans are ongoing and initial reports (as yet unpublished) are encouraging. If reports of low toxicity and

efficacy are substantiated, this factor is likely to play a role in supporting platelet counts postallograft, with the proviso that all cytokines require the presence of adequate numbers of their target cell population, and so patients with established graft failure are unlikely to benefit. Another promising agent for platelet recovery is IL-11 [247]. Other haemopoietic growth factors that act on uncommitted haemopoietic progenitors, such as stem cell factor and flt-3 ligand, are still undergoing *in vitro* and early *in vivo* study. Their theoretical potential to encourage engraftment and *in vivo* and *ex vivo* expansion of marrow cells is great, but it is unlikely that clinical studies in allogeneic BMT will take place until their use in autografts and stem cell mobilization is determined.

Indications for and results of allogeneic bone marrow transplantation

Major advances have occurred over the past 5 or more years in the management of patients undergoing BMT. These developments have encouraged the use of allogeneic BMT in older patients (certainly up to 55 years), and for a wider range of diagnoses. The use of unrelated donors has increased markedly, and is likely to increase further as improvements in the accuracy of tissue matching [248] affect post-transplant outcome. Using relatives other than siblings produces successful outcomes which depend on the degree of tissue match, with overall survival with minor mismatches not being affected [249,250]. Certainly, unrelated donor BMT has a higher complication and mortality rate [251] than family donor procedures. The results and techniques appear to be improving over time however [252–254].

Acute myeloid leukaemia

This group of disorders is also described as acute nonlymphoblastic leukaemia, in recognition of the inclusion of some cases of acute leukaemia which do not express either myeloid or lymphoid differentiation markers and which, conventionally, are included with the myeloid leukaemias. Management with conventional chemotherapy will produce remissions in about 80% of patients under the age 55 years, which is the group of patients eligible for allogeneic BMT. Until recently, only about 15–25% of patients in this age group became long-term disease-free survivors with conventional treatment (see Chapters 9 and 10). The decision whether to offer allogeneic BMT depends on the perceived benefit in long-term survival over conventional chemotherapy. Therefore, if the results from conventional nontransplant treatment for AML improve, the previously held view that allogeneic BMT is always the treatment of choice in AML has become challenged. The use of high-dose cytarabine as consolidation therapy [255], or of four very intensive cycles of chemotherapy in the UK MRC 10th AML Trial [43], have both improved nontransplant results to approximately 40% in standard-risk cases. These figures are now approaching those for allogeneic BMT, but they have much reduced toxic death rates and morbidity. The EORTC/GIMEMA study compared autologous and allogeneic BMT, and found an improved relapse-free survival for either transplant over conventional therapy, but long-term overall survival was similar because of good complete remission (CR) responses in the conventional group [256].

Patients in whom serious consideration should be given to deferring allogeneic BMT to second CR (CR2) are those with chromosome abnormalities t(8;21) and inv16 [43,44], and probably those with acute promyelocytic leukaemia (APL) who have t15; 17 [43].

If it is now possible to identify good-risk cases among the AML cases, it also appears to be possible to identify poor-risk patients. These will be cases with abnormalities of chromosomes 7 and 8 who respond poorly to the first course of therapy. Such patients are unlikely to be cured with conventional-dose therapy, and they should be offered allogeneic BMT soon after achieving remission. Unrelated donor transplants may also be appropriate for this group of patients if there is no family donor.

The best results from BMT for AML are achieved in first CR (CR1) and, preferably, early in that CR to avoid the risk of subsequent relapse. Patients transplanted at this time will have a 55% chance of long-term disease-free survival [257]. These results can be considered to represent cure, and have remained valid over 15–20 years and this is supported by the plateaux in both International and European Bone Marrow Transplant Registries which appear stable (Fig. 22.4). Late relapses occasionally occur, however, and in most cases these are in recipient cells. However, occasional relapses have been described in which the relapsing leukaemia has been of donor cell origin [258]. Approximately 40% of those patients who fail to become long-term survivors will relapse and subsequently die of their leukaemia, or the complications of its treatment. The risk of relapse is highly dependent on the status of disease at the time of transplantation (Fig. 22.5). The remainder of deaths are a result of pneumonitis or other infectious complications or those related to GVHD. The impact of GVHD is probably rather greater than this, however, because a significant proportion of those patients who die of pneumonitis or other infections also have GVHD which contributes to their immune suppression.

Data have been presented from the Seattle Group suggesting that BMT in early first relapse of AML gives long-term results which are as good as those for patients transplanted in CR1 [259].

For those people who relapse and then receive further induction therapy, the long-term results following allogeneic BMT in second remission will offer only a 30% long-term survival. For the patient already in a stable second CR, allogeneic BMT offers the best, and perhaps only, opportunity for cure. Most patients who relapse with AML do so within a year of entering CR, so the time available for making these decisions is

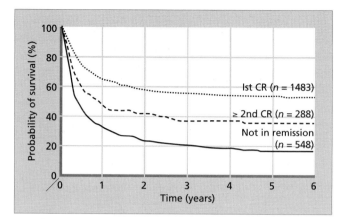

Fig. 22.4 Probability of leukaemia-free survival for up to 6 years after HLA-identical sibling BMT for AML: 1987–94. The data show a 55% chance of survival for patients transplanted in the first CR. The results of transplants during the second CR are still good at >35% and a substantial improvement over conventional therapy. (Data from the IBMTR and the ABMTR of North America.) *P* = 0.0001.

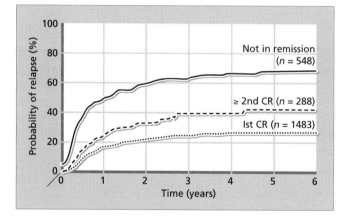

Fig. 22.5 Probability of relapse after HLA-identical sibling BMT for AML: 1987–94. Results show that about half of the treatment failures are a result of relapse is the first CR transplants, whereas nearly all the deaths were relapse related in the patients who were not in remission. Relapse is unusual beyond 2 years post-BMT in first CR patients, whereas for later disease status the risk continues until about 4 years post-BMT. (Data from the IBMTR and the ABMTR of North America.) *P* = 0.0001.

not long. Combining this with the difficulties of achieving second remission, and the usual deterioration in the physical condition of the patient, makes first remission the optimum time to transplant patients.

Unrelated donor transplants for AML have, in the main, been confined to CR2, although there is a good case for offering such transplants in CR1 to those with especially high-risk disease. Again, the National Marrow Donor Program (NMDP) data is most informative [254]. First or second CR patients did well, with 2-year disease-free survival (DFS) at 45%. Beyond CR2, only 19% survived 2 years, but even this result is probably better than might be expected by conventional therapy, given that any patients with a sibling donor would already have had an allograft by such a late stage. Because the median duration for CR2 of AML is short, it is important that the donor search is carried out promptly and the transplant proceeded with as quickly as possible.

A recent series from Seattle [34] suggests similarly encouraging results in CR2 of 31%, with CR1 better at 55% DFS at 3 years. Even third or later remissions had a 26% chance of survival. However, similar results can be obtained in these patient groups with autologous procedures. Both the Seattle Group and the European Group for BMT (EBMT) have compared results in matched patients treated with either MUD or autologous transplant [41,42]. The Seattle series showed a small advantage for the MUD procedure, whereas there was no difference at all in the EBMT study. The cause of death was different, however, with more transplant-related deaths in the MUD BMTs and more relapse deaths in the autografts.

It is clear that a patient who has completed their initial courses of chemotherapy now has a range of options available. Those in the better prognostic groups may prefer to wait, and consider transplantation in CR2. For standard-risk AML—the majority — allogeneic BMT from a family donor will be the treatment of choice in CR1. If no family donor is available, then usually an autograft, or perhaps a course of high-dose cytarabine, will be advised, unless there are especially poor prognostic features, in which case an unrelated donor transplant will be considered. Finally, in the absence of an unrelated donor and perhaps with no useful autologous marrow for an autograft, recent results from Aversa *et al.* [36] suggest that, with appropriate T-cell depletion and immune suppression of the patient, haplo-identical marrow can engraft and provide acceptable short-term results. However, the results of conventional therapy are improving decade by decade, and it is entirely possible that in the future allografting for AML will be confined to patients in relapse or CR2, or those with a known poor outlook with chemotherapy alone.

Acute lymphoblastic leukaemia

Acute lymphoblastic leukaemia in adults is a less common disorder than AML and initial treatment to CR tends to be more successful, with about 90% achieving remission [260,261]. However, long-term disease-free survivals are very disappointing, being in the order of 15–25% depending on the particular study [262]. Although there are subgroups with a particularly poor outlook, especially Philadelphia (Ph) Chromosome positive disease and t(4;11), B-ALL and those patients presenting with central nervous system (CNS) involvement, all adults have a poor prognosis when compared to children with ALL. In children between the ages of 2 and 12 years, over 60% long-term DFS will be achieved with modern intensive chemotherapy without marrow transplantation [261] (see Chapter 5). Therefore, allogeneic BMT should be considered only for those

children who have particularly poor-risk disease, whereas survival in adults with ALL is poor, and a good case can be made for offering a family donor BMT in CR1.

For those patients without a related allogeneic BMT donor, matched unrelated donors should be considered for CR2 transplants, unless there is a Ph chromosome or t(4;11), in which case MUD transplant is advised in CR1 [263].

The alternative intensive treatment in CR1 or CR2 would be an autologous procedure. Studies of autologous procedures in ALL have tended to be less extensive [264] than those for AML, and interpretation is complicated by the much greater use of monoclonal antibody purging of autologous marrow. However, autologous procedures appear likely to be competitive with matched unrelated donor allogeneic BMT in ALL. The management of ALL has been reviewed recently [265]. A current study organized by the Eastern Cooperative Oncology Group and the UK MRC intends to answer the question of the role of autografting, allografting and conventional therapy in a large multination trial.

Current results of allogeneic BMT in ALL from the IBMTR are shown in Figs 22.6 & 22.7. There remains a significant risk of relapse and, overall, the long-term survivals are similar to AML. GVHD prevention regimens incorporating corticosteroids appear to offer added survival benefit for BMT in ALL [266]. A major risk factor for a poor outcome is late-stage disease [266,267], and the decision to proceed with transplantation must be weighed carefully with the risk of shortening the patient's life.

Chronic myeloid leukaemia

Conventional treatment produces no cures in CML, whereas

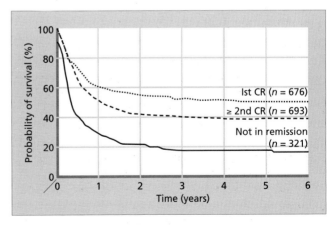

Fig. 22.6 Probability of leukaemia-free survival after HLA-identical sibling BMT for ALL: 1987–94. The results indicate that half of those patients with ALL who have a sibling allogeneic BMT will be alive and disease free 6 years later. The results for second CR are also good at just below 40%, especially as this group of patients is incurable by conventional therapy. (Data from the IBMTR and the ABMTR of North America.) *P* = 0.0001.

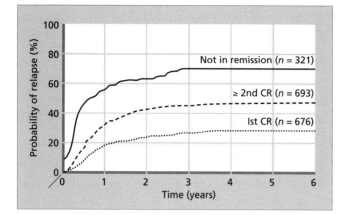

Fig. 22.7 Probability of relapse after HLA-identical sibling BMT for ALL: 1987–94. The risk of relapse is higher than for AML for all remission status groups shown. Few relapses occur after 4 years. (Data from the IBMTR and the ABMTR of North America.) *P* = 0.0001.

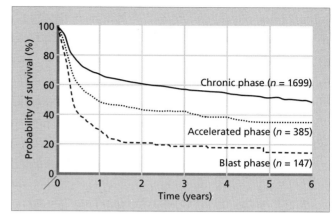

Fig. 22.8 Probability of leukaemia-free survival after HLA-identical sibling BMT for CML: 1987–94. Although 50% of patients were transplanted in the first chronic phase, there is no plateau of survival, suggesting that relapses continue to occur beyond 9 years post-BMT. (Data from the IBMTR and the ABMTR of North America.) *P* = 0.0001.

allogeneic BMT can do so regularly [21,268]. Therefore, in patients under the age of 55 with Ph+ CML, who have a related allogeneic BMT donor, the question is not whether to offer transplantation but when to offer it [269]. The first chronic phase of CML can last for any time from weeks up to 9–10 years. Since the quality of life during the first chronic phase is excellent, ideally, one would wish to maximize the duration of this phase before proceeding with transplantation. However, data from the Seattle Group suggest that patients transplanted in the first year of diagnosis do significantly better than those transplanted later in the first chronic phase [270].

The overall results in CML for transplantation from sibling donors are somewhat disappointing (Figs 22.8 & 22.9), and these data may still reflect the impact of T-cell-depleted allogeneic BMT which was used particularly in the middle years of the 1980s. For non-T-cell-depleted transplants, a figure of at least 50–60% DFS for good-risk patients transplanted early in the first chronic phase should now be achieved. Late relapse after allogeneic bone marrow transplantation for CML may still occur however [271], and vigilance is required to ensure that early intervention can be made with donor lymphocyte infusions [26,272]. Such infusions appear likely to dramatically reduce the number of second transplants performed for relapse in CML [273].

Because of the prolonged nature of the first chronic phase of CML, the time available to search for matched unrelated donors is more often adequate than for AL. Furthermore, since patients who fail to respond adequately to alpha interferon alpha (IFNα) are known to be incurable by any other means, patients in the first chronic phase of CML are excellent candidates for matched unrelated donor transplants, and for this reason CML has become the most frequent indication for unrelated donor transplantation. The results of matched unrelated donor transplants in the first chronic phase vary between

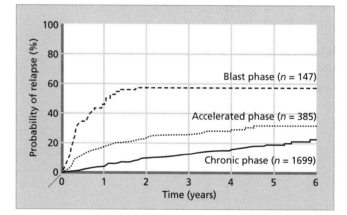

Fig. 22.9 Probability of relapse after HLA-identical sibling BMT for CML: 1987–94. Paradoxically, relapses appear to be rare after 4 years in patients transplanted with advanced-stage CML. Since these data are confined to patients transplanted after 1987, there is likely to be a continuing contribution of T-cell-depleted BMT to the relapse figures. (Data from the IBMTR and the ABMTR of North America.) *P* = 0.0001.

different studies, with DFS between 27 and 52%, depending on the age and degree of HLA matching [274,275]. The results from the NMDP [275] showed that for patients under 30 years with a full HLA match, a 43% DFS was obtained, while a single HLA locus mismatch reduced this to 31%. Older patients did less well, with 27% with a full match and only 14% with one antigen mismatch surviving long term. Overall, it appears reasonable to expect between 35 and 43% DFS at about 3 years for a full match graft, although a smaller series has shown better results [276]. Acute GVHD incidence varies widely, and although it is lower in the series that used T-cell depletion [276], there is no evidence that this translates into improved survival [275,277]. Managing accelerated-phase

CML with a MUD BMT seems a reasonable approach, because two studies have found no worse an outlook than for CP1 [276,278]. These studies also suggest that the results in blast crisis are poor.

Although significant numbers of unrelated transplants have now been carried out for CML, the number in proportion to related allogeneic BMT is still small. Because of the effect of selection, it is difficult to compare the results directly, and there is still a tendency for poorer-risk patients in younger age groups to be considered for matched unrelated donor procedures. For patients without a family donor and who are under 45 years of age, a MUD transplant may be considered the treatment of choice, despite the higher risk [279].

The monitoring of patients post-transplant with highly sensitive probes for *BCR/ABL* is proving to be most helpful. The detection of the BCR/ABL hybrid gene product by PCR [105], ideally quantitative PCR [280], post-transplant may not signify a definite relapse if present early post-BMT, but if present at more than 1 year afterwards, or with evidence of increasing gene copies (using quantitative PCR) or cytogenetic detection, then intervention is necessary or clinical relapse is inevitable. The use of donor lymphocyte infusions to treat relapse is discussed later in this chapter.

The recent use of high-dose IFNα early in the disease leads to a reduction in the Ph chromosome metaphases in a significant proportion of CML patients [281]. However, although all patient groups in the recent MRC Trial [282] had improved survival with IFNα rather than hydroxyurea, it appears now that only those patients who achieve a substantial reduction or complete loss of Ph chromosomes actually enjoy a prolonged survival. Therefore it would seem appropriate for patients having such a cytogenetic response to delay transplantation until cytogenetic relapse or resistance occur. For the majority of patients who are either unable to tolerate IFNα or who do not respond to it, then allogeneic BMT offers the only prospect of cure, although it may be some years before the survival benefit of allogeneic BMT outweighs the procedural risk [283].

In the past few years autografting has been used increasingly in CML [284–286]. Although this approach appears to be a useful and less hazardous alternative to unrelated donor BMT for some patients, it is unlikely to lead to a cure. Autografting for CML is discussed in more detail in Chapter 23.

Lymphomas

Conventional chemotherapy for non-Hodgkin's and Hodgkin's lymphomas is satisfactory for most histological subtypes and, therefore, it is only rarely that patients are considered for allogeneic BMT [287,288]. Most patients considered for allogeneic BMT have high-grade non-Hodgkin's lymphomas with involvement of blood or marrow at diagnosis and with a morphology and phenotype similar to ALL. Lymphomas in which the bone marrow is spared are usually amenable to treatment with high-dose chemo/radiotherapy and autologous marrow rescue.

For this reason, patients in whom BMT for lymphoma is considered should be referred to a centre with substantial experience in high-dose consolidation treatments, so that the appropriate decision between autologous and allogeneic BMT can be made. Relatively few data are available to enable comparison between allogeneic and autologous grafting for lymphoma. The effects of time censoring, stage of disease, effect of purging/CD34 selection and different histologies make an individual decision at an experienced centre essential.

Myeloma

Multiple myeloma is an incurable disease with a poor prognosis. Most patients are elderly, and so data on allogeneic BMT is limited in terms of the numbers of patients. Most patients thus treated will be young and fit, and all usually have normal renal function, and this group has a relatively good prognosis with conventional therapy [289]. However, dissatisfaction with the certainty of eventual progression and death with either conventional melphalan and prednisone or other combination chemotherapy has lead to a number of studies using intensification. For allogeneic BMT patients up to 55 years with good performance status, who have active disease, would be considered. Ideally allogeneic transplantation should be performed as part of a planned approach to initial therapy, and not at the relapse or resistant stage. What sort of results can be expected in this group? It has to be acknowledged that because of procedural mortality rates, which tend to be high in multiple myeloma [290], the 5-year survival postallograft may be no better than that seen in autografts or even with conventional therapy. Allogeneic BMT is potentially curative, however, and improved long-term survivals seem to be better, with about 30% of patients alive beyond 7 years [291]. Different subtypes have different outlooks, with patients with IgA myeloma, low beta-2-microglobulin levels and GVH grades 0–II doing better. Recent results, suggesting that autologous transplantation for multiple myeloma is superior to conventional therapy in younger patients [292], may encourage greater use of allogeneic BMT for this disease. Experience with unrelated donors remains anecdotal.

Myelodysplasia and myelofibrosis

Most of these patients are too old for consideration of allogeneic BMT. However, the younger patients may well be best treated in this way, and an increasing number of protocols use intensive AML-type therapy followed by BMT.

Myelodysplastic syndrome

This is a heterogeneous group of disorders of uncertain aetiology. The severity of the condition can be determined depending on the severity of pancytopenia and the presence or absence of blast cells in blood and bone marrow. These prognostic indicators have been summarized in the Bournemouth Score [293]; this enables the prediction of survival with conventional management, which may vary between 10 months and 10 years. The various classifications of myelodysplasia have been summarized by the FAB Classification, which is based principally on morphological rather than functional grounds [294]. Acute transformation is relatively uncommon, and there is usually time in which to plan transplantation. Because of the intrinsic defect in the bone marrow, autologous procedures are problematical, although recently these have been attempted following initial chemotherapy [295]. Existing myelodysplasia is known to lead to a poor outlook following conventional chemotherapy, however, and the risk is that some patients may not regenerate after intensive AML-type treatment. However, allogeneic BMT may be more successful, particularly in patients who have more advanced myelodysplasia (refractory anaemia with excess blasts (RAEB), or RAEB in transformation (RAEB-t)), if cytoreduction of blast cell numbers is attempted beforehand. BMT is also best carried out before multiple transfusions lead to iron overload, hepatitis C and other virus infections. Patients with pancytopenia and increasing numbers of blast cells in blood or bone marrow should be candidates for early BMT, however. Although extensive series are not available, the results would be expected to be similar to those for allogeneic BMT in early relapse of AML. The results have been reviewed recently in relation to pretreatment variables [296] and other factors relevant to outcome [297]. In this later study, Sutton *et al.* obtained a 32% event-free survival at 7 years for *de novo* myelodysplastic syndromes. The median age was 37 years and the transplant mortality high at 39%. Unrelated donor BMT may also be contemplated for selected patients [298]. For a full discussion of myelodysplastic syndromes and secondary leukaemias see Chapters 11 and 12.

Myelofibrosis

There are few data on allogeneic BMT in this disorder [299]. Conditioning with TBI is known to reverse myelofibrosis in patients with CML [300] and is worthwhile for young patients. It should be considered early in the course of the disease, before the spleen size becomes unmanageable.

Nonmalignant disorders

Allogeneic BMT for acquired nonmalignant disorders such as SAA has been undertaken for many years and is well established (Fig. 22.10) [15,16,31]. Transplantation for inherited disorders of the bone marrow is carried out regularly for thalassaemia [72] and less frequently for sickle cell disease [301]. In both of these disorders the benefits of transplantation are relative and the subject of controversy. Other rare disorders,

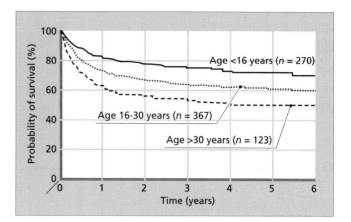

Fig. 22.10 Probability of survival after HLA-identical sibling BMT for aplastic anaemia: 1987–94. The results of BMT for aplastic anaemia are highly dependent on the age of the patient. Patients with very severe aplastic anaemia are likely to benefit from BMT, even in the older age groups, in which 50% will survive 6 years. (Data from the IBMTR and the ABMTR of North America.) *P* = 0.0001.

such as severe combined immunodeficiency and metabolic disorders [302,303], have also been successfully transplanted from family and unrelated donors (see ref. [304] for a review).

Patient selection

The results of allogeneic BMT must be interpreted cautiously because of the problem of patient selection. For example, there may be selective referral of only the youngest and fittest patients to the BMT centre or, conversely, only those with an especially poor outlook may progress through the screening system in local hospitals. Recent randomized studies such as the 10th, and now the 12th (AML 12), UK MRC AML Trial are addressing this problem.

Time censoring is also a particular problem in analysing BMT data. Patients may be referred for allogeneic BMT 6 months into remission, during which time other patients may have already relapsed. Therefore, by the time transplants are carried out 9–12 months into first remission, a significant proportion of such patients may already be cured or are likely to be long-term disease-free survivors. Only by following cohorts of patients from diagnosis to relapse or death can the true impact of BMT, whether autologous or allogeneic, be assessed.

Age and marrow transplantation

In addition to the primary indication for BMT, the fitness of the patient to undergo such a demanding and hazardous procedure must be considered. Age is a significant limiting factor for allogeneic BMT. Patients over 20 years do less well, but transplants can be negotiated successfully well beyond 45 years of age [305,306]. Depending on the indication, patients may be considered for allogeneic BMT up to the age of 55 years. The use of PBSC in allogeneic BMT [1,59] has speeded up engraftment and encouraged the move towards offering allografts to older patients.

The age and sex of the donor may also have a significant bearing on the outcome of the transplant, and female donors who have had children appear to cause more GVHD [307], presumably because of the stimulation of the immune system by the HLA haplotype not shared by the mother.

Relapse after allogeneic bone marrow transplantation

The management of relapse after allogeneic BMT is one area in which great advances are being made. Why do patients relapse after allografting, and when can they be reassured that the risk of relapse is past [308]? Clearly, residual disease has survived the conditioning, but relapses are not confined to patients who are transplanted in advanced states of leukaemia, although it is more common in that situation. The recognition that CML patients transplanted with T-cell-depleted grafts had a very high relapse rate [21,22] was an early clue to the importance of immune surveillance in the cure of residual leukaemia after allogeneic BMT [3,309]. It was found intriguing that such an effect is seen much less in acute leukaemia, suggesting that mechanisms of cure owe more to the conditioning in acute leukaemia than in CML. The awareness of the importance of immune competent cells to continued remission of CML postallogeneic BMT lead to preliminary studies in which patients relapsing after allogeneic BMT received infusions of peripheral blood cells from the original donor. Such infusions (donor lymphocyte infusions, (DLI)) were found to induce clinical, cytogenetic and molecular remissions [2]. The complications in the original series were major however, particularly as a result of graft failure and the induction of severe GVHD. Graft failure was a particular problem if the DLI were given when the patient was in clinical relapse. Further work by Mackinnon *et al.* [26] has shown that there is a dose–response curve for the number of lymphocytes infused, and that by treating patients in early relapse (molecular or cytogenetic) with a known dose of T cells, cytogenetic and molecular remission of CML can be reinduced in the absence of significant GVHD or graft failure.

The antitumour effect of DLI has been confirmed in a few patients with myeloma relapsing after allografts [27], and it seems likely that such developments will be extended to other disorders in the near future. The dissection of the GVL effect into its constituent components is also a high priority for research in the next few years, and it seems likely that, eventually, the precise dose of T cells, and their specific phenotype, will be defined. Clearly, the ideal situation would be to develop a 'vaccine' approach where a specific tumour antigen might be targeted by a population of T cells specifically stimulated to attack them. Such an approach is actively being sought, and preliminary data suggests that it should be effective [310].

Prevention of relapse

At present, however, the best way to prevent relapse after allogeneic BMT is to transplant the patients in the first remission of acute leukaemia or in the first stable chronic phase of CML, using a regimen which does not include T-cell depletion. The use of methotrexate to prevent GVHD has an intrinsic antileukaemic effect [311], whereas high-dose cyclosporin appears to have an increased relapse risk [24]. The body of evidence suggests that the more vigorously and effectively GVHD is prevented, then the higher will be the rate of relapse [312]. Inducing GVHD after autologous BMT has been used in an attempt to reduce recurrent leukaemia rates [313]. The possibility that some form of maintenance therapy, whether chemotherapy [314] or cytokines [315], might prevent relapse has not been fully tested in controlled trials.

Management of relapse

If patients with acute leukaemia relapse more than 1 year after BMT, reinduction of remission of the primary disease is often successful [316]. However, early relapses are likely to be resistant to further therapy, particularly if the patient was transplanted in an early relapse or in a second or subsequent remission. Second transplants have a high mortality and morbidity and should be reserved for selected patients only, those who had at least 1 year's remission prior to relapse, and who have no adverse features to suggest that toxicity related to the conditioning will be particularly severe [317]. The detailed options for therapy have been reviewed recently [318,319].

Second malignancies

Over the past decade, attention has been focused on some of the late complications of BMT that can affect long-term survivors. It is clear that the risk of a second neoplasm is considerable [320], such that patients should be advised of the risk before the transplant. How much contribution the transplant makes, rather than the underlying disease or prior chemotherapy, is not clear. For instance, it is known that patients with aplastic anaemia treated with immunotherapy rather than BMT have a higher risk for second malignancy, so the degree of immune suppression may be important. This is certainly true in EBV-associated B-cell lymphoproliferative disorders occurring after BMT [37,321].

In a recent report, Bhatia *et al.* [35] studied over 2000 transplant survivors, of whom 51 developed a malignancy against an expected number of 4.3. The actuarial risk was 9.9% at 13 years post-transplant.

EBV-associated lymphomas may respond to infusions of donor lymphocytes [322], which in a novel gene-marking experiment gave responses that were confirmed to be due to the infused cells [323].

Support for patients and staff

Patients who are being considered for BMT will require advice, information and counselling in order to assist them in making the decision whether to proceed. There should be sufficient time for the advice and counselling to take place, within the limits imposed by the underlying disorder. Patients should be fully informed of the risks and benefits of marrow transplantation and give their written consent to the transplant [324]. A combination of written information and structured interviews is an appropriate way of ensuring that all patients receive comprehensive advice. Information by video also has the benefit of not requiring high literacy skills. The Internet provides a rich source of information about BMT, although not all is presented in an impartial way. Over the next few years it is likely that many patients will be arriving at BMT units armed with such information.

During the transplant, support should continue to be available, because most patients are highly anxious as they undergo this life-threatening procedure [325]. Support may come from the physicians, nurses and counselling staff, who may be either social workers or lay counsellors, and for those severely disturbed people clinical psychology or even psychiatric support may be appropriate. There is value in patients having access to a counsellor who is seen to be independent of the clinical care team.

Continuing care of the patient after BMT should not be confined to physical problems. Long-term psychological morbidity can occur [325] and suicide may be a risk [326]. Evidence is beginning to accumulate about the incidence and severity of sexual dysfunction after BMT. This appears to be worse after allogeneic BMT if patients have continuing GVHD, but any form of transplant seems to induce more morbidity in this group of patients than in patients who receive intensive chemotherapy only [327].

Whereas allogeneic BMT may be carried out at specialized units many miles from the patient's home, the care of the relapsed patient is best carried out near to their home.

Staff support should not be overlooked in any marrow transplant programme. Nursing staff are required to spend many hours with individual patients with whom they will develop mutually supportive relationships. Staff working on marrow transplant units have major vested interests in the success of their procedures and will suffer when these treatments fail. It is important that staff support systems are available, both for the group as a whole and also, if necessary, for individual counselling.

Conclusion

Allogeneic BMT has a major place in the management of CML, and is the only reliable hope for cure in patients in second complete remission of acute leukaemia. The improved results of conventional intensive therapy of AML mean that good-risk

patients may wish to defer BMT until early relapse or second remission. Randomized trials, such as the UK MRC AML 12th Study, appear fully justified in attempting to randomize for allogeneic as well as autologous BMT. Adults with ALL have a poor outlook, and all but the best prognostic groups should be offered allogeneic BMT in first remission. Other groups, such as those with myelodysplastic syndromes, multiple myeloma and other lymphoid neoplasms, should be considered for allogeneic BMT within the context of study protocols in which data collection will allow an assessment of value.

BMT remains, however, a hazardous and expensive procedure [328] that is extremely demanding on the patient and their family and of medical, nursing and ancillary staff resources. Improvements in engraftment seen with PBSC allografts will, hopefully, translate into improved DFS. Unrelated donor transplants are now an established part of the therapy for selected patients with leukaemia, and the introduction of umbilical cord blood cells to replace adult marrow will ensure that allogeneic BMT will be producing interesting information in the very near future. Techniques utilizing adoptive immunotherapy to prevent, or treat early, relapse will also be fully tested, and seem set to transform the outlook after both allogeneic and autologous BMT over the next decade. Above all, the need to maintain support for long-term survivors [329] over many years, in order to maximize their quality of life [330,331] and minimize serious complications, will become more and more important over the next decade.

References

1 Goldman J.M. (1995) Peripheral blood stem cells for allografting. *Blood*, **85**, 1413–1416.
2 Porter D.L., Roth M.S., McGarigle C., Ferrara J.L. & Antin J.H. (1994) Induction of graft-versus-host disease as immunotherapy for relapsed chronic myeloid leukaemia. *New England Journal of Medicine*, **330**, 100–106.
3 Antin J.H. (1993) Graft-versus-leukaemia: no longer an epiphenomenon. *Blood*, **82**, 2273–2277.
4 Santos G.W. (1987) History of bone marrow transplantation. *Clinics in Haematology*, **12**, 611–639.
5 Gale R.P. & Reisner Y. (1988) The role of bone marrow-transplants after nuclear accidents. *Lancet*, **i**, 923–926.
6 Thomas E.D., Lochte H.L. Jr, Lu W.D. *et al.* (1957) Intravenous infusion of bone marrow in patients receiving radiation and chemotherapy. *New England Journal of Medicine*, **257**, 491–496.
7 Lorenz E., Uphoff D., Reid T.R. *et al.* (1951) Modification of irradiation injury in mice and guinea pigs by bone marrow injections. *Journal of the National Cancer Institute*, **12**, 197–201.
8 Thomas E.D., Buckner C.D., Rudolph R.H. *et al.* (1971) Allogeneic marrow grafting for hematologic malignancy using HL-A matched donor-recipient sibling pairs. *Blood*, **38**, 267–287.
9 Thomas E.D., Storb R., Clift R.A. *et al.* (1975) Bone marrow transplantation. *New England Journal of Medicine*, **292**, 832–843, 895–902.
10 Powles R.L., Clink H.M., Spence D. *et al.* (1980) Cyclosporin A to prevent graft-versus-host disease. *Lancet*, **i**, 327–329.
11 Biggs J.C., Atkinson K., Hayes J. *et al.* (1982) After allogeneic

bone marrow transplantation, cyclosporin A is associated with faster engraftment, less mucositis and three distinct syndromes of nephrotoxicity when compared to methotrexate. *Transplantation Proceedings*, **15**, 1487–1489.

12 Irle C., Deeg H.J., Buckner C.D. *et al.* (1985) Marrow transplantation for leukemia following fractionated total body irradiation. A comparative trial of methotrexate and cyclosporine. *Leukemia Research*, **9**, 1255–1261.

13 Storb R., Deeg H.J., Whitehead J. *et al.* (1986) Methotrexate and cyclosporine compared with cyclosporine alone for prophylaxis of acute graft versus host disease after marrow transplantation for leukaemia. *New England Journal of Medicine*, **314**, 728–735.

14 Storb R., Deeg H.J., Pepe M. *et al.* (1989) Methotrexate and cyclosporine versus cyclosporine alone for prophylaxis of graft-versus-host disease in patients given HLA-marrow grafts for leukemia: long-term follow-up of a controlled trial. *Blood*, **6**, 1729–1734.

15 Storb R., Thomas E.D., Buckner C.D. *et al.* (1982) Marrow transplantation with or without donor buffy coat cells for 65 transfused aplastic anemia patients. *Blood*, **59**, 236–246.

16 Champlin R.E., Horowitz M.M., van Bekkum D.W. *et al.* (1989) Graft failure following bone marrow transplantation for severe aplastic anemia: risk factors and treatment results. *Blood*, **73**, 606–613.

17 Korngold R. & Sprent J. (1978) Lethal graft-versus-host disease after bone marrow transplantation across minor histocompatibility barriers in mice. Prevention by removing mature T cells from marrow. *Journal of Experimental Medicine*, **148**, 1687–1698.

18 Reisner Y., Kapoor N., Kirkpatrick D. *et al.* (1981) Transplantation for acute leukaemia with HLA-A and B non-identical parental marrow cells fractionated with soy-bean agglutinin and sheep red blood cells. *Lancet*, **ii**, 327–331.

19 Martin P.J., Hansen J.A., Storb R. *et al.* (1985) A clinical trial of *in vitro* depletion of T cells in donor marrow for prevention of graft-versus-host disease (GVHD). *Transplantation Proceedings*, **17**, 486–488.

20 Reinherz E., Geha R., Rappeport J.M. *et al.* (1982) Reconstitution after transplantation with T-lymphocyte depleted HLA haplotype-mismatched bone marrow for severe combined immunodeficiency. *Proceedings of the National Academy of Sciences, USA*, **79**, 6047–6051.

21 Goldman J.M., Gale R.P., Horowitz M.M. *et al.* (1988) Bone marrow transplantation for chronic myelogenous leukemia in chronic phase. Increased risk of relapse associated with T-cell depletion. *Annals of Internal Medicine*, **108**, 806–814.

22 Apperley J.F., Mauro F., Goldman J.M. *et al.* (1988) Bone marrow transplantation for chronic myeloid leukaemia in chronic phase: importance of a graft-versus-leukaemia effect. *British Journal of Haematology*, **69**, 239–245.

23 Slavin S., Ackerstein A., Naparstek E. *et al.* (1990) The graft-versus-leukemia (GVL) phenomenon: is GVL separable from GVHD. *Bone Marrow Transplantation*, **6**, 155–161.

24 Bacigalupo A., van Lint M.T., Occhini D. *et al.* (1991) Increased risk of leukemic relapse with high-dose cyclosporine A after allogeneic marrow transplantation for acute leukemia. *Blood*, **77**, 1423–1428.

25 Aschan J., Ringden O., Sundberg B. *et al.* (1991) Methotrexate combined with cyclosporin A decreases graft-versus-host disease, but increases leukemic relapse compared to monotherapy. *Bone Marrow Transplantation*, **7**, 107–112.

26 Mackinnon S., Papadopoulos E.B., Carabasi M.H. *et al.* (1995) Adoptive immunotherapy evaluating escalating doses of donor leucocytes for relapsed chronic myeloid leukaemia after allogeneic bone marrow transplantation—separation of graft-versus-host leukaemia responses from graft-versus-host disease. *Blood*, **86**, 1261–1268.

27 Tricot G., Vesole D.H. Jagannath S. *et al.* (1996) Graft versus myeloma effect—proof of principle. *Blood*, **87**, 1196–1198.

28 Bensinger W.I., Weaver C.H., Appelbaum F.R. *et al.* (1995) Transplantation of allogeneic peripheral blood stem cells mobilized by recombinant human granulocyte colony-stimulating factor. *Blood*, **85**, 1655–1658.

29 Schmitz N., Dreger P., Suttorp M. *et al.* (1995) Primary transplantation of allogeneic peripheral blood progenitor cells mobilized by filgrastim (granulocyte colony-stimulating-factor). *Blood*, **85**, 1666–1672.

30 Storek J., Gooley T., Siadak M. *et al.* (1997) Allogeneic peripheral blood stem cell transplantation may be associated with a high risk of chronic graft-versus-host disease. *Blood*, **90**, 4705–4709.

31 Hows J.M., Yin J., Marsh D. *et al.* (1986) Histocompatible unrelated volunteer donors compared with HLA non-identical family donors in marrow transplantation for aplastic anemia and leukemia. *Blood*, **68**, 1322–1328.

32 Gingrich R.D., Gonder G., Goeken N.E. *et al.* (1988) Allogeneic marrow grafting with partially mismatched, unrelated marrow donors. *Blood*, **71**, 1375–1381.

33 McCullough J., Hansen J., Perkins H. *et al.* (1989) The National Marrow Donor Program; how it works, accomplishments to date. *Oncology*, **3**, 63–72.

34 Sierra J., Storer B. & Hansen J. (1995) Unrelated donor marrow transplants for acute leukaemia. *Blood*, **86**(Suppl. 1), 1146.

35 Bhatia S., Ramsay N.K.C., Steinbuch M. *et al.* (1996) Malignant neoplasms following bone marrow transplantation. *Blood*, **87**, 3633–3639.

36 Aversa F., Tabilio A., Terenzi A. *et al.* (1994) Successful engraftment of T-cell-depleted haploidentical three-loci incompatible transplants in leukemia patients by addition of recombinant human granulocyte colony-stimulating-factor mobilized peripheral blood progenitor cells to bone marrow inoculum. *Blood*, **84**, 3948–3955.

37 Shapiro R.S., McClain K., Frizzera G. *et al.* (1988) Epstein–Barr virus associated B-cell lymphoproliferative disorders following bone marrow transplantation. *Blood*, **71**, 1234–1243.

38 Bortin M.M. & Rimm A.A. (1989) Increasing utilization of bone marrow transplantation. II Results of 1985–1987 survey. *Transplantation*, **48**, 453–458.

39 Gratwohl A., Hermans J. & Baldomero H. (1996) Hematopoietic precursor cell transplants in Europe: activity in 1994. Report from the European Group for Blood and Marrow Transplantation (EBMT). *Bone Marrow Transplantation*, **17**, 137–148.

40 Armitage J.O. (1994) Bone marrow transplantation. *New England Journal of Medicine*, **330**, 827–838.

41 Gorin N.C., Labopin M. & Fouillard C. (1995) Autologous (ABMT) versus unrelated (MUD) marrow transplantation for acute leukaemia. A retrospective survey from the European Cooperative Group for Blood and Marrow Transplantation (EBMT). *Blood*, **86**(Suppl. 1), 617 (abstract).

42 Busca A., Anasetti C., Anderson G. *et al.* (1994) Unrelated donor or autologous marrow transplantation for treatment of acute leukemia. *Blood*, **83**, 3077–3084.

43 Burnett A.K., Goldstone A. & Stevens R.F. (1994) The role of

BMT in addition to intensive chemotherapy in AML in first CR: the results of the AML X trial. *Blood*, **84**(Suppl. 1), 252 (abstract).

44 Bloomfield C.D., Lawrence D., Arthur D.C. *et al.* (1994) Curative impact of intensification with high-dose cytarabine (HiDAC) in acute myeloid leukaemia (AML) varies by cytogenetic group. *Blood*, **84**(Suppl. 1), 111 (abstract).

45 Schmitz N., Gratwohl A., Goldman J.M. for the Accreditation Sub-committee of the European Group for Blood and Marrow Transplantation (EBMT) (1996) Allogeneic (allo) and autologous (auto) transplantation for haematological diseases, solid tumours and immune disorders—current practice in Europe in 1996 and proposals for an operational classification. *Bone Marrow Transplantation*. (In press.)

46 Rowe J.M., Ciobanu N., Ascensao J. *et al.* (1994) Recommended guidelines for the management of autologous and allogeneic bone marrow transplantation. *Annals of Internal Medicine*, **120**, 143–158.

47 Bensinger W.I. (1992) Supportive care in marrow transplantation. *Current Opinion in Oncology*, **4**, 614–623.

48 British Committee for Standards in Haematology Clinical Haematology Task Force (1995) Guidelines on the provision of facilities for the care of adult patients with haematological malignancies (including leukaemia and lymphoma and severe bone marrow failure). *Clinical and Laboratory Haematology*, **17**, 3–10.

49 Petersen F.B., Clift R.A., Hickman R.O. *et al.* (1986) Hickman catheter complications in marrow transplant recipients. *Journal of Parenteral and Enteral Nutrition*, **10**, 58–62.

50 Haire W.D., Lieberman R.P., Lund G.B. *et al.* (1991) Thrombotic complications of silicone rubber catheters during autologous marrow and peripheral stem cell transplantation: prospective comparison of Hickman and Groshong catheters. *Bone Marrow Transplantation*, **7**, 57–59.

51 Bortin M.M., Ringden O., Horowitz M.M. *et al.* (1989) Temporal relationship between the major complications of bone marrow transplantation for leukemia. *Bone Marrow Transplantation*, **4**, 339–344.

52 Buckner C.D., Clift R.A., Sanders J.E. *et al.* (1984) Marrow harvesting from normal donors. *Blood*, **64**, 630–634.

53 Bortin M.M. & Buckner C.D. (1983) Major complications of marrow harvesting for transplantation. *Experimental Hematology*, **11**, 916–921.

54 Bacigalupo A., Tong J., Podesta M. *et al.* (1992) Bone marrow harvest for marrow transplantation: effect of multiple small (2 ml) or large (20 ml) aspirates. *Bone Marrow Transplantation*, **9**, 467–470.

55 Jones R. & Burnett A.K. (1992) How to harvest bone marrow for transplantation. *Journal of Clinical Pathology*, **45**, 1053–1057.

56 Thorne A.C., Stewart M. & Gulati S.C. (1993) Harvesting bone marrow in an outpatient setting using newer anesthetic agents. *Journal of Clinical Oncology*, **11**, 320–323.

57 Abrahams C. & Catchatourian R. (1983) Bone fragment emboli in the lungs of patients undergoing bone marrow transplantation. *American Journal of Clinical Pathology*, **79**, 360–363.

58 Russell N.H., Hunter A., Rogers S. *et al.* (1993) Peripheral blood stem cells as an alternative to marrow for allogeneic transplantation (letter). *Lancet*, **341**, 1482.

59 Russell N.H., Gratwohl A. & Schmitz N. (1996) The place of blood stem cells in allogeneic transplantation. *British Journal of Haematology*, **93**, 747–753.

60 Silberstein L.E. & Jefferies L.C. (1996) Placental-blood banking—a new frontier in transfusion medicine. *New England Journal of Medicine*, **335**, 199–201.

61 Laporte J-P., Gorin N-C. & Rubinstein P. (1996) Cord-blood transplantation from an unrelated donor in an adult with chronic myelogenous leukaemia. *New England Journal of Medicine*, **335**, 167–170.

62 Wagner J.E., Kernan N.A., Broxmeyer H.E. & Gluckman E. (1994) Transplantation of umbilical cord blood in 50 patients: analysis of the Registry data. *Blood*, **84**, 395a.

63 Kurtzberg J., Laughlin M., Graham M.L. *et al.* (1996) Placental blood as a source of hematopoietic stem cells for transplantation into unrelated recipients. *New England Journal of Medicine*, **335**, 157–166.

64 Thomas E.D., Buckner C.D., Banaji M. *et al.* (1977) One hundred patients with acute leukemia treated by chemotherapy, total body irradiation, and allogeneic marrow transplantation. *Blood*, **49**, 511–533.

65 Thomas E.D., Storb R. & Buckner C.D. (1976) Total body irradiation in preparation for marrow engraftment. *Transplantation Proceedings*, **8**, 591–593.

66 Thomas E.D., Clift R.A., Hersman J. *et al.* (1982) Marrow transplantation for acute nonlymphoblastic leukemia in first remission using fractionated or single-dose irradiation. *International Journal of Radiation Oncology and Biological Physics*, **8**, 817–821.

67 Brochstein J.A., Kernan N.A., Groshen S. *et al.* (1987) Allogeneic Bone Marrow Transplantation after hyperfractionated total-body irradiation and cyclophosphamide in children with acute leukemia. *New England Journal of Medicine*, **317**, 1618–1624.

68 Bortin M.M., Kay H.E.M., Gale R.P. *et al.* (1982) Factors associated with interstitial pneumonitis after bone marrow transplantation for acute leukemia. *Lancet*, **i**, 437–439.

69 Ehrlich R.M., Freedman A., Goldsobel A.B. *et al.* (1984) The use of sodium 2-mercaptoethane to prevent cyclophosphamide cystitis. *Journal of Urology*, **131**, 960–962.

70 Biggs J.C., Szer J., Crilley P. *et al.* (1992) Treatment of chronic myeloid leukaemia with allogeneic bone marrow transplantation after preparation with BuCy2. *Blood*, **80**, 1352–1357.

71 Clift R.A., Buckner C.D., Thomas E.D. *et al.* (1994) Marrow transplantation for chronic myeloid leukaemia: a randomised study comparing cyclophosphamide and total body irradiation with busulfan and cyclophosphamide. *Blood*, **84**, 2036–2043.

72 Lucarelli G., Galimberti M., Polchi P. *et al.* (1990) Bone marrow transplantation in patients with thalassemia. *New England Journal of Medicine*, **322**, 417–421.

73 Morgan M., Dodds A., Atkinson K. *et al.* (1991) The toxicity of busulphan and cyclophosphamide as the preparative regimen for bone marrow transplantation. *British Journal of Haematology*, **77**, 529–534.

74 Bearman S.I. (1995) The syndrome of hepatic veno-occlusive disease after marrow transplantation. *Blood*, **85**, 3005–3020.

75 Powles R.L., Milliken S. & Helenglass G. (1989) The use of melphalan in conjunction with total body irradiation as treatment for acute leukaemia. *Transplantation Proceedings*, **21**, 2955–2957.

76 Blume K.G., Forman S.J., O'Donnell M.R. *et al.* (1987) Total body irradiation and high-dose etoposide: a new preparatory regime for bone marrow transplantation in patients with advanced hematologic malignancies. *Blood*, **69**, 1015–1020.

77 Bostrom B., Weisdorf D.J., Kim T. *et al.* (1990) Bone marrow transplantation for advanced acute leukemia: a pilot study of high energy total body irradiation, cyclophosphamide and continuous infusion etoposide. *Bone Marrow Transplantation*, **5**, 83–89.

78 Demirer T., Weaver C.H., Buckner C.D. *et al.* (1995) High-dose cyclophosphamide, carmustine, and etoposide followed by allo-

geneic bone marrow transplantation in patients with lymphoid malignancies who had received prior dose-limiting radiation therapy. *Journal of Clinical Oncology*, **13**, 596–602.

79 Brown R.A., Wolff S.N., Fay J.W. *et al.* (1995) High-dose etoposide, cyclophosphamide, and total body irradiation with allogeneic bone marrow transplantation for patients with acute myeloid leukaemia in untreated first relapse: a study by the North American Marrow Transplant Group. *Blood*, **85**, 1391–1395.

80 Kantarjian H.M., Talpaz M., Andersson B. *et al.* (1994) High doses of cyclophosphamide, etoposide and total body irradiation followed by autologous stem cell transplantation in the management of patients with chronic myelogenous leukaemia. *Bone Marrow Transplantation*, **14**, 57–61.

81 Przepiorka D., Ippoliti C., Giralt S. *et al.* (1994) A phase I–II study of high-dose thiotepa, busulfan and cyclophosphamide as a preparative regimen for allogeneic marrow transplantation. *Bone Marrow Transplantation*, **14**, 449–453.

82 UCLA Bone Marrow Transplantation Group (1997) Bone marrow transplantation with intensive combination chemotherapy/radiation therapy (SCARI) in acute leukemia. *Annals of Internal Medicine*, **86**, 155–161.

83 Woods W.G., Ramsay N.K.C., Weisdorf D.J. *et al.* (1990) Bone marrow transplantation for acute lymphoblastic leukaemia utilizing total body irradiation followed by high doses of cytosine arabinoside: lack of superiority over cyclophosphamide containing regimes. *Bone Marrow Transplantation*, **6**, 9–16.

84 Aurer I. & Gale R.P. (1991) Are new conditioning regimens for transplants in acute myelogenous leukemia better? *Bone Marrow Transplantation*, **7**, 255–261.

85 Bandini G., Belardinelli A., Rosti G. *et al.* (1994) Toxicity of high-dose busulphan and cyclophosphamide as conditioning therapy for allogeneic bone marrow transplantation in adults with haematological malignancies. *Bone Marrow Transplantation*, **13**, 577–581.

86 Przepiorka D., Dimopoulos M., Smith T. *et al.* (1994) Thiotepa, busulfan, and cyclophosphamide as a preparative regimen for marrow transplantation: risk factors for early regimen-related toxicity. *Annals of Hematology*, **68**, 183–188.

87 Bianco J., Nemunaitis J., Almgren J. *et al.* (1990) Pentoxifylline (PTX) diminishes regimen related toxicity (RRT) in patients undergoing bone marrow transplantation (BMT). *Blood*, **76**(Suppl. 1), 528a.

88 Clift R.A., Bianco J.A., Appelbaum F.R. *et al.* (1993) A randomized controlled trial of pentoxifylline for the prevention of regimen-related toxicities in patients undergoing allogeneic marrow transplantation. *Blood*, **82**, 2025–2030.

89 Attal M., Huguet F., Rubie H. *et al.* (1993) Prevention of regimen-related toxicities after bone marrow transplantation by pentoxifylline: a prospective randomized trial. *Blood*, **82**, 732–736.

90 Stockschlader M., Kalhs P., Peters S. *et al.* (1993) Intravenous pentoxifylline failed to prevent transplant-related toxicities in allogeneic bone marrow transplant recipients. *Bone Marrow Transplantation*, **12**, 357–362.

91 van der Jagt R.H., Pari G., McDiarmid S.A. *et al.* (1994) Effect of pentoxifylline on regimen-related toxicity in patients undergoing allogeneic or autologous bone marrow transplantation. *Bone Marrow Transplantation*, **13**, 203–207.

92 Cunningham D., Pople A., Ford H.T. *et al.* (1987) Prevention of emesis in patients receiving cytotoxic drugs by GR38032F, a selective 5HT3 receptor antagonist. *Lancet*, **i**, 1461–1462.

93 Perez E.A. (1995) Review of the preclinical pharmacology and comparative efficacy of 5-hydroxytryptamine-3 receptor antagonists for chemotherapy-induced emesis. *Journal of Clinical Oncology*, **13**, 1036–1043.

94 Labar B., Mrsic M., Pavletic Z. *et al.* (1993) Prostaglandin E2 for prophylaxis of oral mucositis following BMT. *Bone Marrow Transplantation*, **11**, 379–382.

95 Kwan-Hwa C., Chen-Hsin C., Wing-Kai C. *et al.* (1995) Effect of granulocyte macrophage colony stimulating factor on oral mucositis in head and neck cancer patients after cisplatin, fluorouracil, and leucovorin chemotherapy. *Journal of Clinical Oncology*, **13**, 2620–2628.

96 Hinterberger-Fischer M., Kier P., Kalhs P. *et al.* (1991) Fertility, pregnancies and offspring complications after bone marrow transplantation. *Bone Marrow Transplantation*, **7**, 5–9.

97 Apperley J.F. & Reddy N. (1995) Mechanism and management of treatment-related gonadal failure in recipients of high dose chemoradiotherapy. *Blood Reviews*, **9**, 93–116.

98 Giri N., Vowels M.R., Barr A.L. *et al.* (1992) Successful pregnancy after total body irradiation and bone marrow transplantation for acute leukaemia. *Bone Marrow Transplantation*, **10**, 93–95.

99 Atkinson H.G., Apperley J.F., Dawson K. *et al.* (1994) Successful pregnancy after allogeneic bone marrow transplantation for chronic myeloid leukaemia. *Lancet*, **344**, 199 (letter).

100 Pakkala S., Lukka M., Helminen P. *et al.* (1994) Paternity after bone marrow transplantation following conditioning with total body irradiation. *Bone Marrow Transplantation*, **13**, 489–490.

101 Sanders J.E., Pritchard S., Mahoney P. *et al.* (1986) Growth and development following marrow transplantation for leukemia. *Blood*, **68**, 1129–1135.

102 Urban C., Schwingshandl J., Slavc I. *et al.* (1988) Endocrine function after bone marrow transplantation without the use of preparative total body irradiation. *Bone Marrow Transplantation*, **3**, 291–296.

103 Hershman J.M., Eriksen E., Kaufman N. *et al.* (1990) Thyroid function tests in patients undergoing bone marrow transplantation. *Bone Marrow Transplantation*, **6**, 49–52

104 Ugozzoli L., Yam P., Petz G.B. *et al.* (1991) Amplification by the polymerase chain reaction of hypervariable regions of the human genome for evaluation of chimerism after bone marrow transplantation. *Blood*, **77**, 1607–1615.

105 Lin F., van Rhee F., Goldman J.M. & Cross N.C.P. (1996) Kinetics of increasing BCR-ABL transcript numbers in chronic myeloid leukaemia patients who relapse after bone marrow transplantation. *Blood*, **87**, 4473–4478.

106 McDonald G.B., Sharma P., Matthews *et al.* (1985) The clinical course of 53 patients with venocclusive disease of the liver after marrow transplantation. *Transplantation*, **39**, 603–608.

107 McDonald G.B., Hinds M.S., Fisher L.D. *et al.* (1993) Veno-occlusive disease of the liver and multi-organ failure after bone marrow transplantation: a cohort study of 355 patients. *Annals of Internal Medicine*, **118**, 255–267.

108 Bearman S.I., Hinds M.S., Wolford J.L. *et al.* (1990) A pilot study of continuous infusion heparin for the prevention of hepatic veno-occlusive disease after bone marrow transplantation. *Bone Marrow Transplantation*, **5**, 407–411.

109 Attal M., Huguet F., Rubie H. *et al.* (1992) Prevention of hepatic veno-occlusive disease after bone marrow transplantation by continuous infusion of low dose heparin; a prospective, randomised trial. *Blood*, **79**, 2149–2150.

110 Ringden O., Wennberg L., Ericzon B-G. *et al.* (1992) Alteplase for hepatic veno-occlusive disease after bone marrow transplantation. *Lancet*, **340**, 546–547 (letter).

111 Baglin T.P., Harper P. & Marcus R.E. (1990) Veno-occlusive

disease of the liver complicating ABMT successfully treated with recombinant tissue plasminogen activator (rt-PA). *Bone Marrow Transplantation*, **5**, 439–441.

112 Reed E.C., Myerson D., Corey L. *et al.* (1991) Allogeneic marrow transplantation in patients positive for hepatitis B surface antigen. *Blood*, **77**, 195–200.

113 Kolho E., Ruutu P. & Ruutu T. (1993) Hepatitis C infection in BMT patients. *Bone Marrow Transplantation*, **11**, 119–123.

114 Brink N.S., Chopra R., Perrons C.J. *et al.* (1993) Acute hepatitis C infection in patients undergoing therapy for haematological malignancies: a clinical and virological study. *British Journal of Haematology*, **83**, 498–503.

115 McKay P., Murphy J., Cameron S. *et al.* (1996) Survivors after allogeneic or autologous bone marrow transplantation have markedly increased serum ferritin associated with liver dysfunction responsive to venesection. *Bone Marrow Transplantation*, **17**, 63–66.

116 Levine L.A. & Jarrard D.F. (1993) Treatment of cyclophosphamide-induced hemorrhagic cystitis with intravesical carboprost tromethamine. *Journal of Urology*, **149**, 719–723.

117 Ambinder R., Burns W., Forman M. *et al.* (1986) Hemorrhagic cystitis associated with adenovirus infection in bone marrow transplantation. *Archives of Internal Medicine*, **146**, 1400–1401.

118 Miyamura K., Takeyama K., Kojima S. *et al.* (1989) Hemorrhagic cystitis associated with urinary excretion of adenovirus type 11 following allogeneic bone marrow transplantation. *Bone Marrow Transplantation*, **4**, 533–535.

119 Deeg H.J., Flournoy N., Sullivan K.M. *et al.* (1984) Cataracts after total body irradiation and marrow transplantation — a sparing effect of dose fractionation. *International Journal of Radiation, Oncology, Biology and Physics*, **10**, 957–964.

120 Editorial (1989) Lung disease following allogeneic marrow transplantation. *Lancet*, **ii**, 1368–1369.

121 Paradis I.L., Grgurich W.F., Dummer J.S. *et al.* (1988) Rapid detection of cytomegalovirus pneumonia from lung lavage cells. *American Review of Respiratory Disease*, **138**, 697–701.

122 Miller W., Flynn P., McCullough J. *et al.* (1986) Cytomegalovirus infection after bone marrow transplantation: an association with graft-versus-host disease. *Blood*, **67**, 1162–1167.

123 Schmidt G.M., Horak D.A., Niland J.C. *et al.* (1991) A randomized, controlled trial of prophylactic ganciclovir for cytomegalovirus pulmonary infection in recipients of allogeneic bone marrow transplants. *New England Journal of Medicine*, **324**, 1005–1011.

124 Atkinson K., Downs K., Golenia M. *et al.* (1991) Prophylactic use of ganciclovir in allogenic bone marrow transplantation: absence of clinical cytomegalovirus infection. *British Journal of Haematology*, **79**, 57–62.

125 Kaplan E.B., Wodell R.A., Wilmott R.W. *et al.* (1994) Late effects of bone marrow transplantation on pulmonary function in children. *Bone Marrow Transplantation*, **14**, 613–621.

126 Kadakia M.P., Rybka W.B., Stewart J.A. *et al.* (1996) Human herpesvirus 6: infection and disease following autologous and allogeneic bone marrow transplantation. *Blood*, **87**, 5341–5354.

127 Storring R.A., Jameson B., McElwain T.J. *et al.* (1977) Oral non-absorbed antibiotics prevent infection in acute non-lymphoblastic leukaemia. *Lancet*, **ii**, 837–840.

128 Starke I.D., Donelly J.P., Catovsky D. *et al.* (1982) Cotrimoxazole alone for the prevention of bacterial infection in patients with acute leukaemia. *Lancet*, **ii**, 5–6.

129 de Pauw B.E., Donelly J.P., de Witte T. *et al.* (1990) Options and limitations of long term oral ciprofloxacin as antibacterial prophylaxis in allogeneic bone marrow transplant recipients. *Bone Marrow Transplantation*, **5**, 179–182.

130 Lew M.A., Kehoe K., Ritz J. *et al.* (1995) Ciprofloxacin versus trimethoprim/sulfamethoxazole for prophylaxis of bacterial infections in bone marrow transplant recipients: a randomized, controlled trial. *Journal of Clinical Oncology*, **13**, 239–250.

131 Sayer H.G., Longton G., Bowden R. *et al.* (1994) Increased risk of infection in marrow transplant patients receiving methylprednisolone for graft-versus-host disease prevention. *Blood*, **84**, 1328–1332.

132 Goodman J.L., Winston D.J., Greenfield R.A. *et al.* (1992) A controlled trial of fluconazole to prevent fungal infections in patients undergoing bone marrow transplantation. *New England Journal of Medicine*, **326**, 845–851.

133 Alangaden G., Chandrasekar P.H., Bailey E. *et al.* (1994) Antifungal prophylaxis with low-dose fluconazole during bone marrow transplantation. *Bone Marrow Transplantation*, **14**, 919–924.

134 Beyer J., Schwartz S., Barzen G. *et al.* (1994) Use of amphotericin B aerosols for the prevention of pulmonary aspergillosis. *Infection*, **22**, 143–148.

135 Hann I.M., Prentice H.G., Corringham R. *et al.* (1983) Acyclovir prophylaxis against herpes virus infections in severely immunocompromised patients: randomised double blind trial. *British Medical Journal*, **287**, 384–388.

136 Prentice H.G., Gluckman E., Powles R.L. *et al.* (1994) Impact of long-term acyclovir on cytomegalovirus infection and survival after allogeneic bone marrow transplantation. *Lancet*, **343**, 749–753.

137 Bowden R.A., Ayers M., Flournoy N. *et al.* (1986) Cytomegalovirus immune globulin and seronegative blood products to prevent primary cytomegalovirus infection after marrow transplantation. *New England Journal of Medicine*, **314**, 1006–1010.

138 Miller W.J., McCullough J., Balfour H.H. *et al.* (1991) Prevention of cytomegalovirus infection following bone marrow transplantation: a randomized trial of blood product screening. *Bone Marrow Transplantation*, **7**, 227–234.

139 de Graan-Hentzen Y.C.E., Gratma J.W., Mudde G.C. *et al.* (1989) Prevention of primary cytomegalovirus infection in patients with hematologic malignancies by intensive leukocyte depletion of blood products. *Transfusion*, **29**, 757–760.

140 Meyers J.D., Reed E.C., Shepp D.H. *et al.* (1988) Acyclovir for prevention of cytomegalovirus infection and disease after allogeneic bone marrow transplantation. *New England Journal of Medicine*, **318**, 70–75.

141 Reed E.C., Bowden R.A., Dandliker P.S. *et al.* (1988) Treatment of cytomegalovirus pneumonia with ganciclovir and intravenous cytomegalovirus immunoglobulin in patients with bone marrow transplants. *Annals of Internal Medicine*, **109**, 783–788.

142 Ringden O., Pihlstedt P., Volin L. *et al.* (1987) Failure to prevent cytomegalovirus infection by cytomegalovirus hyperimmune plasma: a randomized trial by the Nordic Bone Marrow Transplantation Group. Bone Marrow Transplantation, **2**, 299–305.

143 Bowden R.A. & Meyers J.D. (1990) Prophylaxis of cytomegalovirus infection. *Seminars in Hematology*, **27**(Suppl. 1), 17–21.

144 Przepiorka D., Ippoliti C., Panina A. *et al.* (1994) Ganciclovir three times per week is not adequate to prevent cytomegalovirus reactivation after T cell-depleted marrow transplantation. *Bone Marrow Transplantation*, **13**, 461–464.

145 Goodrich J.M., Mori M., Gleaves C.A. *et al.* (1993) Ganciclovir prophylaxis to prevent cytomegalovirus disease after allogeneic marrow transplantation. *Annals of Internal Medicine,* **118,** 173–178.

146 Winston D.J., Ho W.G., Bartoni K. *et al.* (1993) Ganciclovir prophylaxis of cytomegalovirus infection and disease in allogeneic bone marrow transplant recipients. Results of a placebo-controlled, double blind trial. *Annals of Internal Medicine,* **118,** 179–184.

147 Meyers J.D., Pifer L.L., Sale G.E. *et al.* (1979) Value of *Pneumocystis carinii* antibody and antigen detection for diagnosis of *Pneumocystis carinii* pneumonia after marrow transplantation. *American Review of Infectious Diseases,* **120,** 1283–1289.

148 Leoung G.S., Feigal D.W., Montgomery A.B. *et al.* (1990) Aerosolized pentamidine for prophylaxis against *Pneumocystis carinii* pneumonia. The San Francisco Community prophylaxis trial. *New England Journal of Medicine,* **323,** 769–775.

149 Przepiorka D., Selvaggi K., Rosenzweig P.Q. *et al.* (1991) Aerosolized pentamidine for prevention of pneumocystis pneumonia after allogeneic marrow transplantation. *Bone Marrow Transplantation,* **7,** 324–325.

150 Slavin M.A., Meyers J.D., Remington J.S. *et al.* (1994) *Toxoplasma gondii* infection in marrow transplant recipients: a 20 year experience. *Bone Marrow Transplantation,* **13,** 549–557.

151 Foot A.B., Garin Y.J., Ribaud P., *et al.* (1994) Prophylaxis of toxoplasma infection with pyrimethamine/sulfadoxine (Fansidar) in bone marrow transplant recipients. *Bone Marrow Transplantation,* **14,** 241–245.

152 Han C.S., Miller W., Haake R. & Weisdorf D. (1994) Varicella zoster infection after bone marrow transplantation: incidence, risk factors and complications. *Bone Marrow Transplantation,* **13,** 277–283.

153 Shields A., Hackman R., Fife K. *et al.* (1985) Adenovirus infection in patients undergoing bone marrow transplantation. *New England Journal of Medicine,* **312,** 344–347.

154 Fielding A.K. (1994) Prophylaxis against late infection following splenectomy and bone marrow transplant. *Blood Reviews,* **8,** 179–191.

155 Peterson F.B., Bowden R.A., Thornquist M. *et al.* (1987) The effect of prophylactic intravenous immune globulin on the incidence of septicemia in marrow transplant recipients. *Bone Marrow Transplantation,* **2,** 141–147.

156 Sullivan K.M., Kopecky K.J., Jocom J. *et al.* (1990) Immunomodulatory and antimicrobial efficacy of intravenous immune globulin in bone marrow transplantation. *New England Journal of Medicine,* **323,** 705–712.

157 Siadak M.F., Kopechy K. & Sullivan K.M. (1994) Reduction in transplant-related complications in patients given intravenous immunoglobulin after allogeneic marrow transplantation. *Clinical Experimental Immunology,* **97**(Suppl. 1), 53–57.

158 Guglielmo B.J., Wong-Beringer A. & Linker C.A. (1994) Immune globulin therapy in allogeneic bone marrow transplant: a critical review. *Bone Marrow Transplantation,* **13,** 499–510.

159 Marcus R.E. & Goldman J.M. (1986) Management of infection in the neutropenic patient. *British Medical Journal,* **293,** 406–408.

160 Lang E., Schmid J. & Fauser A.A. (1990) A clinical trial on efficacy and safety of teicoplanin in combination with beta-lactams and aminoglycosides in the treatment of severe sepsis of patients undergoing allogeneic/autologous bone marrow transplantation. *British Journal of Haematology,* **76,** 14–18.

161 Attal M., Schlaifer D., Rubie H. *et al.* (1991) Prevention of gram positive infections after bone marrow transplantation by systemic vancomycin. *Journal of Clinical Oncology,* **9,** 865–870.

162 Meyers J.D. & Thomas E.D. (1988) Infection complicating bone marrow transplantation. In: *Clinical Approach to Infection in the Compromised Host* (eds R.H. Rubin & L.S. Young), pp. 525–556, Plenum, New York.

163 Tollemar J., Ringden O. & Tyden G. (1990) Liposomal amphotericin B (AmBisome) treatment in solid organ and bone marrow transplant recipients. Efficacy and safety evaluation. *Clinical Transplantation,* **4,** 167–175.

164 Ringden O., Andstrom E., Remberger M. *et al.* (1994) Safety of liposomal amphotericin B (AmBisome) in 187 transplant recipients treated with cyclosporin. *Bone Marrow Transplantation,* **14**(Suppl. 5), S10–14.

165 Hiemenz J.W., Lister J., Anaisse E.J. *et al.* (1995) Emergency use amphotericin B lipid complex (ABLC) in the treatment of patients with aspergillosis: historical control comparison with amphotericin B. *Blood,* **86**(Suppl. 1), 3383.

166 Ljungman P., Duraj V. & Magnius L. (1991) Response to immunisation against polio after allogeneic marrow transplantation. *Bone Marrow Transplantation,* **7,** 89–94.

167 Ljungman P., Fridell E., Lonnqvist B. *et al.* (1989) Efficacy and safety of vaccination of transplant recipients with a live attenuated measles mumps and rubella vaccine. *Journal of Infectious Disease,* **159,** 610–615.

168 Oksanen K. & Elonen E. (1993) Impact of leucocyte-depleted blood components on the haematological recovery and prognosis of patients with acute myeloid leukaemia. *British Journal of Haematology,* **84,** 639–647.

169 Buckner C.D., Clift R.A., Sanders J.E. *et al.* (1978) ABO incompatible marrow transplants. *Transplantation,* **26,** 233–241.

170 Blacklock H.A., Gilmore M.J.M.L., Prentice H.G. *et al.* (1982) ABO-incompatible bone-marrow transplantation: removal of red blood cells from donor marrow avoiding recipient antibody depletion. *Lancet,* **ii,** 1061–1064.

171 Fearon T.C. & Luban N.L.C. (1986) Practical dosimetric aspects of blood and blood product irradiation. *Transfusion,* **26,** 457–459.

172 Moroff G., George V.M., Siegl A.M. *et al.* (1986) The influence of irradiation on stored platelets. *Transfusion,* **26,** 453–456.

173 Editorial (1989) Transfusions and graft-versus-host disease. *Lancet,* **i,** 529–530.

174 Williamson L.M. & Warwick R.M. (1995) Transfusion-associated graft versus host disease and its prevention. *Blood Reviews,* **9,** 251–261.

175 Young L.S. (1983) The role of granulocyte transfusions in treating and preventing infection. *Cancer Treatment Reports,* **67,** 109–111.

176 Bensinger W.I., Price T.H., Dale D.C. *et al.* (1993) The effects of daily recombinant human granulocyte colony-stimulating-factor administration on normal granulocyte donors. *Blood,* **81,** 1883–1888.

177 British Committee for Standards in Haematology Blood Transfusion Task Force (1992) Platelet transfusions. *Transfusion Medicine,* **2,** 311–318.

178 Hows J., Beddow K., Gordon-Smith E.C. *et al.* (1986) Donor-derived red blood cell antibodies and immune hemolysis after allogeneic bone marrow transplantation. *Blood,* **67,** 177–181.

179 Bierling P., Cordonnier C., Fromont P. *et al.* (1985) Acquired autoimmune thrombocytopenia after allogeneic bone marrow transplantation. *British Journal of Haematology,* 643–646.

180 Klumpp T.R., Caligiuri M.A., Rabinowe S.N. *et al.* (1990) Autoim-

mune pancytopenia following allogeneic bone marrow transplantation. *Bone Marrow Transplantation*, **6**, 445–447.

181 Ferrara J.L.M. & Deeg H.J. (1991) Graft-versus-host disease. *New England Journal of Medicine*, **324**, 667–674.

182 Glucksberg H., Storb R., Fefer A. *et al.* (1974) Clinical manifestations of graft-versus-host disease in human recipients of marrow from HL-A-matched sibling donors. *Transplantation*, **18**, 295–304.

183 Lazarus H.M., Coccia P.F., Herzig R.H. *et al.* (1984) Incidence of acute graft-versus-host disease with and without methotrexate prophylaxis in allogeneic bone marrow transplant patients. *Blood*, **64**, 215–220.

184 Storb R., Prentice R.L., Sullivan K.M. *et al.* (1983) Graft-versus-host disease and survival in patients with aplastic anemia treated with marrow grafts from HLA-identical siblings. *New England Journal of Medicine*, **308**, 302–307.

185 Deeg H.J. & Henslee-Downey P.J. (1990) Management of acute graft-versus-host disease. *Bone Marrow Transplantation*, **6**, 1–8.

186 Saurat J.H. (1981) Cutaneous manifestations of graft-versus-host disease. *International Journal of Dermatology*, **20**, 249–256.

187 Shulman H.M., Sharma P., Amos D. *et al.* (1988) A coded histologic study of hepatic graft-versus-host disease after human bone marrow transplantation. *Hepatology*, **8**, 463–470.

188 Shulman H.M., Sullivan K.M., Weidan P.L. *et al.* (1980) Chronic graft-versus-host disease in man. A long-term clinicopathologic study of 20 Seattle patients. *American Journal of Medicine*, **69**, 204–217.

189 Sullivan K.M., Witherspoon R.P., Storb R. *et al.* (1988) Prednisone and azathiaprine compared with prednisone and placebo for the treatment of chronic graft-versus-host disease: a prognostic influence of thrombocytopenia after allogeneic bone marrow transplantation. *Blood*, **72**, 546–554.

190 Vogelsang G.B. & Hess A.D. (1994) Graft-versus-host disease: new directions for a persistent problem. *Blood*, **84**, 2061–2067.

191 Atkinson K., Horowitz M.M., Biggs J.C. *et al.* (1988) The clinical diagnosis of graft-versus-host disease: a diversity of views amongst marrow transplant centers. *Bone Marrow Transplantation*, **3**, 5–10.

192 Sullivan K.M., Deeg H.J., Sanders J. *et al.* (1986) Hyperacute graft-versus-host disease in patients not given immunosuppression after allogeneic marrow transplantation. *Blood*, **67**, 1172–1175.

193 Powles R.L., Morgenstern G.R., Kay H.M. *et al.* (1983) Mismatched family donors for Bone-Marrow Transplantation as treatment for acute leukaemia. *Lancet*, **i**, 612–615.

194 Gale R.P., Bortin M.M., van Bekkum D.W. *et al.* (1987) Risk factors for acute graft-versus-host disease. *British Journal of Haematology*, **67**, 397–406.

195 Sviland L., Dickinson A.M., Carey P.J. *et al.* (1990) An *in vitro* predictive test for clinical graft-versus-host disease in allogeneic bone marrow transplant recipients. *Bone Marrow Transplantation*, **5**, 105–109.

196 Fussell S.T., Donnellan M., Cooley M.A. & Farrell C. (1994) Cytotoxic T lymphocyte precursor frequency does not correlate with either the incidence or severity of graft-versus-host disease after matched unrelated donor bone marrow transplantation. *Transplantation*, **57**, 673–676.

197 Bishara A., Brautbar C., Nagler A. *et al.* (1994) Prediction by a modified mixed leukocyte reaction assay of graft-versus-host disease and graft rejection after allogeneic bone marrow transplantation. *Transplantation*, **57**, 1474–1479.

198 Weisdorf D., Filipovich A., McGlave P. *et al.* (1993) Combination graft-versus-host disease prophylaxis using immunotoxin (anti-

CD5-RTA [Xomazyme-CD5]) plus methotrexate and cyclosporine or prednisone after unrelated donor marrow transplantation. *Bone Marrow Transplantation*, **12**, 531–536.

199 Phillips G.L., Nevill T.J., Spinelli J.J. *et al.* (1995) Prophylaxis for acute graft-versus-host disease following unrelated donor bone marrow transplantation. *Bone Marrow Transplantation*, **15**, 213–219.

200 Hale G. & Waldmann H. (1994) CAMPATH-1 monoclonal antibodies in bone marrow transplantation. *Journal of Hematotherapy*, **3**, 15–31.

201 Hale G. & Waldmann H. (1994) Control of graft-versus-host disease and graft rejection by T cell depletion of donor and recipient with Campath-1 antibodies. Results of matched sibling transplants for malignant diseases. *Bone Marrow Transplantation*, **13**, 597–611.

202 Ringden O., Pihlstedt P., Markling L. *et al.* (1991) Prevention of graft-versus-host disease with T cell depletion or cyclosporin and methotrexate. A randomized trial in adult leukemic marrow recipients. *Bone Marrow Transplantation*, **7**, 221–226.

203 Horowitz M.M., Gale R.P., Sondel P.M. *et al.* (1990) Graft-versus-leukemia reactions following bone marrow transplantation in humans. *Blood* **75**, 555–562.

204 Johnson B.D. & Truitt R.L. (1995) Delayed infusion of immunocompetent donor cells after bone marrow transplantation breaks graft-host tolerance and allows for persistent antileukemic reactivity without severe graft-versus-host disease. *Blood*, **85**, 3302–3312.

205 Verdonck L.F., Dekker A.W., de Gast G.C. *et al.* (1994) Allogeneic bone marrow transplantation with a fixed low number of T cells in the marrow graft. *Blood*, **83**, 3090–3096.

206 Leelasiri A., Greer J.P., Stein R.S. *et al.* (1995) Graft-versus-host-disease prophylaxis for matched unrelated donor bone marrow transplantation: comparison between cyclosporine-methotrexate and cyclosporine-methotrexate-methylprednisolone. *Bone Marrow Transplantation* **15**, 401–405.

207 Fay J.W., Nash R.A., Wingard J.R. *et al.* (1995) FK506-based immunosuppression for prevention of graft versus host disease after unrelated donor marrow transplantation. *Transplantation Proceedings*, **27**, 1374.

208 Koehler M., Hurwitz C.A., Krance R.A. *et al.* (1994) XomaZyme-CD5 immunotoxin in conjunction with partial T cell depletion for prevention of graft rejection and graft-versus-host disease after bone marrow transplantation from matched unrelated donors. *Bone Marrow Transplantation*, **13**, 571–575.

209 Przepiorka D., Ippoliti C., Koberda J. *et al.* (1994) Interleukin-2 for prevention of graft-versus-host disease after haploidentical marrow transplantation. *Transplantation*, **58**, 858–860.

210 Holler E., Kolb H.J., Mittermuller J. *et al.* (1995) Modulation of acute graft-versus-host disease after allogeneic bone marrow transplantation by tumor necrosis factor (TNF-α) released in the course of pretransplant conditioning: role of conditioning regimens and prophylactic application of a monoclonal antibody neutralizing human TNF-α (MAK 195F). *Blood*, **86**, 890–899.

211 Durie F.H., Aruffo A., Ledbetter J. *et al.* (1994) Antibody to the ligand of CD40, gp39, blocks the occurrence of the acute and chronic forms of graft-vs.-host disease. *Journal of Clinical Investigation*, **94**, 1333–1338.

212 Blaise D., Olive D., Michallet M. *et al.* (1995) Impairment of leukaemia-free survival by addition of interleukin-2-receptor. *Lancet*, **345**, 1144–1146.

213 Deeg H.J., Spitzer T.R., Cottler-Fox M. *et al.* (1991) Conditioning-related toxicity and acute graft-versus-host disease in patients given methotrexate/cyclosporine prophylaxis. *Bone Marrow Transplantation*, **7**, 193–198.

214 Essell J.H., Thompson J.M., Harman G.S. *et al.* (1992) Marked increase in veno-occlusive disease of the liver associated with methotrexate use for graft-versus-host disease prophylaxis in patients receiving busulfan/cyclophosphamide. *Blood*, **79**, 2784–2788.

215 International Bone Marrow Transplant Registry (1989) Effect of methotrexate on relapse after bone-marrow transplantation for acute lymphoblastic leukaemia. *Lancet*, **i**, 535–537.

216 Sullivan K.M., Witherspoon R.P., Storb R. *et al.* (1988) Alternating-day cyclosporin and prednisone for treatment of high-risk chronic graft-v-host disease. *Blood*, **72**, 555–561.

217 Gluckman E., Devergie A., Varin F. *et al.* (1984) Treatment of steroid resistant severe acute graft-versus-host disease with a monoclonal pan T OKT3 antibody. *Experimental Hematology*, **12**, 66–67.

218 Marmont A.M., Horowitz M.M., Gale R.P. *et al.* (1991) T-cell depletion of HLA-identical transplants in leukemia. *Blood*, **78**, 2120–2130.

219 Champlin A.E., Horowitz M.M., van Bekkum D.W. *et al.* (1989) Graft failure following bone marrow transplantation for severe aplastic anemia: risk factors and treatment results. *Blood*, **73**, 606–613.

220 Drobyski W.R., Ash R.C., Casper J.T. *et al.* (1994) Effect of T-cell depletion as graft-versus-host disease prophylaxis on engraftment, relapse, and disease free survival in unrelated marrow transplantation for chronic myelogenous leukaemia. *Blood*, **83**, 1980–1987.

221 Deeg H.J., Loughran T.P., Storb R, *et al.* (1985) Treatment of human graft-versus-host disease with anti-thymocyte globulin and cyclosporine with or without methylprednisolone. *Transplantation*, **401**, 162–166.

222 Anasetti C., Hansen J.A., Waldmann T.A. *et al.* (1994) Treatment of acute graft-versus-host disease with humanised anti-Tac: an antibody that binds to the interleukin-2 receptor. *Blood*, **84**, 1320–1327.

223 Sykes M., Harty M.W., Szot G.L. & Pearson D.A. (1994) Interleukin-2 inhibits graft-versus-host disease-promoting activity of CD4+ cells while preserving CD4– and CD-8 mediated graft-versus-leukemia effects. *Blood*, **83**, 2560–2569.

224 Kernan N.A., Byers V., Scannon P.J. *et al.* (1988) Treatment of steroid resistant graft-versus-host disease by *in vivo* administration of an anti-T-cell ricin-A-chain immunotoxin. *Journal of the American Medical Association*, **259**, 3154–3157.

225 Kennedy M.S., Deeg H.J., Storb R. *et al.* (1985) Treatment of acute graft-versus-host disease after allogeneic marrow transplantation. *American Journal of Medicine*, **78**, 978–983.

226 Sullivan K.M., Mori M., Witherspoon R. *et al.* (1990) Alternating-day cyclosporine and prednisone (csp/pred) treatment of chronic graft-versus-host disease (GVHD): predictors of survival. *Blood*, **76**(Suppl. 1), 568a.

227 Saurat J.H., Camenzind M., Helg C. *et al.* (1988) Thalidomide for graft-versus-host disease after bone marrow transplantation. *Lancet*, **ii**, 359.

228 Heney D., Norfolk D.R., Wheeldon J. *et al.* (1991) Thalidomide treatment for chronic graft-versus-host disease. *British Journal of Haematology*, **78**, 23–27.

229 Gryn J. & Crilley P. (1990) Tretinoin for the treatment of cuta-

neous graft-versus-host disease. *Bone Marrow Transplantation*, **5**, 279–280.

230 Atkinson K., Weller P., Ryman W. *et al.* (1986) PUVA therapy for drug resistant graft-versus-host disease. *Bone Marrow Transplantation*, **1**, 227–236.

231 Sieber F. (1993) Phototherapy, photochemotherapy and bone marrow transplantation. *Journal of Hematotherapy*, **2**, 43–62.

232 Siadak M. & Sullivan K.M. (1994) The management of chronic graft versus host disease. *Blood Reviews*, **8**, 154–160.

233 Storb R., Prentice R.L., Sullivan K.M. *et al.* (1983) Predictive factors in chronic graft-versus-host disease in patients with aplastic anemia treated by marrow transplantation from HLA-identical siblings. *Annals of Internal Medicine*, **98**, 461–466.

234 Ochs L.A., Miller W.J., Filipovich A.H. *et al.* (1994) Predictive factors for chronic graft-versus-host disease after histocompatible sibling donor bone marrow transplantation. *Bone Marrow Transplantation*, **13**, 455–460.

235 Martin P.J. (1990) The role of donor lymphoid cells in allogeneic marrow engraftment. *Bone Marrow Transplantation*, **6**, 283–289.

236 Roberts M.M., To L.B., Gillis D. *et al.* (1993) Immune reconstitution following peripheral blood stem cell transplantation, autologous bone marrow transplantation and allogeneic bone marrow transplantation. *Bone Marrow Transplantation*, **12**, 469–475.

237 Ugozzoli L., Yam P., Petz G.B. *et al.* (1991) Amplification by the polymerase chain reaction of hypervariable regions of the human genome for evaluation of chimerism after bone marrow transplantation. *Blood*, **77**, 1607–1615.

238 Katz, F., Hann I, Kinsey S. *et al.* (1993) Assessment of graft status following allogeneic bone marrow transplantation for haematological disorders in children using locus-specific minisatellite probes. *British Journal of Haematology*, **83**, 473–479.

239 Mackinnon S., Barnett L., Heller G. & O'Reilly R.J. (1994) Minimal residual disease is more common in patients who have mixed T cell chimerism after bone marrow transplantation for chronic myelogenous leukemia. *Blood*, **83**, 3409–3416.

240 Jackson N. & Franklin I.M. (1986) Successful treatment of late graft failure following T cell depleted bone marrow transplantation. *British Journal of Haematology*, **63**, 207–209.

241 Horowitz M.M., Mrsic M., Gale R.P. *et al.* (1990) Second bone marrow transplants for graft failure. *Blood*, **76**(Suppl. 1), 546a.

242 Lazarus H.M. & Rowe J.M. (1994) Clinical use of haemopoietic growth factors in allogeneic bone marrow transplantation. *Blood Reviews*, **8**, 169–178.

243 Ganser A., Lindemann A., Seibelt G. *et al.* (1991) Effects of recombinant human interleukin-3 in patients with normal hematopoiesis and in patients with bone marrow failure. *Blood*, **76**, 666–676.

244 Khwaja A. & Goldstone A.H. (1991) Haemopoietic growth factors. *British Medical Journal*, **302**, 1164–1165.

245 de Sauvage F., Hass P., Spencer S. *et al.* (1994) Stimulation of megakaryopoiesis and thrombopoiesis by the c-mpl ligand. *Nature*, **369**, 533–538.

246 Molineux G., Hartley C., McElroy P. *et al.* (1996) Megakaryocyte growth and development factor acelerates platelet recovery in peripheral blood progenitor cell transplant recipients. *Blood*, **88**, 366–376.

247 Tepler I, Elias L., Smith J.W. *et al.* (1996) A randomized placebo-controlled trial of recombinant human interleukin-11 in cancer patients with severe thrombocytopenia due to chemotherapy. *Blood*, **87**, 3607–3614.

248 Speiser D.E., Tiercy J-M., Rufer N. *et al.* (1996) High resolution HLA matching associated with decreased mortality after unrelated bone marrow transplantation. *Blood*, **87**, 4455–4462.

249 Ash R.C., Horowitz M.M., Gale R.P. *et al.* (1991) Bone marrow transplantation from related donors other than HLA-identical siblings: effect of T-cell depletion. *Bone Marrow Transplantation*, **7**, 443–452.

250 Beatty P.G., Clift R.A., Mickelson E.M. *et al.* (1985) Marrow transplantation from related donors other than HLA-identical siblings. *New England Journal of Medicine*, **313**, 765–771.

251 Bearman S.I., Mori M., Beatty P.G. *et al.* (1994) Comparison of morbidity and mortality after marrow transplantation from HLA-genotypically identical siblings and HLA-phenotypically identical unrelated donors. *Bone Marrow Transplantation*, **13**, 31–35.

252 Schiller G., Feig S.A., Territo M. *et al.* (1994) Treatment of advanced acute leukaemia with allogeneic bone marrow transplantation from unrelated donors. *British Journal of Haematology*, **88**, 72–78.

253 Ash R.C., Casper J.T., Chitambar C.R. *et al.* (1990) Successful allogeneic transplantation of T-cell-depleted bone marrow from closely HLA-matched unrelated donors. *New England Journal of Medicine*, **322**, 485–494.

254 Kernan N.A., Bartsch G., Ash R.C. *et al.* (1993) Analysis of 462 transplantations from unrelated donors facilitated by the National Marrow Donor Program. *New England Journal of Medicine*, **328**, 593–602.

255 Bloomfield C.D., Lawrence D., Arthur D.C. *et al.* (1994) Curative impact of intensification with high-dose cytarabine (HiDAC) in acute myeloid leukaemia (AML) varies by cytogenetic group. *Blood*, **84**(Suppl. 1), 111 (abstract).

256 Zittoun R.A., Mandelli F., Willemze R. *et al.* (1995) Autologous or allogeneic bone marrow transplantation compared with intensive chemotherapy in acute myelogenous leukemia. European Organization for Research and Treatment of Cancer (EORTC) and the Gruppo Italiano Malattie Ematologiche Maligne dell'Aduto (GIMEMA) Leukemia Cooperative Groups. *New England Journal of Medicine*, **332**, 217–223.

257 Clift R.A., Buckner C.D., Appelbaum F.R. *et al.* (1990) Allogeneic marrow transplantation in patients with acute myeloid leukemia in first remission. *Blood*, **76**, 1867–1871.

258 Boyd C.N., Ramberg R.C. & Thomas E.D. (1982) The incidence of recurrence of leukemia in donor cells after allogeneic bone marrow transplantation. *Leukemia Research*, **6**, 833–837.

259 Appelbaum F.R., Clift R.A., Buckner C.D. *et al.* (1983) Allogeneic marrow transplantation for acute nonlymphoblastic leukaemia after first relapse. *Blood*, **61**, 949–953.

260 Hoelzer D. (1994) Treatment of acute lymphoblastic leukaemia. *Seminars in Hematology*, **31**, 1–15.

261 Chessells J.M., Bailey C. & Richards S.M. (1995) Intensification of treatment and survival in all children with lymphoblastic leukaemia: results of UK Medical Research Council trial UKALL X. Medical Research Council Working Party on Childhood Leukaemia. *Lancet*, **345**, 143–148.

262 Copelan E.A. & McGuire E.A. (1995) The biology and treatment of acute lymphoblastic leukemia in adults. *Blood*, **85**, 1151–1168.

263 Barrett A.J. (1994) Bone marrow transplantation for acute lymphoblastic leukaemia. *Baillière's Clinical Haematology*, **7**, 377–401.

264 Jackson G.H., Taylor P.R.A., Lennard A.L. & Proctor S.J. (1994) Autologous bone marrow transplantation in acute lymphoblastic leukaemia. *Blood Reviews*, **8**, 161–168.

265 Preti A. & Kantarjian H.M. (1994) Management of adult acute lymphocytic leukemia: present issues and key challenges. *Journal of Clinical Oncology*, **12**, 1312–1322.

266 Barrett A.J., Horowitz M.M., Gale R.P. *et al.* (1989) Marrow transplantation for acute lymphoblastic leukemia: factors affecting relapse and survival. *Blood*, **74**, 862–871.

267 Weisdorf D.J., Woods W.G., Nesbit M.E. Jr *et al.* (1994) Allogeneic bone marrow transplantation for acute lymphoblastic leukaemia: risk factors and clinical outcome. *British Journal of Haematology*, **86**, 62–69.

268 Kantarjian H.M., O'Brien S., Anderlini P. & Talpaz M. (1996) Treatment of chronic myelogenous leukaemia: current status and investigational options. *Blood*, **87**, 3069–3081.

269 Sokal J.E., Baccarini M., Tura S. *et al.* (1985) Prognostic discrimination among younger patients with chronic granulocytic leukemia: relevance to bone marrow transplantation. *Blood*, **66**, 1352–1357.

270 Thomas E.D., Clift R.A., Fefer A. *et al.* (1986) Marrow transplantation for the treatment of chronic myelogenous leukemia. *Annals of Internal Medicine*, **104**, 155–163.

271 Enright H., Davies S.M., DeFor T. *et al.* (1996) Relapse after non-T-cell depleted allogeneic bone marrow transplantation for chronic myeloid leukaemia: early transplantation, use of an unrelated donor, and chronic graft-versus-host disease are protective. *Blood*, **88**, 714–720.

272 van Rhee F., Lin F., Cullis J.O. *et al.* (1994) Relapse of chronic myeloid leukaemia after allogeneic bone marrow transplant: the case for giving donor leukocyte transfusions before the onset of hematologic relapse. *Blood*, **83**, 3377–3383.

273 Cullis J.O., Schwarer A.P., Hughes T.P. *et al.* (1992) Second transplants for patients with chronic myeloid leukaemia in relapse after original transplant with T-depleted donor marrow: feasibility of using busulphan alone for re-conditioning. *British Journal of Haematology*, **80**, 33–39.

274 McGlave P.B., Beatty P., Ash R. & Hows J.M. (1990) Therapy for chronic myelogenous leukemia with unrelated donor bone marrow transplantation: results in 102 cases. *Blood*, **75**, 1728–1732 [erratum in *Blood*, 1990, **76**, 654].

275 McGlave P., Bartsch G., Anasetti C. *et al.* (1993) Unrelated donor marrow transplantation therapy for chronic myelogenous leukemia: initial experience of the National Marrow Donor Program. *Blood*, **81**, 543–550.

276 Drobyski W.R., Ash R.C., Casper J.T. *et al.* (1994) Effect of T-cell depletion as graft-versus-host disease prophylaxis on engraftment. Relapse and disease free survival in unrelated marrow transplantation for chronic myelogenous leukaemia. *Blood*, **83**, 1980–1987.

277 Devergie A., Labopin M., Apperly J. *et al.* for the EMBT Chronic Leukaemia Working Party (1994) Matched unrelated donor (MHD) transplant for chronic myeloid leukaemia (CML) in Europe. Report of 299 cases and analysis of prognosis factors. *Experimental Haematology*, **22**, 715 (abstract).

278 Clift R.A. Anasetti C., Petersdorf F.E. *et al.* (1993) Marrow transplants from unrelated donors for chronic myelogenous leukaemia—the Seattle Experience. *Experimental Haematology*, **21**, 1111 (abstract).

279 Marks D.I., Cullis J.O., Ward K.N. *et al.* (1993) Allogeneic bone marrow transplantation for chronic myeloid leukemia using sibling and volunteer unrelated donors. A comparison of complications in the first 2 years. *Annals of Internal Medicine*, **119**, 207–214.

280 Cross N.C.P. (1995) Quantitative PCR techniques and applications. *British Journal of Haematology*, **89**, 693–697.

281 The Italian Cooperative Study Group on Chronic Myeloid Leukaemia (1994) Interferon-alpha2a as compared with conventional chemotherapy for the treatment of chronic myeloid leukaemia. *New England Journal of Medicine*, **330**, 820–825.

282 Allan N.C., Richards S.M. & Shepherd P.C. (1995) UK Medical Research Council randomised, multicentre trial of interferon-alpha-nl for chronic myeloid leukaemia: improved survival irrespective of cytogenetic response. The UK Medical Research Council's Working Parties for Therapeutic Trials in Adult Leukaemia. *Lancet*, **345**, 1392–1397.

283 Italian Cooperative Study Group on Chronic Myeloid Leukaemia (1993) Evaluating survival after allogeneic bone marrow transplant for chronic myeloid leukaemia in chronic phase: a comparison of transplant versus no-transplant in a cohort of 258 patients first seen in Italy between 1984 and 1986. *British Journal of Haematology*, **85**, 292–299.

284 O'Brien S.G. & Goldman J.M. (1994) Autografting in chronic myeloid leukaemia. *Blood Reviews*, **8**, 63–69.

285 McGlave P.B., De Fabritiis P, Deisseroth A. *et al.* (1994) Autologous transplants for chronic myelogenous leukaemia: results from eight transplant groups. *Lancet*, **343**, 1486–1488.

286 Reiffers J., Goldman J.M., Meloni G. *et al.* (1994) Autologous stem cell transplantation in chronic myelogenous leukaemia: a retrospective analysis of the European Group for Bone Marrow Transplantation. *Bone Marrow Transplantation*, **14**, 407–410.

287 Bandini G., Michallet M., Rosti G. *et al.* (1991) Bone marrow transplantation for chronic lymphocytic leukemia. *Bone Marrow Transplantation*, **7**, 251–253.

288 Shepherd J.D., Barnett M.J., Connors J.M. *et al.* (1993) Allogeneic bone marrow transplantation for poor prognosis non-Hodgkin's lymphoma. *Bone Marrow Transplantation*, **12**, 591–596.

289 Alexanian R. (1985) Ten year survival in multiple myeloma. *Archives of Internal Medicine*, **145**, 2073–2074.

290 Gahrton G., Tura S., Ljungman P. *et al.* (1991) Allogeneic bone marrow transplantation in multiple myeloma. *New England Journal of Medicine*, **325**, 1267–1273.

291 Gahrton G., Tura S., Ljungman P. *et al.* (1995) Prognostic factors in allogeneic bone marrow transplantation for multiple myeloma. *Journal of Clinical Oncology*, **13**, 1312–1322.

292 Attal M., Harousseau J-L., Stoppa A-M. *et al.* (1996) A prospective randomized trial of autologous bone marrow transplantation and chemotherapy in multiple myeloma. *New England Journal of Medicine*, **335**, 91–97.

293 Mufti G.J., Stevens J.R., Oscier D.G. *et al.* (1985) Myelodysplastic syndromes: a scoring system with prognostic significance. *British Journal of Haematology*, **59**, 425–433.

294 Bennett J.M., Catovsky D., Daniel M.T., *et al.* (1982) Proposals for the classification of the myelodysplastic syndromes. *British Journal of Haematology*, **51**, 189–199.

295 De Witte T., Gratwohl A., Niederweiser D. *et al.* (1994) Allogeneic bone marrow transplantation for patients with myelodysplastic syndromes or leukaemia following MDS treated with remission induction therapy. *Bone Marrow Transplantation*, **14**(Suppl. 1), 95 (abstract).

296 Appelbaum F.R., Barrall J., Storb R. *et al.* (1990) Bone marrow transplantation for patients with myelodysplasia. Pretreatment variables and outcome. *Annals of Internal Medicine*, **112**, 590–597.

297 Sutton L., Chastang C., Ribaud P. *et al.* (1996) Factors influencing outcome in *de novo* myelodysplastic syndromes treated by allogeneic bone marrow transplantation: a long term study of 71 patients. *Blood*, **88**, 358–365.

298 Arnold R., de Witte T. & Van Beizen A.E. (1995) Matched unrelated donor BMT in myelodysplasia/secondary AML: an EBMT survey. *Blood*, **86**(Suppl. 1), 368a.

299 O'Donnell M.R., Nademanee A.P., Snyder D.S. *et al.* (1987) Bone marrow transplantation for myelodysplastic and myeloproliferative disorders. *Journal of Clinical Oncology*, **5**, 1822–1826.

300 Rajantie J., Sale G.E., Deeg H.J. *et al.* (1986) Adverse effect of severe marrow fibrosis on hematologic recovery after chemoradiotherapy and allogeneic bone marrow transplantation. *Blood*, **67**, 1693–1697.

301 Kodish E., Lantos J., Siegler M. *et al.* (1991) Bone marrow transplantation for sickle cell disease. A study of parents' decisions. *New England Journal of Medicine*, **325**, 1349–1353.

302 Fischer A., Landais P., Friedrich W. *et al.* (1990) European experience of bone-marrow transplantation for severe combined immune deficiency. *Lancet*, **ii**, 850–854.

303 Kernan N.A., Bartsch G., Ash R.C. *et al.* (1993) Retrospective analysis of 462 unrelated marrow transplants facilitated by the National Marrow Donor Program (NMDP) for treatment of acquired and congenital disorders of the lymphohemopoietic system and congenital metabolic disorders. *New England Journal of Medicine*, **328**, 593–602.

304 Thomas E.D. (1985) Marrow transplantation for non-malignant disorders. *New England Journal of Medicine*, **312**, 46–48.

305 Klingemann H-G., Storb R., Fefer A. *et al.* (1986) Bone marrow transplantation in patients aged 45 years and older. *Blood*, **67**, 770–776.

306 Aschan J., Ringden O., Tollemar J. *et al.* (1990) Improved survival in marrow recipients above 30 years of age with better prevention of graft-versus-host disease. *Transplantation Proceedings*, **1**, 195–197.

307 Atkinson K., Farrell C., Chapman G. *et al.* (1986) Female marrow donors increase the risk of acute GVHD; effect of donor age and parity and analysis of cell subpopulations in the donor marrow innoculum. *British Journal of Haematology*, **63**, 231–239.

308 Frassoni F., Labopin M., Gluckman E. *et al.* (1994) Are patients with acute leukaemia, alive and well 2 years post bone marrow transplantation cured? A European survey. Acute leukaemia Working Party of the European Group for Bone Marrow Transplantation (EBMT). *Leukemia*, **8**, 924–928.

309 Barrett A.J. & Malkovska V. (1996) Graft-versus-leukaemia: understanding and using the alloimmune response to treat haematological malignancies. *British Journal of Haematology*, **93**, 754–761.

310 Kwak L.W., Taub D.D., Duffey P.L. *et al.* (1995) Transfer of myeloma idiotype-specific immunity from an actively immunized marrow donor. *Lancet*, **345**, 1016–1020.

311 Horowitz M.M., Gale R.P., Barrett A.J. *et al.* (1989) Effect of methotrexate on relapse after bone marrow transplantation for acute lymphoblastic leukaemia. *Lancet*, **i**, 535–537.

312 Weaver C.H., Clift R.A., Deeg H.J. *et al.* (1994) Effect of graft-versus-host disease prophylaxis on relapse in patients transplanted for acute myeloid leukemia. *Bone Marrow Transplantation*, **14**, 885–893.

313 Jones R.J., Vogelsang G.B., Hess A.D. *et al.* (1989) Induction of graft-versus-host disease after autologous bone marrow transplantation. *Lancet*, **i**, 754–757.

314 Barrett A.J., Joshi R., Kendra J.R. *et al.* (1986) Prediction and prevention of relapse of acute lymphoblastic leukaemia after

bone marrow transplantation. *British Journal of Haematology*, **64**, 179–186.

315 Soiffer R.J., Murray C., Gonin R. & Ritz J. (1994) Effect of low-dose interleukin-2 on disease relapse after T-cell-depleted allogeneic bone marrow transplantation. *Blood*, **84**, 964–971.

316 Wagner J.E., Vogelsang G.B., Zehnbauer B.A. *et al.* (1992) Relapse of leukemia after bone marrow transplantation: effect of second myeloablative therapy. *Bone Marrow Transplantation*, **9**, 205–209.

317 Radich J.P., Sanders J.E., Buckner C.D. *et al.* (1993) Second allogeneic marrow transplantation for patients with recurrent leukemia after initial transplant with total body irradiation-containing regimens. *Journal of Clinical Oncology*, **11**, 304–313.

318 Boiron J-M., Cony-Makhoul P., Mahon F-X. *et al.* (1994) Treatment of haematological malignances relapsing after allogeneic bone marrow transplantation. *Blood Reviews*, **8**, 234–240.

319 Kumar L. (1994) Leukemia: management of relapse after allogeneic bone marrow transplantation. *Journal of Clinical Oncology*, **12**, 1710–1717.

320 Witherspoon R.P., Fisher L.D., Schoch G. *et al.* (1989) Secondary cancers after bone marrow transplantation for leukemia or aplastic anemia. *New England Journal of Medicine*, **321**, 784–789.

321 Zutter M.M., Martin P.J., Sale G.E. *et al.* (1988) Epstein–Barr virus lymphoproliferation after bone marrow transplantation. *Blood*, **72**, 520.

322 Papadopoulos E.B., Ladanyi M., Emanuel D. *et al.* (1994) Infusions of donor leukocytes as treatment of Epstein–Barr virus associated lymphoproliferative disorders complicating allogeneic marrow transplantation. *New England Journal of Medicine*, **330**, 1185–1191.

323 Rooney C.M., Smith C.A., Ng C.Y.C. *et al.* (1995) Use of gene-modified virus-specific T lymphocytes to control Epstein–Barr virus-related lymphoproliferation. *Lancet*, **345**, 9–13.

324 Singer D.A., Donnelly M.B. & Messerschmidt G.L. (1990) Informed consent for bone marrow transplantation; identification of relevant information by referring physicians. *Bone Marrow Transplantation*, **6**, 431–437.

325 Hengeveld M.W., Houtman R.B & Zwaan F.E. (1988) Psychological aspects of bone marrow transplantation: a retrospective study of 17 long-term survivors. *Bone Marrow Transplantation*, **3**, 69–75.

326 Jenkins P.L. & Roberts D.J. (1991) Suicidal behaviour after bone marrow transplantation. *Bone Marrow Transplantation*, **7**, 159–161.

327 Lesko L.M. (1994) Bone marrow transplantation: support of the patient and his/her family. Support. *Care Cancer*, **2**, 35–49.

328 Dufoir T., Saux M.C., Terraza B. *et al.* (1992) Comparative cost of allogeneic bone marrow transplantation and chemotherapy in patients with acute myeloid leukaemia in first remission. *Bone Marrow Transplantation*, **10**, 323–329.

329 Syrjala K.L., Chapko M.K., Vitaliano P.P. *et al.* (1993) Recovery after allogeneic marrow transplantation: prospective study of predictors of long term physical and psychosocial functioning. *Bone Marrow Transplantation*, **11**, 319–327.

330 Bush N.E., Haberman M., Donaldson G. & Sullivan K.M. (1995) Quality of life of 125 adults surviving 6–18 years after bone marrow transplantation. *Social Science and Medicine*, **40**, 479–490.

331 Baker F., Wingard J.R., Curbow B. *et al.* (1994) Quality of life of bone marrow transplant long-term survivors. *Bone Marrow Transplantation*, **13**, 589–596.

23 Autologous Blood and Marrow Transplantation

J. Mehta and R.L. Powles

Introduction

Myelosuppression is the dose-limiting side effect of radiation and most cytotoxic drugs. However, high-dose chemotherapy or chemo/radiotherapy in myeloablative or severely myelo-suppressive doses, which do not cause irreversible dysfunction of any other organ, can be used for treatment of malignant diseases if followed by haematopoietic stem cell rescue. This mode of therapy is now commonly utilized in the management of malignant haematological diseases which exhibit steep dose–response curves.

The origin of the haematopoietic stem cells may be syngeneic (identical twin), allogeneic (related or unrelated) or autologous (patient). The applicability of syngeneic transplants is limited by the rarity of patients with identical twins. Allogeneic transplantation, despite the advantage of immunological graft-vs-tumour reactions [1], is limited by the availability of suitable HLA-matched donors, and the morbidity and mortality associated with the procedure which restrict its use to patients under the age of 55 years. Stem cells of autologous origin were first used to support high-dose treatment of refractory and advanced solid tumours, lymphoma, and leukaemia [2–6].

Haematopoietic stem cells

Source of haematopoietic support

Traditionally, bone marrow has been used to provide haematopoietic support [7]. Peripheral blood was first used as the source of haematopoietic support in a patient with chronic myeloid leukaemia (CML) in blast crisis, who received previously cryopreserved chronic-phase blood cells in an attempt to re-establish the chronic phase [8]. Körbling et al. collected Philadelphia (Ph) chromosome-negative progenitors from the blood during recovery from chemotherapy-induced myelosuppression in a patient with CML and used these for an autograft in blast crisis [9]. Juttner et al. reported prompt, but incomplete, haematopoietic reconstitution with blood-derived autologous cells collected in early remission in patients with acute myeloid leukaemia (AML) after high-dose chemotherapy or chemo/radiotherapy [10].

Peripheral blood is the only suitable source of haematopoietic support with marrows that are fibrotic and inaspirable as a result of previous irradiation [11] or because of the underlying disease [12]. Marrow with overt metastatic disease is not considered suitable for transplantation, because of the risk of contamination of the harvested marrow with malignant cells and reinfusion of disease. However, peripheral blood stem cells have been used under these circumstances, with prolonged disease-free survival in some patients [13]. The avoidance of general anaesthesia eliminates a small but definite risk related to a bone marrow harvest [7]. Recovery of haematopoiesis is usually faster after infusion of blood cells than after marrow, with a shortened period of post-transplant pancytopenia because of infusion of haematopoietic progenitors at all stages of development. The faster haematological recovery results in a decreased incidence of infection, blood-product requirements, stay in hospital and cost of the procedure [14,15].

In addition to haematopoietic progenitors, the mononuclear cell fraction collected from the peripheral blood for transplantation is rich in immunocompetent lymphocytes and NK cells [16]. Reconstitution of the immune system is also faster after peripheral blood stem cell transplantation (PBSCT) than after autologous bone marrow transplantation (ABMT) [17]. These may result in immunologic antitumour effects, or may permit graft-vs-tumour reactions to be elicited by appropriate immunomodulating agents, with a consequent decrease in the risk of relapse [1]. As a result of these advantages, the use of peripheral blood as an alternative to autologous marrow has been steadily increasing.

There is a striking difference between marrow and blood stem cell doses; the total number of cells collected from the blood and reinfused during the transplant are far higher than the number of cells in a marrow graft [18]. There is concern that this may result in higher relapse rates after autografting for AML, as a result of reinfusion of more residual disease [18,19].

Tumour cells are detectable in peripheral blood collections in lymphoma [20] and myeloma [21] as well, but their significance is uncertain. A case-controlled analysis of lymphoma patients undergoing PBSCT or ABMT, from the European Group for Blood and Bone Marrow Transplantation (EBMT), showed that while PBSCT recipients had faster engraftment and less toxicity, the progression-free survival of the two groups was comparable [22]. The Nebraska Group have shown significantly better progression-free survival in lymphoma patients undergoing PBSCT compared with ABMT [23], but differences in conditioning regimens (more PBSCT patients receiving irradiation) could have contributed to the effect.

Harvesting haematopoietic stem cells

Bone marrow

A detailed description of the technique of harvesting, processing and cryopreserving bone marrow is beyond the scope of this chapter, and has been dealt with comprehensively elsewhere [7,24–26]. Briefly, marrow is aspirated from both posterior iliac crests through multiple punctures under general or regional anaesthesia and sterile conditions. The aspirated material is anticoagulated with heparin or acid-citrate-dextrose and collected in a sterile steel jar or a blood bag. After filtration to remove bony chips, aggregates and large fat particles, the marrow is ready for further manipulation or cryopreservation. Usually $1–5 \times 10^8$/kg nucleated cells are collected (average 2×10^8/kg).

Peripheral blood stem cells

Blood-derived stem cells are harvested by leukapheresis using a cell separator programmed to collect low-density mononuclear cells or lymphocytes [7]. This setting results in collection of haematopoietic progenitors in addition to lymphocytes, monocytes and NK cells. Neutrophil contamination is minimized, but the extent of the purity of the product varies from machine to machine, and also depends on the ease of blood flow and operator skill. Continuous-flow machines (e.g. Cobe Spectra) are faster than intermittent-flow machines (e.g. Haemonetics MCS-3P) and yield a purer product [27], but the latter require only one site of vascular access. Vascular access has to be obtained with large-bore cannulas or rigid in-dwelling catheters. Between 7 and 10 litres of blood (150–250% calculated blood volume) are processed over 2–4 hours at each harvest session on 1–4 consecutive days.

Leukapheresis in the basal haematopoietic state with normal blood counts required between eight and 10 harvest sessions for an adequate number of progenitor cells to be collected, and has now been largely abandoned. The number of haematopoietic progenitors circulating in the blood is greatly increased during recovery from myelosuppressive chemotherapy and after the administration of growth factors [7,10,15,28–31]. This reduces the number of apheresis sessions required to between one and four.

Chemotherapy may be administered specially for stem cell mobilization (e.g. a single dose of cyclophosphamide; 1.5–7 g/m²), or stem cells may be harvested after disease-specific chemotherapy [10,28,29]. The addition of a growth factor such as granulocyte (G-CSF) or granulocyte macrophage (GM-CSF) colony-stimulating factor at a dose of 3–10 μg/kg at the nadir of the leucocyte count improves cell yields further. Cell yields are highest when chemotherapy and growth factor treatment are combined. The best time to start harvesting is variable, and can be accurately determined by the proportion of CD34+ cells in the peripheral blood. Daily flow cytometric monitoring, however, is not convenient, and starting leukapheresis when the recovering total leucocyte count is approximately 1×10^9/l is usually adequate.

The disadvantage of using chemotherapy for mobilization is variability in the recovery of counts, with some degree of unpredictability in harvest dates. Additionally, thrombocytopenia and infections can make apheresis difficult. Growth factors alone administered in the basal state (i.e. without chemotherapy) also yield adequate cells for transplantation. Typical mobilization regimens utilize 5–16 μg/kg or 250 μg/m² daily of G-CSF or GM-CSF for a period of 4–7 days, with harvests on 1–4 consecutive days starting on day 4 or 5 [12,15,30,31]. Other cytokines used for mobilization include stem cell factor, PIXY, IL-3 and erythropoietin; singly or in various combinations.

Peripheral blood stem cells are increasingly being utilized for allogeneic transplantation as well, and cells are mobilized using 5–16 μg/kg G-CSF [32–34]. This yields adequate cells for a transplant in between one and three apheresis procedures, depending on the weight disparity between the donor and the recipient. The number of T-lymphocytes in the harvest is approximately 1 log higher than in bone marrow, but preliminary results suggest there is no increase in the incidence or severity of graft-vs-host disease [32–34].

Ex vivo purging

Standard pretransplant conditioning regimens are incapable of eradicating leukaemic cells completely from the body, because relapses are seen even after allogeneic BMT, where the infused haematopoietic progenitors are free of malignant cells and graft-vs-leukaemia effects eliminate some of the malignant cells surviving the chemo/radiotherapy. It is therefore logical to assume that in most cases of relapse after autografting, where the reinfused marrow was microscopically free of disease and was harvested in remission, persistent disease within the host is responsible for relapse. However, using gene-marking techniques, Brenner *et al.* showed that reinfused marrow contributed to relapse after autografting in two patients with AML [35]. It is likely that some cases of relapse do originate from clonogenic tumour cells in the autologous cells infused after myeloablative therapy.

In a study of 114 patients with B-cell non-Hodgkin's lymphoma (NHL) autografted with marrow purged by monoclonal antibodies [36], Gribben *et al.* provided indirect evidence of the utility of purging. Disease-free survival was significantly higher in 57 patients, whose marrow contained no detectable residual t(14;18) on PCR after purging, than in those whose marrow contained detectable residual lymphoma.

Tumour load in the harvested material can be minimized, by the use of multiple courses of intensive consolidation chemotherapy (*in vivo* purging) or by treatment of the harvested cells (*ex vivo* purging). Purging is clearly not universally necessary, because a number of patients survive in continuous remission long-term after varying intensities of consolidation therapy and unpurged autografts. The development of better techniques to detect minimal residual disease would allow the identification of persistent disease within the patient or the harvested marrow, and permit selection of appropriate patients for purging.

The ideal purging agent should be selectively toxic to malignant cells, while sparing normal haematopoietic progenitors at concentrations used *ex vivo*. Its activity should not be dependent upon the cell cycle, and the effect should be achieved with a short exposure. The agent should be easily inactivated or removed before infusion of the treated marrow, or should be nontoxic at the concentrations infused.

A number of different pharmacological, immunological and physical methods have been utilized to remove ('purge') occult malignant cells from autologous marrow. Some of the purging agents and techniques which have been used in clinical practice are shown in Table 23.1 [36–73].

The benefits of purging are difficult to evaluate in practice. No randomized studies have been performed to assess the role of purging. Purging with pharmacological agents usually damages normal progenitors as well, resulting in significantly delayed granulocyte and platelet recovery. Increased morbidity and mortality from the resultant infectious and haemorrhagic complications counteract the decreased relapse rate, to some extent. Drugs such as amifostine, which can selectively protect normal cells during purging with 4-hydroperoxycyclophosphamide (4-HC), prevent delayed haematopoietic reconstitution [74], and may increase the interest in pharmacological purging techniques.

The cyclophosphamide derivatives 4-HC and mafosfamide (Asta-Z 7557) have been most widely used clinically—mafosfamide mainly in Europe [41–44], and 4-HC in the USA [37–40]. However, the availability of 4-HC has recently become uncertain.

The development of monoclonal antibodies to cell-surface antigens enables separation of distinct cell populations. The CD34 antigen is expressed on primitive haematopoietic cells and is not expressed on most nonhaematopoietic cells. Its expression on haematopoietic cells appears to decrease with maturation or differentiation. The selection of CD34+ cells using an avidin-biotin affinity column (Ceprate, CellPro) can, potentially, purge malignant cells by concentrating progenitor cells (positive selection). This is feasible in myeloma and lymphoma [75], but leukaemic cells often express CD34, and thus the applicability of the positive selection technique to autografting in leukaemia may be limited.

In a study of different freezing techniques, Allieri *et al.* showed that the recovery of AML progenitor colony-forming units (CFUs) was significantly lower than normal granulocyte macrophage colony-forming units (GM-CFUs) and erythroid burst-forming units (E-BFUs) after thawing, and that freezing reduced the cloning efficiency of AML-CFU significantly [76]. However, in a study of prognostic factors affecting the outcome of 74 patients undergoing unpurged ABMT for AML, Mehta *et al.* could find no effect of cryopreservation on relapse rates or disease-free survival [77].

Conditioning regimens

Conditioning regimens for autologous transplantation, unlike those used for allogeneic BMT, do not need to be immunosuppressive. There is greater flexibility in designing protocols which can provide maximally intensive therapy to eradicate the malignant disease being treated. Autograft recipients are not at risk of graft-vs-host disease (GVHD), and serious infections (especially viral) are rare because immune reconstitution following autografts is faster [17]. Autograft recipients, therefore, can tolerate more intensive regimens than allograft recipients, with relatively limited regimen-related toxicity [78].

Most conditioning regimens for the leukaemias utilize total body irradiation (TBI), usually in combination with cyclophosphamide. The variables determining the biological effects of TBI include total dose, dose rate, fraction size and fractionation interval. Although TBI is usually fractionated in an attempt to reduce toxicity, it is possible to utilize single-fraction TBI delivered at a low dose without increasing the toxicity significantly. Increasing the TBI dose decreases relapse rates, but does not appreciably increase survival because of the greater toxicity [79–81].

Newer methods of delivering TBI, hyperfractionation and better shielding techniques, especially for the lungs, may allow escalation of the dose without a significant increase in toxicity. Table 23.2 shows some commonly used conditioning regimens which utilize TBI [42,46,77,82–88].

The use of radiolabelled monoclonal antibodies directed at surface antigens specific to malignant cells or to haematopoietic cells, or bone-seeking radionuclide chelates, can selectively irradiate medullary, or medullary as well as extramedullary, haematopoietic tissues. This minimizes the exposure of normal organs and tissues to irradiation [89–92].

Table 23.1 Clinical use of purging agents and techniques.

Technique/agent	Disease	References
Pharmacological		
4-Hydroperoxycyclophosphamide	AML	Korbling et al., 1983 [37], Kaizer et al., 1983 [38]
	ALL	Yeager et al., 1990 [39]
	Myeloma	Reece et al., 1993 [40]
	NHL	Kaizer et al., 1983 [38]
Mafosfamide	AML	Herve et al., 1984 [41], Gorin et al., 1986 [42]
	ALL	Gorin et al., 1986 [42]
	CML	Carlo-Stella et al., 1994 [43]
	NHL	Sweetenham et al., 1994 [44]
Deoxycoformycin + deoxyadenosine	T-ALL	Cahn et al., 1986 [45]
Vincristine + prednisone	ALL	Colleselli et al., 1991 [46]
1-O-octadecyl-2-O-methyl-rac-glycero-3-phosphocholine (Edelfosine)	AML	Vogler et al., 1992 [47]
4-HC + etoposide	Acute biphenotypic leukaemia	Chao et al., 1993 [48]
Immunological		
IL-2	AML	Klingemann et al., 1994 [49]
Interferon-τ	CML	McGlave et al., 1990 [50]
Anti-CD10 (J5) + C	C-ALL	Ritz et al., 1982 [51]
Murine MoAb T 101 + Ricin A-chain	T-ALL	Gorin et al., 1985 [52]
Anti-lacto-N-fucopentaose III S4-7 antibody + C	AML	Ferrero et al., 1987 [53]
Anti-CD15 (PM-81) and/or Anti-CD14 (AML-2-23) + C	AML	Ball et al., 1986 [54]
Anti-CD9 (BA-2) + Anti-CD10 (BA-3) + Anti-CD24 (BA-1) + C	B/C-ALL	Kersey et al., 1987 [55]
Anti-CD3 (UCHT1) + Anti-CD5 (T101) + Anti-LFA (TA-1) + Ricin	T-ALL	Kersey et al., 1987 [55]
Anti-CD7 (WT1) + Ricin A-chain	T-ALL	Preijers et al., 1989 [56]
Neuraminidase + Anti-CD15 (PM-81) + C	AML	Ball et al., 1990 [57]
Anti-CD9 (DuALL-1) + Anti-CD10 (WCMH15.14) + Anti-CD19 (HD-37) + Magnabeads	C-ALL	Janssen et al., 1990 [58]
Anti-CD33 + C	AML	Robertson et al., 1992 [59]
Anti-CD9 (J2) + Anti-CD10 (J5) + C	ALL	Billett et al., 1993 [60]
Anti-CD10 (ALB1, ALB2) + Anti-CD19 (CLB-B4) + Anti-CD24 (ALB9) + Anti-CD19 coated magnetic beads	B/C-ALL	Schmid et al., 1993 [61]
Anti-CD10 + Anti-CD20 + Anti-B5 + C	CLL	Rabinowe et al., 1993 [62]
	NHL	Gribben et al., 1991 [36]
Anti-CD19 + Magnetic beads	CLL	Khouri et al., 1994 [63]
Anti-CDw52 (Campath-1M) + C	ALL	Tiley et al., 1993 [64]
Phorbol esters	AML	Abrahm et al., 1986 [65]
Short-term culture	CML	Barnett et al., 1994 [66]
	AML	Ranson et al., 1991 [67]
Hyperthermia	AML	Herrmann et al., 1992 [68]
Serum-free liquid culture	Ph + ALL	Fabrega et al., 1993 [69]
Antisense oligonucleotides	CML	Luger et al., 1994 [70]
Combinations		
Anti-CD5 (Tp67) + Anti-CD7 (Tp41) + Ricin + 4-HC	T-ALL	Uckun et al., 1990 [71]
Hyperthermia + Interferon-α	ALL	Higuchi et al., 1991 [72]
Anti-CD9 (BA-2) + Anti-CD10 (BA-3) + Anti-CD24 (BA-1) + C + 4-HC	B/C-ALL	Uckun et al., 1992 [73]

ALL = acute lymphoblastic leukaemia; AML = acute myeloblastic leukaemia; CLL = chronic lymphocytic leukaemia; CML = chronic myeloid leukaemia; NHL = non-Hodgkin's lymphoma.

Table 23.2 Conditioning regimens with total body irradiation (TBI).

Drugs/TBI	Dose	References
Cyclophosphamide fTBI	120–200 mg/kg 1200–1670 cGy	Stewart *et al.*, 1985 [82]; Körbling *et al.*, 1989 [83]
Cyclophosphamide ufTBI	120 mg/kg 1000 cGY	Gorin *et al.*, 1986 [42]
Cyclophosphamide Busulfan fTBI	60 mg/kg 8 mg/kg 1200 cGy	Petersen *et al.*, 1993 [84]
Melphalan ufTBI	110–140 mg/m^2 950–1150 cGy	Mehta *et al.*, 1995 [77]; Schroeder *et al.*, 1991 [85], Powles *et al.*, 1995 [86]
Etoposide fTBI	60 mg/kg 1200 cGy	Schmid *et al.*, 1993 [61]
Cytarabine Melphalan fTBI	24 g/m^2 140 mg/m^2 1200 cGy	Cahn *et al.*, 1991 [87]
Vincristine Cyclophosphamide fTBI	4 mg/m^2 3600 mg/m^2 1200 cGy	Colleselli *et al.*, 1991 [46]
Cytarabine ufTBI	36 g/m^2 850 cGy	Woods *et al.*, 1990 [88]

fTBI = fractionated total-body irradiation; ufTBI = unfractionated total-body irradiation.

Irradiation contributes significantly to the acute toxicity of the transplant procedure [78], and is also associated with a number of adverse long-term consequences [93]. Therefore conditioning regimens not containing TBI are more attractive, although compromised efficacy is a potential problem. The original busulphan-cyclophosphamide (BuCy4) regimen [94] has been modified, with the addition and the substitution of several drugs such as thiotepa, etoposide, cytarabine, and melphalan, but none of the regimens has been found to be more effective. Table 23.3 shows some conditioning regimens which utilize chemotherapy alone [48,86,94–104].

No conditioning regimen for autografting has been clearly shown to be superior to another in a randomized study, and the regimen chosen for a particular patient is likely to be determined by the availability of TBI, the importance of potentially preserving fertility and physician preference.

Clinical results

Critical evaluation of clinical results

Most patients are referred for BMT to specialist transplant centres after having received the initial chemotherapy elsewhere. This usually results in patient selection, because only 'good-risk' patients (relatively young patients in good physical condition) tend to be referred and accepted for BMT.

Patients who relapse before transplantation are excluded from reports of BMT in first-remission acute leukaemia. With continuing remission, the probability of relapse decreases with the passage of time, irrespective of the subsequent therapy administered. Therefore the later in their first remission patients are autografted, the better the probability of disease-free survival. This 'time-censoring' effect biases the results of almost all single-centre reports of ABMT significantly, and studies with longer median remission–transplant intervals tend to show better results.

The only reasonable way to evaluate the impact of BMT (autologous or allogeneic) on survival is to consider the outcome of an entire group of unselected, consecutive patients, rather than the outcome of only the transplanted patients [105]. Other than large, randomized multicentre studies [106–110] comparing chemotherapy and BMT prospectively, few reports consider the denominator of eligible patients while reporting their results [105,111,112].

Large, multicentre randomized studies solve some, but not all, of the problems associated with the evaluation of autografting. A significant proportion of patients entering large studies do not reach the point of randomization. In the UK Medical Research Council's (MRC) AML 10 study, of all first remission patients without HLA-identical siblings eligible for randomization to autografting versus no further treatment, 91 patients relapsed or died in remission before being randomized, 63 chose ABMT, 302 elected to have no ABMT and only 357 patients were actually randomized [107].

Negative results from large studies need to be evaluated cautiously as well. The design of two recent multicentre studies,

Table 23.3 Conditioning regimens without TBI.

Drugs	Dose	References
Busulphan Cyclophosphamide (BuCy4)	16 mg/kg 200 mg/kg	Yeager *et al.*, 1986 [94]
Busulphan Cyclophosphamide (BuCy2)	16 mg/kg 120 mg/kg	Beelen *et al.*, 1989 [95]
Cyclophosphamide BCNU Etoposide (CBV)	4.5–6 g/m² 300 mg/m² 600–750 mg/m²	Zander *et al.*, 1981 [96], Spinolo *et al.*, 1990 [97]
Busulpan	16 mg/kg	Mehta *et al.*, 1996 [98]
Busulphan Melphalan	16 mg/kg 140 mg/m²	Mehta *et al.*, 1993 [99]
Melphalan	200 mg/m²	Mehta *et al.*, 1993 [99], 1995 [100]
Melphalan Methylprednisolone	200 mg/m² 7.5 g	Cunningham *et al.*, 1994 [101]
Busulphan Etoposide	16 mg/kg 60 mg/kg	Chao *et al.*, 1993 [48], Linker *et al.*, 1993 [102]
BCNU Amsacrine Etoposide Cytarabine (BAVC)	800 mg/m² 450 mg/m² 450 mg/m² 900 mg/m²	Meloni *et al.*, 1990 [103]
BCNU Etoposide Cytarabine Melphalan (BEAM)	300 mg/m² 400–800 mg/m² 800–1600 mg/m² 140 mg/m²	Mills *et al.*, 1995 [104]

which showed no survival benefit with autografting compared to chemotherapy, may have resulted in a lack of exploitation of any potential benefit of ABMT [107,108]. It has been shown that patients receiving a nucleated cell dose of less than 2 × 10⁸/kg are at a significantly greater risk of transplant-related mortality [113,114] and poorer disease-free survival than those receiving greater than 2 × 10⁸ cells/kg [77]. Both the multicentre studies specified 1 × 10⁸ nucleated cells/kg as the target harvest quantity [107,108]. This may have resulted in a higher transplant-related mortality, which could have diminished the potential benefit of the autograft procedure. However, data on the effect of the nucleated cell dose on mortality are not available for these studies. In one of these studies [108], patients received only one course of consolidation therapy before marrow harvest and unpurged ABMT. This could have resulted in inadequate *in vivo* purging of the marrow and higher relapse rates; adequate *in vivo* purging may require two courses of consolidation therapy [77]. In the MRC AML 10 Study, on the other hand, patients received up to three courses of consolidation chemotherapy before being

autografted [107]. This quantity of pretransplant chemotherapy may make the contribution, if any, made by an autograft procedure hard to discern, except with a very large number of patients. This problem has been rectified in the MRC AML 12 Study, which should be able to address the question of the quantity of pretransplant chemotherapy. However, the AML 12 Study includes optional peripheral blood progenitor support during consolidation therapy, which may result in reinfusion of malignant cells [18,19].

Unlike the acute leukaemias, the natural course of myeloma and low-grade lymphoma tends to be slowly progressive. Encouraging preliminary results of autografting therefore need to be interpreted with caution, because much longer follow-up is required before the long-term impact of this procedure on survival and disease-free survival can be determined [115].

Acute myeloid leukaemia

The role of autografting in first remission continues to remain

Table 23.4 Autografting for AML in first remission.

Patients (no.)	Age (years) Median	Age (years) Range	Conditioning regimen	Purging	Median CR-BMT interval (months)	Patients with good-risk disease*	Actuarial probability of DFS	Actuarial probability of relapse	References
20	40	16–53	BuCy2	—	6	10%†	55%, 3 yr	38%, 3 yr	Beelen et al., 1989 [95]
12	38	18–53	Cy-TBI	—	6	8.3%†	58%, 3 yr	NS (n = 5)	Burnett et al., 1984 [117]
55	37	12–62	Cy-TBI	—	5	27%†	49%, 5 yr	43%, 5 yr	Carella et al., 1992 [118]
39‡	36	18–51	BuCy4	4-HC	2	38%†	54%, 3 yr§	NS (n = 15)§	Cassileth et al., 1993 [119]
21	36	17–58	Melphalan-etoposide-TBI	—	10	NS	58%, 4 yr	39%, 4 yr	Keating & Crump, 1992 [120]
20§	41	5–48	Cy-TBI	—	3.5	10%†	35%, 2 yr	NS (n = 14)	Körbling et al., 1989 [83]
23	33	17–50		Mafosfamide	4	13%†	51%, 2 yr	NS (n = 11)	
64	36	16–53	Cy-TBI	Mafosfamide	5	NS	58%, 5 yr	25%, 5 yr	Laporte et al., 1994 [121]
32	39	17–59	Bu-etoposide	4-HC	3	47%†	76%, 4 yr	22%, 4 yr	Linker et al., 1993 [102]
82¶	40	16–57	BCNU-cytarabine-Cy-thiguanine-doxorubicin	—	5	10%†	53%, 5 yr	48%, 5 yr	McMillan et al., 1990 [122]
74	31	5–53	Melphalan-TBI	—	4	20%†	34%, 5 yr	53%, 5 yr	Mehta et al., 1995 [77]
25	20	5–40	BCNU-amsacrine-etoposide-cytarabine (BAVC)	—	6	4%†	48%, 4 yr	NS (n = 12)	Meloni et al., 1989 [123]
14	30	19–48	Cy-TBI	—	5	14%†	67%, 4 yr	NS (n = 1)	
11**	10	1–16	Melphalan	—	4	0%†	55.7%, 2 yr	44.3%, 2 yr	Michel et al., 1988 [124]
18	35	21–51	Cy-BCNU-etoposide (CBV)	—	6	39%	56%, 4 yr	NS (n = 8)	Spinolo et al., 1990 [97]
24§	40	14–62	BuCy4	—	4	4%	35%, 2 yr	60%, 2 yr	Sanz et al., 1993 [125]
24	7	0–14	Melphalan/BuCy2	—	4	46%	87%, 5 yr	13%, 5 yr	Tiedemann et al., 1993 [126]

CR = complete remission; DFS = disease-free survival; NS = not specified; yr = year.

* Defined as FAB-M3, inv(16), or t(8;21).

† Incomplete cytogenetic data.

‡ Intent-to-treat analysis; includes four patients relapsing before ABMT.

§ Peripheral blood stem cell transplantation.

¶ 26 patients received double autografts.

** Double transplants; marrow for the second ABMT harvested after the first ABMT.

controversial because a number of chemotherapeutic regimens, especially those containing high-dose cytarabine, result in excellent long-term disease-free survival of selected groups of patients [116].

Table 23.4 shows the results of autografting for AML in first remission from different transplant teams using a variety of conditioning regimens with or without purging [77,83,95,97,102,117–126]. As the table shows, the remission–transplant interval and the proportion of patients with good-risk disease vary considerably between series, confounding interpretation of the data. Additionally, few studies provide information on the amount of consolidation chemotherapy administered before harvesting the marrow, which may affect the outcome of the transplant procedure significantly [78]. The estimates of survival range from 34 to 87%, and relapse rates from 13 to 60%.

A recent analysis from the International Bone Marrow Transplant Registry (IBMTR) and the North American Auto-logous Blood and Marrow Transplant Registry (NAABMTR), showed leukaemia-free survival after ABMT and allogeneic BMT from matched siblings for AML in first remission to be comparable [127]. For 432 patients autografted with purged or unpurged marrow in first remission, the actuarial 2-year probabilities of disease-free survival and relapse were 55 and 36% respectively. EBMT data shows allografting to be superior to autografting for AML, with lower relapse rates, higher transplant-related mortality and better disease-free survival in both adults and children [128]. For 598 adults autografted in first remission, the disease-free survival and relapse were 42% and 27% respectively, and younger age, FAB-M3 subtype and a longer remission–transplant interval were found to affect the outcome favourably. For 113 children autografted in first remission, the disease-free survival was 47%, with purging affecting the outcome favourably.

In an earlier EBMT analysis of 671 AML patients autografted in first remission [129], patients with no high risk factor had a

462   *Chapter 23*

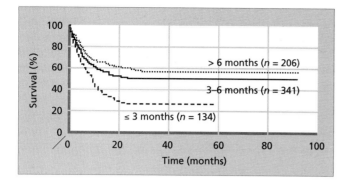

Fig. 23.1 Effect of the remission–transplant interval on disease-free survival after autografting for AML in first remission (*P* < 0.0001). LFS = leukaemia-free survival. (From Gorin *et al.*, 1991 [129], with permission.)

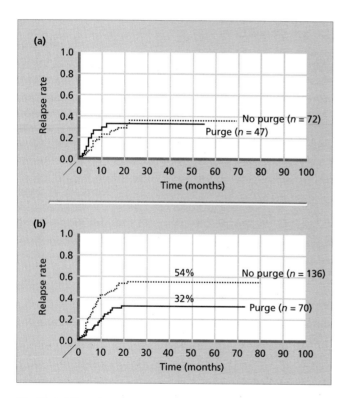

Fig. 23.2 Effect of purging on relapse rates of AML patients transplanted in first remission after conditioning regimens containing TBI. (a) Patients attaining remission within 40 days (*P* = NS). (b) Patients attaining remission in more than 40 days (*P* = 0.005). (From Gorin *et al.*, 1991 [129], with permission.)

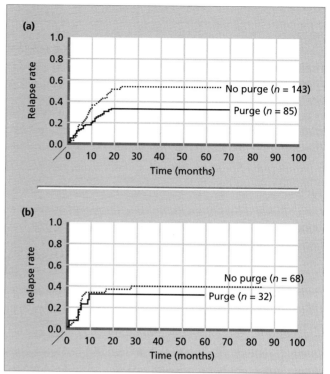

Fig. 23.3 Effect of purging on relapse rates of AML patients transplanted in first remission after conditioning regimens containing TBI. (a) Patients autografted within 6 months of attaining remission (*P* = 0.02). (b) Patients autografted beyond 6 months of attaining remission (*P* = NS). (From Gorin *et al.*, 1991 [129], with permission.)

7-year disease-free survival of 48% and a relapse rate of 41%. Secondary leukaemia was associated with a significantly poorer disease-free survival (19% at 1 year) and a higher relapse rate (76%). The results with conditioning regimens, with or without TBI, were comparable. Patients attaining remission within 40 days had a better disease-free survival (53 vs 42%, *P* = 0.03) and a lower relapse rate (46 vs 57%, *P* =

0.03). With remission–transplant intervals of less than 3 months, 3–6 months and more than 6 months, the disease-free survival was 26, 49 and 55% respectively, and the relapse rates 63, 38 and 36% (*P* < 0.0001; Fig. 23.1). In patients conditioned with TBI-containing regimens, purging was found to decrease relapse in patients who required more than 40 days to attain remission (Fig. 23.2) and in those transplanted within 6 months of attaining remission (Fig. 23.3). Purging of the marrow showed apparently superior results in patients transplanted before 1988, but the magnitude of the advantage decreased when patients transplanted in 1988–89 were included. One explanation for this may be improved chemotherapy, which may eliminate the disease from the patient more effectively. This would be expected to benefit only patients receiving unpurged grafts.

The European Organization for Research and Treatment of Cancer (EORTC) and the Gruppo Italiano Malattie Ematologiche Maligne Dell'Adulto (GIMEMA) cooperative group recently reported the results of a prospective study evaluating BMT [108]. Consolidation therapy, with intermediate-dose cytarabine and amsacrine, was given to 623 patients attaining remission after daunorubicin and cytarabine. At this stage, 168 patients with an HLA-identical sibling were assigned to

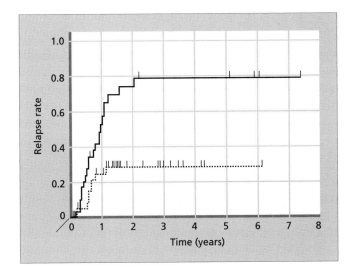

Fig. 23.4 Effect of the number of courses of consolidation chemotherapy on relapse after unpurged autografting in 74 patients with AML in first remission ($P = 0.0011$). Patients underwent either less than two courses (—) or two or more courses (---). (From Mehta *et al.*, 1995 [130], with permission.)

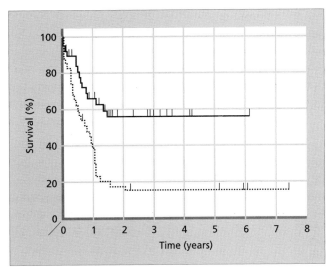

Fig. 23.5 Effect of the number of courses of consolidation chemotherapy on disease-free survival after unpurged autografting in 74 patients with AML in first remission ($P = 0.0008$). Patients underwent either less than two courses (---) or two or more courses (—). (From Mehta *et al.*, 1995 [130], with permission.)

undergo allogeneic BMT, and 254 were randomly assigned to unpurged ABMT or a second course of consolidation chemotherapy with daunorubicin and high-dose cytarabine. Ninety-five patients actually underwent ABMT, and 104 received intensive consolidation chemotherapy. The relapse rate was higher in the chemotherapy group than in the ABMT group, whereas the treatment-related mortality was higher in the ABMT group. The actuarial 4-year disease-free survival with ABMT was significantly better than that with chemotherapy (48 vs 30%). However, the overall survival was similar in both groups, because some of the patients relapsing after chemotherapy became disease-free survivors with ABMT in second remission.

In a single-centre study of 74 first-remission patients [77], Mehta *et al.* [130] showed that the 5-year probability of relapse for patients receiving two or more courses of consolidation chemotherapy before the marrow harvest was significantly lower than that for patients receiving less than two courses (28.2 vs 78.2%, $P = 0.0011$) (Fig. 23.4). The 5-year probability of disease-free survival for patients receiving two or more courses of consolidation chemotherapy was significantly higher than that for patients receiving less than two courses (55.6 vs 15.1%, $P = 0.0008$) (Fig. 23.5). Although multivariate analysis identified the number of courses of chemotherapy as the only significant factor affecting relapse, the remission–transplant duration was closely linked to the number of courses of consolidation chemotherapy. The median remission–transplant intervals for patients receiving less than two and two or more courses of consolidation chemotherapy were 85 days and 147 days, respectively. It was concluded that the effects of time-censoring (remission–transplant interval)

and intensity of consolidation chemotherapy were intimately intertwined, and would be very difficult to separate.

Haematopoietic reconstitution after ABMT for AML is very slow, and platelet recovery often takes months [77]. In order to hasten the recovery of the blood counts, Sanz *et al.* employed PBSCT after busulphan-cyclophosphamide in 24 patients with AML in first remission [125]. Among the 22 patients evaluable for engraftment, neutrophil recovery to 0.5×10^9/l occurred at a median of 13 days (range 10–17 days), and platelets reached 50×10^9/l at a median of 19 days (range 12–213 days). However, the stem cells were collected immediately after remission was reached, before any consolidation chemotherapy. This resulted in a relatively high actuarial 4-year relapse rate of 66% with a 30% disease-free survival. The next 12 patients received a course of consolidation therapy before the stem cell harvest, and a second course of consolidation chemotherapy after the harvest before the transplant [131]. The disease-free survival of the latter group, with a shorter follow-up, is better at 60%, with a relapse risk of 31%.

Apart from historical comparisons within the EBMT database [128,129], evidence to support *ex vivo* purging is limited. Rowley *et al.* [132] used the GM-CFU content of the graft after 4-HC treatment as a measure of the efficacy of *ex vivo* purging of leukaemic cells from autologous marrow grafts in 45 AML patients. Patients who relapsed after ABMT had 4.2% GM-CFU survival after purging, compared with 1.1% in patients who remained in remission ($P = 0.06$). Conversely, the 23 patients with a greater than 1% GM-CFU content had a significantly lower disease-free survival than the 22 patients with a 1% or less GM-CFU content (12 vs 36%, $P = 0.006$).

These results suggest that the effective purging of the marrow is important.

Double autografts, where the marrow for the second procedure is harvested after the first graft, may maximize antileukaemic effects by harvesting better quality marrow after an *in vivo* purge (first graft) and decreasing the procedure-related toxicity by dividing drug delivery into two stages. Twenty-eight of the 82 patients treated by McMillan *et al.* received double autografts [122]. The projected leukaemia-free survival for these patients was 67%, compared with 40% for those receiving a single graft. Not all the patients eligible for a second graft could receive it because of early relapse, poor haematopoietic recovery after the first graft, or refusal.

There appears to be more consensus on the value of autografting for AML beyond the first remission. Long-term disease-free survival of patients with advanced disease (second remission or beyond) who receive chemotherapy only is very poor. High-dose therapy and autografting can result in prolonged disease-free survival in a number of these patients. The occurrence of remission inversion, i.e. a longer disease-free survival after autografting than before, is a measure of the efficacy of the procedure in an individual patient transplanted beyond the first remission. Table 23.5 summarizes the results of autografting for AML beyond the first remission [84,102,103,121,133–137]. The estimates of disease-free survival range from 19 to 61%, and relapse from 25 to 70%. The results of most of these studies are likely to be biased by biological patient selection, as the proportion of relapsing patients who reach the stage of an autograft is likely to be small.

Schiffman *et al.* harvested and cryopreserved marrow in 98 AML patients at a median of 6 months after achieving first remission, with the intention of performing an ABMT early in the first untreated relapse [138]. Sixty-five of the 98 patients relapsed at a median of 7 months (range 1–53 months) after marrow storage. Thirty-eight (58%) of these proceeded to ABMT in the first untreated relapse, and had a 4-year disease-free survival of 13%. However, the 3-year survival of the 17 most recent patients autografted after busulphan-containing conditioning regimens was 41%. The actuarial 2-year and 4-year survival for the entire group of 65 relapsing patients was 22 and 8% respectively. The relatively poor results of this prospectively studied, unselected group of patients suggests that there certainly is some patient selection with other single-centre reports.

The better disease-free survival seen in patients with advanced AML treated with busulphan-containing regimens [138] is similar to the earlier observations of Chopra *et al.*, who reported 33% disease-free survival and 44% survival at 3 years after busulphan-cyclophosphamide conditioning in 34 patients transplanted with unpurged marrow in the first untreated relapse or second remission [133]. Meloni *et al.* [103] reported a 5-year disease-free survival of 53% among 21 AML patients transplanted in second remission with unpurged marrow after BAVC conditioning (Table 23.3). Remission inversion was seen in all the long-term survivors. It is possible than busulphan- or chemotherapy-based conditioning regimens are better than TBI-containing regimens beyond the first remission.

Table 23.5 Autografting for AML beyond first remission.

Patients (no.)	Age (years) Median	Range	Stage	Conditioning regimen	Purging	Actuarial probability of DFS	Actuarial probability of relapse	References
9*	33	21–62	Rel1	BuCy2/BuCy4	—	30%, 3 yr	NS (*n* = 6)	Chopra *et al.*, 1991 [133]
25†	40	21–60	CR2		—	48%, 3 yr	NS (*n* = 9)	
20	32	17–53	CR2	Cy-TBI	Mafosfamide	34%, 5 yr	48%, 5 yr	Laporte *et al.*, 1994 [121]
13	5	1–13	CR2	BuCy4	4-HC	61%, 3 yr	NS (*n* = 5)	Lenarsky *et al.*, 1990 [134]
26	38	15–58	CR2/3 (21) CR1 (5)‡	Bu-etoposide	4-HC	56%, 4 yr	25%, 4 yr	Linker *et al.*, 1993 [102]
21	24	1–47	CR2	BAVC	—	52%, 4 yr	45%, 4 yr	Meloni *et al.*, 1990 [103]
21	35	4–54	Rel1	BuCy/BuCy-TBI	4-HC (62%)	45%, 3 yr	30%, 3 yr	Petersen *et al.*, 1993 [84]
26	37	2–54	CR2		4-HC (54%)	32%, 3 yr	44%, 3 yr	
24	33	10–61	≥CR2	BuCy/Cy-TBI/ BuCy-cytarabine	4-HC§	19%, 3 yr	70%, 3 yr	Rosenfeld *et al.*, 1989 [135]
45	36	11–57	CR2/3	Cy-TBI/BuCy2	MAbs	31%, 5 yr	52% 5 yr	Selvaggi *et al.*, 1994 [136]
24	7	1–15	CR2	BuCy4	4-HC	40%, 3 yr	56%, 3 yr	Yeager *et al.*, 1990 [137]

CR = complete remission; DFS = disease-free survival; MAbs = monoclonal antibodies; NS = not specified; Rel = relapse; yr = year.

* Two patients received peripheral blood stem cells in addition to marrow.

† One patient received peripheral blood stem cells in addition to marrow.

‡ Five patients who were refractory to high-dose cytarabine-containing induction therapy but attained CR with other salvage therapy have been classified as having 'advanced disease'.

§ Unpurged back-up marrow infused in seven patients.

Chopra *et al.* showed that the timing of the marrow harvest (first or second remission), the stage of the disease at ABMT (relapse or second remission), the type of chemotherapy after the first relapse (high-dose cytarabine or not, and consolidation chemotherapy or not) or the conditioning regimen (BuCy4 or BuCy2) made no significant impact on the outcome [133].

As in the first remission, IBMTR and NAABMTR data show leukaemia-free survival after ABMT and allogeneic BMT from matched siblings to be comparable in AML in second remission [127]. For 175 patients autografted in second remission with purged or unpurged marrow, the 2-year actuarial probabilities of disease-free survival and relapse were 39 and 53%, respectively [127]. For 190 adults autografted in second remission in the EBMT, the disease-free survival and relapse were 30 and 63% respectively [128].

The results of allogeneic BMT cannot be easily compared with those of ABMT, because of immunological graft-vs-leukaemia reactions which contribute significantly to the control of minimal residual disease [1]. Biologically, syngeneic marrow can be considered the ideal autologous graft, as it is tumour-free and it has not been compromised by the action of chemotherapy or purging. However, the number of leukaemia patients with identical twin donors is limited, and only 69 syngeneic transplants for acute leukaemia in first remission were reported to the IBMTR between 1978 and 1990 [139]. Three-year probabilities of disease-free survival and relapse after syn-

geneic BMT for AML in first remission were 42 and 52% respectively [139]. Although no direct comparisons are available, these results do not appear to be significantly better than most reports of unpurged autografting. They emphasize that while leukaemic contamination of infused marrow may contribute to relapse in some cases [35], most relapses occur as a result of incomplete eradication of the malignant clone from the patient, and that purging of autologous marrow is probably unnecessary in the majority of patients.

Acute lymphoblastic leukaemia

While conventional treatment of childhood acute lymphoblastic leukaemia (ALL) results in cure of the disease in a significant proportion of patients, relapse and death are the most likely outcomes after conventional combination chemotherapy of adult ALL, despite remission rates of up to 90%. Characteristics associated with a poor prognosis, apart from age, include a high leucocyte count at diagnosis, unfavourable karyotypes, extramedullary disease at presentation, B-cell lineage and prolonged time (over 4 weeks) to the achievement of remission [140]. Most reported studies of autografting in ALL, therefore, involve high-risk patients in the first remission or patients beyond the first remission who do not have suitable allogeneic donors. One of the earliest reported autografts was performed in a patient with relapsed refractory ALL almost four decades ago [3].

Table 23.6 Autografting for ALL in first remission.

Patients (no.)	Age (years) Median	Age (years) Range	Conditioning regimen	Purging	Median CR–BMT interval (months)	Patients with Ph+ disease	Actuarial probability of DFS	Actuarial probability of relapse	References
10	28	2–45	Cy-TBI/etoposide-TBI	MAbs (n = 7)	NS (>6)	NS	50%, 3 yr	27%, 3 yr	Doney *et al.*, 1993 [141]
95*	NS	69% ⩽ 35	Cy-TBI	Mafosfamide/ MAbs (n = 52)	4	3%†	39%, 3 yr*	NS	Fière *et al.*, 1993 [106]
27	18	11–45	Cy-TBI/cytarabine-Cy-TBI	MAbs	2	4%†	32%, 5 yr	67%, 5 yr	Gilmore *et al.*, 1991 [142]
35	29	17–55	Cy-TBI	Mafosfamide	5	9%†	56%, 5 yr	37%, 5 yr	Laporte *et al.*, 1994 [121]
50‡	26	15–58	Melphalan-TBI/melphalan	MAbs (n = 7)	2	10%†	53%, 5 yr	31%, 5 yr	Powles *et al.*, 1995 [86]
10	35	15–50	Melphalan-TBI	—	NS (>6)	NS	30%, 3 yr	NS (n = 5)	Proctor *et al.*, 1988 [143]
34	29	16–59	Cy-TBI/melphalan-TBI	MAbs/4-HC/ mafosfamide/ etoposide (n = 24)	5.5	3%†	27%, 5 yr	65%, 5 yr	Vey *et al.*, 1994 [144]

CR = complete remission; DFS = disease-free survival; MAbs, monoclonal antibodies; NS = not specified.

* Intent-to-treat analysis; includes 32 patients not receiving ABMT in first CR.

† Incomplete data.

‡ 12 patients received peripheral blood stem cells and all eligible patients received 6-mercaptopurine and methotrexate post-transplant.

The results of autografting in ALL depend on the age of the patient, the stage of the disease at the time of the transplant, the karyotype and the response to previous therapy. The best results for high-risk patients are obtained in the first remission, and for others beyond the first remission. Tables 23.6 and 23.7 show the results of autografting for ALL in first remission [86,106,121,141–144] and beyond the first remission [46,60,61,85,136,141,145], respectively. In the absence of detailed data on most other prognostic features, Ph+ disease has been considered the main high-risk factor in Table 23.6. The probability of leukaemia-free survival for patients autografted in first remission ranges from 27 to 56%, and for relapse from 27 to 67%; the corresponding figures for patients transplanted for advanced disease are from 0 to 58% and from 40 to 100%.

Monoclonal antibodies and pharmacological agents have been utilized extensively in purging autologous marrow before transplantation in ALL (Tables 23.1, 23.6 & 23.7), but relapse continues to be the main problem. Uckun *et al.* autografted 28 patients with high-risk ALL, using marrow purged with a combination of monoclonal antibodies (B-lineage) or immunotoxins (T-lineage) and 4-HC [71,73]. In both these groups of patients, minimal residual disease was quantitated in the pretransplant remission marrow and in the purged marrow with a combination of fluorescence-activated multiparametric flow cytometry and leukaemic progenitor cell assays. High numbers of residual leukaemic progenitors detected in the remission marrow samples before transplant predicted relapse, whereas the efficacy of purging and the number of leukaemic progenitors remaining in the graft after purging did not. These results suggest that the main reason for relapse in the population studied was inadequate elimination of disease from the patient by the conditioning regimen, rather than inefficient purging.

Maintenance chemotherapy with 6-mercaptopurine and methotrexate is an integral part of the conventional therapy of childhood ALL to prevent early relapse, and is presumed to be useful in adult ALL because its omission has been associated with high relapse rates [146]. As an autograft procedure is essentially very intensive consolidation therapy, it is logical to administer prolonged maintenance chemotherapy afterwards to decrease relapse rates. However, this strategy has been adequately evaluated by only one group [64,86,100]. Powles *et al.* have pioneered the approach of maintenance chemotherapy with oral 6-mercaptopurine and methotrexate for a period of 2 years after autografting in ALL [86]. Despite a short median remission–transplant interval of 2 months, the relatively low 5-year relapse rate of 31% seen in their group of adult ALL patients may be attributable to the post-transplant therapy.

Fière *et al.* compared ABMT to conventional chemotherapy in first remission in adult patients under the age of 50 years who did not have HLA-identical siblings [106]. Based on

Table 23.7 Autografting for ALL beyond first remission.

Patients (no.)	Age (years) Median	Age (years) Range	Stage	Conditioning regimen	Purging	Actuarial probability of DFS	Actuarial probability of relapse	Reference
51	9	3–18	CR2 (*n* = 31) CR3 (*n* = 19) CR4 (*n* = 1)	Cytarabine-TBI/ teniposide-Cy-cytarabine-TBI	MAbs	58%, 3 yr	NS (*n* = 18)	Billett *et al.*, 1993 [60]
56	11	4–19	CR2 (*n* = 36) CR > 2 (*n* = 20)	Vincristine-Cy-TBI/Cy-TBI/ BuCy	Vincristine-Prednisolone (*n* = 32), Mafosfamide (*n* = 16)	21%, 4 yr	NS (*n* = 25)	Colleselli *et al.*, 1991 [46]
27	18	4–44	CR2	Cy-TBI	MAbs (*n* = 18)	27%, 3 yr	69%, 3 yr	Doney *et al.*, 1993 [141]
25	12	2–46	CR > 2	Etoposide-TBI	MAbs (*n* = 12)			
27*	19	6–47	Rel		MAbs/4-HC (*n* = 12)	8%, 3 yr	90%, 3 yr	
22	5	1–16†	≥CR2	Etoposide-TBI	MAbs	18%, 3 yr	80%, 3 yr	Schmid *et al.*, 1993 [61]
24	NS	<16	CR2 (*n* = 17) CR3 (*n* = 7)	Melphalan-TBI	MAbs (*n* = 6)	45%, 3 yr	NS (*n* = 8)	Schroeder *et al.*, 1991 [85]
22‡	28	18–54	≥CR2	Cy-TBI/ cytarabine-Cy-TBI	MAbs	20%, 3 yr	NS (*n* = 13)	Soiffer *et al.*, 1993 [145]
9	9	3–15	CR2	Cy-TBI	4-HC	0%, 1.5 yr	100%, 1.5 yr	Yeager *et al.*, 1990 [137]

CR = complete remission; MAbs = monoclonal antibodies; NS = not specified; Rel = relapse.

* 7 patients received interferon after ABMT.

† Age at diagnosis; 12 patients received IFN-τ and IL-2 after ABMT.

‡ Includes one patient in first CR.

an intention-to-treat analysis, ABMT (95 patients) and chemotherapy (96 patients) resulted in comparable 3-year disease-free survival rates (39 vs 32%). However, late relapses after 36 months were mainly observed in the chemotherapy arm, and early post-transplant relapse remained an important cause of treatment failure. It is possible that post-transplant maintenance chemotherapy in a setting like this may reduce the incidence of early post-transplant relapse, thus improving the disease-free survival.

Graft-vs-leukaemia reactions are least marked after allografting for ALL in first remission [1]. In view of this, to avoid the morbidity and mortality associated with allogeneic BMT, Mehta *et al.* have developed a sequential approach to the treatment of adult ALL [100]. In their sequential high-dose therapy programme, patients aged 15 years and over who were in first remission after standard induction and intensification therapy underwent PBSCT after high-dose melphalan ($200 \, mg/m^2$), irrespective of the availability of HLA-identical siblings. Two-year maintenance chemotherapy with daily 6-mercaptopurine was begun when the leucocytes reached $3 \times 10^9/l$ and the platelets $100 \times 10^9/l$. Relapsing patients underwent allografts from matched siblings or unrelated donors in the second remission after high-dose VP-16 (60 mg/kg) and TBI (1050 cGy as a single fraction). Of the 16 patients treated between 1993 and 1995, 12 were alive in continuous remission after PBSCT, and three of four relapsing patients were alive after sibling allografts in second remission. With limited follow-up, the projected 2-year survival and disease-free survival were 85.7 and 68.4%, respectively (Fig. 23.6).

The outcome of Ph+ ALL remains disappointing with conventional chemotherapy [147,148]. There are anecdotal reports of long-term leukaemia-free survival after autografting in Ph+ ALL [149,150]. Carella *et al.* have harvested Ph-peripheral blood stem cells in patients with Ph+ ALL during haematopoietic recovery after myelosuppressive chemotherapy [151]. However, with adequate induction chemotherapy, a number of patients with Ph+ ALL can attain cytogenetic remissions which are sustained long enough for marrow or blood cells to be harvested. Therefore, the exact utility of the approach suggested by Carella *et al.* remains to be defined. Interferon alpha (IFNα) can suppress the malignant clone in CML, but data on its efficacy in Ph+ ALL are limited. It is possible, in cases of minimal residual disease after ABMT, prolonged maintenance therapy with IFNα may eradicate the malignant clone, and this is being explored in the current MRC UKALL 12 Adult ALL Study.

Chronic myeloid leukaemia

There is a considerable amount of evidence to show that normal stem cells are present in CML patients: intensive chemotherapy in CML patients with exclusively Ph+ haematopoiesis can result in restoration of partial or complete Ph negativity [152], and IFNα treatment can result in partial or complete cytogenetic remission [153]. These data suggest that autografting in CML could result in remission and prolongation of the natural course of the disease, without being curative.

Autologous BMT was initially used in CML to re-establish a short-lived second chronic phase in patients with advanced disease [6]. Autografting in the chronic phase has been shown to result in improved survival, as a result of prolongation of the natural history of the disease [154].

McGlave *et al.* reported 200 CML patients who were autografted using blood or marrow at one of eight centres over a period of 7 years [154]. In 21 patients, the marrow was cultured *ex vivo* before infusion [66], and in 23, the marrow was incubated with recombinant human interferon gamma [50] to select normal haematopoietic progenitors. At the time of the report, 125 of the 200 patients were alive after transplant, with a follow-up of 1–91 months (median 30 months). The survival after transplantation of the chronic-phase patients ($n = 142$) was significantly superior ($P < 0.0001$) to those transplanted in the accelerated phase ($n = 30$) or in blast crisis or in the second chronic phase ($n = 28$). Not a single blast-crisis patient survived beyond 2.5 years, whereas the actuarial survival of chronic-phase patients was 58% at 4 years. Interestingly, the last of the 36 deaths in the chronic-phase group occurred at 43.3 months, resulting in a plateau in the survival curve beyond this time (Fig. 23.7). Although these data provide good evidence that autografting prolongs the survival of patients with CML considerably, the apparent survival plateau must be interpreted with some caution, because some patients with CML do tend to survive for long periods of time on conventional or no therapy. Additionally, interferon therapy confers a significant survival benefit without an autograft. Data on post-transplant

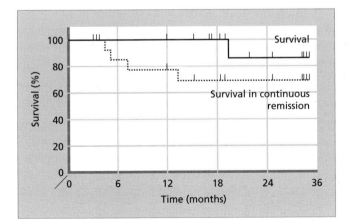

Fig. 23.6 Outcome of 16 adult patients with ALL receiving sequential high-dose chemotherapy at the Royal Marsden Hospital. The disease-free survival curve represents 12 patients in continuous remission after a peripheral blood stem cell autograft. The overall survival curve includes three additional patients who are alive without disease after sibling allografts in second remission.

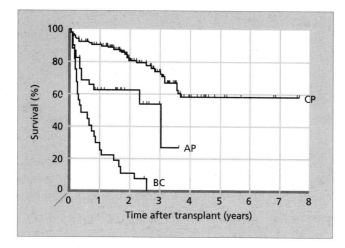

Fig. 23.7 Overall survival of patients receiving autologous transplants for CML by disease stage at transplant. AP = accelerated phase; BC = blast crisis or second chronic phase; CP = chronic phase. (From McGlave *et al.*, 1994 [154], with permission. © The Lancet Ltd.)

maintenance therapy with interferon in the surviving patients in this series were not available.

The marrow or blood used for autografting may be Ph+, or partially or completely Ph−. Infusion of Ph+ cells can also result in establishment of transiently Ph− haematopoiesis [155]. Infusion of Ph− cells may result in long-lasting restoration of Ph− haematopoiesis. Relapse after autografting in CML may be caused by persistent leukaemia in the patient and/or leukaemic cells in the infused autologous marrow or blood. Deisseroth *et al.* [156] used retroviral gene-marking techniques to show, in two CML patients autografted in blast crisis with marked cells, that sufficient numbers of leukemia cells remained in the infused marrow to contribute to systemic relapse. Talpaz *et al.* [157] showed that the extent of Ph negativity seen after autografting depended on the extent of the suppression of the malignant clone in the harvested material after the myelosuppressive chemotherapy used to mobilize the cells. These data argue in favour of using partially or totally Ph− 'normal' cells for autografting in order to obtain cytogenetic remissions after transplantation. In patients who show no cytogenetic response to IFNα, a number of techniques have been utilized to obtain normal progenitor cells.

The Vancouver Group have autografted 22 CML patients (16 in the first chronic phase and six beyond the first chronic phase) with marrow cultured *ex vivo* to establish Ph− haematopoiesis after myeloablative therapy [66]. During haematopoietic recovery post-transplant, the marrow was 100% Ph− in 13 patients and 75–94% Ph− in three. Five patients required an infusion of back-up unmanipulated Ph+ cells because of failure of neutrophil recovery by 6 weeks. Ph+ cells became detectable at a median of 1 year (4–36 months) post-transplant in all surviving patients who had attained Ph negativity post-transplant.

Carella *et al.* have developed the approach of harvesting

Ph− progenitor cells by leukapheresis during recovery from chemotherapy-induced myelosuppression in patients with CML [158]. Forty patients with Ph+ CML received intensive combination chemotherapy with idarubicin, cytarabine and etoposide (ICE), followed by G-CSF. Four to eight leukaphereses were performed early during recovery from marrow hypoplasia when the leucocyte count was 0.5–2.0 × 10⁹/l and increasing. In seven of 10 patients with chronic-phase disease, the harvests were cytogenetically normal, and in five they were *BCR/ABL* negative by PCR. Mehta *et al.* [98] obtained 33 cytogenetically evaluable harvests in 10 patients after ICE chemotherapy. Six of these showed few or no metaphases, while seven were 100% Ph−, four more than 50% Ph−, seven less than 50% Ph− and nine 100% Ph+. None of the harvests evaluated was negative for *BCR/ABL* by PCR. Four of six patients harvested in the first chronic phase showed significant cytogenetic response, compared with none of four harvested beyond the first chronic phase (*P* = 0.036). Nine of 19 harvests from first-chronic-phase patients were significantly Ph−, compared with two of 14 from patients with advanced disease (*P* = 0.047).

Other approaches to chemotherapy-induced mobilization of Ph− cells have utilized high-dose hydroxyurea [159], daunorubicin-cytarabine [160] or fludarabine-cytarabine-mitoxantrone [160].

Engraftment is usually prompt and consistent with unmanipulated Ph+ marrow [154], but failure of engraftment may be a problem with Ph− cells. Two of four patients autografted by Mehta *et al.* engrafted rapidly, but a third had slow recovery of platelets and a fourth died of graft failure [98]. Two of 12 patients transplanted by Carella *et al.* failed to engraft with mobilized cells, and subsequent rescue with unmanipulated marrow was unsuccessful [158]. O'Brien *et al.* had to reinfuse back-up Ph+ marrow in two of six patients; one patient required three rescue infusions before showing haematopoietic reconstitution [161]. This could be because of quantitatively or qualitatively poor cells in the apheresis product, or a stromal cell defect, or a combination of the two.

Two of three chronic-phase patients transplanted by Carella *et al.* with Ph− cells were alive with Ph− and *BCR/ABL*-negative haematopoiesis 3 and 10 months post-transplant [158]. The two patients transplanted with Ph− cells by Mehta *et al.* were Ph− in the early stages after autografting, but relapsed within a year despite post-transplant maintenance therapy with IFNα [98]. Therefore, longer follow-up on patients who are Ph− soon after transplantation is required, before the exact place of this procedure in the treatment of CML can be defined. Immunomodulation with IL-2 or roquinimex may have a role in attaining or maintaining Ph negativity after autografting [162].

The management of a newly diagnosed patient with CML who is ineligible for an allograft presents a dilemma. Commencement of IFNα treatment confers a significant survival benefit [153], but in the 1–2 years it takes for nonresponders to be identified [163], it may be too late for chemotherapy-induced mobilization of normal progenitors to succeed. On the other hand, the use of severely myelosuppressive chemotherapy which may be associated with significant complications, including death [160], may be difficult to justify in a newly diagnosed patient.

Chronic lymphocytic leukaemia

Conventional therapy of chronic lymphocytic leukaemia (CLL) rarely results in remission and is not curative. Allogeneic and autologous BMT have been shown to result in molecular remission in CLL [62,63]. However, most patients with CLL are unlikely to be eligible for allogeneic BMT, because of their advanced age or a lack of suitable HLA-identical donors.

Treatment with purine analogues, such as fludarabine, can result in an excellent response (CR or nodular CR) in 50–60% of patients, enabling adequate quantities of normal haematopoietic progenitors to be harvested. This autologous material can then be used to consolidate the response to fludarabine with high-dose chemotherapy or chemo/radiotherapy. It is also easy to monitor for minimal residual disease in the harvested material and *in vivo* post-transplantation using flow cytometry for cells coexpressing CD5 and CD19/CD20 (the CLL phenotype) and Southern blotting for monoclonal immunoglobulin (Ig) gene rearrangement.

Bastion *et al.* [164] harvested peripheral blood progenitor cells from two extensively pretreated patients, who were in nodular complete remission after fludarabine therapy. Cells were mobilized with cyclophosphamide and GM-CSF. Both were conditioned with cyclophosphamide, etoposide and fractionated TBI. One patient had rapid myeloid recovery and slow platelet engraftment, and was alive with no microscopic evidence of disease 11 months after the transplant. The other patient had a poor harvest (0.98×10^8 mononuclear cells/kg and 0.9×10^4 GM-CFU/kg), and died of failed engraftment at 3 months.

The Dana-Farber group have treated 32 CLL patients under 60 years of age with poor prognostic features with cyclophosphamide-TBI and monoclonal antibody-purged autologous marrow [62,165]. All patients had attained minimal disease status (<10% marrow involvement, <2 cm lymph nodes and no organomegaly) pretransplant, but they all had molecular evidence of residual disease with persistent monoclonal Ig gene rearrangements. Approximately half the patients did not show cells coexpressing CD5 and CD20. Three patients died as a result of transplant-related causes, three had persistent disease postautograft and one relapsed. Twenty-six patients were alive in remission 1–52 months (median 12 months) post-transplant at the last follow-up [165]. Three patients evaluated at 1 year or beyond did not have detectable monoclonal Ig gene rearrangements [62].

Khouri *et al.* [63] used purged (seven patients) or unpurged (four patients) autografts in 11 patients with advanced CLL who relapsed after fludarabine therapy. The marrow was collected during a previous fludarabine-induced remission. Six

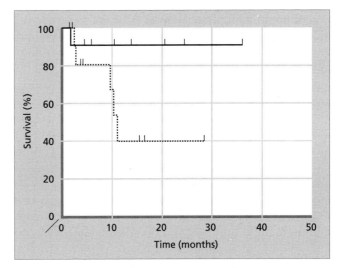

Fig. 23.8 Probability of survival after allogeneic (——) or autologous (----) BMT for CLL. (From Khouri *et al.*, 1994 [63], with permission.)

patients achieved complete remission, four nodular complete remission and one partial remission. Two patients relapsed, and three developed Richter's transformation. Six of the 11 patient were alive in remission at 2–29 months. Unlike the experience of the Dana-Farber group, where allogeneic and autologous BMT resulted in similar disease-free survival, there was a trend towards lower disease-free survival with autografting in the MD Anderson series (Fig. 23.8).

Autografting for CLL is associated with an unusually high rate of opportunistic infections [165], as it is with allogeneic BMT for CLL [166]. It is felt that earlier transplantation, and less aggressive use of purine analogues before the transplantation, may decrease the high rate of infections [165]. This may be easier with allografting, but not so easy with autografting, because purine analogue therapy is essential to achieve a minimal disease state.

Multiple myeloma

McElwain & Powles [167] showed that high-dose melphalan administered without haematopoietic rescue could result in complete remission in myeloma and plasma cell leukaemia. Since then, a large number of myeloma patients have received high-dose chemotherapy or chemo/radiotherapy in nonrandomized studies with autologous haematopoietic support, in order to maximize disease response. Unlike acute leukaemia, where a complete remission is a prerequisite for harvesting autologous stem cells, most myeloma patients are harvested in partial remission (plateau phase), and most complete remissions are attained only *after* the autograft. The attainment of remission and clearance of paraprotein are gradual, and occur over a period of up to 6 months [168].

Table 23.8 shows results of autografting in myeloma [40,75,101,169–173]. The wide variation in outcomes is the result of a variation in pretransplant induction chemotherapy, the different criteria for defining response and the different strategies for maintaining remission after transplantation. It is noteworthy that the average duration of response is only 20–24 months, because with longer follow-up, most patients tend to relapse [101].

Barlogie *et al.* [174] have described a total therapy approach for myeloma where three noncross-resistant chemotherapy regimens are utilized for initial cytoreduction, and are followed by two autografts (or one autograft and one allograft) and maintenance therapy with IFNα. For the first 142 patients followed up for at least 1 year from presentation, the median survival and progression-free survival are 47 and 39 months respectively.

The Royal Marsden Hospital Group have performed a randomized study of maintenance IFNα after high-dose therapy in 84 patients [175,176]. The median progression-free survival was 46 months in the IFNα group and 27 months in the control group (P = 0.03) (Fig. 23.9). Although there appeared to be a small but significant survival advantage for the IFNα group initially [175], with a longer follow-up (median 55 months) this was no longer apparent [176]. One of the reasons for this may be that patients in the control arm were then treated with IFNα at the time of disease progression, resulting in a narrowing of the survival difference between the two groups. Another interesting observation in this study was that the benefit of IFNα was confined to patients attaining complete remission [176], although IFNα administration did not influence the probability of attaining remission [168].

Complete remissions in myeloma, seen after high-dose therapy but rarely with conventional therapy, are associated with the resolution of bone lesions and symptoms. The resultant improvement in the quality of life makes autografting worthwhile, despite the procedure being not curative. Strategies are required to increase the number of patients attaining remission after autografting, and to evolve better post-transplant strategies to maintain the remission.

Hodgkin's disease

The majority of patients with Hodgkin's disease (HD) attain sustained remissions with combination chemotherapy or radiotherapy, and a large proportion become long-term survivors. Patients failing to remit with the initial therapy and those relapsing after achieving remission respond to conven-

Table 23.8 Autografting for multiple myeloma.

Patients (no.)	Age (years) Median	Age (years) Range	Conditioning of cells	Source	Purging	CR after transplant*	Overall CR†	Toxic deaths	Interferon post BMT	Actuarial overall survival	Actuarial progression-free survival	Reference
26	47	35–59	Melphalan-TBI/ Cy-TBI	BM	MAbs	42%	44%	4%	±	52%, 3 yr	38%, 3 yr	Anderson *et al.*, 1991 [169]
15	49	40–57	Melphalan	BM	—	42%	50%	7%	–	NS	78%, 2 yr	Björkstrand *et al.*,
11			Melphalan-TBI	PBSC	—	40%	73%	—	±			1995 [170]
53	52	30–69	Melphalan-methylpred-nisolone	BM	—	72%	77%	2%	–	63%, 3 yr	30%, 3 yr	Cunningham *et al.*, 1994 [101]
40	49	34–64	Thiotepa-Bu-Cy	BM/PBSC	±‡	29%	29%	13%	+	NS	88%, 1 yr§	Dimopoulos *et al.*,
										NS	55%, 1 yr¶	1993 [171]
										NS	0%, 1 yr**	
81	55	26–66	Various ± TBI	BM	—	27%	37%	3%	NS	47%, 4 yr	26%, 4 yr	Harousseau *et al.*,
51	49	36–65		PBSC	—	37%	40%	6%	NS	49%, 4 yr	47%, 4 yr	1995 [172]
75††	50	28–69	Melphalan/ melphalan-TBI	BM + PBSC	—	8%	20%	0%	NS	88%, 1 yr	78%, 1 yr	Jagannath *et al.*, 1992 [173]
14	48	24–60	Bu-Cy-melphalan	BM	4–HC	50%‡‡	57%‡‡	21%	–	10%, 3 yr	10%, 3 yr	Reece *et al.*, 1993 [40]
37	51	34–65	BuCy2	PBSC	CD4+	15%‡‡	15%‡‡	14%	+§§	68%, 1 yr	67%, 1 yr	Schiller *et al.*, 1995 [75]

BM = bone marrow; CR = complete remission; MAbs = monoclonal antibodies; NS = not specified; PBSC = peripheral blood stem cells; yr = year.
* Excludes patients in CR before transplantation and toxic deaths.
† Includes patients in CR before transplantation but excludes toxic deaths.
‡ CD19-coated magnabeads.
§ Patients in partial remission at transplant.
¶ Patients with primary refractory disease at transplant.
** Patients with refractory relapse at transplant.
†† 60 patients reached transplantation; response and mortality figures apply to transplanted patients only, but the survival probabilities apply to the whole group.
‡‡ Includes two patients dying of toxicity who were assessible for response to therapy.
§§ Dexamethasone was also administered (4 days a month).

tional second-line therapy, and some may become long-term survivors. However, the majority of them eventually die of the disease or of treatment-related toxicity. High-dose therapy has been used to salvage relapsed or refractory patients with HD [177–182].

As shown in Table 23.9, varying prognostic factors have been used to identify patients who are likely to benefit from

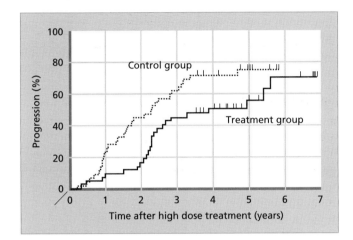

Fig. 23.9 Effect of maintenance therapy with IFNα on progression-free survival after high-dose therapy in multiple myeloma. (From Powles *et al.*, 1994 [175], with permission.)

autografting [177–181]. Anderson *et al.* reported on 127 patients undergoing myeloablative therapy, followed by autologous, allogeneic or syngeneic marrow transplantation for relapsed or refractory HD in Seattle [182]. The 5-year actuarial probabilities of event-free survival, relapse and treatment-related mortality for the entire group were 21, 18, 65 and 49%, respectively. In multivariate analysis, a higher performance status and an absence of bulky disease were associated with a better event-free survival and a decreased relapse, while fewer previous treatment regimens were associated with an improved event-free survival and a lower treatment-related mortality. These data, and those from the table, indicate that outcome is better if transplantation is performed early after relapse, when the disease burden is less, tumour chemosensitivity is greater and the patient's general condition is better.

Much of the past concern over high-dose therapy for the lymphomas has been due to the morbidity, mortality and expense associated with the procedure. All of these have improved considerably over the past few years, because of technical advances, increased experience and better patient selection. At the University of Nebraska, over a 5-year period from 1987 to 1991, the mortality associated with autografting for lymphoma fell from 20–29% to 0–4%, the average hospitalization from 45–51 days to 32–38 days, and the cost from US$ 91–96 000 to 55–74 000 [183].

Carella *et al.* treated 15 patients with very poor prognosis HD in first remission with high-dose chemotherapy and ABMT

Table 23.9 Autografting for Hodgkin's disease.

Patients (no.)	Age (years) Median	Age (years) Range	Stage at transplant	Conditioning regimen	Toxic deaths	Subgroups analysed for outcome	Actuarial overall survival	Actuarial progression-free survival	Reference
155	29	14–54	Refractory/ relapsed	BEAM	10%	All Chemoresistant Chemosensitive Untested	55%, 5 yr	50%, 5 yr 32%, 5 yr 52%, 5 yr 78%, 5 yr	Chopra *et al.*, 1993 [177]
56	32	17–51	Relapsed	CBV	7%	All Marrow involved Marrow not involved	56%, 3 yr	37%, 3 yr 27%, 3 yr 47%, 3 yr	Kessinger *et al.*, 1991 [178]
85	32	16–56	Refractory/ relapsed	Etoposide-Cy-TBI/CBV	13%	All 1–2 prior regimens ≥3 prior regimens	76%, 2 yr	58%, 2 yr 75%, 2 yr 45%, 2 yr	Nademanee *et al.*, 1995 [179]
58	29	13–51	Relapsed	CBV ± cisplatin	5%	All 0 poor prognostic factors* 1 poor prognostic factor 2 poor prognostic factors 3 poor prognostic factors	72%, 3 yr	64%, 3 yr 100%, 3 yr 81%, 3 yr 40%, 3 yr 0%, 1 yr	Reece *et al.*, 1994 [180]
47	27	12–48	Refractory/ relapsed	Total lymphoid irradiation-etoposide-Cy	17%	All Refractory Relapsed	NS	50%, 4 yr 33%, 4 yr 79%, 4 yr	Yahalom *et al.*, 1993 [181]

NS = not specified; yr = years.

* 'B' symptoms at relapse, length of remission <1 year, extranodal disease at relapse.

[184]. Thirteen of these patients (86.6%) were alive in remission at a median of 36 months post-transplant, compared with eight (33%) of a historic control group of 24 first-remission patients with the same poor prognostic factors who were not autografted. The encouraging results of this pilot study must be confirmed in a prospective randomized study, evaluating high-dose therapy consolidation for high-risk disease in first remission.

Non-Hodgkin's lymphoma

Approximately 30–40% of patients with non-Hodgkin's lymphoma (NHL) do not achieve a complete remission with initial chemotherapy, and 40–50% relapse after attaining a remission. Conventional-dose salvage chemotherapy results in responses in 20–60% of patients, but the remissions are rarely sustained. However, as Table 23.10 shows [23,44,104,185–187], high-dose chemotherapy or chemo/radiotherapy with autologous haematopoietic support results in long-term survival of selected groups of patients. Most of these reports have evaluated prognostic factors which may be able to identify patients who are likely to derive significant benefit from high-dose therapy.

Usually chemosensitive disease tends to respond to high-dose therapy. However, whether to give relapsed patients salvage chemotherapy to determine chemosensitivity or to proceed straight into an autograft is debatable. Among those patients failing to attain a complete remission with initial therapy, patients achieving a partial response may benefit from high-dose therapy, but those with primary refractory disease usually do not.

Autografting in first remission in high-risk lymphomas is controversial, and two recent studies have cast doubt on the utility of early autografting. A randomized study by a French cooperative group evaluated high-dose chemotherapy consolidation of intermediate- and high-grade lymphoma in first remission [109]. Two hundred and thirty patients received CBV (cyclophosphamide, BCNU, etoposide) and autograft, and 234 received sequential conventional-dose chemotherapy (ifosfamide, etoposide, asparaginase, cytarabine). With a median follow-up duration of 28 months, the 3-year survival and disease-free survival in the chemotherapy arm (71%

Table 23.10 Autografting for non-Hodgkin's lymphoma.

Patients (no.)	Age (years) Median	Age (years) Range	Histological grade (stage)	Conditioning regimen	Toxic deaths	Subgroups analysed for outcome	Actuarial overall survival	Actuarial progression-free survival	References
107	38	16–64	Intermediate/high (Refractory/relapsed)	BEAM	7%	All Chemoresistant Chemosensitive Untested	41%, 5 yr	35%, 5 yr 13%, 5 yr 49%, 5 yr 57%, 2 yr	Mills *et al.*, 1995 [104]
53	NS	>40	Intermediate/high (42), low (11) (Refractory/relapsed)	BCNU-etoposide-cytarabine-Cy/other ± TBI	NS	All Bulky disease Minimal disease	NS	40%, 2 yr 48%, 2 yr 25%, 2 yr	Rapoport *et al.*, 1993 [185]
121*	43	24–61	Low (relapsed)	Cy-TBI	3%	All	68%, 4 yr	50%, 4 yr	Rohatiner *et al.*, 1994 [186]
102†	39	17–58	High (first remission)	Various	4%	All Small noncleaved Other high-grade	70%, 5 yr 46%, 5 yr 72%, 5 yr	70%, 5 yr	Sweetenham *et al.*, 1994 [44]
105‡ 53§	36 44	3–68 21–60	Intermediate/high (Refractory/relapsed)	Various	NS	All ABMT PBSCT Poor prognosis Good prognosis	NS	29%, 3 yr 23%, 3 yr 40%, 3 yr 10%, 3 yr 45%, 3 yr	Vose *et al.*, 1993 [23]
78	43	16–66	Intermediate/high (Refractory/relapsed)	CBV	8%	All Intermediate/immunoblastic Other high grade	52%, 3 yr	42%, 3 yr 48%, 3 yr 0%, 1 yr	Wheeler *et al.*, 1993 [187]

ABMT = autologous bone marrow transplant; NS = not specified; PBSCT = peripheral blood stem cell transplant; yr = years.
* Monoclonal antibody-purged marrow.
† 17% received monoclonal antibody- or mafosfamide-purged marrow.
‡ Bone marrow.
§ Peripheral blood stem cells.

and 52%) were not significantly different from those in the autograft arm (69% and 59%).

A Dutch cooperative study addressed the issue of autografting in patients with aggressive NHL, with a slow response to the initial phase of first-line chemotherapy, who are at high risk of relapse [110]. Patients with complete responses after three courses of CHOP (cyclophosphamide, vincristine, doxorubicin, prednisolone), and those with partial response but with persistent tumour in the marrow, received five more courses of CHOP. Patients with partial response but tumour-free marrow were randomized to autografting or five courses of CHOP. One hundred and six of 286 patients were slow responders; 69 of these were randomized to further CHOP or autografting. The remission rates (74 vs 68%), and 4-year overall (85 vs 56%) and event-free (53 vs 41%) survival, were not significantly different between the CHOP and the transplantation groups.

The issue of effective marrow purging and the significance of detection of residual disease remains unresolved. In contrast to the findings reported by Gribben *et al.* [36], Johnson *et al.* [188] showed that PCR positivity t(14;18), after purging, did not correlate with the probability of disease progression after ABMT using similar purging and conditioning. Additionally, 26 of 27 patients studied showed persistent t(14;18) by PCR 3 months to 7 years after ABMT; 13 were in complete remission clinically.

Adequate follow-up is essential to interpret data accurately, especially in diseases such as low-grade NHL with a protracted natural course. The Dana-Farber Group reported [189] that low-grade NHL patients in complete remission at the time of the autograft had significantly superior disease-free survival compared with patients in partial remission (Fig. 23.10a), but with an additional follow-up of 2 years [115], the difference was no longer obvious (Fig. 23.10b).

The development of myelodysplasia and secondary AML is increasingly being encountered in medium- to long-term survivors of autografts for lymphoma [190,191]. This is probably the result of exposure of haematopoietic stem cells to alkylating agents during the initial therapy of the disease, and argues in favour of one or more of the following: earlier use of transplantation, some change in the type of initial chemotherapy used, and the use of allogeneic marrow where feasible.

Postautograft strategies to reduce relapse

High-dose chemo/radiotherapy in safely tolerated doses does not eradicate malignant cells completely. Treatment after an autograft, in a minimal residual disease state, might be expected to control or eliminate surviving malignant cells and decrease relapse. Post-transplant treatment may be cytotoxic chemotherapy [64,86,100] or biological response modifiers. The latter may be administered for their direct antimalignancy activity, such as IFNα for CML [98] or myeloma [175], and for immunomodulation to evoke graft-vs-tumour reactions in the autologous setting [61,141,162,192–200].

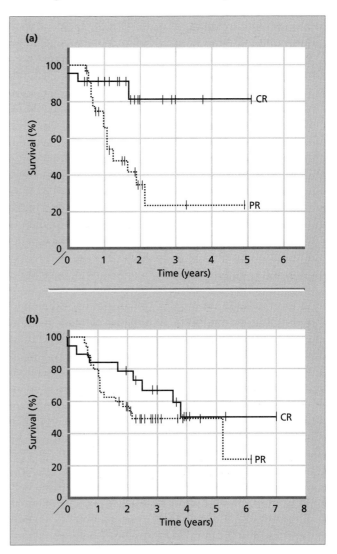

Fig. 23.10 Effect of the stage at autograft on disease-free survival in 51 patients with low-grade NHL. (a) Analysis in January 1991. The difference is significant (*P* < 0.05). (b) Analysis with 2 additional years of follow-up. The difference is not significant. CR = complete remission; PR = partial remission. (From Freedman & Nadler, 1993 [115], with permission.)

Immunomodulating agents used singly or in combination after autografting include cyclosporin [192–195], IFNα [61,141,197,198], IL-2 [61,196–200], roquinimex [162], allogeneic lymphocytes [196] and autologous lymphokine-activated killer cells [199,200], in varying combinations.

Under normal circumstances, immunoregulatory mechanisms play an important role in controlling antiself responses during T-cell ontogeny following autologous transplantation. It is possible to disrupt these mechanisms with cyclosporin administration for a short period following an autograft. The cessation of cyclosporin results in a syndrome histologically and clinically resembling cutaneous GVHD [192–195]. Unfortunately, all human studies on cyclosporin-induced autologous GVHD for control of residual disease have been phase I studies, which have not shown any direct evidence of anti-tumour effects or improvement in disease-free survival.

Similarly, while most studies have shown that immuno-modulatory agents, notably IL-2, can enhance killer cell activity after autografting, no data are yet available on the efficacy of these approaches. As peripheral blood stem cell collections contain a large number of immunocompetent lymphocytes and mononuclear cells [201], immunotherapy may be more successful.

Management of advanced disease

Relapse of the underlying disease is the main cause of failure of autografting for high-risk or advanced leukaemia. This risk reduces considerably with HLA-matched unrelated or HLA-mismatched family donor transplants. The main problem with alternative allogeneic donors is transplant-related mortality. As supportive measures become more refined, the toxicity of these procedures is likely to reduce, which may improve survival.

Busca *et al.* [202] compared 43 acute leukaemia patients transplanted from HLA-matched unrelated donors with 77 disease-, stage- and age-matched patients who were auto-grafted during the same period. The cumulative proportion of patients discharged alive (79 vs 77%) was similar for unrelated and autologous transplants. For patients transplanted in remission, relapse occurred in 27% of the unrelated graft recipients and in 55% of the autograft recipients ($P = 0.08$). For patients transplanted with active disease, the relapse rates were 48 and 63% respectively ($P =$ NS). Disease-free survival rates were 33% for unrelated and 25% for autologous trans-plants in remission ($P =$ NS), and 12 and 5% for transplants in relapse ($P =$ NS). These data suggest that unrelated donor transplants are as effective as autografts in patients with advanced leukaemia. Further studies are warranted to assess the relative effectiveness of unrelated and autologous trans-plantation for standard-risk leukaemia.

Unlike the leukaemias and the lymphomas, there is currently no evidence that autografting is curative in myeloma. Allogeneic BMT, therefore, may be preferable in younger patients with HLA-identical sibling donors, because this procedure can result in molecular remissions and may be curative in a proportion of the patients.

Allogeneic BMT in NHL and HD is associated with an immunological graft-vs-lymphoma effect which decreases the probability of disease progression [181,203,204]. The increased transplant-related morbidity may be tolerated reasonably well in younger patients, who may benefit from an allograft rather than an autograft [181,204,205].

Conclusion

Autografting is an integral part of the management of leukaemia and other haematological malignancies, although

selection of the right candidates who would benefit from the procedure continues to be controversial. Transplant-related morbidity and mortality have decreased progressively with increasing experience and technical advances, and relapse of the disease is the main cause of failure. An improvement in the existing conditioning regimens, along with novel post-transplant chemotherapeutic or immunotherapeutic strategies, are essential to improve the outcome.

Note added in proof

Since the original chapter was written, the following key developments have occurred.

Acute myeloid leukaemia: The MRC AML 10 study [107], with longer follow-up, showed a survival advantage for AML patients autografted in first CR in comparison with those treated with chemotherapy only [206]. Karyotype was found to dominate the prognosis of autografted AML patients [207,208]. Contrary to their previous report [129], a new EBMT study found no beneficial effect for purging [208].

Multiple myeloma: A French cooperative randomized study showed the superiority of autotransplantation over conventional chemotherapy [209]. Karyotype was shown to dominate the prognosis of auto-grafted myeloma patients [210,211].

Hodgkin's disease: A matched-pair analysis of blood versus marrow transplantation from the EBMT showed a significantly higher rate of progression amongst HD patients autografted with blood than with marrow [212]. The progression rates were comparable for NHL patients [212]; this needs further study.

Non-Hodgkin's lymphoma: The final report of the Parma study showed that high-dose chemotherapy with ABMT increased event-free and overall survival in patients with chemotherapy-sensitive NHL in relapse compared with conventional chemotherapy [213]. An update [214] of a French cooperative randomized study [109] showed that, with longer follow-up, consolidative autotransplantation was superior to continued chemotherapy in patients with higher-risk aggressive NHL in first CR. Sequential induction and high-dose chemotherapy were found to result in superior response rates and event-free survival compared with MACOP-B in patients with diffuse large-cell lymphoma [215]. There was a trend towards improved survival.

References

1 Mehta J. (1993) Graft-versus-leukemia reactions in clinical bone marrow transplantation. *Leukemia and Lymphoma*, **10**, 427–432.

2 Kurnick N.B., Montano A., Gerdes J.C. & Feder B.H. (1958) Preliminary observations on the treatment of postirradiation hematopoietic depression in man by the infusion of stored autogenous bone marrow. *Annals of Internal Medicine*, **49**, 973–986.

3 McGovern J., Russell P. & Atkins Webster E.W. (1959) Treatment of terminal leukemic relapse by total-body irradiation and intravenous infusion of stored autologous bone marrow obtained during remission. *New England Journal of Medicine*, **260**, 675–683.

4 McFarland W., Granville N.B. & Dameshek W. (1959) Autologous bone marrow infusion as an adjunct in therapy of malignant disease. *Blood*, **14**, 503–521.

5 Clifford P., Clift R.A. & Duff J.K. (1961) Nitrogen-mustard therapy combined with autologous marrow infusion. *Lancet*, **i**, 687–690.

6 Buckner C.D., Clift R.A., Fefer A., Neiman P.E., Storb R. &

Thomas E.D. (1974) Treatment of blastic transformation of chronic granulocytic leukemia by high dose cyclophosphamide, total body irradiation and infusion of cryopreserved autologous marrow. *Experimental Hematology*, **2**, 138–146.

7 Treleaven J.G. & Mehta J. (1992) Bone marrow and peripheral stem cell harvesting. *Journal of Hematotherapy*, **1**, 215–223.

8 Goldman J.M., Catovsky D. & Galton D.A.G. (1978) Reversal of blast-cell crisis in C.G.L. by transfusion of stored autologous buffy-coat cells. *Lancet*, **i**, 437–438.

9 Körbling M., Burke P., Braine H., Elfenbein G., Santos G. & Kaizer H. (1981) Successful engraftment of blood derived normal hemopoietic stem cells in chronic myelogenous leukemia. *Experimental Hematology*, **9**, 684–690.

10 Juttner C.A., To L.B., Haylock D.N., Branford A. & Kimber R.J. (1985) Circulating autologous stem cells collected in very early remission from acute non-lymphoblastic leukaemia produce prompt but incomplete haemopoietic reconstitution after high dose melphalan or supralethal chemoradiotherapy. *British Journal of Haematology*, **61**, 739–745.

11 Körbling M., Holle R., Haas R. *et al.* (1990) Autologous blood stem-cell transplantation in patients with advanced Hodgkin's disease and prior radiation to the pelvic site. *Journal of Clinical Oncology*, **8**, 978–985.

12 Mehta J., Powles R.L., Shepherd V., Dainton M. & Treleaven J. (1993) Transplantation of autologous peripheral blood stem cells mobilized using GM-CSF for acute leukemia with myelofibrosis *Leukaemia and Lymphoma*, **11**, 157–158.

13 Kessinger A., Vose J.M., Bierman P.J. & Armitage J.O. (1991) High-dose therapy and autologous peripheral stem cell transplantation for patients with bone marrow metastases and relapsed lymphoma: an alternative to bone marrow purging. *Experimental Hematology*, **19**, 1013–1016.

14 To L.B., Roberts M.M., Haylock D.N. *et al.* (1992) Comparison of haematological recovery times and supportive care requirements of autologous recovery phase peripheral blood stem cell transplants, autologous bone marrow transplants and allogeneic bone marrow transplants. *Bone Marrow Transplantation*, **9**, 277–284.

15 Peters W.P., Rosner G., Ross M. *et al.* (1993) Comparative effects of granulocyte-macrophage colony-stimulating factor (GM-CSF) and granulocyte colony-stimulating factor (G-CSF) on priming peripheral blood progenitor cells for use with autologous bone marrow after high-dose chemotherapy. *Blood*, **81**, 1709–1719.

16 Talpaz M. & Spitzer G. (1984) Low natural killer cell activity in the bone marrow of healthy donors with normal natural killer cell activity in the peripheral blood. *Experimental Hematology*, **12**, 629–632.

17 Roberts M.M., To L.B., Gillis D. *et al.* (1993) Immune reconstitution following peripheral blood stem cell transplantation, autologous bone marrow transplantation and allogeneic bone marrow transplantation. *Bone Marrow Transplantation*, **12**, 469–475.

18 Mehta J., Powles R., Singhal S. & Treleaven J. Peripheral blood stem cell transplantation may result in increased relapse of acute myeloid leukaemia due to reinfusion of a higher number of malignant cells. *Bone Marrow Transplantation*, **15**, 652–653.

19 Körbling M., Fliedner T.M., Holle R. *et al.* (1991) Autologous blood stem cell (ABSCT) versus purged bone marrow transplantation (pABMT) in standard risk AML: influence of source and cell composition of the autograft on hemopoietic reconstitution and disease-free survival. *Bone Marrow Transplantation*, **7**, 343–349.

20 Gribben J.G., Neuberg D., Barber M. *et al.* (1994) Detection of residual lymphoma cells by polymerase chain reaction in peripheral blood is significantly less predictive for relapse than detection in bone marrow. *Blood*, **83**, 3800–3807.

21 Corradini P., Voena C., Astolfi M. *et al.* (1995) High-dose sequential chemoradiotherapy in multiple myeloma: residual tumor cells are detectable in bone marrow and peripheral blood cell harvests and after autografting. *Blood*, **85**, 1596–1602.

22 Liberti G., Pearce R., Taghipour G., Majolino I. & Goldstone A.H. (1994) Comparison of peripheral blood stem-cell and autologous bone marrow transplantation for lymphoma patients: a case-controlled analysis of the EBMT Registry data. *Annals of Oncology*, **5**(Suppl. 2), S151–S153.

23 Vose J.M., Anderson J.R., Kessinger A. *et al.* (1993) High-dose chemotherapy and autologous hematopoietic stem-cell transplantation for aggressive non-Hodgkin's lymphoma. *Journal of Clinical Oncology*, **11**, 1846–1851.

24 Thomas E.D. & Storb R. (1970) Technique for human marrow grafting. *Blood*, **36**, 507–515.

25 Gorin N.C. (1986) Collection, manipulation and freezing of haemopoietic stem cells. *Clinical Haematology*, **15**, 19–48.

26 Hutchinson R.M., Bell A.J., Duguid J.K.M. *et al.* (1994) Guidelines for the collection, processing and storage of human bone marrow and peripheral stem cells for transplantation. *Transfusion Medicine*, **4**, 165–172.

27 Mehta J., Powles R., Cabral S. *et al.* (1995) Comparison of Cobe Spectra and Haemonetics MCS-3P cell separators for harvesting peripheral blood stem cells. *Bone Marrow Transplantation*, **16**, 707–709.

28 Shimazaki C., Oku N., Ashihara E. *et al.* (1992) Collection of peripheral blood stem cells mobilized by high-dose Ara-C plus VP-16 or aclarubicin followed by recombinant human granulocyte-colony stimulating factor. *Bone Marrow Transplantation*, **10**, 341–346.

29 Pettengell R., Morgenstern G.R., Woll P.J. *et al.* (1993) Peripheral blood progenitor cell transplantation in lymphoma and leukemia using a single apheresis. *Blood*, **82**, 3770–3777.

30 Bensinger W., Singer J., Appelbaum F. *et al.* (1993) Autologous transplantation with peripheral blood mononuclear cells collected after administration of recombinant granulocyte stimulating factor. *Blood*, **81**, 3158–3163.

31 Mehta J., Powles R., Singhal S., Shepherd V., Cabral S. & Treleaven J. (1985) Peripheral blood stem cell autografts for acute lymphoblastic leukemia: effect of G-CSF dose and harvest schedule on cell yields. *British Journal of Haematology*, **89**(Suppl. 1) 19.

32 Schmitz N., Dreger P., Suttorp M. *et al.* (1995) Primary transplantation of allogeneic peripheral blood progenitor cells mobilized by filgrastim (granulocyte colony-stimulating factor). *Blood*, **85**, 1666–1672.

33 Bensinger W.I., Weaver C.H., Appelbaum F.R. *et al.* (1995) Transplantation of allogenic peripheral blood stem cells mobilized by recombinant human granulocyte colony-stimulating factor. *Blood*, **85**, 1655–1658.

34 Körbling M., Przepiorka D., Huh Y.O. *et al.* (1995) Allogeneic blood stem cell transplantation for refractory leukemia and lymphoma: potential advantage of blood over marrow allografts. *Blood*, **85**, 1659–1665.

35 Brenner M.K., Rill D.R., Moen R.C. *et al.* (1993) Gene-marking to trace origin of relapse after autologous bone-marrow transplantation. *Lancet*, **341**, 85–86.

36 Gribben J.G., Freedman A.S., Neuberg D. *et al.* (1991) Immunologic purging of marrow assessed by PCR before autologous bone marrow transplantation for B-cell lymphoma. *New England Journal of Medicine*, **325**, 1525–1533.

37 Körbling M., Dorken B., Tischbirek K. *et al.* (1983) Autologous transplantation of a bone marrow graft manipulated by chemoseparation to eliminate residual tumor cells. *Blut*, **46**, 89–93.

38 Kaizer H., Tutschka P., Stuart R. *et al.* (1983) Autologous bone marrow transplantation in acute leukemia and non-Hodgkin's lymphoma: a phase I study of 4-hydroperoxycyclophosphamide (4HC) incubation of marrow prior to cryopreservation. *Hamatologia Bluttransfusion*, **28**, 90–91.

39 Yeager A.M., Rowley S.D., Kaizer H. & Santos G.W. (1990) *Ex vivo* chemopurging of autologous bone marrow with 4-hydroperoxycyclophosphamide to eliminate occult leukemic cells. Laboratory and clinical observations. *American Journal of Pediatric Hematology/Oncology*, **12**, 245–256.

40 Reece D.E., Barnett M.J., Connors J.M. *et al.* (1993) Treatment of multiple myeloma with intensive chemotherapy followed by autologous BMT using marrow purged with 4-hydroperoxycyclophosphamide. *Bone Marrow Transplantation*, **11**, 139–146.

41 Herve P., Cahn J.Y., Plouvier E. *et al.* (1984) Autologous bone marrow transplantation for acute leukemia using transplant chemopurified with metabolite of oxazaphosphorines (ASTA Z 7557, INN mafosfamide). First clinical results. *Investigational New Drugs*, **2**, 245–252.

42 Gorin N.C., Douay L., Laporte J.P. *et al.* (1986) Autologous bone marrow transplantation using marrow incubated with Asta Z 7557 in adult acute leukemia. *Blood*, **67**, 1367–1376.

43 Carlo-Stella C., Mangoni L., Almici C. *et al.* (1994) Autologous transplant for chronic myelogenous leukemia using marrow treated *ex vivo* with mafosfamide. *Bone Marrow Transplantation*, **14**, 425–432.

44 Sweetenham J.W., Proctor S.J., Blaise D. *et al.* (1994) High-dose therapy and autologous bone marrow transplantation in first complete remission for adult patients with high-grade non-Hodgkin's lymphoma: the EBMT experience. *Annals of Oncology*, **5**(Suppl. 2), S155–S159.

45 Cahn J.Y., Herve P., Flesch M. *et al.*(1986) Autologous bone marrow transplantation (ABMT) for acute leukaemia in complete remission: a pilot study of 33 cases. *British Journal of Haematology*, **63**, 457–470.

46 Colleselli P., Dini G., Andolina M. *et al.* (1991) Autologous bone marrow transplantation for acute lymphoblastic leukemia: the high dose vincristine study of AIEOP BMT group. *Bone Marrow Transplantation*, **7**(Suppl. 3), 28–30.

47 Vogler W.R., Berdel W.E., Olson A.C., Winton E.F., Heffner L.T. & Gordon D.S. (1992) Autologous bone marrow transplantation in acute leukemia with marrow purged with alkyl-lysophospholipid. *Blood*, **80**, 1423–1429.

48 Chao N.J., Stein A.S., Long G.D. *et al.* (1993) Busulfan/etoposide — initial experience with a new preparatory regimen for autologous bone marrow transplantation in patients with acute non-lymphoblastic leukemia. *Blood*, **81**, 319–323.

49 Klingemann H.G., Eaves C.J., Barnett M.J. *et al.* (1994) Transplantation of patients with high risk acute myeloid leukemia in first remission with autologous marrow cultured in interleukin-2 followed by interleukin-2 administration. *Bone Marrow Transplantation*, **14**, 389–396.

50 McGlave P.B., Arthur D., Miller W.J., Lasky L. & Kersey J. (1990) Autologous transplantation for CML using marrow treated *ex vivo* with recombinant human interferon gamma. *Bone Marrow Transplantation*, **6**, 115–120.

51 Ritz J., Sallan S.E., Bast R.C. *et al.* (1982) Autologous bone-marrow transplantation in CALLA-positive acute lymphoblastic leukemia after *in-vitro* treatment with J5 monoclonal antibody and complement. *Lancet*, **ii**, 60–63.

52 Gorin N.C., Douay L., Laporte J.P. *et al.* (1985) Autologous bone marrow transplantation with marrow decontaminated by immunotoxin T 101 in the treatment of leukemia and lymphoma: first clinical observations. *Cancer Treatment Reports*, **69**, 953–959.

53 Ferrero D., De Fabritiis P., Amadori S. *et al.* (1987) Autologous bone marrow transplantation in acute myeloid leukemia after *in-vitro* purging with an anti-lacto-N-fucopentaose III antibody and rabbit complement. *Leukemia Research*, **11**, 265–272.

54 Ball E.D., Mills L.E., Coughlin C.T., Beck J.R. & Cornwell G.G. (1986) Autologous bone marrow transplantation in acute myelogenous leukemia: *in vitro* treatment with myeloid cell-specific monoclonal antibodies. *Blood*, **68**, 1311–1315.

55 Kersey J.H., Weisdorf D., Nesbit M.E. *et al.* (1987) Comparison of autologous and allogeneic bone marrow transplantation for treatment of high-risk refractory acute lymphoblastic leukemia. *New England Journal of Medicine*, **317**, 461–467.

56 Preijers F.W., De Witte T., Wessels J.M. *et al.* (1989) Autologous transplantation of bone marrow purged *in vitro* with anti-CD7-(WT1-) ricin A immunotoxin in T-cell lymphoblastic leukemia and lymphoma. *Blood*, **74**, 1152–1158.

57 Ball E.D., Vredenburgh J.J., Mills L.E. *et al.* (1990) Autologous bone marrow transplantation for acute myeloid leukemia following *in vitro* treatment with neuraminidase and monoclonal antibodies. *Bone Marrow Transplantation*, **6**, 277–280.

58 Janssen W.E., Lee C., Johnson K.S. *et al.* (1990) Immunomagnetic microsphere mediated purging of cALLa positive leukemic cells from bone marrow for autologous reinfusion. *Progress in Clinical and Biological Research*, **333**, 285–292.

59 Robertson M.J., Soiffer R.J., Freedman A.S. *et al.* (1992) Human bone marrow depleted of CD33-positive cells mediates delayed but durable reconstitution of hematopoiesis: clinical trial of MY9 monoclonal antibody-purged autografts for the treatment of acute myeloid leukemia. *Blood*, **79**, 2229–2236.

60 Billett A.L., Kornmehl E., Tarbell N.J. *et al.* (1993) Autologous bone marrow transplantation after a long first remission for children with recurrent acute lymphoblastic leukemia. *Blood*, **81**, 1651–1657.

61 Schmid H., Henze G., Schwerdtfeger R. *et al.* (1993) Fractionated total body irradiation and high-dose VP-16 with purged autologous bone marrow rescue for children with high risk relapsed acute lymphoblastic leukemia. *Bone Marrow Transplantation*, **12**, 597–602.

62 Rabinowe S.N., Soiffer R.J., Gribben J.G. *et al.* (1993) Autologous and allogeneic bone marrow transplantation for poor prognosis patients with B-cell chronic lymphocytic leukemia. *Blood*, **82**, 1366–1376.

63 Khouri I.F., Keating M.J., Vriesendorp H.M. *et al.* (1994) Autologous and allogeneic bone marrow transplantation for chronic lymphocytic leukemia: preliminary results. *Journal of Clinical Oncology*, **12**, 748–758.

64 Tiley C., Powles R., Treleaven J. *et al.* (1993) Feasibility and efficacy of maintenance chemotherapy following autologous bone marrow transplantation for first remission acute lymphoblastic leukaemia. *Bone Marrow Transplantation*, **12**, 449–455.

65 Abrahm J.L., Gerson S.L., Hoxie J.A., Tannenbaum S.H., Cassileth P.A. & Cooper R.A. (1986) Differential effects of phorbol esters on normal myeloid precursors and leukemia cells: basis for autologous bone marrow reconstitution in acute nonlymphocytic leukemia using phorbol ester-treated bone marrow from patients in remission. *Cancer Research*, **46**, 3711–3716.

66 Barnett M.J., Eaves C.J., Phillips G.L. *et al.* (1994) Autografting with cultured marrow in chronic myeloid leukemia: results of a pilot study. *Blood,* **84,** 724–732.

67 Ranson M.R., Scarffe J.H., Morgenstern G.R. *et al.* (1991) Post consolidation therapy for adult patients with acute myeloid leukaemia. *British Journal of Haematology,* **79,** 162–169.

68 Herrmann R.P., O'Reilly J., Meyer B.F. & Lazzaro G. (1992) Prompt haemopoietic reconstitution following hyperthermia purged autologous marrow and peripheral blood stem cell transplantation in acute myeloid leukaemia. *Bone Marrow Transplantation,* **10,** 293–295.

69 Fabrega S., Laporte J.P., Giarratana M.C. *et al.* (1993) Polymerase chain reaction: a method for monitoring tumor cell purge by long-term culture in BCR/ABL positive acute lymphoblastic leukemia. *Bone Marrow Transplantation,* **11,** 169–173.

70 Luger S.M., Ratajczak M.Z., Stadtmauer E.A. *et al.* (1994) Autografting for chronic myelogenous leukemia (CML) with c-myb antisense oligonucleotide purged bone marrow. *Blood,* **84**(Suppl. 1), 151a.

71 Uckun F.M., Kersey J.H., Vallera D.A. *et al.* (1990) Autologous bone marrow transplantation in high-risk remission T-lineage acute lymphoblastic leukemia using immunotoxins plus 4-hydroperoxycyclophosphamide for marrow purging. Blood, **76,** 1723–1733.

72 Higuchi W., Moriyama Y., Kishi K. *et al.* (1991) Hematopoietic recovery in a patient with acute lymphoblastic leukemia after an autologous marrow graft purged by combined hyperthermia and interferon *in vitro. Bone Marrow Transplantation,* **7,** 163–166.

73 Uckun F.M., Kersey J.H., Haake R., Weisdorf D. & Ramsay N.K. (1992) Autologous bone marrow transplantation in high-risk remission B-lineage acute lymphoblastic leukemia using a cocktail of three monoclonal antibodies (BA-1/CD24, BA-2/CD9, and BA-3/CD10) plus complement and 4-hydroperoxycyclophosphamide for *ex vivo* bone marrow purging. *Blood,* **79,** 1094–1104.

74 Shpall E.J., Stemmer S.M., Hami L. *et al.* (1994) Amifostine (WR-2721) shortens the engraftment period of 4-hydroperoxycyclophosphamide-purged bone marrow in breast cancer patients receiving high-dose chemotherapy with autologous bone marrow support. *Blood,* **83,** 3132–3137.

75 Schiller G., Vescio R., Freytes C. *et al.* (1995) Transplantation of CD34+ peripheral blood progenitor cells after high-dose chemotherapy for patients with advanced myeloma. *Blood,* **86,** 390–397.

76 Allieri M.A., Lopez M., Douay L., Mary J.Y., Nguyen L. & Gorin N.C. (1991) Clonogenic leukemic progenitor cells in acute myelocytic leukemia are highly sensitive to cryopreservation: possible purging effect for autologous bone marrow transplantation. *Bone Marrow Transplantation,* **7,** 101–105.

77 Mehta J., Powles R., Singhal S. *et al.* (1995) Autologous bone marrow transplantation for acute myeloid leukemia in first remission: identification of modifiable prognostic factors. *Bone Marrow Transplantation,* **16,** 499–506.

78 Bearman S.I., Appelbaum F.R., Buckner C.D. *et al.* (1988) Regimen-related toxicity in patients undergoing bone marrow transplantation. *Journal of Clinical Oncology,* **6,** 1562–1568.

79 Clift R.A., Buckner C.D., Appelbaum F.R. *et al.* (1990) Allogeneic marrow transplantation in patients with acute myeloid leukemia in first remission: a randomized trial of two irradiation regimens. *Blood,* **76,** 1867–1871.

80 Clift R.A., Buckner C.D., Appelbaum F.R. *et al.* (1991) Allogeneic marrow transplantation in patients with chronic myeloid leukemia in the chronic phase: a randomized trial of two irradiation regimens. *Blood,* **77,** 1660–1665.

81 Petersen F.B., Deeg H.J., Buckner C.D. *et al.* (1992) Marrow transplantation following escalating doses of fractionated total body irradiation and cyclophosphamide — a phase I trial. *International Journal of Radiation, Oncology, Biology, Physics,* **23,** 1027–1032.

82 Stewart P., Buckner C.D., Bensinger W. *et al.* (1985) Autologous marrow transplantation in patients with acute nonlymphocytic leukemia in first remission. *Experimental Hematology,* **13,** 267–272.

83 Körbling M., Hunstein W., Fliedner T.M. *et al.* (1989) Disease-free survival after autologous bone marrow transplantation in patients with acute myelogenous leukemia. *Blood,* **74,** 1898–1904.

84 Petersen F.B., Lynch M.H.E., Clift R.A. *et al.* (1993) Autologous marrow transplantation for patients with acute myeloid leukemia in untreated first relapse or in second complete remission. *Journal of Clinical Oncology,* **11,** 1353–1360.

85 Schroeder H., Pinkerton C.R., Powles R.L. *et al.* (1991) High dose melphalan and total body irradiation with autologous marrow rescue in childhood acute lymphoblastic leukaemia after relapse. *Bone Marrow Transplantation,* **7,** 11–15.

86 Powles R., Mehta J., Singhal S. *et al.* (1995) Autologous bone marrow or peripheral blood stem cell transplantation followed by maintenance chemotherapy for adult acute lymphoblastic leukemia in first remission: 50 cases from a single center. *Bone Marrow Transplantation,* **16,** 241–247.

87 Cahn J.Y., Bordigoni P., Souillet G. *et al.* (1991) The TAM regimen prior to allogeneic and autologous bone marrow transplantation for high-risk acute lymphoblastic leukemias: a cooperative study of 62 patients. *Bone Marrow Transplantation,* **7,** 1–4.

88 Woods W.G., Ramsay N.K., Weisdorf D.J. *et al.* (1990) Bone marrow transplantation for acute lymphocytic leukemia utilizing total body irradiation followed by high doses of cytosine arabinoside: lack of superiority over cyclophosphamide-containing conditioning regimens. *Bone Marrow Transplantation,* **6,** 9–16.

89 Appelbaum F.R., Matthews D.C., Eary J.F. *et al.* (1992) The use of radiolabeled anti-CD33 antibody to augment marrow irradiation prior to marrow transplantation for acute myelogenous leukemia. *Transplantation,* **54,** 829–833.

90 Matthews D.C., Appelbaum F.R., Eary J.F. *et al.* (1995) Development of a marrow transplant regimen for acute leukemia using targeted hematopoietic irradiation delivered by ^{131}I-labeled anti-CD45 antibody, combined with cyclophosphamide and total body irradiation. *Blood,* **85,** 1122–1131.

91 Press O.W., Eary J.F., Appelbaum F.R. *et al.* (1993) Radiolabeled-antibody therapy of B-cell lymphoma with autologous bone marrow support [see comments]. *New England Journal of Medicine,* **329,** 1219–1224.

92 Bierman P.J., Vose J.M., Leichner P.K. *et al.* (1993) Yttrium 90-labeled antiferritin followed by high-dose chemotherapy and autologous bone marrow transplantation for poor-prognosis Hodgkin's disease. *Journal of Clinical Oncology,* **11,** 698–703.

93 Deeg H.J. (1990) Delayed complications and long-term effects after bone marrow transplantation. *Hematology/Oncology Clinics of North America,* **4,** 641–657.

94 Yeager A.M., Kaizer H., Santos G.W. *et al.* (1986) Autologous bone marrow transplantation in patients with acute nonlymphocytic leukemia, using *ex vivo* marrow treatment with 4-hydroperoxycyclophosphamide. *New England Journal of Medicine,* **315,** 141–147.

95 Beelen D.W., Quabeck K., Graeven U., Sayer H.G., Mahmoud H.K. & Schaefer U.W. (1989) Acute toxicity and first clinical results of intensive postinduction therapy using a modified busulfan and cyclophosphamide regimen with autologous bone

marrow rescue in first remission of acute myeloid leukemia. *Blood*, **74**, 1507–1516.

96 Zander A.R., Vellekoop L., Spitzer G. *et al.* (1981) Combination of high-dose cyclophosphamide, BCNU, and VP-16-213 followed by autologous marrow rescue in the treatment of relapsed leukemia. *Cancer Treatment Reports*, **65**, 377–381.

97 Spinolo J.A., Dicke K.A., Horwitz L.J. *et al.* (1990) Double intensification with amsacrine/high dose ara-C and high dose chemotherapy with autologous bone marrow transplantation produces durable remissions in acute myelogenous leukemia. *Bone Marrow Transplantation*, **5**, 111–118.

98 Mehta J., Mijovic A., Powles R. *et al.* (1996) Myelosuppressive chemotherapy to mobilize normal stem cells in chronic myeloid leukemia. *Bone Marrow Transplantation*, **17**, 25–29.

99 Mehta J., Powles R.L., Treleaven J. & Milan S. (1993) Busulfan-melphalan conditioning prior to bone marrow transplantation for poor-risk leukemia. *European Journal of Cancer*, **29A**(Suppl. 6), S152.

100 Mehta J., Powles R., Singhal S. *et al.* (1995) Sequential high-dose therapy of adult acute lymphoblastic leukemia: role of maintenance chemotherapy after peripheral blood stem cell transplantation in first remission. In: *Autologous Marrow and Blood Transplantation: Proceedings of the Seventh International Symposium, Arlington, Texas* (eds K.A. Dicke & A. Keating), pp. 135–144. The Cancer Treatment Research and Educational Institute, Arlington.

101 Cunningham D., Paz-Ares L., Milan S. *et al.* (1994) High-dose melphalan and autologous bone marrow transplantation as consolidation in previously untreated myeloma. *Journal of Clinical Oncology*, **12**, 759–763.

102 Linker C.A., Ries C.A., Damon L.E., Rugo H.S. & Wolf J.L. (1993) Autologous bone marrow transplantation for acute myeloid leukemia using busulfan plus etoposide as a preparative regimen. *Blood*, **81**, 311–318.

103 Meloni G., De Fabritiis P., Petti M.C. & Mandelli F. (1990) BAVC regimen and autologous bone marrow transplantation in patients with acute myelogenous leukemia in second remission. *Blood*, **75**, 2282–2285.

104 Mills W., Chopra R., McMillan A., Pearce R., Linch D.C. & Goldstone A.H. (1995) BEAM chemotherapy and autologous bone marrow transplantation for patients with relapsed or refractory non-Hodgkin's lymphoma. *Journal of Clinical Oncology*, **13**, 588–595.

105 Powles R., Singhal S., Mehta J. *et al.* (1995) A package of treatment options for total therapy of acute myeloid leukaemia. *Bone Marrow Transplantation*, **15**(Suppl. 2), S62.

106 Fière D., Lepage E., Sebban C. *et al.* (1993) Adult acute lymphoblastic leukemia: a multicentric randomized trial testing bone marrow transplantation as postremission therapy. *Journal of Clinical Oncology*, **10**, 1990–2001.

107 Burnett A.K., Goldstone A.H., Stevens R.F. *et al.* (1994) The role of BMT in addition to intensive chemotherapy in AML in first CR: results of the MRC AML-10 trials. *Blood*, **84**(Suppl. 1) 252a.

108 Zittoun R.A., Mandelli F., Willemze R. *et al.* (1995) Autologous or allogeneic bone marrow transplantation compared with intensive chemotherapy in acute myelogenous leukemia. *New England Journal of Medicine*, **332**, 217–223.

109 Haioun C., Lepage E., Gisselbrecht C. *et al.* (1994) Comparison of autologous bone marrow transplantation with sequential chemotherapy for intermediate-grade and high-grade non-Hodgkin's lymphoma in first complete remission: a study of 464 patients. *Journal of Clinical Oncology*, **12**, 2543–2551.

110 Verdonck L.F., van Putten W.L., Hagenbeek A. *et al.* (1995) Comparison of CHOP chemotherapy with autologous bone marrow transplantation for slowly responding patients with aggressive non-Hodgkin's lymphoma. *New England Journal of Medicine*, **332**, 1045–1051.

111 Ferrant A., Doyen C., Delannoy A. *et al.* (1991) Allogeneic or autologous bone marrow transplantation for acute non-lymphocytic leukemia in first remission. *Bone Marrow Transplantation*, **7**, 303–309.

112 Mitus A.J., Miller K.B., Schenkein D.P. *et al.* (1995) Improved survival for patients with acute myelogenous leukemia. *Journal of Clinical Oncology*, **13**, 560–569.

113 Singhal S., Powles R., Mehta J. *et al.* (1995) Effect of cell dose on transplant-related mortality after autografting for acute myeloid leukemia. *British Journal of Haematology*, **89**(Suppl. 1), 19.

114 Demirer T., Gooley T., Buckner C.D. *et al.* (1995) Influence of total nucleated cell dose from marrow harvests on outcome in patients with acute myelogenous leukemia undergoing autologous transplantation. *Bone Marrow Transplantation*, **15**, 907–913.

115 Freedman A.S. & Nadler L.M.(1993) Which patients with relapsed non-Hodgkin's lymphoma benefit from high-dose therapy and hematopoietic stem-cell transplantation? *Journal of Clinical Oncology*, **11**, 1841–1843.

116 Mayer R.J., Davis R.B., Schiffer C.A. *et al.* (1994) Intensive postremission chemotherapy in adults with acute myeloid leukemia. *New England Journal of Medicine*, **331**, 896–903.

117 Burnett A.K., Tansey P., Watkins R. *et al.* (1984) Transplantation of unpurged autologous bone-marrow in acute myeloid leukaemia in first remission. *Lancet*, **ii**, 1068–1070.

118 Carella A.M., Frassoni F., Damasio E. *et al.* (1992) Allogeneic versus autologous marrow transplantation for patients with acute myeloid leukemia in first marrow remission. An update of the Genoa experience with 159 patients. *Leukemia*, **6**(Suppl. 4) 78–81.

119 Cassileth P.A., Andersen J., Lazarus H.M. *et al.* (1993) Autologous bone marrow transplant in acute myeloid leukemia in first remission. *Journal of Clinical Oncology*, **11**, 314–319.

120 Keating A. & Crump M. (1992) High dose etoposide melphalan, total body irradiation and ABMT for acute myeloid leukemia in first remission. *Leukemia*, **6**(Suppl. 4), 90–91.

121 Laporte J.P., Douay L., Lopez M. *et al.* (1994) One hundred and twenty-five adult patients with primary acute leukemia autografted with marrow purged by mafosfamide: a 10-year single institution experience. *Blood*, **84**, 3810–3818.

122 McMillan A.K., Goldstone A.H., Linch D.C. *et al.* (1990) High-dose chemotherapy and autologous bone marrow transplantation in acute myeloid leukemia. *Blood*, **76**, 480–488.

123 Meloni G., De Fabritiis P., Pulsoni A. *et al.* (1989) Results of two different conditioning regimens followed by ABMT in refractory acute lymphoblastic leukemia. *Haematologica*, **74**, 67–70.

124 Michel G., Maraninchi D., Demeocq F. *et al.* (1988) Repeated courses of high dose melphalan and unpurged autologous bone marrow transplantation in children with acute non-lymphoblastic leukemia in first complete remission. *Bone Marrow Transplantation*, **3**, 105–111.

125 Sanz M.A., De la Rubia J., Sanz G.F. *et al.* (1993) Busulfan plus cyclophosphamide followed by autologous blood stem-cell transplantation for patients with acute myeloblastic leukemia in first complete remission: a report from a single institution. *Journal of Clinical Oncology*, **11**, 1661–1667.

126 Tiedemann K., Waters K.D., Tauro G.P., Tucker D. & Ekert H. (1993) Results of intensive therapy in childhood acute myeloid leukemia, incorporating high-dose melphalan and autologous

bone marrow transplantation in first complete remission. *Blood*, **82**, 3730–3738.

127 Keating A., Rowlings P.A., Horowitz M.M., Dicker K., Gale R.P. & Klein J.P. (1994) Comparison of HLA-identical sibling and autologous bone marrow transplants for acute myelogenous leukemia (AML). *Blood*, **84**(Suppl. 1), 201a.

128 Gorin N.C., Labopin M., Esperou-Bourdeau H. & Gluckman E. (1994) Comparison of allogeneic and autologous bone marrow transplantation for acute myelocytic leukemia (AML) in Europe. An EBMT survey. *Blood*, **84**(Suppl. 1), 211a.

129 Gorin N.C., Labopin M., Meloni G. *et al.* (1991) Autologous bone marrow transplantation of acute myeloblastic leukemia in Europe: further evidence of the role of marrow purging by mafosfamide. European Co-operative Group for Bone Marrow Transplantation (EBMT). *Leukemia*, **5**, 896–904.

130 Mehta J., Powles R., Singhal S. *et al.* (1995) Autologous bone marrow transplantation for acute myeloid leukaemia in first remission: identification of modifiable prognostic factors. *Bone Marrow Transplantation*, **16**, 499–506.

131 De la Rubia J., Sanz G.F., Martínez J. *et al.* (1994) Autologous blood stem cell transplantation in acute myeloblastic leukemia in first remission. *Blood*, **84**(Suppl. 1), 213a.

132 Rowley S.D., Jones R.J., Piantadosi S. *et al.* (1989) Efficacy of *ex vivo* purging for autologous bone marrow transplantation in the treatment of acute nonlymphoblastic leukemia. *Blood*, **74**, 501–506.

133 Chopra R., Goldstone A.H., McMillan A.K. *et al.* (1991) Successful treatment of acute myeloid leukemia beyond first remission with autologous bone marrow transplantation using busulfan/cyclophosphamide and unpurged marrow: the British autograft group experience. *Journal of Clinical Oncology*, **9**, 1840–1847.

134 Lenarsky C., Weinberg K., Petersen J. *et al.* (1990) Autologous bone marrow transplantation with 4-hydroperoxycyclophosphamide purged marrows for children with acute nonlymphoblastic leukemia in second remission. *Bone Marrow Transplantation*, **6**, 425–429.

135 Rosenfeld C., Shadduck R.K., Przepiorka D., Mangan K.F. & Colvin M. (1989) Autologous bone marrow transplantation with 4-hydroperoxycyclophosphamide purged marrows for acute nonlymphocytic leukemia in late remission or early relapse. *Blood*, **74**, 1159–1164.

136 Selvaggi K.J., Wilson J.W., Mills L.E. *et al.* (1994) Improved outcome for high-risk acute myeloid leukemia patients using autologous bone marrow transplantation and monoclonal antibody-purged bone marrow. *Blood*, **83**, 1698–1705.

137 Yeager A.M., Rowley S.D., Kaizer H. & Santos G.W. (1990) *Ex vivo* chemopurging of autologous bone marrow with 4-hydroperoxycyclophosphamide to eliminate occult leukemic cells. Laboratory and clinical observations. *American Journal of Pediatric Hematology/Oncology*, **12**, 245–256.

138 Schiffman K., Clift R., Appelbaum F.R. *et al.* (1993) Consequences of cryopreserving first remission autologous marrow for use after relapse in patients with acute myeloid leukemia. *Bone Marrow Transplantation*, **11**, 227–232.

139 Gale R.P., Horwitz M.M., Ash R.C. *et al.* (1994) Identical-twin bone marrow transplants for leukemia. *Annals of Internal Medicine*, **120**, 646–652.

140 Hoelzer D., Thiel E., Loffler H. *et al.* (1988) Prognostic factors in a multicenter study for treatment of acute lymphoblastic leukemia in adults. *Blood*, **71**, 123–131.

141 Doney K., Buckner C.D., Fisher L. *et al.* (1993) Autologous bone marrow transplantation for acute lymphoblastic leukemia. *Bone Marrow Transplantation*, **12**, 315–321.

142 Gilmore M.J.M.S., Hamon M.D., Prentice H.G. *et al.* (1991) Failure of purged autologous bone marrow transplantation in high risk acute lymphoblastic leukaemia in first complete remission. *Bone Marrow Transplantation*, **8**, 19–26.

143 Proctor S.J., Hamilton P.J., Taylor P. *et al.* (1988) A comparative study of combination chemotherapy versus marrow transplant in first remission in adult acute lymphoblastic leukaemia. *British Journal of Haematology*, **69**, 35–39.

144 Vey N., Blaise D., Stoppa A.M. *et al.* (1994) Bone marrow transplantation in 63 adult patients with acute lymphoblastic leukaemia in first complete remission. *Bone Marrow Transplantation*, **14**, 383–388.

145 Soiffer R.J., Roy D.C., Gonin R. *et al.* (1993) Monoclonal antibody-purged autologous bone marrow transplantation in adults with acute lymphoblastic leukemia at high risk of relapse. *Bone Marrow Transplantation*, **12**, 243–251.

146 Cuttner J., Mick R., Budman D.R. *et al.* (1991) Phase III trial of brief intensive treatment of adult acute lymphocytic leukemia comparing daunorubicin and mitoxantrone: a CALGB Study. *Leukemia*, **5**, 425–431.

147 Bloomfield C.D., Goldman A.I. Alimena G. *et al.* (1986) Chromosomal abnormalities identify high-risk and low-risk patients with acute lymphoblastic leukemia. *Blood*, **67**, 415–420.

148 Fletcher J.A., Lynch E.A., Kimball V.M., Donnelly M., Tantravahi R. & Sallan S.E. (1991) Translocation (9;22) is associated with extremely poor prognosis in intensively treated children with acute lymphoblastic leukemia. *Blood*, **77**, 435–439.

149 Dunlop L.C., Mehta J., Treleaven J. & Powles R. (1995) Results of bone marrow transplantation in Philadelphia chromosome positive acute lymphoblastic leukaemia. *British Journal of Haematology*, **89**(Suppl. 1), 18.

150 Peters S.O., Stockschläder M., Hegewisch-Becker S. *et al.* (1995) Infusion of tumor-contaminated bone marrow for autologous rescue after high-dose therapy leading to long-term remission in a patient with relapsed Philadelphia chromosome-positive acute lymphoblastic leukemia. *Bone Marrow Transplantation*, **15**, 783–784.

151 Carella A.M., Frassoni F., Pollicardo N. *et al.* (1995) Philadelphia-chromosome-negative peripheral blood stem cells can be mobilized in the early phase of recovery after a myelosuppressive chemotherapy in Philadelphia-chromosome-positive acute lymphoblastic leukaemia. *British Journal of Haematology*, **89**, 535–538.

152 Goto T., Nishikori M., Arlin Z. *et al.* (1982) Growth characteristics of leukemic and normal hematopoietic cells in Ph' + chronic myelogenous leukemia and effects of intensive treatment. *Blood*, **59**, 793–808.

153 The Italian Cooperative Study Group on Chronic Myeloid Leukemia (1994) Interferon alfa-2a as compared with conventional chemotherapy for the treatment of chronic myeloid leukemia. *New England Journal of Medicine*, **330**, 820–825.

154 McGlave P.B., De Fabritiis P., Deisseroth A. *et al.* (1994) Autologous transplants for chronic myelogenous leukaemia: results from eight transplant groups. *Lancet*, **343**, 1486–1488.

155 Kantarjian H.M., Talpaz M., LeMaistre C.F. *et al.* (1991) Intensive combination chemotherapy and autologous bone marrow transplantation leads to the reappearance of Philadelphia chromosome-negative cells in chronic myelogenous leukemia. *Cancer*, **67**, 2959–2965.

156 Deisseroth A.B., Zu Z., Claxton D. *et al.* (1994) Genetic marking shows that Ph+ cells present in autologous transplants of chronic

myelogenous leukemia (CML) contribute to relapse after autologous bone marrow in CML. *Blood*, **83**, 3068–3076.

157 Talpaz M., Kantarjian H., Liang J. *et al.* (1995) Percentage of Philadelphia chromosome (Ph)-negative and Ph-positive cells found after autologous transplantation for chronic myelogenous leukemia depends on percentage of diploid cells induced by conventional-dose chemotherapy before collection of autologous cells. *Blood*, **85**, 3257–3263.

158 Carella A.M., Pollicardo N., Pungolino E. *et al.* (1993) Mobilization of cytogenetically 'normal' blood progenitors cells by intensive conventional chemotherapy for chronic myeloid and acute lymphoblastic leukemia. *Leukemia and Lymphoma*, **9**, 477–483.

159 Kuss B.J., Sage R.E., Shepherd K.M., Hardingham J. & Nicola M. (1993) High dose hydroxyurea in collection of Philadelphia chromosome-negative stem cells in chronic myeloid leukaemia. *Leukemia and Lymphoma*, **10**, 73–78.

160 Kantarjian H.M., Talpaz M., Hester J. *et al.* (1995) Collection of peripheral-blood diploid cells from chronic myelogenous leukemia patients early in the recovery phase from myelosuppression induced by intensive-dose chemotherapy. *Journal of Clinical Oncology*, **13**, 553–559.

161 O'Brien S.G., Rule S., Spencer A. *et al.* (1995) Autografting in chronic phase CML using PBPCs mobilized by intermediate-dose chemotherapy. *British Journal of Haematology*, **89**(Suppl. 1), 39.

162 Rowe J.M., Ryan D.H., Nilsson B.I. *et al.* (1994) Chronic myelogenous leukemia treated with autologous bone marrow transplantation followed by roquinimex. *Blood*, **84**(Suppl. 1), 204a.

163 Mehta J. (1994) Interferon alfa-2a for chronic myeloid leukemia. *New England Journal of Medicine*, **331**, 401–402.

164 Bastion Y., Felman P., Dumontet C., Espinouse D. & Coiffier B. (1992) Intensive radiochemotherapy with peripheral blood stem cell transplantation in young patients with chronic lymphocytic leukemia. *Bone Marrow Transplantation*, **10**, 467–468.

165 Bartlett-Pandite L., Soiffer R., Gribben J.G. *et al.* (1994) Autologous and allogeneic bone marrow transplantation for B-cell CLL: balance between toxicity and efficacy. *Blood*, **84**(Suppl. 1), 536a.

166 Zomas A., Mehta J., Powles R. *et al.* (1994) Unusual infections following allogeneic bone marrow transplantation for chronic lymphocytic leukemia. *Bone Marrow Transplantation*, **14**, 799–803.

167 McElwain T.J. & Powles R.L. (1983) High-dose intravenous melphalan for plasma-cell leukaemia and myeloma. *Lancet*, **ii**, 822–824.

168 Singhal S., Powles R., Cunningham D. *et al.* (1995) Clearance of paraprotein after autografting for multiple myeloma. *Bone Marrow Transplantation*, **16**, 537–540.

169 Anderson K.C., Barut B.A., Ritz J. *et al.* (1991) Monoclonal antibody-purged autologous bone marrow transplantation therapy for multiple myeloma. *Blood*, **77**, 712–720.

170 Björkstrand B., Ljungman P., Bird J.M., Samson D & Gahrton G. (1995) Double high-dose chemoradiotherapy with autologous stem cell transplantation can induce molecular remissions in multiple myeloma. *Bone Marrow Transplantation*, **15**, 367–371.

171 Dimopoulos M.A., Alexanian R., Przepiorka D. *et al.* (1993) Thiotepa, busulfan, and cyclophosphamide: a new preparative regimen for autologous marrow or blood stem cell transplantation in high-risk multiple myeloma. *Blood*, **82**, 2324–2328.

172 Harousseau J.L., Attal M., Divine M. *et al.* (1995) Comparison of autologous bone marrow transplantation and peripheral blood stem cell transplantation after first remission induction treatment in multiple myeloma. *Bone Marrow Transplantation*, **15**, 963–969.

173 Jagannath S., Vesole D.H., Glenn L., Crowley J. & Barlogie B. (1992) Low-risk intensive therapy for multiple myeloma with combined autologous bone marrow and blood stem cell support. *Blood*, **80**, 1666–1672.

174 Barlogie B., Jagannath S., Vesole D. *et al.* (1994) Total therapy (TT) for 202 newly diagnosed patients (pts) with multiple myeloma (MM). *Blood*, **84**(Suppl. 1), 386a.

175 Powles R., Cunningham D., Malpas J.S. *et al.* (1994) A randomised trial of maintenance therapy with Intron-A following high-dose melphalan and ABMT in myeloma. *Blood*, **84**(Suppl. 1), 535a.

176 Cunningham D., Powles R., Malpas J. *et al.* A randomised trial of maintenance interferon following high dose chemotherapy in multiple myeloma. (In preparation.)

177 Chopra R., McMillan A.K., Linch D.C. *et al.* (1993) The place of high-dose BEAM therapy and autologous bone marrow transplantation in poor-risk Hodgkin's disease. A single-center eight-year study of 155 patients. *Blood*, **81**, 1137–1145.

178 Kessinger A., Bierman P.J., Vose J.M. & Armitage J.O. (1991) High-dose cyclophosphamide, carmustine, and etoposide followed by autologous peripheral stem cell transplantation for patients with relapsed Hodgkin's disease. *Blood*, **77**, 2322–2325.

179 Nademanee A., O'Donnell M.R., Snyder D.S. *et al.* (1995) High-dose chemotherapy with or without total body irradiation followed by autologous bone marrow and/or peripheral blood stem cell transplantation for patients with relapsed and refractory Hodgkin's disease: results in 85 patients with analysis of prognostic factors. *Blood*, **85**, 1381–1390.

180 Reece D.E., Connors J.M., Spinelli J.J. *et al.* (1994) Intensive therapy with cyclophosphamide, carmustine, etoposide +/– cisplatin, and autologous bone marrow transplantation for Hodgkin's disease in first relapse after combination chemotherapy. *Blood*, **83**, 1193–1199.

181 Yahalom J., Gulati S.C., Toia M. *et al.* (1993) Accelerated hyperfractionated total-lymphoid irradiation, high-dose chemotherapy, and autologous bone marrow transplantation for refractory and relapsing patients with Hodgkin's disease. *Journal of Clinical Oncology*, **11**, 1062–1070.

182 Anderson J.E., Litzow M.R., Appelbaum F.R. *et al.* (1993) Allogeneic, syngeneic, and autologous marrow transplantation for Hodgkin's disease: the 21-year Seattle experience. *Journal of Clinical Oncology*, **11**, 2342–2350.

183 Bennett C.L., Armitage J.L., Armitage G.O. *et al.* (1993) A 'learning curve' exists in autologous transplantation for Hodgkin's disease (HD) and non-Hodgkin's lymphoma (NHL) as evidenced by improvements in cost and in-hospital mortality. *Blood*, **82**(Suppl. 1), 146a.

184 Carella A.M., Carlier P., Congiu A. *et al.* (1991) Autologous bone marrow transplantation as adjuvant treatment for high-risk Hodgkin's disease in first complete remission after MOPP/ABVD protocol. *Bone Marrow Transplantation*, **8**, 99–103.

185 Rapoport A.P., Rowe J.M., Kouides P.A. *et al.* (1993) One hundred autotransplants for relapsed or refractory Hodgkin's disease and lymphoma: value of pretransplant disease status for predicting outcome. *Journal of Clinical Oncology*, **11**, 2351–2361.

186 Rohatiner A.Z.S., Freedman A., Nadler L., Lim J & Lister T.A. (1994) Myeloablative therapy with autologous bone marrow transplantation as consolidation therapy for follicular lymphoma. *Annals of Oncology*, **5**(Suppl. 2), S143–S146.

187 Wheeler C., Strawderman M., Ayash L. *et al.* (1993) Prognostic factors for treatment outcome in autotransplantation of intermediate-grade and high-grade non-Hodgkin's lymphoma with cyclophosphamide, carmustine, and etoposide. *Journal of Clinical Oncology*, **11**, 1085–1091.

188 Johnson P.W.M., Price C.G.A., Smith T. *et al.* (1994) Detection of

cells bearing the t(14;18) translocation following myeloablative treatment and autologous bone marrow transplantation for follicular lymphoma. *Journal of Clinical Oncology*, **12**, 798–805.

189 Freedman A.S., Ritz J., Neuberg D. *et al.* (1991) Autologous bone marrow transplantation in 69 patients with a history of low-grade B-cell non-Hodgkin's lymphoma. *Blood*, **77**, 2524–2529.

190 Darrington D.L., Vose J.M., Anderson J.R. *et al.* (1994) Incidence and characterization of secondary myelodysplastic syndrome and acute myelogenous leukemia following high-dose chemoradiotherapy and autologous stem-cell transplantation for lymphoid malignancies. *Journal of Clinical Oncology*, **12**, 2527–2534.

191 Miller J.S., Arthur D.C., Litz C.E., Neglia J.P., Miller W.J. & Weisdorf D.J. (1994) Myelodysplastic syndrome after autologous bone marrow transplantation: an additional late complication of curative cancer therapy. *Blood*, **83**, 3780–3786.

192 Talbot D.C, Powles R.L., Sloane J.P. *et al.* (1990) Cyclosporine-induced graft-versus-host disease following autologous bone marrow transplantation in acute myeloid leukaemia. *Bone Marrow Transplantation*, **6**, 17–20.

193 Rizzoli V., Carella A.M., Carlo-Stella C. & Mangoni L. (1990) Autologous marrow transplantation in acute lymphoblastic leukemia: control of residual disease with mafosfamide and induction of syngeneic GVHD with cyclosporin. The Italian Mafosfamide Study Group. *Bone Marrow Transplantation*, **6**(Suppl. 1), 76–78.

194 Carella A.M., Gaozza E., Raffo M.R. *et al.* (1991) Therapy of acute phase chronic myelogenous leukemia with intensive chemotherapy, blood cell autotransplant and cyclosporine A. *Leukemia*, **5**, 517–521.

195 Yeager A.M., Vogelsang G.B., Jones R.J. *et al.* (1992) Induction of cutaneous graft-versus-host disease by administration of cyclosporine to patients undergoing autologous bone marrow transplantation for acute myeloid leukemia. *Blood*, **79**, 3031–3035.

196 Nagler A., Ackerstein A., Or R. *et al.* (1992) Adoptive immunotherapy with mismatched allogeneic peripheral blood lymphocytes (PBL) following autologous bone marrow transplantation (ABMT). *Experimental Hematology*, **20**, 705.

197 Slavin S., Or R., Kapelushnik Y. *et al.* (1992) Immunotherapy of minimal residual disease in conjunction with autologous and allogeneic bone marrow transplantation (BMT). *Leukemia*, **6**(Suppl. 1), 164–166.

198 Morecki S., Revel Vilk S., Nabet C. *et al.* (1992) Immunological evaluation of patients with hematological malignancies receiving ambulatory cytokine-mediated immunotherapy with recombinant human interferon-alpha 2a and interleukin-2. *Cancer Immunology and Immunotherapy*, **35**, 401–411.

199 Benyunes M.C., Massumoto C., York A. *et al.* (1993) Interleukin-2 with or without lymphokine-activated killer cells as consolidative immunotherapy after autologous bone marrow transplantation for acute myelogenous leukemia. *Bone Marrow Transplantation*, **12**, 159–163.

200 Fefer A., Benyunes M., Higuchi C. *et al.* (1993) Interleukin-2 +/– lymphocytes as consolidative immunotherapy after autologous bone marrow transplantation for hematologic malignancies. *Acta Haematologica*, **89**(Suppl. 1), 2–7.

201 Neubauer M.A., Benyunes M.C., Thompson J.A. *et al.* (1994) Lymphokine-activated killer (LAK) precursor cell activity is present in infused peripheral blood stem cells and in the blood after autologous peripheral blood stem cell transplantation. *Bone Marrow Transplantation*, **13**, 311–316.

202 Busca A., Anasetti C., Anderson G. *et al.* (1994) Unrelated donor or autologous marrow transplantation for treatment of acute leukemia. *Blood*, **83**, 3077–3084.

203 Chopra R., Goldstone A.H., Pearce R. *et al.* (1992) Autologous versus allogeneic bone marrow transplantation for non-Hodgkin's lymphoma: a case-controlled analysis of the European Bone Marrow Transplant Group Registry data. *Journal of Clinical Oncology*, **10**, 1690–1695.

204 Ratanatharathorn V., Uberti J., Karanes C. *et al.* (1994) Prospective comparative trial of autologous versus allogeneic bone marrow transplantation in patients with non-Hodgkin's lymphoma. *Blood*, **84**, 1050–1055.

205 Lundberg J.H., Hansen R.M., Chitambar C.R. *et al.* (1991) Allogeneic bone marrow transplantation for relapsed and refractory lymphoma using genotypically HLA-identical and alternative donors. *Journal of Clinical Oncology*, **9**, 1848–1859.

206 Burnett A.K. (1997) Evaluation of chemotherapy, allogeneic and autologous bone marrow transplants for the treatment of AML. *Bone Marrow Transplant*, **19**(Suppl. 1), S160.

207 Burnett A.K., Goldstone A.H., Stevens R., Hann I., Rees J.K. & Wheatley K. (1995) Biological characteristics of disease determine the outcome of allogeneic and autologous BMT in CR1. *Blood*, **86**(Suppl. 1), 616a.

208 Ferrant A., Labopin M., Frassoni F. *et al.* (1997) Karyotype in acute myeloblastic leukemia: prognostic significance for bone marrow transplantation in first remission: a European Group for Blood and Marrow Transplantation study. *Blood*, **90**, 2931–2938.

209 Attal M., Harousseau J.L., Stoppa A.M. *et al.* (1996) A prospective, randomized trial of autologous bone marrow transplantation and chemotherapy in multiple myeloma. Intergroupe Francais du Myelome. *New England Journal of Medicine*, **335**, 91–97.

210 Vesole D.H., Tricot G., Jagannath S. *et al.* (1996) Autotransplants in multiple myeloma: what have we learned? *Blood*, **88**, 838–847.

211 Singhal S., Mehta J., Barlogie B. (1997) Advances in the treatment of multiple myeloma. *Current Opinion in Hematology*, **4**, 291–297.

212 Majolino I., Pearce R., Taghipour G. & Goldstone A.H. (1997) Peripheral blood stem-cell transplantation versus autologous bone marrow transplantation in Hodgkin's and non-Hodgkin's lymphomas: a new matched-pair analysis of the European Group for Blood and Marrow Transplantation Registry Data. Lymphoma Working Party of the European Group for Blood and Marrow Transplantation. *Journal of Clinical Oncology*, **15**, 509–517.

213 Philip T., Guglielmi C., Hagenbeek A. *et al.* (1995) Autologous bone marrow transplantation as compared with salvage chemotherapy in relapses of chemotherapy-sensitive non-Hodgkin's lymphoma. *New England Journal of Medicine*, **333**, 1540–1545.

214 Haioun C., Lepage E., Gisselbrecht C. *et al.* (1997) Benefit of autologous bone marrow transplantation over sequential chemotherapy in poor-risk aggressive non-Hodgkin's lymphoma: updated results of the prospective study LNH87-2. Groupe d'Etude des Lymphomes de l'Adulte. *Journal of Clinical Oncology*, **15**, 1131–1137.

215 Gianni A.M., Bregni M., Siena S. *et al.* (1997) High-dose chemotherapy and autologous bone marrow transplantation compared with MACOP-B in aggressive B-cell lymphoma. *New England Journal of Medicine*, **336**, 1290–1297.

24 Supportive Care: Blood Products

J.A.F. Napier

Introduction

Leukaemic disorders in general are characterized by hypoplasia of normal haemopoesis and accelerated consumption or destruction of circulating functional blood cells. As a result, severely symptomatic anaemia, thrombocytopenia and neutropenia are potential major causes of morbidity and mortality. Maintenance of an acceptable level of haematological functionality is therefore an essential cornerstone of management. Patients with leukaemia are heavily dependent on the transfusion centre output of blood products and certainly account for the majority of platelet concentrate usage. The efforts of all involved in transfusion therapy must therefore be directed towards ensuring that an adequate supply of safe and effective materials is always available for patients in need. As a consequence, most transfusion services have responded by dramatically increasing the provision of blood components for transfusion support. This seemingly successful cooperative arrangement has not come about easily. Clinical demands have always tended to exceed supplies, hence shortages are likely. Platelet products in particular have a limited shelf life and therefore cannot be stored to any significant extent; an unexpected reduction in demand will therefore contribute to these expensive materials becoming outdated.

Platelet transfusion

The success of modern intensive chemotherapy or bone marrow transplantation (BMT) regimens, which entail haemopoetic ablation, depends very much on the ability to control the risk of haemorrhage by platelet transfusions. This very success in the use of platelet therapy has led to further problems being identified. The capacity of platelet concentrates, for example, to transmit cytomegalovirus (CMV) infection, to cause graft vs host disease (GVHD) in immunocompromised recipients and, more seriously, the frequent induction of refractoriness, a state of immune-mediated unresponsiveness to platelet therapy, have all necessitated

preventative action. Even today, when there are active attempts to develop synthetic alternatives to many of the current human-based transfusion products, there is no prospect of any substitute for platelet concentrates derived from voluntary blood donations.

To achieve the most effective use of this valuable resource, it is necessary to define the proper indications for platelet therapy. In particular, it is important to identify and take preventative measures for patients who would be difficult to manage if they became unresponsive to conventional treatment, and to improve serological procedures for providing compatible platelets for those who do become refractory. Because the management of the refractory state is such a difficult problem, simple, effective and economical measures for reducing the immunogenicity of platelet concentrates are also a high priority.

The preparation and storage of platelets must be improved, so that functional effectiveness is preserved, but without increasing the risks of bacterial contamination. There is also a need for better *in vitro* measures of potential clinical efficacy which could be incorporated into quality control programmes.

Structural and functional aspects

Normal platelets have a discoid structure of approximate diameter 2–4 μm and volume 5.8–8.7 fl. Suspended in plasma, they impart a characteristic opalescent appearance. Progressive metabolic deterioration during the artificial conditions of storage leads to spherical transformation and the development of multiple spicular protuberances from the platelet surface. These features are indicative of loss of platelet viability.

The plasma membrane bounding the platelet surface is invaginated to form an intricate labyrinthine internal tubular system—the tubules each leading to the external surface. This system serves as a pathway for secreted materials. Running circumferentially within the disc perimeter is a bundle-shaped microtubular structure which maintains the discoid shape. A further functionally separate darkly staining dense tubular system occupies the cytoplasmic interior, and this appears to function as a calcium-storage organelle and for prostaglandin synthesis. The platelet surface membrane is highly absorptive for a variety of plasma proteins, including factor VIII, von Willebrand complex, fibrinogen and other coagulation factors. The platelet cytoplasm contains large numbers of secretory granules related to its haemostatic function. Alpha granules are most numerous and are apparently the storage site for many platelet-secreted proteins, for example, beta-thromboglobin, P-F4, platelet-derived growth factor and various clotting factors. Smaller numbers of densely staining granules contain ATP, ADP, calcium and serotonin. Immediately beneath the inner cytoplasmic membrane lies a network of actin fibres which, together with the circumferential band of microtubules, assists in the maintenance of the discoid shape.

Damage to the vascular endothelial lining, particularly where collagen fibres are exposed, is quickly followed by recruitment of platelets from the circulating blood to plug the site of injury and leakage. The haemostatic process begins with platelet adhesion to the site of injury. Platelets then undergo rapid conversion from a discoid to a spherical structure with multiple pseudopodia—this process appears to follow contraction of actin, myosin and other contractile cytoskeletal components in the platelet cytoplasm. The pseudopodia appear to facilitate adhesion and mutual attachment of adjacent platelets. Discharge of alpha-granule and dense-body contents occurs, further reinforcing the local adhesion/aggregation stimulus and recruiting further platelets. This mass of adherent aggregating platelets quickly spreads to cover the area of vascular surface injury. Additional platelet membrane changes occur to make available clot-promoting platelet factor 3 activity, which facilitates development of a coagulant plug to reinforce the original platelet plug. Thrombin formation, probably formed in part on the platelet surface, completes the transformation of the mixture of adherent platelets and developing fibrin meshwork into the beginning of a more haemostatically robust fibrin clot.

Platelet kinetics

Platelet counts within the normal population may vary from 150 to 450×10^9/l. The range seems remarkably wide for such an important blood constituent, but platelet size also varies widely and the two variables correlate inversely, i.e. larger platelets are found in individuals with lower counts and vice versa [1]. This has led to the concept of total functional platelet mass [2], a product of the platelet count and mean platelet volume [3,4] akin to total red cell mass determination. The total platelet mass seems to show less variation among individuals, and it may be that this parameter provides the signal for homeostatic feedback control [2]. This being the case, it might be reasonable to suppose that total platelet mass could be used as a potentially better predictor of haemostatic risk than the platelet count in thrombocytopenic states alone. Although

there is a general impression that the risk of bleeding seems somewhat less in thrombocytopenias with higher mean platelet volumes, these observations are not yet sufficiently well substantiated to be clinically helpful.

Platelets are constantly required for the maintenance of vascular integrity. Small injuries resulting from the normal pattern of daily trauma must be sealed instantly. This process of aggregation and adhesion, sealing sites of vascular injury, consumes a proportion of the daily platelet turnover. Based on the normal lifespan of around 8–11 days, about 10–12% of the total circulating pool will be destroyed daily. Assuming a 5-litre blood volume, this amounts to a replacement rate of around $75–225 \times 10^9$ platelets daily. Hanson & Slichter [5] demonstrated that in both normal and in hypoplastic thrombocytopenic subjects, platelet lifespan became shorter as the platelet count fell. Their studies provided evidence for a fixed platelet requirement which they assumed was that required for maintenance of normal haemostasis and amounted to around 7.1×10^9/l per day. This appeared to be a rapid random consumptive process but which corresponded to no more than 18% of the daily turnover in normal subjects. The remaining platelets were presumed to be destroyed by a slower process of senescence. In hypoplastic thrombocytopenia, the haemostatically consumed fraction occupies a progressively greater proportion of total platelet turnover as platelet counts fall. Under these circumstances, symptoms would not be expected until platelet production falls below the calculated 7.1×10^9/l daily requirement for haemostasis. This would amount to 35×10^9 total platelets for an adult with a blood volume of 5 litres. These figures are relevant to the determination of dosages for prophylactic support.

Production and quality control of platelet concentrates

Therapeutic doses of platelets are supplied as concentrates prepared either from random volunteer blood donations or from a variety of apheresis procedures.

Platelets from random donors

Random donor platelets must be prepared from whole blood which has not been cooled below 20°C [6]. It is conventionally accepted that separation and concentrate production should be accomplished within 8 hours of collection [7], although protocols for a preprocessing hold for upto 24 hours have been validated [8]. Traditional methods have involved first-step preparation of platelet-rich plasma [9] by centrifugation of whole blood. After careful removal of the platelet-rich plasma from the sedimented red cells, further centrifugation can be used to sediment platelets together with an unavoidable number of contaminating red cells and leucocytes. Finally, most of the supernatant plasma is removed to leave a platelet concentrate together with about 50 ml of plasma. An increasing number of laboratories are now utilizing an alternative procedure, whereby a high-speed spin ($3000g$) is used to demarcate the buffy coat layer between red cells and plasma. After decanting the supernatant platelet-depleted plasma, the buffy coats can then be removed, pooled with others to make an appropriate therapeutic dose, and then subjected to a further spin to permit removal of most of the contaminating red cells and leucocytes. Although technically more cumbersome, this latter method may cause less traumatic damage to the platelets and result in a more pure product [10]. Nominally, each single donation is assumed to contain 7.0×10^9 platelets. Quality control requirements usually specify that more than 75% should have platelet counts in excess of 5.5×10^9 [7,11].

Platelets from apheresis procedures

Most transfusion services supply a proportion of routine platelets by apheresis procedures. These offer certain logistic benefits, because they are collected in more predictable numbers and often in close proximity to the transfusion centre. They are especially advantageous for special donor requirements, for example when CMV-negative or HLA-typed donations must be met from designated panels of donors. Plateletpheresis is now a highly efficient means of high-quality platelet procurement. Machines such as the COBE spectre and Fenwall CS3000 are capable of collecting $5–6 \times 10^{11}$ platelets with much lower leucocyte contamination than previously used apheresis procedures and conventional random donor products [12,13]. Preselection of donors is important, the best yields are obtained if donors with lower than average platelet counts are excluded. Apheresis machines are microprocessor controlled and, if provided with figures for donor body weight and platelet count, will calculate the optimum operating conditions necessary to ensure the desired yield. The use of both arms (for blood collection and return) and the need to spare the 100 or so minutes necessary for the collection has not been found to discourage most donors. It is normally possible to collect two patient dose equivalents, the platelet components will have negligible red cell contamination and white cell count can also be very low; a proportion may even meet leucocyte-depleted product requirements ($<5 \times 10^6$ per random donor equivalent). If products are to be issued as leuco-depleted, it is essential to confirm by quality control counting that each donation reaches the specified standard. Leucocyte numbers are generally too low for counting by conventional blood cell analysers; use of the specially designed Nageotte counting chamber [14] or flow cytometry [15,16] is necessary.

Storage of platelet concentrates

Platelet concentrates are now invariably stored at $22 \pm 2°C$ — this temperature results in optimal post-transfusion recovery and survival. Platelet survivals ($t_{\frac{1}{2}}$) of around 5 days are to be expected under normal circumstances. It does, however, appear that recovery of full haemostatic function may not be achieved until a few hours following transfusion [17–20].

The logistics of maintaining platelet banking have been improved, following greater understanding of the storage needs of platelets. The observation of platelets during storage demonstrated that post-transfusion viability was worst in packs showing a low Po_2; these changes being associated with anaerobic glycolysis, lactate accumulation, glucose depletion, low pH and high Pco_2. These adverse changes could be averted by the use of storage packs manufactured from plastics with better gas-exchange characteristics [21–24]. These plastics permit escape of CO_2 and transfer of O_2 and, as a result, more efficient (in terms of ATP generation) aerobic glycolysis. Less glucose is utilized, less lactate is generated and the pH is maintained at higher levels. These newer plastics are now in widespread use for random donor platelet concentrates and are also being incorporated as part of the harnesses for plateletpheresis machines. Platelet storage life for random donations has, as a result of these developments, been extended from 3 to 5 days postcollection. Adequate metabolic function and survival characteristics can in fact be maintained for 7 days, and this was originally permitted for platelet storage until increasing reports of severe microbial contamination led to reversion to the shorter storage period.

Platelets have, until recently, been stored in the same plasma-anticoagulant preservative solution that had been designed for optimal preservation of red cells. Recognition of the metabolic problems encountered by stored platelets, as well as realization that platelet cytoplasm still retains the efficient Krebs citric acid cycle phase of glycolysis, has opened up the possibility of designing specifically tailored platelet preservation solutions [25,26]. Platelets, through the citric acid glycolytic cycle, are able to utilize a far wider range of energy substrates than red cells. Acetate in particular has been shown to be a good energy source. It seems likely that in the near future, therapeutic platelets will be provided as a suspension in an optimally designed artificial storage medium rather than, as now, in the plasma-anticoagulant solution designed for red cell storage.

Quality control and laboratory assessment of platelets for transfusion

Unlike transfusion of red cells or many other transfusion materials, it is less easy to be confident that a platelet transfusion will produce a sustained increment restoring normal function. Not only is the collection and preparation of platelet concentrates an inherently more variable process, but platelets are also liable to mechanical or metabolic damage during their preparative manipulations. Even after successful preparation, poor storage may lead to premature deterioration and loss of clinical efficacy. There has been no shortage of means for assessing platelet function, but relatively few parameters provide a reliable guide to the likely efficacy of transfused platelets.

The deterioration of platelet morphology during storage does equate with poor post-transfusion survival [27,28] and is generally associated with a fall in pH to 6.0 or below [24]. Objective measurement of the disc to sphere transformation can be made either by careful microscopic examination of platelet suspensions and scoring the degree of abnormality [29], or by measurement of light transmission through an agitated platelet suspension [29–31]. Optical measurements of platelet quality are not, however, in widespread use. Most transfusion services routinely measure pH change in a proportion of platelet concentrates — storage conditions should be such that pH remains above 6.4 throughout. The response of platelets to hypotonic shock [32] is also claimed to be an accurate measure of potential *in vivo* effectiveness, although in other studies its value has been less convincing [33,34]. Hypotonic shock causes abrupt spherical transformation. The capacity of platelets to recover their previous discoid shape is an index of their metabolic state and, presumably, *in vivo* viability.

Aggregation tests involving ADP, collagen, or other aggregating agents have not generally been found to be helpful as markers of clinical efficacy, nor have measurements of serotonin uptake and ATP content. Assay of lactic dehydrogenase and thromboglobulin release into the surrounding media give an indication of the degree of mechanical disruption and may be helpful in comparing the damaging effect of various preparative manipulations.

Inappropriate platelet activation, caused either by mechanical handling during preparation or by storage-related deterioration, has been shown to result in poor post-transfusion recovery. Activation results in expression of an alpha granule membrane protein GMP-140 on the platelet surface [35,36]. The proportion of the platelets expressing GMP-140 can be measured by flow cytometry using monoclonal anti GMP-140 and the results seem promising as a quality control measure for platelet control production storage.

More reliable *in vivo* assessment of likely efficacy is obtained by measurements of platelet survival and bleeding time correction. Post-transfusion survival of radiolabelled platelets (^{51}Cr or ^{111}In oxine are the usual labels) are used to validate changes in collection, storage or preparative conditions. These assessments are usually performed by the use of autologous transfusions in volunteers. The techniques are not applicable in the clinical setting, as in most patients extraneous factors such as alloimmunization, blood loss and sepsis cause shortened survival and negate the value of the investigation. The measurement of template bleeding time correction should, in theoretical terms, provide useful confirmation that a clinically successful transfusion has occurred. In practice, during the management of oncology patients, bleeding time measurements have little value and would be an unnecessarily distressing intrusion [37]. Bleeding times will be invariably prolonged at pretreatment platelet count levels and it is presumed that if an acceptable increment can be achieved post-transfusion, then haemostatic improvement will occur.

Bacterial contamination is a much-feared complication of platelet therapy, and monitoring sterility of a small proportion of platelet concentrates is often done to confirm that collection and preparative procedures are aseptically sound.

Clinical indications for platelet therapy

Platelets are used either for treatment of thrombocytopenic bleeding, or for prophylaxis where there is a risk of bleeding. The relationship between the risk of bleeding and low platelet counts was first clearly demonstrated by Duke in 1910 [38]. The bleeding time lengthens as the platelet count falls, although this relationship is only true for counts below 100×10^9/l [39,40]. Although spontaneous bleeding will not occur at the higher level, it is now generally agreed that, in actively bleeding patients with a platelet count around 50×10^9/l, thrombocytopenia is at least playing a contributory role and requires correction. At lower counts, bleeding may occur in the absence of trauma, but the precise point at which there is a significant increase in risk has been difficult to obtain. The danger of life-threatening haemorrhage or irreversible damage secondary to bleeding means careful attention should be paid to devising safe prophylactic transfusion policies. For each patient, these require accurate assesment of the bleeding risk at given low platelet counts, recognizing that factors other than the platelet count influence the degree of risk.

Haemorrhage is more likely in patients with anaemia. Reduction of the bleeding risk of thrombocytopenic patients following transfusion was recorded, even in the original studies of Duke [38]. Further evidence was provided 50 years later by Hellem *et al.* [41], and more recently by others [42,43], showing that the bleeding time correlated inversely with the haematocrit. Loss of the platelet aggregation promoting effect of red cell ADP was considered as a possible factor to explain this phenomenon. A rheological explanation now seems more tenable. During blood flow, at normal haematocrit, red cells crowding in the axial stream displace platelets to the periphery and thus closer contact with the vascular endothelium [44–46]. This effect is lost during anaemia and platelets may therefore be less able to adhere and aggregate to damaged areas.

The mean age of circulating platelets may determine their haemostatic capacity. At any given platelet count, the bleeding predisposition seems less for high turnover states with an active regenerative element. Patients with marrow recovery appear less vulnerable than those with falling platelet counts. This may be linked to changes in platelet volume, which are larger during bone marrow regeneration. Roy *et al.* [47] noted that for the same platelet count, recently transfused patients experience less bleeding than untransfused patients. It was suggested that the younger transfused platelets are functionally more effective.

Sepsis and fever also appear to increase the risk of bleeding [48,49]. Increased platelet turnover has been observed and loss of the expected post-transfusion increments is a well-recognized phenomenon [50]. These effects have been claimed to be worse with stored platelets compared to fresh platelets [51].

Concomitant drug therapy must always be considered in thrombocytopenic patients. Apart from the numerous and well-recognized platelet-damaging effects of drug therapy, there are several drugs that are specific to the management of patients with leukaemia. Commonly used antibiotics, particularly those of the synthetic penicillin category [52], impair platelet function. This may also be true for several cytotoxic agents, including vincristine, L-asparaginase, daunorubicin and cyclophosphamide [52,53].

Prophylactic therapy and the risk of spontaneous bleeding

The rationale for prophylactic platelet therapy is based on the premise that serious thrombocytopenic bleeding—that liable to cause distress, irreversible injury or even death—can occur without sufficient warning for early treatment of the symptoms to be effective. This view has generally prevailed in the management of haematological malignancies, although the argument that prophylactic therapy actually improves overall survival is controversial [54] Murphy *et al.* [55] randomized

children with acute leukaemia into a treatment group for whom platelets were provided only for bleeding episodes, was compared with a group for whom prophylaxis was given for platelet counts below 20 × 10⁹/l. Those given prophylaxis showed a significantly longer symptom-free phase prior to their first bleeding episode, but there was no difference in survival rate between the two groups (Figs 24.1 & 24.2). Using a similar prophylactic transfusion policy, Roy *et al.* [47] were able to demonstrate that a 58% incidence of bleeding episodes could be reduced to 8%. Despite the rather conflicting conclusions from available studies [56], most haematologists favour the institution of prophylactic platelet transfusion for patients with platelet counts falling to about 20 × 10⁹/l [57–59].

Prophylactic therapy has been claimed to have been instrumental in the dramatic reduction of haemorrhage, particularly cerebal haemorrhage, as a cause of death. There are however disadvantages, platelet transfusion adds to the overall cost of treatment, increased donor exposure may accelerate the appearance of refractoriness and will certainly multiply the infection transmission risk. A second point of contention concerns the platelet count level at which prophylactic therapy should be started. It has been difficult to determine the precise point at which a discernible change in risk level occurs. Gaydos *et al.* [60] recognized a gradual increase in symptoms as throm-

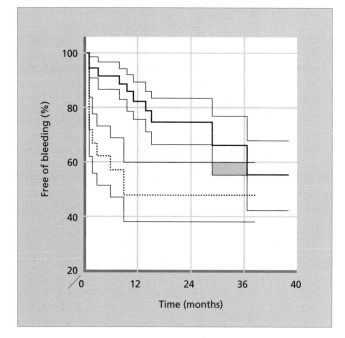

Fig. 24.1 Percentage of patients free of bleeding at intervals after randomization. The thin black lines represent ±1 standard deviation (68% confidence limit). The cross-hatched region is the region that the areas have in common. The percentage of patients remaining free of bleeding at intervals after randomization is increased in the prophylactic (——) as opposed to the therapeutic (----) group. See text for further description. (From Murphy *et al.*, 1982 [55], with permission.)

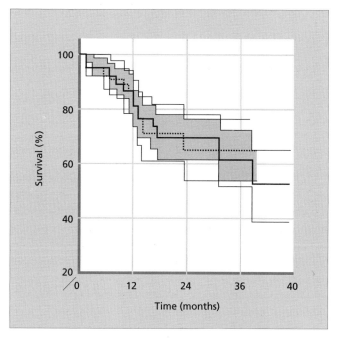

Fig. 24.2 Life-table analysis of patients treated with prophylactic (——) or therapeutic (----) platelet transfusion. As in Fig. 24.1, the cross-hatched region represents the region that the two 68% confidence limits have in common. There is no difference in survival for the two regimens for the total group (shown above) or for ALL analysed separately. See text for further description. (From Murphy *et al.*, 1982 [55], with permission.)

bocytopenia became more severe, but substantial increases in bleeding risk were not seen until counts fell to below 20 × 10^9/l, and serious episodes of haemorrhage occurred only in the range 5–10 × 10^9/l. Roy *et al.* [47], studying acute lymphatic leukaemia in children, identified the earliest evidence of minor bleeding in the form of cutaneous and mucous membrane haemorrhage or epistaxes at counts below 50 × 10^9/l. Severe bleeding, however, occurred in 4% of their patients at counts between 30 and 50 × 10^9/l, but the incidence rose to 26% for severely thrombocytopenic patients with counts below 10 × 10^9/l. Freireich *et al.* [61] calculated the incidence of days with gross haemorrhage in thrombocytopenic patients and observed a significant increase only in those with counts below 5 × 10^9/l. These observations are supported by radiolabelled blood loss studies, which confirmed the view that substantial risk was confined to patients with counts below 5 × 10^9/l. Intracranial haemorrhage is the most severe complication of thrombocytopenia, and this has been largely restricted to patients with platelet counts below 5 × 10^9/l, with the exception of those with high blast counts in whom bleeding may be associated with intracerebral infiltrates [62–64] likewise identified patients at serious risk of bleeding only below 5 × 10^9/l.

Thresholds for the institution of prophylactic therapy have varied according to institutional practices. It now seems to be becoming generally accepted that prophylaxis may not be necessary until platelet counts have fallen to 10 × 10^9/l, unless there are other complicating problems such as fever, sepsis, disseminated intravascular coagulation (DIC), or sites of tissue injury [65]. If there are such risk factors for bleeding, target values approaching 50 × 10^9/l might be more appropriate.

Bone marrow transplantation and platelet transfusion

Because of the fear of a higher risk of future graft rejection as a consequence of minor HLA sensitization, it is generally believed that family members should not be used as platelet donors for patients with aplastic anaemia who are anticipating BMT. However, this has not been shown to be disadvantageous in the case of patients with leukaemia [66]. Allogeneic BMT may well not lead to substantially different platelet transfusion requirements when compared to chemotherapy [67–70]. The position for autologous bone marrow transplants may be different. Smith *et al.* [71] claims significantly greater needs for platelet support during autologous compared to allogeneic transplants. The use of autologous peripheral blood stem cell transplants for marrow rescue is increasing. Thrombopoietic recovery is faster with peripheral blood stem cell transplant, and the duration of platelet support is correspondingly reduced. CMV infections [72] and GVHD [73] are both recognized as causing increased platelet needs. There is some evidence that platelet needs can be influenced by the use of haemopoietic growth factors, such as granulocyte macrophage colony-stimulating factor (GM-CSF), which might be expected

to have some thrombopoietic effect [74–76]. Studies of combinations with IL-3, IL-6 and IL-7 appear to produce some platelet count increases. Both GM-CSF and G-CSF have been shown to accelerate the recovery of neutrophil function and to reduce the vulnerability to infection [76], although overall survival may not be improved [77,78]. The recent identification and cloning of thrombopoietin [79] opens up exciting possibilities for therapeutic enhancement of platelet production. The success of thrombopoietic growth factor treatment will, of course, be contingent on the presence of sufficient numbers of growth factor-sensitive megakaryocyte precursor cells.

The refractory state

Compared to red cells, conventional platelet transfusions are highly immunogenic and a large proportion of patients eventually show evidence of immunization to platelet-borne antigens. This phenomenon, known as refractoriness, shows itself both as a loss of the clinically beneficial effect as well as a failure to obtain the expected post-transfusion elevation of the recipient's platelet count. Post-transfusion platelet counts, in particular the corrected count increment (CCI), provide the most reliable guide to expected efficacy. The CCI [80] is calculated as follows:

$$CCI = \left(\text{post-transfusion}-\text{pretransfusion count}\right) \\ \times \text{body surface area (m}^2) \\ / \text{number of platelets transfused} \left(\times 10^{11}\right)$$

Increments are conventionally measured either at 1 hour or at 24 hours, or at both times [81]. The occurrence of two consecutive 1-hour CCIs below 7.5 × 10^9, in the absence of other factors known to diminish platelet recovery, are usually taken as evidence of alloimmunization and the refractory state. Ten-minute increments have been claimed to be equally valuable as a clinical indicator of likely efficacy [82], and are often more convenient. Assessment of the success of transfusion is complicated by the imperfect correlation between results at 1 hour and those at 24 hours. Drawing a parallel with post-transfusion red cell survival in alloimmunized patient studies, it would be reasonable to assume that the differences in post-transfusion survival reflect quantitative and qualitative aspects of antibody function or underlying differences in the phagocytic capacity of the recipient's reticuloendothelial system.

Although alloimmune-mediated platelet destruction attracts the greatest attention as a cause of the refractory state, it is most important that the patient be assessed carefully for the presence of other contributing factors. Fever, sepsis, active bleeding, disseminated intravascular coagulation (DIC) and splenomegaly are now well-recognized factors associated with the loss of post-transfusion efficacy [50,83,84]. Various estimates have been made of the relative proportion of immune and nonimmune causes of the refractory state. It seems that nonimmune causes may well contribute the greater proportion of apparently unresponsive patients. Estimates of the likelihood of developing immune refractoriness during platelet transfusion support range from 24 to 90% [50,64,85–87]. In the majority of cases the immune refractory state reflects sensitization to human leucocyte antigens (HLA) of transfused cellular products. A history of previous transfusion or pregnancies [86,88] is generally agreed to predispose to refractoriness. Conversely, chemotherapy-induced immunosuppression is likely to retard its appearance [87]. Certainly, patients with acute leukaemia do not develop platelet unresponsiveness as readily as those with aplastic anaemia [87], in whom virtually all eventually become highly refractory. Patients with acute lymphoblastic leukaemia (ALL) appear less liable to become refractory than those with acute myeloid leukaemia (AML) [89].

It has been important to attempt to answer certain questions relevant to the appearance of immunization. There is uncertainty about how much the phenomenon is related to the dose of platelet therapy administered. A strong dose–response relationship would be a constraint to the use of prophylactic therapy. A number of studies have shown that refractoriness often takes some months to appear, and is related to the dose of blood products administered [86,90–92]. In these studies, refractoriness only rarely arose to complicate the first remission induction phase of patients with acute leukaemia. Howard & Perkins [86] also showed a progressive increase in the proportion of patients immunized over the first 2 months of transfusion therapy. In contrast, Sintnicolaas *et al.* [90] showed platelet recoveries diminished even by the second transfusion episode, and became steadily worse as transfusions continued. In the series of Dutcher *et al.* [93], most of the patients who became refractory also did so early in their treatment programme, 38% within a few weeks of therapy, some even becoming refractory after only four donor exposures. The more general experience suggests that exposure to between 10 and 20 or so donors seems sufficient to identify predisposed patients [86,94]. Patients who do not become sensitized within the first 3 months rarely do so later. In these studies, most patients who became refractory developed cytotoxic HLA antibodies, these being assumed to be causative.

Common to almost all studies is the observation that 30% or more patients never show alloimmunization and refractoriness, however long transfusion support is maintained [86,93]. Even patients who do become immunized may sometimes show loss of HLA antibodies and recover therapeutic responsiveness [89]. This has been observed not only in patients in whom therapy was discontinued, but also in others receiving further transfusions of mismatched donations [83,87].

Development of the refractory state

Alternative approaches to the prevention of alloimmunization became apparent when it was recognized that, in several species, including man, pure platelets are not on their own capable of inducing HLA sensitization [95,96]. Although platelets carry HLA-Class I antigens, thus explaining their post-transfusion destruction in alloimmunized patients, they lack the HLA-Class II products which are necessary for induction of the anti-HLA immune response. HLA immunization appears to be due to the HLA-Class II antigens of contaminating leucocytes (predominantly B-lymphocytes and monocytes), which are invariably present in platelet concentrates produced under normal conditions. Leucocytes carrying Class II products are capable of presenting their foreign Class I-HLA gene products to T-helper cells of the recipient. This process is followed by T-helper-cell secretion of growth factors, which activate B cells of the recipient and thereby initiate alloimmune responses to the donor HLA-Class I products. Contaminating leucocytes bearing Class II products therefore serve as a catalyst permitting immunization to Class I products.

Based on animal studies [96,97] showing that purified platelet suspensions do not stimulate alloimmunization, clinical trials of leucocyte-depleted transfusion regimens were established and these have, in general, confirmed the clinical utility of this approach. Large numbers of studies have been conducted since the early 1980s, and it has become progressively clear that the better the quality of leucodepletion, the more successfully alloimmunization can be prevented. Modern leucocyte depletion filters are capable of a greater than 99.9% reduction of leucocytes from both red cells and platelet products and appear to virtually prevent alloimmunization in patients who have not been previously sensitized by transfusion or pregnancy [98]. However, the feasibility of the successful wider-scale application of filtration procedures cannot be assumed [99].

Leucocyte depletion of blood components

Platelets stated to be leucocyte depleted should, by common definition, contain below 5×10^6 leucocytes for each transfusion. This is most reliably achieved by filtration using the modern third-generation leucocyte-depleted filters. If these are to be used in the context of a programme to prevent alloimmunization, quality-control leucocyte counting must be performed on each donation. For reasons, which are not fully understood, occasional relative failures of filtration occur and transfusion of these substandard components could undermine the entire prophylactic effort for the patient concerned. Leucocyte removal should be carried out under standardized laboratory conditions, the practice of 'bedside' filtration, although superficially convenient and attractive, has proved unreliable. Leucocyte removal by filtration appears to be a complex process involving, to a variable extent, filtration, adhesion of leucocytes to the filter matrix and cell-to-cell adhesion. The nature of the blood component, its temperature and flow rate, are all important variables which must be standardized as far as possible. Filtered red cells should show a greater than 99% leucocyte removal, with no more than 15% red cell loss [100,101]. Platelet concentrates can be prepared with less than 5×10^6 leucocytes and less than 5–10% loss of platelets [102–104].

Although filtration has been found to be a most reliable way of achieving leucocyte depletion, some platelet apheresis machines, in particular the COBE spectra, now reach 'leucocyte depletion' levels of purity. Leucocyte-depleted products are considerably more costly than their routine counterparts, but this has to be balanced against the very expensive problem of managing patients refractory to conventional treatment. Filtration of platelets appears to cause little,if any, discernible damage [105]. Platelet morphology is little affected and aggregation and hypotonic shock responses and clot retraction are all comparable to unfiltered platelets [106]. Filter systems do not appear to damage *in vivo* platelet function or viability, as judged by bleeding time correction, post-transfusion increments or survival [106]. Holme *et al.* [107] studied a range of both *in vivo* and *in vitro* platelet viability parameters and found no substantial differences, apart from a slight but significant evidence of complement C3a activation.

There is currently very little information that would help in a cost–benefit based decision to utilize leucocyte-depleted components. It is likely that prevention of clinical immunization would be most successful in patients not previously transfused or pregnant; it may not be preventable for patients with previous exposure to blood or blood products. Widely performed studies, showing benefits in terms of morbidity, inpatient stay or improvements in overall survival [108], are not yet available. It does seem likely, however, that some patients, in particular those who for serological reasons could not be supported by matched platelets should immunization occur, would benefit under a leucodepleted blood programme.

Reduction of HLA immunogenicity using ultraviolet irradiation

It has been shown experimentally that platelet concentrates can be made incapable of stimulating HLA immunization by the apparently simple process of exposure to ultraviolet (UV) irradiation. Alloimmunization has been prevented by this means in canine transfusion studies [109,110]. Animal studies have also shown that induction of both *in vitro* and *in vivo* HLA sensitization requires the interaction between antigen-presenting cells and dendritic cells [111–113]. UV B irradiation (wavelength range 280–340 nm) destroys dendritic cell function and the cluster-forming activity between antigen-presenting cells is prevented. Lymphocytes from UV-irradiated human platelet concentrates do not respond to phytohaemagglutinin [113]. *In vitro* mixed lymphocyte culture (MLC) responses, and subsequent interleukin production, are also prevented. Fortunately, at the dose levels adequate for lymphocyte inactivation, *in vitro* platelet function seems unim-

paired [113,114], and platelet half-life and recovery are equivalent to nonirradiated controls [115]. However, conventional platelet storage containers transmit UV light poorly [114–116] —many plastics with better UV permeability do not meet the pack-pliability and gas-transport requirements for platelet storage. The potential value of a relatively inexpensive, noninvasive procedure for negating the immunogenicity of platelet concentrates is enormous, and it is to be hoped that the residual practical problems will eventually be overcome. Clearly, concurrent transfusions of red cells must not contain viable leucocytes and should be filtered. UV irradiation of red cell preparations is not feasible; red cells in their own right absorb virtually all the UV irradiation, leaving lymphocytes unaffected.

Management of the refractory state

Patients who appear to be refractory to conventional random donations present a difficult therapeutic problem. In view of the expense and the logistical difficulties of attempting to seek compatible donations, it is most important to establish conclusively that apparent unresponsiveness is a result of alloimmunization. The importance of other causes of poor response, such as fever, splenomegaly and DIC, must not be overlooked [50,117]. In all patients, regular monitoring of post-transfusion increments is essential.

Provided that satisfactory samples can be obtained, the opportunity should be taken to determine the HLA phenotype of patients in whom long-term platelet support is anticipated. In addition, regular serum screening for the presence of lymphocytotoxic antibodies should be carried out. When the diagnosis of refractoriness due to alloimmunization has been made, several approaches may be considered. As an initial measure, dose sizes or frequencies are sometimes increased [118]. More logically, efforts should be made to identify immunologically compatible platelets, either from HLA-matched donors or from donations which are lymphocytotoxicity crossmatch or platelet crossmatch compatible.

Provision of HLA-matched platelets

The provision of HLA-matched platelets represents the earliest, and is probably still the most widely practised, approach to the treatment of refractory patients [119]. It is only necessary to match for HLA-A and B antigens; those of the C locus seem unimportant in this respect. Several studies have confirmed the generally beneficial effects of fully HLA-matched transfusions. Tosato *et al.* [120], studying transfusion support of alloimmunized patients with aplastic anaemia, showed clearly a correlation between transfusion responses and the degree of HLA matching. Of donors fully matched for the recipient A and B loci, 28% provided excellent responses, while only 17% of those mismatched for two or more antigens were successful. Conversely, only 18% of fully matched transfusions were categorized as poor, while for two mismatched donor antigens 46% were regarded as failures. Very similar findings were reported by Lohrmann [121]; both fully matched donations and those with one of the recipient HLA antigens not identified in the donation were associated with satisfactory increments. Noteworthy in both these and subsequent studies is the very considerable variability of response occurring at all antigen matching levels. Both full A- and B-locus matching and complete mismatches will have successes as well as failures. The preponderance of clinical successes (approximately 65%), however, lies with fully matched donations. More recently, McFarland *et al.* [50], conducting a careful clinical and immunological evaluation of refractory patients, obtained nearly 100% clinical success rates for fully matched donations, provided that nonimmune factors were excluded and that proof of HLA immunization in the form of lymphocytotoxic antibodies could be demonstrated (Fig. 24.3). Unrelated HLA matches are less likely to be as closely identical as HLA-matched sibling donations, and it seems likely that unidentified minor histocompatibility antigen differences account for the poorer responses in some unrelated transfusions. In other instances, subtle but significant differences between apparently identical HLA-Class I phenotypes may be important. The presence of reactions to platelet-specific antigens is an additional possibility, explaining the poor responsiveness following fully matched donations.

Conversely, donations that would appear to be mismatched, for example those with one or two antigens novel to the recipient, may nevertheless still elicit adequate responses. In part, this may be a result of the existence of crossreactive groups, for example recipients of HLA-A2 may accept A28 donations. Similarly, B18 and B16 may be acceptable to B5 crossreactive group recipients, B5 in B18 and B22 and B7 in the B7 crossreactive group [122]. Conversely, MacPherson found intragroup antibody formation to be common within the HLA-A1 crossreactive group (HLA-AL, A3, A10, A11), suggesting that, for transfusion within the group, failures would be likely but not invariable [123]. Broadly similar findings were obtained by Dahlke & Weiss [122], although differences in detail between the two studies suggests that intragroup incompatibility varies in importance. The strength of HLA-Class I antigen expression on platelets is also believed to vary widely [124–128]. HLA-B8 and B12 are sometimes poorly expressed on platelets [125]; HLA-B12, for example, being up to 35 times more abundant on the platelets of some individuals than on others [128]. Variations in clinical responses to transfusions mismatched for B12 or for antigen splits B44/B45 have been observed [129]. Therefore, it is possible that some unexpectedly favourable responses may be ascribed to poor antigen expression in donor platelets. In other instances, apparent mismatches may not be incompatible with the antibody specificities actually present in the recipient's serum. Rather more puzzling is the observation that even over relatively short periods of time, the same donor–recipient pairs

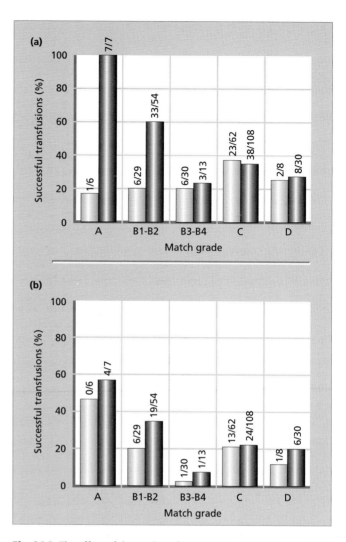

Fig. 24.3 The effect of the quality of HLA match on (a) 1-hour and (b) 18–24-hour transfusion success rates (*n* = 347 transfusion events in 36 patients refractory to random platelet concentrates). The dark bars represent transfusions to recipients whose serum demonstrated less than 20% reactivity against a panel of random lymphocytes. The lighter bars represent transfusions to recipients whose serum reacted with greater than 20% of the panel of random lymphocytes in the microlymphocytotoxicity assay. The ratio in each column compares the number of successful transfusions to the total number of transfusions in each category. (From McFarland *et al.*, 1989 [50], with permission.)

may, at times, produce good responses and, at other times, be unsuccessful [61,120].

Donor panels for HLA-matched donations

Because of the highly polymorphic nature of the HLA system, the provision of matched donations only becomes possible if large panels of HLA-typed donors willing to provide apheresis donations are established. In the UK this activity is integrated with the expanding British Bone Marrow and Platelet Donor

Panel, which in 1995 amounted to about 100 000 potential volunteers. Local regional transfusion services may therefore use their own contribution of recruited volunteers for this purpose. Recent estimates suggest that between 3000 [130] and 25 000 [131] donors may be necessary to form an effective panel. The latter study demonstrated the relationship between genetic heterogeneity of the population and the size of the donor panel that may be required. Takahashi *et al.* [131] found that their resident Japanese population could be matched adequately from a panel of 5000 donors, only a fifth of that estimated to be required to meet the needs of North American Caucasoid populations. The required donor panel size is largely influenced by the matching objectives of the transfusion service. Estimates must be made of the likely number of donations per patient, of the potential donor availability and the acceptable degree of mismatching in donor selection. In addition to fully matched donations, it may be convenient to utilize donors with only two or three out of the four possible identified recipient antigens on the assumption that homozygosity exists at the unpaired antigen locus. This assumption seems generally true, because post-transfusion responses for these two groups are similar. Panels of HLA-phenotyped donors are expensive to establish and maintain. Many of the volunteer donors will have uncommon phenotypes which would be rarely needed while, conversely, matched donations will not be readily available for recipients with uncommon phenotypes. The provision of platelet support can be facilitated if donors with antigens crossreactive to those in the recipient can be used, and computer-searching programs making use of acceptable degrees of mismatch can be helpful [132].

Schiffer *et al.* [133] showed the matching position to be most favourable for the 60–70% of patients with the most common phenotypes. A high proportion of those remaining could not be adequately supported, even with substantial increases in panel size. For some patients with rare phenotypes, only family-member donations were available. It seems logical that these patients should be a priority for the use of leucocyte-depleted products as a prophylactic measure to prevent alloimmunization.

Selection of platelet donations according to HLA lymphocytotoxic antibody specificity

Since lymphocytotoxic antibodies seem to be associated with most instances of alloimmune refractoriness [93], it seems logical to select donations according to the profile of the individual patient's current lymphocytotoxic antibody specificity. Patients' sera are customarily screened against panels of 60 or more fully typed cells in order to determine their reaction frequency and, if possible, their specificity. Individual sera may react with either very few or virtually all of the panel cells. Where high panel reactivity is found, the chances of providing compatible platelet donations is clearly small. However, if antibodies with a more restricted specificity are present, it may be

possible to select donors whose lymphocytes are unreactive with the recipients' serum. Under these circumstances, it may be possible to select a wider range of HLA phenotypes than would normally be selected by HLA phenotypic matching. For all patients, except those whose sera react with a very high proportion of panel cells, crossmatching has been used as an effective means of identifying suitable donations. Successful transfusions can be predicted on about 60–70% of occasions following negative lymphocytotoxicity crossmatches [134]. However, both unexpected successes and failures occur. The crossmatch only reflects cytotoxic HLA antibodies, and positive crossmatches may still be associated with successful transfusion outcomes. This may be ascribed to the previously mentioned phenomenon of diminished expression of HLA antigens on the donor platelets. Conversely, lymphocytotoxicity testing will not recognize noncomplement-fixing HLA antibodies or platelet-specific alloimmunization, and these may account for a proportion of crossmatch-compatible transfusions which appear to be unsuccessful.

Platelet-reactive antibodies and platelet crossmatching

Direct compatibility testing against donor platelets undoubtedly permits exclusion of incompatible transfusions that may not be identified by means of lymphocytotoxicity tests [91]. It seems possible that some of these represent instances of alloimmunization to platelet-specific antigens, either alone or coexisting with a background of HLA immunization. However, these antibodies have only occasionally been shown to react with recognized platelet-specific antigens [135,136]. The reaction frequencies of sera do not generally conform to those expected of the currently known platelet alloantigen systems, most of which are biallelic systems where one antigen is present at a relatively high frequency. Under such circumstances, platelet antigen-specific alloimmunization would be found in relatively few patients and there would be equally low chances of finding compatible donors. In most instances in which conclusions of platelet specificity have been reached, there has been no proof of association with recognized systems of platelet antigens [137]. Clarification of the nature of this platelet-specific alloantigenicity is therefore still awaited.

Immunological reactivity of sera against platelets has been investigated in a variety of ways, with a view to developing tools for understanding the alloimmune response. Initial approaches to platelet antibody detection used techniques such as complement fixation, platelet aggregation, platelet factor 3 liberation or serotonin release. These techniques proved neither sufficiently sensitive, nor reliable, nor convenient to serve as a basis for compatibility selection. They have now been superseded by test procedures based on immunoglobulin binding either by intact platelets or by immobilized platelet antigens, the most widely used being the platelet-specific immunofluorescence test (PSIFT) [84,138] but others include platelet-reactive antiglobulin tests

[139], solid phase red cell adherence tests [140] and enzyme immunoassays (ELISA) [141–143]. Platelets carry Class I-HLA antigens, therefore the test results will reflect both HLA and platelet-specific reactions. This, of course, does not debar their use in compatibility selection, but it does hamper the understanding of the immunological basis for the refractory state. During use of the PSIFT, pretreatment of the test platelets with chloroquine has been claimed to remove HLA-Class I products [144] and sera reacting with chloroquine-treated platelets are therefore presumed to contain platelet-specific alloantibodies. Lymphocytotoxicity assays and platelet crossmatching tests can be clinically effective when used in combination to identify platelet donations which are likely to give acceptable post-transfusion increments. Donations may be identified even among donors who are HLA mismatched [145]. Under these circumstances, the patients' sera are presumed to contain antibodies either of restricted HLA specificity, or of platelet specificity alone, or the chosen platelet donations may show very weak expression of the Class I-HLA products. Confidence in the predictive nature of platelet crossmatching procedures has grown, to the extent that they have even been proposed as the preferred basis of platelet donor selection for the treatment of alloimmunized patients [146–148] in contrast to the conventional, but expensive, alternative of establishing HLA-typed donor panels. Certain crossmatching techniques, in particular ELISA techniques and solid-phase red cell adherence methods, are claimed to be relatively inexpensive and suitable for rapid screening of large number of potential donations [139]. Indeed, these platelet crossmatching techniques have even been used to screen random platelet donations for the support of refractory patients [145].

Platelet compatibility selection procedures are ultimately judged in terms of their success in the prediction of post-transfusion increments (Fig. 24.4). Numerous studies have demonstrated the high predictive value of the various immunoglobulin-binding-based crossmatch procedures. Their value in improving the odds of a successful transfusion outcome in alloimmunized refractory patients, without super-added nonimmune factors for refractoriness, is not in doubt. There is even evidence that crossmatching is helpful for those more typical patients in whom alloimmunization is complicated by sepsis, bleeding and splenomegaly [140,143,149]. Although several studies have attempted to rank test procedures in terms of their capacity to accurately predict transfusion outcomes, there is no clear indication that any one of the currently popular assays is overwhelmingly superior to any of the others. The basic principles of immunoglobulin binding assays are common to several methods; any apparent advantages presumably result as much from local expertise and minor technical variations than from any fundamental superiority. Bearing this in mind, the rather poor concordance of these assays of 40–60% with each other is surprising [145]. It might, however, be expected that lymphocytotoxicity assays show a lesser degree of agreement with immunoglobulin

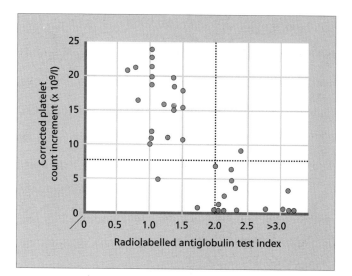

Fig. 24.4 The transfusion outcome 1 hour after transfusion in relation to the crossmatch result is shown. The horizontal dotted line at $7.5 \times 10^9/l$ notes the lower limit of an acceptable 1-hour increment. The vertical dotted line marks an index of 2, which is a positive test result. (Modified from Kickler *et al.*, 1988 [148], with permission.)

binding assays [91] and may be less capable, than platelet crossmatch procedures, of identifying incompatible transfusions [91,134]. While lymphocytotoxicity assays are clearly responsive to complement-dependent HLA antibodies, the antigen specificities detected by immunoglobulin binding assays are by no means established. Generally, it seems agreed that noncomplement-dependent HLA antibodies and also, possibly, multispecific antibodies reacting against platelet glycoproteins, account for reactivity in platelet crossmatch tests. Because of the uncertainty about the antigen specificities of these reactions, the term 'platelet reactive antibodies' is preferred [91].

Choice of compatibility procedures

Probably because of the heterogeneity in the alloimmune responses no single approach to compatibility selection is true for all patients. Moroff *et al.* [150] found the best results in general high-grade HLA matches (avoiding possible crossreactive incompatibilities), with crossmatch-compatible platelets being an acceptable alternative. In order to determine the most cost-effective approach to providing compatible platelet transfusion, Freedman *et al.* [151] conducted a careful cost-evaluation study, comparing various combinations of approach in popular use. These included HLA-matched single donor platelets, crossmatch-compatible pooled random-donor or single-donor platelets. Their crossmatch methods included lymphocytotoxicity tests (LCT), PSIFT, platelet radioactive antiglobulin tests (PRAT) and ELISA. In their study, the cost–benefit assessment ranked order was PRAT > LCT > PSIFT

> ELISA, but all were superior and much cheaper than HLA matching. However, these calculations of cost effectiveness were influenced by their rather higher than usual chances (50%) of finding crossmatch-compatible platelets among their panel of donors. Of the various combinations of compatibility tests for provision of platelet support in alloimmunized patients, single donor HLA-matched LCT- and PRAT-compatible donations were the most successful. These had a 95% success rate in predicting effective transfusion, but they were the most costly. Single (but not HLA-matched) LCT and PRAT crossmatch-compatible donations were almost as effective (93% successful) at a much lower cost. These authors clearly show, however, that this cost advantage diminishes if the proportion of crossmatch-compatible donations falls from their assumed figure of 50% towards the more common estimate of 10–20%. The maintenance of large HLA-matched panels to meet the needs of patients with multispecific antibodies (e.g. <2% donor/s compatible) was shown to be very expensive. Even the costing of HLA-matched platelets was shown to be markedly influenced by the size of the donor pool. Costs were 60% greater per transfusion with a panel of 3000 donors compared to when a pool of only 1000 donors is maintained. These studies show the difficulties of discovering the most cost effective approach.

Accumulating evidence from various approaches to the provision of platelets for alloimmunized patients suggests that the underlying immunological cause of refractoriness may be complex and multifactorial. Certainly, HLA antibodies, both complement fixing and possibly noncomplement fixing, against Class I products, and possibly also minor histocompatibility antigens, seem to be important. Non-HLA platelet-reactive antibodies are claimed to be demonstrable in up to 25% of patients [84,152], or in other studies in a far lower proportion [147]. Only a few examples conform to recognized platelet-specific antigens [135,136]. ABO incompatibility (see below) seems to be unimportant before the refractory state develops, but should be avoided where possible once refractoriness has been established [153,154]. In managing the provision of platelets for alloimmunized patients, the majority view now appears to favour the use of a validated platelet crossmatch technique combined with lymphocytotoxicity crossmatching. Where HLA-typed panels of donors are available, crossmatch-compatible or HLA-matched donations are equally effective. Interestingly, Heal *et al.* [143] demonstrated that even in crossmatch-negative transfusions, platelet increments varied according to the degree of HLA matching and ABO compatibility, an observation which illustrates the limitations of current compatibility procedures. From this evidence, HLA matching still appears to be important, even in crossmatch-negative transfusions.

ABO, Rh compatibility and platelet transfusion

The logistic difficulties experienced by transfusion centres in supplying platelets to meet expanding clinical demand have led to a common practice of disregarding ABO incompatibility — there is reasonably good evidence that ABO-mismatched platelets could be almost equally effective. ABO antigens do not seem to be intrinsic constituents of the platelet surface membrane but appear to be largely adsorbed from plasma in proportion to their plasma concentration [155]. A proportion of ABO-incompatible transfused platelets may have a reduced survival, the remainder seeming to persist in the circulation normally. The increasing problem of platelet refractoriness, while predominantly a result of HLA alloimmunization, has prompted re-examination of the role of ABO compatibility. It now seems apparent that while initial transfusion of ABO-mismatched platelets is usually effective, repeated mismatched transfusions may provoke an ABO-related refractory state, in parallel with increases in A or B isoagglutinin titres [154] and also HLA allosensitization [153]. It has also been suggested that immune complexes formed between soluble ABH antigens and alloantibodies may damage circulating platelets by an innocent bystander mechanism [143]. Following transfusion of ABO-incompatible platelets, the presence of immune anti-A and, to a lesser extent, anti-B can be demonstrated by immunofluorescence tests on transfused platelets [156]. Under these circumstances, group A platelets will be tolerated by group O recipients significantly less well than group B platelets [157]. The antigenicity of group A2 platelets is much less than those from group A1 donors, and these appear to be acceptable in group O recipients [158]. Group O platelets, particularly from apheresis donors, are commonly used for patients of other ABO groups. It has been shown that provision of up to 350 ml of group O plasma to A recipients is tolerated, patients may show a positive direct antiglobulin test, but clinical haemolysis does not usually occur [159]. Occasionally, however, severely haemolytic reactions do follow the use of incompatible plasmas (see 'Adverse reactions' below). ABO matching should therefore be considered as a possibility in the management of refractory patients and compliance with ABO compatibility may sometimes enable effective transfusions. While supply and demand problems are always likely to necessitate consideration of the use of ABO mismatches, it seems prudent to minimize the practice in those patients for whom the need for long-term support is anticipated.

In contrast, the use of Rh-incompatible platelets carries no risk of refractoriness. The consequences of possible Rh immunization should, however, be considered. This was formerly not regarded as a significant problem [160], because recipients are frequently highly immunosuppressed, platelets do not carry the Rh D antigen and the dose of Rh D-positive red cells should be very low. Furthermore, only a proportion of Rh D-positive recipients form anti-D in response to Rh D antigen, and the phenomenon is very much dose related. However, recently, Rh D immunization has been reported in transfused patients with haematological malignancies [161]. The possibility of future pregnancies should therefore be borne in mind for Rh D-negative females. For such patients, Rh D-negative platelets would be preferred; alternatively, intravenous preparations of anti-D immunoglobulin can be given or, if that is not available, 250 iu of an intramuscular preparation can be given subcutaneously to prevent Rh D immunization [162].

Use of IV immunoglobulin for refractory patients

Despite occasional apparent successes, the majority view is now that IV immunoglobulin is not effective at improving the results of platelet therapy for refractory patients [163–165]. Anti-D immunoglobulin, sometimes used successfully for the treatment of autoimmune thrombocytopenic purpura in Rh D-positive patients, does also not seem to benefit post-transfusion refractoriness [166].

Clinical problems associated with platelet therapy

Adverse reactions

Platelet transfusions are often given in relatively large numbers over many weeks or months and it is not altogether surprising that recipients experience a relatively high frequency of adverse reactions. Nonhaemolytic febrile reactions, which have usually been ascribed to alloimmunization to leucocytes or platelet antigens, are by far the most common problem, but less frequent causes of reaction include haemolytic reactions following ABO-incompatible plasma and septicaemic shock as a result of bacterial contamination of platelet packs. Highly immunocompromised patients are vulnerable to GVHD mediated by viable lymphocytes in platelet transfusions.

Approximately 1% of all transfusion recipients experience febrile reactions during transfusion of blood or the various labile blood components [167]. Platelet recipients in general experience these reactions much more frequently, this may be a consequence of their accumulating immunological exposure to foreign leucocyte or platelet antigens. Overall incidences of up to 35% have been reported [168,169]. Most commonly, the symptoms consist of mild, low-grade febrile reactions. Diagnostic criteria vary but in general require a temperature rise of 1°C or more above the basal pretransfusion temperature. This should subside within 48 hours and there should be no evidence of other clinical causes of fever. In addition to fever, some patients experience chills and rigors, and pruritis and urticaria may be present. A small proportion show more severe symptoms: nausea, vomiting, back or chest pain and severe respiratory distress symptoms. Platelet reactions may thus contribute significantly to overall patient morbidity. In some patients symptoms appear to result from histamine release following antibody–antigen reaction or immune mediated neutrophil degranulation. In the latter case, the release of proteolytic enzymes, or the allergic reaction byproducts

C3a and C5a, are believed to damage pulmonary capillaries, causing respiratory distress.

Serological investigation of such patients has revealed a wide diversity in cell-specific immunological changes [167,170–172] but rather poor evidence of correlation with clinical symptoms. Most patients show positive reactions to HLA antibodies, both by lymphocytotoxicity and by platelet immunofluorescence tests. In some patients, platelet-reactive antibodies are found. Granulocyte-specific antibodies have traditionally been considered to be the principal cause for febrile nonhaemolytic transfusion reactions. The immunological hypothesis appeared to be confirmed by reports that the reaction rates depended on the diversity of the HLA antigenic challenge and the widely shared observation that nonhaemolytic transfusion reactions could generally be reduced by the use of leucocyte-depleted blood products. Attempts to confirm the benefits of leucodepletion in platelet transfusion have shown that the problem may be more complex than first thought. A UK multicentre trial of bedside leucocyte depletion clearly demonstrated the ineffectiveness of this procedure. Febrile transfusion reaction rates of over 30% were seen, irrespective of the use of filtration [168], and a similar experience has been reported from the USA [173,174]. Although failure of filter performance during bedside use is now widely appreciated to be a problem, the most illuminating observation has been made that febrile haemolytic transfusion reactions (FHTRs) can be effectively reduced by early (prestorage) leucocyte depletion, but the benefit is much reduced if filtration is delayed. Adverse clinical reactions can be clearly linked to the appearance of cytokines (e.g. principally TNF, IL-6) in platelet supernatant plasma [175]. The leucocytes commonly contaminating conventional platelet products are recognized to cause a number of problems, in particular their consumption of metabolites contributes to lactic acid accumulation and the fall in pH accelerates the deterioration of platelet concentrate quality. Leucocytes, principally granulocytes and monocytes, liberate cytokines and proteases into the supernatant plasma during storage of platelet concentrates. Infusion of the plasma alone from such concentrates has been shown to replicate FHTR symptoms [176]. The most effective means of abrogating adverse reactions in repeatedly transfused platelet recipients appears to be the use of prestorage leucocyte depletion [175] and the possible future use of synthetic platelet storage media in place of plasma is likely to give even better clinical results.

ABO haemolytic transfusion reactions have, on rare occasions, caused clinically dramatic and life-threatening episodes. These occur against a background recognition that ABO compatibility can be disregarded for most platelet transfusions and only merits particular attention for patients showing evidence of refractoriness. In this context, there are too few ABO-incompatible red cells in platelet donations to cause a problem. However, group O platelet donations containing exceptionally high anti-A or anti-B alloantibodies have caused symptoms typical of severe intravascular haemolysis, circulatory collapse and renal failure [177–180]. Implicated donations had sera with exceptionally high titres of haemolytic, agglutinating and antiglobulin-reactive antibodies. The problem is most acute for group O single donor platelet pheresis donations to group A patients. In such circumstances, screening to identify high-titre donations has been advised [178,180]. In general, the rarity of these events, coupled with the almost universal difficulties of maintaining adequate supplies, justify the continued use of group O random donations as determined by clinical need. It is, however, necessary to be aware of this uncommon, but serious, possibility.

Septicaemia from platelet transfusion. Septicaemia from bacterial contamination of blood units has always been recognized as a rare though serious possibility. During the mid 1980s, a series of reports began to implicate platelet transfusion with a disproportionate frequency [146,181,182]. Causative organisms were mainly Gram-negative, for example *Salmonella* sp. [182], but Gram-positive *Staphylococcus epidermis* [182] and beta-haemolytic streptococci [180] were also involved. Slight microbial contamination of blood is an unavoidable but rare risk during blood collection, despite the most scrupulous attention to asepsis. Sterility checks performed by transfusion centres on blood components show only very low rates of contamination [183], suggesting a probable self-sterilizing capacity of donor blood.

Two factors appear to have contributed to the emergence of contamination as a serious concern during platelet transfusion, these being the adoption of 22°C for storage and the opportunity to extend the storage period to 7 days following the introduction of gas-permeable containers. Inoculation studies [146,182] showed that bacteria typically exhibited logarithmic growth in platelet concentrates and that clinically serious proliferation levels were less likely to occur if storage was limited to 5 days [184,185]. Accordingly, this is now the required storage limit for platelet concentrates. Greater risks of infection are still associated with platelet transfusions and it behoves staff administering platelets to be vigilant. Typical symptoms of transfusion septicaemia include chills, fever and hypotension, usually leading to profound circulatory collapse and, frequently, death. It is clearly of the utmost importance to recognize the possibility and to institute appropriate measures. These include stopping the infusion, maintaining intravenous plasma volume support, pressor agents, corticosteroids and broad-spectrum antibacterial chemotherapy. Blood cultures are essential, as is retention of all transfusion material for microbiological examination.

Transfusion-associated graft vs host disease. This is a serious well-recognized hazard but, because of its low incidence, it has not been easy to define precisely the circumstances in which the use of irradiated products should be obligatory. Recommendations for use, together with a review, are provided in the British Committee for Standards in Haematology 'Guidelines for Use of Irradiated Blood Products' [186]. It has now been agreed that cellular blood products should receive a minimum of 25 Gy — the most agreed recommendations for the use of irradiated blood products include all donations from first- or second-degree relatives, irrespective of the risk status of the recipient. Irradiation is not required for the general support of adults or children with leukaemia, although the case has been made where HLA-matched platelets are to be used.

Recipients of allogeneic marrow should receive irradiated products from the time of conditioning until evidence of lymphopoietic regeneration, or when GVHD prophylaxis is no longer necessary. In addition, it is common practice to irradiate blood products given to potential autologous BMT or peripheral blood stem cell recipients before harvesting (to prevent the possibility of third party engraftment) and to continue this policy until clear evidence of engraftment is seen. Patients with Hodgkin's disease (but not non-Hodgkin's lymphomas) also appear to be at enhanced risk of transfusion-associated (TA) GVHD.

Transfusion of red cells

Anaemia, like thrombocytopenia in leukaemic states, is multifactorial in origin. Repeated, often subclinical, bleeding is common; monitoring haemoglobin levels and being alert to possible causes for accelerated red cell loss is an important part of patient management. The complexities of blood product support during BMT introduce various possibilities of immune haemolytic destruction of red cells which may show in the form of declining haemoglobin values, biochemical evidence of haemolysis or a positive antiglobulin test. Under these circumstances, expert serological help will be necessary. Red cells should be transfused to maintain haemoglobin levels above levels which, for each patient, are known to be associated with anaemic symptoms. The long-established concept of a transfusion trigger value (e.g. Hb 10.0/Hct 0.3) as mandating red cell transfusion has now been abandoned, in favour of a more individualized approach. Anaemia is sometimes corrected in the belief supported by some experimental studies that it exaggerates the bleeding risk [41–43]. This belief requires confirmation in modern clinical treatment.

Granulocyte therapy

The enthusiasm for the use of granulocytes for the support of neutropenic infection of a decade or more ago has largely evaporated. Evidence was always controversial that production of a therapeutically effective dose was possible. Fortunately, modern antibiotic regimens, the use of recombinant myeloid growth factors [78,77] and, where appropriate, peripheral blood stem cell transplantation [187], have each the potential to help patients to survive phases of severe neutropenia.

Cytomegalovirus transmission

Cytomegalovirus (CMV) infection is recognized as one of the most serious causes of mortality and morbidity in patients transplanted for haematological malignancy. Accordingly, transfusion services now endeavour to provide seronegative blood donations for seronegative recipients of seronegative marrow grafts and the practice has substantially reduced the incidence of CMV infection in recipients [188]. The seriousness of CMV infection dictates that CMV-negative support should be provided for all susceptible patients anticipating BMT. In addition to the now well-recognized clinical sequelae of post-transplantation infection, there is also evidence that CMV-infected patients show delayed restoration of platelet counts following BMT [72].

In most of Europe and North America, close to half the donor population are seronegative for CMV and this enables provision of CMV-negative donations in the required quantity to be a manageable problem. However, it must be recognized that arrangements for selection of donors previously known to be CMV negative, so that their donations can be reconfirmed as seronegative before issue, adds complications and potential delays to an already demanding area of transfusion-centre activity. The overriding concern is to establish an agreed CMV-negative transfusion support policy, to identify individual recipients in such a way that their support with noninfective products is securely maintained. It is also important to ensure that CMV-negative blood products in short supply are not given inadvertently to unintended recipients.

Seronegativity of donations is usually established by ELISA, latex agglutination or haemagglutination assays. Results from these assays do not show complete concordance, and it has to be accepted that around 1–2% of samples will be positive by only one assay system and not by others [188]. Screening assays conventionally detect IgG CMV antibody; however, it appears that only a minority of seropositive-identified donations are capable of transmitting infection. Assays based on the detection of IgM antibodies, supposedly indicative of recent infection, have not so far been found to be a reliable alternative.

There is general agreement about the necessity to ensure supplies of CMV-seronegative components to seronegative donors receiving seronegative bone marrow grafts. Widening the policy to include other categories carries the risk of depleting stocks such that the agreed most vulnerable recipients are placed in jeopardy. A case could be made, where supplies permit, for supplying CMV-negative products to all recipients who have received marrow grafts from CMV-seropositive donors, on the basis that infection from the graft should not be a foregone conclusion, irrespective of their own CMV serological status. However, proof of the validity of this approach is awaited. Seropositive patients are recognized to be at risk of CMV reactivation, possibly precipitated by the immune challenge from allogeneic blood products [189]. However, experience from renal transplantation recipients has also demonstrated the possibility of reinfection by a second strain of CMV infection [189,190].

Leucocytes in blood components constitute the transmission vehicle and it has been shown that leucocyte depletion using methods capable of greater than 99% removal can prevent CMV transmission. Accordingly, red cells and platelets which are leucocyte depleted can be used in circumstances where CMV-seronegative products are unavailable [191].

References

1 O'Brien J.R. & Jamieson S. (1974) A relationship between platelet volume and platelet number. *Thrombosis of Diathesis Haemorrhagica (Stuttgart)*, **31**, 363–365.

2 Thompson C.B. & Jakubowski J.A. (1988) The pathophysiology and clinical relevance of platelet heterogeneity. *Journal of the American Society of Hematology*, **72**, 1–8.

3 Giles C. (1981) The platelet count and mean platelet volume. *British Journal of Haematology*, **48**, 31–37.

4 Lippi U. & Cappelletti P. (1984) Mean platelet volumes and platelet counts in hospitalized patients. *American Journal of Clinical Pathology*, **81**, 406.

5 Hanson S.R. & Slichter S.J. (1985) Platelet kinetics in patients with bone marrow hypoplasia: evidence for a fixed platelet requirement. *Blood*, **66**, 1105–1109.

6 Loos J.A., Blok-Schut B., van Doorn R. *et al.* (1976) A method for the recognition and separation of human blood monocytes on density gradients. *Blood*, **48**, 731–742.

7 UK Blood Transfusion Services/National Institute for Biological Standards and Control Liaison Group (1997) *Guidelines for the Blood Transfusion Service*, 3rd edn. HMSO, London.

8 Reesink H.W. (1993) What is the optimal storage temperature for whole blood prior to preparation of blood components. *Vox Sanguinis*, **65**, 320–327.

9 Slichter S.J. & Harker L.A. (1976) Preparation and storage of platelet concentrates. I. Factors influencing the harvest of viable platelets from whole blood. *British Journal of Haematology*, **34**, 395–402.

10 Prins H.K., de Bruijn J.C.G.H., Henrichs H.P.J. *et al.* (1980) Prevention of microaggregate formation by removal of 'buffycoats'. *Vox Sanguinis*, **39**, 48–51.

11 Aster R.H. (1981) Which are the parameters to be controlled in platelet concentrates in order that they may be offered to the medical profession as a standardized product with specific properties? *Vox Sanguinis*, **40**, 115–126.

12 Burgstaler E.A., Pineda A.A. & Brecher M.A. (1993) Plateletpheresis: comparison of platelet yields, processing time, and white cell content with two apheresis systems. *Transfusion*, **33**, 393–398.

13 Olthuis H.P., Stienstra S., Puylaert C.E.N.M. *et al.* (1993) Preparation of random donor leukocyte-poor platelets by cytapheresis. *Transfusion Science*, **14**, 195–197.

14 Masse M., Naegelen C., Pellegrini N. *et al.* (1992) Validation of a simple method to count very low white cell concentrations in filtered red cells or platelets. *Transfusion*, **32**, 565–571.

15 Sheckler V.L. & Loken M.R. (1993) Routine quantitation of white cells as low as 0.001 per I L in platelet components. *Transfusion*, **33**, 256–261.

16 Vachula M., Simpson S.J., Martinson J.A. *et al.* (1993) A flow cytometric method for counting very low levels of white cells in blood and blood components. *Transfusion*, **33**, 262–267.

17 Slichter S.J. & Harker L.A. (1976) Preparation and storage of platelet concentrates. II. Storage variables influencing platelet viability and function. *British Journal of Haematology*, **34**, 403–419.

18 Kahn R.A. & Meryman K.T. (1976) Storage of platelet concentrates. *Transfusion*, **16**, 13–16.

19 Becker G.A., Tuccelli M., Kunicki T. *et al.* (1973) Studies of platelet concentrates stored at 22°C and 4°C. *Transfusion*, **13**, 61–68.

20 Owens M., Holme S., Haeton A. *et al.* (1992) Post-transfusion recovery of function of 5 day stored platelet concentrates. *British Journal of Haematology*, **80**, 539–544.

21 Rock G., Sherring V.A. & Tittley P. (1984) Five-day storage of platelet concentrates. *Transfusion*, **24**, 147–152.

22 Archer G.T., Grimsley P.G., Jindra J. *et al.* (1982) Survival of transfused platelets collected into new formulation plastic packs. *Vox Sanguinis*, **43**, 223–230.

23 Koerner K. (1984) Platelet function of room temperature platelet concentrates stored in a new plastic material with high gas permeability. *Vox Sanguinis*, **47**, 406–411.

24 Murphy S. & Gardner F.H. (1975) Platelet storage at 22°C: role of gas transport across plastic containers in maintenance of viability. *Blood*, **46**, 209–218.

25 Beutler E. (1993) Letter to the Editor: artificial preservatives for platelets. *Transfusion*, **33**, 279–280.

26 Eriksson L., Shanwell A., Gulliksson H. *et al.* (1993) Platelet concentrates in an additive solution prepared from pooled buffy coats. *Vox Sanguinis*, **64**, 133–138.

27 Slichter S.J. (1981) *In vitro* measurements of platelet concentrates stored at 4°C and 22°C: correlation with posttransfusion platelet viability and function. *Vox Sanguinis*, **40**(Suppl. 1), 72–86.

28 Holme S. & Murphy S. (1978) Quantitative measurements of platelet shape by light transmission studies; application to storage of platelets for transfusion. *Journal of Laboratory and Clinical Medicine*, **92**, 53–64.

29 Kunicki T.J., Tuccelli M., Becker G.A. *et al.* (1975) A study of variables affecting the quality of platelets stored at room temperature. *Transfusion*, **15**, 414–421.

30 Trenchard P.M. (1986) Continuous monitoring of platelet morphology during small-scale *in vitro* storage. *Vox Sanguinis*, **51**, 185–191.

31 Bellhouse E.L., Inskip M.J., Davis I.G. *et al.* (1987) Pre-transfusion non-invasive quality assessment of stored platelet concentrates. *British Journal of Haematology*, **66**, 503–508.

32 Kim B.K. & Baldini M.G. (1974) The platelet response to hypotonic shock. Its value as an indicator of platelet viability after storage. *Transfusion*, **14**, 130–138.

33 Valeri C.R., Feingold H. & Marchionni L.D. (1974) The relation between response to hypotonic stress and the 5'Cr recovery *in vivo* of preserved platelets. *Transfusion*, **14**, 331–337.

34 Odink J. & Brand A. (1977) Platelet preservation. V. Survival, serotonin uptake velocity, and response to hypotonic stress of fresh and cryopreserved human platelets. *Transfusion*, **17**, 203–209.

35 Rinder H.M., Murphy M., Mitchell J.G. *et al.* (1991) Progressive platelet activation with storage: evidence for shortened survival of activated platelets after transfusion. *Transfusion*, **31**, 409–414.

36 Triulzi D.J., Kickler T.S. & Braine H.G. (1992) Detection and significance of alpha granule membrane protein 140 expression on platelets collected by apheresis. *Transfusion*, **32**, 529–533.

37 Lind S.E. (1991) The bleeding time does not predict surgical bleeding. *Blood*, **77**, 2547–2552.

38 Duke W.W. (1910) The relation of blood platelets to hemorrhagic disease. *Journal of the American Medical Association*, **60**, 1185–1192.

39 O'Brien J.R. (1951) The bleeding time in normal and abnormal subjects. *Journal of Clinical Pathology*, **4**, 272–285.

40 Harker L.A. & Slichter S.J. (1972) The bleeding times as a screening test for evaluation of platelet function. *New England Journal of Medicine*, **287**, 155–159.

41 Hellem A.J., Borchgrevink C.F. & Ames S.B. (1961) The role of red cells in haemostasis: the relation between haematocrit, bleeding time and platelet adhesiveness. *British Journal of Haematology*, **7**, 42–50.

42 Livio M., Gotti E., Marchesi D. *et al.* (1982) Uraemic bleeding: role of anaemia and beneficial effect of red cell transfusion. *Lancet*, **ii**, 1013–1015.

43 Small M., Lowe G.D.O., Cameron E. *et al.* (1983) Contribution of the haematocrit to the bleeding time. *Haemostasis*, **13**, 379–384.

44 Goldsmith H.L. (1971) Red cell motions and wall interactions in tube flow. *Federation Proceedings*, **30**, 1578–1588.

45 Turitto V.T. & Baumgartner H.R. (1975) Platelet interaction with subendothelium in a perfusion system: physical role of red blood cells. *Microvascular Research*, **9**, 335–344.

46 Escolar G., Garrido M., Mazzara R. *et al.* (1988) Experimental basis for the use of red cell transfusion in the management of anemic-thrombocytopenia patients. *Transfusion*, **28**, 406–411.

47 Roy A.J., Jaffe N. & Djerassi I. (1973) Prophylactic platelet transfusions in children with acute leukemia: a dose response study. *Transfusion*, **13**, 283–290.

48 Pisciotta A.V. & Schultz E.J. (1955) Fibrinolytic purpura in acute leukemia. *American Journal of Medicine*, **19**, 824–828.

49 Freeman G. & Buckley E.S. Jr (1954) Serum polysaccharide and fever in thrombocytopenic bleeding of leukemia. *Blood*, **9**, 586–594.

50 McFarland J.G., Anderson A.J. & Slichter S.J. (1989) Factors influencing the transfusion response to HLA-selected apheresis donor platelets in patients refractory to random platelet concentrates. *British Journal of Haematology*, **73**, 380–386.

51 Norol F., Kuentz M., Cordonnier C. *et al.* (1994) Influence of clinical status on the efficiency of stored platelet transfusion. *British Journal of Haematology*, **86**, 125–129.

52 George J.N. & Shattil S.J. (1991) Medical progress: the clinical importance of acquired abnormalities of platelet function. *New England Journal of Medicine*, **324**, 27–38.

53 Panella T.J., Peters W., White I.G. *et al.* (1990) Platelets acquire a secretion defect after high-dose chemotherapy. *Cancer*, **65**, 1711–1716.

54 Baer M.R. & Bloomfield C.D. (1992) Controversies in transfusion medicine. Prophylactic platelet transfusion therapy: pro. *Transfusion*, **32**, 377–385.

55 Murphy S., Litwin S., Herring L.M. *et al.* (1982) Indications for platelet transfusion in children with acute leukemia. *American Journal of Hematology*, **12**, 347–356.

56 Solomon J., Bofenkamp T., Fahey J.L. *et al.* (1978) Platelet prophylaxis in acute non-lymphoblastic leukaemia. *Lancet*, **i**, 267.

57 Murphy S. (1988) Guidelines for platelet transfusion. *Journal of the American Medical Association*, **259**, 2453–2454.

58 Consensus Conference (1987) Platelet transfusion therapy. *Journal of the American Medical Association*, **257**, 1777–1780.

59 Aderka D., Praff G., Santo M. *et al.* (1986) Bleeding due to thrombocytopenia in acute leukemias and reevaluation of the prophylactic platelet transfusion policy. *American Journal of Medicine, Science,* **291**, 147–151.

60 Gaydos L.A., Freireich E.J. & Mantel N. (1962) The quantitative relation between platelet count and hemorrhage in patients with acute leukemia. *New England Journal of Medicine,* **266**, 905–909.

61 Freireich E.J., Kliman A., Gaydos L.A. *et al.* (1963) Response to repeated platelet transfusions from the same donor. *Annals of Internal Medicine,* **59**, 277–287.

62 Freireich E.J., Thomas L.B. Frei E. III *et al.* (1960) Distinctive type of intracerebral hemorrhage associated with 'blastic crisis' in patients with leukemia. *Cancer,* **13**, 146–154.

63 Fritz R.D., Forkner C.E. Jr, Freireich E.J. *et al.* (1959) Association of fatal intracranial hemorrhage and 'blastic crisis' in patients with acute leukemia. *New England Journal of Medicine,* **261**, 59–64.

64 Gmur J., von Felten A., Osterwalder B. *et al.* (1983) Delayed alloimmunization using random single donor platelet transfusions: a prospective study in thrombocytopenic patients with acute leukemia. *Blood,* **62**, 743–749.

65 BCSH Guidelines: Murphy M.F., Brozovic B., Murphy W. *et al.* (1992) Guidelines for platelet transfusions. *Transfusion Medicine,* **2**, 311–318.

66 Ho W.G., Champlin R.E., Winston D.J. *et al.* (1987) Bone marrow transplantation in patients with leukaemia previously transfused with blood products from family members. *British Journal of Haematology,* **67**, 67–70.

67 Watson J.G., Powles R.L., Clink H.M. *et al.* (1981) Acute myeloid leukaemia: comparison of support required during initial induction of remission and marrow transplantation in first remission. *Lancet,* **ii**, 957–959.

68 Welch H.G. & Larson E.B. (1989) Cost effectiveness of bone marrow transplantation in acute nonlymphocytic leukaemia. *New England Journal of Medicine,* **321**, 807–812.

69 McCullough J. (1983) Role of blood bank in bone marrow transplantation. In: *Bone Marrow Transplantation* (eds R.S. Weiner, E. Hackel & C.A. Schiffer), pp. 101–121. American Association of Blood Banks, Bethesda, Maryland.

70 Osterwalder D., Gratwohl A., Reusser P. *et al.* (1988) Hematological support in patients undergoing allogeneic bone marrow transplantation. *Recent Results in Cancer Research,* **108**, 44–52.

71 Smith O.P., Prentice H.G., Hazlehurst G. *et al.* (1991) Blood product support in patients undergoing chemotherapy and autologous or allogeneic bone marrow transplantation for haematological malignancies. *Clinical and Laboratory Haematology,* **13**, 107–114.

72 Verdonk L.F., van Heugten H. & de Gast G.C. (1985) Delay in platelet recovery after bone marrow transplantation: impact of cytomegalovirus infection. *Blood,* **66**, 921–925.

73 Bensinger W., Petersen F.B., Banaji M. *et al.* (1989) Engraftment and transfusion requirement after allogeneic marrow transplantation for patients with acute non-lymphocytic leukemia in first complete remission. *Bone Marrow Transplantation,* **4**, 409–414.

74 Vadhan-Raj S., Buescher S., LeMaistre A. *et al.* (1988) Stimulation of hematopoiesis in patients with bone marrow failure and in patients with malignancy by recombinant human granulocyte macrophage colony-stimulating factor. *Blood,* **72**, 134–141.

75 Powles R., Smith C., Milan S. *et al.* (1990) Human recombinant GM-CSF in allogeneic bone-marrow transplantation for leukaemia: double-blind, placebo-controlled trial. *Lancet,* **336**, 1417–1420.

76 Kodo H., Tajika K., Takahashi S. *et al.* (1988) Acceleration of neutrophilic granulocyte recovery after bone-marrow transplantation by administration of recombinant human granulocyte colony-stimulating factor. *Lancet,* **ii**, 38–39.

77 Dombret H., Chastang C., Fenaux P. *et al.* (1995) A controlled study of recombinant human granulocyte colony-stimulating factor in elderly patients after treatment for acute myelogenous leukemia. *New England Journal of Medicine,* **332**, 1678–1683.

78 Stone R.M., Berg D.T., George S.L. *et al.* (1995) Granulocyte-macrophage colony-stimulating factor after initial chemotherapy for elderly patients with primary acute myelogenous leukemia. *New England Journal of Medicine,* **332**, 1671–1677.

79 Schick B.P. (1994) Clinical implications of basic research. Hope for treatment of thrombocytopenia. *New England Journal of Medicine,* **331**, 875–876.

80 Brubaker D.B. (1993) Correction of the corrected count increment units. *Transfusion,* **33**, 358–359.

81 Bishop J.F., Matthews J.P., Uuen K. *et al.* (1992) The definition of refractoriness to platelet transfusions. *Transfusion Medicine,* **2**, 35–41.

82 O'Connell B., Lee E.J. & Schiffer C.A. (1988) The value of 10-minute posttransfusion platelet counts. *Transfusion,* **28**, 66–67.

83 Messerschmidt G.L., Makuch R., Appelbaum F. *et al.* (1988) A prospective randomized trial of HLA matched versus mismatched single-donor platelet transfusions in cancer patients. *Cancer,* **62**, 790–801.

84 Pegels J.G., Bruynes E.C.E., Engelfriet C.P. *et al.* (1982) Serological studies in patients on platelet and granulocyte substitution therapy. *British Journal of Haematology,* **52**, 59–68.

85 Kickler T.S., Ness P.M., Braine H.G. *et al.* (1990) The expression of IgG allotypes and on platelets immunization to IgG allotypes in multitransfused thrombocytopenic patients. *Blood,* **76**, 849–852.

86 Howard J.E. & Perkins H.A. (1978) The natural history of alloimmunization to platelets. *Transfusion,* **18**, 496–503.

87 Holohan T.V., Terasaki P.I. & Deisseroth A.B. (1981) Suppression of transfusion-related alloimmunization in intensively treated cancer patients. *Blood,* **58**, 122–128.

88 Brand A., Claas F.H.J., Voogt P.J. *et al.* (1988) Alloimmunization after leukocyte-depleted multiple random donor platelet transfusions. *Vox Sanguinis,* **54**, 160–166.

89 Lee E.J. & Schiffer C.A. (1987) Serial measurement of lymphocytotoxic antibody and response to nonmatched platelet transfusions in alloimmunized patients. *Blood,* **70**, 1727–1729.

90 Sintnicolaas K., Sizoo W., Haije W.G. *et al.* (1981) Delayed alloimmunisation by random single donor platelet transfusions: a randomised study to compare single donor and multiple donor platelet transfusions in cancer patients with severe thrombocytopenia. *Lancet,* **i**, 750–754.

91 Brubaker D.B. & Romine M. (1987) Relationship of HLA and platelet-reactive antibodies in alloimmunized patients refractory to platelet therapy. *American Journal of Haematology,* **26**, 341–352.

92 Shulman N.R. (1966) Immunological considerations attending platelet transfusion. *Transfusion,* **6**, 39–49.

93 Dutcher J.P., Schiffer C.A. & Aisner J. (1981) Alloimmunization following platelet transfusion: the absence of a dose-response relationship. *Blood,* **57**, 395–398.

94 Lee M., Kim B.K., Park S. *et al.* (1988) Refractoriness to platelet transfusion after single-donor consecutive platelet transfusions and its relationship to platelet antibodies. *Journal of Korean Medical Science,* **3**, 143–149.

95 Frangoulis B., Besluau D., Chopin M. *et al.* (1988) Immune response to H-2 class I antigens on platelets. I. immunogenicity of platelet class I antigens. *Tissue Antigens*, **32**, 46–54.

96 Welsh K.I., Burgos H. & Batchelor J.R. (1977) The immune response to allogeneic rat platelets; Ag-B antigens in matrix form lacking 1a. *European Journal of Immunology*, **7**, 267–272.

97 Claas F.H.J., Smeenk R.J.T., Schmidt R. *et al.* (1981) Alloimmunization against the MHC antigens after platelet transfusions is due to contaminating leukocytes in the platelet suspension. *Experimental Hematology*, **9**, 84–89.

98 Oksanen K., Kekomaki R., Ruutu T. *et al.* (1991) Prevention of alloimmunization in patients which acute leukemia by use of white cell-reduced blood components — a randomized trial. *Transfusion*, **31**, 588–594.

99 Kao K.J., Mickel M., Braine H.G. *et al.* (1995) White cell reduction in platelet concentrates and packed red cells by filtration: a multicenter clinical trial. *Transfusion*, **35**, 13–19.

100 Barker J., Patterson H., Brown S. *et al.* (1987) Preparation of leukocyte-poor red blood cells by filtration (Abstract). *Transfusion*, **27**, 510.

101 Pietersz R.N.I., Dekker W.J.A. & Reesink H.W. (1989) A new cellulose acetate filter to remove leukocytes from buffy-coat-poor red cell concentrates. *Vox Sanguinis*, **56**, 37–39.

102 Patten E. & Patel S. (1989) Preparation of leukocyte-poor platelet concentrates. *Transfusion*, **29**, 562–563.

103 Sirchia G., Parravicini A., Rebulla P. *et al.* (1983) Preparation of leukocyte-free platelets for transfusion by filtration through cotton wool. *Vox Sanguinis*, **44**, 115–120.

104 Koerner K. & Kubanek B. (1987) Comparison of three different methods used in the preparation of leukocyte-poor platelet concentrates. *Vox Sanguinis*, **53**, 26–30.

105 Bertolini F., Rebulla P., Porretti L. *et al.* (1990) Comparison of platelet activation and membrane glycoprotein Ib and IIb–IIIa expression after filtration through three different leukocyte removal filters. *Vox Sanguinis*, **59**, 201–204.

106 Brecher M.E., Pineda A.A., Zylstra-Halling V.W. *et al.* (1990) *In vivo* viability and functional integrity of filtered platelets. *Transfusion*, **30**, 718–721.

107 Holme S., Ross D. & Heaton W.A. (1989) *In vitro* and *in vivo* evaluation of platelet concentrates after cotton wool filtration. *Vox Sanguinis*, **57**, 112–115.

108 International Forum: Reesink H.W. & Nydegger U.E. (1992) Should all platelet concentrates issued be leukcoyte-poor? *Vox Sanguinis*, **62**, 57–64.

109 Slichter S.J., Deeg H.J. & Kennedy M.S. (1987) Prevention of platelet alloimmunization in dogs with systemic cyclosporine and by UV-irradiation or cyclosporine-loading of donor platelets. *Blood*, **69**, 414–418.

110 Deeg H.J., Aprile J., Graham T.C. *et al.* (1986) Ultraviolet irradiation of blood prevents transfusion-induced sensitization and marrow graft rejection in dogs. *Blood*, **67**, 537–539.

111 Deeg H.J., Aprile J., Storb R. *et al.* (1988) Functional dendritic cells are required for transfusion induced sensitization in canine marrow graft recipients. *Blood*, **71**, 1138–1140.

112 Aprile J. & Deeg H.J. (1986) Ultraviolet irradiation of canine dendritic cells prevents mitogen induced cluster formation and lymphocyte proliferation. *Transplantation*, **42**, 653–660.

113 Andreu G., Boccaccio C., Lecrubier C. *et al.* (1990) Ultraviolet irradiation of platelet concentrates: feasibility in transfusion practice. *Transfusion*, **30**, 401–406.

114 Pamphilon D.H., Corbin S.A., Saunders J. *et al.* (1989) Applications of ultraviolet light in the preparation of platelet concentrates. *Transfusion*, **29**, 379–383.

115 Pamphilon D.H., Potter M., Cutis M. *et al.* (1990) Platelet concentrates irradiated with ultraviolet light retain satisfactory *in vitro* storage characteristics and *in vivo* survival. *British Journal of Haematology*, **75**, 240–244.

116 van Prooijen H.C., van Marwijk Kooy M., van Weelden H. *et al.* (1990) Evaluation of a new UVB source for irradiation of platelet concentrates. *British Journal of Haematology*, **75**, 573–577.

117 Panzer S., Maier F., Hocker P. *et al.* (1987) Thrombocyte transfusion: increase in platelets in relation to clinical and immunologic pre-requisites. *Infusionstherapie und Klinische Ernahrung*, **14**(Suppl. 2), 10–14.

118 Nagasawa T., Kim B.K. & Baldini M.G. (1978) Temporary suppression of circulating antiplatelet alloantibodies by the massive infusion of fresh, stored, or lyophilized platelets. *Transfusion*, **18**, 429–435.

119 Yankee R.A., Grumet F.C. & Rogentine G.N. (1969) Platelet transfusion therapy: the selection of compatible platelet donors for refractory patients by lymphocyte HL-A typing. *New England Journal of Medicine*, **281**, 1208–1212.

120 Tosato G., Appelbaum F.R. & Deisseroth A.B. (1978) HLA-matched platelet transfusion therapy of severe aplastic anemia. *Blood*, **52**, 846–854.

121 Lohrmann H-P., Bull M.I., Decter J.A. *et al.* (1974) Platelet transfusions from HL-A compatible unrelated donors to alloimmunized patients. *Annals of Internal Medicine*, **80**, 9–14.

122 Dahlke M.B. & Weiss K.L. (1984) Platelet transfusion from donors mismatched for crossreactive HLA antigens. *Transfusion*, **24**, 299–302.

123 MacPherson B.R. (1989) HLA antibody formation within the HLA-AL crossreactive group in multitransfused platelet recipients. *American Journal of Hematology*, **30**, 228–232.

124 Liebert M. & Aster R.H. (1977) Expression of HLA-B12 on platelets, on lymphocytes and in serum. A quantitative study. *Tissue Antigens*, **9**, 199–208.

125 Duquesnoy R.J., Filip D.J. & Rodey G.E. (1977) Successful transfusion of platelets 'mismatched' for HLA antigens to alloimmunized thrombocytopenic patients. *American Journal of Hematology*, **2**, 219–226.

126 Aster R.H., Szatkowski N., Liebert M. *et al.* (1977) Expression of HLA-B12, HLA-B9, w4, and w6 on platelets. *Transplantation Proceedings*, **9**, 1695–1696.

127 McElligot M.C., Menitove J.E., Duquesnoy R.J. *et al.* (1982) Effect of HLA Bw4/Bw6 compatibility on platelet transfusion responses of refractory thrombocytopenic patients. *Blood*, **59**, 971–975.

128 Szatkowski N.S. & Aster R.H. (1980) HLA antigens of platelets: IV. Influence of 'private' HLAB locus specificities on the expression of Bw4 and Bw6 on human platelets. *Tissue Antigens*, **15**, 361–368.

129 Schiffer C.A., O'Connel B. & Lee E.J. (1989) Platelet transfusion therapy for alloimmunized patients: selective mismatching for HLA B12, an antigen with variable expression on platelets. *Blood*, **74**, 1172–1176.

130 Bolgiano D.C., Larson E.B. & Slichter S.J. (1989) A model to determine required pool size for HLA typed community donor apheresis program. *Transfusion*, **29**, 306–310.

131 Takahashi K., Juji T. & Miyazaki H. (1989) Determination of an appropriate size of unrelated donor pool to be registered for HLA-matched bone marrow transplantation. *Transfusion*, **29**, 311–316.

132 Jorgensen D.W., McFarland J.G., Hillman R.S. *et al.* (1984) Plateletpheresis program: II. Computer selection of HLA compatible donors. *Transfusion,* **24**, 292–298.

133 Schiffer C.A., Keller C., Dutcher J.P. *et al.* (1983) Potential HLA-matched platelet donor availability for alloimmunized patients. *Transfusion,* **23**, 286–289.

134 Kakaiya R.M., Gudino M.D., Miller M.V. *et al.* (1984) Four cross-match methods to select platelet donors. *Transfusion,* **24**, 35–41.

135 Saiji H., Maruya E., Fujii H. *et al.* (1989) New platelet antigen, Siba, involved in platelet transfusion refractoriness in a Japanese man. *Vox Sanguinis,* **56**, 283–287.

136 Ikeda H., Mitani T., Ohnuma M. *et al.* (1989) A new platelet-specific antigen, Naka, involved in the refractoriness of HLA-matched platelet transfusion. *Vox Sanguinis,* **57**, 213–217.

137 Herman J.H., Kickler T.S. & Ness P.M. (1985) Western blot analysis of HLA compatible platelet transfusion failures (abstract). *Blood,* **66**, 279.

138 Myers T.J., Kim B.K., Steiner M. *et al.* (1981) Selection of donor platelets for alloimmunized patients using a platelet-associated IgG assay. *Blood,* **58**, 444–450.

139 Kickler T.S., Braine H. & Ness P.M. (1985) The predictive value of crossmatching platelet transfusion for alloimmunized patients. *Transfusion,* **25**, 385–389.

140 Rachel J.M., Summers T.C., Sinor L.T. *et al.* (1988) Use of solid phase red blood cell adherence method for pretransfusion platelet compatibility testing. *American Journal of Clinical Pathology,* **90**, 63–68.

141 Gudino M. & Miller W.V. (1981) Application of the enzyme linked immunospecific assay (ELISA) for the detection of platelet antibodies. *Blood,* **57**, 32–37.

142 Sintnicolaas K., van der Steuijt K.J.B., van Putten W.L.J. *et al.* (1987) A microplate ELISA for the detection of platelet alloantibodies: comparison with platelet immunofluorescence test. *British Journal of Haematology,* **66**, 363–367.

143 Heal J.M., Blumberg N. & Masel D. (1987) An evaluation of crossmatching, HLA, and ABO matching for platelet transfusions to refractory patients. *Blood,* **70**, 23–30.

144 Nordhagen R. & Flaathen S.T. (1985) Chloroquine removal of HLA antigens from platelets for the platelet immunofluoresence test. *Vox Sanguinis,* **48**, 156–159.

145 Freedman J., Garvey M.B., de Friedberg S. *et al.* (1988) Random donor platelet crossmatching: comparison of four platelet antibody detection methods. *American Journal of Haematology,* **28**, 1–7.

146 Braine H.G., Kickler T.S., Charache P. *et al.* (1986) Bacterial sepsis secondary to platelet transfusion: an adverse effect of extended storage at room temperature. *Transfusion,* **26**, 391–393.

147 Millard F.E., Tani P. & McMillan R. (1987) A specific assay for anti-HLA antibodies: application to platelet donor selection. *Blood,* **70**, 1495–1499.

148 Kickler T.S., Ness P.M. & Braine H.G. (1988) Platelet crossmatching: a direct approach to the selection of platelet transfusions for the alloimmunized thrombocytopenic patient. *American Journal of Clinical Pathology,* **90**, 69–72.

149 Kieckbusch M.E., Moore S.B., Koenig V.A. *et al.* (1987) Platelet crossmatch evaluation in refractory hematologic patients. *Mayo Clinic Proceedings,* **69**, 595–600.

150 Moroff G., Garratty G., Heal J.M. *et al.* (1992) Selection of platelets for refractory patients by HLA matching and prospective crossmatching. *Transfusion,* **32**, 633–640.

151 Freedman J., Gafni A., Garvey M.B. *et al.* (1989) A cost-effectiveness evaluation of platelet crossmatching and HLA matching in the management of alloimmunized thrombocytopenic patients. *Transfusion,* **29**, 201–207.

152 Murphy M.F. & Waters A.H. (1985) Immunological aspects of platelet transfusions. *British Journal of Haematology,* **60**, 409–414.

153 Carr R., Hutton J.L., Jenkins J.A. *et al.* (1990) Transfusion of ABO-mismatched platelets leads to early platelet refractoriness. *British Journal of Haematology,* **75**, 408–413.

154 Lee E.J. & Schiffer C.A. (1989) ABO compatibility can influence the results of platelet transfusion: results of a randomized trial. *Transfusion,* **29**, 384–389.

155 Kelton J.G., Hamid C., Aker S. *et al.* (1982) The amount of blood group A substance on platelets is proportional to the amount of plasma. *Blood,* **59**, 980–985.

156 Brand A., Sintnicolaas K., Claas F.H. *et al.* (1986) ABH antibodies causing platelet transfusion refractoriness. *Transfusion,* **26**, 463–466.

157 Heal J.M., Mullin A. & Blumberg N. (1989) The importance of ABH antigens in platelet crossmatching. *Transfusion,* **29**, 514–520.

158 Okogen B., Rosseb Hansen B., Husebekk A. *et al.* (1988) Minimal expression of blood group A antigen on the thrombocytes from A2 individuals. *Transfusion,* **28**, 456–459.

159 Shanwell A., Ringden O., Wiechel B *et al.* (1991) A study of the effect of ABO incompatible plasma in platelet concentrates transfused to bone marrow transplant recipients. *Vox Sanguinis,* **160**, 23–27.

160 Lichtiger B., Surgeon J. & Rhorer S. (1983) Rh-incompatible platelet transfusion therapy in cancer patients: a study of 30 cases. *Vox Sanguinis,* **45**, 139–143.

161 Lichtiger B. & Hester J.P. (1986) Transfusion of Rh-incompatible blood components to cancer patients. *Haematologia (Budapest),* **19**, 81–88.

162 Heim M.U., Bock M. & Mempel W. (1993) Dose of anti-D immunoglobulin for the prevention of RhD immunisation after RhD-incompatible platelet transfusions. *Vox Sanguinis,* **65**, 74.

163 Kickler T., Braine H.G., Piantadosi S. *et al.* (1990) A randomized, placebo-controlled trial of intravenous gammaglobulin in alloimmunized thrombocytopenic patients. *Blood,* **75**, 313–316.

164 Schiffer C.A., Hogge D.E., Aisner J. *et al.* (1984) High-dose intravenous gammaglobulin in alloimmunized platelet transfusion recipients. *Blood,* **64**, 937–940.

165 Lee E.J., Norris D. & Schiffer C.A. (1987) Intravenous immune globulin for patients alloimmunized to random donor platelet transfusion. *Transfusion,* **27**, 245–247.

166 Heddle N.M., Klama L., Kelton J.G. *et al.* (1995) The use of anti-D to improve post-transfusion platelet response: a randomized trial. *British Journal of Haematology,* **89**, 163–168.

167 Decary F., Ferner P., Giavedoni L. *et al.* (1984) An investigation of nonhemolytic transfusion reactions. *Vox Sanguinis,* **46**, 277–285.

168 Williamson L.M., Copplestone J.A., Wimperis J.A. *et al.* (1994) Bedside filtration of blood products in the prevention of HLA alloimmunization. A prospective randomized study. *Blood,* **83**, 3028–3035.

169 Chambers L.A., Kruskall A.S., Pacini D.G. *et al.* (1990) Febrile reactions after platelet transfusion: the effect of single versus multiple donors. *Transfusion,* **30**, 219–221.

170 Heinrich D., Mueller-Eckhardt C. & Stier W. (1973) The specificity of leukocyte and platelet alloantibodies in sera of patients with nonhemolytic transfusion reactions. *Vox Sanguinis,* **25**, 442–456.

171 Bashir H. (1980) Adverse reactions due to leukocyte and platelet antibodies. *Anaesthesia and Intensive Care*, **8**, 132–138.

172 de Rie M.A., van der Plas-van Dalen C.M., Engelfriet C.P. *et al.* (1985) The serology of febrile transfusion reactions. *Vox Sanguinis*, **49**, 126–134.

173 Goodnough L.T., Riddell J. IV & Lazarus H. (1993) Prevalence of platelet transfusion reactions before and after implementation of leukocyte-depleted platelet concentrates by filtration. *Vox Sanguinis*, **65**, 103–107.

174 Dzieckowski J.S., Barrett B.B., Nester D. *et al.* (1995) Characterization of reactions after exclusive transfusion of white cell-reduced cellular blood components. *Transfusion*, **35**, 20–25.

175 Brand A. (1994) Passenger leukocytes, cytokines, and transfusion reactions. Letter to the Editor. *New England Journal of Medicine*, **331**, 670–671.

176 Heddle N.M., Klama L., Singer J. *et al.* (1994) The role of the plasma from platelet concentrates in transfusion reactions. *New England Journal of Medicine*, **331**, 625–628.

177 McLeod B.C., Sassetti R.I., Weens J.H. *et al.* (1982) Haemolytic transfusion reaction due to ABO incompatible plasma in a platelet concentrate. *Scandinavian Journal of Haematology*, **28**, 193–196.

178 Pierce R.N., Reich L.M. & Mayer K. (1985) Hemolysis following platelet transfusions from ABO-incompatible donors. *Transfusion*, **25**, 60–62.

179 Reis M.D. & Coovadia A.S. (1989) Transfusion of ABO-incompatible platelets causing severe haemolytic reaction. *Clinical and Laboratory Haematology*, **11**, 237–240.

180 Winter P.M., Amon M. & Hacker P. (1988) Febrile transfusion reaction caused by ABO-incompatible platelet transfusion. *Infusionstherapie*, **15**, 251–253.

181 Douglas D., Sorace J.M. & Kickler T. (1987) Betahemolytic streptococcus contamination of a platelet unit (abstract). *Transfusion*, **27**, 512.

182 Heal J.M., Singal S., Sardisco E. *et al.* (1986) Bacterial proliferation in platelet concentrates. *Transfusion*, **26**, 388–390.

183 Illert W.E., Sanger W. & Weise W. (1995) Bacterial contamination of single-donor blood components. *Transfusion Medicine*, **5**, 57–61.

184 Anderson K.C., Lew M.A., Gorgone B.C. *et al.* (1986) Transfusion-related sepsis after prolonged platelet storage. *American Journal of Medicine*, **81**, 405–411.

185 Punsalang A., Heal J.M. & Murphy P.J. (1989) Growth of Gram-positive and Gram-negative bacteria in platelet concentrates. *Transfusion*, **29**, 596–599.

186 British Committee for Standards in Haematology (1996) Guidelines on gamma irradiation of blood components for the prevention of transfusion-associated-graft-versus-host disease. *Transfusion Medicine*, **6**, 261–271.

187 McCullough J. (1995) The new generation of blood components. *Transfusion*, **35**, 374–377.

188 Bowden R.A., Sayers M., Gleaves C.A. *et al.* (1987) Cytomegalovirus-seronegative blood components for the prevention of primary cytomegalovirus infection after marrow transplantation. Considerations for blood banks. *Transfusion*, **27**, 478–481.

189 Cheung K.S. & Lang D.J. (1977) Transmission and activation of cytomegalovirus with blood transfusion: a mouse model. *Journal of Infectious Disease*, **135**, 841–845.

190 Chou S. (1986) Acquisitions of donor strains of cytomegalovirus by renal-transplant recipients. *New England Journal of Medicine*, **314**, 1418–1423.

191 Verdonk L.F., de Graan-Hentzen Y.C., Dekker A.W. *et al.* (1987) Cytomegalovirus seronegative platelets and leukocyte-poor red blood cells from random donors can prevent primary cytomegalovirus infection after bone marrow transplantation. *Bone Marrow Transplantation*, **2**, 73–78.

25   Supportive Care: Infection
J.A. Liu Yin

Introduction

Infection is a major problem in the management of leukaemic patients and remains a common cause of morbidity and mortality. Leukaemic patients have an increased susceptibility to infectious complications as they commonly have impaired defence mechanisms, of which neutropenia is probably the most important. In patients with acute leukaemia, neutropenia is almost invariable and may result from either the disease itself or the treatment administered. Similarly, neutropenia can occur in chronic leukaemias, as for example in advanced chronic lymphocytic leukaemia, hairy cell leukaemia and chronic granulocytic leukaemia in blast crisis. Thus in discussing the management of infection in the leukaemic patient, emphasis will be placed on its prevention, diagnosis and treatment in relation to the patient with severe neutropenia resulting from bone marrow failure. In addition, because different patterns of infection can occur in the chronic leukaemias, these will be discussed in the appropriate sections. While it is not proposed to review separately the infectious complications specific to bone marrow transplant patients however, where relevant, these will be discussed within the context of the severely immunocompromised host.

Infection as a cause of morbidity and mortality in acute leukaemia

Only three decades ago, the most common cause of death in patients with acute leukaemia was haemorrhage. With improvements in platelet support, the mortality from haemorrhagic complications has fallen significantly, while that from infective causes has risen proportionately. Such a trend is reflected by the experience at the National Cancer Institute, in the USA, between the years 1955 and 1971. Between 1955 and 1963 the mortality rate from infection alone in patients with acute leukaemia was 38%, whereas in the subsequent period between 1965 and 1971 it had increased to 69% in patients with haematological malignancies, including acute leukaemia [1,2]. The difference in mortality in the two series can be primarily accounted for by the decline in the proportion of deaths associated with haemorrhage. Another recent series also showed that infection alone is responsible for some 70% of deaths from acute leukaemia, while haemorrhage, as a primary cause, accounted for another 15% [3].

In an attempt to achieve a radical cure for leukaemia, increasingly intensive chemotherapeutic regimens and other procedures, including bone marrow transplantation (BMT), are being used. These manoeuvres have led to a further compromise of the host's defence mechanisms, rendering these patients more susceptible to infections by a wide spectrum of pathogens. Patients with prolonged periods of treatment-related neutropenia are at increased risk of infectious complications, while in BMT patients, infection with cytomegalovirus (CMV) remains a major cause of death. Furthermore, a new pattern of opportunistic infections from microorganisms, which were hitherto considered to be nonpathogenic, has emerged and become an important cause of morbidity and mortality. Thus despite major advances in the management of leukaemic patients, which have resulted in significantly prolonged survival for many and probable cure for some, infection nevertheless remains an important determinant of survival.

Predisposing factors associated with infection

Multiple defects in host-defence mechanisms may increase the susceptibility to infection in the leukaemic patient. Cellular or humoral defects may occur singly or in combination, along with breaches in physical barriers which normally provide protection against infecting organisms. Indeed, the patient with acute leukaemia represents, *par excellence*, such a compromised host. The main predisposing factors are listed in Table 25.1.

Anatomical barriers to entry of microorganisms

The intact skin is an effective physical barrier to the entry of

502

Table 25.1 Main factors predisposing to infection in acute leukaemia patients.

Cellular defects	Humoral defects	Anatomical factors
Neutropenia and neutrophil dysfunction	Impaired antibody production	Stomatitis
Lymphopenia and lymphocyte dysfunction	Decreased complement activity	Pharyngitis
		Gastrointestinal ulceration
		Venepunctures
Monocytopenia		Vascular catheters
Defective antibody-dependent cellular cytotoxicity		Urinary cathethers
		Endotracheal aspiration
		Bone marrow aspiration
Defective natural killer cellular cytotoxicity		Decreased ciliary activity of respiratory tract

microorganisms, but in patients with acute leukaemia it is frequently broken down by the use of needles and intravascular catheters. The broken integument can thus become a potential site and source of infection. In leukaemic patients the prolonged use of indwelling intravascular catheters is often required, and this is often associated with the development of bacteraemias by skin commensals such as *Staphylococcus epidermidis* and *Corynebacteria* species. One study showed that up to 80% of patients receiving intravenous fluids through indwelling catheters develop catheter-related septicaemia, and that the risk increased directly with the length of time the catheter is left *in situ* [4]. The use of the large-bore right atrial catheter (e.g. Hickman), which provides ready venous access in leukaemic or BMT patients, has been a major advance in the management of such patients. However, this has led to a sharp increase in bacteraemia caused by Gram-positive organisms, especially coagulase-negative staphylococci, although infections of the exit site and subcutaneous tunnel through which the catheter is brought out do also occur [5].

Damage to the mucous membranes of the gastrointestinal tract is an important factor in the development of infection, as it offers a portal of entry for infecting organisms. Oropharyngeal and gastrointestinal ulceration are frequent side effects of the cytotoxic agents (e.g. anthracyclines) used during intensive remission-induction chemotherapy for acute leukaemia. For patients undergoing BMT, further damage to the mucous membrane is caused by radiotherapy. Damaged sites can be colonized by bacterial and fungal organisms, which can subsequently invade the blood stream. Common sites of infection in the alimentary tract are the oropharynx, the oesophagus and the perianal region. Poor oral hygiene with underlying periodontal disease may also predispose to the development of oral infections. Similarly, perianal or perirectal infections are not infrequent, and these probably arise from a combination of two factors, namely damaged anal mucosa and the high pressure generated during defaecation.

Within the respiratory tract, the mucosa and ciliary function of the endothelial cells are similarly damaged by chemothera-

peutic agents and this is partly responsible for the frequent development of pneumonias in leukaemic patients. Procedures such as bronchoscopy and endotracheal intubation, which are sometimes necessary in the management of such patients, can further predispose to infection. The introduction of mechanical tubes in the trachea or bronchi not only disrupts natural barriers but can also cause spread of contaminated materials into the lungs. The genitourinary tract can also become a source of invasive infection if urethral catheters are introduced and left *in situ*, as the risks of bacteriuria and Gram-negative septicaemia are then significantly increased [6].

Cellular defects

Neutropenia and neutrophil dysfunction

Neutropenia is undoubtedly the most important factor responsible for the increased frequency of infectious complications in the leukaemic patient. Bodey has demonstrated an adverse relationship between the number of circulating neutrophils and the risk of infections, which rises sharply as the neutrophil count drops to below 0.5×10^9/l, and is highest when the count is below 0.1×10^9/l [7]. In a study of 52 patients with acute leukaemia, Bodey showed that there were 43 episodes of major infection per 1000 days when the neutrophil count was less than 0.1×10^9/l, compared to only four episodes per 1000 days when the count was greater than 0.1×10^9/l [7]. The risk of infection becomes greater with increasing duration of neutropenia. The importance of the neutrophil count in determining the response to antibiotics, and hence survival, in neutropenic patients has also been shown. In the first EORTC Trial comparing different antibiotic combinations, if the organism was susceptible to the antibiotic regimen, 88% of patients whose neutrophil count increased to more than 0.1×10^9/l improved, whereas only 22% of those whose neutrophil count did not rise got better [8].

In addition, leukaemic patients may also have qualitative neutrophil defects, such as impairment of bone marrow mobilization, chemotaxis, phagocytosis and intracellular killing [9,10]. In patients with acute lymphoblastic leukaemia (ALL), some functional impairment of neutrophils was noted even when remission had been achieved [11]. In another study the frequency of infection in children with ALL increased as the impairment in bactericidal function of neutrophils became more severe [12].

Lymphopenia and lymphocyte dysfunction

The role of lymphocytes in providing immunity against infections is well established. The complex cooperative functions of several classes of lymphocytes and their interactions with monocytes are being slowly unravelled. Cell-mediated immunity is frequently impaired in patients with lymphocytic leukaemias and in those receiving chemotherapy or radiotherapy and steroid treatment. Such patients are at risk of developing infections by intracellular parasites such as protozoa or mycobacteria and viruses of which herpes simplex, herpes zoster and CMV are the commonest. Many of these infections are believed to represent reactivation of latent organisms. Among the protozoal infections, *Pneumocystis carinii* pneumonia and toxoplasmosis are important, while infection with the yeast *Cryptococcus neoformans* is also occasionally seen.

Monocytopenia

Patients with hairy cell leukaemia, in addition to being neutropenic, commonly have monocytopenia. This may therefore explain their susceptibility to develop not only pyogenic but also mycobacterial and other opportunistic infections [13].

Humoral immune defects

The humoral immune response, through the action of antibodies and complement, plays an essential role against infection. Impaired antibody production may result from either the disease itself as, for example, in chronic lymphocytic leukaemia (CLL), or following chemo/radiotherapy for acute leukaemia. Thus as a result of therapy, the leukaemic patient may suffer from impairment of both cellular and humoral immunity. IgG and IgM are particularly important immunoglobulins, because they not only promote phagocytosis through opsonization but they can also fix complement and lead to direct bacterial lysis [14]. In addition, deficiency of IgA may facilitate invasion of organisms through mucosal surfaces which may be already compromised [15]. As a consequence of hypogammaglobulinaemia, these patients are particularly prone to repeated infections by encapsulated Gram-positive organisms, such as *Streptococcus pneumoniae*.

While serum complement activity is within the normal range in patients in remission from acute leukaemia, it is reduced in those undergoing induction chemotherapy and also in those with relapsed leukaemia [16]. Patients with rare isolated complement deficiencies, for example C3, are known to have an increased susceptibility to infections [17].

Effects of immunosuppressive drugs

Most leukaemic patients with impairment of both cellular and humoral immunity are receiving cytotoxic drugs and/or corticosteroids. Corticosteroids which are used during remission induction for ALL, and in the treatment of CLL, have a profound effect on the immune system in man. They cause a marked but transient lymphopenia and monocytopenia [18] and, in addition, they have been shown to suppress the bactericidal activity of monocytes [19]. It has been clearly demonstrated that in experimental infections the use of corticosteroids has deleterious effects on the outcome. For example, in one study the administration of cortisone increased the mortality rate in mice infected with *Candida albicans* from 11 to 83% [20]. In clinical practice, patients being treated with steroids appear to have increased frequency and severity of infections caused by a multitude of organisms including bacteria, viruses, fungi and protozoa [21].

Independently of myelosuppression, cytotoxic drugs may cause immunosuppression by interfering with functions such as cytotoxicity mediated by leucocytes. Recent work has been carried out on the phenomenon of cytotoxicity *in vitro* mediated by leucocytes against virus-infected cells, bacteria, fungi and parasites [22]. Bolivar *et al.* [23] have demonstrated that antineoplastic drugs, such as doxorubicin, cyclophosphamide, procarbazine, vincristine and prednisolone, when tested *in vitro*, can decrease human leucocyte-mediated, antibody-dependent cellular cytotoxicity and NK cytotoxicity against target cells infected with herpes simplex. These findings suggest that chemotherapeutic agents used in the treatment of leukaemia may impair cell-mediated cytotoxicity against viruses, and possibly against other nonviral organisms as well.

Postsplenectomy state

The spleen plays a vital role in protecting the host from filterable encapsulated organisms and may also be responsible for the early production of IgM antibodies directed against these organisms [24]. Some patients with chronic leukaemias may require splenectomy as part of the management of their disease. The main danger following splenectomy, especially in immunocompromised hosts, is overwhelming sepsis and the organisms most frequently involved are pneumococci, meningococci, *E. coli, Haemophilus influenzae* and staphylococci [25]. It has been estimated that after splenectomy approximately 5% of patients, over their lifetime, will develop sepsis, resulting in a mortality of about 50% [25]. However, with an increased awareness of the postsplenectomy state and the use of pneumococcal and other vaccines, mortality from overwhelming sepsis should now be a very rare event.

Diagnosis of infection

While fever is the hallmark of infection, it is not specific. Fever in patients with leukaemia and lymphomas can be a manifestation of the underlying disease itself or it can result from a hypersensitivity reaction if such patients, as is often the case, are receiving multiple drug combinations or blood products.

Thus, a new fever associated with a generalized rash arising in a patient who is already taking antibiotics, is often suggestive of a drug allergy. On the other hand, serious infection can occur in the absence of fever, and it is well worth remembering that fever in the presence of infection can be masked by the concurrent use of large doses of steroids.

The neutropenic patient is not capable of mounting an adequate inflammatory response to infection. Fever may be the only sign and the other classical signs of inflammation may be absent, thus making the diagnosis of infection difficult. For example, pneumonia is a common infection which has a high mortality rate in neutropenic patients, and yet its diagnosis in the early stages may not be obvious. The usual signs, such as crepitations, pulmonary consolidation and X-ray changes, may be minimal or delayed. Similarly, while the only clues for infective lesions such as cellulitis or perianal sepsis may be minimal erythema, tenderness or pain in the affected areas, such an infection may have progressed to a septicaemic phase with accompanying fever and rigors. Accordingly, reliance must be placed on the actual isolation of the infecting organism in blood cultures.

In practice, the terms septicaemia and bacteraemia are used interchangeably and the distinction between the two terms often becomes a matter of semantics. While bacteraemia can be transient, for example following a dental extraction, septicaemia implies systemic colonization of the blood stream and systemic spread of infection. Evidence for septicaemia comes not only from positive blood cultures or blood smears, but also from histological evidence of disseminated infection in soft tissues, muscle, bone marrow, skin and other organs.

Colonization and infection

Numerous studies have demonstrated the importance of colonization by microorganisms and the subsequent risk of infection. Infections occurring in neutropenic patients may be caused by organisms already present in the patient's endogenous flora or by those acquired from the hospital environment. For example, in one series of 87 patients undergoing chemotherapy for acute leukaemia, the carrier state for *Pseudomonas* species was shown to increase from 25% on admission to 54% after 4 weeks of hospitalization [26]. The acquisition of these organisms contributed to the high incidence of *Pseudomonas* infection in these patients. Another study showed that leukaemic patients, while in hospital, have altered oropharyngeal and faecal flora even without the administration of antibiotics, and that their parental use was associated with a reduction in normal flora followed by colonization by Gram-negative bacilli [27]. In addition, acquired potential pathogens were more likely to cause infections than those which comprised the patient's endogenous flora.

Schimpff *et al.* [28] have demonstrated that over 80% of infections are caused by organisms already present at, or adjacent to, the site where infection would eventually develop. The major sites of infection in patients with acute leukaemia are the oropharynx, the lower oesophagus, the perianal area, the lungs and the skin. The enteric organisms which commonly cause infections are the Gram-negative bacilli, *E. coli*, *Pseudomonas aeruginosa* and *Klebsiella pneumoniae*. In the leukaemic patient these organisms also frequently colonize the oropharynx and it is therefore not surprising that most cases of life-threatening pneumonias are caused by Gram-negative bacilli. In addition, further changes in the microbial flora occur as a result of antibiotic therapy. The suppression of normal flora allows the emergence and colonization of yeasts in the oropharynx and facilitates the growth of filamentous fungi,

Table 25.2 Frequent and recently recognized organisms causing infection in patients with leukaemia.

Bacteria	
Gram-negative	*E. coli*, *Klebsiella–Enterobacter–Serratia* group, *Pseudomonas aeruginosa* and other species, *Proteus* species, *Aeromonas hydrophilia*, *Acinobacter* species, *Legionella pneumophilia*
Gram-positive	*Steptococcus pneumoniae*, *Strep. faecalis*, vancomycin-resistant enterococci *Staphylococcus aureus*, *Staph. epidermidis*, diphtherthoids, *Listeria monocytogenes*, *Bacillus cereus*
Anaerobes	*Clostridium difficile*, *Cl. perfringens*, *Bacteroides* species
Nonbacterial pathogens	
Fungi	*Candida* species, *Torulopsis glabrata*, *Aspergillus* species, *Mucor*, *Trichosporum cutaneum*, *Cryptococcus neoformans*
Protozoa/parasites	*Pneumocystis carinii*, *Toxoplasma gondii*, *Strongyloides stercolaris*
Viruses	Herpes simplex, herpes zoster, cytomegalovirus, hepatitis A, B, and C, measles

such as *Aspergillus*, in the nasal passages. Consequently in these patients, colonization by fungal organisms increases the risk of invasive disease.

The major organisms causing infection in leukaemic patients are shown in Table 25.2.

Bacterial infections

During the 1950s the majority of fatal infections in patients with acute leukaemia were caused by *Staphylococcus aureus* [1]. The introduction of antistaphylococcal penicillins has produced a dramatic reduction in the incidence of fatal septicaemia caused by this organism, which is now less than 5%. As a result, the Gram-negative bacilli have become the predominant organisms causing fatal infections. *Pseudomonas aeruginosa*, *E. coli* and organisms of the *Klebsiella–Enterobacter–Serratia* group are responsible for most of the fatal cases of pneumonia and septicaemia. In one study of patients with acute leukaemia, pneumonia and systemic infections of bacterial origin accounted for 67% of all deaths from infective causes [3]. Similarly, Bodey *et al.* [29] have shown that septicaemia and pneumonia together were responsible for 69% of the total episodes of documented infection in leukaemic patients, although not all with a fatal outcome, and that the great majority of infecting organisms were Gram-negative bacilli.

Gram-negative bacilli

Pseudomonas aeruginosa remains a major pathogen in the patient with acute leukaemia and in many studies it has been a leading cause of mortality [30,31]. The lung is a common site of infection and *Pseudomonas* pneumonia carries a particularly poor prognosis [32,33]. Ecthyma gangrenosum is a characteristic skin lesion of *Pseudomonas* septicaemia and is often found in the perineal, axillary and inframammary areas. The organism can be cultured from these lesions, which classically have a bluish-purple necrotic centre surrounded by an erythematous halo. Untreated, *Pseudomonas* septicaemia can cause death very rapidly, sometimes within 24 hours.

The introduction of carbenicillin as a *Pseudomonas*-specific antibiotic has resulted in a decline in mortality from *Pseudomonas* infection in patients with acute leukaemia, and consequently other Gram-positive organisms, such as *E. coli* and the *Klebsiella–Enterobacter–Serratia* group, have emerged as frequent causes of fatal infections. It is important to note that, unless prompt treatment is instituted, these organisms can cause deaths equally rapidly as *Pseudomonas* species can. It is also likely that as more antibiotics with increasing potency against *Pseudomonas* and other Gram-negative bacilli become available, the pattern of serious and fatal infections in the compromised host will continue to change. In this respect, the increasing incidence of infections with nosocomially acquired organisms, yeasts and other fungi has become quite alarming.

Changing patterns of infection

Several organisms considered in the past to be nonpathogenic have now become important causes of infection in leukaemic patients. The aerobic Gram-positive cocci are now a major cause of nosocomially acquired infections [34,35]. Although *Staph. aureus*, causing fatal infection, is much less frequently encountered nowadays, strains which are resistant to methicillin have been reported and could pose problems in some institutions. The skin commensal *Staph. epidermidis* has now become an increasingly common cause of bacteraemia in patients undergoing BMT or intensive chemotherapy for acute leukaemia. This changing spectrum of infection has resulted from the use of long-term indwelling venous catheters in these patients. Fortunately, *Staph. epidermidis* infections can be readily treated with vancomycin, although this antibiotic is potentially nephrotoxic. An alternative antibiotic, effective against coagulase-negative staphylococci, is teicoplanin; this antibiotic has the potential advantages of once-daily administration and of being non-nephrotoxic [36,37]. In addition, several species of *Corynebacterium* and other diphtheroids, which are normally skin organisms, have been shown to cause septicaemia and pneumonia in immunocompromised patients [35,38]. Untreated, these infections may prove fatal, but they usually respond to vancomycin [38]. Other organisms which have been considered to be essentially nonpathogenic, but which can cause infections in leukaemic patients, include *Aeromonas hydrophilia* and *Bacillus* species [38,39]. More recently, the emergence of vancomycin-resistant enterococci in leukaemic patients has given much cause for concern. These enterococci, which can give rise to septicaemia, are resistant to most antibiotics and are very difficult to eradicate. Some organisms are sensitive to chloramphenicol but the risk of resistance developing is very high.

Two other pathogens that can be found in the compromised host, deserve mention. The anaerobe, *Clostridium difficile*, can cause pseudomembranous colitis, a severe form of diarrhoea, usually in patients receiving antibiotics. However, it can also occur in patients receiving cytotoxic drugs and the organism is sensitive to oral vancomycin. The fastidious bacterium *Legionella pneumophilia* is now recognized to be a cause of atypical pneumonia, which can occur either as an epidemic or as sporadic cases [40,41]. Several other species of *Legionella* have since been characterized. Transmission is believed to be airborne and the organisms may be spread by air-conditioning systems. Legionellosis is a severe multisystem disease, characterized by fever, myalgia, changes in the mental state and pneumonia. Erythromycin is the drug of choice for treating *Legionella* pneumonia and rifampicin should be added in non-responsive cases.

Fungal infections

The incidence of invasive fungal infections has increased

significantly over the last three decades and these have now become an important cause of morbidity and mortality in the immunocompromised host [42]. This trend has coincided with the use of increasingly intensive immuno-suppression, long-term indwelling venous catheters and broad-spectrum antibiotics in patients who are now surviving longer. The major fungal pathogens include *Candida* and *Aspergillus* species, the Mucoraceae and *Cryptococcus neoformans*.

Candida infections

Candida organisms, which are normal commensals in the oropharynx, intestinal tract and vagina, are the most common cause of fungal infection in neutropenic patients. Of the different species, *C. albicans* and *C. tropicalis* are the most frequently associated with invasive candidiasis [43]. While patients with neutropenia and neutrophil dysfunction tend to develop systemic candidiasis, those with defects of cell-mediated immunity are prone to mucocutaneous disease. In leukaemic patients, in addition to cellular defects, local factors such as mucosal and skin damage, indwelling venous catheters and parenteral feeding, predispose to candidal infections and systemic spread. Clinical syndromes include focal infection of the gastrointestinal tract such as oropharyngeal candidiasis, and *Candida* septicaemia with dissemination to multiple organs. While oropharyngeal infection presents with the characteristic exudates adherent to the underlying mucosa, oesophageal candidiasis commonly presents with dysphagia and retrosternal pain. Candida septicaemia with multiple-organ involvement is the most serious type of infection and carries a high mortality. The organs most frequently involved are the kidneys, lungs, heart and liver [44]. The diagnosis should be suspected when there is unexplained fever in the ill neutropenic patient receiving broad-spectrum antibiotics. Cutaneous lesions in the form of discrete multiple erythematous nodules may aid in the diagnosis. These lesions should be biopsied and cultured. In addition, retinal lesions appearing as white exudates can be visualized directly with the ophthalmoscope.

The diagnosis of systemic candidiasis is often difficult to make, because blood cultures are often negative and conventional serological tests are of limited value. A definite diagnosis can be established by histological demonstration of *Candida* in tissue or positive cultures from a sterile body site or fluid. A positive culture from blood taken from a venous catheter may imply colonization of the catheter and does not always indicate systemic infection. The detection of circulating *Candida* antigens and metabolites appears to be more valuable than conventional antibody tests, and many such tests, using a variety of investigational methods, have been evaluated [43,45,46]. The need for a rapid, sensitive and specific test which can be used to confirm the diagnosis of systemic disease remains a clinical priority [46].

Aspergillus infections

Aspergillus infections are the second most common type of invasive fungal infections and are an important cause of death in neutropenic patients [47]. *Aspergillus fumigatus* is the commonest species, followed by *A. flavus*, *A. niger* and *A. glavius*. Outbreaks of *Aspergillus* infection in leukaemic patients can arise from contamination of hospital ventilation systems or in wards near construction sites. The most frequent clinical presentation is pulmonary infection. Invasive pulmonary aspergillosis is characterized by necrotizing haemorrhagic bronchopneumonia, consolidation, followed by cavitation, abscess formation and aspergillomas [48]. The upper lobes are often involved and X-ray changes may show characteristic well-defined round opacities (Fig. 25.1). *Aspergillus* organisms tend to invade blood vessels and erosion of a major blood vessel in a cavity wall can sometimes result in fatal haemoptysis. Disseminated aspergillosis frequently complicates pulmonary infection. The main organs are the brain, gastrointestinal tract, liver, kidneys, heart and spleen, but unfortunately, in most cases, the extent of the disease is only established at autopsy.

The most reliable way of making a definitive diagnosis is by

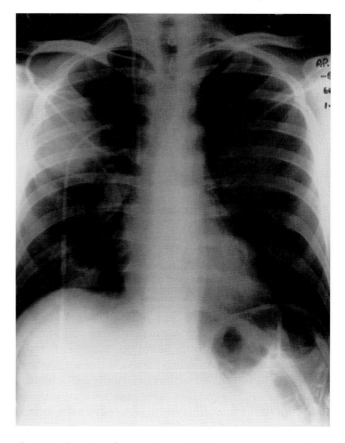

Fig. 25.1 Chest X-ray from a patient with refractory acute myeloid leukaemia. *Aspergillus* pneumonia of the right upper lobe.

the demonstration of the *Aspergillus* organism by culture and histological examination of pulmonary tissue obtained by bronchoscopy or open lung biopsy. However, *Aspergillus* isolated in a sputum culture does not necessarily imply invasive disease and may simply indicate colonization of the upper respiratory tract [49]. Detection of antibodies against *Aspergillus* may be of value but appears to be a relatively insensitive test for invasive aspergillosis [50]. Early diagnosis of invasive aspergillosis is important, as it would lead to prompt institution of the appropriate therapy and may improve the generally poor outlook associated with such infection. Although radioimmunoassay and latex agglutination methods for the detection of circulating *Aspergillus* antigens are available, there still remains an urgent need to develop a rapid and specific test to diagnose invasive disease [46,51]. In this respect, the recent report that determination of plasma $(1 \rightarrow 3)$-B-D-glucan, a characteristic fungal cell-wall constituent, is a highly sensitive and specific test for invasive deep mycosis and fungal febrile episodes appears promising [52].

The Mucoraceae and *Cryptococcus neoformans*, which can cause infection in the leukaemic patient, will also be mentioned here. The Mucoraceae usually cause pneumonias, but they may invade the nasopharynx and spread to the nasal and paranasal sinuses, the orbit and the frontal lobes of the brain. The ubiquitous organism *Cryptococcus neoformans* has been reported to be the most common cause of fungal infection of the central nervous system in the cancer patient with impaired cell-mediated immunity. The lung is the next most common site of cryptococcal infection. A detailed description of these infections can be found in the comprehensive review by Hawkins & Armstrong [42]

Pneumocystis carinii infections

Pneumocystis carinii is a cause of severe, rapidly progressive, bilateral interstitial pneumonia in the immunocompromised host. In one study reported by Hughes *et al.* [53], *P. carinii* pneumonia occurred in approximately 6.5% of patients with acute leukaemia. However, the incidence of *Pneumocystis* infection in children with ALL appears to be related to the intensity of immunosuppression given during maintenance therapy [54]. It also occurs in patients with CLL and in recipients of BMT, although in the latter group it can now be effectively prevented by co-trimoxazole prophylaxis. Dyspnoea is the common symptom of *Pneumocystis* pneumonia; other clinical features include fever, cyanosis and a dry nonproductive cough. A lack of auscultatory findings in the chest is often characteristic. Typically the radiographic picture is a perihilar infiltrate in the early stages, which progresses to a diffuse alveolar infiltrate involving all areas of the lung. However, atypical patterns may appear as unilateral infiltrate, lobar or segmental consolidation (Fig. 25.2) [55]. A definitive diagnosis is made by demonstrating the typical cysts in material obtained from the lung. Numerous methods to obtain specimens have been

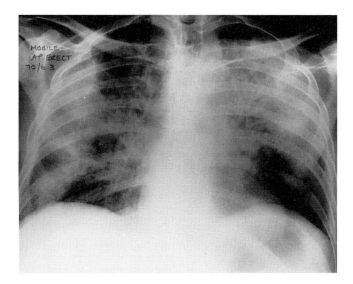

Fig. 25.2 Proven *Pneumocystis carinii* pneumonia in a patient with CLL.

described: these include fibreoptic bronchoscopy with endobronchial brushing or transbronchial biopsy [56,57] and, more recently, bronchoalveolar lavage, percutaneous needle biopsy [58] and open-lung biopsy [59]. Open lung biopsy is the most invasive of these procedures, but it ensures that an adequate specimen of lung tissue is obtained for histological and microbiological examination. However, with newer diagnostic techniques such as the application of monoclonal antibodies and specific DNA probes, combined with the polymerase chain reaction (PCR), it may be possible to make the diagnosis of *Pneumocystis* infections with greater accuracy on material such as induced sputum or bronchoalveolar lavage fluid.

Viral infections

Viral infections remain an important cause of morbidity and mortality in the immunocompromised patient. The herpes group, herpes simplex, varicella zoster and CMV are clinically the more important pathogens, although infections such as hepatitis and measles pose a particular threat to the leukaemic patient. With the advent of effective treatment with acyclovir, the clinical course of herpes simplex and varicella zoster infections has changed dramatically, although CMV pneumonitis remains a major cause of deaths in bone marrow transplant recipients. Following chemo/radiotherapy in leukaemic and BMT patients, herpes simplex infections most commonly present as herpes labialis and gingivostomatitis and, occasionally, as herpes genitalis. Patients with impairment of cell-mediated immunity, for example in CLL, ALL and following BMT, may have reactivation of latent herpes zoster and develop shingles with the subsequent risk of dissemination. In BMT patients the incidence of herpes zoster infection is about 40%, of which 20–40% will disseminate; the mortality from herpes

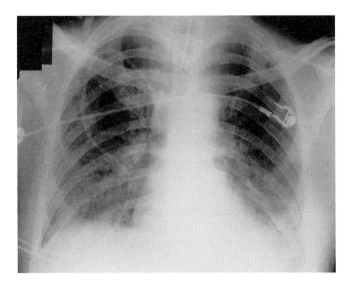

Fig. 25.3 Diffuse interstitial CMV pneumonitis in a patient, 30 days postallogeneic BMT.

zoster infections was reported at 5–8%, with pneumonia being the most frequent cause of death [60]. However, with the early use of acyclovir, death from herpes zoster is now preventable.

In the child with ALL, measles can be a severe infection and can run a fulminating course. The use of prophylactic normal human immunoglobulin for leukaemic patients who have been in contact with measles has been disappointing, and it may be worth considering the use of larger doses of immunoglobulins given intravenously, because better preparations are now available [61]. Leukaemic patients who require frequent support with blood or blood products are at risk of developing viral hepatitis, including hepatitis B and C. They may be more susceptible to fulminant infection, associated with acute liver atrophy, or they may later develop chronic liver disease [38].

Cytomegalovirus infection

Cytomegalovirus can produce a variety of clinical syndromes, including pneumonitis, hepatitis and retinitis. The BMT recipient is at particular risk and CMV infection may account for up to 20% of deaths following BMT. It is responsible for 50–70% of all cases of pneumonitis in BMT patients [60]. Symptoms include fever, malaise, anorexia, myalgia and night sweats. Dry cough and tachypnoea suggest pulmonary involvement, and radiographic changes may show symmetrical bilateral interstitial infiltrates or lobar consolidation (Fig. 25.3). Attention has focused on methods for detecting the virus, and these have included the use of probes to identify viral DNA, monoclonal antibodies which allow the detection of viral antigens either in tissue section or in culture [62–64] and, more recently, PCR-based techniques for detecting viral DNA in blood and urine [65–68]. These techniques, which can provide

an answer within 24 hours, have greatly facilitated the early diagnosis of CMV infection and, consequently, can influence the clinical management of infected patients.

Infection prophylaxis

Prevention of nosocomial infection: total protective environment

The most efficient way of providing a pathogen-free environment is by the use of high-efficiency particulate air (HEPA) filters, through which air is forced in a laminar or unidirectional flow. These filters remove particles greater than 0.3 μm, which include all bacteria and fungi and some larger viruses [69]. The use of laminar air flow in a standard hospital room can reduce potential pathogens from about 3000 per 1000 ft³ (28.34 m³) of air to virtually zero, [70]. However, for total protective isolation to be effective, all items brought into the room must be sterile or nearly sterile—this includes food and water, medical and personal items. Before entering the room, personnel and visitors must wash their hands thoroughly, using an antiseptic such as chlorhexidine or povidone iodine, and wear gloves, masks, hair and shoe covers. In addition, regular decontamination of floors and surfaces with disinfectants is essential. Ideally patients should have undergone endogenous decontamination before admission to the sterile environment.

The use of total protection isolation within laminar air flow rooms should, in theory, reduce the rate of infections by about 50%, because half of the infections in neutropenic patients are caused by organisms acquired from the hospital environment. There are, unfortunately, only a few studies which have been carried out to evaluate the effectiveness of the total protective environment without the concurrent use of nonabsorbable antibiotics to suppress the endogenous microbial flora. Nevertheless, the controlled studies of Dietrich *et al.* [71] and Yates & Holland [72] appear to suggest that the protected environment can indeed reduce the rate of infection by about 50%.

Several prospective controlled studies of laminar air flow rooms, or similar isolation rooms, in conjunction with the use or oral nonabsorbable antibiotics, have been carried out against control groups which incorporated neither protective isolation nor oral nonabsorbable antibiotics. All these studies showed that this combination achieved a substantial reduction in the incidence of all infections, including pneumonias, soft tissue infections and Gram-negative bacteraemia [70–77]. An additional consistent benefit resulting from the use of laminar air flow filtration was the elimination of *Aspergillus* infections.

The use of a total protective environment (TPE) not only involves considerable expenses in the setting up and running of LAF units but it also imposes physical and psychological isolation of patients who, in addition, are subjected to the discomfort of having to take unpalatable oral antibiotics. Thus it is pertinent to ask whether its use significantly improves patient survival, to justify the constraints and costs it incurs. Certainly a good case can be made for treating BMT recipients in such facilities, as these patients have relatively long periods of neutropenia. Moreover, a study by Storb *et al.* [78] has indicated that the TPE, combined with gut decontamination, reduced the incidence and severity of graft vs host disease (GVHD) and increased the survival in patients with severe aplastic anaemia treated by BMT. When laminar air flow facilities are not available, isolation rooms fitted with HEPA filters appear to be an adequate substitute.

Nevertheless, it is at present difficult to justify the use of the TPE for treating leukaemic patients. Indeed, the use of TPE has not significantly improved the complete remission rate or survival of patients undergoing chemotherapy for acute leukaemia [79]. Furthermore, there are many leukaemia units which manage their patients without any facilities for protective isolation or air filtration and appear to do as well as centres equipped with LAF units [80]. It may be argued that TPE, through a reduction in infectious complications, may permit the escalation of chemotherapy doses and result in increased remission rates, duration of remission and survival, but this hypothesis, in the context of the treatment of acute leukaemia, still requires testing.

Care of the skin

The skin is a source of potential pathogens, which in the neutropenic patient can cause local infections and give rise to septicaemia. To minimize such risks, skin and hair should be washed regularly with an antiseptic such as chlorhexidine or povidone-iodine, and particular attention should be paid to the axillae, groins and perineum. Any procedure which results in a breach of the skin, for example the insertion of an intravenous cannula or bone marrow aspiration, should be carried out under strictly aseptic conditions. In the neutropenic patient it is advisable to give antibiotic cover (e.g. vancomycin) before and shortly after the insertion of the indwelling right atrial catheter of the Hickman/Broviac type. Since the use of such long-term venous catheters has resulted in a dramatic increase in the incidence of infections caused by skin commensals, it is essential that aseptic techniques for catheter care are applied at all times.

A programme of bacteriological surveillance (including nose, throat, axillary, groin and perianal swabs, and urine and stool culture) may reveal the presence of potential pathogens. For example, surveillance swabs may reveal nasal carriage of *Staph. aureus* or *Aspergillus* species—a situation known to lead to subsequent infection in the neutropenic patient [81]. Eradication of the carrier state by local measures is frequently unsuccessful and, for *Staph. aureus*, the use of systemic therapy has been advocated [82]. However, the usefulness of surveillance cultures in the routine management of neutropenic patients has been questioned, although in certain groups of patients (e.g. those receiving prophylactic antibiotics) limited surveillance can provide useful information.

Diet and fomites

Food and water are an important source of infecting organisms in the neutropenic patient. Uncooked leafy vegetables, for example lettuce, may contain high counts of Gram-negative bacilli, such as *E. coli*, *Klebsiella pneumoniae* and *Pseudomonas aeruginosa*. For this reason salads, fresh fruits and tap water must be avoided. A low-microbial diet can be achieved by providing freshly cooked foods, commercially sterilized foods and sterile water. Such a diet is also an integral part of any programme of gastrointestinal decontamination [79].

To reduce the risk of cross-infection in the protected environment, fomites such as thermometers and medical instruments should be sterilized before introduction into the room and sterilized again after use. These should be left in the room and cleaned with 70% alcohol to remove any organic debris after each use.

It is worth making the point that for effective prevention of nosocomial infection, patients should be isolated from the time of hospital admission, and standard reverse isolation procedures should be observed at all times. Unless the measures discussed above are adhered to, the practice of 'simple' protective isolation, often carried out in hospital side rooms, is unlikely to be more effective than careful hand washing before entering the rooms.

Infection prophylaxis and prevention of infection from endogenous flora

Oral nonabsorbable antibiotics for gastrointestinal decontamination

Since the gastrointestinal tract is a major source of pathogens, one direct approach to infection prevention is to suppress organisms colonizing the alimentary tract. However, gastrointestinal decontamination, although extensively practised in the past, remains an area of controversy. Two modalities, namely 'total' versus 'selective' gastrointestinal decontamination, have been used and will be discussed here.

Total decontamination is not achieved in practice but the oral nonabsorbable antibiotics (ONA) are very effective in suppressing the gut flora. Some of the oral antibiotics regimens used are shown in Table 25.3. Assessment of the value of ONA in the prevention of infection in neutropenic patients from published data is fraught with difficulties. These studies have included relatively small numbers of patients and have used widely different oral antibiotics and cytotoxic regimens. In addition, multiple variables, including cutaneous antisepsis, low pathogen diet and protective environment, were employed but were not always strictly controlled [75,83–85]. Lastly, compliance with these unpalatable drugs was most likely an important factor but it was not always adequately evaluated. Hence it is not surprising that studies to data have failed to show a consistent benefit of ONA when used in the

Table 25.3 Oral antibiotic regimens used for infection prophylaxis.

Eponym	Drug	Dosage
GVN	Gentamicin suspension	200 mg 4 hourly
	Vancomycin suspension	250–500 mg 4 hourly
	Nystatin tablets	4 Mu 4 hourly
	Nystatin suspension	1 Mu 4 hourly
FRACON	Framycetin	0.5 g q.d.s.
	Colistin sulphate	1.5 Mu q.d.s.
	Nystatin	2.4 Mu/day
NEOCON	Neomycin sulphate	0.5 g b.d.
	Colistin sulphate	1.5 Mu b.d.
	Nystatin tablets	0.5 Mu b.d.
	Nystatin suspension	0.1 Mu b.d.
	Amphotericin lozenges	10 mg q.d.s.
TSN	Co-trimoxazole	320–480 mg/day
	Nystatin	30 Mu/day

absence of a protected environment. Indeed, studies by Yates & Holland [72] failed to show any benefit, either with or without a protected environment. On the other hand, Schimpff et al. [75] demonstrated that, irrespective of protective isolation, ONA were effective when compliance with medication was good. Levine et al. [74] showed that the use of ONA was beneficial and that this was more marked when ONA were combined with protective isolation.

The GVN combination is expensive, unpleasant to take and has led to the emergence of multiple resistant organisms [86]. Consequently, alternative regimens such as FRACON and NEOCON (Table 25.3) were studied, and both have been found to be effective in reducing the incidence of infection in patients treated in a protected environment [87,88]. With FRACON, the benefit was most marked when the neutrophil count was less than 0.1 × 10⁹/l. NEOCON is cheaper than FRACON and, in addition, there are fewer tablets to take.

Selective gastrointestinal decontamination

Another approach to prophylaxis in the neutropenic patient makes use of selective gastrointestinal decontamination (SGD). This is aimed at exploiting the concept of 'colonization resistance', whereby the preservation of the intestinal anaerobic flora protects against overgrowth of aerobic pathogens. The formulation of this concept was based on the experimental animal work performed by Van der Waaij et al. [89]. Antibiotics like co-trimoxazole, nalidixic acid and polymyxin B selectively depress the aerobic flora and thus preserve the host's colonization resistance, which is normally lost with the use of penicillin and aminoglycosides.

Attempts at exploiting SGD in patients with acute leukaemia have used oral antimicrobial regimens which included neomycin, polymyxin, nalidixic acid and amphotericin B. Two

such studies showed that SGD was effective in reducing major infections in treated compared to control groups [90,91]; however, no difference in remission rates was seen in the study by Guiot et al. [91]. The use of SGD, either with co-trimoxazole or other antibiotic combinations, has considerable advantages over ONA which frequently cause gastrointestinal intolerance and, in particular, diarrhoea. Compliance with ONA has consequently been poor and the need for a simpler and better tolerated regimen became obvious.

Co-trimoxazole prophylaxis

The beneficial effect of co-trimoxazole was first suggested by Hughes et al. [92], when he noted that children with acute leukaemia who received co-trimoxazole for prophylaxis of *Pneumocystis carinii* had fewer infections when compared to a placebo. Since then several studies have been carried out to test the efficacy of co-trimoxazole alone, or in combination with other antibiotics, for infection prophylaxis in neutropenic patients. Initial encouraging reports led to the widespread use of co-trimoxazole and nystatin in routine practice, and it is therefore useful to critically review the role of co-trimoxazole in infection prophylaxis for patients with acute leukaemia.

In a study by Gurwith et al. [93], co-trimoxazole was compared with placebo in a mixed group of patients with acute leukaemia and solid tumours undergoing induction chemotherapy. A significant decrease in infections, including bacteraemias, was demonstrated in the co-trimoxazole-treated group. Benefit was also shown in a randomized study by Enno et al. [94], in which patients receiving FRACON and co-trimoxazole developed fewer infections than those on FRACON alone. However, the infection rate in the FRACON group (control) was unusually high. When co-trimoxazole was compared with NEOCON in patients undergoing BMT or remission induction for acute nonlymphocytic leukaemia, a significant reduction in infection and in the need for further antibiotic treatment was observed in the co-trimoxazole group [95]. The EORTC have also carried out a large multicentre trial of co-trimoxazole versus placebo in patients with acute leukaemia and solid tumours [96]. A benefit was only seen in a subgroup of patients with lung cancer and none in patients with acute leukaemia.

The widespread use of co-trimoxazole prophylaxis has led to the emergence of resistant organisms. Thus, in a study of patients with acute leukaemia, Dekker et al. [97] found an increased incidence of infections caused by co-trimoxazole-resistant organisms in their treatment group, although the total number of infections was lower compared to the control group. Similarly, two other groups of workers have shown that although co-trimoxazole prophylaxis was beneficial, there was no difference in the number of febrile days between treated and control groups and, in addition, an increased colonization by co-trimoxazole-resistant organisms was noted [98,99].

Pizzo et al. [100] have compared a combination of co-trimoxazole and erythromycin vs placebo in patients with acute leukaemia and solid tumours. Although no overall benefit was observed in the treated groups, in a subgroup of patients with acute leukaemia in whom compliance with medication was excellent, a significant benefit was observed. Finally, then co-trimoxazole was compared with nalidixic acid (both used with nystatin), there was a significant delay in the onset of first documented infection but, at the same time, significantly longer neutropenia in the co-trimoxazole group [101].

In summary, the above results suggest that, overall, prophylaxis with co-trimoxazole alone, or in combination with other agents, reduces the incidence of infection, including bacteraemia. However, in two of these studies, the need for intervention with systemic antibiotics is not altered by the use of co-trimoxazole prophylaxis. There are, however, no convincing data to suggest that co-trimoxazole prophylaxis offers any survival benefit to patients with chemotherapy-induced neutropenia [102].

Although co-trimoxazole is generally well tolerated, it not infrequently causes allergic rashes and has to be discontinued. In addition, co-trimoxazole may delay bone marrow recovery and its use may also lead to the emergence of resistant organisms [98,101]. In patients with sulphonamide hypersensitivity, trimethoprim may be used as an alternative to co-trimoxazole. It thus became apparent that there was still a need for further evaluation of potentially useful antibiotics for gut decontamination.

Quinolone prophylaxis

The newer 4-quinolones have good activity against Gram-negative bacteria, especially the Enterobacteriaceae and *P. aeruginosa*. Furthermore, they have virtually no activity against anaerobes and enterococci and would therefore not compromise any putative 'colonization resistance'. Ciprofloxacin and norfloxacin are two examples of the new generation of fluorinated quinolones which have been used for infection prophylaxis.

In one study ciprofloxacin was more effective than the combination of co-trimoxazole and colistin for the prevention of infections caused by Gram-negative bacilli in patients with acute leukaemia [103]. Similar results were obtained with norfloxacin prophylaxis in patients with neutropenia [104]. Both antibiotics are well tolerated and are relatively inexpensive. However, while they offer effective prophylaxis against Gram-negative septicaemia, their use may not reduce the need for parenteral broad-spectrum antibiotics in granulocytopenic patients [103]. Furthermore, the emergence of resistance to quinolones remains a significant clinical issue. There have already been reports of ciprofloxacin-resistant strains, and the experience of cystic fibrosis patients on long-term prophylaxis must also give cause for concern. In the neutropenic patient, however, one approach to reduce the risk of resistant strains emerging might be to include colistin in the ciprofloxacin-

containing prophylactic regimen. Thus, the routine use of quinolone prophylaxis in neutropenic patients remains a controversial issue.

Fungal prophylaxis

The overgrowth of pathogenic fungi results from the use of oral nonabsorbable or parenteral antibiotics and therefore exposes the neutropenic patient to the particular risk of invasive fungal disease. It is therefore important to institute appropriate antifungal prophylaxis in the patient with prolonged bone marrow failure. The two nonabsorbable antifungal agents extensively used are nystatin and amphotericin B. Nystatin alone, even in large doses, may not provide adequate prophylaxis, whereas oral amphotericin B has been shown to be effective in reducing the incidence of systemic candidal infections [105,106].

Ketoconazole, of the imidazole group, is available as an oral preparation and has been shown to be effective in the treatment of chronic mucocutaneous fungal infection [107]. Although it appears to reduce the overgrowth of *C. albicans* in the gastrointestinal tract, its efficacy in preventing invasive candidiasis, at higher doses than previously used, is not known [108,109]. However, ketoconazole should be used with caution, as it can cause serious liver damage which, in some cases, has proved fatal [110,111]. Transient abnormalities of liver function have been reported in a small percentage of patients and the incidence of symptomatic hepatitis has been estimated to be one in 10000 patients receiving ketoconazole [112]. Ketoconazole is poorly absorbed in the presence of antacids and H2 receptor antagonists, and when used concurrently with cyclosporin A, the dose of the latter should be reduced [113]. Ketoconazole is not active against *Candida tropicalis*, *Candida glabrata* and *Aspergillus* species.

In recent years, two triazoles with excellent activity against *Candida* organisms have become available. Fluconazole, as an oral preparation, offers effective prophylaxis against candidal infections in immunocompromised hosts and has the advantages of low toxicity and once-daily administration [114]. Fluconazole (50 mg daily) has been shown to reduce oral and faecal colonization and oral infection with all candida species, apart from *C. glabrata* and *C. krusei*. However, it offers no protection against *Aspergillus* infection although in animal models high doses may help prevent aspergillosis [115]. In a recent randomized placebo-controlled double-blind trial, Winston *et al.* [116] showed that prophylactic fluconazole (400 mg daily) prevents colonization and superficial infections by *Candida* species other than *C. krusei* in patients undergoing chemotherapy for acute leukaemia. However, fluconazole could not be clearly shown to be effective for preventing invasive fungal infections, reducing the use of amphotericin B or decreasing the number of deaths. On the other hand, Goodman *et al.* [117] showed that prophylactic administration of fluconazole (400 mg daily) to recipients of bone marrow transplants reduced the incidence of both systemic and superficial infections.

Itraconazole has the added benefit of being active against *Aspergillus* species and, at a dose of 400 mg daily, does appear to help prevent the development of aspergillosis in neutropenic patients [118,119]. However, absorption of the drug from the gastrointestinal tract is erratic but the new liquid formulation may lead to improved absorption, in addition to being better tolerated. Its use is recommended in units where there is a high incidence of *Aspergillus* infections, for example where building works are being undertaken.

Prophylaxis of viral infections

Herpes simplex infections, which are common in both BMT patients and those undergoing intensive chemotherapy for acute leukaemia, can be completely prevented by the use of either intravenous or oral acyclovir [120,121]. Acyclovir is used extensively for both prophylactic and therapeutic purposes, but with its widespread use, the possibility of resistant strains emerging needs to be borne in mind. The resistant strains detected in patients so far have been thymidine kinase-deficient and also appear to be less pathogenic [122,123]; constant vigilance is therefore necessary. The other common viral infection in the immunocompromised host, for which prophylaxis should be considered, is varicella zoster infection. In patients who have no antibody to the virus and have been exposed to it, high-titre zoster immune globulin (ZIG) is effective in modifying the course of the infection, provided it is given within 72 hours of exposure [124].

In BMT patients, CMV is still a major cause of death, despite the promising reports from the use of the combination of ganciclovir and intravenous hyperimmune immunoglobulin in established CMV pneumonitis [125–128]. Thus attention remains focused on prophylaxis. Several measures have been shown to offer protection against the development of CMV disease. Transmission of infection can be eliminated by the use of seronegative blood products in seronegative recipients of marrows from seronegative donors [129]. Another approach is the use of newer generation filters to extract the majority of contaminating leucocytes from blood products, thereby reducing the risk of CMV transmission [130]. The passive administration of CMV hyperimmune globulin or conventional immunoglobulin preparations in seronegative BMT patients has also been shown to be effective prophylaxis, but its benefit in seropositive patients remains uncertain [131–134]. CMV hyperimmune globulin administration would also be useful in seronegative patients receiving marrow from seropositive donors.

Although acyclovir is ineffective for treating established CMV pneumonitis, its role as a prophylactic agent has been investigated. In one study from Seattle, the use of intravenous acyclovir was shown to significantly reduce the frequency of CMV pneumonitis in seropositive patients, although some uncertainty still remains as to its true effectiveness [135,136]. Ganciclovir has now been shown to be effective in preventing CMV infection in BMT patients [137,138], but its use is expensive and is not always successful, and it is sometimes complicated by myelosuppression. Thus a strategy based on 'preemptive' therapy with ganciclovir in at-risk patients would be very useful, assuming that CMV infection could be detected early enough. Early therapy based on rapid culture techniques has reduced the risk of CMV pneumonitis, but failures as a result of disease development before initiation of treatment occurred in up to 15% of patients [137,139]. Optimization of this strategy would clearly depend on improving the accuracy of the tests used to detect CMV infection. Over the last few years, new methodologies to detect CMV antigen or DNA in the blood have been developed to improve earlier detection of CMV disease [65]. Among them, viral DNA detection by PCR techniques in BMT patients appears to be most promising as a method for routine laboratory use [68]. In fact, the PCR method allows earlier detection of viral infection in urine samples [66]. However the very high sensitivity of PCR used in various studies did not allow sufficient discrimination between the presence of the virus and CMV disease. For this reason, the application of semiquantitative PCR for viral DNA in peripheral blood leucocytes may be more useful in clinical management [140].

Prophylaxis of *Pneumocystis* infection

Pneumocystis carinii pneumonia can be effectively prevented by the prophylactic use of co-trimoxazole. Infection usually arises from endogenous reactivation of the latent organism, although exogenous transmission can also occur. In BMT patients, the institution of co-trimoxazole prophylaxis has resulted in a virtual elimination of *Pneumocystis* infections, but protocols for prophylaxis have used different schedules for both the dosage and the frequency of co-trimoxazole administration [141,142]. A regimen of co-trimoxazole 960 mg three times a week appears to be suitable and effective. It is generally recommended to continue prophylaxis for up to 120 days post-BMT. As discussed previously, co-trimoxazole may have several undesirable side effects and thus the indications for its routine use for other high-risk groups should take into account the frequency with which this infection is encountered in a particular institution. For patients with ALL, some treatment protocols include co-trimoxazole prophylaxis during the entire duration of therapy, as for example in the Medical Research Council UKALL 12 Trial.

Enhancement of host defences

Active immunization

The risk of overwhelming pneumococcal infection in postsplenectomy patients has already been mentioned. Immunization against the pneumococcus is desirable, but unfortunately the antibody response of splenectomized patients is impaired [143]. Patients with chronic leukaemias, for example CLL, may already be immunosuppressed either from the disease itself or from chemotherapy, so that antibody responses are likely to be impaired even before splenectomy. It is recommended that, following splenectomy, patients should stay on life-long penicillin prophylaxis, because serotypes causing infection may not be incorporated into the polyvalent vaccine or be sufficiently immunogenic.

Interest in developing a *Pseudomonas* vaccine arose from the hope that it would be useful in preventing infection in neutropenic patients. Although such vaccines have been of value in burns patients, they were ineffective in patients with malignant disease and in children with leukaemia [144,145]. Failure of the vaccine in these studies was related to both low levels of opsonizing antibodies and the absence of neutrophils.

Passive immunization

Another useful approach to the prevention and management of *Pseudomonas* infections involves the use of an antiserum directed against the common core glycolipid antigen of Gram-negative bacteria. This antiserum is raised against a rough mutant of *E. coli*, known as J5, and crossreacts against a wide range of Gram-negative pathogens, including *Pseudomonas*. Studies in neutropenic rabbits have demonstrated that the J5 antiserum has antitoxic and protective properties against Gram-negative bacteraemia [146]. Clinical trials have also shown that human J5 antiserum is effective in combatting the endotoxaemic effects of Gram-negative bacteraemia and also in the prophylaxis of such infections in high-risk surgical patients [147,148]. However, a trial of J5 antiserum for prophylaxis of Gram-negative infections in severely neutropenic patients failed to demonstrate any benefit, although it is possible that the dose of J5 was inadequate [148]. Recently a human monoclonal antibody (HA-1A) against endotoxin has become available and, in a randomized, double-blind trial, it was shown to be effective for the treatment of patients with Gram-negative bacteraemia and septic shock [149]. Unfortunately, as a result of reported adverse effects, the HA-IA antibody has now been withdrawn from use.

Other manoeuvres and immunomodulation

Lithium carbonate was noted to induce a leucocytosis in patients treated for depressive illnesses [150]. This apparently results from the enhancement of colony-stimulating activity for committed granulocyte-macrophage precursors [151]. However, the use of lithium therapy in neutropenic patients has been largely unrewarding; it has been shown to reduce infection in neutropenic patients having chemotherapy in only one study [152–154].

One of the most exciting developments in recent years has been the application of recombinant colony-stimulating factors (CSFs) to accelerate haemopoietic recovery in patients undergoing chemotherapy or BMT. The use of specific cytokines to modulate and enhance immune responses will require further investigation. The role of haemopoietic growth factors such as granulocyte CSF (G-CSF) and granulocyte-macrophage CSF (GM-CSF) in modifying the neutropenic phase in leukaemic and BMT patients is discussed below.

Treatment of infection in the neutropenic patient

General principles

It has already been pointed out that infections in the neutropenic patient, especially those caused by Gram-negative bacilli, can be rapidly fatal unless prompt treatment with antibiotics is instituted. Cognizance of this fact, and the institution of early empirical antibiotic therapy before an infecting pathogen is known, have resulted in a marked decrease in early deaths from infection in granulocytopenic patients. Fever in the neutropenic patient is presumed to be infective in origin unless there is some other obvious cause, as for example during transfusion of blood or blood products, in which case rapid defervescence is expected when the transfusion is stopped. A neutropenic patient who has a temperature above 39.0°C on one single reading, or above 38.0°C on two successive readings within a period of 2 hours, is considered to have significant pyrexia and qualifies for empirical antibiotic treatment. In the cancer patient, neutropenia is usually defined as an absolute neutrophil count of less than 1×10^9/l. Treatment with antibiotics may still be indicated, even if the neutrophil count is above this cut-off point for neutropenia. For example, it is important to consider empirical antibiotic treatment in febrile patients with acute leukaemia, whose neutrophil count may still be above 1×10^9/l, but continues to fall rapidly as a result of intensive chemotherapy. Conversely, the absence of fever does not rule out infection, especially in patients receiving corticosteroids. Clinical signs such as tachypnoea, tachycardia, hypotension and shock indicate a Gram-negative septicaemia which requires prompt treatment.

In the neutropenic patient who develops a fever, a thorough search for a source of infection is required. Blood, urine and swabs from any appropriate sites should be collected and cultured for both aerobic and anaerobic bacteria and fungi. Ideally three sets of blood cultures should be taken before antibiotic treatment is started and daily blood cultures should be repeated if fever persists. In addition, a chest X-ray should be performed, even in the absence of the clinical signs of pneumonia.

Documented infection

In the neutropenic patient, the reported success rate of finding an infective organism during a febrile episode varies from series to series. Recent studies have shown that the incidence of documented infection was in the range 24–66% [155,156]. Undoubtedly, the yield rate of microbiologically documented infection will vary according to how actively the search for a putative infective organism is carried out. In general, it can be expected that a specific microbiological diagnosis can be made in about 50% of febrile neutropenic patients, of whom half will have bacteraemias [157]. Another 20% or so of patients will have clinically documented infection but no organism can be isolated. The remainder may have possible infections or other causes of fever. However, in such patients the response to empirical antibiotic treatment, judged by resolution of fever and unequivocal clinical improvement, suggests, retrospectively, that infection was the likely cause of fever.

Empirical antibiotic treatment

In the absence of bacteriological data, the aim of an empirical antibiotic regimen for the treatment of a presumed infection is to provide adequate cover against a broad spectrum of pathogens. The use of antibiotic combinations with activity against the major pathogens, in particular the Gram-negative bacilli and Gram-positive cocci, has been the mainstay of empirical treatment for the febrile neutropenic patient. One important advantage of using a combination of antibiotics lies in the exploitation of synergistic activity against infecting organisms. Several workers have clearly demonstrated the usefulness of synergistic combinations [158,159]. In one study, when the antibiotic combination had synergistic activity against the infecting organism, the cure rate was 80%, compared to 49% when synergistic activity was absent [160]. In addition, Klastersky *et al.* [160] have shown that Gram-negative infections respond better if the serum bactericidal activity is 1 : 8 or greater, and that synergistic combinations are more likely to produce such bactericidal activity than non-synergistic ones.

The exact choice of antibiotics to be used in any particular institution often depends on the types of organisms most frequently isolated and of the known antibiotic resistances of endemic strains. Thus close collaboration between clinicians and bacteriologists is indeed essential. Combinations of the three classes of antibiotics, namely the semisynthetic penicillins, the aminoglycosides and cephalosporins, have been extensively evaluated as empirical treatment in the neutropenic patient. Most of the antibiotic regimens have consisted of either two or three drug combinations of a semisynthetic penicillin (carbenicillin or ticarcillin), and aminoglycoside (gentamicin, tobramycin or amikacin) and a cephalosporin (cephalothin or cefazolin). Since there have been numerous reports on the efficacy of such combinations, it is intended to review only the main studies.

In the first European Organization for the Research and Treatment of Cancer (EORTC) Trial, three antibiotic combinations (carbenicillin + cephalothin, carbenicillin + gentamicin, cephalothin + gentamicin) were evaluated for the treatment of presumed infections in the neutropenic cancer patient. The main organisms isolated were *Staph. aureus*, *E. coli*, *K. pneumo-*

niae and *P. aeruginosa*. All three regimens were generally equally effective, with response rates of over 40% [8]. However, the combination of carbenicillin and cephalothin was less effective against Gram-negative bacteria and, in addition, the gentamicin/cephalothin combination was the more nephrotoxic of the three regimens. Furthermore, the response of Gram-negative bacteraemia depended primarily on the recovery of neutrophils, provided that the organism was sensitive to the antibiotics used. In the second EORTC Trial, the efficacy of a two-drug (carbenicillin + amikacin) versus a three-drug (carbenicillin + amikacin + cephazolin) combination was tested. There was no significant difference in the response to treatment in the two groups when all infections were considered or when only bacteraemias were analysed [161]. The overall response rate was again greater than 70% and only 5% of deaths were caused by the presenting infection.

In the third EORTC Trial, the combinations of amikacin + azlocillin and amikacin + cefotaxime (as a third-generation cephalosporin) were compared with the standard regimen of amikacin + ticarcillin. Preliminary results suggested that the azlocillin + amikacin combination might be more effective for bacteraemic infections [148]. A significant difference was found when the two arms containing azlocillin and ticarcillin were compared: the response rates were 61 and 45%, respectively. However, this difference could be accounted for by the high frequency of ticarcillin-resistant organisms in that study [162]. Two other studies, using either carbencillin or ticarcillin in combination with an aminoglycoside, have also confirmed the usefulness of these combinations in febrile neutropenic patients. A response rate of greater than 80% was seen in Gram-negative septicaemia when the pathogen was susceptible to both antibiotics (reviewed by Young [163]). Thus the synergistic combination of an antipseudomonal penicillin and an aminoglycoside is a proven effective regimen in the initial empirical therapy of the febrile neutropenic patient. Furthermore, the use of a double beta-lactam combination with an aminoglycoside does not appear to be any more effective and indeed some double beta-lactam combinations may be antagonistic. A brief description of the main antibiotics in current use is therefore appropriate at this stage.

Antipseudomonal penicillins

As newer antibiotics with claims of increasing potency against Gram-negative organisms become available, the choice among the penicillins and the cephalosporins becomes wider still. A critical appraisal of the newer antibiotics is therefore necessary (Table 25.4). One of the extensively used earlier penicillins, carbenicillin, is no less efficacious than ticarcillin, but the latter can be given with a reduced sodium load, thereby minimizing the problems of fluid retention and hypokalaemia. The three N-acyl derivatives of ampicillin, namely mezlocillin, piperacillin and azlocillin, are highly active broad-spectrum

Table 25.4 Antibiotics used in the treatment of febrile neutropenic patients.

Antibiotics	Comments
Anti-pseudomonal penicillins	
Carbenicillin	High sodium content, fluid retention, hypokalaemia
Ticarcillin	About twice as potent as carbenicillin
Mezlocillin	Some anti-*Klebsiella* activity
Piperacillin	Monosodium salt: potent anti-pseudomonal and some anti-*Klebsiella* activity
Azlocillin	Monosodium salt: potent anti-pseudomonal activity
Piperacillin/tazobactam	Added benefit of good activity against Gram-positive organisms including *Staph. epidermidis*
Aminoglycosides	
Gentamicin	Least expensive but rising incidence of resistant organisms, especially in Europe and USA
Tobramycin	Most active against *P. aeuruginosa*
Netilmicin	Lower incidence of nephrotoxicity
Amikacin	Most resistant to enzymatic inactivation: useful for other aminoglycoside-resistant organisms
Cephalosporins	
Cefotaxime	Weak anti-pseudomonal activity: good CNS penetration
Ceftizoxime	Potent Gram-negative activity except for *Pseudomonas*
Ceftazidime	Potent anti-*Pseudomonas* activity: may be used as monotherapy
Moxalactam	Good anaerobic cover: associated hypoprothrombinaemia and antiplatelet aggregation activity
Quinolone	
Ciprofloxacin	Most active against Gram-negative organisms: no cross-hypersensitivity to beta-lactam antibiotics. Available in oral and intravenous formulations
Carbapenem	
Imipenem/cilastatin	Broad-spectrum activity including anaerobic cover. May be used as monotherapy
Meropenem	Broad-spectrum activity; may be used as monotherapy: well tolerated

antibiotics especially against *Klebsiella* species, when compared to the earlier penicillins. Azlocillin, in addition, shows substantially greater activity against *P. aeruginosa in vitro* than carbenicillin or ticarcillin. Mezlocillin and piperacillin used alone as single-drug therapies in neutropenic patients have yielded disappointing results [164], but the combination of piperacillin or azlocillin with amikacin appears to be as equally effective as other combinations of the carboxy-penicillins (carbenicillin and ticarcillin) and an aminoglycoside [164–166]. Piperacillin and azlocillin are monosodium salts, and are therefore less likely to cause fluid retention and electrolyte imbalance than the earlier di-sodium penicillins (e.g. carbenicillin). Moreover, in institutions where ticarcillin-resistant strains or *Klebsiella* species are prevalent, the combination of piperacillin or azlocillin with an aminoglycoside is more suitable as empirical therapy in neutropenic patients [164].

In view of the continuous change in the type of microorganisms causing infection in the neutropenic patient, there has been a need to reassess the efficacy of the standard combination of aminoglycoside and ureidopenicillin. Tazobactam is a substituted penicillin sulphone which inhibits a wide variety of beta-lactamases. It not only synergizes with piperacillin to increase the activity of this antibiotic against a number of Gram-negative pathogens, but this combination also has an excellent activity against Gram-positive organisms, including *Staph. epidermidis*. The EORTC data on the usage of

piperacillin/tazobactam in combination with amikacin vs ceftazidime plus amikacin as empirical therapy for fever in granulocytopenic patients with cancer showed a shorter duration of fever, less need for added vancomycin and a lower frequency of superinfection [167].

Aminoglycosides

Several prospective randomized studies have compared the efficacy of the various aminoglycosides (gentamicin, amikacin, tobramycin, sisomycin and netilmicin), when used in combination with carbenicillin or ticarcillin. In some studies, aminoglycosides were administered as a continuous infusion. The results of these trials showed that, for general usage, all aminoglycosides appear to be equally effective (reviewed by Bodey *et al.* [38]). All aminoglycosides are potentially ototoxic and nephrotoxic but there are some differences which may be clinically important. A published literature review suggested that netilmicin may be less nephrotoxic than other aminoglycosides [168]. Amikacin is resistant to bacterial enzymes which destroy gentamicin and tobramycin, and it is therefore a useful agent against resistant Gram-negative organisms. When using aminoglycosides it is important to monitor the renal function and to check serum levels at frequent intervals, to ensure that therapeutic levels are achieved, and toxic levels are avoided. For routine use gentamicin and netilmicin are the aminoglycosides of choice. However, gentamicin is cheaper than netilmicin but the latter may be preferred in patients who are receiving other nephrotoxic drugs, for example BMT patients on cyclosporin A.

Cephalosporins

The 'third-generation' cephalosporins, which include moxolactam, cefotaxime, cefoperazone and ceftazidime, have superior activity against most Enterobacteriacae over the earlier cephalosporins [169]. These have been used both as single-agent monotherapy or in combination with other beta-lactam antibiotics or aminoglycosides. Ceftazidime used alone for empirical treatment in neutropenic patients had given response rates between 43% and 79% and, in one study, appeared to be as effective as the combination of carbenicillin, cephalothin and gentamicin [164,170].

Similarly, a small randomized prospective trial of ceftazidime vs a combination of netilmicin, piperacillin and cefotaxime as initial therapy of febrile episodes in neutropenic patients, with acute leukaemia, showed no significant differences in response rates between the two treatment groups [171]. Recently, in a large randomized trial comparing ceftazidime alone with a combination of cephalothin, gentamicin and carbenicillin in cancer patients with fever and neutropenia, Pizzo *et al.* [172] showed that initial therapy with ceftazidime was a safe alternative to a standard combination antibiotic therapy, although some patients were likely to require additional or modified treatment.

Data for the clinical activity of combinations of the new cephalosporins and other antibiotics are rather scanty. The combination of cefotaxime and amikacin in a previous EORTC Trial gave a response of 47% in bacteriologically documented infections [164]. Caution must, however, be exercised in using beta-lactam combinations in neutropenic patients, as those tested are not superior to other regimens (e.g. beta-lactam + aminoglycosides) and, as mentioned previously *in vitro* testing has shown that some combinations appear to be antagonistic.

Quinolones and carbapenems

Newer antibiotics, like ciprofloxacin, imipenem/cilastin and meropenem, are recent useful additions to the therapeutic armamentarium. These agents have a broad spectrum of activity against both Gram-positive and Gram-negative organisms, including *P. aeruginosa*. Ciprofloxacin as a single agent, used in the relatively high dose of 300 mg intravenously twice a day, has been shown to be safe and as effective as a combination of azlocillin and netilmicin in the initial empirical treatment of febrile neutropenic patients [173,174]. Similarly, imipenem/cilastin monotherapy appears to be as effective as a standard combination regimen in the empirical treatment of febrile episodes in granulocytopenic patients [175–178]. Furthermore, monotherapy with meropenem, a new carba-

penem with a broad-spectrum activity similar to that of imipenem/cilastatin, has been shown to be as effective as ceftazidime for empirical treatment of febrile neutropenic patients [179]. Meropenem was very well tolerated, with no gastrointestinal toxicity. A recent EORTC Study confirmed that monotherapy with meropenem was as effective as the combination of ceftazidime and amikacin for the empirical treatment of fever in persistently granulocytopenic cancer patients [180]. While monotherapy with these new antibiotics has the advantages of simplicity and reduced toxicity, caution must be exercised in their widespread usage, as clearly there is a risk of resistant organisms emerging which would thus limit their value as monotherapy.

Length of antibiotic treatment

The optimum duration of antibiotic treatment in the neutropenic patient who responds to therapy is not known, and the decision to continue or stop antibiotics is often an arbitrary one. Too short a course of antibiotics may result in recrudescence of infection, as shown in some series [181], whereas prolonged courses are costly, increase the risk of serious toxicity and predispose the patient to fungal infection [8]. In addition, there is probably no merit in continuing antibiotics in the responsive neutropenic patient until recovery of the granulocyte count (>0.5 × 10^9/l) [182]. The length of antibiotic treatment in various studies has been widely different; for example, in the third EORTC Trial a 9-day course was used, whereas other workers have advocated a 14-day course for the persistently neutropenic patient with septicaemia [183]. Clearly no universally accepted guidelines are available at present. In the patient with a pyrexia of unknown origin, who becomes afebrile on empirical antibiotic treatment, it is our practice to continue antibiotics for an additional 3 days. A minimum of 5 days treatment is recommended. Similarly, in patients with a septicaemia or some other serious documented infection, it would appear sensible to continue antibiotics until the infection has resolved and the temperature has returned to normal for at least 3 days. It is clear that there is a need to develop tests which would allow the detection of residual bacterial infection in the neutropenic patient. Until such tests or results of prospective trials become available, the question what constitutes an adequate course of antibiotic treatment in the responsive neutropenic patient remains unanswered.

Management of the patient with a persistent fever

The neutropenic patient who fails to respond to antibiotic treatment remains a difficult management problem. Some 30% of neutropenic patients will remain pyrexial after 3–4 days of initial empirical antibiotic treatment and thus will require changes to their management. If a pathogen has been isolated, it would be logical to adjust the initial antibiotic treatment with regard to the *in vitro* sensitivity pattern of the organism. If there is no resolution of a documented life-threatening bacterial infection, in spite of appropriate antibiotic treatment, granulocytes' transfusion is indicated. However, with the availability of recombinant growth factors, the use of G-CSF or GM-CSF to accelerate granulocyte recovery may, indeed, be life saving.

A major difficulty arises in the patient who has no microbiologically documented infection and shows no resolution of fever after 3–4 days of empirical antibiotic treatment. Several courses of action can be considered at this stage. If the patient remains well and has no clinical evidence of infection, it may be safe to stop all antibiotics, repeat cultures and watch the patient very carefully. At this stage other adjuncts to diagnosis, for example C-reactive protein, may help in distinguishing between a bacterial and a nonbacterial cause of fever (see below). Some workers have pointed out the danger of a 'rebound' septicaemia in febrile patients, when antibiotics have been stopped, and it is therefore essential that the clinical condition of such patients is constantly monitored and that antibiotics are promptly reinstituted at the earliest signs of deterioration.

However, the febrile patient who remains ill requires a different approach. The various alternatives include the addition of another (usually a third) antibiotic, on the assumption that the infecting organism may be resistant to the current antibiotic regimen, or the institution of antifungal therapy to treat an occult fungal infection. An additional antibiotic may be appropriate if surveillance cultures from stools or other sites reveal a resistant organism. Metronidazole should be considered if an anaerobic infection is suspected, as for example in the presence of severe oropharyngeal ulceration, abdominal or perianal sepsis. In the patient with prolonged neutropenia, fungal infection should always be considered. The presence of yeasts, such as *Candida albicans*, in the mouth or stools raises the possibility of invasive candidiasis. There is plenty of evidence to suggest that many patients have occult fungal infections which, unfortunately, are only diagnosed at postmortem [44]. Hence for neutropenic patients who remain unresponsive to multiple antibiotics, the index of suspicion for an occult fungal infection must remain high and, in these cases, it is advisable to start empirical antifungal treatment with amphotericin B earlier rather than later. Moreover, there are some data to suggest that early specific treatment achieves better control of fungal infections [184].

Management of pulmonary infiltrates

The neutropenic patient with pulmonary infiltration who fails to respond to empirical antibiotic therapy, or who develops pulmonary changes while being treated with antibiotics, presents another challenging problem. Radiological changes may reveal localized or diffuse infiltrates and may provide no clues about the pathogenesis. Examination of sputum, when available, is often negative. In the leukaemic or BMT patient, non-

infectious causes of pulmonary infiltrates, such as haemorrhage and toxicity, from chemo/radiotherapy, should be considered, but pneumonias of a nonbacterial origin are a more frequent problem. Atypical bacteria, fungi, CMV and *Pneumocystis carinii* are potential pathogens.

Two options are available: either to use blind therapy aimed at treating one or more potential pathogens or further investigation to make a specific diagnosis. The decision about which option to adopt will depend on the type of pulmonary infiltration, the patient's clinical condition, the availability of expertise in invasive or bronchoscopic procedures and of prompt microbiological diagnostic facilities. In the individual patient, the risks of an invasive procedure must be carefully weighed against the potential toxic effects of polypharmacy. An early definitive diagnosis allows specific treatment to be given and may therefore obviate the need for using an empirical combination of toxic drugs. In the thrombocytopenic patient, all diagnostic procedures, especially invasive ones, carry certain risks, of which haemorrhage is important. Moreover, the choice of procedures is still a matter of controversy. While it is generally agreed that open lung biopsy provides the most reliable way of making a diagnosis, this may not be suitable for the very ill patient. Bronchoscopy with transbronchial biopsy and/or bronchoalveolar lavage is a suitable alternative in these patients [185,186]. Indeed, there may be a case for attempting these less invasive procedures in the first instance in all patients, and to proceed to open lung biopsy only in those in which a diagnosis could not be made.

In the neutropenic patient already receiving broad-spectrum antibiotics, the appearance of a localized pulmonary infiltrate is highly suggestive of a fungal superinfection and, if a diagnostic procedure is not feasible, empirical treatment with amphotericin B is indicated. Similarly, if there is a high suspicion of an atypical bacterial pneumonia (e.g. *Legionella* species), erythromycin should be added. Opinion is still divided over the management of the patient with progressive diffuse pulmonary infiltration suggestive of *P. carinii* pneumonia. Initial empirical treatment with high-dose co-trimoxazole has been advocated, with the option of undertaking open lung biopsy in nonresponsive cases. It must, however, be remembered that the response to treatment may take 3–4 days and that mixed infections can occur, and therefore additional cover with other potentially toxic drugs may be required. On the other hand, a diagnostic procedure performed when the patient is still relatively well may be less risky and may reveal one or more pathogens for which appropriate treatment can be confidently given.

C-reactive protein

It is likely that up to 20% of neutropenic patients who develop fevers and are started on empirical antibiotic treatment are not infected and are therefore receiving antibiotics unnecessarily [187]. In this group of patients it would be most useful to have other parameters which may help in the exclusion of a bacterial infection. C-reactive protein (CRP) is an acute-phase protein which, in the neutropenic patient, has been shown to rise quickly with the onset of a bacterial infection [188–190]. Values of over 100 mg/ml correlate well with the presence of bacterial infection while smaller changes may occur with other causes of fever, for example drug allergy, transfusion reactions or viral infections [191]. Although CRP measurements may be high in neoplastic conditions such as lymphomas, they are not raised or affected by disease activity in acute leukaemia or by cell death following chemotherapy [192]. Unfortunately a raised CRP level (>100 mg/ml) does not differentiate between a bacterial and an invasive fungal infection [193].

Thus in neutropenic patients with acute leukaemia and unexplained fever, CRP measurements offer a potentially useful, albeit indirect, method for excluding the presence of a bacterial infection. However, caution must be exercised in the interpretation of CRP measurements. A single CRP measurement is of limited value, whereas it is the trend of serial levels which is likely to be most informative. The availability of rapid and reliable methods of CRP measurements means that the results can be made available on a daily basis [194,195]. Used in conjunction with clinical and bacteriological data, CRP measurements can extend the diagnostic repertoire currently available in the management of febrile episodes. In addition, CRP measurements can be used to monitor the resolution of infection. A persistently high CRP level, in the absence of fever, may indicate residual infection and caution against the early cessation of antimicrobial therapy.

Treatment of fungal infections

Candida infections

Oropharyngeal candidiasis can usually be treated successfully with topical antifungal agents. A combination of oral nystatin suspension (2 mU/day in divided doses) and amphotericin B lozenges (200 mg four times a day) is usually effective. Oral ketoconazole at a dose of 200 mg/m²/day for 2 weeks has also been used with some success in cancer patients [196], but it should be used with caution because of its potential hepatotoxic effects. Fluconazole 50–100 mg once daily, for 1–2 weeks or longer, has also proved to be effective in immunocompromised patients, and is probably the treatment of choice nowadays [197]. However, caution must be exercised in its liberal usage, as there are increasing reports of candidal resistance developing. For resistant oropharyngeal candidiasis, small doses of intravenous amphotericin B (e.g. 10 mg daily) given for 1–2 weeks are effective in eradicating infection. Mild oesophageal candidiasis may be treated with oral nystatin suspensions (10 mU daily in divided doses) or fluconazole, but it is advisable to institute intravenous amphotericin B at a dose of 0.3–0.4 mg/kg/day if symptoms are severe, or if there is no response to oral treatment.

The risk of candidaemia with the use of long-term indwelling intravenous catheters and parenteral feeding is well recognized. In immunocompromised patients, catheter-related candidaemia may frequently lead to invasive disease. Hence if a catheter is the source of candidaemia and there is no evidence of systemic spread, it should be removed, and a short course of intravenous amphotericin B (200–300 mg) is recommended. In the neutropenic patient, treatment should continue until the neutrophil count returns to normal and it is advisable to give a total dose of 0.5–1 g [42]. For invasive candidiasis, amphotericin B remains the treatment of choice. Alternatively, intravenous fluconazole may be used, especially in the presence of renal impairment. Treatment is often unsuccessful if it is delayed or if the patient's bone marrow fails to recover. The optimum length of therapy with amphotericin B is not known, but a total dose of 1–2 g over a period of 4–6 weeks is usually recommended.

Complications arising from the use of amphotericin B include fever, chills, hypotension, bronchospasm, hypokalaemia and renal impairment. Previous administration of hydrocortisone usually controls fever and chills and amiloride is also useful in reducing renal potassium loss. A maintenance daily dose of 0.5–1 mg/kg/day can be used, but an alternate-day regime is also effective. Animal work has shown that amphotericin B in combination with 5-fluorocytosine (5FC) has an additive and possibly a synergistic effect on *C. albicans* infections [198]. This combination has also been used in the treatment of systemic *Candida* infections in man [199], but unfortunately the use of 5FC is limited by its haematological and gastrointestinal toxicity. 5-Fluorocytosine should never be used as a single agent for treating systemic candidiasis, as both primary and acquired resistance to the drug can occur [200]. Ketoconazole is not recommended and miconazole is generally ineffective for the treatment of invasive candidal infection.

Liposomal amphotericin B (AmBisome) and other lipid-based formulations of amphotericin B (Abelcet, Amphocil) are now available and can be used to deliver high levels of the drug without many of the toxic effects of conventional amphotericin B therapy. The results of treatment of deep-seated fungal infections with liposomal amphotericin B are quite encouraging [201–204] and cumulative evidence suggests that the lipid-based formulations offer a safe and effective alternative to conventional amphotericin B. However, at present, the high costs of these new agents are likely to limit their widespread use in clinical practice.

Aspergillus infections

In previous years, amphotericin B was the only effective treatment for systemic *aspergillus* infections. As with candidiasis, the outcome depends on early treatment and recovery of granulocytes. The total dose and length of treatment are not known; in practice, a dose of 1–3 g given over 4–6 weeks appears to be effective. Combinations of amphotericin B with 5FC or rifampicin for treatment of invasive aspergillosis have been tried in a small number of patients, but their use needs further evaluation [205,206]. However, with the availability of liposomal amphotericin B, more effective treatment can now be given [203,204]. In addition, itraconazole appears to be effective against *Aspergillus* infections and has the added advantage of oral administration [207]. In the persistently neutropenic patient with invasive pulmonary aspergillosis, surgical excision of the affected segments may be required to ensure eradication of the disease. There is now evidence that monocytic function is important in combating invasive mycoses, and this is supported by anecdotes of successful treatment of aspergillosis with a combination of GM-CSF and amphotericin B in neutropenic patients. The value of GM-CSF, combined with amphotericin B, in treating invasive mycoses in neutropenic patients is being currently assessed.

Treatment of *Pneumocystis carinii* pneumonia

High-dose co-trimoxazole and pentamidine are equally effective for the treatment of *P. carinii* pneumonia (PCP), but co-trimoxazole is preferred as it is less toxic. The dose of co-trimoxazole is trimethoprim 20 mg/kg/day and sulpha-methoxazole 100 mg/kg/day, and it is given intravenously in divided doses every 6–8 hours. In the immunocompromised patient, a course of 10–14 days is usually adequate. In patients who are allergic to sulphonamides or who fail to respond to co-trimoxazole, pentamidine can be used and is given as a single dose of 4 mg/kg/day intramuscularly or intravenously.

Granulocyte transfusions

Because the risk of infection is directly related to the severity and duration of neutropenia, and its resolution is largely dependent on the recovery of neutrophils, it would appear logical to attempt either to prevent or treat infection with the transfusion of exogenous granulocytes. As experience with the use of granulocytes has accumulated over the years, it is therefore useful to take a critical look at their usage in the management of infection in the neutropenic patient.

Source and collection of granulocytes

The early success of Freireich's group [208], in demonstrating the effectiveness of granulocytes from chronic granulocytic leukaemia (CGL) donors in infected neutropenic patients, gave the impetus for the development of techniques for the collection of large numbers of granulocytes from normal donors. A variety of cell separators is now available and these use the principle of differential density centrifugation to separate the granulocyte buffy coats from the red cells and plasma. Three machines, the IBM-2997 (now replaced by Cobe Spectra), the Aminco celltrifuge 1 and the Fenwal CS-3000,

use continuous-flow centrifugation, whereas the Haemonetics Model 30 is an intermittent-flow centrifuge. The separation of buffy coats can be improved by the addition of hydroxyethyl starch, dextran or plasmagel to the donor blood, all of which act by enhancing the sedimentation of red cells. A further increase in granulocyte yield can be achieved by prior donor stimulation with corticosteroids.

Another technique for collecting granulocytes is based on their property of reversible adhering to nylon fibres. In 'filtration leucopheresis', heparinized blood is passed through disposable nylon fibres to which the granulocytes adhere, and these can be subsequently eluted with a calcium chelating agent such as ACD or EDTA [209]. This procedure, however, has been abandoned because of adverse toxic reactions in both donor and recipient.

Granulocytes can also be obtained by pooling buffy coats from separate units of fresh blood packs collected at blood donor sessions; this service is available from some UK regional transfusion centres. However, this approach is rather inefficient as the yield of granulocytes is low (much less than the minimum of 1.5×10^{10} granulocytes recommended) and, in addition, there is excessive red cell contamination and large volumes of buffy coats are required for transfusion.

Lastly, patients with CGL and high white cell counts are a useful source of granulocytes. It is likely that the large number of cells usually available more than compensate for any mild functional defects of the neutrophils [210]. CGL granulocytes stored at 4°C can be expected to be still functional for periods up to 72 hours after collection and are therefore a ready source of granulocytes when required [211]. It is, however, necessary to irradiate CGL cells to prevent inadvertent lymphoid engraftment in the immunosuppressed patient, which can result in fatal GVHD. A dose of 2.5 Gy is recommended.

Therapeutic granulocyte transfusions

The exact role of granulocyte transfusions in the treatment of established infection in the neutropenic patient is still a matter of controversy. While the results of previous studies have favoured the usefulness of granulocyte transfusions, a later trial has cast some doubts on the earlier findings. Of seven controlled studies carried out between 1972 and 1982, five had randomized controls and all, except the study by Winston *et al.*, showed significant improvement in survival in the group of patients receiving granulocytes [212–218]. In particular, patients with Gram-negative septicaemia who had delayed recovery of neutrophils appeared to have benefited most. In contrast to most of the other studies, the UCLA Study [219] did not perform any crossmatching to detect lymphocytotoxic antibodies or leucoagglutinins. However, the main difference between this and previous studies was the high rate of survival in the nontransfused group of patients. The conclusions from all these studies have to be interpreted with caution, because these trials have included relatively small numbers of patients who were necessarily a very heterogeneous group. Thus the results of such trials would be influenced by the interplay of several factors, such as the potency of available antibiotics, the type of bacterial infection, the dose of granulocytes transfused and the selection of donors.

Prophylactic granulocyte transfusions

The role of granulocyte transfusions as prophylaxis against infection has also been examined. Two studies have shown no benefit from their prophylactic use [219,220], whereas three other randomized trials in BMT patients have demonstrated their effectiveness in preventing infections [221–223]. The study by Schiffer *et al.* [224] in patients with acute leukaemia had to be abandoned because of the unacceptable risk of alloimmunization which adversely affected platelet transfusion therapy. Winston *et al.* [220] showed that patients undergoing induction therapy for acute nonlymphocytic leukaemia did not benefit from granulocyte transfusions, whereas another cooperative study demonstrated that, although prophylactic granulocytes offered protection against septicaemia, they did not influence the remission rate or survival [225]. Similarly, the controlled study by Clift *et al.* [221] in BMT patients showed a reduction in the incidence of infection in the transfused group but failed to show an improvement in survival.

Adverse effects

The transfusion of granulocytes is often accompanied by adverse side effects, some of which can be quite serious. Fever and chills are common but can be abrogated by prior administration of hydrocortisone and chlorpheniramine. Adverse reactions may be related to the presence of HLA antibodies or leucoagglutinins in the recipient. However, the major complications of granulocyte transfusions are pulmonary toxicity and transmission of CMV. Pulmonary complications presenting as bilateral infiltrates and respiratory distress are rare with granulocyte transfusions alone but lethal pulmonary reactions have been described with the combined use of amphotericin B [226].

An increased incidence of CMV infection has also been reported in (CMV) seronegative BMT recipients. Lastly, GVHD arising from the transfusion of immunocompetent lymphocytes is a real risk in BMT patients, but its incidence in patients receiving intensive chemotherapy for acute leukaemia is probably very low. This can be effectively prevented by irradiating cellular blood products with 2.5 Gy.

Role of granulocyte transfusions

What then is the role of granulocyte transfusions in the management of infection in the neutropenic patient? The collection of granulocytes is expensive and time-consuming and often involves healthy volunteer donors being subjected to a procedure not without some, albeit very small, risks. It is therefore important to restrict their use to patients who are most likely to benefit from them. In clinical practice the prophylactic use of granulocytes transfusion is not recommended, as no study has demonstrated that it alters the mortality of patients at risk. There are, however, very few situations where therapeutic granulocyte transfusions may be indicated; these should be reserved for the severely neutropenic patient with a documented bacterial infection that is unresponsive to antibiotic therapy and they are also useful in the treatment of severe soft tissue infections, for example in patients with perianal sepsis. Transfusions should consist of a minimum number of 1.5×10^{10} granulocytes and should be given daily for at least 4 days. The therapeutic role of granulocyte transfusions in the management of patients with fungal infections has not been fully assessed, although experimental *Candida* infections in dogs have responded to granulocyte transfusions [227]. In patients with established invasive candidal infections, who fail to respond to optimal antifungal therapy, it would appear reasonable to give granulocyte transfusions. When granulocytes and amphotericin B are used in combination, it is advisable to space their times of infusion as widely as possible to minimize the risk of pulmonary complications, although the reported toxicity has not been confirmed in all studies [228]. It is, however, likely that with the use of growth factors (G-CSF, GM-CSF) to accelerate granulocyte recovery, the need for granulocyte transfusions will become increasingly small.

Donor selection

Donor selection is clearly an important consideration. There is evidence to suggest that recipient alloimmunization may be responsible for poor clinical responses to granulocyte transfusions [229]. In addition to HLA antigens, granulocytes have a number of specific antigens against which alloantibodies can react. Testing for granulocyte-specific antigens and antibodies is not generally available for routine use, whereas testing for HLA compatibility can be more readily carried out. In the alloimmunized patients, HLA matching between donor and recipient appears to be the minimum necessary requirement. Thus to ensure effective clinical responses from granulocyte transfusions, it is important to avoid using donors against whom the recipient is already sensitized. When providing granulocytes for transfusion purpose, HLA-identical siblings (not a potential bone marrow donor if BMT is contemplated) would be the first-choice donors. The next best choice are haploidentical family donors, provided that the cytotoxic cross-match between the donor and the recipient is negative. Moreover, in the nonimmunized recipient, granulocytes from mismatched donors are known to be effective and can therefore be used. Hence it is useful to screen the serum of potential recipients for, at least, the presence of HLA alloantibodies. The practice of using unmatched random donors in strongly immunized recipients is to be avoided. However, the logistical problems of providing sufficient HLA-compatible unrelated donors, who are also ABO compatible, remain at present considerable.

Haemopoietic growth factors

The haemopoietic growth factors are glycoproteins that regulate the proliferation and differentiation of haemopoietic progenitor cells and the function of mature blood cells [230–232]. Growth factors which control the proliferation of granulocytes and macrophages have been purified, molecularly cloned and produced as recombinant proteins.

G-CSF has a preferential action on neutrophil granulocytes, while GM-CSF has effects on the neutrophil, eosinophil and macrophage lineages. The effects of the CSFs are mediated by cells bearing receptors for these factors. Thus any agents which are capable of accelerating recovery of granulocytes from chemotherapy-induced myelosuppression, may be potentially beneficial to the neutropenic patient. In preclinical studies, CSF administration has been shown to improve survival from experimental infections. G-CSF administration reversed the neutropenia in cyclophosphamide-treated mice and prevented death from inoculation with bacterial and fungal organisms. Furthermore, a synergistic effect with antibiotics was observed for experimental *Pseud. aeruginosa* infections [233]. In another study, infusion of GM-CSF to primates undergoing total body irradiation and rescue with autologous bone marrow, accelerated haemopoietic recovery [234]. The results of such studies suggested that G-CSF and GM-CSF, by shortening the period of neutropenia, would be effective in reducing the morbidity and mortality associated with infection in patients undergoing chemotherapy or BMT. In phase I and II clinical studies of G-CSF and GM-CSF in cancer patients, both CSFs were shown to accelerate neutrophil recovery after chemotherapy and this resulted in a beneficial effect on several parameters of sepsis [235–241].

Clinical use of the two commercially available CSFs (G-CSF and GM-CSF) has had a remarkable impact on the treatment of patients with haematological malignancies. One current application for granulocyte growth factors is for the prevention or reduction of the severity of neutropenia and associated complications in patients undergoing cytotoxic chemotherapy or BMT. In patients with nonmyeloid malignancies, treated with intensive chemotherapy and in whom there is severe and prolonged neutropenia, with or without accompanying fever, the use of growth factors is appropriate [242]. In these circumstances, the use of growth factors may reduce the need for antibiotics and shorten the hospital stay.

The ability of growth factors to improve neutropenia following autologous bone marrow transplantation (ABMT) has been shown in a number of studies using G-CSF and GM-CSF [243,244]. In a nonrandomized study of CSF in ABMT for nonmyeloid malignancies, a reduction in both the duration of neutropenia and the use of parenteral antibiotics was noted [244]. Similarly, the use of CSFs in allogeneic BMT has been explored [245]. In a randomized placebo-controlled phase III trial of lenograstim in patients undergoing BMT, Gisselbrecht *et al.* [246] showed that G-CSF-treated patients had a shorter duration of neutropenia, fewer days of infection and of antibiotic administration, and also spent less time in hospital. However, clinical and microbiological sepsis was similar in both treated and placebo groups. It is now generally accepted that the use of growth factor post transplantation is potentially useful in accelerating haemopoietic recovery. However, it is not known what is the optimal time for starting growth factors administration. A common practice is to start G-CSF or GM-CSF on day + 7 post bone marrow infusion. Growth factors should be given until there is stable engraftment. This has been defined by some authorities as three consecutive days on which the neutrophil count exceeds $0.1 \times 10^9/l$ [242]. In practice, growth factor administration is continued until the neutrophil count reaches at least $0.5 \times 10^9/l$. The type of growth factor used is not thought to make a difference, although GM-CSF causes more side effects. Growth factors are also indicated in cases of graft failure.

As acquisition costs for G-CSF and GM-CSF are relatively high, it is important to evaluate the cost effectiveness of these agents. Several studies have recently addressed the pharmacoeconomic implications of using growth factors for chemotherapy-induced neutropenia. Data from these studies indicate that the clinical benefits from growth factors, in terms of reducing antibiotic usage, parenteral nutrition and shortening hospital stay, lead to a reduction in overall health-care costs. These cost savings in general, partially or completely outweigh the cost of the growth factors [247–249]. Furthermore, growth factors can improve the quality of life of patients undergoing chemotherapy, by reducing the incidence and severity of infections. In bone marrow transplantation, however, the cost–benefit implications of using growth factors also need to be established.

The use of growth factors in AML has been limited by theoretical concerns about their ability to stimulate the growth of myeloid leukaemia, since these agents have been shown to stimulate the proliferation of leukaemic blasts *in vitro* [250–252]. However, early phase I/II studies with G-CSF and GM-CSF given after chemotherapy in AML patients gave promising results and indicated no effect on leukaemia regrowth or recurrence. These results provided the basis for randomized clinical studies of G-CSF and GM-CSF in patients with AML. Several randomized trials have now been reported, in which myeloid growth factors have been used as an adjunct to remission induction chemotherapy in patients with AML. Four studies used GM-CSF [253–256] and three used G-CSF [257–259]. All of these, except one [259], were confined to older patients. The two largest studies [255,259] showed no impact of growth factor on complete remission rates. In fact, in most studies, survival was not significantly improved in patients receiving growth factors. However, these studies did confirm that growth factors did not stimulate leukaemia regrowth in AML. The study carried out by Heil *et al.* [259] in 521 adult AML patients demonstrated that filgrastim was a safe and effective adjunct in AML treatment (both induction and consolidation). Filgrastim reduced the duration of neutropenia, fever, use of parenteral antibiotics and hospitalization. On the basis of the latter benefits, which could translate into cost savings, a case could therefore be made for the prophylactic use of G-CSF following chemotherapy in AML patients. The determination of optimal dosage schedules (for example starting G-CSF on day +7 post chemotherapy instead of day +1) in AML, may help reduce the costs of treatment further. Clearly detailed studies of the cost–benefit ratio for the use of growth factors in this setting still need to be carried out.

Growth factors can also be used to develop new schedules of chemotherapy. Because neutropenia and its consequences can be ameliorated by CSF administration, it may therefore be possible to administer higher doses of cytotoxic agents to cancer patients in an attempt to increase tumour-kill, possibly resulting in increased rates of long-term survival and cure. Similarly, as myelotoxicity is often the dose-limiting toxicity for many cytotoxic agents, the use of growth factors may obviate the need for dose reduction in planned chemotherapy, and allow the shortening of cycle time. Their use may permit the escalation of chemotherapy doses and this approach has been evaluated in patients with solid tumours [240]. However, with dose escalation, it is likely that other dose-limiting toxicities, such as thrombocytopenia and cardiac damage, will be identified.

Finally, the use of recombinant thrombopoietin or megakaryocytic growth and development factor may hold some promise for the future in the treatment of thrombocytopenia.

References

1 Hersh E.M., Bodey G.P. & Nies B.A. (1965) Cause of death in acute leukemia. *Journal of the American Medical Association*, **193**, 105–109.

2 Levine A.S., Schimpff S.C., Graw R.G. Jr *et al.* (1974) Haematologic malignancies and other marrow failure states: progress in the management of complicating infections. *Seminars in Haematology*, **11**, 141–202.

3 Chang H.-Y., Rodriguez V., Narboni G. *et al.* (1976) Causes of death in adults with acute leukaemia. *Medicine*, **55**, 259–268.

4 Maki D.G., Goldman D.A. & Rhame F.S. (1973) Infection control in intravenous therapy. *Annals of Internal Medicine*, **79**, 867–887.

5 Press O.W., Ramsey P.G., Larson E.B. *et al.* (1984) Hickman catheter infections in patients with malignancies. *Medicine*, **63**, 189–200.

6 Stamm W.E. (1975) Guidelines for prevention of catheter associated urinary tract infections. *Annals of Internal Medicine*, **82**, 386–390.

7 Bodey G.P., Buckley B.A., Sathe Y.S. *et al.* (1966) Quantitative

8 EORTC International Antimicrobial Therapy Project Group (1978) Three antibiotic regimens in the treatment of infection in febrile granulocytopenic patients with cancer. *Journal of Infectious Diseases*, **137**, 14–29.

9 Gregory L., Williams R. & Thompson E. (1972) Leucocyte function in Down's syndrome and acute leukaemia. *Lancet*, **i**, 1359–1361.

10 Holland J.F., Sen J.J. & Bannerjee T. (1971) Quantitative studies of localized leucocyte mobilisation in acute leukemia. *Blood*, **37**, 499–511.

11 Pickering L.K., Anderson D.C. & Choi S. *et al.* (1975) Leukocyte function in children with malignancies. *Cancer*, **35**, 1365–1371.

12 Thompson E.N. & Williams R. (1974) Bactericidal capacity of peripheral blood leukocytes in relation to bacterial infections in acute lymphoblastic leukaemia in childhood. *Journal of Clinical Pathology*, **27**, 906–910.

13 Stewart D.J. & Bodey G.P. (1981) Infection in hairy cell leukaemia (leukaemic-reticuloendotheliosis). *Cancer*, **47**, 801–805.

14 Natvig J.B. & Kunkel H.G. (1973) Human immunoglobulins: classes, subclasses, genetic variants and idiotypes. *Advances in Immunology*, **16**, 1–59.

15 Waldman R.H. & Ganguly R. (1976) Role of immune mechanisms on secretory surfaces in prevention of infection. In: *Infection in the Compromised Host* (ed. J.G. Allen), pp. 29–48. Williams & Wilkins, Baltimore.

16 Nedelkova M., Bacolova S. & Georgieva B. (1981) Infections complications and host immune defense in acute leukaemia. *European Journal of Cancer*, **17**, 617–622.

17 Agnello V. (1978) Complement deficiency states. *Medicine*, **57**(i), 1–23.

18 Fauci A.S. & Dale D.G. (1974) The effect of *in vivo* hydrocortisone on subpopulations of human lymphocytes. *Journal of Clinical Investigation*, **53**, 240–246.

19 Rinehart J.J., Sagone A.L., Balcerzak S.P. *et al.* (1975) Effect of corticosteroid therapy on monocyte function. *New England Journal of Medicine*, **292**, 236–241.

20 Louria D.B., Fallon N. & Brown H.G. (1960) The influence of cortisone on experimental fungus infections in mice. *Journal of Clinical Investigation*, **39**, 1435–1449.

21 Dale D. (1981) Defects in host defense mechanism in compromised patients. In: *Clinical Approach to Infection in the Compromised Host* (eds R.H. Bubin & L.S. Young), pp. 35–74. Plenum Medical Book Company, New York.

22 Lowell G.H., MacDermott R.P., Summers P.L. *et al.* (1980) Antibody-dependent cell mediated antibacterial activity: K lymphocyte, monocytes and granulocytes are effective against shigella. *Journal of Immunology*, **125**, 2778–2784.

23 Bolivar R., Kohl S., Pickering L.K. *et al.* (1980) Effect of antineoplastic drugs on antibody dependent cellular cytotoxicity mediated by human leukocytes against Herpes simplex. *Cancer*, **46**, 1555–1561.

24 Ellis E.F. & Smith R.T. (1966) The role of the spleen in immunity with special reference to the post-splenectomy problems in infants. *Pediatrics*, **37**, 111–119.

25 Singer D.B. (1973) Post-splenectomy sepsis. In: *Perspectives in Pediatric Pathology*, Vol. 1 (eds H.S. Rosenberg & R.P. Bolande), pp. 285–311. Year Book Medical Publishers, Chicago.

26 Bodey G.P. (1970) Epidemiological studies of *Pseudomonas* species

7 Bodey G.P., Buckley B.A., Sathe Y.S. *et al.* (1966) Quantitative relationships between circulating leucocytes and infection in patients with acute leukaemia. *Annals of Internal Medicine*, **64**, 328–340.

in patients with leukemia. *American Journal of the Medical Sciences*, **260**, 82–89.

27 Fainstein V., Rodriguez V., Turck M. *et al.* (1981) Patterns of oropharyngeal and fecal flora in patients with acute leukemia. *Journal of Infectious Diseases*, **144**, 10–18.

28 Schimpff S.C., Aisner J. & Wiernik P.H. (1979) Infection in acute nonlymphocytic leukaemia: The alimentary tract as a major source of pathogens. In: *New Criteria for Antimicrobial Therapy: maintenance of digestive tract colonization resistance* (eds D. van der Waaij & J. Verhoen), pp. 12–19. Excerpta Medica, Amsterdam.

29 Bodey G.P., Rodriguez V. & Chang H-Y. (1978) Fever and infection in leukemia patients. *Cancer*, **41**, 1610–1622.

30 Hughes W.T. (1971) Fatal infections in childhood leukemia. *American Journal of Diseases in Childhood*, **122**, 283–287.

31 Armstrong D., Young L.S., Meyer R.D. *et al.* (1971) Infectious complications of neoplastic disease. *Medical Clinics of North America*, **55**, 729–745.

32 Pennington J.E., Reynolds H.Y. & Carbone P.P. (1973) Pseudomonas pneumonia: retrospective study of 36 cases. *American Journal of Medicine*, **55**, 155–160.

33 Sickles E.A., Young V.M., Greene W.H. *et al.* (1973) Pneumonia in acute leukaemia. *Annals of Internal Medicine*, **79**, 528–534.

34 Kilton L.J., Fossieck B.E., Cohen M.H. *et al.* (1979) Bacteremia due to Gram-positive cocci in patients with neoplastic disease. *American Journal of Medicine*, **66**, 596–602.

35 Watson J.G. (1983) Problems of infection after bone marrow transplantation. *Journal of Clinical Pathology*, **36**, 683–692.

36 Smith S.R., Cheesbrough J., Spearing R. *et al.* (1989) Randomised prospective study comparing vancomycin with teicoplanin in the treatment of infections associated with Hickman catheters. *Antimicrobial Agents and Chemotherapy*, **33**, 1193–1197.

37 Smith S.R., Cheesbrough J., Harding I. *et al.* (1990) Role of glycopeptide antibiotics in the treatment of febrile neutropenic patients. *British Journal of Haematology*, **76**(Suppl. 2), 54–56.

38 Bodey G.P., Bolivar R. & Fainstein V. (1982) Infectious complications in leukaemic patients. *Seminars in Haematology*, **19**, 193–226.

39 Ihde C.C. & Armstrong D. (1973) Clinical spectrum of infection due to *Bacillus* species. *American Journal of Medicine*, **55**, 839–845.

40 Fraser D.W., Tsai J.F., Orensrein W. *et al.* (1977) Legionnaires' disease. Description of an epidemic of pneumonia. *New England Journal of Medicine*, **297**, 1189–1197.

41 Haley C.E., Cohen M.L., Halter J. *et al.* (1979) Nosocomial Legionnaires' disease: a continuing common-source epidemic in Wadsworth Medical Centre. *Annals of Internal Medicine*, **90**, 583–586.

42 Hawkins C. & Armstrong D. (1984) Fungal infections in the immunocompromised host. *Clinics in Haematology*, **13**, 599–630.

43 Meunier-Carpentier F., Kiehn T.E. & Armstrong D. (1981) Fungemia in the immunocompromised host. *American Journal of Medicine*, **71**, 363–370.

44 Hart P.D., Russell E. Jr & Remington J.S. (1969) The compromised host and infection. II. Deep fungal infection. *Journal of Infectious Diseases*, **120**, 169–191.

45 Lew M.A., Siber G.R., Donahue D.M. *et al.* (1982) Enhanced detection from an enzyme linked immunosorbent assay of candida mannan in antibody-containing serum after heat extraction. *Journal of Infectious Diseases*. **145**, 45–56.

46 Burnie J.P. (1991) Developments in the serological diagnosis of opportunistic fungal infections. *Journal of Antimicrobial Chemotherapy*, **28**(Suppl. A), 23–33.

47 DeGregorio M.W., Lee W.F., Linker C.A. *et al.* (1982) Fungal

infections in patients with acute leukaemia. *American Journal of Medicine*, **73**, 543–548.

48 Young R.C., Bennett J.E., Vogel C.L. *et al.* (1970) Aspergillosis the spectrum of disease in 98 patients. *Medicine*, **49**, 147–173.

49 Fisher B.D., Armstrong D., Yu B. *et al.* (1981) Invasive aspergillosis: progress in early diagnosis and treatment. *American Journal of Medicine*, **71**, 571–577.

50 Gold J.W.M., Fisher B., Yu B. *et al.* (1980) Diagnosis of invasive aspergillosis by passive haemagglutination assay of antibody. *Journal of Infectious Diseases*, **142**, 87–94.

51 Weiner M.H., Talbot G.H., Gerson S.L. *et al.* (1983) Antigen detection in the diagnosis of invasive aspergillosis. *Annals of Internal Medicine*, **99**, 777–782.

52 Obayashi T., Toshida M., Mori T. *et al.* (1995) Plasma (1–3)-B-D-glucan measurement in diagnosis of invasive deep mycosis and fungal febrile episodes. *Lancet*, **345**, 17–20.

53 Hughes W.T., Price R.A., Kim H.K. *et al.* (1973) *Pneumocystis carinii* pneumonia in children with malignancies. *Journal of Paediatrics*, **82**, 404–415.

54 Hughes W.T., Feldman S., Aur R.J.A. *et al.* (1975) Intensity of immunosuppressive therapy and the incidence of *Pneumocystis carinii* pneumonitis. *Cancer*, **36**, 2004–2009.

55 Hughes W.T. (1976) Protozoan infections in haematological diseases. *Clinics in Haematology*, **5**, 329–345.

56 Repsher L.H., Schroter G. & Hammon W.S. (1972) Diagnosis of *Pneumocystis carinii* pneumonitis by means of endobronchial brush biopsy. *New England Journal of Medicine*, **287**, 340–341.

57 Hodgkin J.E., Anderson H.A. & Rosenow E.C. (1973) Diagnosis of *Pneumocystis carinii* pneumonia by transbronchoscopic lung biopsy. *Chest*, **64**, 551–554.

58 Gentry L.O., Ruskin J. & Remington J.S. (1972) *Pneumocystis carinii* pneumonia: problems in diagnosis and therapy in 24 cases. *California Medicine*, **116**, 6–14.

59 Rosen P.P., Martini N. & Armstrong D. (1975) *Pneumocystis carinii* penumonia: diagnosis by lung biopsy. *American Journal of Medicine*, **58**, 794–802.

60 Saral R., Burns W.H. & Prentice H.G. (1984) Herpes virus infections: clinical manifestations and therapeutic strategies in immunocompromised patients. *Clinics in Haematology*, **13**, 645–660.

61 Kay H.E.M. & Rankin A. (1984) Immunoglobulin prophylaxis of measles in acute lymphoblastic leukaemia. *Lancet*, **i**, 901–902.

62 Volpi A., Whitley R.J., Ceballos R. *et al.* (1983) Rapid diagnosis of pneumonia due to cytomegalovirus with specific monoclonal antibodies. *Journal of Infectious Diseases*, **147**, 1119–1120.

63 Chou S. & Merigan T.C. (1983) Rapid detection and quantitation of human cytomegalovirus in urine through DNA hybridisation. *New England Journal of Medicine*, **308**, 921–925.

64 Griffiths P.D. (1984) Diagnostic techniques for cytomegalovirus infection. *Clinics in Haematology*, **13**, 631–644.

65 The T.H., Van der Ploeg M., Van den Berg A.P. *et al.* (1992) Direct detection of cytomegalovirus in peripheral blood leucocytes: a review of the antigenaemia assay and polymerase chain reaction. *Transplantation*, **54**, 193–198.

66 Cassol S.A., Poon M., Pal R. *et al.* (1989) Primer-mediated enzymatic amplification of cytomegalovirus (HCMV) DNA. Application to the early diagnosis of HCMV infection in marrow transplant recipients. *Journal of Clinical Investigation*, **83**, 1109–1115.

67 Jiwa N.M., Van Gemert G.W., Raap A.K. *et al.* (1989) Rapid detection of human cytomegalovirus DNA in peripheral blood leuco-

cytes of viremic transplant recipients by the polymerase chain reaction. *Transplantation*, **48**, 72–76.

68 Imbert-Marcille B.M., Milpied N., Coste-Burel M. *et al.* (1995) Clinical and practical value of human cytomegalovirus DNAaemia detection by semi-nested PCR for follow up of BMT recipients. *Bone Marrow Transplantation*, **15**, 611–617.

69 Perry S. & Penland W.Z. (1970) The portable laminar flow isolator. New unit for patient protection in a germ-free environment. In: *Recent Results in Cancer Research* (ed. G. Mathe), pp. 34–40. Springer, New York.

70 Bodey G.P. & Johnston D. (1971) Microbiological evaluation of protected environments during patients occupancy. *Applied Microbiology*, **22**, 828–836.

71 Deitrich M., Gaus W., Vossen J. *et al.* (1977) Protective isolation and antimicrobial decontamination in patients with high susceptibility to infection. A prospective co-operative study of gnotobiotic care in acute leukaemia patients. I Clinical results. *Infection*, **5**, 107–114.

72 Yates J.W. & Holland J.F. (1973) A controlled study of isolation and endogenous microbial suppression in acute myelocytic leukaemia patients. *Cancer*, **32**, 1490–1498.

73 Jameson B., Gamble D.R., Lynch J. *et al.* (1971) Five year analysis of protective isolation. *Lancet*, **i**, 1034–1040.

74 Levine A.S., Seigel S.E., Schreiber A.D. *et al.* (1973) Protected environments and prophylactic antibiotics. A prospective controlled study of their utility in the therapy of acute leukaemia. *New England Journal of Medicine*, **288**, 477–483.

75 Schimpff S.C., Greene W.H., Young V.M. *et al.* (1975) Infection prevention in acute non-lymphocytic leukaemia. Laminar air flow room reverse isolation with oral non-absorbable antibiotic prophylaxis. *Annals of Internal Medicine*, **82**, 351–358.

76 Buckner C.D., Clift R.A., Sanders J.E. *et al.* (1978) Protective environment for marrow transplant recipients. A prospective study. *Annals of Internal Medicine*, **89**, 893–901.

77 Bodey G.P. (1979) Treatment of acute leukaemia in protected environment units. *Cancer*, **44**, 431–436.

78 Storb R., Prentice R.L., Buckner C.D. *et al.* (1983) Graft versus host disease and survival in patient with aplastic anaemia treated by bone marrow grafts from HLA-identical siblings. *New England Journal of Medicine*, **308**, 302–306.

79 Pizzo P.A. & Levine A.S. (1977) The utility of protected-environment regimens for the compromised host: a critical assessment. In: *Progress in Hematology* (ed. H. Brawn), pp. 311–332. Grune and Stratton, New York.

80 Gale R.P. & Cline M.J. (1977) High remission induction rate in acute myeloid leukaemia. *Lancet*, **i**, 497–500.

81 Schimpff S.C. (1982) Protected environments for the treatment of high risk cancer patients. In: *Controversies in Oncology* (ed. P.H. Wiernik), pp. 247–265. Wiley, New York.

82 Sande M.A. & Mandell G.L. (1975) Effect of rifampicin on nasal carriage of *Staph. aureus*. *Antimicrobial Agents and Chemotherapy*, **7**, 294–297.

83 Bodey G.P., Gehan E.A., Freireich E.J. *et al.* (1971) Protected environment prophylactic antibiotic program in the chemotherapy of acute leukaemia. *American Journal of the Medical Sciences*, **262**, 138–151.

84 Lohner D., Debusscher L., Prevost J.M. *et al.* (1979) Comparative randomised study of protected environment plus oral antibiotics versus oral antibiotics alone in neutropenic patients. *Cancer Treatment Report*, **63**, 363–368.

85 Rodriguez V., Bodey G.P., Freireich E.J. *et al.* (1978) Randomised trial of protected environment prophylactic antibiotics. *Medicine*, **57**, 253–266.

86 Hahn D.M., Schimpff S.C., Fortner C.C. *et al.* (1978) Infection in acute leukaemia patients receiving oral non-absorbable antibiotics. *Antimicrobial Agents and Chemotherapy*, **13**, 958–964.

87 Storring R.A., Jameson B., McElwain J.J. *et al.* (1977) Oral non-absorbed antibiotics prevent infection in acute non-lymphoblastic leukaemia. *Lancet*, **ii**, 837–840.

88 Watson J.G. & Jameson B. (1979) Antibiotic prophylaxis for patients in protective isolation. *Lancet*, **i**, 1183.

89 Van der Waaij D., Berghuis J.M. & Lekkerkerk J.E.F. (1972) Colonisation resistance of the digestive tract of mice during systemic antibiotic treatment. *Journal of Hygiene*, **70**, 605–610.

90 Sleijfer D.T., Mulder N.H., de Vries-Hospers H.G. *et al.* (1980) Infection of prevention in granulocytopenic patients by selective decontamination of the digestive tracts. *European Journal of Cancer*, **16**, 859–869.

91 Guiot H.F.L., Van der Brock P.J., Van der Meer J.W.M. *et al.* (1983) Selective antimicrobial decontamination of the intestinal flora of patients with acute non-lymphocytic leukaemia. *Journal of Infectious Diseases*, **147**, 615–623.

92 Hughes W.T., Kuhn S., Chaudhary S. *et al.* (1977) Successful prophylaxis for *Pneumocystis carinii* pneumonia. *New England Journal of Medicine*, **297**, 1419–1426.

93 Gurwith M.J., Brunton J.L., Lank B.A. *et al.* (1979) A prospective controlled investigation of prophylactic trimethoprim-sulfamethoxazole in hospitalised granulocytopenic patients. *American Journal of Medicine*, **66**, 248–256.

94 Enno A., Darrell J. & Hows J. (1978) Co-trimoxazole for prevention of infection in acute leukaemia. *Lancet*, **ii**, 395–397.

95 Watson J.G., Jameson B., Powles R.L. *et al.* (1982) Co-trimoxazole versus non-absorbable antibiotics in acute leukaemia. *Lancet*, **i**, 6–9.

96 Zinner S.H. (1993) Prophylaxis of bacterial infections with oral antibiotics in neutropenic patients. *Schweizerische Medizinische Wochenschrift*, **14**(Suppl. 14), 7–14.

97 Dekker A., Rozenberg-Arska M., Sixman J.J. *et al.* (1981) Prevention of infection by TMP/SMZ plus amphotericin B in patients with acute non-lymphocytic leukaemia. *Annals of Internal Medicine*, **95**, 555–559.

98 Kaufman C.A., Leipman M.K., Bergman A.G. *et al.* (1983) Trimethoprim-sulfamethoxazole prophylaxis in neutropenic patients. Reduction of infections and effect on bacterial and fungal flora. *American Journal of Medicine*, **74**, 599–607.

99 Gualitieri R.J., Donowitz G.R., Kaiser C.E. *et al.* (1983) Double-blind randomised study of prophylactic trimethoprim-sulfamethoxazole in granulocytopenic patients with haematologic malignancies. *American Journal of Medicine*, **74**, 934–940.

100 Pizzo P.A., Robichaud K.J., Edwards B.K. *et al.* (1983) Oral antibiotic prophylaxis in patients with cancer. A double-blind randomised placebo controlled trial. *Journal of Paediatrics*, **102**, 125–133.

101 Wade J.C., de Jough C.A., Newman K.A. *et al.* (1983) Selective antimicrobial modulation as prophylaxis against infection during granulocytopenia: TMP/SMZ versus nalidixic acid. *Journal of Infectious Diseases*, **147**, 624–634.

102 Cotton D.J. & Pizzo P.A. (1985) Prevention of infection in patients with haematologic malignancy. In: *Neoplastic Diseases of the Blood* Vol. 2 (eds P.H. Wernick *et al.*), pp. 919–941. Churchill Livingstone, Edinburgh.

103 Dekker A.W., Rozenberg-Arska M. & Verhoef J. (1987) Infection

prophylaxis in acute leukaemia: a comparison of ciprofloxacin with trimethoprim — sulfamethoxazole and colistin. *Annals of Internal Medicine*, **106**, 7–12.

104 Karp J.E., Merz W.G., Hendricksen C. *et al.* (1987) Oral norfloxacin for prevention of gram-negative bacterial infections in patients with acute leukaemia and granulocytopenia: a randomised, double-blind, placebo-controlled trial. *Annals of Internal Medicine*, **106**, 1–7.

105 Pizzo P.A. (1983) Antimicrobial prophylaxis in the immunosuppressed cancer patient. In: *Current Clinical Topics in Infectious Diseases* (eds J.S. Remington & M.N. Scharz), pp. 153–185. McGraw Hill, New York.

106 Ezdindi E.Z., O'Sullivan D.D., Wasser L.P. *et al.* (1979) Oral amphotericin for candidiasis in patients with haematological neoplasia. *Journal of American Medical Association*, **224**, 258–269.

107 Heel R.C. (1982) Chronic mucocutaneous candidiasis. In: *Ketoconazole in the Management of Fungal Disease* (ed. H.N. Levine), pp. 103–108. Adis Press, New York.

108 Hann I.M., Prentice H.G., Corringham R. *et al.* (1982) Ketoconazole versus nystatin plus amphotericin B for fungal prophylaxis in severely immunocompromised patients. *Lancet*, **i**, 826–829.

109 Meunier-Carpentier F. (1983) Prophylaxis of fungal infections in neutropenic cancer patients. *Schweizerische Medizinsche Wochenschrift*, **113**(Suppl. 14), 15–19.

110 Lewis J.H., Zimmerman H.J., Benson G.D. *et al.* (1984) Hepatic injury associated with ketoconazole therapy. Analysis of 33 cases. *Gastroenterology*, **86**, 503–513.

111 Duarte P.A., Chow C.C., Simmons F. *et al.* (1984) Fatal hepatitis associated with ketoconazole therapy. *Archives of Internal Medicine*, **144**, 1069–1070.

112 Janssen P.A.J. & Symeons J.E. (1983) Hepatic reactions during ketaconazole treatment. *American Journal of Medicine*, **74**, 80–85.

113 Morgenstern G.R., Powles R., Robinson B. *et al.* (1982) Cyclosporin interaction with ketoconazole and melphalan. *Lancet*, **ii**, 1342.

114 De Wit S., Weerts D., Goosens H. *et al.* (1989) Comparison of fluconazole and ketoconazole for oropharyngeal candidiasis in AIDS. *Lancet*, **i**, 746–747.

115 Patterson T.F., Miniter P., Andriole V.T. *et al.* (1990) Efficacy of fluconazole in experimental invasive aspergillosis. *Reviews of Infectious Diseases*, **12**(Suppl. 3), 5281–5285.

116 Winston D.J., Chandrasekar P.H., Lazarus H.M. *et al.* (1993) Fluconazole prophylaxis of fungal infections in patients with acute leukaemia. *Annals of Internal Medicine*, **118**, 495–503.

117 Goodman J.L., Winston D.J., Greenfield R.A. *et al.* (1992) A controlled trial of fluconazole to prevent fungal infections in patients undergoing bone marrow transplantation. *New England Journal of Medicine*, **326**, 845–851.

118 Richardson M.D. & Warnock D.W. (1993) Antifungal drugs. In: *Fungal Infection, Diagnosis and Management*, pp. 17–43. Blackwell Scientific Publications, Oxford.

119 Espinel-Ingroff A., Shadomy S. & Gebhart R.J. (1984) *In vitro* studies with R51211 (itraconazole). *Antimicrobial Agents and Chemotherapy*, July 5–9.

120 Hann I.M., Prentice H.G., Blacklock H.A. *et al.* (1983) Acyclovir prophylaxis against herpes virus infections in severely compromised patients: a randomised double-blind trial. *British Medical Journal*, **87**, 375–392.

121 Gluckman E., Devergie A., Melo R. *et al.* (1983) Prophylaxis of herpes infections after bone marrow transplantation by oral acyclovir. *Lancet*, **ii**, 706–708.

122 Burns W.H. & Saral R. Chemotherapy of herpes simplex virus infections. In: *Human Immunity to Viruses* (ed. F.A. Ennis), pp. 203–218. Academic Press, New York.

123 Field H.J. & Darby G. (1980) Pathogenicity of thymidine kinase-deficient mutants of herpes simplex virus in mice. *Antimicrobial Agents and Chemotherapy*, **17**, 209–216.

124 Brunell P.A., Ross A., Miller L.H. *et al.* (1969) Prevention of varicella by zoster immune globulin. *New England Journal of Medicine*, **280**, 1191–1194.

125 Emanuel D., Cunningham I. & Jules-Elysee K. (1988) Cytomegalovirus pneumonia after bone marrow transplantation successfully treated with the combination of ganciclovir and high-dose intravenous immunoglobulin. *Annals of Internal Medicine*, **109**, 777–782.

126 Reed E.C., Bowden R.A., Dandliker P.S. *et al.* (1988) Treatment of cytomegalovirus pneumonia with ganciclovir and intravenous cytomegalovirus immunoglobulin in patients with bone marrow transplants. *Annals of Internal Medicine*, **109**, 783–788.

127 Schmidt G.M., Kovacs A. & Zaia J.A. (1988) Ganciclovir/immunoglobulin combination therapy for the treatment of human cytomegalovirus-associated interstitial pneumonia in bone marrow allograft recipients. *Transplantation*, **464**, 905–907.

128 Verdonck L.F., de Gast G.C. & Dekker A.W. (1989) Treatment of cytomegalovirus immunoglobulin combined with ganciclovir. *Bone Marrow Transplantation*, **4**, 187–189.

129 Mackinnon S., Burnett A.K., Crawford R.J. *et al.* (1988) Seronegative blood products prevent primary cytomegalovirus infection after bone marrow transplantation. *Journal of Clinical Pathology*, **41**, 948–950.

130 Ciararella D. & Snyder E. (1988) Clinical use of blood transfusion devices. *Transfusion Medicine Review*, **2**, 95–111.

131 Meyers J.D., Leszcynski J. & Zaia J.A. (1983) Prevention of cytomegalovirus infection by cytomegalovirus immune globulin after marrow transplantation. *Annals of Internal Medicine*, **98**, 442–446.

132 Condie R.M. & O'Reilly R.J. (1984) Prevention of cytomegalovirus infection by prophylaxis with an intravenous, hyperimmune, native, unmodified cytomegalovirus globulin. Randomised trial in bone marrow transplantation recipients. *American Journal of Medicine*, **76**, 134–141.

133 Winston D.J., Ho W.G. & Lin C.H. (1987) Intravenous immune globulin for prevention of cytomegalovirus infection and interstitial pneumonia after bone marrow transplantation. *Annals of Internal Medicine*, **106**, 12–18.

134 Sullivan K.M., Kopecky K.J., Jocom J. *et al.* (1990) Immunomodulatory and antimicrobial efficacy of intravenous immunoglobulin in bone marrow transplantation. *New England Journal of Medicine*, **323**, 705–712.

135 Meyers J.D., Reed E.C. & Shepp D.H. (1988) Acyclovir for prevention of cytomegalovirus infection and disease after allogeneic marrow transplantation. *New England Journal of Medicine*, **318**, 70–75.

136 Wingard J.R. (1990) Advances in the management of infectious complications after bone marrow transplantation. *Bone Marrow Transplantation*, **6**, 371–383.

137 Goodrich J.M., Bowden R.A., Fisher L. *et al.* (1993) Ganciclovir prophylaxis to prevent cytomegalovirus disease after allogeneic marrow transplant. *Annals of Internal Medicine*, **118**, 173–178.

138 Winston D.J., Ho W.G., Bartoni K. *et al.* (1993) Ganciclovir prophylaxis of cytomegalovirus infection and disease in allogeneic

bone marrow transplant recipients. *Annals of Internal Medicine*, **118**, 179–184.

139 Schmidt G.M., Horak D.A., Niland J.C. *et al.* (1991) A randomised, controlled trial of prophylactic ganciclovir for cytomegalovirus pulmonary infection in recipients of allogeneic bone marrow transplants. The City of Hope-Stanford-Syntex CMV Study Group. *New England Journal of Medicine*, **324**, 1005–1011.

140 Ljungman P., Lore K., Aschan J. *et al.* (1996) Use of a semi-quantitative PCR for cytomegalovirus DNA as a basis for pre-emptive antiviral therapy in allogeneic bone marrow transplant patients. *Bone Marrow Transplantation*, **17**, 583–587.

141 Meyers J.D. & Thomas E.D. (1981) Infection complicating bone marrow transplantation. In: *Clinical Approach to Infection in the Compromised Host* (eds R.H. Rubin & L.S. Young), pp. 507–551. Plenum Medical Book Company, New York.

142 Young J.S. (1984) An overview of infection in bone marrow transplant recipients. *Clinics in Haematology*, **13**, 661–678.

143 Hosea S.W., Burch C.G., Brown E.J. *et al.* (1981) Impaired immune response of splenectomised patients to polyvalent pneumococcal vaccine. *Lancet*, **ii**, 804–807.

144 Haghbin M, Armstrong D. & Murphy M.L. (1973) Controlled prospective trial of *Pseudomonas aeruginosa* vaccine in children with acute leukaemia. *Cancer*, **32**, 761–766.

145 Young L.S., Meyer R.D. & Armstrong D. (1973) *Pseudomonas aeruginosa* vaccine in cancer patients. *Annals of Internal Medicine*, **79**, 518–527.

146 Ziegler E.J., Douglas H., Sherman J.E. *et al.* (1973) Treatment of *E. coli* and *Klebsiella* bacteremia in agranulocytic animals with anti-serum to a UDP-GAL epimerase-deficient mutant. *Journal of Immunology*, **111**, 433–439.

147 Ziegler E.N., McCutchan J.A., Fiercer J. *et al.* (1982) Treatment of gram-negative bacteremia and shock with human antiserum to a mutant *Escherichia coli*. *New England Journal of Medicine*, **307**, 1225–1230.

148 Glauser M.P., McCutchan J.A. & Ziegler E. (1984) Immunoprophylaxis and immunotherapy of gram-negative infections in the immuno-compromised host. *Clinics in Haematology*, **13**, 549–555.

149 Ziegler E.J., Fisher C.J., Sprung C.L. *et al.* (1991) Treatment of gram-negative bacteremia and septic shock with HA-1A human monoclonal antibody against endotoxin. *New England Journal of Medicine*, **324**, 429–436.

150 Fawcett J. (1980) Lithium carbonate in medicine and psychiatry. In: *Lithium Effects in Granulopoiesis and Immune Function* (eds. A.H. Rossof & W.A. Robinson) pp. 1–13. Plenum Press, New York.

151 Boggs D.R. & Joyce R.A. (1983) The hematopoietic effects of lithium. *Seminars in Hematology*, **20**, 129–138.

152 Lyman G.H. (1980) The use of lithium carbonate to reduce infection and leukopenia during systemic chemotherapy. *New England Journal of Medicine*, **302**, 257–260.

153 Stein R.S., Beaman C., Ali M.Y. *et al.* (1977) Lithium carbonate attenuation of chemotherapy-induced neutropenia. *New England Journal of Medicine*, **297**, 430–431.

154 Stein R.S., Vogler W.R. & Lefante J. (1981) Failure of lithium to limit neutropenia during induction therapy of acute myelogenous leukaemia. *Proceedings of the American Association of Cancer Research/American Society of Clinical Oncology*, **22**, 423.

155 Goodhall P.T. & Vosti K.L. (1975) Fever in acute myelogenous leukaemia. *Archives of Internal Medicine*, **135**, 1197–1203.

156 Prentice H.G. & Hann I.M. (1985) The prophylaxis and treatment of infections in patients with bone marrow failure. *Recent Advances in Haematology*, **4**, 199–219.

157 Pizzo P.A., Robichaud K.J., Wesley R. *et al.* (1982) Fever in the paediatric and young adult patient with cancer. A prospective study of 1001 episodes. *Medicine*, **61**, 153–165.

158 Anderson E.T., Young L.S. & Hewitt W.L. (1978) Anti-microbial synergism in the therapy of gram-negative rod bacteremia. *Chemotherapy*, **24**, 45–54.

159 Klastersky J. & Zinner S.H. (1982) Synergistic combinations of antibiotics in gram-negative infections. *Review of Infectious Diseases*, **4**, 294–301.

160 Klastersky J., Cappel R., Swings G. *et al.* (1971) Bacteriological and Clinical activity of the ampicillin/gentamicin and cephalothin/gentamicin combinations. *American Journal of the Medical Sciences*, **262**, 283–290.

161 Gaya H. (1984) Rational basis for the choice of regimens for empirical therapy of sepsis in granulocytopenic patients. *Clinics in Haematology*, **13**, 573–586.

162 Klastersky J. (1983) The role of the new penicillins and cephalosporins in the management of infection in granulocytopenic patients. *Schweizerische Medizinsche Wochenschrift*, **113**(Suppl. 14), 64–69.

163 Young L.S. (1985) Treatment of established bacterial and fungal infections in patients with haematological malignancy. In: *Neoplastic Diseases of the Blood*, Vol. 2 (eds P.H. Wiernick *et al.*), pp. 943–960. Churchill Livingstone, Edinburgh.

164 Klastersky J. (1984) New antibacterial agents: the role of new penicillins and cephalosporins in the management of infection in granulocytopenic patients. *Clinics in Haematology*, **13**, 587–598.

165 Wade J.C., Schimpff S.C., Newman K.A. *et al.* (1981) Piperacillin or ticarcillin plus amikacin. A double-blind prospective comparison of empiric antibiotic therapy for febrile granulocytopenic cancer patients. *American Journal of Medicine*, **71**, 983–990.

166 Winston D.J., Ho W.G., Young L.S. *et al.* (1981) Piperacillin plus amikacin therapy versus carbenicillin plus amikacin therapy in febrile, granulocytopenic patients. *Archives of Internal Medicine*, **142**, 1663–1667.

167 Cometta A., Zinner S., de Bock R. *et al.* (1995) Piperacillin-tazobactam plus amikacim versus ceftazidime plus amikacim as empiric therapy for fever in granulocytopenic patients with cancer. *Antimicrobial Agents and Chemotherapy*, **39**, 445–452.

168 Dashlager J.I. (1980) The effect of netilmicin and other aminoglycosides on renal function: a survey of literature on the nephrotoxicity of netilmicin. *Scandinavian Journal of Infectious Diseases*, Suppl. 23, 96–102.

169 Cunha B.A. & Ristuccia A.M. (1982) Symposium on antimicrobial therapy. Third generation cephalosporins. *Medical Clinics of North America*, **66**, 283–291.

170 Ramphal R., Kramer B.S., Rand K.H. *et al.* (1983) Early results of comparative trial of ceftazidime versus cephalothin, carbenicillin and gentamicin in the treatment of febrile granulocytopenic patients. *Journal of Antimicrobial Chemotherapy*, **12**(Suppl. A), 81–88.

171 Donnelly J.P., Marcus R.E., Goldman J.M. *et al.* (1985) Ceftazidime as a first-line therapy for fever in acute leukaemia. *Journal of Infection*, **11**, 205–215.

172 Pizzo P.A., Hathorn J.W., Hiemanz J. *et al.* (1986) A randomised trial comparing ceftazidime alone with combination antibiotic therapy in cancer patients with fever and neutropenia. *New England Journal of Medicine*, **315**, 525–528.

173 Johnson P.R.E., Liu Yin J.A. & Tooth A.J. (1989) Randomised

study of ciprofloxacin versus azlocillin and netilmicin in the empirical treatment of febrile episodes in neutropenic patients. In: *Proceedings of the 16th International Congress of Chemotherapy*, pp. 233.1–233.2.

174 Johnson P.R.E., Liu Yin J.A. & Tooth J.A. (1990) High dose intravenous ciprofloxacin in febrile neutropenic patients. *Journal of Antimicrobial Chemotherapy*, **26**(Suppl. F), 101–107.

175 Norrby S.R., Vandercam B., Lovie T. *et al.* (1987) Imipenem/cilastin versus amikacin plus piperacillin in the treatment of infections in neutropenic patients: a prospective, randomised, multi-clinic study. *Scandinavian Journal of Infectious Diseases*, Suppl. 52, 65–78.

176 Leyland M.J., Bayston K.E., Cohen J. *et al.* (1992) A comparative study of imipenem versus piperacillin plus gentamicin in the initial management of febrile neutropenic patients with haematological malignancies. *Journal of Antimicrobial Chemotherapy*, **30**, 843–854.

177 Liang R., Yung R., Chiu E. *et al.* (1990) Ceftazidime versus imipenem-cilastatin as initial monotherapy for febrile neutropenic patients. *Antibicrobial Agents and Chemotherapy*, **34**, 1336–1341.

178 Rolston K.V.I., Berkey P., Bodey G.P. *et al.* (1992) A comparison of imipenem to ceftazidime with or without amikacin as empiric therapy in febrile neutropenic patients. *Archives of Internal Medicine*, **152**, 283–291.

179 The Meropenem Study Group of Leuven, London and Nijmegen (1995) Equivalent efficacies of meropenem and ceftazidime as empirical monotherapy of febrile neutropenic patients. *Journal of Antimicrobial Chemotherapy*, **36**, 185–200.

180 Cometta A., Calandra T., Gaya H. *et al.* (1996) Monotherapy with meropenem versus combination therapy with ceftazidime plus amikacin as empiric therapy for fever in granulocytopenic patients with cancer. *Antimicrobial Agents and Chemotherapy*, **40**, 1108–1115.

181 Pizzo P.A., Robichaud J.K., Gill F.A. *et al.* (1979) Duration of empiric antibiotic therapy in granulocytopenic patients with cancer. *American Journal of Medicine*, **67**, 194–200.

182 Klastersky J. (1983) A co-operative trial of empirical treatment in febrile neutropenic patients. The Third EORTC Trial. In: *The International Chemotherapy Congress*, pp. 33–35, abstract 71.

183 Hiemenz J.W. & Pizzo P.A. (1985) New developments in the etiology, diagnosis, treatment and prevention of infectious complications in patients with leukaemia. In: *Chronic and Acute Leukaemias in Adults* (ed. D.C. Bloomfield), pp. 283–337. Martinus Nijhoff Publishers, Dordrecht.

184 Pizzo P.A., Robichaud K.J., Gill F.A. *et al.* (1982) Empiric antibiotic and antifungal therapy for cancer patients with prolonged fever and granulopoiesis. *American Journal of Medicine*, **72**, 101–111.

185 Puksa S., Hutcheon M.A. & Hyland R.H. (1983) Usefulness of transbronchial biopsy in immunosuppressed patients with pulmonary infiltrates. *Thorax*, **38**, 146–150.

186 Yung J.A., Hopkin J.M. & Cuthbertson W.P. (1984) Pulmonary infiltrates in immunocompromised patients; diagnosis by cytological examination of bronchoalveolar lavage fluid. *Journal of Clinical Pathology*, **37**, 390–397.

187 Schimpff S.C. (1983) Infection in the leukaemic patient. In: *Diagnosis, Therapy and Prevention in Leukaemia* (eds F.W. Gunz & E.S. Henderson), pp. 799–822. Grune and Stratton, New York.

188 Mackie P.H., Crockston R.A. & Stuart J.R. (1979) C-reactive protein for rapid diagnosis of infection in leukaemia. *Journal of Clinical Pathology*, **32**, 1253–1256.

189 Rose P.E., Johnson S.A., Meakin M. *et al.* (1981) Serial study of C-reactive protein during infection in leukaemia. *Journal of Clinical Pathology*, **34**, 263–266.

190 Schofield K., Voulgari F., Gozzard D.I. *et al.* (1982) C-reactive protein concentration as a guide to antibiotic therapy in acute leukaemia. *Journal of Clinical Pathology*, **35**, 866–869.

191 Gozzard D.I., French E.A., Blecher T.E. *et al.* (1985) C-reactive protein levels in neutropenic patients with pyrexia. *Laboratory and Clinical Haematology*, **7**, 307–315.

192 Peltola H., Saarinen U.M. & Slimes M.A. (1983) C-reactive protein in the rapid diagnosis and follow-up of bacterial septicaemia in children with leukaemia. *Paediatric Infectious Diseases*, **2**, 370–373.

193 Kostiala I. (1984) C-reactive response induced by fungal infections. *Journal of Infection*, **8**, 212–220.

194 Harris R.I., Stone P.C.W., Hudson A.G. *et al.* (1984) C-reactive protein rapid assay techniques for monitoring resolution of infection in immunocompromised patients. *Journal of Clinical Pathology*, **37**, 821–825.

195 O'Callaghan C., Franklin P., Elliott T. *et al.* (1984) C-reactive protein levels in neonates: determined by a latex-enhanced immunoassay. *Journal of Clinical Pathology*, **37**, 1027–1028.

196 Hughes W.T., Bartley D.L., Patterson G.G. *et al.* (1983) Ketoconazole and candidiasis: a controlled study. *Journal of Infectious Diseases*, **147**, 1060–1063.

197 Meunier F., Gerain J., Snoeck R. *et al.* (1987) Fluconazole therapy of oropharyngeal candidiasis in cancer patients. In: *Recent Trends in the Discovery, Development and Evaluation of Antifungal Agents* (ed. R.A. Fromtling), pp. 169–174. JR Prous Science Publishers, South Africa.

198 Rabinovich S., Shaw B.D., Bryant T. *et al.* (1974) Effect of 5-fluorocytosine and amphotericin-B on *Candida albicans* infection in mice. *Journal of Infectious Diseases*, **130**, 28–31.

199 Bennett J.E. (1977) Flucytosine. *Annals of Internal Medicine*, **86**, 319–322.

200 Medoff G. & Kobayashi G.S. (1980) Strategies in the treatment of systemic fungal infections. *New England Journal of Medicine*, **302**, 145–155.

201 Tollemar J., Ringden O. & Tyden G. (1990) Liposomal amphotericin-B (Ambisome) treatment in solid organ and bone marrow transplant recipients. Efficacy and safety evaluation. *Clinical Transplantation*, **4**, 167–175.

202 Katz N.M., Pierce P.F. & Anzeck R.A. (1990) Liposomal amphotericin-B for treatment of pulmonary aspergillosis in a heart transplant patient. *Journal of Heart Transplantation*, **9**, 14–17.

203 Ringden O., Meunier F., Tollemar J. *et al.* (1991) Efficacy of amphotericin B encapsulated in liposomes (AmBisome) in the treatment of invasive fungal infections in immunocompromised patients. *Journal of Antimicrobial Chemotherapy*, **28**(Suppl. B), 73–82.

204 Mills W., Chopra R., Linch D.C. & Goldstone A.H. (1994) Liposomal amphotericin B in the treatment of fungal infections in neutropenic patients: a single-centre experience of 133 episodes in 116 patients. *British Journal of Haematology*, **86**, 754–760.

205 Atkinson G.W. & Israel H.I. (1973) 5-Fluorocytosine treatment of meningeal and pulmonary aspergillosis. *American Journal of Medicine*, **55**, 496–504.

206 Ribner B., Keusch G.T., Hanna B.A. *et al.* (1976) Combination amphotericin-B/rifampicin therapy for pulmonary aspergillosis in leukaemic patients. *Chest*, **70**, 681–683.

207 Denning D.W., Tucker R.M., Hanson L.H. *et al.* (1989) Treatment

of invasive aspergillosis with itraconazole. *American Journal of Medicine*, **86**, 791--800.

208 Freirich E.J., Levin E.H., Whang J. *et al.* (1964) The function and fate of transfused leukocytes from donors with chronic myelocytic leukaemia in leukopenic recipients. *Annals of the New York Academy of Sciences*, **113**, 1081–1089.

209 Djerassi I., Kim J.S., Mitrakul C. *et al.* (1970) Filtration leukapheresis for separation of concentration of transfusable amounts of normal human granuloctyes. *Journal of Medicine (Basel)*, **1**, 358–364.

210 Goldman J.M. (1977) Granulocyte transfusions. *Recent Advances in Haematology*, **2**, 127–143.

211 McCollough J., Carter S.J. & Qule P.G. (1974) Effects of anticoagulants and storage on granulocyte function in bank blood. *Blood*, **43**, 207–217.

212 Graw R.G. Jr, Herzig G., Perry S. *et al.* (1972) Normal granulocyte transfusion therapy. Treatment of septicaemia due to Gram-negative bacteria. *New England Journal of Medicine*, **287**, 367–371.

213 Higby D.J., Yates J.W., Henderson E.S. *et al.* (1975) Filtration leukapheresis for granulocyte transfusion therapy. *New England Journal of Medicine*, **292**, 761–766.

214 Fortuny I.E., Bloomfield C.D., Hadlock D.C. *et al.* (1975) Granulocyte transfusion: a controlled study in patients with acute non-lymphocytic leukaemia. *Transfusion*, **15**, 548–558.

215 Herzig R.H., Herzig G.P., Graw R.G. Jr *et al.* (1977) Successful granulocyte transfusion: a controlled study. *New England Journal of Medicine*, **296**, 702–705.

216 Alavi J.B., Root R.K., Djerassi I. *et al.* (1977) A randomised clinical trial of granulocyte transfusions for infection in acute leukaemia. *New England Journal of Medicine*, **296**, 706–711.

217 Vogler W.R. & Winton E.F. (1977) A controlled study of the efficacy of granulocyte transfusions in patients with neutropenia. *New England Journal of Medicine*, **63**, 548–554.

218 Winston D.J., Ho W.J. & Gale R.P. (1982) Therapeutic granulocytic transfusions for documented infections. *Annals of Internal Medicine*, **97**, 509–515.

219 Winston D.J., Ho W.J., Young L.S. *et al.* (1980) Prophylactic granulocyte transfusions during human bone marrow transplantation. *American Journal of Medicine*, **68**, 893–897.

220 Winston D.J., Ho W.G. & Gale R.P. (1981) Prophylactic granulocyte transfusions during chemotherapy of acute non-lymphocytic leukaemia. *Annals of Internal Medicine*, **94**, 622–626.

221 Clift R.A., Sanders J.E., Thomas E.D. *et al.* (1978) Granulocyte transfusions for the prevention of infection in patients receiving bone marrow transplants. *New England Journal of Medicine*, **298**, 1052–1057.

222 Buckner C.D., Clift R.A., Thomas E.D. *et al.* (1983) Early infectious complications in allogeneic marrow transplant recipients with acute leukaemia: effects of prophylactic measures. *Infection*, **11**, 243–250.

223 Navari R.M., Buckner C.D., Clift R.A. *et al.* (1984) Prophylaxis of infection in patients with aplastic anaemia receiving allogeneic marrow transplants. *American Journal of Medicine*, **76**, 564–572.

224 Schiffer C.A., Aisner J., Daly P.A. *et al.* (1979) Alloimmunization following prophylactic granulocyte transfusion. *Blood*, **54**, 766–774.

225 Strauss R.G., Connett J.E., Gale R.P. *et al.* (1981) A controlled trial of prophylactic granulocyte transfusions during initial induction chemotherapy for acute myelogenous leukaemia. *New England Journal of Medicine*, **305**, 597–602.

226 Wright D.G., Robichaud K.J., Pizzo P.A. *et al.* (1981) Lethal pul-

monary reactions associated with the combined use of amphotericin B and leukocyte transfusions. *New England Journal of Medicine*, **304**, 1185–1189.

227 Ruthe R.C., Anderson B.R., Cunningham B.L. *et al.* (1978) Efficacy of granulocyte transfusions in the control of systemic candidiasis in the leukopenic host. *Blood*, **52**, 493–498.

228 Buckner C.D. & Clift R.A. (1984) Prophylaxis and treatment of infection of the immunocompromised host by granulocyte transfusions. *Clinics in Haematology*, **13**, 557–572.

229 Dahlke M.B., Keashen M.A., Alavi J.B. *et al.* (1980) Response to granulocyte transfusions in the alloimmunised patient. *Transfusion*, **20**, 555–558.

230 Metcalf D. (1985) The granulocyte-macrophage colony-stimulating factors. *Science*, **229**, 16–22.

231 Clark S.C. & Kamen R. (1987) The human haemopoietic colony-stimulating factors. *Science*, **236**, 1229–1237.

232 Sieff C.A. (1987) Haematopoietic growth factors. *Journal of Clinical Investigation*, **79**, 1549–1557.

233 Ono M., Matsumoto M., Matsubara S. *et al.* (1988) Protective effect of human granulocyte colony-stimulating factor on bacterial and fungal infection in neutropenic mice. *Behring Institute Mitteilungen*, **83**, 216–221.

234 Nienhuis A.W., Donahue R.E., Karlson S. *et al.* (1987) Recombinant human granulocyte-macrophage colony-stimulating factor (GM-CSF) shortens the period of neutropenia after autologous bone marrow transplantation in a primate model. *Journal of Clinical Investigation*, **80**, 573–577.

235 Bronchud M.H., Scarffe J.W., Thatcher N. *et al.* (1987) Phase I/II study of recombinant human granulocyte colony-stimulating factor in patients receiving intensive chemotherapy for small cell lung cancer. *British Journal of Cancer*, **56**, 809–813.

236 Morstyn G., Campbell L., Souza L.M. *et al.* (1988) Effect of granulocyte colony-stimulating factor on neutropenia induced by cytotoxic chemotherapy. *Lancet*, **i**, 667–672.

237 Morstyn G., Campbell L., Lieschke G.J. *et al.* (1989) Abrogation of chemotherapy induced neutropenia by subcutaneously administered granulocyte colony-stimulating factor (G-CSF) with optimization of dose and duration of therapy. *Journal of Clinical Oncology*, **7**, 1554–1562.

238 Gabrilove J.L., Jakubowski A., Scher H. *et al.* (1988) Effect of granulocyte colony-stimulating factor on neutropenia and associated morbidity due to chemotherapy for transitional cell carcinoma of the urothelium. *New England Journal of Medicine*, **318**, 1414–1422.

239 Niedhart J., Kohler B., Castillo A. *et al.* (1988) Recombinant human granulocyte colony-stimulating factor (rhG-CSF) shortens duration of granulocytopenia and thrombocythaemia following intensive chemotherapy dosing. *Proceedings of the American Association of Cancer Research*, **29**, 356 (abstract).

240 Bronchud M.H., Howell A., Crowther D. *et al.* (1989) The use of granulocyte colony-stimulating factor to increase the intensity of treatment with doxorubicin in patients with advanced breast and ovarian cancer. *British Journal of Cancer*, **60**, 121–125.

241 Autman K.S., Griffin J.D., Elias A. *et al.* (1988) Effects of recombinant human granulocyte-macrophage colony-stimulating factor on chemotherapy-induced myelosuppression. *New England Journal of Medicine*, **319**, 593–598.

242 Boogaerts M., Cavalli F., Cortes-Funes H. *et al.* (1995) Granulocyte growth factors: achieving a consensus. *Annals of Oncology*, **6**, 237–244.

243 Brandt S.J., Peters W.P., Atwater S.K. *et al.* (1988) Effect of

recombinant human granulocyte-macrophage colony-stimulating factor on hematopoietic reconstitution after high dose chemotherapy and autologous bone marrow transplantation. *New England Journal of Medicine*, **318**, 869–875.

244 Sheridan W.P., Morstyn G., Wolf M. *et al.* (1989) Granulocyte colony-stimulating factor and neutrophil recovery after high-dose chemotherapy and autologous bone marrow transplantation. *Lancet*, **ii**, 891–895.

245 Powles R., Smith C., Milan S. *et al.* (1990) Human recombinant GM-CSF in allogeneic bone marrow transplantation for leukaemia: double-blind, placebo-controlled trial. *Lancet*, **336**, 1417–1420.

246 Gisselbrecht G., Prentice H.G., Bacigalupo A. *et al.* (1994) Placebo-controlled phase III trial of lenograstim in bone marrow transplantation. *Lancet*, **343**, 696–700.

247 Faulds D., Lewis N.J.W., Milne R.J. *et al.* (1992) Recombinant granulocyte colony-stimulation factor (rG-CSF). Pharmacoeconomic considerations in chemotherapy-induced neutropenia. *Pharmacoeconomics*, **1**, 231–249.

248 Glaspy J.A., Bleecker G., Crawford J. *et al.* (1993) The impact of therapy with filgrastim (recombinant granulocyte colony-stimulating factor) on the health care costs associated with cancer chemotherapy. *European Journal of Cancer*, **29A**(Suppl. 7), 523–530.

249 Goa K.L. & Bryson H.M. (1994) Recombinant granulocyte macrophage colony-stimulating factor (rGM-CSF). An appraisal of its pharmacoeconomic status in neutropenia associated with chemotherapy and autologous bone marrow transplant. *Pharmacoeconomics*, **5**, 56–57.

250 Vellenga E., Young D.C., Wagner K. *et al.* (1987) The effects of GM-CSF and G-CSF in promoting growth of clonogenic cells in acute myeloblastic leukaemia. *Blood*, **69**, 1771–1776.

251 Griffin J.D. & Lowenberg B. (1986) Clonogenic cells in acute myeloblastic leukaemia. *Blood*, **68**, 1185–1195.

252 Griffin J.D., Young D., Herrmann F. *et al.* (1986) Effects of recombinant human GM-CSF on proliferation of clonogenic cells in acute myeloblastic leukaemia. *Blood*, **67**, 1448–1453.

253 Zittoun R., Mandelli F., De Witte T. *et al.* (1994) Recombinant human granulocyte-macrophage colony stimulating factor (GM-CSF) during induction treatment of acute myelogenous leukaemia: a randomised trial from EORTC-GIMEMA Leukaemia Cooperative Groups. *Blood*, **84**(Suppl. 1), 231a (abstract).

254 Rowe J.M., Andersen J.W., Mazza J.J. *et al.* (1995) A randomised, placebo-controlled phase III study of granulocyte-macrophage colony-stimulating factor in adult patients (>55–70 years of age) with acute myelogenous leukaemia. A study of the Eastern Cooperative Oncology Group. *Blood*, **86**, 457–462.

255 Stone R.M., Berg D.T., George S.L. *et al.* (1995) Granulocyte-macrophage colony-stimulating factor after initial chemotherapy for elderly patients with primary acute myelogenous leukaemia. *New England Journal of Medicine*, **332**, 1671–1677.

256 Lowenberg B., Suciu S., Zittoun R. *et al.* (1995) GM-CSF during as well as after induction chemotherapy in elderly patients with acute myeloid leukaemia. The EORTC-HOVON phase III trial (AML 11). *Blood*, **86**(Suppl. 1), abstract 1719.

257 Godwin J.E., Kopecky K.J., Head D.R. *et al.* (1995) A double-blind placebo-controlled trial of G-CSF in elderly patients with previously untreated acute myeloid leukaemia. A Southwest Oncology Group study. *Blood*, **86**(Suppl. 1), abstract 1723.

258 Dombret H., Chastang C., Fenaux P. *et al.* (1995) A controlled study of recombinant human granulocyte colony stimulating factor in elderly patients after treatment for acute myelogenous leukaemia. *New England Journal of Medicine*, **332**, 1678–1683.

259 Heil G., Hoelzer D., Sanz M.A. *et al.* (1995) Results of a randomised, double-blind, placebo-controlled, phase III study of Filgrastim in remission induction and early consolidation therapy for adults with de-novo acute myeloid leukaemia. *Blood*, **86**(Suppl. 1), abstract 1053.

26   Haemostasis and Thrombosis

P.H. Roddie and C.A. Ludlam

Normal haemostasis

The maintenance of normal haemostasis involves a complex interaction between blood vessels, platelets and coagulation factors. The controlled production of fibrin, and its subsequent dissolution, depends on three separate, but interrelated, systems: the coagulation pathway, the coagulation–inhibitory system and the fibrinolytic system. Pathological disturbances in any of these systems can lead to a haemorrhagic tendency or to intravascular coagulation.

Our understanding of the process of coagulation initially stemmed from the testing of the time taken for blood to clot in glass tubes following the addition of certain activators. On the basis of these relatively simple tests of coagulation, two main pathways were suggested: the extrinsic pathway and the contact or intrinsic pathway. For a time the contact system was perceived to be of most physiological relevance. This involves the activation of factor XII by kallikrein, a reaction accelerated by high-molecular-weight kininogen (HMWK). The activated factor XII subsequently leads to activation of factor XI, the sequence continuing through factors IX, VIII and X and, finally, to the generation of thrombin which acts on fibrinogen to produce fibrin. However the fact that patients with deficiencies of factor XII, prekallikrein and HMWK had no bleeding tendency called into doubt the *in vivo* significance of this pathway. Attention was then centred on the extrinsic pathway. The initiating step in this is the binding of factor VII or factor VIIa to tissue factor (TF). This complex is a potent activator of factor X which causes cascade activation and thrombin generation. With the discovery that TF:factor VIIa also activates factor IX, the two pathways of coagulation were linked (Fig. 26.1) [1].

It has now become accepted that TF is the main initiator of coagulation *in vivo*. Blood can come into contact with TF, either through damage to the vessel wall leading to exposure of the subendothelium or by the expression of TF on the cell surfaces of endothelial cells or monocytes. The latter can occur following stimulation, for example by tumour necrosis factor, endo-toxin or interleukin-1 [2]. Factor VII or factor VIIa binds to TF to form the complex TF:factor VII. It is not clear whether coagulation is initiated by factor VII, which has a low proteolytic activity, or by the presence of small amounts of factor VIIa circulating in the plasma [3]. The TF:factor VII is rapidly activated, probably through the action of factor Xa. Thrombin and factor Xa generated during coagulation exert positive feedback, through their ability to activate the TF:factor VIIa complex. The TF:factor VIIa complex then activates factors IX and X. The importance of TF in the initiation of coagulation can be inferred from a knowledge of factor VII. Patients with severe factor VII deficiency (<2%) have a high incidence of early haemorrhagic deaths [4]. The only known role for factor VII is in the activation of factors IX and X, which is known only to occur at appreciable rates in the presence of TF. This confirms the vital role that TF plays in the initiation of coagulation.

The importance of factors IX and VIII in normal haemostasis, and the reason why haemophiliacs bleed, may be because, in tissues with low levels of TF and high levels of tissue factor pathway inhibitor (TFPI), these coagulation proteins are important in maintaining factor Xa formation. Such a situation occurs in the joints, which could be why this site has a predilection for bleeding in haemophiliacs [5].

Thrombin activates both factors VIII and V to factors VIIIa and Va respectively. Factor VIIIa complexes with factor IXa and phospholipid to produce a complex that can activate factor X. Similarly, factor Va forms a complex with factor Xa and phospholipid to produce prothrombinase, which converts prothrombin to thrombin. Thrombin also acts to promote coagulation through its effects on platelets. Platelets release factor V and von Willebrand's factor (vWF) under the influence of thrombin. Another effect of thrombin is to induce platelets to undergo a change in their membrane whereby phosphatidylserine becomes externalized. This provides a site for binding Ca^{2+}, which in turn binds prothrombin and factors IX and X, thus facilitating the rapid generation of thrombin locally. Platelets also contribute to haemostasis through the

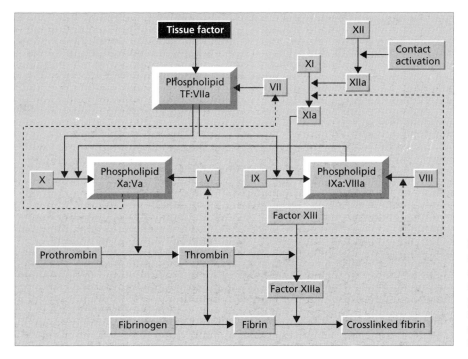

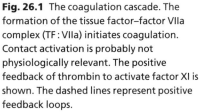

Fig. 26.1 The coagulation cascade. The formation of the tissue factor–factor VIIa complex (TF : VIIa) initiates coagulation. Contact activation is probably not physiologically relevant. The positive feedback of thrombin to activate factor XI is shown. The dashed lines represent positive feedback loops.

reactions of adhesion and aggregation. Platelets adhere to the subendothelial matrix exposed at the site of endothelial damage. This is mediated by the platelet glycoprotein receptors gp Ia/IIa and Ib/IX, which are able to bind to collagen and vWF. Aggregation follows the activation of platelets, which are stimulated by a variety of agonists, including thrombin, ADP and collagen. Activated platelets release ADP and thromboxane, in addition to factor V and vWF, which in turn promotes further platelet activation and aggregation, leading to the formation of a platelet plug at the site of tissue injury. Platelet aggregation is mediated by gp IIb/IIIa receptors which form bridges with fibrinogen to other platelets (Fig. 26.2).

The final step in coagulation is the conversion of soluble fibrinogen to fibrin. Thrombin cleaves fibrinopeptides A and B leaving fibrin monomers. Cross-linking of these monomers takes place under the action of factor XIII, activated by thrombin, and leads to the formation of a stable fibrin plug.

The above scheme of coagulation does not explain why patients with factor XI deficiency should have a haemorrhagic tendency, as factor XI is not activated by the TF : factor VIIa complex. However, it is now known that thrombin can activate FXI [6]. If this positive feedback loop operates *in vivo*, this would then be compatible with the current theory of blood coagulation.

Inhibition of coagulation

A variety of mechanisms are in place in order to prevent uncontrolled coagulation. Tissue factor is a membrane-bound protein and it therefore acts as an anchor to localize coagula-

tion to its own vicinity, i.e. the site of tissue damage. A number of naturally occurring anticoagulants exist whose role is to limit excessive thrombin generation (Fig. 26.3). Antithrombin III is a serine protease inhibitor that inhibits factor Xa and thrombin, but it also has activity against factors IXa and XIa. Heparin cofactor II is a specific thrombin inhibitor but its physiological importance is uncertain. Thrombin also acts itself to limit the process of coagulation. At the site of tissue injury, thrombin binds to thrombomodulin on the surface of intact endothelium. This leads to a change in thrombin such that it is no longer a procoagulant protein but, instead, it acts as an inhibitor of coagulation. The thrombin–thrombomodulin complex activates protein C which, in combination with its cofactor protein S, cleaves and inactivates factors Va and VIIIa, thus preventing further factor X activation. Protein C also inactivates plasminogen activator inhibitor-1 (PAI-1), the major inhibitor of tissue plasminogen activator (tPA), which leads to enhanced fibrinolysis. Tissue factor pathway inhibitor (TFPI) is a Kunitz-type protein which forms a complex with factor Xa; this complex then binds to TF : factor VIIa, rendering an inactive enzyme (Fig. 26.4) [7]. Its main role appears to be inhibiting small amounts of TF, which is probably essential in the maintenance of normal haemostatic balance.

Fibrinolysis

The process of fibrinolysis must ensure that fibrin dissolution occurs locally at the site of thrombus formation, in synchrony with vessel healing, but without the development of systemic fibrinolysis (Fig. 26.5). Plasmin is the enzyme which is able to

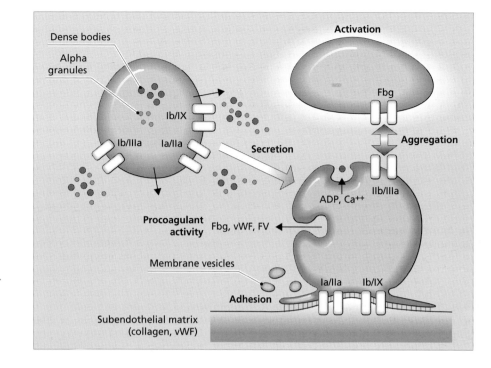

Fig. 26.2 The role of platelets in homeostasis. Following activation, platelets have a number of methods by which they promote homeostasis. Secretion takes place from the dense bodies and alpha granules. Aggregation to other platelets occurs via gpIIb/IIIa receptors in conjunction with fibrinogen. Platelet adhesion to subendothelial structures is mediated via gpIa/IIa and Ib/IX receptors. ADP = adenosine diphosphate; Fbg = fibrinogen; FV = factor V; vWF = von Willebrand's factor.

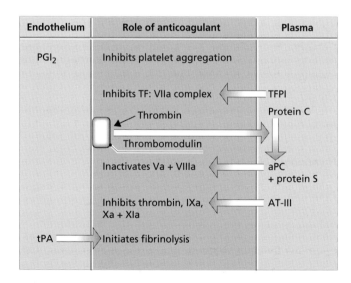

Endothelium	Role of anticoagulant	Plasma
PGI$_2$	Inhibits platelet aggregation	
	Inhibits TF: VIIa complex	TFPI
	Thrombin	Protein C
	Thrombomodulin	
	Inactivates Va + VIIIa	aPC + protein S
	Inhibits thrombin, IXa, Xa + XIa	AT-III
tPA	Initiates fibrinolysis	

Fig. 26.3 The natural anticoagulants—endothelial and plasma-derived inhibitors of thombosis. aPC = activated protein C; AT-III = antithrombin III; PGI2 = prostacyclin; TF = tissue factor; TFPI = tissue factor pathway inhibitor; tPA = tissue plasminogen activator.

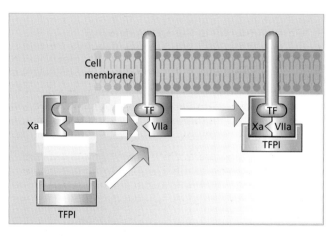

Fig. 26.4 Inhibition of the TF : factor VIIa complex by TFPI. TFPI first binds to factor Xa, the resulting complex then binds to the TF : factor VIIa complex and inactivates it in the process.

lyse fibrin. The conversion of the inactive plasminogen to plasmin occurs through the action of the plasminogen activators tPA and urokinase (uPA). Urokinase is released from the kidney and helps to maintain urothelial patency. tPA is released from endothelial cells in response to a variety of stimuli, including local thrombin and fibrin formation and venous stasis. During clotting, a proportion of the circulating plasminogen binds to fibrin and becomes incorporated into the thrombus. tPA also binds to fibrin, which increases its ability to convert the bound plasminogen to plasmin. The initial plasmin degradation of fibrin accelerates further fibrinolysis in a positive feedback mechanism. Premature clot dissolution is prevented by inhibitors of plasmin and plasminogen activators. Circulating α$_2$ antiplasmin, the main plasmin inhibitor, is not efficient at inhibiting fibrin-bound plasmin, but it rapidly inactivates any free plasmin. This favours fibrin degradation while preventing systemic plasminaemia. PAI-1 is present in small amounts in the plasma but it is also present in platelets and endothelial cells. A rise in its plasma concentration occurs as part of the acute-phase response to inflammatory stimuli. PAI-

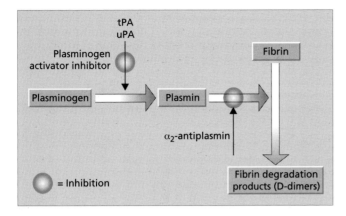

Fig. 26.5 Fibrinolytic activators and inhibitors. tPA = tissue plasminogen activator; uPA = urokinase.

1 bound to fibrin can inibit both tPA and uPA. Congenital deficiency of PAI-1 results in a serious bleeding disorder [8]. The process of fibrinolysis leads to the formation of a variety of fibrin degradation products. The presence of X-linked fibrin fragments can be detected in the plasma of patients with disseminated intravascular coagulation (DIC).

Role of tissue factor in the pathogenesis of disseminated intravascular coagulation

Tissue factor is present in most tissues, and many cells that are not normally in contact with plasma constitutively express TF [9]. As previously mentioned, endothelial cells and monocytes can be induced to synthesize TF under certain stimuli. It is thought that TF expressed in cancer cells, leukaemia cells, stimulated endothelial cells and monocytes plays an important role in the pathogenesis of DIC [10].

Increased tissue factor activity has been demonstrated for leukaemia cells in both acute myeloblastic leukaemia (AML) and acute lymphoblastic leukaemia (ALL) [11]. Tissue factor activity in leukaemia cells from AML (M1–M5) has 24–210 times more activity than that of intact mononuclear cells from normal subjects. Tissue factor activity is also elevated in leukaemia cells from patients with ALL, although to a lesser degree. The relationship between high TF activity and the development of DIC has been investigated. In a study of patients with AML, development of DIC was closely linked not only with high TF contents in leukaemia cells but also with elevated plasma TF concentrations [12]. In a more heterogeneous population with DIC, raised plasma levels of TF were found in only approximately 50% of patients, but these were predominately those with haematological solid tumours and leukaemias [13].

In addition to those patients with leukaemia who have raised TF at presentation, who are known to be at high risk of developing DIC early in the course of their admission, it might be possible to predict those at risk of DIC following the start

of chemotherapy. In a study looking at the TF activity of leukaemia cells in patients with newly diagnosed leukaemia, a group of patients had low TF activity, but this became elevated following the incubation of the leukaemia cells with endotoxin [14]. These patients subsequently developed DIC following the start of chemotherapy, whereas those patients with low TF activity, which failed to rise after endotoxin stimulation, did not go on to develop DIC. The induction of TF activity on leukaemia cells by incubation with endotoxin may be a useful predictor to patients at risk of developing DIC during chemotherapy.

The mechanism by which patients develop DIC at presentation is thought to result from high levels of TF expression on the leukaemia cells, with the subsequent release of TF into the circulation, leading to extrinsic pathway activation and thrombin generation. Following chemotherapy, cell lysis leads to further cytoplasmic release of TF and similarly induces DIC. Although DIC is a well-recognized feature of AML, in particular acute promyelocytic leukaemia and acute monocytic leukaemias, it has been perceived to be less of a clinical problem in ALL. However, some authors have suggested that this is not in fact the case, with DIC being detected in seven out of 58 patients with ALL before the initiation of chemotherapy and in 35 out of 45 patients during remission induction [15]. L-Asparaginase was not used during remission induction in this group of patients. As previously stated, leukaemia cells in ALL do have increased levels of TF expression, although not to the same degree as that in AML. Current evidence suggests that TF expression by leukaemia cells is likely to play an important role in the pathogenesis of DIC in patients with AML and, possibly, ALL.

Haemostatic defects in leukaemia

Platelets

Thrombocytopenia

The most frequent cause of haemorrhage in patients with leukaemia is secondary to thrombocytopenia. The causes are usually a result of leukaemic infiltration of the bone marrow or the myelosuppressive effects of cytotoxic chemotherapy. Rarely, thrombocytopenia may be autoimmune in nature following allogenic bone marrow transplantation (BMT). In this situation, bone marrow aspirate has plentiful megakaryocytes in association with a reduced platelet count.

Serious spontaneous bleeding is unlikely to occur at platelet counts above 30×10^9/l, whereas at platelet counts below 5×10^9/l significant increases in gastrointestinal blood loss can be demonstrated using ^{51}Cr-labelled red cells [16]. Prophylactic platelet transfusions are often given when the platelet count has fallen to between 10 and 20×10^9/l, the exact threshold varying between centres. At any platelet count the risk of bleeding is increased by fever, septicaemia, coagulation abnormalities, a rapidly falling platelet count and a high circulating blast count [17]. The concomitant administration of drugs should also be taken into account in deciding on the need for prophylactic platelet transfusion. Amphotericin B, commonly used to treat systemic fungal infection in neutropenic patients, has been shown to induce injury in stored platelets and could have *in vivo* effects on platelet function [18]. Beta-lactam antibiotics are known to cause platelet dysfunction associated with a prolonged bleeding time. An inhibitory effect on agonist-stimulated calcium influx in platelets can be shown to occur following exposure to these antibiotics [19].

Platelet function

Mucocutaneous bleeding with a normal platelet count, coagulation and fibrinolytic systems may indicate a defect in platelet function. Such abnormalities are most commonly observed in AML, myelodysplasia and myeloproliferative disorders, and are less common in the lymphoid leukaemias [20,21]. Acquired storage pool defects and, in particular, dense granule defects have been described. The possible causes may be either the presence of a factor which activates platelets, leading to discharge of the contents of their granules, or a chromosomal defect which results in the production of an abnormal protein critical to dense granule formation. Most authorities favour platelet activation as a cause of storage pool deficiency in leukaemia and myelodysplasia, and this view is supported by the fact that elevated levels of platelet alpha-granule proteins can be found in the plasma of these patients [22]. Further evidence comes from studies in patients transfused autologous platelets labelled with ^{14}C-serotonin (serotonin being taken up by dense granules), which had a shorter apparent half-life than those labelled with ^{51}Cr, suggesting that the platelets were activated *in vivo* and preferentially lost the contents of their dense granules [23]. Others workers have suggested that primary megakaryocyte abnormalities can lead to an inability to store platelet granules properly. Certainly dysplastic megakaryocytes are common in myelodysplasia and are not infrequently encountered in AML [24]. Circulating platelets also often have a bizarre morphology, which includes giant forms, decreased microtubules and reduced granulation. Evidence to support the fact that platelet dense granule deficiency may be related to chromosome defects comes from the report of a family with an inherited dense granule defect in which seven members of the family went on to develop leukaemia [25]. Cytogenetic studies were performed on two of the patients, one had monosomy 7 and the other had an extra G chromosome. The authors speculate that a chromosome alteration in the megakaryocyte cell line could affect genes involved in dense granule formation and also predispose to the development of leukaemia.

A variety of well-defined functional platelet abnormalities have been described in leukaemias, for example decreased aggregation to ADP or collagen, impaired nucleotide release and decreased thromboxane B_2 production [20,26]. The underlying biochemical abnormalities causing the disordered cell function mostly remain obscure. Also, some of the *in vitro* characteristics may in fact be caused by the presence of leukaemic cells contaminating the platelet preparations [27].

Another cause of acquired platelet function disorders is in association with paraproteinaemias. This occurs in approximately one-third of patients with IgA myeloma or Waldenström's macroglobulinaemia, in 15% of patients with IgG myeloma and, occasionally, in patients with benign monoclonal gammopathy [28]. A variety of defects may result, including a prolonged bleeding time, reduced platelet aggregation, granule secretion and abnormal procoagulant activity. Although in most cases the paraprotein inteferes with platelet function in a nonspecific manner, some specific abnormalities related to the paraprotein have been reported. These include an IgGκ myeloma protein, which was shown to bind to platelet membrane gpIIIa, causing an acquired thrombasthenia [29].

The treatment of patients with gross impairment in platelet function, who may bleed at relatively normal counts, is by platelet transfusion. In such individuals transfusions may have to be given prophylactically, as the platelet count may not be a good indicator of the haemorrhagic potential.

Acute promyelocytic leukaemia

Acute promyelocytic leukaemia (APL) is a distinct subtype of AML which is associated with a life-threatening haemorrhagic diathesis, the pathogenesis of which is incompletely understood.

The consistently observed coagulation abnormalities include thrombocytopenia, prolongation of the activated partial thromboplastin time (APTT) and thrombin time, minimal prolongation or normal prothrombin time (PT), raised fibrin degradation products (FDPs) and hypofibrinogenaemia [30]. Both DIC and primary fibrinolysis can give rise to this pattern of abnormality, with the thrombocytopenia being attributable to leukaemic infiltration of the bone marrow. There is controversy about which is the predominant mechanism, with a variety of evidence suggesting both DIC and fibrinolysis play a part in the coagulopathy associated with APL. The laboratory features of DIC with secondary fibrinolysis are compared and contrasted with those of primary fibrinolysis in Table 26.1.

Excessive fibrinolysis has been implicated, on the basis that patients with the coagulopathy have reduced levels of plasminogen and α_2 plasmin inhibitor, a protein that binds free plasmin in the circulation [31]. Also leukaemic promyelocytes have been shown to release plasminogen activators as well as elastases, which can inactivate α_2 plasmin inhibitors [32]. Raised levels of uPA and tPA have been found in the plasma of some patients with APL [33,34].

Using the HL60 APL cell lines, both high levels of procoagulant activity (PCA) and proteolytic activity have been found

Table 26.1 Comparison of laboratory features of disseminated intravascular coagulation (DIC) accompanied by secondary fibrinolysis with primary fibrinolysis.

	Fibrinogen	PT	APTT	ATIII	ATIII thrombin complexes	Plasminogen	α_2-Anti-plasmin	α_2-M	PAI-1	Plasmin α_2-antiplasmin complexes
DIC with secondary fibrinolysis	↓	↑	↑	↓	↑	↓	↓	↓	↓	↑
Primary fibrinolysis	N	N	N	N	—	↓	↓	N	↓	↑

α_2-M = macroglobulin; APTT = activated partial thromboplatin time; ATIII = antithrombin III; PAI-1 = plasminogen activator inhibitor; PT = prothrombin time.

[35]. When the cells were differentiated along monocytic or granulocytic lineages, there was a decrease in proteolytic activity and PCA respectively. This indicates that the maturation state of the promyelocyte is unique in exhibiting the combination of strong PCA and proteolytic activity. The proteolytic activity is thought to reside in the cell granules, where there are high concentrations of proteases which are capable of degrading fibrinogen, thus bringing about fibrinolysis [36]. The PCA of the promyelocytes may well be caused by TF. Earlier in the chapter it was suggested that the high levels of TF, and the subsequent release into the plasma of TF, are important events in the initiation of DIC. The PCA of the APL cells closely resembles TF, because it appears to activate coagulation through the extrinsic pathway [37]. APL cells have high levels of TF expression which would be consistent with the high incidence of coagulopathy among patients with APL.

Before the advent of all-*trans* retinoic acid (ATRA) treatment, the coagulopathy was treated with appropriate plasma product replacement, with some authorities advocating the use of heparin [38]. ATRA treatment for patients with APL and coagulopathy has been shown, in a number of studies, to lead to the rapid improvement of haemostatic parameters [39–41]. In the largest of these studies, the mean time to resolution of the coagulopathy was 4.2 days, with none of the patients dying of haemorhage [40]. One of the mechanisms by which ATRA may control DIC in APL is through its effects on TF and thrombomodulin expression on leukaemia cells. ATRA has been demonstrated to upregulate thrombomodulin expression and reduce TF expression in APL cell lines, thereby reducing the procoagulant activity of these cells — further evidence which suggests it is a valuable agent in the treatment and prevention of the coagulopathy associated with APL [42].

There have, however, been a number of reports of thromboembolic complications occurring among patients treated with ATRA [43,44]. The reason for this may be because of the persistence of procoagulant activity of the APL cells after treatment with ATRA. This was demonstrated in two patients who developed ATRA-induced hyperleukocytosis where rapid correction of fibrinogenolysis was contrasted with the persistence of procoagulant activity, thus predisposing to the development of thrombosis [45].

Haemostatic defects associated with multiple myeloma and paraproteinaemias

It has long been recognized that haemostatic abnormalities can be detected in patients with myeloma and Waldenström's macroglobulinaemia, and that there is a significant predisposition to bleeding as a consequence. The pathophysiology of the bleeding diathesis is usually multifactorial, however paraproteinaemia often plays an important role in its development. Causes other than paraproteinaemia include thrombocytopenia secondary to bone marrow infiltration or cytotoxic chemotherapy, renal failure and uraemic platelet dysfunction and DIC.

Paraproteins may intefere with normal haemostasis in a variety of ways. They can inhibit vWF, act as circulating anticoagulants or intefere with fibrin polymerization. Amyloid deposits, consisting of the light-chain fragments of immunoglobulin, can affect local tissue integrity and impair the normal vascular response to injury, thus preventing the control of haemorrhage. They may also reduce plasma factor X levels. Finally, paraproteins may intefere with platelet function, as previously described in this chapter (Table 26.2).

Acquired von Willebrand's (vWD) disease is known to occur in patients with myeloma, Waldenström's macroglobulinaemia, monoclonal gammopathy of unknown significance, hairy cell leukaemia, chronic lymphocytic leukaemia (CLL) and non-Hodgkin's lymphoma. The pattern of bleeding is similiar to that seen in congenital vWD, with mucosal-type bleeding such as epistaxis being common. Both types 1 and 2 vWD have been described [46,47]. There appear to be several mechanisms involved in the development of vWD; the majority are due to the increased clearance of vWF from the plasma with the normal release of vWF from platelet and endothelial stores. How this occurs could be a result of the interaction of the paraprotein with an epitope of the vWF molecule involved in its binding, thus inactivating it. Less commonly, the paraproteins may form immune complexes that nonspecifically bind to vWF, facilitating Fc-receptor-mediated clearance by phagocytes. The bleeding tendency associated with acquired vWD is variable, with many patients having no haemorrhagic manifestations. Treatment is usually directed at the underlying

Table 26.2 Causes of bleeding in patients with paraproteinaemias and associated conditions.

General
Thrombocytopenia
DIC
Renal failure

Secondary to the presence of a paraprotein
Acquired von Willebrand's disease
Amyloid tissue infiltration
Acquired factor X deficiency
Platelet function defects
Impaired fibrin polymerization
Acquired heparin sulphate anticoagulant

---

disorder which, if successful, will usually lead to resolution of the vWD. In patients with bleeding DDAVP, plasma exchange or IV immunoglobulin followed by vWF replacement with appropriate concentrates have been used and have been shown to be effective [48].

Amyloidosis complicates up to 10% of cases of myeloma. There is a high incidence of bleeding complications in these patients, including extensive bruising, gastrointestinal bleeding and bleeding from biopsy sites. Infiltration of tissues by amyloid leads to an increased fragility and affects the normal vascular response to injury. Amyloid can also lead to acquired coagulation protein deficiencies, most notably factor X deficiency [49]. The mechanism by which this arises is through the absorption of factor X onto the amyloid fibrils, which leads to a marked fall in its plasma half-life. The treatment of this acquired factor X deficiency is often problematical and control of the underlying myeloma does not necessarily lead to its resolution. In patients with extensive splenic involvment by amyloid, removal of the spleen may lead to a rise in factor X levels [50].

Impaired fibrin polymerization can result from the interference of circulating paraprotein and this can be a feature of both myeloma and Waldenström's macroglobulinaemia. The severity, in terms of risk of bleeding, is quite variable, with many patients having no haemorrhagic manifestations. If treatment is required then plasmapheresis, followed by the administration of fibrinogen concentrates, may be employed.

Rarely bleeding in patients with myeloma has been associated with the presence of a circulating heparin sulphate anticoagulant [51].

Thrombosis

Thrombosis in patients with acute leukaemia may occur in a number of different clinical settings. Individuals with DIC are at major risk of large vessel thrombosis. Bone marrow transplantation is associated with a number of conditions, which are characterized by vascular occlusion and thrombosis, and may itself represent a prothrombotic state. In the syndrome of hyperleucocytosis, patients are at increased risk of haemorrhage and thrombosis. Indwelling central venous catheters may act as a nidus for thrombus formation. L-Asparaginase used in the treatment of patients with ALL can lead to falls in the levels of natural anticoagulants, which in turn predisposes to thrombosis.

Is there a hypercoagulable state following bone marrow transplantation?

There are a number of thrombotic conditions which may occur early in the post-transplant procedure. These include pulmonary endothelial leak syndrome, bone marrow transplant-associated thrombotic microangiography (BMT-TM), venous thrombosis and hepatic veno-occlusive disease (VOD).

Although the aetiology of these conditions is probably multifactorial, investigators have examined various haemostatic parameters to determine if a procoagulant state is present following BMT. In one group of 30 patients undergoing allogenic and autologous BMT, no significant alterations were found in the levels of the natural anticoagulants (protein C and S, AT-III) or the fibrinolytic system (plasminogen, α_2 antiplasmin, tPA, PAI-1, D-dimers) following transplantation. However, significant elevations of plasma thrombin–antithrombin complex (TAT) and prothrombin fragments F1 + 2, sensitive markers of blood hypercoagulability, were found compared with normal controls [52]. They concluded that a hypercoagulable state did exist following BMT which was not related to an impairment of the anticoagulant or fibrinolytic system.

Other groups have, however, shown falls in the levels of natural anticoagulants post-BMT, particularly protein C [53,54]. In one study low levels of protein C and protein S post-BMT were accompanied by similar reductions in factors VII and IX [55]. It was inferred, from this study, that no overall procoagulant state existed and the changes were predominantly the result of hepatic dysfunction induced by chemo/radiotherapy. Another explanation for the high incidence of thrombotic changes following BMT is that endothelial cell activation leads to thrombogenic changes on the cell surface. Plasma levels of endothelium-derived proteins increase after high-dose cytoreductive therapy. Elevated levels of von Willebrand factor and thrombomodulin, which are both markers for endothelial activation, have been reported in patients undergoing BMT [56,57].

Hepatic veno-occlusive disease

Veno-occlusive disease is characterized by hepatomegaly, fluid retention and hyperbilirubinaemia, and occurs as a result of high-dose cytoreductive therapy. The initial sites of injury are believed to be the endothelium and hepatocytes in zone 3 of the liver acinus. Immunohistochemical studies of liver specimens from patients with VOD show deposition of factor

VIII and fibrinogen in the subendothelial zone of affected venules and sinusoids. The end result is obstruction to sinusoidal blood flow, sinusoidal hypertension and further hepatocyte injury.

The pathogenesis of VOD is not completely understood, but factors possibly involved in its development are changes in the procoagulant activity of plasma, as previously described, and circulating cytokines such as TNFα. This cytokine is known to promote procoagulant activity and suppress endothelial cell surface anticoagulant activity by blocking the protein C pathway through the suppression of thrombomodulin synthesis. In a study of 30 patients undergoing BMT, two individuals went on to develop VOD and they were found to have raised levels of TNFα before the onset of VOD [58]. Elevated TNFα levels at the time of preparation for BMT, and in the early transplant period, may be of value in predicting those patients who subsequently develop VOD.

Reported incidences vary from 0 to 70%, but experience from a large transplant centre gave an incidence of VOD of 53%, with an overall mortality of 15% [59]. Risk factors for the development of severe VOD include pretransplant hepatitis, certain intensive conditioning regimens, persistent fever during the pretransplant and early transplant period and mismatched or unrelated donor transplants. Diagnosis is usually established on clinical grounds using criteria proposed by the Seattle and Baltimore groups [60,61] (Table 26.3). The high risk of haemorrhage, particularly as patients are often platelet refractory, precludes the use of percutaneous liver biopsy, however transvenous liver biopsies are relatively safe and can be combined with the measurement of hepatic venous pressure measurements. They may be useful when the diagnosis is in doubt and consideration is being given to aggressive intervention with, for example, rtPA.

Prophylaxis of VOD has been attempted with a diversity of agents with variable success. Intravenous heparin infusions have been used and equivocal results have been reported [62,63]. Prostaglandin E$_1$ is a vasodilatory prostaglandin with mild antithrombotic activity. While an initial study gave some promising results, a phase I/II trial conducted in patients with a high risk of VOD was associated with an unacceptable level of toxicity and failed to demonstrate any benefit in terms of reduced development of VOD [64,65]. Ursodeoxycholic acid, a nonhuman bile acid, has been shown to reduce the incidence of VOD in a prospective randomized trial [66]. The mechanism of its action is unknown.

Treatment of VOD is usually directed at relieving the fluid accumulation caused by sodium retention while, at the same time, maintaining intravascular volume. This requires careful monitoring of fluid and electrolyte balance and judicious use of red cells and volume expanders to maintain the intravascular volume. Paracentesis may be required to relieve the respiratory embarrassment caused by tense ascites. Recombinant tissue plasminogen activator (rtPA) has been shown to be effective in the treatment of VOD, but its use has been associ-

Table 26.3 Clinical criteria for VOD diagnosis.

Baltimore criteria
Hyperbilirubinaemia greater than or equal to 34 μmol/l before day 21 after transplant and, at least, two of the following data:
    Hepatomegaly usually painful
    Ascites
    Weight gain greater than 5% from baseline

Modified Seattle criteria
Presence before day 14 after transplant of at least two of the following features:
    Bilirubin greater than or equal to 34 μmol/l
    Hepatomegaly and right upper quandrant pain
    Ascites and/or unexplained weight gain greater than 2%

ated with catastrophic haemorrhage [67]. A review of the outcome of using rtPA and heparin to treat 42 patients with VOD showed that an objective response was obtained in 12 patients (29%), as defined by a fall in bilirubin by 50% within 10 days of starting treatment. However, severe bleeding occurred in 10 patients and was clearly fatal in three of these. The authors of the review conclude that the benefits of using rtPA and heparin are unproven for the treatment of VOD, and its use should therefore be restricted to those with a high probability of fatal outcome from their VOD and who have no accompanying renal or pulmonary dysfunction [68].

Bone marrow transplant-associated thrombotic microangiopathy

Bone marrow transplant-associated thrombotic microangiopathy (BMT-TM) forms part of the spectrum of disease which includes haemolytic uraemic syndrome (HUS) and thrombotic thrombocytopenic purpura (TTP). It differs from the latter two conditions in that its development is usually multifactorial in origin and it is frequently refactory to therapy. The pathophysiology of all types of thrombotic microangiography is a combination of vascular endothelial damage, platelet aggregation and red cell fragmentation caused by microangiographic haemolysis. Bone marrow transplant-associated thrombotic microangiopathy is now a well recognized, although probably underdiagnosed, complication of BMT. Diagnosis may be difficult because many of the cardinal features of thrombotic microangiopathies, such as pyrexia, renal impairment and thrombocytopenia, are common sequelae following BMT. The presence of red cell fragmentation is a valuable indicator of the development of BMT-TM. The incidence of the disease varies from series to series, but overall it is reported as 6.8% [69]. It occurs more commonly following allogeneic BMT as compared with autologous transplant. The mortality rates are also variable, reflecting the varying severity of this condition, but it is reported as 23% overall. Many of the survivors will go on to develop chronic and progressive renal impairment.

The pathogenesis of BMT-TM, as previously stated, is multi-factorial and includes vascular endothelial damage, platelet activation and changes in coagulation proteins which promote thrombogenesis. These changes are caused by a combination of circumstances that exist following BMT, which includes the use of cyclosporin A, alterations in coagulation proteins favouring a prothrombotic state, GVHD, TBI and sepsis. Cyclosporin A has a number of effects which predispose to the development of BMT-TM. It can directly damage the endothelium, and the increased capillary permeability which has been demonstrated following BMT has been attributed to this effect [70]. This may even culminate in a 'capillary leak' syndrome. In addition, cyclosporin has been linked with a number of alterations in coagulation proteins and increased platelet aggregabilty, all of which favour thrombogenesis. BMT itself appears to induce a hypercoagulable state as a result of changes in the coagulation proteins, as discussed in a previous section. In acute GVHD, allogeneic T-lymphocytes become activated through recognition of nonself HLA molecules in the recipient, leading to their production of interferon gamma (IFNγ). The IFNγ causes activation of monocytes, which in turn produce IL-1 and TNF. These cytokines induce endothelial cells to express tissue factor, as do the monocytes. High levels of tissue factor, in combination with the endothelial damage caused by cyclosporin A, provide a suitable environment in which thrombotic microangiopathy may develop. Total body irradiation (TBI) is known to cause radiation nephritis. The pathogenesis of this condition is of endothelial cell damage and death, vasoconstriction and decreased production of prostacyclin by endothelial cells, and it therefore has many parallels with BMT-TM [71]. It is likely therefore that TBI, when used as transplant conditioning, can predispose to the subsequent occurrence of BMT-TM. Infection is also an important factor in the development of BMT-TM and often the most fulminant forms of the disease occur in a septic patient. Childhood haemolytic uraemic syndrome is caused by verotoxin-producing *E. coli*. The verotoxin is capable of directly damaging the endothelium, thus initiating the thrombotic microangiopathic process. In the post-transplant period, infection with organisms that similarly cause endothelial damage may also predispose to BMT-TM. Active CMV infection can stimulate the development of BMT-TM, as it is often associated with a worsening severity GVHD with its attendant endothelial damage and tissue factor expression.

The management of BMT-TM is currently unsatisfactory, with no universally effective therapy available. A variety of different therapeutic approaches have been tried and those with no proven benefit include antiplatelet drugs such as aspirin and dipyridamole, heparin, corticosteroids and other immunosuppresive drugs, and prostacyclin. Some cases of BMT-TM which arise primarily as a result of cyclosporin A, respond to reduction or withdrawal of this drug. This is less likely to be effective in the more fulminant multifactorial form, but nonetheless cyclosporin A should still be stopped and alternative immuosuppresion given if required. Unlike classical TTP where plasma exchange with fresh-frozen plasma is effective in the majority of cases, with remissions frequently being durable, in BMT-TTP response rates are only about 50% and relapse is common. This encouraged some investigators to try a different approach, whereby plasma exchange with cryosupernatant is alternated on a daily basis with protein A immunoadsorption over a 2-week period. This regimen in 13 patients with severe BMT-TM lead to a response, as judged by a fall in LDH and a reduction in the proportion of fragmented red cells on a blood film, in 62%. Five of the responders remained alive at a median follow-up of 90 days (range 21–464). All the nonresponders died of multiorgan failure within a short period of time following the development of BMT-TM [72]. The investigators suggest that this therapeutic approach should be subjected to a randomized clinical trial.

Hyperleucocytosis

Hyperleucocytosis, which may be arbitrarily defined as a white cell count greater than $100 \times 10^9/l$, occurs in 20–25% of patients with AML, particularly in FAB subtypes M5:AML and M4:AML [73]. Its presence is associated with the development of leucostasis in the lung, central nervous system (CNS) and/or gastrointestinal tract. Symptoms of leucostasis in the brain include headaches and blurred vision and intracranial haemorrhage may result. Disturbance of the circulation to the sensory organs may result in blurring of vision, diplopia, retinal haemorrhages, tinnitus and deafness. Slowing in the pulmonary circulation causes tachypnoea, dyspnoea, cyanosis and pulmonary infiltrates.

The symptoms of hyperviscosity arise from a variety of causes, including occlusion of small vessels by large numbers of leucocytes, some of which aggregate into clumps. Endothelial damage, as well as tissue invasion and high oxygen consumption, increase the risk of thrombosis and tissue hypoxia [74].

Hyperleucocytosis is associated with a less favourable prognosis because of its association with CNS haemorrhage, CNS involvement and a higher relapse rate [75]. Management entails prompt recognition of the syndrome as a medical emergency and instituting immediate therapy to reduce the white cell count. Therapeutic options to decrease the white cell count include leucapheresis, large doses of hydroxyurea and/or induction chemotherapy. Early cranial irradiation has been recommended for children who are too small to have leucapheresis or for adults with severe CNS manifestations. Red cell transfusions should be minimized initially because of the risk of increasing blood viscosity. Platelet transfusions are however often required to decrease the risk of haemorrhage, especially when leucapheresis is used, as this will tend to exacerbate thrombocytopenia. Although there are no controlled trials to indicate optimal management of this syndrome, most authorities recommend leucapheresis if symptoms of leucostasis are present.

Treatment should also include measures to prevent the development of the tumour lysis syndrome, such as maintaining adequate hydration, alkalinizing the urine and giving allopurinol.

Asparaginase

L-Asparaginase is a highly effective chemotherapeutic agent used in the treatment of ALL. Its use is associated with a number of serious side effects, which include an increased risk of thromboembolic events. The reported incidence of these varies from 1 to 14%, but the true incidence is likely to be higher, as a large number of clinically asymptomatic but clinical significant thromboembolic events are probably unnoticed [76]. The development of thromboembolism is closely related to the administration of asparaginase, with the overwhelming majority of cases occurring either during or immediately after treatment. The main site for thromboembolism is in the CNS, with 67% of events occurring there; deep vein thrombosis and pulmonary embolism comprise 16%, with the remaining 17% being variously distributed and including intravenous catheter-associated thrombosis [76].

The increased incidence of thrombosis is related to a number of factors. Asparaginase causes a complex coagulopathy associated with deficiencies of many anticoagulant proteins, but particularly protein C, protein S, plasminogen and AT-III. Levels of AT-III are markedly reduced and are similar or lower than those found in congenital AT-III deficiency. Congenital AT-III is known to be associated with an increased risk of thrombosis. Why AT-III should be affected more than other coagulation proteins is not clear. It is probably a result of a combination of reduced protein synthesis and increased utilization for thrombin inhibition.

Other factors also contribute to the development of thromboembolism. There is evidence for increased thrombin generation (raised F1 + 2, TATs) during the first few months of treatment for ALL. The fall in plasma coagulation proteins caused by asparaginase does not appear to interfere with this ability to generate thrombin. A hypercoagulable state, in combination with low levels of AT-III, therefore predisposes these patients to the development of thromboembolic complications.

AT-III concentrates have been used in an attempt to prevent the asparaginase-induced coagulopathy. In 25 patients undergoing treatment for ALL, AT-III concentrates were administered for 10 days from the beginning of asparaginase therapy. AT-III levels were maintained at supranormal levels and there was no increase in the markers of hypercoagulability [77]. The authors conclude that AT-III supplementation could prevent the associated coagulopathy and thus prevent the development of thromboembolic complications. The small numbers involved in this study are, however, insufficient to allow definite clinical benefit to be seen in terms of a reduction in thromboembolic events, and larger numbers would be needed to demonstrate that this occurs.

Thrombosis associated with indwelling central venous catheters

Indwelling central venous catheters are commonly used in patients being treated for leukaemia. They avoid the problems of phlebitis induced by vesicant chemotherapy given into peripheral veins and allow simultaneous administration of various therapeutic agents, including antibiotics and blood products. In certain treatments, such as during BMT, they are virtually indispensable. However their use is associated with complications. The two main complications are infections and thrombosis, and both may be linked. Following insertion of a central venous catheter it quickly becomes engulfed by a fibrin sheath which can promote adherence of staphylococcal and *Candida* species [78]. Staphylococci produce coagulase enzymes which could promote thrombogenesis and enhance further their ability to adhere to catheters. Clinical thrombosis leading to catheter removal is about 10%. In a large series where all catheters were inserted by a single surgeon, thrombosis necessitating removal was associated with large-bore, i.e. triple-lumen, catheters and with tip placement above the level of T3 [79]. However, subclincal thrombosis is much more common and when catheters have been prospectively screened radiographically, in the absence of the clinical evidence of thrombosis, the rates of thrombosis have been found to be higher. Fifty-seven patients with central venous catheters were screened by phlebography and incomplete thrombosis was detected in 26 (45.5%) and complete thrombosis in six (10.5%) [80]. If the clinical consequences of the thrombosis are just occlusion of the catheter, with no evidence of major venous obstruction and in the absence of catheter sepsis, then an attempt can be made to dissolve the clot by instilling urokinase down the catheter. A 10 000 unit bolus of urokinase, repeated if necessary, will restore catheter function in around 60% of cases. Because of the inconvenience of replacing occluded catheters, rtPA has been used, in a lower dose than is normally employed to treat major thrombosis, to try to restore catheter function. In a randomized trial comparing 10 000 units urokinase with 2 mg rtPA, catheter function was restored in 59 and 89% of episodes of catheter thrombosis respectively [81]. However, rtPA is an expensive drug and a 20-mg vial is the lowest commercially available dosage, thus most of the drug is wasted. The cost may be partly offset by saving on the expense and inconvenience entailed in catheter removal and replacement. In additon to just occlusion, catheter thrombosis may be more extensive. Major thrombosis can occur in the veins in which the catheter is inserted, leading to a superior vena caval syndrome or to the obstruction of the subclavian or brachiocephalic veins. The management of these episodes usually entails removal of the catheter and administration of heparin to prevent extension of the thrombus or embolization. Treatment is often complicated by the fact that patients are thrombocytopenic or have preexisting coagulation abnormalities. rtPA has been used as thrombolysis in the treatment of the superior vena caval syndrome and is effective. However, even when given in a reduced dose, it can be associated with severe haemorrhage in some individuals [82].

Because of the relatively high incidence of thrombosis associated with indwelling catheter use, prophylaxis has been attempted. Therapeutic warfarinization maintaining the INR at between 2 and 3 would be problematical in patients undergoing intensive chemotherapy. Low-dose warfarin at a dose of 1 mg daily has therefore been tried. At this dose no prolongation of prothrombin time or reduction in the levels of the vitamin K-dependent coagulation factors are obtained. However, patients receiving low-dose warfarin do have a reduced incidence of catheter vein thrombosis, as detected by venography [83]. Therefore there may be a useful role for low-dose warfarin as prophlaxis against central venous catheter thrombosis.

References

1 Osterud B. & Rapaport S.I. (1977) Activation of factor IX by the reaction product of tissue factor and factor VII. *Proceedings of the National Academy of Sciences USA*, **74**, 5260–5264.

2 Carson S.D. & Brozna J.P. (1993) The role of tissue factor in the production of thrombin. *Blood Coagulation and Fibrinolysis*, **4**, 281–292.

3 Andree H.A.M. & Nemerson Y. (1995) Tissue factor: regulation of activity by flow and phospholipid surfaces. *Blood Coagulation and Fibrinolysis*, **6**, 189–197.

4 Triplett D.A. (1984) The extrinsic system. *Clinics in Laboratory Medicine*, **4**, 221–244.

5 Brinkmann T., Kahnert H., Prohaska W., Nordfang O. & Kleesiek K. (1994) Synthesis of tissue factor pathway inhibitor in human synovial cells and chondrocytes makes joints the predilected site of bleeding in haemophiliacs. *European Journal of Clinical Chemistry and Clinical Biochemistry*, **32**, 313–317.

6 Gailani D. & Broze G.J. Jr (1991) Factor XI activation in a revised model of blood coagulation. *Science*, **253**, 909–912.

7 Lindahl A.K., Sandset P.M. & Abildgaard U. (1992) The present status of tissue factor pathway inhibitor. *Blood Coagulation and Fibrinolysis*, **3**, 439–449.

8 Schleef R.R., Higgins D.L., Pillemer E. & Levitt L.J. (1989) Bleeding diathesis due to decreased functional activity of type 1 plasminogen activator inhibitor. *Journal of Clinical Investigation*, **83**, 1747–1752.

9 Fleck R.A., Rao L.V.M., Rapaport S.I. & Nissi V. (1990) Localisation of human tissue factor antigen by immunostaining with monospecific, polyclonal anti-human tissue factor antibody. *Thrombosis Research*, **57**, 765–781.

10 Muller-Berghaus G. (1989) Pathophysiologic and biochemical events in disseminated intravascular coagulation: dysregulation of procoagulant and anticoagulant pathways. *Seminars in Thrombosis and Haemostasis*, **15**, 58–87.

11 Tanaka M. & Yaminishi H. (1992) The expression of tissue factor antigen and activity on the surface of leukaemia cells. *Leukaemia Research*, **17**, 103–111.

12 Kubota T., Andoh K., Sadakata H., Tanaka H. & Kobayashi N. (1991) Tissue factor released from leukaemia cells. *Thrombosis and Haemostasis*, **65**, 59–63.

13 Takahashi H., Satoh N., Wada K., Takakuwa E., Seki Y. & Shibata A. (1994) Tissue factor in plasma of patients with disseminated intravascular coagulation. *American Journal of Haematology*, **46**, 333–337.

14 Naitoh M., Andoh K., Sadakata H., Tanaka H. & Kobayashi N. (1994) Prediction of disseminated intravascular coagulation in patients with leukaemia. *Internal Medicine*, **33**, 131–135.

15 Sarris A.H., Kempin S., Berman E. *et al.* (1992) High incidence of disseminated intravascular coagulation during remission induction of adult patients with acute lymphoblastic leukaemia. *Blood*, **79**, 1305–1310.

16 Slichter S.J. & Harker L.A. (1978) Thrombocytopenia: mechanisms and management of defects in platelet production. *Clinical Haematology*, **7**, 523–531.

17 Gaydos L.A., Freireich E.J. & Mantel N. (1962) The quantitative relation between platelet count and haemorrhage in patients with acute leukaemia. *New England Journal of Medicine*, **266**, 905–909.

18 McGrath K., Bertram J.F., Houghton S., Boothman J., Manderson J.A. & Minchinton R. (1992) Amphotericin-B induced injury in stored platelets. *Transfusion*, **32**, 46–80.

19 Burroughs S.F. & Johnson G.J. (1993) Beta-lactam antibiotics inhibit agonist stimulated platelet calcium influx. *Thrombosis and Haemostasis*, **69**, 503–508.

20 Cowan D.H., Graham R.C. Jr & Baunach D. (1975) The platelet defect in leukaemia. Platelet ultrastructure, adenine nucleotide metabolism, and the release reaction. *Journal of Clinical Investigation*, **56**, 188–200.

21 Pui C.H., Kackson C.W. & Chesney C. (1991) Normal platelet function after therapy for acute lymphocytic leukaemia. *Archives of Internal Medicine*, **143**, 73–74.

22 Najean Y., Poirier O. & Lokiec F. (1983) The clinical significance of beta-thromboglobulin and platelet factor-4 in polycythaemic patients. *Scandinavian Journal of Haematology*, **31**, 298–304.

23 Malpass T.W., Savage B., Hanson S.R., Slichter S.J. & Harker L.A. (1984) Correlation between bleeding time and depletion of platelet dense granule ADP in patients with myelodysplastic myeloproliferative disorders. *Journal of Laboratory and Clinical Medicine*, **103**, 894–904.

24 Wong K.F. & Cham J.K.C. (1991) Are dysplastic and hypogranular megakaryocytes specific markers for the myelodysplastic syndrome? *British Journal of Haematology*, **77**, 509–514.

25 Gerrard J.M. & McNicol A. (1992) Platelet storage pool deficiency, leukaemia, and myelodysplastic syndromes. *Leukaemia and Lymphoma*, **8**, 277–281.

26 Woodcock B.E., Cooper P.C., Brown P.R., Pickering C., Winfield D.A. & Preston F.E. (1984) The platelet defect in acute myeloid leukaemia. *Journal of Clinical Pathology*, **37**, 1339–1342.

27 Zawilska K., Komarnicki M., Trepinska E., Sokolowski K. & Wysocki K. (1991) The effect of isolated leukaemic blasts on platelet aggregation. *Haemostasis*, **10**, 233–244.

28 Lackner H. (1973) Haemostatic abnormalities associated with dysproteinaemias. *Seminars in Haematology*, **10**, 125–133.

29 DiMinno G., Coraggio F., Cerbone A.M. *et al.* (1986) A myeloma paraprotein with specificity for platelet glycoprotein IIIa in a patient with a fatal bleeding disorder. *Journal of Clinical Investigation*, **77**, 157–164.

30 Rand J.J., Moloney W.D. & Sise H.S. (1969) Coagulation defects in acute promyelocytic leukaemia. *Archives of Internal Medicine*, **123**, 39–47.

31 Kahle L.H., Avvisati G., Lampling R.J., Moretti T., Mandelli F. & Cate J.W. (1985) Turnover of α_2 antiplasmin in patients with acute promyelocytic leukaemia. *Scandinavian Journal of Clinical and Laboratory Investigation*, **45**(Suppl. 178), 75–80.

32 Velasco F., Torres A., Andres P., Martinez F. & Gomez P. (1984) Changes in the plasma levels of protease and fibrinolytic inhibitors induced by treatment of acute myeloid leukaemia. *Thrombosis and Haemostasis*, **52**, 81–84.

33 Bennett B., Booth N.A., Croll A. & Dawson A.A. (1989) The bleeding disorder in acute promyelocytic leukaemia: fibrinolysis due to u-PA rather than defibrination. *British Journal of Haematology*, **71**, 511–517.

34 Wilson E.L., Jacobs P. & Dowdle E.B. (1983) The secretion of plasminogen activators by human myeloid leukaemic cells *in vitro*. *Blood*, **61**, 568–574.

35 Wijermans P.W., Rebel V.I., Ossenkoppele G.J., Huijgens P.C. & Langenhuijsen M.M.A.C. (1989) Combined procoagulant activity and proteolytic activity of acute promyelocytic leukaemia cells: reversal of the bleeding disorder by cell differentiation. *Blood*, **73**, 800–805.

36 Ohlsson K. & Olsson I. (1974) The neutral proteases of human granulocytes. Isolation and partial characterisation of granulocyte elastase. *European Journal of Biochemistry*, **42**, 519–527.

37 Gralnick H.R. & Abrell E. (1973) Studies of the procoagulant and fibrinolytic activity of promyelocytes in acute promyelocytic leukaemia. *British Journal of Haematology*, **24**, 89–99.

38 Hoyle C.F., Swirsky D.M., Freedman L. & Hayhoe F.G.J. (1988) Beneficial effect of heparin in the management of patients with APL. *British Journal of Haematology*, **68**, 283–289.

39 Huang M.E., Ye Y.C. & Chen S.R. (1988) Use of all-*trans* retinoic acid in the treatment of acute promyelocytic leukaemia. *Blood*, **72**, 567–572.

40 Chen X., Xue Y., Zhang R. *et al.* (1991) A clinical and experimental study on all-*trans* retinoic acid treated acute promyelocytic leukaemia patients. *Blood*, **78**, 1413–1419.

41 Kawai Y., Watanabe K., Kizaki M. *et al.* (1994) Rapid improvement of coagulopathy by all-*trans* retinoic acid in acute promyelocytic leukaemia. *American Journal of Haematology*, **46**, 184–188.

42 Koyoma T., Hirosawa S., Kawamata N., Tohda S. & Aoki N. (1994) All-*trans* retinoic acid upregulates thrombomodulin and downregulates tissue factor expression in acute promyelocytic leukaemia cells: distinct expression of thrombomodulin and tissue factor in human leukaemia cells. *Blood*, **84**, 3001–3009.

43 Runde V., Aul C., Heyll A. & Schneider W. (1992) All-*trans* retinoic acid: not only a differentiating agent, but also an inducer of thromboembolic events in patients with M_3 leukaemia. *Blood*, **79**, 534–535.

44 Brouns M.C., Deloughery T.C. & Nichols M.J. (1994) Fatal thrombosis complicating all *trans* retinoic acid (ATRA) therapy in acute promyelocytic leukaemia (APL). *Blood*, **84**(Suppl), 616.

45 Dombret H., Scrobohaci M.L., Zini J.M., Daniel M.T., Castaigne S. & Degos L. (1993) Coagulation disorders associated with acute promyelocytic leukaemia; corrective effect of all-*trans* retinoic acid treatment. *Leukaemia*, **7**, 2–9.

46 Goudemand J., Samor B., Caron C., Jude B., Gosset D. & Mazurier C. (1988) Acquired type II von Willebrand's disease: demonstration of a complexed inhibitor of the von Willebrand factor–platelet interaction and response to treatment. *British Journal of Haematology*, **68**, 277–283.

47 Meyer D., Frommel D., Larrieu M.J. & Zimmerman T.S. (1979) Selective absence of large forms of factor VIII/von Willebrand factor in acquired von Willebrand's syndrome. Response to transfusion. *Blood*, **54**, 600–606.

48 Glaspy J.A. (1992) Haemostatic abnormalities in multiple myeloma and related disorders. *Haematology-Oncology Clinics of North America*, **6**, 1301–1314.

49 Furie B., Greene E. & Furie B.C. (1977) Syndrome of acquired factor X deficiency and systemic amyloidosis: *in vivo* studies of the metabolic fate of factor X. *New England Journal of Medicine*, **297**, 81–85.

50 Greipp P.R., Kyle R.A. & Walter Bowie E.J. (1979) Factor X deficiency in primary amyloidosis: resolution after splenectomy. *New England Journal of Medicine*, **301**, 1050–1051.

51 Palmer R.N., Rick M.E., Rick P.D., Zeller J.A. & Gralnick H.R. (1984) Circulating heparin sulphate anticoagulant in a patient with a fatal bleeding disorder. *New England Journal of Medicine*, **310**, 1696–1699.

52 Catani L., Gugliotta L., Mattioli Belmonte M. *et al.* (1993) Hypercoagulability in patients undergoing autologous or allogeneic BMT for haematological malignancies. *Bone Marrow Transplantation*, **12**, 253–259.

53 Gordon B., Haire W., Kessinger A., Duggan M. & Armitage J. (1991) High frequency of antithrombin III and protein C deficiency following autologous bone marrow transplantation for lymphoma. *Bone Marrow Transplantation*, **8**, 497–502.

54 Harper P.L., Jarvis J., Jennings I., Luddington R. & Marcus R.E. (1990) Changes in natural anticoagulants following bone marrow transplantation. *Bone Marrow Transplantation*, **5**, 39–42.

55 Collins P., Roderick A., O'Brein D. *et al.* (1994) Factor VIIa and other haemostatic variables following bone marrow transplantation. *Thrombosis and Haemostasis*, **72**, 28–32.

56 Collins P., Gutteridge C., O'Driscoll A. *et al.* (1992) Von Willebrand factor as a marker of endothelial cell activation following bone marrow transplantation. *Bone Marrow Transplantation*, **10**, 499–506.

57 Bearman S.I., Lefkowitz J.B., Mones R.B., Shpall E.J. & Stemmer S.M. (1993) Thrombomodulin increases in patients receiving high dose chemotherapy with autologous progenitor cell support. *Blood*, **82**(Suppl.), 614.

58 Gugliotta L., Catani L., Vianelli N. *et al.* (1994) High plasma levels of tumour necrosis factor-α may be predictive of veno-occlusive disease in bone marrow transplantation. *Blood*, **83**, 2385–2386.

59 McDonald G.B., Hinds M.S., Fisher L.D. *et al.* (1993) Venocclusive disease of the liver and multi-organ failure following marrow transplantation: a cohort study of 355 patients. *Annals of Internal Medicine*, **118**, 255–267.

60 Jones R.J., Lee K.S., Beschorner W.E. *et al.* (1987) Venocclusive disease of the liver following bone marrow transplantation. *Transplantation*, **44**, 778–783.

61 McDonald G.B., Sharma P., Matthews D.E., Shulman H.M. & Thomas D.E. (1984) Venocclusive disease of the liver after bone marrow transplantation: diagnosis, incidence and predisposing factors. *Hepatology*, **4**, 116–122.

62 Attal M., Huguet F., Rubie H. *et al.* (1992) Prevention of hepatic veno-occlusive disease after bone marrow transplantation by continuous infusion of low-dose heparin: a prospective randomized trial. *Blood*, **79**, 2834–2840.

63 Bearman S.I., Hinds M.S., Wolford J.L. *et al.* (1990) A pilot study of continuous infusion heparin for the prevention of hepatic veno-occlusive disease after bone marrow transplantation. *Bone Marrow Transplantation*, **5**, 407–411.

64 Gluckman E., Jolivet I., Scrobohaci M.L. *et al.* (1990) Use of prostaglandin E₁ for prevention of liver veno-occlusive disease in leukaemic patients treated by allogenic bone marrow transplantation. *British Journal of Haematology*, **74**, 277–281.

65 Bearman S.I., Shen D.D., Hinds M.S., Hill H.A. & McDonald G.B. (1993) A phase I/II study of prostaglandin E₁ for the prevention of hepatic venocclusive disease after bone marrow transplantation. *British Journal of Haematology*, **84**, 724–730.

66 Essell J., Schroeder M., Thompson J., Harman G., Halvorson R. & Callander N. (1994) A randomised double-blind trial of prophylactic ursodeoxycholic acid vs placebo to prevent venocclusive disease of the liver on patients undergoing allogenic bone marrow transplantation. *Blood*, **84**(Suppl.), 250.

67 Bearman S.I., Shuhart M.C., Hinds M.S. & McDonald G.B. (1992) Recombinant human tissue plasminogen activator for the treatment of established severe venocclusive disease of the liver after bone marrow transplantation. *Blood*, **80**, 2458–2462.

68 Bearman S.I., Lee J.L., Barón A.E. & MacDonald G.B. (1997) Treatment of hepatic venocclusive disease with recombinant human tissue plasminogen activator and heparin in 42 marrow transplant patients. *Blood*, **89**, 1501–1506.

69 Pettitt A.R. & Clark R.E. (1994) Thrombotic microangiopathy following bone marrow transplantation. *Bone Marrow Transplantation*, **14**, 495–504.

70 Peters A.M., Vassilarou D.S., Hows J.M. & Ballardie F.W. (1991) Bone marrow transplantation: effects of conditioning and cyclosporin prophylaxis on microvascular permeability to a small solute (technetium-99m diethylene triamine penta-acetic acid). *European Journal of Nuclear Medicine*, **18**, 199–202.

71 Chappell M.E., Keeling D.M., Prentice H.G. & Sweny P. (1988) Haemolytic uraemic syndrome after bone marrow transplantation: an adverse effect of total body irradiation? *Bone Marrow Transplantation*, **3**, 339–347.

72 Zeigler Z.R., Shadduck R.K., Nath R. & Andrews D.F. (1996) Pilot study of combined cryosupernatant and protein A immunoadsorption exchange in the treatment of grade 3–4 bone marrow transplant-associated thrombotic microangiopathy. *Bone Marrow Transplantation*, **17**, 81–86.

73 Bunin N.J. & Pui C. (1985). Differing complications of hyperleukocytosis in children with acute lymphoblastic or acute non-lymphoblastic leukaemia. *Journal of Clinical Oncology*, **3**, 1590–1595.

74 Lichtman M.A. & Rowe J.M. (1982) Hyperleukocytic leukaemias: rheological, clinical and therapeutic considerations. *Blood*, **60**, 280–283.

75 Dutcher J.P., Schiffer C.A. & Wiernik P.H. (1987) Hyperleukocytosis in adult nonlymphocytic leukaemia: impact on remission rate and duration and survival. *Journal of Clinical Oncology*, **5**, 1364–1372.

76 Andrew M., Brooker L. & Mitchell L. (1994) Acquired antithrombin III deficiency secondary to asparaginase therapy in childhood acute lymphoblastic leukaemia. *Blood Coagulation and Fibrinolysis*, **5**(Suppl.), 24–36.

77 Mazzucconi M.G., Gugliotta L., Leone G. *et al.* (1994) Antithrombin III infusion suppresses the hypercoagulable state in adult acute lymphoblastic leukaemia patients treated with a low dose of *Escherichia coli* L-asparaginase. *Blood Coagulation and Fibrinolysis*, **5**, 23–28.

78 Raad I.I., Luna M., Khalil S.A.M., Costerton J.W., Lam C. & Bodey G.P. (1994) The relationship between the thrombotic and infectious complications of central venous catheters. *Journal of the American Medical Association*, **271**, 1014–1016.

79 Eastridge B.J. & Lefor A.T. (1995) Complications of indwelling venous access devices in cancer patients. *Journal of Clinical Oncology*, **13**, 233–238.

80 Balestreri L., De Cicco M., Matovic M., Coran F. & Morassut S. (1995) Central venous catheter-related thrombosis in clinically asymptomatic oncological patients: a phlebographic study. *European Journal of Radiology*, **20**, 108–111.

81 Haire W.D., Atkinson J.B., Stephens L.C. & Kotulak G.D. (1994) Urokinase versus recombinant tissue plasminogen activator in thrombosed central venous catheters: a double-blinded, randomized trial. *Thrombosis and Haemostasis*, **72**, 543–547.

82 Rodenhuis S., van't Hek L.G.F.M., Vlasveld L.T., Kroger R., Dubbleman R. & van Tol R.G.L. (1993) Central venous catheter associated thrombosis of major veins: thrombolytic treatment with recombinant tissue plasminogen activator. *Thorax*, **48**, 558–559.

83 Bern M.M., Lokich J.J., Wallach S.R. *et al.* (1990) Very low doses of warfarin can prevent thrombosis in central venous catheters. *Annals of Internal Medicine*, **112**, 423–428.

27 Design of Clinical Trials

H.S. Cuckle

Introduction

This chapter provides a practical guide for those intending to carry out randomized clinical trials of therapeutic regimens for haematological malignancies. It should also be useful reading for those who wish to enhance their critical appreciation of the published results of leukaemia trials, as many of the pitfalls associated with trial design and analysis are discussed. Nonetheless, this is not a complete account of trial design and method of statistical analysis. The interested reader might refer to one of several reviews on the subject [1–6].

Knowledge of specific statistical tests is not assumed, and whenever possible technical statistical terms are avoided. However, two technicalities are unavoidable: these are the 'power' of a study and the 'level of significance'. One way of understanding these notions is as the analogue of the true-positive rate and the false-positive rate, respectively, of a biochemical test. Carrying out a study is rather like performing a test and the power of the study is the probability of it demonstrating an effect when one truly exists (compare finding a positive test result when the patient has the disease being tested for). The level of significance is the probability of the study demonstrating an effect when one does not in fact exist (compare finding a positive test result when the patient does not have the disease being screened for).

Just as an increase in a test's true-positive rate can only be achieved at the expense of increasing its false-positive rate, so for a given trial size, power is a function of level of significance.

Trial design

Regimens

The choice of which regimen to test in a trial is of course largely dependent on the results of pilot studies and clinical considerations. However, there are also statistical factors that need to be considered. These mainly relate to the maximization of statistical power.

A trial which compares two regimens will in general be more powerful than where three are being compared. An exception to this is when the three regimens are effectively different intensities of a single regimen and the extent of intensity can be quantified; for example, when three multidrug regimens differ only by the addition of one of the drugs in varying amounts. Such a trial maintains its power by testing for a dose–response relationship rather than comparing the arms of the trial singly. When three completely different regimens are to be compared, power might still be maintained by adopting a factorial design which is described in more detail below.

When an intensive regimen is being compared with a less intensive one, maximum power would be ensured by making the former as intensive as is possible, consistent with acceptable toxicity. Sometimes two multidrug regimens may appear to differ in intensity, but on closer examination they do so only under certain untested assumptions; for example, that an increase in the number of fractions in which a drug is given will increase the effective dose. It is worthwhile considering in advance how such a trial will be interpreted if it does not demonstrate an effect, and ensuring that this cannot be attributed to there being little difference in the actual regimens which are being compared.

When a multicentre study is undertaken, the number of different clinicians who will be administering treatments can be quite large. This can tend to increase disagreement at the design stage about the optimal treatment and a compromise regimen may be tested as a result, rather than the one which will maximize statistical power.

Endpoints

Ultimately, the efficacy of a regimen must be measured by its ability to alter some endpoint. The simplest endpoint to study is death, because it is not open to subjective interpretation. However, while the event of death will not be doubted in an individual trial patient, the cause of death might. For this reason, when conducting trials in diseases such as acute leukaemia in adults, where most deaths will be a result of the disease, it is better to compare total mortality in the different regimens rather than just leukaemia mortality. In other diseases the 'dilution effect' of including all deaths might be so great that a separate analysis may be necessary.

Other endpoints such as remission, relapse or blast crisis are inevitably subjective to some extent. It may be possible, in some trials, to make special arrangements designed to avoid the possibility of bias in establishing the endpoints. For example, a 'blind' review of records, in at least a sample of cases, could be considered. Such procedures will not, however, deal with bias which is built into the protocol itself. This might occur if two regimens being compared require a marrow biopsy at the end of each treatment cycle, but one regimen has short cycles and the other long cycles. In that case the former will be able to establish remission earlier and artefactually produce longer durations of remission.

Number of patients

The statistician, when asked the seemingly simple question of how many patients are needed in the trial which compares a new with an existing regimen, invariably replies by posing a string of questions. What is the mortality rate (or rate of other endpoints) using the current regimen? By what percentage would you expect the rate to be reduced using the new regimen? How great a risk are you willing to accept for the trial to produce a spuriously positive finding (i.e. what will the level of significance be)? Or a spuriously negative finding (what will the power be)?

The first question is not usually difficult to answer. The last two questions are conventionally answered by 5 and 80% respectively. Roughly, to increase the level of significance to 1% requires a doubling of the trial size, and to reduce the power to 50%, would require only half the trial size.

The second question presents greater difficulties. How can it be answered objectively before the trial has been carried out? Perhaps the results of pilot studies might be used to estimate the benefit of the new regimen, but this argument is circular. If the pilot study was unbiased enough to estimate the extent of benefit then there is no need to carry out the trial. In practice, whether consciously or not a slightly different question is often substituted: how large would the benefit need to be before it was considered medically useful (i.e. the trial result would change medical practice)? It is natural to suppose that such benefits are large but this is unrealistic. In fact, most medical advances have been relatively small and, despite that, they are useful as part of the process of improving treatment. Several small advances, if independent, can be concatenated with a resultant dramatic change overall. The tendency for medical advances to be modest is further compounded by the fact that regimens which are overwhelmingly better than current practice will be obviously so in the pilot stages of development. Such regimens are unlikely to be tested in randomized trials. Thus it is prudent to assume that the benefit in the trial will be small. The trial organizers may need to convince their colleagues to change practice when even a modest benefit is found, provided it is not associated with more toxicity than current regimens.

Once the four questions above have been answered and the statistician has estimated the numbers required, the trial organizers will need to be realistic about their ability to recruit that many patients. It is probably advisable for them to aim for a considerably greater rate of recruitment than needed, in the expectation that this will not be completely fulfilled. If it is, then the trial will end sooner.

Multicentre trials

The number of patients needed to test the efficacy of potentially moderately beneficial regimens is so great that a single centre alone would only accumulate that number over many years, by which time the efficacy may have been established by others. In normal practice a clinician will have experienced improvement in therapy when they have only been tried on a small series of his or her patients. While this experience will be counterbalanced by the many times apparent improvement has not been sustained, this will have been less memorable than when it was sustained.

Not only is the single-centre small trial low in power, it also has a high chance of showing an apparent improvement when there is none. False-negative results from individual centres represent a waste of time and resources, but this is a less unfortunate outcome than even a single false-positive. The latter may generate considerable further investigation in an attempt to replicate the results. While it is sometimes possible to pool the results of small trials in a 'meta-analysis' (see below) and reach an unambiguous conclusion, this is not always the case. Moreover, a cooperative attempt to launch a multicentre trial initially would have led to an earlier answer.

Naturally, the organizational difficulties of multicentre trials are greater than single-centre trials. In the UK it is fortunate that there is an infrastructure to facilitate collaboration in leukaemia trials within the Medical Research Council. As well as providing facilities for collaborators to meet in the planning, execution and analysis phases of the trial, it provides a central statistical office.

Apart from the organizational difficulties, it is often felt that there is some statistical loss in aggregating data from many centres, some of which are specialist referral centres in teaching hospitals, others having less experience in treating haematological malignancies. This is not necessarily the case, and provided the randomization procedure is designed so that no centre is over-represented in those treated with any one of the regimens, then the result will not be biased. Moreover, the technique of retrospective stratification can remove between-centre variability as a source of random error, and so maintain the trial's power. Indeed, it could be argued that since leukaemias and lymphomas are treated in a diverse range of centres, only a trial which is representative of that range will produce a reliable estimate of the practical benefits of the therapy.

The need for randomization

The need for random allocation of treatment arises because the potential benefits of new regimens are likely to be small. The need is even greater if the new treatment is a modified version of an existing regimen. Such new treatments are sometimes evaluated not by randomization but, instead, by switching over at a particular time from the routine use of some standard protocol to the routine use of that same protocol plus the new treatment (historically controlled trials). The idea is that the new treatment can be assessed by comparing the outcome of the more recent patients with that of the earlier patients. However, any apparent benefit of the new treatment might be due to an underlying trend for improved outcome, even with existing treatments. This might result from, possibly unnoticed, changes in the extent and quality of supportive care or in the extent of compliance with the treatment protocol.

Evaluation of a new treatment by comparing the patient outcome at centres that have elected to use it routinely with that at other centres (geographical controls) is presumably also potentially misleading, because the same factors which can bring about differences in outcome over time are also likely to operate between centres. Thus, both forms of nonrandomized evaluation appear to contain potential biases that may be of the same order of magnitude as the type of moderate effect one might reasonably hope to discover.

Methods of randomization

The mechanics of generating random allocations are straightforward, a random number table being the usual one employed, but a pocket calculator can also be used. However, the questions of who does it and when, as well as whether and how the randomization should be stratified, are important considerations.

There is little point in allowing blind chance to play a part in treatment allocation if it is not seen to be doing so. For this reason, the act of randomization is best done by someone who is unconnected with the individual patient, certainly not by the doctor who is treating the patient. Ideally, a list of treatments in random order should be kept by a third party who is telephoned with the patient details and then reveals the next allocation on the list. This can lead to problems outside of normal office hours, and those responsible for carrying out the randomization might need to make special arrangements for this time.

When donor transplantation of, say, a bone marrow is being considered as a treatment option, a form of randomization not involving a list of allocations is possible as the consideration of whether or not the donated marrow is compatible is effectively a random event. For example, each potential marrow transplant patient, with his or her potential sibling donor, could be registered in a trial. Then tissue typing would be done and those who had a compatible sibling would have been effectively randomized to have a transplant and the rest to avoid it.

The timing of the allocation is best done immediately before treatment begins. However, that might be some time after presentation, for example when regimens for maintenance are being compared, and in that case it might be more acceptable both for the patient and the clinician to know at the time of presentation what treatment is to be used if and when remission is achieved. Provided remission can be established in an unbiased manner, then patients could be randomized at presentation and only included in the trial if they remit.

Random allocation should select groups of patients who have the same prior prognosis. But the play of chance could lead to imbalance with the allocation of, say, older patients to one group rather than the other. If the trial is large enough imbalance is unlikely and can be corrected for by retrospective stratification (see below). It can be avoided in smaller trials by having separate random lists of treatments for each age group, or for any other major prognostic factor, thus creating automatic balance. Provided that the prognostic information required for this 'stratified' randomization is readily available at the time of entry to the trial, there is little lost in doing this, even for large trials.

Factorial design

Even if a considerable proportion of newly diagnosed leukaemia patients were to enter a national trial of some new treatment, it would still be some years before its efficacy could be established. Therefore, only a limited number of new treatment options can ever be tested, using the conventional trial design. While simple trial designs are to be recommended, where two or more treatments can be administered concurrently, the so-called factorial design allows them all to be tested at once without increasing the trial size.

As an example, two new treatment modifications to some standard regimen, A and B, which can be administered separately or together or not at all, will be considered. The patients are allocated at random into four groups representing all the possible combinations:

		Treatment B	
		Present	Absent
Treatment A	Present	Group 1	Group 2
	Absent	Group 3	Group 4

Groups 1 and 2 can be combined and compared with groups 3 and 4 combined to evaluate treatment A. Similarly, groups 1 and 3 combined compared with groups 2 and 4 combined will evaluate B. In addition, where appropriate, it is possible to investigate whether the use of A and B together is more effective than A alone or B alone, although this aspect of the study will have a relatively low power.

The use of a factorial design to test more than one new treatment without loss of power is subject to the assumption that the treatments have different modes of action. In other words, the effect of A should be expected to be the same in the presence of B as when B is not administered; and the same for B in relation to A. While this will not, in general, be known in advance of the trial, provided that treatments which are different enough are considered any interaction will be minimal.

Exclusion rules

General rules which exclude from the trial patients who might be difficult to follow up (e.g. foreign residents) or those who have been previously treated for the disease will increase statistical power overall, provided that not too many patients are involved. However, the adoption of an upper age limit for eligibility needs careful consideration, as it will limit the numbers of patients in the trial. The fear that the regimen may not be as effective in older patients does not necessitate such a rule. Indeed, the only way to establish an interaction between age and efficacy is to allow older patients entry into the trial and to analyse their results separately.

Stopping rules

Consideration should be given in advance as to when the trial results are to be analysed. The power calculations will have been based on achieving a certain number of endpoint events (e.g. deaths).

In most trials the principle endpoints occur only after all the patients have been entered. Sometimes, however, one of the treatments is more effective than anticipated and sufficient patient data accumulate to answer the principle question before all the intended patients have been entered into the trial. Therefore, it would seem sensible to perform repeated early analyses of the trial, stopping entry as soon as a statistically significant result arises, and thus avoiding having to allocate patients an inferior treatment unnecessarily. This is the group sequential design [5]. It must be stressed that the interim analyses should be planned before the trial starts, so that advice can be sought about statistical defects of repeated significance testing. The number of analyses is usually restricted, because the number of significance tests increases the probability of at least one incorrect result occurring by chance. In other words the level of significance increases [7]. This is particularly obvious at the beginning of a trial, when chance imbalances between the outcomes in the small number of patients on each treatment can easily occur and be reversed as more data accumulate. In order to maintain the overall level of significance, more stringent levels of significance must be adopted for each individual significance test.

A more sophisticated method of repeat analysis can be adopted, in which the results are monitored constantly [8]. In practice, such a design has serious disadvantages, and the group sequential designs are more favoured.

Whatever approach is taken, there is usually some pressure to analyse the results early. The trial should be as short as possible, in order to avoid the results being overtaken by new potential developments in treatment derived from pilot studies. However, there is also a danger that the desire for an early end to the trial will lead to misleading conclusions being drawn.

Data collection

It is advisable to keep the amount of information collected in a trial to a minimum, particularly if it is a multicentre trial. The following are sufficient: (i) patient identification; (ii) treatment allocation; (iii) date of allocation; (iv) presence or absence of the endpoint. The full name and date of birth will usually uniquely identify a patient. In the UK, for the purpose of determining an individual's vital status using the National Health Service (NHS) Central Register, it is preferable, but not necessary, to also know the NHS number. For a small per capita fee, patients in the trial can be 'flagged' on the Central Register so that in the event of them dying a copy of the death certificate is automatically forwarded to the investigator. Permission to do this must be obtained from the British Medical Association Ethics Committee. In acute leukaemia a proportion of patients will die in the first few weeks of the trial, so it may be best to flag only those who are still alive at the first follow-up enquiry. If the endpoint is other than death, then the establishment of its presence or absence may itself require considerable collection of data. For example, 'blast crisis' in the study of chronic granulocytic leukaemia might require the collection of complete patient charts so that an independent panel could review them and decide if, and when, it had occurred.

The collection of information on known prognostic factors measured at the time of presentation may increase statistical power. By taking into account predictable variations in prognosis, there is more chance of the experimentally controlled factor, the treatment difference, being demonstrable. This data might also be of value in identifying subgroups of particularly high-risk or low-risk patients who react differently to the regimen. In some cases a regimen may have little effect among patients as a whole but it may have a large benefit in a particular subgroup.

Another reason for collecting information on prognostic factors at presentation is the chance of imbalance between the two regimens with respect to the factors. This can then be adjusted for in the statistical analysis.

In the treatment of individual patients, examination of the charts and indeed the whole patient record may be of prognostic value. However, when whole series of such charts are collected in a randomized trial, it is difficult to know how to analyse the data statistically. The problems of assessing completeness and verification of data are likely to outweigh any extra information gained on the efficacy of treatment. A more appropriate way of analysing such data might be outside the context of a clinical trial.

It is often assumed that detailed information should be collected on the extent of compliance with the regimen. However, this is primarily of interest only if the trial fails to show a difference between the treatments. Provided that the information is available retrospectively, it might be best to collect compliance data if the trial result indicates this. If the trial does show a difference between treatments and it is still felt desirable to describe the compliance rate, then inspecting a small sample of records may be sufficient.

Trial forms

The careful design of forms can help to avoid the considerable effort required during progress of the trial to obtain missing information or in the clarification of ambiguous results. Simplicity should be aimed for, provided this does not lead to errors.

For example the instruction on a form to circle 'YES' if a specific factor is present is prone to error, because it assumes that an uncircled 'YES' means that the factor is not present, whereas there is the possibility that the question was overlooked. A better instruction would be to circle 'YES', NO' or 'DON'T KNOW' as appropriate. Where numerical data are being collected, providing a separate box for each digit will lead to fewer errors than allowing the results to be written on a dotted line.

It is worthwhile trying out all the study forms on a pilot basis before the trial begins, preferably with colleagues who do not know the details of the trial, especially as some of the forms may well be completed by junior doctors who may be in a similar position.

Printing forms on copy paper which does not require carbon can save time and reduces the reliance on breakdown-prone photocopiers. Although such paper is costly, compared with the total costs of the trial the expense will be relatively small.

Keeping a register

There are advantages to instituting a system in participating hospitals for registering with the trial every newly diagnosed patient with the type of haematological malignancy being studied, even though some would not actually be entered into the trial. The main function is to be able to describe in the trial report how the patients entering the trial differ from those who were eligible but were not entered. This may influence the interpretation of trial results. A further useful consequence of collecting eligibility data for such a register is that fewer patients are liable to be left out of the trial by default.

Economic analysis

In the NHS there is now increasing pressure to make explicit the financial costs of new technologies and treatments. Those designing clinical trials might want to consider assessing costs as an integral part of the trial. Such investigations are particularly important when one of the treatments being compared is likely to cost much more than standard practice. However, this might not be straightforward. For example, the circumstances of the trial may mean that costs are greater than they would be in routine clinical practice. The Department of Health has produced a guide for those wishing to undertake an economic analysis as part of a trial [9].

Ethics committees

In a multicentre trial it is necessary to seek approval from every local ethics committee where patients may be treated. This will inevitably introduce a delayed start for some centres. The same protocol may be approved almost without discussion by one committee and judged to be severely flawed by another. There will then be a protracted period of discussion, possibly ending with the protocol being amended.

While there are no general rules guaranteeing an easy passage through this process, care should be taken that certain broad ethical principles have been adhered to. Clearly, the study must be technically sound in so far as it should be capable of giving an unambiguous answer to a clinically important question. The prime necessary condition which justifies the randomization of patients between different treatments is the 'null hypothesis', i.e. that there is no reason to believe that one is more effective than the other. In such a state of 'equipoise', the patient has nothing to lose in agreeing to enter the trial, and may gain if allocated a new treatment which turns out to be superior. Even if the null hypothesis is confirmed, simply being in the trial may, of itself, confer some psychological benefit to participants and future patients will benefit from the trial result.

Randomized trials are now so widespread in medicine that this principle has become almost self evident. Unfortunately, closer examination of it reveals greater ethical complexity than is usually appreciated [10]. For example, there are two kinds of equipoise, namely a balance of preference between two treatments by individual clinicians and a balance within the profession as a whole, or an expert subgroup ('collective equipoise'). There can be collective equipoise even when each clinician has a strong preference, with half favouring one treatment and the rest favouring the second treatment. In these circumstances some clinicians would still want to enter a patient into the trial because of a contribution to the 'greater good'. Indeed some have argued that collective norms should take precedence, as they do in issues of medical negligence. There is a conflict of interest here between the welfare of future and present patients, and it is debatable whether it is ethically acceptable to trade-off between the two. Moreover, patient–doctor trust could be jeopardized by so doing.

Another problem is that the null hypothesis is a one-dimensional statement referring to better or worse prognosis. In practice there are other dimensions, such as the side effects and financial costs. A small benefit in terms of prognosis may be offset by insuperable costs or severe adverse side effects. Individual patients may differ in their judgement about whether the side effects are worth enduring for the potential benefits. To allow for this, 'preference' trials can be conducted, where the patient has the choice of either one of the competing treatments or entry into a randomized trial.

Analysis of results

Exclusions and reallocations

A fundamental principle of clinical trial analysis is that patients should not be excluded from the analysis once randomized, neither should they be reallocated to a different arm of the trial. This more than any other aspect of the trial is likely to be misunderstood, for example when a proportion of those randomly allocated to a particular treatment do not actually receive it.

Common sense would suggest that these patients are excluded from the statistical analysis. Moreover, if some of them actually received the other trial treatment then the temptation might be to put them in the other arm of the trial in the analysis. Nonetheless, in both cases this action might lead to an erroneous trial result as a result of selection bias. Consider a trial in which a more intensive regimen is being compared with a less intensive one. In such a trial patients who are randomized to the intensive regimen, but are judged to be unable to tolerate the treatment and are reallocated to the less intensive one, will tend to be a selected group of patients who are so unwell as to have a relatively poor prognosis; thus, removing them from the intensive group will yield an apparent improvement in results for this group and transferring them to the other group will further increase the difference in outcome between the groups by worsening prognoses for the less intensive regimen. These biases are avoided by leaving patients in their original groups in the statistical analyses, regardless of the treatment they actually received.

Another way of describing the principle is 'analysis by intention to treat'. It can be argued that this not only avoids bias but, more correctly, approximates to normal practice, so that any improvements in prognosis observed in the trial will reflect what can be expected when the regimen comes into more general use. In spite of this, some would argue that the trial is not designed to answer this practical question but rather the theoretical questions of which treatment can *in principle* provide better results. Once that is known, it is argued, the treatment can then be refined to make it more practical for routine use. That may be so, but if many withdrawals and reallocations of treatment are made in the analysis, the trial will effectively revert to a nonrandomized comparison, raising the question whether the magnitude of the bias introduced is small in comparison with the observed difference in outcome between the treatments.

There are situations where exclusions after randomization can be made without bias, for example when the patient has been entered in error because of failure to fulfil some entry criteria. Provided individuals are excluded systematically by checking the entry criteria of all patients, this is acceptable. To be absolutely sure that there is no bias, the data necessary to judge whether a person is eligible should have been collected before randomization was made. Another example in leukaemia trials concerns patients entered into a trial of AML, say, who are subsequently found to have ALL. It is difficult to see how withdrawal from the trial would lead to bias and inclusion in the trial appears absurd. Again, if histopathological material was collected before randomization, then a systematic check of all patients can be made with appropriate exclusions.

Lifetables and survival curves

The simplest way to present the trial results is in the form of the probability of attaining the endpoint after varying time intervals, either in tabular or graphical form. If no patient is lost to follow-up and the analysis is restricted to the follow-up period of the last patient to enter the trial, this probability is simply the observed percentage of patients who have actually survived. Such a restriction is obviously wasteful of information and so methods have been devised to use all the data. The Kaplan–Meier method, a simple technique frequently used in clinical trials [11], takes the probability of surviving to a given day of the trial and multiplies it by the observed survival rate for that day among those patients who have been followed long enough. The series of multiplications carry on until the follow-up time of the patient who has been in the trial the longest is reached. As this time is approached in the analysis, the estimate of the daily survival rate will be less accurate. A single death in the few patients contributing to the estimate at an extended time interval can cause the survival rate to fall dramatically and this should be remembered when looking at survival curves.

Log rank test and Cox's proportional hazards model

Once a survival curve has been constructed for each group of patients, a method of comparing the curves is required. The simplest method is the log rank test, which is essentially a chi-square test for comparing the observed deaths in the groups with the numbers of deaths that would be expected on the assumption that the treatments are equally effective [12].

The log rank test can be adapted to take into account the effect of qualitative prognostic factors (e.g. performance status) on the treatments for each value of the factor, and combining these to form a single chi-square. The result compares the treatments allowing for this factor. If the prognostic factor is quantitative, the values can be grouped and treated similarly to a qualitative factor. Alternatively, each individual value can be taken into account using Cox's proportional hazard model

[13], which is rather like a multiple regression analysis with survival as the dependent variable. The use of the Cox model will reduce possible bias caused by the investigator grouping the factor in different ways until one which shows a treatment difference is found. However, like all statistical models, it has the disadvantage of basing the result on assumptions which may not be testable in the study itself.

Prognostic factors

If a factor which is a strong determinant of prognosis can be measured at the time of recruitment to a trial, then statistical methods are available to compare the treatments among individuals with similar values of this factor (a stratum). As mentioned above, this stratification serves many purposes. Firstly, it will redress any chance imbalance between the groups allocated to each regimen with respect of the factor. Secondly, it will reduce, to some extent, the 'noise' of factors other than the treatment which determine prognosis and will allow the treatment effect to emerge.

As well as considering single prognostic factors by themselves, they can be combined to define groups of patients with an even more extreme *a priori* prognosis. Major prognostic factors are often highly correlated, but insofar as they are not completely correlated their combination will produce more information than each alone.

Because of systematic differences between different series of patients, a definition of prognostic groups appropriate to one series may not apply so well to another. Even in the absence of such systematic differences, prognostic groups which have been constructed to fit the results from one study will, in general, provide less strong discrimination when applied to another. This is because they will have been made to fit the chance features of that particular series as well as the real ones. This effect is especially true when information on several factors is combined to define the prognostic groups. The smaller the number of factors needed to define prognostic groupings in a particular series of patients, the more robust these groupings are likely to be when used in other series, although even the relationship of single variables to prognosis is sometimes only moderately reproducible from one series to another.

Retrospective stratification can also be used to see if one of the regimens is effective in some subgroup of patients but not in others. However, there is need for caution in such analyses, unless there is some *a priori* reason to expect such a specific treatment effect. As mentioned above in connection with sequential analysis, the laws of statistics are such that if several analyses are done there is an increased probability of obtaining a statistically significant result, even when no differences exist. It is probably safest to avoid looking at subgroups in this way unless the overall effect of treatment interpretation is statistically strongly significant. An overall marginal treatment effect can easily, by chance, produce an apparent strong effect in favour of one treatment in some subgroup and the opposite effect in the remaining patients.

Interpretation of results

Familiarity with new treatments

A not uncommon situation in clinical trials is that the current widely used regimen is compared with a radically different one. This can present a problem, because the clinicians using the new treatment may have had no experience with it before the trial. This of itself might render the potential advantages of the new regimen ineffective. Indeed, it could even produce much worse results than the old treatment, even when it was intrinsically better. One way of overcoming this might be to have a period during which centres familiarize themselves with the new treatment by accepting patients for it but not entering them into the trial. Another solution would be to begin randomization immediately but to exclude the first ten or so patients from each centre in the statistical analysis.

Applicability of results

As trials often take place in specialist centres among groups of patients partly selected by the eligibility criteria in the protocol and also in ways less easy to define, it is reasonable to suppose that the trial results may not apply generally. Insofar as the trial aims to show that one regimen yields a better prognosis than another, this should not be of concern. However, one of the trial aims will be to determine *how much* better the new regimen is, and this will be determined by patient selection. The analysis of prognostic factors measured at presentation will allow some quantification of any interactions between such factors and treatment effects. However, other factors leading to patient selection, or indeed other aspects of treatment not being tested, will not be so well defined and the interactions will remain unknown.

Comparison with other series

Sometimes when a trial demonstrates improved prognosis for a new treatment over standard practice the magnitude of the effect is compared with that obtained in trials of other treatment regimens. However, such comparisons are no more valid than historically or geographically controlled studies. If the outcome is similar for the common standard treatment arm of the trials that may lend some weight to the comparison, but even then the possibility of bias cannot be excluded.

The situation is somewhat different when trials of the same new treatment are being compared. It is important to set the observed results of any study in the context of other similar publications and, increasingly, this is being done by carrying out a formal meta-analysis. As mentioned above, this method of combining trials can be used to draw meaningful conclusions from a set of studies which are individually too small. This has been done, for example, in adjuvant tamoxifen and chemotherapy for breast cancer [14], for antiplatelet treatment [15], beta-blockers after myocardial infarction [16] and vitamin E in the prevention of retinopathy in very low birth weight infants [17]. Even when a trial of sufficient power yields a statistically significant result, this may still be a result of the chance allocation of better-prognosis patients to one of the arms. The possibility of the result being a false-positive will be reduced if a meta-analysis is carried out for all trials of the same treatment.

Meta-analysis can be done in one of two ways. The first approach involves examination of the published reports of the individual studies. Where possible an odds ratio is estimated for each usually quantifying the extent to which the mortality rate is reduced given the new treatment. The odds ratios are then averaged across the trials after appropriate weighting according to the number of events (e.g. deaths) in each trial. The second approach is to pool all the raw data and analyse them as though each trial is a different strata of the same study. This is often difficult to achieve in practice. With both approaches the validity of the analysis depends on the similarity in design of the individual trials which can be tested formally. If there is statistically significant heterogeneity, one or more of the trials may need to be excluded. The credibility of a meta-analysis rests on its completeness and so it is important to only exclude trials if there is a strong reason to do so and to make the reason explicit. Another possible pitfall arises from a publication bias, such that there is less chance of getting a study published if it does not indicate that a new treatment is beneficial. Every effort should be made to discover unpublished studies when carrying out a meta-analysis.

Conclusion

When only moderate treatment effects are expected, large collaborative randomized clinical trials are needed. Provided certain safeguards are taken, simple statistical methods are available to derive a valid conclusion from these trials. There might sometimes be difficulties of interpretation, but these are no greater than for nonrandomized trials, which are, in addition, associated with the possibility of severe bias.

References

1 Peto R., Pike M.C., Armitage P. *et al.* (1976) Design and analysis of randomised clinical trials requiring prolonged observation of each patient. *British Journal of Cancer*, **34**, 585; **35**, 1.

2 Schwartz D., Flamant R. & Lellouch J. (1980) *Clinical Trials.* Academic Press, London.

3 Friedman L.M., Furberg C.D. & DeMets D.L. (1980) *Fundamentals of Clinical Trials.* John Wright, Boston.

4 Gore S.M. & Altman D.G. (1982) *Statistics in Practice.* British Medical Association, London.

5 Pocock S.J. (1983) *Clinical Trials, A Practical Approach.* John Wiley, Chichester.

6 Kay H.E.M. (1983) Planning and comparisons in clinical trials. *British Journal of Cancer*, **47**, 315–318.

7 McPherson K. (1974) Statistics: the problem of examining accumulating data more than once. *New England Journal of Medicine*, **289**, 501–502.

8 Armitage P. (1975) *Sequential Medical Trials.* Blackwell Scientific Publications, Oxford.

9 Drummond M. (1994) *Economic Analysis Alongside Controlled Trials.* Department of Health, London.

10 Lilford R.J & Jackson J. (1995) Equipoise and the ethics of randomisation. *Journal of the Royal Society of Medicine*, **88**, 552–554.

11 Kaplan E.L. & Meier P. (1958) Nonparametric estimation from incomplete observations. *Journal of the American Statistical Association*, **53**, 457–481.

12 Peto R. & Peto J. (1972) Asymptotically efficient rank invariant test procedures. *Journal of the Royal Statistical Society*, A, **135**, 185–206.

13 Cox D.R. (1972) Regression models and life tables (with discussion). *Journal of the Royal Statistical Society*, B, **34**, 187–202.

14 Early Breast Cancer Trialists' Collaborative Group (1992) Systemic treatment of early breast cancer by hormonal, cyto-toxic or immune therapy 133 randomized trials involving 31 000 recurrences and 24 000 deaths among 75 000 women. *Lancet*, **339**, 1–15, 71–85.

15 Antiplatelet Trialists' Collaboration (1988) Secondary prevention of vascular disease by prolonged antiplatelet treatment. *British Medical Journal*, **296**, 320–331.

16 Yusof S., Peto R., Lewis J. *et al.* (1984) Beta-blockade during and after myocardial infarction: an overview of the randomized trials. *Progress in Cardio-vascular Disease*, **27**, 335–371.

17 Law MR, Wijewardene K. & Wald N.J. (1990) Is routine vitamin E administration justified in very low-birthweight infants? *Developmental Medicine and Child Neurology*, **32**, 442–450.

28 Gene Transfer in Leukaemia and Related Disorders

M.K. Brenner

Introduction

The concept of using somatic cell gene transfer to express a new gene in the somatic cells of an individual has excited fervid interest, speculation and hyperbole. The inevitable backlash against promises that are far from being fulfilled has led to considerable confusion about the current aims and achievements of gene transfer. There is a lurking suspicion that the entire field is simply a 'South Sea Bubble' waiting to burst. Hence, this chapter will attempt to provide a balanced account of the current status of gene transfer as applied to leukaemia and related disorders and to review the accomplishments of the field and the impediments to progress. Most importantly, it will try to give an idea of the incremental way in which gene transfer technologies will supplement, long before they supplant, current therapeutic approaches to hamatological malignancy.

Gene transfer to haemopoietic stem cells

Leukaemic cells derive ultimately from haemopoietic stem cells (HSC), so that many therapeutic approaches to haematological malignancy will, ultimately, have to target these cells. There is widespread interest in the HSC as a target for gene transfer, even outside the field of haematological malignancy, because inherited and acquired genetic disorders of a wide variety of cell types originating from marrow could be corrected by stem cell modification. Moreover, the cells are readily obtained and returned to the host and, in principle, the return of a single-gene-modified stem cell could repopulate an entire patient for life. However, at present the HSC is an elusive target. It has not been phenotypically defined and there are no *ex vivo* assays to establish its function. Hence, it is impossible to discern whether or not a stem cell has been transduced or to determine the likely effects of the transferred gene without returning the putatively transduced stem cell to the patient. This is a matter of some concern. Without knowing the efficiency of transfer or of gene expression, it is impossible to assess the likely benefits of a therapy. Because no

gene transfer protocol can be devoid of risks (as discussed below), this means the risk:benefit ratio is unsatisfactory. Therefore, for pragmatic reasons, most clinical protocols using gene transfer for haematological malignancy have focused on the modification of committed cells, in which it is possible to validate the efficiency of the process. However, as our techniques for gene transfer improve and as our knowledge of the biology of the HSC increases, it is likely that the ability of these cells to provide long-lived repopulation of the patient will make them the favoured targets for many of the strategies to be described.

Applications of gene transfer to the therapy of haematological malignancy

To date, four major strategies have been adopted for incorporating gene transfer into the therapy of leukaemia and lymphoma.
1 Modifying the tumour cell itself, by one of the following: (i) 'repairing' one or more of the genetic defects associated with the malignant process; (ii) introducing a gene that will trigger an antitumour immune response; (iii) delivering a pro-drug metabolizing enzyme that will render the tumour sensitive to the corresponding cytotoxic agent.
2 Modifying the immune response to the tumour, by altering the specificity or effector function of immune system cells.
3 Decreasing the sensitivity of normal host tissue by delivering cytotoxic drug-resistance genes to marrow precursor cells and thereby increasing the therapeutic index of cytotoxic agents.
4 Marking normal and malignant haemopoietic cells, to more closely monitor the efficacy of conventional therapies.

Of these approaches, 1 and 2 target committed cells, 3 targets the HSC and 4 targets committed cells and the HSC as well.

Limitations of current vectors

The limitations of current gene-transfer techniques represent a major constraint on any of the strategic approaches for gene therapy of haematological malignancies, as outlined above. Only four classes of gene transfer vectors have entered clinical study to date, retroviruses [1–4], adenoviruses [5,6], adeno-associated virus [7,8] and liposomes [9]. All have severe limitations.

Retrovirus vectors

Figure 28.1(a) shows the structure of a classical retrovirus vector [10]. The structural and replicative genes (*gag*, *pol* and *env*) of a murine retrovirus are replaced by one or more genes of interest, driven either by the retroviral promoter in the 5' long terminal repeat (LTR) or by an internal promoter. The retroviral constructs are made in cell lines in which the missing retrovirus genes are present *in trans*, and thus reproduce and

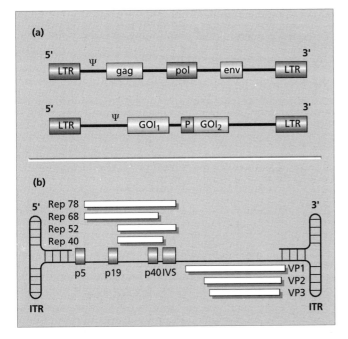

Fig. 28.1 (a) Retrovirus and retrovirus vector. The gag (reverse transcriptase), polymerase and envelope coding sequences are removed, and supplied in trans by a producer cell. One or more genes of interest (GOI) are inserted, driven from the viral long terminal repeat (LTR) promoter or from an internal promoter (P). The viral packaging signal (ψ) remains in the vector, so that it is appropriately packaged by the producer cell. (b) Structure of adeno-associated vector (AAV). The AAV genome is a linear single-stranded DNA molecule. The viral genome is transcribed in three overlapping regions, producing seven primary transcripts. The transcripts obtained from each gene are shown as black lines. The virus has two palindromic inverted terminal repeats (ITR) which, in combination with products of the rep region, are responsible for site-specific integration. The rep products are also required for replication during coinfection with adenovirus. VP1-3 encode the viral capsid proteins. Promoter regions for these genes are boxed (p5, p19, p40, IVS).

package a vector that is not replication competent. Retrovirus vectors have a wide target cell range, and the genetic information they convey is integrated into the host cell DNA. Thus, the transferred gene not only survives for the entire life span of the transduced cell, but is also present in that cell's progeny. Hence, these vectors are ideal for transferring genes into a rapidly dividing cell population (e.g. gene marking of tumour cells or lymphocytes), or for gene therapy in which HSC are the intended target. Provided that replication-competent virus is absent, the vector preparations appear to be nontoxic. However, retroviral vectors have several disadvantages. Expression of the transferred gene requires integration, which occurs only in dividing cells. Hence, the efficiency of transfer to many cell types may be low [3]. Further, because the integration events themselves occur at largely random sites in the host cell DNA, regulatory genes could conceivably be damaged, contributing to later oncogenesis [11]. Finally, retrovirus vectors are not well suited for use *in vivo* [12], because they are generally unstable in primate complement and cannot be targeted to specific cell types.

Adenovirus vectors

Most adenovirus vectors are E1 (early protein) deletion mutants and therefore are not replication competent [5,6]. Early genes in the E3 region may also be deleted to increase the 'space' for new genes to be inserted [6]. Adenoviruses also infect a wide range of cell types and, unlike retrovirus vectors, can transfer genes into nondividing cells. The vectors are reasonably stable *in vivo* and can be used to infect cells *in situ*. Examples include gene transfer into respiratory epithelium (the CFTR gene in cystic fibrosis [6]) or liver (factors VIII and IX for haemophilia A or B [13]). However, adenovirus vectors are generally nonintegrating, so that the gene products are expressed from episomal DNA [5]. The episome is often lost after cell division and can be inactivated or lost even in a non-dividing cell [13]. Thus, adenovirus vectors are unsuited to any application that requires long-term expression in a short-lived cell population, or transfer into a stem cell and expression in that cell's progeny. Another limitation is that most adenovirus vectors are immunogenic. Immune responses are generated against the vector proteins themselves, and often prevent readministration of the vector — an obvious strategy for overcoming the transient nature of adenovirus-mediated gene transfer. More significantly, cellular and humoral immune responses may be generated against low levels of adenovirus proteins expressed even when cells are transduced by defective viruses [13]. In addition, the entry of adenoviruses into many cell types will trigger release of cytokines such as IL-8, which recruit a nonspecific, but potentially highly destructive, local inflammatory response [14]. While these immunostimulatory attributes of adenoviruses may render them inherently unsuited to chronic application in diseases such as haemophilia A or B, they may be an asset when the intent is to prepare a tumour vaccine (see below), emphasizing the importance of matching vector characteristics to intended use. Aside from issues of immunostimulation, there are also concerns about recombination with endogenous adenoviruses, potentially leading to the release of novel variants into the environment. Finally, the wide host cell range of adenovirus vectors may hinder *in vivo* targeting to a specific cell type [5,6].

Liposomes and other physical methods

Clinical experience with the available physical methods of gene transfer has primarily involved cationic liposome–DNA complexes [9,15,16], which fuse with the cell membrane and enter the endosomal uptake pathway. DNA released from these endosomes may then pass through the nuclear membrane and be expressed. The main advantage of liposomes is that they are nontoxic and can be given repeatedly. In some cell types, high levels of gene transfer have been obtained [9]. Liposomes are unstable *in vivo* and cannot effectively be given systemically, but liposomal transfer by local injection of human melanoma cells *in situ* has resulted in expression of a new gene (HLA-B7) [9]. However, the DNA transferred by liposomes is nonintegrating, and despite the incorporation of a variety of ligands into the liposome–DNA complex [16], the ability to target these vectors is still quite limited.

Adeno-associated vector

Adeno-associated virus (AAV) [7] (Fig. 28.1b) is a 'dependovirus', that can replicate only when an AAV-infected cell is coinfected with adenovirus or herpes virus. Structurally, AAV is a DNA parvovirus, containing two palindromic inverted terminal repeats (ITRs) (Fig. 28.1b). Together with two gene products from the *REP* gene region, these ITRs favour site-specific integration of the AAV in chromosome 19 [8]. Thus, AAV, like retroviruses, should be present for the entire life span of the host cell and in its progeny. Because integration of AAV is relatively site specific, the possibilities of oncogenesis should be reduced. Moreover, it had been claimed that integration would occur in nondividing cells, so that, in contrast to retroviruses, AAV should be permanently expressed even in resting or postmitotic cells. Unfortunately, as more has been learned about the biology of AAV, many of these putative advantages have proved illusory. For example, the REP gene products that contribute to site-specific integration are toxic to virus producer cells and are usually deleted from vectors. However, rep-deficient vectors appear to lose almost all their ability to integrate, regardless of site [7]. Finally, it has proved difficult to develop high-titre producer cell lines, free of contaminating helper adenoviruses. Hence, the introduction of AAV into clinical use has been delayed and is only now beginning.

Other vectors

While a number of other viral and physical methods of gene transfer have been proposed as future substitutes for currently available vector systems, most investigators now accept that no naturally occurring virus and no simple physical vector will ever prove suitable for all gene therapy purposes. Ultimately, therefore, entirely new synthetic or semisynthetic vectors will have to be developed [17]. Possibilities include the generation of hybrid viral vectors, which may combine, for example, the *in vivo* stability of adenoviruses and the integrating capacity of retroviruses. Alternative, fully synthetic vectors will be developed, combining multiple components from multiple different vectors, allowing safe, efficient and specific gene transfer and regulation (Table 28.1). For the foreseeable future, however, gene-therapy protocols for leukaemia will require the investigator to circumvent the limitations of current vectors and to choose their agent on the basis of the most important feature required. For example, a requirement for long-term expression in the progeny of HSC dictates a retroviral vector; transient expression in cells transduced *in vivo* may favour an adenovirus.

Current uses of gene transfer for leukaemia and related disorders

Because clinical studies of gene therapy have to show that the potential benefits outweigh the potential risks, most gene-therapy protocols for malignancy are open only to patients with advanced disease, in whom the risk to benefit ratio is most likely to be favourable. It must be emphasized that these patients are unlikely, ultimately, to be the most suitable group

Table 28.1 Novel vectors.

Vector type	Potential advantages
HIV VISNA D-type viruses	Integrate in nondividing cells
Pseudotyped retroviruses incorporating novel proteins in viral envelope	1. Increased stability for purification 2. Increased resistance to primate complement 3. Altered target cell specificity/efficiency of transfection
Hybrid vectors Virosomes (virus coats containing plasmid DNA) Liposomes + ligands Liposomes + viral components/DNA sequences	1. High efficiency transfer by avoidance of endosomal degradation 2. Specific targeting 3. Integration of transferred DNA

for gene therapy. Instead, many of the gene-therapy approaches to be described are likely to be most valuable for the eradication of minimal residual disease remaining after conventional therapies.

Modification of the tumour

Leukaemia/lymphoma correction

There is an attractive elegance to the strategy of introducing genetic material into a haematological malignancy to correct the specific genetic defects contributing to the malignant phenotype. A number of mutant oncogenes and fusion transcripts have been described in leukaemia and lymphoma that are certainly specific to the malignant clone and frequently form a critical component of the malignant process [18]. Unfortunately, this approach is technologically extremely demanding. All malignancies are the result of a multiplicity of genetic abnormalities. Unless correction of a single defect is subsequently lethal for the malignant cell, transfer of an individual gene to a patient with 10^{11} or 10^{12} leukaemia or lymphoma cells will leave many cells that are effectively premalignant, with a high risk of later transformation. Moreover, many relevant gene defects produce molecules with 'transdominant' effects that will continue to produce a malignant phenotype even if a wild-type gene is introduced. Such genes could only be neutralized by antisense RNA, by a ribozyme or by homologous recombination with a wild-type gene [19–21]. None of these approaches are fully evolved. Finally, present methods of gene transfer are inefficient [1,22]. While adenovirus vectors may produce gene transfer to 90% or more of certain target cells, even this would be insufficient to produce more than transient clinical benefit in most haematological malignancies.

Notwithstanding the above limitations, several protocols have been proposed in the use of the tumour correction approach. In spite of the polygenic aetiology of cancer, it is hoped that certain individual genetic abnormalities will be both pivotal to the malignant process and amenable to correction. For example, efforts are being made to neutralize fusion transcripts such as BCR-ABL or activated oncogenes such as C-MYB (chronic myeloid leukaemia), using ribozymes, antisense RNA or wild-type genes respectively [23,24] (Table 28.2). Similarly, nonfunctional antioncogenes such as *p53* may be replaced by wild-type genes in patients with acute myeloid leukaemia or myelodysplasia [25]. Interest is also increasing in targeting the gene pathways involved in regulating apoptosis. Experimental models suggest that even minor perturbations in these pathways can greatly modify the sensitivity of cancer cells to chemotherapy [26]. Finally, it has been suggested that tumour correction may best be used preventively, for patients in whom known single-gene defects predispose to subsequent mutagenesis and cancer.

Pro-drug metabolizing enzymes

Instead of introducing genes that modify genetic defects in tumours, efforts have been made to insert genes that will encode enzymes able to convert harmless pro-drugs into lethal cytotoxins. For this approach to be cancer selective, either the vector or the prodrug product must be targeted to the malignant cell. The first clinical studies have aimed for both types of selectivity, by introducing a thymidine kinase gene into a tumour cell using a retroviral vector [27,28]. On exposure to ganciclovir, the transduced cells will phosphorylate the drug. If the cell then divides, the product will be incorporated into DNA with lethal consequences, while nondividing cells are unaffected. Initial therapeutic study of Tk gene transfer was made in patients with primary and secondary brain tumours; in this context, there is a particularly clear distinction between tumour cells which divide and will be killed by the ganciclovir and normal neurones which do not divide and should escape unharmed. In this system, retroviral vectors offer additional tumour specificity because they function only in dividing cells, and therefore do not transduce normal neurones. Such selectivity cannot occur when the malignant progeny of HSC are the target, because normal cells derived from HSC are also rapidly dividing. In haematological disease, therefore, the approach will probably be used to incorporate a suicide gene into genetically modified effector cells, providing a means of controlling any undesirable effects of the modified cells (see below).

One of the most puzzling features of the preclinical Tk-retrovirus system was that it worked so well. Even when fewer than 10% of tumour cells were transduced, ganciclovir produced nearly 100% tumour cell death [27,28]. This advantage over the tumour correction protocols described above appears to result from a 'bystander' effect. Thus, cells which lack the pro-drug metabolizing gene can be killed if they are adjacent to transduced cells. The bystander effect is most evident in tumour cells that have gap junctions, so it probably represents the transfer of a toxic metabolite or of an apoptosis signal [29,30]. The potency of the bystander effect is likely to be much lower among the 'gapless' cells of haematological malignancy. However, an immunological bystander effect may also occur *in vivo*: after the cell is killed by the toxic metabolite, it is processed and presented by host antigen presenting cells, immunizing the host [29,30] (see below).

Additional pro-drug enzyme systems. Cytosine deaminase [31,32] converts 5-fluorocytosine to 5-fluorouracil and will be investigated in an imminent trial in the UK. In this study in patients with recurrent c-erb2B-positive nodular breast cancer, specific expression of the enzyme will be achieved both by injecting the retroviral vector directly into the nodules and by driving the contained cytosine deaminase gene by the c-erb2B promoter, which should be inactive in normal breast cells. More

Table 28.2 Tumour correction studies.

Cancer patient population	Transferred nucleic acids	Protocol	Institution/country
AML	p53 antisense	Phase I Study of p53 antisense oligodeoxyribonucleotide (OL(1) p53 for refractory or relapsed acute myelogenous leukaemia and myelodysplastic syndrome	University of Nebraska Medical Center Omaha, NE, USA
Breast	C-FOS antisense C-MYC antisense	Gene therapy for the treatment of metastatic breast cancer by in vivo injection with breast-targeted retroviral vectors expressing antisense C-FOS or antisense C-MYC RNA	Vanderbilt University Nashville, TN, USA
CML	BCR/ABL antisense (B3/A2)	High-dose therapy with antisense purged peripheral stem cell transplantation for chronic myelogenous leukaemia	University of Nebraska Medical Center, Omaha, NE, USA
CML	C-MYB Antisense	Autologous CD34+ bone marrow cells purged with C-MYB antisense transplanted into chronic or accelerated phase CML patients prepared with busulphan and cyclophosphamide	Hospital of the University of Pennsylvania, Philadelphia, PA, USA
Lung: non-small cell	p53 K-RAS antisense	Modification of oncogene and tumour suppressor gene expression in non-small cell lung cancer using a retroviral vector	University of Texas, MD Anderson Cancer Center, Houston, TX, USA
Lung: non-small cell	p53	Modification of tumour suppressor gene expression and induction of apoptosis in non-small cell lung cancer using an adenovirus vector	University of Texas, MD Anderson Cancer Center, Houston, TX, USA

than a dozen other pro-drug systems have been described over the past few decades. Of these, the P450-2B1 (converts cyclophosphamide to 4-hydroperoxycyclophosphamide) [33] and the bacterial nitroreductase system [34] (reduces CB1954 to the more active 4-hydroxylamine) are closest to application for gene therapy. However, application of these and other agents [35,36] to haematological malignancy will require improved methods of targeting their expression to malignant cells [37]. While this may ultimately be achieved by coupling tumour-specific ligands to the chosen vector, or by incorporation of tumour-specific promoters (as in the cytosine deaminase studies described above), at present the lack of specificity renders the approach poorly suited to leukaemia or lymphoma.

Generation of tumour vaccines

In an attempt to enhance immune recognition of poorly immunogenic tumours, investigators have evaluated the effect of transducing tumour cells with cytokine genes [38], with allogeneic MHC molecules [9] or with costimulatory molecules such as B7.1 or CD40 ligand [39,40] that activate cytotoxic T cells after engaging their surface ligands or counter receptors.

In murine systems, transfection of tumour cell lines with these molecules has augmented immunogenicity. The injection of neoplastic cells (including those derived from lymphoid and myeloid malignancies) in doses that would normally establish a tumour, instead recruits immune system effector cells and eradicates injected tumour cells [41–47]. Often the animal is then resistant to challenges by further local injections of nontransduced parental tumour. The transduced tumour has therefore acted like a vaccine. In some models, established nontransduced parental malignant cells are also eradicated [43,44].

There are several potential problems in translating these approaches to human haematological malignancy. One recent study has suggested that the same effect is attained if tumour cells are admixed with nonspecific adjuvants, such as *Corynebacterium parvum* [48]. Because adjuvant dependent cancer immunotherapy has had limited success in treating human cancer, there is a concern that the cytokine gene-transfer model in animals will translate no better than any other rodent tumour immunotherapy model [49]. Secondly, the primary malignant cells of many haematological malignancies are highly resistant to transduction by currently available vectors. Finally, the neoplastic cells of many haematological malignancies show considerable phenotypic heterogeneity. A vaccine made from a small proportion of these cells, obtained from one site, may not express the full array of antigens present in the patient as a whole.

From December 1995, the available tumour vaccine approaches were being evaluated in more than 50 different clinical trials, although problems with limited transduction efficiency meant that few of them have, as yet, included haematological disease. Initial results have been presented for melanoma, renal cell carcinoma and neuroblastoma. They suggest that IL-2, gramulocyte macrophage colony-stimulating factor (GM-CSF) or HLA-B7 transduced tumour cells can be given safely, and will frequently produce immuno-modulatory effects, including peripheral blood eosinophilia, a rise in NK and AK cell number and activity, and the development of tumour-specific T cells. In a minority of patients, partial responses have occurred, with the disappearance of some distant metastases [9]. However, other metastases have continued to grow (perhaps because their phenotypic heterogeneity allows them to evade an immune response as described above) and no patients have yet been cured of their disease. In future studies, the vaccines will be used as adjuvants to prevent relapse in patients with presumed minimal residual disease (MRD). Ultimately, it is likely that maximum antitumour immune responses will be obtained when several different immunostimulatory genes are introduced into the tumour. Certainly, in animal and human preclinical studies, combinations of IL-2 and CD40L (for example) can cause regression of pre-established leukaemia, even when either agent alone is inadequate (unpublished data).

Modification of the host immune system

Gene-modified cytotoxic T cells

There is now considerable evidence that the immune system does have the potential to eradicate leukaemia and perhaps lymphoma [50,51]. This effect is most clearly seen in patients who have received bone marrow allografts for the treatment of haematological malignancy. In these patients, the presence of graft vs host disease (GVHD) may reduce the risk of subsequent relapse, while measures that reduce GVHD, such as T-cell depletion or the use of an identical twin allograft, are associated with an increased risk of disease recurrence. This so-called graft vs leukaemia (GVL) effect may simply be another manifestation of GVHD, in which both normal and malignant host cells share the same host-specific polymorphisms that are a target for alloreactive T-lymphocytes [52]. However, it is also possible that malignancy-reactive normal host reactive T cells may be recognizing discrete target antigens. Cytotoxic T-lymphocytes (CTL) recognize processed intracellular proteins presented as short peptide fragments together with MHC molecules on the cell surface. Hence, internal proteins unique to the malignant clone may act as tumour-specific antigens for CTL. Several human malignancies contain novel proteins, such as mutated oncogenes or fusion proteins generated by chromosomal translocations [52,53]. Some lymphomas may express immunogenic proteins encoded by the Epstein–Barr virus (EBV) [54]. Finally, even normal proteins can elicit CTL responses if they are expressed in very high quantities, for example the MAGE

protein in melanoma cells [55]. If tumour cells are able to process and present these tumour-specific peptides, then it is possible that a malignancy-specific response could be generated in the absence of any other host reactivity. Exploration of this possibility and of the effector mechanisms involved is easiest when the target antigens have been identified. Gene transfer, once characterized, affords a mechanism for enhancing or amplifying this effector function.

EBV-driven immunoblastic lymphoma is a useful model system for evaluating the antitumour activity of gene-modified tumour cells in haematological malignancy. EBV is a herpes virus that infects most individuals and persists in an asymptomatic state by a combination of chronic replication in the mucosa and latency in peripheral blood B cells [56]. These EBV-infected B cells are highly immunogenic and normally susceptible to killing by specific cytotoxic T-lymphocytes. However, in immunocompromised patients, the infected B cells may grow unchecked, producing a rapidly progressive lymphoproliferative disease, that usually appears histologically as an immunoblastic lymphoma. This complication occurs in 1–30% of patients receiving immunosuppression after allografts and has a high mortality [54].

If these cells are only able to flourish because of the absence of functional EBV-reactive CTL, then administration of normal peripheral blood lymphocytes from EBV immune donors to patients with lymphoproliferative disease (LPD) should produce resolution. In fact, administration of donor peripheral blood mononuclear cells to recipients after marrow allografting can produce complete clinical and histological responses [51], presumably because of virus-specific T cells within the bulk lymphocyte population. However, since the population also contains many alloreactive T cells, such treatment may also induce severe GVHD [51].

A safer alternative should be to use T cells which are specific only for the viral antigens expressed by the tumour cells. EBV-specific cytotoxic T-lymphocytes lines have therefore been adoptively transferred to patients following marrow allografts, to see whether they behave as a safe and effective prophylaxis and treatment for EBV–LPD [54]. To learn more about the survival, distribution and activity of these cells after administration, they can first be marked with the neomycin-resistance gene (*Neo*) using a retroviral vector [54]. Study of the first 20 patients showed that the infused CTL produced no adverse effects and that the infused cells were long lived; the *Neo* gene has been detected in EBV-specific CTL for up to 18 months. In patients with EBV disease, administration of EBV-specific CTL was rapidly followed by a 1000-fold fall in EBV DNA levels and the resolution of biopsy-proven immunoblastic lymphoma [54]. The approach is now being tested in EBV-positive Hodgkin's disease. It may now be possible to generate a 'universal' T cell with a hybrid receptor that recognized its target independently of MHC molecules but retained the ability to signal T-cell activation [57,58]. Such activity can be generated experimentally by combining the variable region of an antibody molecule with the zeta chain of the T-cell receptor. These cells could be used to target a wide variety of leukaemia/lymphoma-specific antigens.

Genetic modification to enhance antitumour immunity

An alternative way of enhancing the antitumour activity of immunocytes is to increase the levels of cytotoxic cytokines (such as TNF) which they produce at local tumour sites. This approach is being evaluated in studies with tumour-infiltrating lymphocytes (TILs) [4]. The problems with this strategy are that it has been difficult to persuade TIL cells to secrete high levels of cytokines and that only scanty data support the belief that reinfused human TIL cells selectively home to tumour sites. The first six patients treated with TNF TIL have shown few side effects and one patient has had a sustained response [4].

Modification of host cytotoxic drug sensitivity

The increased understanding of cytotoxic drug resistance has suggested gene-therapy approaches to protect normal host tissues from the toxicity of chemotherapy. For example, if haemopoietic stem cells could be rendered resistant to one or more cytotoxic drugs, it might enable them to resist the myelosuppressive effects of cytotoxic drugs during cancer therapy, allowing longer or more intensive therapy that might cure more patients [59–61].

The *MDR1* gene has been the most widely considered for human therapy. The product of the *MDR1* gene, P-glycoprotein, functions as a drug efflux pump and confers resistance to many chemotherapeutic agents [62]. The feasibility of using the *MDR1* gene to protect haemopoietic cells has been shown by transgenic mouse experiments [63,64]. In addition, retroviral transfer of *MDR1* to murine clonogenic progenitors resulted in drug resistance *in vitro* and *in vivo* [65]. These experiments with *MDR1*-containing vectors prove the principle that drug-resistance genes can be used to attenuate drug-induced myelosuppression. It is probable that other drug-resistance genes may function analogously. DNA-methylguanine methyltransferases (MGMT) are enzymes that repair DNA damage done by the nitrosoureas, a class of cancer chemotherapeutic alkylating agents. Preliminary data suggests that retroviral-mediated gene transfer of the human MGMT gene to mouse bone marrow cells results in protection of murine progenitors from BCNU toxicity. Other drug-resistance genes, including dihydrofolate reductase and topoisomerase II, are also under consideration for clinical trial.

Clinical application of drug-resistance gene transfer has several potential pitfalls. The low stem cell transduction efficiencies observed with current clinical protocols predict that amelioration of drug-induced myelosuppression will not occur unless dramatic *in vivo* selection can be enacted. There is also the risk of transferring drug-resistance genes to neoplastic cells that contaminate the HSC graft and produce a drug-resistant relapse. Finally, toxicity to nonprotected organs, including the gut, heart and lungs, may rapidly supervene when marrow resistance allows intensification of cytotoxic drug dosages.

These objections notwithstanding, three trials using transfer of the *MDR1* gene to bone marrow or peripheral blood stem cells in patients with a solid malignancy have now been approved. Patients will be treated with taxol after transplantation, as clinically indicated. The endpoints of these trials are: (i) to test if *MDR1* gene transfer results in toxicity specific to gene transfer; (ii) to test if the *MDR1* vector can be transferred to human haemopoietic stem cells; (iii) to test if *MDR1* can be used as a dominant selectable marker *in vivo*; (iv) to test if *MDR1* gene transfer will result in amelioration of taxol-induced myelosuppression.

Gene marking of haemopoietic progenitor cells

Not all the applications of gene transfer to patients with malignant disease are directly therapeutic in intent. Gene marking of haemopoietic cells provides no immediate benefit to patients. However, information gained from these studies is proving to be valuable for improving the outcome of therapies that incorporate autologous HSC transplantation as a device for eradicating haematological malignancies [3].

While the dose intensification allowed by autologous HSC rescue has shown promise as an effective treatment for leukaemias and lymphomas (and perhaps for some solid tumours) [66–70], disease recurrence remains the major cause of treatment failure. When the malignancy originates from or involves the marrow, relapse could originate from malignant cells persisting in the patient, in the rescuing HSC, or in both [2,66–71]. Concern that the HSC may contain residual malignant cells has led to extensive evaluation of techniques for purging these cells [72–75]. However, no method has been unequivocally shown to reduce the risk of relapse in naturally occurring disease [76–78], and purging techniques usually slow engraftment due to damage to normal progenitor cells.

In gene-marking studies, gene transfer is used to answer biological questions in bone marrow transplantation (BMT) and it allows clinically relevant issues to be addressed even with the limited efficiency of gene transfer available with current vectors. Gene transfer has been used after autologous BMT, to determine the source of relapse and to learn more about the biology of normal marrow reconstitution and how best to accelerate this process.

Gene marking studies after autologous bone marrow transplantation

Source of relapse after autologous bone marrow transplantation. While autologous BMT (ABMT) appears to result in an improvement in survival in many malignant diseases, relapse remains the major cause of treatment failure. The possibility that reinfused malignant cells may contribute to relapse has led to extensive evaluation of techniques for purging marrow to eliminate residual malignant cells, although it has been unclear whether such manoeuvres are necessary [2]. One way of resolving this issue is to mark the marrow at the time of harvest with a retroviral vector, and then find out if the marker gene is present in malignant cells at the time of a subsequent relapse [2].

In the initial acute myeloid study, four of the 12 patients relapsed [2], and in two the malignant cells contained the marker gene. Similar results have been obtained in CML [79]. These data show definitively that marrow harvested in apparent clinical remission may contain residual tumourigenic cells and that these cells can contribute to disease recurrence. The implication is that effective purging will be one requirement for improving the outcome of ABMT.

Gene transfer to normal cells. The efficiency of gene transfer and expression into normal marrow progenitor cells can also be obtained from these marker studies. By phenotype (neomycin resistance) and by genotype (PCR amplification), the gene was present in about 2–15% of haemopoietic progenitor cells after ABMT in children. In adults the levels were somewhat lower. The marker gene continued to be detected and expressed for up to 3 years in the mature progeny of marrow precursor cells, including peripheral blood T and B cells and neutrophils. These results imply that true stem cells are being transduced [3]. Overall, these results are encouraging, particularly in the paediatric population, because the levels of transfer are higher than those predicted from animal models. This discrepancy may be attributed to the fact that marrow was harvested during regeneration after intensive chemotherapy, when a higher than normal proportion of stem cells are in cycle.

Purging studies. Second-generation studies of marrow marking have now begun. Two distinguishable gene markers in two related retroviral vectors can be used in each patient to compare either marrow purging vs no purging, or two different purging techniques within a single patient. If the patient should subsequently relapse, detection of either marker will indicate if either of these purging techniques is effective.

Ex vivo *expansion studies.* Double gene marking is also being used to determine directly which *ex vivo* or *in vivo* combination of cytokines will increase the entry of long-term marrow repopulating cells into the cell cycle and thereby reduce the period of marrow hypoplasia and immunodeficiency that follows autologous stem cell transplantation [3,80,81]. In humans, it certainly appears possible to use growth factors such as IL-1, IL-3 and stem cell factor to increase the numbers of haemopoietic progenitor cells by 10- to 50-fold and to increase the efficiency of gene transfer to levels which may exceed 50% [80,81]. Unfortunately, it is not certain that such

ex vivo data will be reflected by results *in vivo*. In primate and human studies, transplantation of marrow treated *ex vivo* with the growth factor combinations shown to greatly augment both progenitor numbers and gene transfer rates, have been followed by disconcertingly low levels of long-term gene expression *in vivo* [81]. The likeliest explanation for this apparent paradox is that many of the growth factors intended only to induce cycling in marrow stem cells also induce their differentiation and the loss of their self-renewal capacity.

Without any proven *ex vivo* surrogate method for studying the effects of growth factors on stem cell expansion and transducibility, it is possible to use the marker-gene technique to evaluate whether any increase in progenitor cell numbers and transducibility produced by growth factor combinations and cell culture devices *ex vivo* has an effect *in vivo*. Once again, the use of two distinguishable vectors to mark each patient's marrow allows comparison of treatment regimens *within* a patient, reducing the study size required. This technique is also being used to compare the short- and long-term reconstitution of haemopoiesis using peripheral blood and marrow-derived haemopoietic progenitor cells.

Safety of gene transfer

To date, more than 200 patients have received genetically modified cells. Although most of these patients received irradiated gene-modified tumour cells which would be expected to carry little risk, more than 60 patients have received genetically modified haemopoietic progenitor cells. With a maximum follow up of 4.5 years, and a total patient follow up of more than 100 patient years, no adverse events attributable to the gene-transfer process have been reported. In particular, there has been no evidence of any lymphoproliferative disorder. It is of potential concern, however, that preliminary reports are showing a cellular immune response directed against a transferred gene product (of the thymidine kinase gene) on T cells. Clearly, if an immune response is regularly generated against the product of any transferred gene, this will severely circumscribe the value of gene therapy. Fortunately, there is no evidence to suggest a similar problem for marrow cells transduced with *Neo* or with ADA. Prolonged follow-up of patients receiving genetically modified cells is essential at this early stage of development of the technology.

Conclusion

There is still same way to go before the extraordinary potential of gene transfer for therapy of haematological malignancy can be fully exploited. However, it is important to remember that most advances in medicine are made incrementally, and that gene transfer can be used to complement, rather than replace, conventional modalities of therapy. Gene transfer is already contributing in this complementary way to the therapy of haematological malignancy. The benefits of the technology can only increase as current limitations are progressively — albeit slowly—surmounted.

Acknowledgements

Some of the work described in this chapter was supported by NIH Grant CA 20180, HL55703, CA 61384, Cancer Center Support CORE Grant CA 21765, and by the American Lebanese Syrian Associated Charities (ALSAC). We would like to thank Genetic Therapy, Inc. for providing the clinical grade vectors described in the section on Gene Marking, and Nancy Parnell for word processing.

References

1 Anderson W.F. (1990) The ADA human gene therapy clinical protocol. *Human Gene Therapy*, **1**, 327–362.

2 Brenner M.K., Rill D.R., Moen R.C. *et al.* (1993) Gene-marking to trace origin of relapse after autologous bone marrow transplantation. *Lancet*, **341**, 85–86.

3 Brenner M.K., Rill D.R., Holladay M.S. *et al.* (1993) Gene marking to determine whether autologous marrow infusion restores long-term haemopoiesis in cancer patients. *Lancet*, **342**, 1134–1137.

4 Rosenberg S.A. (1992) Gene therapy for cancer. *Journal of the American Medical Association*, **268**, 2416–2419.

5 Engelhardt J.F., Yang Y., Stratford-Perricaudet L.D. *et al.* (1993) Direct gene transfer of human CFTR into human bronchial epithelia of xenografts with E1-deleted adenoviruses. *Nature Genetics*, **4**, 27–34.

6 Le Gal La Salle G., Robert J.J., Berrard S. *et al.* (1993) An adenovirus vector for gene transfer into neurons and glia in the brain. *Science*, **259**, 988–990.

7 Muzyczka N. (1992) Use of adeno-associated virus as a general transduction vector for mammalian cells. *Current Topics in Microbiology and Immunology*, **158**, 97–129.

8 Weitzman M.D., Kyostio S.R.M., Kotin R.M. & Owens R.A. (1998) Adeno-associated virus (AAV) rep proteins mediated complex formation between AAV DNA and the human integration site. *Nature Genetics*. (In press.)

9 Nabel G.J., Nabel E.G., Yang Z.Y. *et al.* (1993) Direct gene transfer with DNA–liposome complexes in melanoma: expression, biologic activity, and lack of toxicity in humans. *Proceedings of the National Academy of Sciences USA*, **90**, 11307–11311.

10 Bender M.A., Palmer T.D., Gelinas R.E. & Miller A.D. (1987) Evidence that the packaging signal of Moloney Murine Leukemia Virus extends into the gag region. *Journal of Virology*, **61**, 1639–1646.

11 Donahue R.E., Kessler S.W., Bodine D. *et al.* (1992) Helper virus induced T cell lymphoma in nonhuman primates after retroviral mediated gene transfer. *Journal of Experimental Medicine*, **176**, 1125–1135.

12 Cornetta K., Morgan R.A. & Anderson W.F. (1991) Safety issues related to retrovirus-mediated gene transfer in humans. *Human Gene Therapy*, **2**, 5–14.

13 Smith T.A., Mehaffey M.G., Kayda D.B. *et al.* (1993) Adenovirus mediated expression of therapeutic plasma levels in human factor IX in mice. *Natural Genetics*, **5**, 397–402.

14 Amin R., Wilmott R., Schwarz Y., Trapnell B. & Stark J. (1995) Replication-deficient adenovirus induces expression of inter-leukin-8 by airway epithelial cells *in vivo*. *Human Gene Therapy*, **6**, 145–154.

15 Gao X. & Huang L. (1991) A novel cationic liposome reagent for efficient transfection of mammalian cells. *Biochemical and Biophysical Research Communications*, **179**, 280–285.

16 Trubetskoy V.S., Torchilin V.P., Kennel S.J. & Huang L. (1992) Cationic liposomes enhance targeted delivery and expression of exogenous DNA mediated by N-terminal modified poly-L-lysine-antibody conjugate in mouse lung endothelial cells. *Biochimica et Biophysica Acta*, **1131**, 311–313.

17 Schofield J.P. & Caskey C.T. (1995) Non-viral approaches to gene therapy. *British Medical Bulletin*, **51**, 56–71.

18 Brenner M.K. & Heslop H.E. (1991) Graft versus leukemia effects after marrow transplantation in man. *Ballière's Clinical Haematology*, **4**, 727–749.

19 Snyder D.S., Wu Y., Wang J.L. *et al.* (1993) Ribozyme-mediated inhibition of *bcr-abl* gene expression in Philadelphia chromosome-positive cell line. *Blood*, **82**, 600–605.

20 Scanlon K.J., Jiao L., Funato T. *et al.* (1991) Ribozyme-mediated cleavage of *c-fos* mRNA reduces gene expression of DNA synthesis enzymes and metallothionein. *Proceedings of the National Academy of Sciences USA*, **88**, 10591–10595.

21 Ratajczak M.Z., Kant J.A., Luger S.M. *et al.* (1992) *In vivo* treatment of human leukemia in a scid mouse model with c-myb antisense oligodeoxynucleotides. *Proceedings of the National Academy of Sciences USA*, **89**, 11823–11827.

22 Miller A.D. (1992) Human gene therapy comes of age. *Nature*, **357**, 455–460.

23 Rossi J.J. (1995) Therapeutic antisense and ribozymes. *British Medical Bulletin*, **51**, 217–225.

24 Zhang Y., Mukhopadhyay T., Donehower L.A., Georges R.N. & Roth J.A. (1993) Retroviral vector-mediated transduction of K-*ras* antisense RNA into human lung cancer cells inhibits expression of the malignant phenotype. *Human Gene Therapy*, **4**, 451–460.

25 Fujiwara T., Grimm E.A., Cai D.W., Owen-Schaub L.B. & Roth J.A. (1993) A retroviral wild-type p53 expression vector penetrates human lung cancer spheroids and inhibits growth by inducing apoptosis. *Cancer Research*, **53**, 4129–4133.

26 Wang J., Bucana C.D., Roth J.A. & Zhang W. (1995) Apoptosis induced in human osteosarcoma cells is one of the mechanisms for the cytocidal effect of Ad5CMV-p53. *Cancer Gene Therapy*, **2**, 9–18.

27 Culver K.W., Ram Z., Wallbridge S., Ishii H., Oldfield E.H. & Blaese R.M. (1992) *In vivo* gene transfer with retroviral vector-producer cells for treatment of experimental brain tumors. *Science*, **256**, 1550–1552.

28 Ram Z., Culver K.W., Walbridge S. *et al.* (1993) *In situ* retroviral-mediated gene transfer for the treatment of brain tumors in rats. *Cancer Research*, **53**, 83–88.

29 Bi W.L., Parysek L.M., Warnick R. & Stambrook P.J. (1993) *In vitro* evidence that metabolic cooperation is responsible for the bystander effect observed with HSV tk retroviral gene therapy. *Human Gene Therapy*, **4**, 725–732.

30 Freeman S.M., Abboud C.N., Whartenby K.A. *et al.* (1993) The 'bystander effect': tumor regression when a fraction of the tumor mass is genetically modified. *Cancer Research*, **53**, 5274–5283.

31 Huber B.E., Austin E.A., Richards C.A., Davis S.T. & Good S.S. (1994) Metabolism of 5-fluorocytosine to 5-fluorouracil in human colorectal tumor cells transduced with the cytosine deaminase gene: significant antitumor effects when only a small percentage of tumor cells express cytosine deaminse. *Proceedings of the National Academy of Sciences USA*, **91**, 8302–8306.

32 Mullen C.A., Coale M.M., Lowe R. & Blaese R.M. (1994) Tumors expressing the cytosine deaminase suicide gene can be eliminated *in vivo* with 5-fluorocytosine and induce protective immunity to wild type tumor. *Cancer Research*, **54**, 1503–1506.

33 Wei M.X., Tamiya T., Chase M. *et al.* (1994) Experimental tumor therapy in mice using the cyclophosphamide-activating cytochrome P450 2B1 gene. *Human Gene Therapy*, **5**, 969–978.

34 Knox R.J., Friedlos F. & Boland M.P. (1993) The bioactivation of CB 1954 and its use as a prodrug in antibody-directed enzyme prodrug therapy (ADEPT). *Cancer Metastasis Reviews*, **12**, 195–212.

35 Mroz P.J. & Moolten F.L. (1993) Retrovirally transduced *Escherichia coli gpt* genes combine selectability with chemosensitivity capable of mediating tumor eradication. *Human Gene Therapy*, **4**, 589–595.

36 Sorscher E.J., Peng S., Bebok Z., Allan P.W., Bennett L.L. & Parker W.B. (1994) Tumor cell bystander killing in colonic carcinoma utilizing the *Escherichia coli* DeoD gene to generate toxic purines. *Gene Therapy*, **1**, 233–238.

37 Huber B.E., Richards C.A. & Austin E.A. (1994) Virus-directed enzyme/prodrug therapy (VDEPT). Selectively engineering drug sensitivity into tumors. *Annals of the New York Academy of Sciences*, **716**, 104–114.

38 Tahara H., Lotze M.T. & Chang P.L. (eds) (1994) Gene therapy for adult cancers: advances in immunologic approaches using cytokines. In: *Somatic Gene Therapy*, Vol. 15, pp. 263–286. CRC Press, Ann Arbor.

39 Chen L., Ashe S., Brady W.A. *et al.* (1992) Costimulation of anti-tumor immunity by the B7 counterreceptor for the T lymphocyte molecules CD28 and CTLA-4. *Cell*, **71**, 1093–1102.

40 Townsend S.E. & Allison J.P. (1993) Tumor rejection after direct costimulation of CD8+ T cells by B7-transfected melanoma cells. *Science*, **259**, 368–370.

41 Tepper R.I., Pattengale P.K. & Leder P. (1989) Murine interleukin-4 displays potent anti-tumor activity *in vivo*. *Cell*, **57**, 503–512.

42 Golumbek P.T., Lazenby A.J., Levitsky H.I. *et al.* (1991) Treatment of established renal cancer by tumor cells engineered to secrete interleukin-4. *Science*, **254**, 713–716.

43 Fearon E.R., Pardoe D.M., Itaya T. *et al.* (1990) Interleukin-2 production by tumor cells bypasses T helper function in the generation of an antitumor response. *Cell*, **60**, 397–403.

44 Gansbacher B., Zier K., Daniels B., Cronin K., Bannerji R. & Gilboa E. (1990) Interleukin 2 gene transfer into tumor cells abrogates tumorigenicity and induces protective immunity. *Journal of Experimental Medicine*, **172**, 1217–1224.

45 Dranoff G., Jaffee E., Lazenby A. *et al.* (1993) Vaccination with irradiated tumor cells engineered to secrete murine GM-CSF stimulates potent, specific, and long lasting anti-tumor immunity. *Proceedings of the National Academy of Sciences USA*, **90**, 9539–9543.

46 Colombo M.P., Ferrari G., Stoppacciaro A. *et al.* (1991) Granulocyte colony-stimulating factor gene transfer suppresses tumorogenicity of a murine adenocarcinoma *in vivo*. *Journal of Experimental Medicine*, **173**, 889–897.

47 Colombo M.P. & Forni G. (1994) Cytokine gene transfer in tumor inhibition and tumor therapy: where are we now? *Immunology Today*, **15**, 48–51.

48 Hock H., Dorsch M., Kunzendorf U. *et al.* (1993) Vaccinations with tumor cells genetically engineered to produce different cytokines: effectivity not superior to a classical adjuvant. *Cancer Research*, **53**, 714–716.

49 Yamada G., Kitamura Y., Sonoda H. *et al.* (1993) Retroviral expression of the human IL-2 gene in a murine T cell line results in cell

growth autonomy and tumorigenicity. *EMBO Journal*, **6**, 2705–2709.

50 Horowitz M.M., Gale R.P., Sondel P.M. *et al.* (1990) Graft-versus-leukemia reactions after bone marrow transplantation. *Blood*, **75**, 555–562.

51 Papadopoulos E.B., Ladanyi M., Emanuel D. *et al.* (1994) Infusions of donor leukocytes to treat Epstein–Barr virus-associated lymphoproliferative disorders after allogeneic bone marrow transplantation. *New England Journal of Medicine*, **330**, 1185–1191.

52 Brenner M.K. & Heslop H.E. (1991) Graft-versus-host reactions and bone marrow transplantation. *Current Opinions in Immunology*, **3**, 752–757.

53 Melief C.J. & Kast W.M. (1993) Potential immunogenicity of oncogene and tumor supressor gene products. *Current Opinions in Immunology*, **5**, 709–713.

54 Rooney C.M., Smith C.A., Ng C. *et al.* (1995) Use of gene-modified virus-specific T lymphocytes to control Epstein–Barr virus-related lymphoproliferation. *Lancet*, **345**, 9–13.

55 van Der Bruggen P., Traversari C., Chomez P. *et al.* (1991) A gene encoding an antigen recognized by cytolytic T lymphocytes on a human melanoma. *Science*, **254**, 1643–1647.

56 Straus S.E., Cohen J.I., Tosato G. & Meier J. (1992) Epstein–Barr virus infections: biology, pathogenesis and management. *Annals of Internal Medicine*, **118**, 45–58.

57 Doherty P.C. (1993) Cell-mediated cytotoxicity. *Cell*, **75**, 607–612.

58 Lanzavecchia A. (1993) Identifying strategies for immune intervention. *Science*, **260**, 937–944.

59 Murphy D., Crowther D., Renninson J. *et al.* (1993) A randomised dose intensity study in ovarian carcinoma comparing chemotherapy given at four week intervals for six cycles with half dose chemotherapy given for twelve cycles. *Annals of Oncology*, **4**, 377.

60 Levin L. & Hryniuk W.M. (1987) Dose intensity analysis of chemotherapy regimens in ovarian carcinoma. *Journal of Clinical Oncology*, **5**, 756–767.

61 Levin L., Simon R. & Hryniuk W. (1993) Importance of multiagent chemotherapy regimens in ovarian carcinoma: dose intensity analysis. *Journal of the National Cancer Institute*, **85**, 1732–1742.

62 Pastan I. & Gottesman M.M. (1991) Multidrug resistance. *Annual Review of Medicine*, **42**, 277–286.

63 Mickisch G.H., Licht T., Merlino G.T., Gottesman M.M. & Pastan I. (1991) Chemotherapy and chemosensitization of transgenic mice which express the human multidrug resistance gene in bone marrow: efficacy, potency, and toxicity. *Cancer Research*, **51**, 5417–5424.

64 Mickisch G.H., Merlino G.T., Galski H., Gottesman M.M. & Pastan I. (1991) Transgenic mice that express the human multidrug-resistance gene in bone marrow enable a rapid identification of agents that reverse drug resistance. *Proceedings of the National Academy of Sciences USA*, **88**, 547–551.

65 McLachlin J.R., Eglitis M.A., Ueda K. *et al.* (1990) Expression of a human complementary DNA for the multidrug resistance gene in murine hematopoietic precursor cells with the use of retroviral gene transfer. *Journal of the National Cancer Institute*, **82**, 1260–1263.

66 Appelbaum F.R. & Buckner C.D. (1986) Overview of the clinical relevance of autologous bone marrow transplantation. *Clinical Haematology*, **15**, 1–18.

67 Burnett A.K., Tansey P., Watkins R. *et al.* (1984) Transplantation of unpurged autologous bone-marrow in acute myeloid leukaemia in first remission. *Lancet*, **ii**, 1068–1070.

68 Goldstone A.H., Anderson C.C., Linch D.C. *et al.* (1986) Autologous bone marrow transplantation following high dose

chemotherapy for the treatment of adult patients with acute myeloid leukaemia. *British Journal of Haematology*, **64**, 529–537.

69 Brugger W., Bross K.J., Glatt M., Weber F., Mertelsmann R. & Kanz L. (1994) Mobilization of tumor cells and hematopoietic progenitor cells into peripheral blood of patients with solid tumors. *Blood*, **83**, 636–640.

70 Shpall E.J. & Jones R.B. (1994) Release of tumor cells from bone marrow. *Blood*, **83**, 623–625.

71 Rill D.R., Santana V.M., Roberts W.M. *et al.* (1994) Direct demonstration that autologous bone marrow transplantation for solid tumors can return a multiplicity of tumorigenic cells. *Blood*, **84**, 380–383.

72 De Fabritiis P., Ferrero D., Sandrelli A. *et al.* (1989) Monoclonal antibody purging and autologous bone marrow transplantation in acute myelogenous leukemia in complete remission. *Bone Marrow Transplantation*, **4**, 669–674.

73 Gambacorti-Passerini C., Rivoltini L., Fizzotti M. *et al.* (1991) Selective purging by human interleukin-2 activated lymphocytes of bone marrows contaminated with a lymphoma line or autologous leukaemic cells. *British Journal of Haematology*, **78**, 197–205.

74 Gorin N.C., Aegerter P., Auvert B. *et al.* (1990) Autologous bone marrow transplantation for acute myelocytic leukemia in first remission: a European survey of the role of marrow purging. *Blood*, **75**, 1606–1614.

75 Santos G.W., Yeager A.M. & Jones R.J. (1989) Autologous bone marrow transplantation. *Annual Review of Medicine*, **40**, 99–112.

76 Gribben J.G., Freedman A.S., Neuberg D. *et al.* (1991) Immunologic purging of marrow assessed by PCR before autologous bone marrow transplantation for B-cell lymphoma. *New England Journal of Medicine*, **325**, 1525–1533.

77 Petersen F.B. & Buckner C.D. (1987) Allogeneic and autologous bone marrow transplantation for acute leukemia and malignant lymphoma: current status. *Hematological Oncology*, **5**, 233–243.

78 Yeager A.M., Kaizer H., Santos G.W. *et al.* (1986) Autologous bone marrow transplantation in patients with acute nonlymphocytic leukemia, using *ex vivo* marrow treatment with 4-hydroperoxycyclophosphamide. *New England Journal of Medicine*, **315**, 141–147.

79 Deisseroth A.B., Zu Z., Claxton D. *et al.* (1994) Genetic marking shows that Ph+ cells present in autologous transplants of chronic myelogenous leukemia (CML) contribute to relapse after autologous bone marrow in CML. *Blood*, **83**, 3068–3076.

80 Moritz T., Mackay W., Feng L.J., Samson L. & Williams D.A. (1993) Gene transfer of O6-methylguanine methyltransferase (MGMT) protects hematopoietic cells (HC) from nitrosourea (NU) induced toxicity *in vitro* and *in vivo*. *Blood*, **82** (Suppl. 1), 118a (abstract).

81 Dunbar C.E., Bodine D.M., Sorrentino B. *et al.* (1994) Gene transfer into hematopoietic cells: implications for cancer therapy. *Annals of the New York Academy of Sciences*, **716**, 216–224.

Index